ADVANCES IN NEURAL INFORMATION PROCESSING SYSTEMS 9

ADVANCES IN NEURAL INFORMATION PROCESSING SYSTEMS

Published by Morgan-Kaufmann

NIPS-1

Advances in Neural Information Processing Systems 1: Proceedings of the 1988 Conference,
David Touretzky, ed., 1989.

NIPS-2

Advances in Neural Information Processing Systems 2: Proceedings of the 1989 Conference,
David Touretzky, ed., 1990.

NIPS-3

Advances in Neural Information Processing Systems 3: Proceedings of the 1990 Conference,
Richard Lippmann, John E. Moody and David S. Touretzky, ed., 1991.

NIPS-4

Advances in Neural Information Processing Systems 4: Proceedings of the 1991 Conference,
John E. Moody, Setphen José Hanson and Richard P. Lippmann, eds., 1992.

NIPS-5

Advances in Neural Information Processing Systems 5: Proceedings of the 1992 Conference,
Stephen JosHanson, Jack D. Cowan and C. Lee Giles, eds., 1993.

NIPS-6

Advances in Neural Information Processing Systems 6: Proceedings of the 1993 Conference,
Jack D. Cowan, Gerald Tesauro and Joshua Alspector, eds., 1994.

Published by The MIT Press

NIPS-7

Advances in Neural Information Processing Systems 7: Proceedings of the 1994 Conference,
Gerald Tesauro, David Touretzky and Todd Leed, eds., 1995.

NIPS-8

Advances in Neural Information Processing Systems 8: Proceedings of the 1995 Conference,
David S. Touretzky, Michael C. Mozer and Michael E. Hasselmo, eds., 1996.

NIPS-9

Advances in Neural Information Processing Systems 9: Proceedings of the 1996 Conference,
Michael C. Mozer, Michael I. Jordan and Thomas Petsche, eds., 1997.

ADVANCES IN NEURAL INFORMATION PROCESSING SYSTEMS 9

Proceedings of the 1996 Conference

edited by
Michael C. Mozer, Michael I. Jordan and Thomas Petsche

A Bradford Book
The MIT Press
Cambridge, Massachusetts
London, England

© 1997 Massachusetts Institute of Technology

All rights reserved. No part of this book may be reproduced in any form by any electronic or mechanical means (including photocopying, recording or information storage and retrieval) without permission in writing from the publisher.

This book was printed and bound in the United States of America.

ISSN: 1049-5258
ISBN: 0-262-10065-7

Contents

Preface xiii

NIPS Committees xv

Reviewers xvii

Part I Cognitive Science

Text-Based Information Retrieval Using Exponentiated Gradient Descent,
Ron Papka, James P. Callan and Andrew G. Barto 3

Why did TD-Gammon Work?, Jordan B. Pollack and Alan D. Blair 10

Neural Models for Part-Whole Hierarchies,
Maximilian Riesenhuber and Peter Dayan 17

Part II Neuroscience

Temporal Low-Order Statistics of Natural Sounds, H. Attias and C. E. Schreiner . 27

Reconstructing Stimulus Velocity from Neuronal Responses in Area MT,
Wyeth Bair, James R. Cavanaugh and J. Anthony Movshon 34

3D Object Recognition: A Model of View-Tuned Neurons,
Emanuela Bricolo, Tomaso Poggio and Nikos Logothetis 41

A Hierarchical Model of Visual Rivalry, Peter Dayan 48

Neural Network Models of Chemotaxis in the Nematode Caenorhabditis Elegans,
Thomas C. Ferrée, Ben A. Marcotte and Shawn R. Lockery 55

Extraction of Temporal Features in the Electrosensory System of Weakly Electric Fish, Fabrizio Gabbiani, Walter Metzner, Ralf Wessel and Christof Koch 62

A Neural Model of Visual Contour Integration, Zhaoping Li 69

Learning Exact Patterns of Quasi-synchronization among Spiking Neurons from Data on Multi-unit Recordings,
Laura Martignon, Kathryn Laskey, Gustavo Deco and Eilon Vaadia 76

Complex-Cell Responses Derived from Center-Surround Inputs: The Surprising Power of Intradendritic Computation,
Bartlett W. Mel, Daniel L. Ruderman and Kevin A. Archie 83

Orientation Contrast Sensitivity from Long-range Interactions in Visual Cortex,
Klaus R. Pawelzik, Udo Ernst, Fred Wolf and Theo Geisel 90

Statistically Efficient Estimations Using Cortical Lateral Connections,
Alexandre Pouget and Kechen Zhang 97

An Architectural Mechanism for Direction-tuned Cortical Simple Cells: The Role of Mutual Inhibition, Silvio P. Sabatini, Fabio Solari and Giacomo M. Bisio 104

Cholinergic Modulation Preserves Spike Timing Under Physiologically Realistic Fluctuating Input,
Akaysha C. Tang, Andreas M. Bartels and Terrence J. Sejnowski 111

A Model of Recurrent Interactions in Primary Visual Cortex,
Emanuel Todorov, Athanassios Siapas and David Somers 118

Part III Theory

Neural Learning in Structured Parameter Spaces — Natural Riemannian Gradient, Shun-ichi Amari 127

For Valid Generalization, the Size of the Weights is More Important than the Size of the Network, Peter L. Bartlett 134

Dynamics of Training, Siegfried Bös and Manfred Opper 141

Multilayer Neural Networks: One or Two Hidden Layers?,
G. Brightwell, C. Kenyon and Hélène Paugam-Moisy 148

Support Vector Regression Machines, Harris Drucker, Chris J.C. Burges, Linda Kaufman, Alex Smola and Vladimir Vapnik 155

Size of Multilayer Networks for Exact Learning: Analytic Approach,
André Elisseeff and Hélène Paugam-Moisy 162

The Effect of Correlated Input Data on the Dynamics of Learning,
Søren Halkjær and Ole Winther 169

Practical Confidence and Prediction Intervals, Tom Heskes 176

Statistical Mechanics of the Mixture of Experts, Kukjin Kang and Jong-Hoon Oh . 183

MLP Can Provably Generalize Much Better than VC-bounds Indicate,
A. Kowalczyk and H. Ferrá 190

Radial Basis Function Networks and Complexity Regularization in Function Learning, Adam Krzyżak and Tamás Linder 197

An Apobayesian Relative of Winnow, Nick Littlestone and Chris Mesterharm ... 204

Noisy Spiking Neurons with Temporal Coding have more Computational Power than Sigmoidal Neurons, Wolfgang Maass 211

On the Effect of Analog Noise in Discrete-Time Analog Computations,
Wolfgang Maass and Pekka Orponen 218

A Mean Field Algorithm for Bayes Learning in Large Feed-forward Neural Networks, Manfred Opper and Ole Winther 225

Removing Noise in On-Line Search using Adaptive Batch Sizes, Genevieve B. Orr . 232

Are Hopfield Networks Faster than Conventional Computers?,
Ian Parberry and Hung-Li Tseng 239

Hebb Learning of Features based on their Information Content,
Ferdinand Peper and Hideki Noda 246

The Generalisation Cost of RAMnets, Richard Rohwer and Michal Morciniec . . . 253

Learning with Noise and Regularizers in Multilayer Neural Networks,
David Saad and Sara A. Solla 260

A Variational Principle for Model-based Morphing,
Lawrence K. Saul and Michael I. Jordan 267

Online Learning from Finite Training Sets: An Analytical Case Study,
Peter Sollich and David Barber 274

Support Vector Method for Function Approximation, Regression Estimation, and Signal Processing, Vladimir Vapnik, Steven E. Golowich and Alex Smola 281

The Learning Dynamcis of a Universal Approximator,
Ansgar H. L. West, David Saad and Ian T. Nabney 288

Computing with Infinite Networks, Christopher K. I. Williams 295

Microscopic Equations in Rough Energy Landscape for Neural Networks,
K. Y. Michael Wong 302

Time Series Prediction using Mixtures of Experts,
Assaf J. Zeevi, Ron Meir and Robert J. Adler 309

Part IV Algorithms and Architecture

Genetic Algorithms and Explicit Search Statistics, Shumeet Baluja 319

Consistent Classification, Firm and Soft, Yoram Baram 326

Bayesian Model Comparison by Monte Carlo Chaining,
David Barber and Christopher M. Bishop 333

Gaussian Processes for Bayesian Classification via Hybrid Monte Carlo,
David Barber and Christopher K. I. Williams 340

Regression with Input-Dependent Noise: A Bayesian Treatment,
Christopher M. Bishop and Cazhaow S. Qazaz 347

GTM: A Principled Alternative to the Self-Organizing Map,
Christopher M. Bishop, Markus Svensén and Christopher K. I. Williams 354

The CONDENSATION Algorithm — Conditional Density Propagation and Applications to Visual Tracking, A. Blake and M. Isard 361

Clustering via Concave Minimization,
P. S. Bradley, O. L. Mangasarian and W. N. Street 368

Improving the Accuracy and Speed of Support Vector Machines,
Chris J.C. Burges and B. Schölkopf 375

Estimating Equivalent Kernels for Neural Networks: A Data Perturbation Approach, A. Neil Burgess 382

Promoting Poor Features to Supervisors: Some Inputs Work Better as Outputs,
Rich Caruana and Virginia R. de Sa 389

Self-Organizing and Adaptive Algorithms for Generalized Eigen-Decomposition,
Chanchal Chatterjee and Vwani P. Roychowdhury 396

Representation and Induction of Finite State Machines using Time-Delay Neural Networks,
Daniel S. Clouse, C. Lee Giles, Bill G. Horne and Garrison W. Cottrell 403

488 Solutions to the XOR Problem, Frans M. Coetzee and Virginia L. Stonick . . . 410

Minimizing Statistical Bias with Queries, David A. Cohn 417

MIMIC: Finding Optima by Estimating Probability Densities,
Jeremy S. de Bonet, Charles L. Isbell, Jr. and Paul Viola 424

On a Modification to the Mean Field EM Algorithm in Factorial Learning,
A. P. Dunmur and D. M. Titterington 431

Softening Discrete Relaxation,
Andrew M. Finch, Richard C. Wilson and Edwin R. Hancock 438

Limitations of Self-organizing Maps for Vector Quantization and Multidimensional Scaling, Arthur Flexer 445

Continuous Sigmoidal Belief Networks Trained using Slice Sampling,
Brendan J. Frey 452

Adaptively Growing Hierarchical Mixtures of Experts,
Juergen Fritsch, Michael Finke and Alex Waibel 459

Balancing Between Bagging and Bumping, Tom Heskes 466

LSTM can Solve Hard Long Time Lag Problems,
Sepp Hochreiter and Jürgen Schmidhuber 473

One-unit Learning Rules for Independent Component Analysis,
Aapo Hyvärinen and Erkki Oja 480

Recursive Algorithms for Approximating Probabilities in Graphical Models,
Tommi S. Jaakkola and Michael I. Jordan 487

Combinations of Weak Classifiers, Chuanyi Ji and Sheng Ma 494

Hidden Markov Decision Trees,
Michael I. Jordan, Zoubin Ghahramani and Lawrence K. Saul 501

Unification of Information Maximization and Minimization, Ryotaro Kamimura . . 508

Unsupervised Learning by Convex and Conic Coding, D. D. Lee and H. S. Seung . 515

ARC-LH: A New Adaptive Resampling Algorithm for Improving ANN Classifiers,
Friedrich Leisch and Kurt Hornik 522

Bayesian Unsupervised Learning of Higher Order Structure,
Michael S. Lewicki and Terrence J. Sejnowski 529

Source Separation and Density Estimation by Faithful Equivariant SOM,
Juan K. Lin, Jack D. Cowan and David G. Grier 536

NeuroScale: Novel Topographic Feature Extraction using RBF Networks,
David Lowe and Michael E. Tipping 543

Ordered Classes and Incomplete Examples in Classification, Mark Mathieson ... 550

Triangulation by Continuous Embedding, Marina Meilă and Michael I. Jordan .. 557

Combining Neural Network Regression Estimates with Regularized Linear Weights, Christopher J. Merz and Michael J. Pazzani 564

A Mixture of Experts Classifier with Learning Based on Both Labelled and Unlabelled Data, David J. Miller and Hasan S. Uyar 571

Learning Bayesian Belief Networks with Neural Network Estimators, Stefano Monti and Gregory F. Cooper 578

Smoothing Regularizers for Projective Basis Function Networks, John E. Moody and Thorsteinn S. Rögnvaldsson 585

Competition Among Networks Improves Committee Performance, Paul W. Munro and Bambang Parmanto 592

Adaptive On-line Learning in Changing Environments, Noboru Murata, Klaus-Robert Müller, Andreas Ziehe and Shun-ichi Amari 599

Using Curvature Information for Fast Stochastic Search, Genevieve B. Orr and Todd K. Leen 606

Maximum Likelihood Blind Source Separation: A Context-Sensitive Generalization of ICA, Barak A. Pearlmutter and Lucas C. Parra 613

A Convergence Proof for the Softassign Quadratic Assignment Algorithm, Anand Rangarajan, Alan Yuille, Steven Gold and Eric Mjolsness 620

Second-order Learning Algorithm with Squared Penalty Term, Kazumi Saito and Ryohei Nakano 627

Monotonicity Hints, Joseph Sill and Yaser S. Abu-Mostafa 634

Training Algorithms for Hidden Markov Models using Entropy Based Distance Functions, Yoram Singer and Manfred K. Warmuth 641

Clustering Sequences with Hidden Markov Models, Padhraic Smyth 648

Fast Network Pruning and Feature Extraction by using the Unit-OBS Algorithm, Achim Stahlberger and Martin Riedmiller 655

Separating Style and Content, Joshua B. Tenenbaum and William T. Freeman ... 662

Early Brain Damage, Volker Tresp, Ralph Neuneier and Hans Georg Zimmermann 669

Probabilistic Interpretation of Population Codes, Richard S. Zemel, Peter Dayan and Alexandre Pouget 676

Part V Implementation

VLSI Implementation of Cortical Visual Motion Detection Using an Analog Neural Computer, Ralph Etienne-Cummings, Jan van der Spiegel, Naomi Takahashi, Alyssa Apsel and Paul Mueller 685

A Spike Based Learning Neuron in Analog VLSI,
Philipp Häfliger, Misha Mahowald and Lloyd Watts 692

An Analog Implementation of the Constant Average Statistics Constraint For Sensor Calibration, John G. Harris and Yu-Ming Chiang 699

Analog VLSI Circuits for Attention-Based, Visual Tracking,
Timothy Horiuchi, Tonia G. Morris, Christof Koch and Stephen P. DeWeerth . . . 706

Dynamically Adaptable CMOS Winner-Take-All Neural Network,
Kunihiko Iizuka, Masayuki Miyamoto and Hirofumi Matsui 713

An Adaptive WTA using Floating Gate Technology,
W. Fritz Kruger, Paul Hasler, Bradley A. Minch and Christof Koch 720

A Micropower Analog VLSI HMM State Decoder for Wordspotting,
John Lazzaro, John Wawrzynek and Richard Lippmann 727

Bangs, Clicks, Snaps, Thuds and Whacks: An Architecture for Acoustic Transient Processing, Fernando J. Pineda, Gert Cauwenberghs and R. Timothy Edwards . . 734

A Silicon Model of Amplitude Modulation Detection in the Auditory Brainstem,
André van Schaik, Eric Fragnière and Eric Vittoz 741

Part VI Speech, Handwriting and Signal Processing

Dynamic Features for Visual Speechreading: A Systematic Comparison,
Michael S. Gray, Javier R. Movellan and Terrence J. Sejnowski 751

Blind Separation of Delayed and Convolved Sources,
Te-Won Lee, Anthony J. Bell and Russell H. Lambert 758

A Constructive RBF Network for Writer Adaptation,
John C. Platt and Nada P. Matić 765

A New Approach to Hybrid HMM/ANN Speech Recognition using Mutual Information Neural Networks, G. Rigoll and C. Neukirchen 772

Neural Network Modeling of Speech and Music Signals, Alex Röbel 779

A Constructive Learning Algorithm for Discriminant Tangent Models,
Diego Sona, Alessandro Sperduti and Antonina Starita 786

Dual Kalman Filtering Methods for Nonlinear Prediction, Smoothing and Estimation, Eric A. Wan and Alex T. Nelson 793

Ensemble Methods for Phoneme Classification, Steve Waterhouse and Gary Cook . 800

Effective Training of a Neural Network Character Classifier for Word Recognition, Larry Yaeger, Richard Lyon and Brandyn Webb 807

Part VII Visual Processing

Viewpoint Invariant Face Recognition using Independent Component Analysis and Attractor Networks, Marian Stewart Bartlett and Terrence J. Sejnowski . . . 817

Contents

Learning Temporally Persistent Hierarchical Representations, Suzanna Becker . . 824

Edges are the "Independent Components" of Natural Scenes,
Anthony J. Bell and Terrence J. Sejnowski 831

Compositionality, MDL Priors, and Object Recognition,
Elie Bienenstock, Stuart Geman and Daniel Potter 838

Learning Appearance Based Models: Mixtures of Second Moment Experts,
Christoph Bregler and Jitendra Malik 845

Spatial Decorrelation in Orientation Tuned Cortical Cells,
Alexander Dimitrov and Jack D. Cowan 852

*Spatiotemporal Coupling and Scaling of Natural Images and Human Visual
Sensitivities*, Dawei W. Dong 859

Selective Integration: A Model for Disparity Estimation, Michael S. Gray,
Alexandre Pouget, Richard S. Zemel, Steven J. Nowlan and Terrence J. Sejnowski   866

ARTEX: A Self-organizing Architecture for Classifying Image Regions,
Stephen Grossberg and James R. Williamson 873

Contour Organisation with the EM Algorithm,
J. A. F. Leite and Edwin R. Hancock 880

Visual Cortex Circuitry and Orientation Tuning,
Trevor Mundel, Alexander Dimitrov and Jack D. Cowan 887

Representing Face Images for Emotion Classification,
Curtis Padgett and Garrison W. Cottrell 894

Rapid Visual Processing using Spike Asynchrony,
Simon J. Thorpe and Jacques Gautrais 901

Interpreting Images by Propagating Bayesian Beliefs, Yair Weiss 908

Salient Contour Extraction by Temporal Binding in a Cortically-based Network,
Shih-Cheng Yen and Leif H. Finkel 915

Part VIII Applications

*An Orientation Selective Neural Network for Pattern Identification in Particle
Detectors*,
Halina Abramowicz, David Horn, Ury Naftaly and Carmit Sahar-Pikielny 925

Adaptive Access Control Applied to Ethernet Data, Timothy X. Brown 932

Predicting Lifetimes in Dynamically Allocated Memory,
David A. Cohn and Satinder Singh 939

Multi-Task Learning for Stock Selection, Joumana Ghosn and Yoshua Bengio . . . 946

*The Neurothermostat: Predictive Optimal Control of Residential Heating
Systems*, Michael C. Mozer, Lucky Vidmar and Robert H. Dodier 953

*Sequential Tracking in Pricing Financial Options using Model Based and Neural
Network Approaches*, Mahesan Niranjan 960

A Comparison between Neural Networks and other Statistical Techniques for Modeling the Relationship between Tobacco and Alcohol and Cancer,
Tony Plate, Pierre Band, Joel Bert and John Grace 967

Reinforcement Learning for Dynamic Channel Allocation in Cellular Telephone Systems, Satinder Singh and Dimitri Bertsekas 974

Spectroscopic Detection of Cervical Pre-Cancer through Radial Basis Function Networks, Kagan Tumer, Nirmala Ramanujam, Rebecca Richards-Kortum and Joydeep Ghosh 981

Interpolating Earth-science Data using RBF Networks and Mixtures of Experts,
Ernest Wan and Don Bone 988

Multi-effect Decompositions for Financial Data Modeling,
Lizhong Wu and John E. Moody 995

Part IX Control, Navigation and Planning

Multidimensional Triangulation and Interpolation for Reinforcement Learning,
Scott Davies 1005

Efficient Nonlinear Control with Actor-Tutor Architecture, Kenji Doya 1012

Local Bandit Approximation for Optimal Learning Problems,
Michael O. Duff and Andrew G. Barto 1019

Reinforcement Learning for Mixed Open-loop and Closed-loop Control,
Eric A. Hansen, Andrew G. Barto and Shlomo Zilberstein 1026

Multi-Grid Methods for Reinforcement Learning in Controlled Diffusion Processes, Stephan Pareigis 1033

Learning from Demonstration, Stefan Schaal 1040

Exploiting Model Uncertainty Estimates for Safe Dynamic Control Learning,
Jeff G. Schneider 1047

Analytical Mean Squared Error Curves in Temporal Difference Learning,
Satinder Singh and Peter Dayan 1054

Learning Decision Theoretic Utilities through Reinforcement Learning,
Magnus Stensmo and Terrence J. Sejnowski 1061

On-line Policy Improvement using Monte-Carlo Search,
Gerald Tesauro and Gregory R. Galperin 1068

Analysis of Temporal-Diffference Learning with Function Approximation,
John N. Tsitsiklis and Benjamin Van Roy 1075

Approximate Solutions to Optimal Stopping Problems,
John N. Tsitsiklis and Benjamin Van Roy 1082

Index of Authors 1089

Keyword Index 1093

Preface

This volume contains the papers presented at the tenth annual conference on Neural Information Processing Systems (NIPS), held in Denver, Colorado, from Dec. 2 to Dec. 5, 1996. These papers cover a wide variety of topics in neural computation, including the design and analysis of learning algorithms, learning theory, neuroscience, vision, speech, control theory and applications in areas such as operations research, finance, applied statistics, and experimental physics.

NIPS consistently receives submissions of the highest quality. This year there were 509 submissions, of which 151 were accepted for oral or poster presentation. Authors received feedback from three reviewers, each of whom provided detailed comments to aid the authors in revising their paper for publication. Authors also had the opportunity to revise their papers after the conference based on feedback they received during their presentations.

The NIPS conference continues to evolve intellectually; novel directions of research arise in each year's conference and are explored in detail in subsequent years. This ongoing evolution is abetted by the high degree of interdisciplinarity and interactiveness that characterize the conference. NIPS is a single track conference, which enhances the exchange of ideas between algorithm developers, theoreticians, implementors and applications-oriented researchers.

Probabilistic methods were particularly in evidence at this year's meeting, continuing a trend that has become increasingly characteristic of NIPS in recent years. Examples include image interpretation via probabilistic propagation (Weiss), maximum likelihood source separation (Pearlmutter and Parra), model combination for regression (Merz and Pazzani), an EM method for spline fitting (Leite and Hancock), model-based morphing (Saul and Jordan), regression via Gaussian processes (Barber and Williams), separable mixture models (Tenenbaum and Freeman), a probabilistic map-forming algorithm (Bishop, Svensen and Williams), and a statistical analysis of lateral connectivity in cortex (Pouget and Zhang). Independent components analysis continued to attract interest (Hyvarinen and Oja; Bell and Sejnowski), as did the topic of function approximation in temporal difference learning (Tsitsiklis and Van Roy).

We want to thank the invited speakers at this year's conference
> Andrew Blake, University of Oxford;
> David Donoho, UC Berkeley and Stanford;
> Eric Enderton, Industrial Light and Magic;
> Stuart Geman, Brown University;
> Henry Markram, The Weizmann Institute for Science; and
> Misha Tsodyks, The Weizmann Institute of Science.

NIPS attendees also benefitted from a strong lineup of tutorial presentations given by
> Frank Eeckman, Lawrence Berkeley National Laboratory;
> Trevor Hastie, Stanford University;
> Dan Jurafsky, University of Colorado at Boulder;
> John Moody, Challenges of Time Series Prediction;
> Brian Ripley, University of Oxford; and
> Richard Sutton, University of Massachusetts.

Finally, a special thanks to all of the people who devote so much of their time to organizing and maintaining the continuity of the conference. Thanks go to the members of the Organizing Committee, the Program Committee, the Publicity Committee, the Board of Directors of the NIPS Foundation, and to all of the 166 referees who reviewed papers for NIPS this year. Particular thanks go to Denise Pruell and Christy Medina, for their stellar work as professional conference administrators and registration coordinators, to Marijke Augusteijn for her devoted efforts with local arrangements, and to the many student volunteers for help with conference logistics. We are also grateful to the Office of Naval Research for providing financial support to allow many graduate students and young investigators to attend the meeting.

Michael C. Mozer, University of Colorado
Michael I. Jordan, Massachusetts Institute of Technology
Thomas Petsche, Siemens Corporate Research, Inc.

January 17, 1997

NIPS Committees

Organizing Committee

General Chair	*Michael C. Mozer*, University of Colorado
Program Chair	*Michael I. Jordan*, MIT
Workshop Co-Chairs	*Steven J. Nowlan*, Motorola, Lexicus Division
	Michael P. Perrone, IBM
Tutorials Chair	*John Lazzaro*, UC Berkeley
Publicity Chair	*Sue Becker*, McMaster University
Publications Chair	*Thomas Petsche*, Siemens Corporate Research Inc.
Treasurer	*Eric Mjolsness*, UC San Diego
Local Arrangements Chair	*Marijke Augusteijn*, University of Colorado

Program Committee

Program Chair	*Michael I. Jordan*, MIT
Algorithms and Architectures	*Christopher Bishop*, Aston University
	Stephen Omohundro, NEC Research Institute
	Robert Tibshirani, University of Toronto
Theory	*Michael Kearns*, AT&T Research
	Sara Solla, AT&T Research
Vision	*David Mumford*, Brown University
Speech and Signal Processing	*Eric Wan*, Oregon Graduate Institute
Control and Navigation	*Andrew Moore*, Carnegie Mellon University
Artificial Intelligence & Cognitive Science	*Stuart Russell*, University of California
Neuroscience	*William Bialek*, NEC Research Institute
Applications	*Anders Krogh*, The Sanger Centre
Implementations	*Fernando Pineda*, The Johns Hopkins University

Publicity Committee

Publicity Chair	*Sue Becker*, McMaster
Liason for Australia, Singapore and India	*Marwan Jabri*, University of Sydney
Liason for Europe	*Joachim Buhmann*, University of Bonn
Liason for Hong Kong, China and Taiwan	*Lei Xu*, Chinese University of Hong Kong
Liason for Isreal	*Hava Siegelmann*, Technion
Liason for Japan	*Kenji Doya*, ATR Research Laboratories
Liason for Turkey	*Ethem Alpaydin*, Bogazici Univesity
Liason for United Kingdom	*Alan Murray*, Edinburgh Univesity
Liason for South America	*Andreas Meier*, Simon Bolivar University
Web Master	*David Redish*, CMU

NIPS Foundation Board Members

President	*Terrence Sejnowski*, The Salk Institute
Vice President for Development	*John Moody*, Oregon Graduate Institute
Treasurer	*Eric Mjolsness*, UC San Diego
Secretary	*Gerald Tesauro*, IBM Watson Labs.
Members	*Scott Kirkpatrick*, IBM Research
	Jack Cowan, University of Chicago
	Stephen J. Hanson, Rutgers
	Richard Lippmann, MIT Lincoln Laboratory
	Dave Touretzky, Carnegie Mellon University
	Gary Blasdel, Harvard Medical School
	Leo Breiman, UC Berkeley
Emeritus	*T.L. Fine*, Cornell University
	Eve Marder, Brandeis University
NIPS*96 General Chair	*Michael Mozer*, University of Colorado, Boulder

Reviewers

Larry Abbott
Naoki Abe
Subutai Ahmad
Ethem Alpaydin
Chuck Anderson
James Anderson
Chris Atkeson
Pierre Baldi
Naama Barkai
Etienne Barnard
Andy Barto
Francoise Beaufays
Sue Becker
Yoshua Bengio
Bill Bialek
Michael Biehl
C.M. Bishop
Leon Bottou
Herve Bourlard
Timothy Brown
Nader Bshouty
Joachim Buhmann
Carmen Canavier
Claire Cardie
Ted Carnevale
Nestor Caticha
Gert Cauwenberghs
David Cohn
Greg Cooper
Corinna Cortes
Gary Cottrell
Marie Cottrell
Bob Crites
Christian Darken
Peter Dayan
Virginia de Sa
Alain Destexhe
Thomas Dietterich
Dawei Dong
Charles Elkan
Ralph Etienne-Cummings
Gary Flake
Paolo Frasconi

Bill Freeman
Yoav Freund
Jerry Friedman
Patrick Gallinari
Stuart Geman
Zoubin Ghahramani
Federico Girosi
Mirta Gordon
Russ Greiner
Vijaykumar Gullapalli
Isabelle Guyon
Lars Hansen
John Harris
Michael Hasselmo
Simon Haykin
David Heckerman
John Hertz
Andreas Herz
Tom Heskes
Geoffrey Hinton
Sean Holden
Don Hush
Nathan Intrator
Tommi Jaakkola
Marwan Jabri
Jeff Jackson
Robbie Jacobs
Chuanyi Ji
Ido Kanter
Bert Kappen
Michael Kearns
Dan Kersten
Ronny Kohavi
Anders Krogh
Alan Lapedes
John Lazzaro
Tai Sing Lee
Todd Leen
Zhaoping Li
Christiane Linster
Richard Lippmann
Michael Littman
David Lowe

David Madigan
Marina Meila
Bartlett Mel
David Miller
Kenneth Miller
Martin Moller
P. Read Montague
Andrew Moore
J. Anthony Movshon
Klaus Mueller
David Mumford
Alan Murray
Ian Nabney
Jean-Pierre Nadal
Ken Nakayama
Ralph Neuneier
Mahesan Niranjan
Peter Norvig
Klaus Obermayer
Erkki Oja
Stephen Omohundro
Genevieve Orr
Art Owen
Barak Pearlmutter
Jing Peng
Fernando Pereira
Pietro Perona
Carsten Peterson
Fernando Pineda
Jay Pittman
Tony Plate
John Platt
Jordan Pollack
Alexandre Pouget
Jose Principe
Adam Prugel-Bennett
Anand Rangarajan
Carl Rasmussen
Steve Renals
Barry Richmond
Peter Riegler
Brian Ripley
David Rohwer

Stuart Russell
David Saad
Philip Sabes
Lawrence Saul
Stefan Schaal
Jeff Schneider
Terrence Sejnowski
Robert Shapley
Patrice Simard
Yoram Singer
Satinder Singh
Padhraic Smyth
Bill Softky
Sara Solla
David Somers

Devika Subramanian
Richard Sutton
Josh Tenenbaum
Michael Thielscher
Sebastian Thrun
Rob Tibshirani
Mike Titterington
Geoffrey Towell
Todd Troyer
Ah Chung Tsoi
Michael Turmon
Joachim Utans
Benjamin VanRoy
Kelvin Wagner
Eric Wan

Raymond Watrous
Yair Weiss
Christopher Williams
Ronald Williams
Robert Williamson
David Willshaw
Ole Winther
David Wolpert
Lei Xu
Alan Yuille
Tony Zador
Richard Zemel
Steven Zucker

ADVANCES IN NEURAL INFORMATION PROCESSING SYSTEMS 9

Part I
Cognitive Science

Text-Based Information Retrieval Using Exponentiated Gradient Descent

Ron Papka, James P. Callan, and Andrew G. Barto [*]
Department of Computer Science
University of Massachusetts
Amherst, MA 01003
papka@cs.umass.edu, callan@cs.umass.edu, barto@cs.umass.edu

Abstract

The following investigates the use of single-neuron learning algorithms to improve the performance of text-retrieval systems that accept natural-language queries. A retrieval process is explained that transforms the natural-language query into the query syntax of a real retrieval system: the initial query is expanded using statistical and learning techniques and is then used for document ranking and binary classification. The results of experiments suggest that Kivinen and Warmuth's Exponentiated Gradient Descent learning algorithm works significantly better than previous approaches.

1 Introduction

The following work explores two learning algorithms – Least Mean Squared (LMS) [1] and Exponentiated Gradient Descent (EG) [2] – in the context of text-based Information Retrieval (IR) systems. The experiments presented in [3] use connectionist learning models to improve the retrieval of relevant documents from a large collection of text. Here, we present further analysis of those experiments. Previous work in the area employs various techniques for improving retrieval [6, 7, 14]. The experiments presented here show that EG works significantly better than widely used ad hoc methods for finding a good set of query term weights.

The retrieval processes being considered operate on a collection of documents, a natural-language query, and a training set of documents judged relevant or non-relevant to the query. The query may be, for example, the information request submitted through a web-search engine, or through the interface of a system with

---

[*] This material is based on work supported by the National Science Foundation, Library of Congress, and Department of Commerce under cooperative agreement number EEC-9209623. Any opinions, findings and conclusions or recommendations expressed in this material are those of the author and do not necessarily reflect those of the sponsor.

domain-specific information such as legal, governmental, or news data maintained as a collection of text. The query, expressed as complete or incomplete sentences, is modified through a learning process that incorporates the terms in the test collection that are important for improving retrieval performance. The resulting query can then be used against collections similar in domain to the training collection.

Natural language query:
An insider-trading case.

IR system query using default weights:
#WSUM(1.0 An 1.0 insider 1.0 trading 1.0 case);

After stop word and stemming process:
#WSUM(1.0 insid 1.0 trade 1.0 case);

After Expansion and learning new weights:
#WSUM(0.181284 insid 0.045721 trade 0.016127 case 0.088143 boesk 0.000001 ivan 0.026762 sec 0.052081 guilt 0.074493 drexel 0.000001 plead 0.003834 fraud 0.091436 takeov 0.018636 lawyer 0.000000 crimin 0.137799 alleg 0.057393 attorney 0.155781 charg 0.024237 scandal 0.000000 burnham 0.000000 lambert 0.026270 investig 0.000000 wall 0.000000 firm 0.000000 illeg 0.000000 indict 0.000000 prosecutor 0.000000 profit 0.000000);

Figure 1: Query Transformation Process.

The query transformation process is illustrated in Figure 1. First, the natural-language query is transformed into one which can be used by the query-parsing mechanism of the IR system. The weights associated with each term are assigned a default value of 1.0, implying that each term is equally important in discriminating relevant documents. The query then undergoes a *stopping and stemming* process, by which morphological stemming and the elimination of very common words, called stopwords, increases both the effectiveness and efficiency of a system [9]. The query is subsequently expanded using a statistical term-expansion process producing terms from the training set of documents. Finally, a learning algorithm is invoked to produce new weights for the expanded query.

2 Retrieval Process

Text-based information retrieval systems allow the user to pose a query to a collection or a stream of documents. When a query q is presented to a collection c, each document $d \in c$ is examined and assigned a value relative to how well d satisfies the semantics of the request posed by q. For any instance of the triple $< q, d, c >$, the system determines an evaluation value attributed to d using the function $eval(q, d, c)$.

The evaluation function $eval(q, d, c) = \frac{\sum_{i=1}^{N} q_i * d_i}{\sum_{i=1}^{N} q_i}$

was used for this work, and is based on an implementation of INQUERY [8]. It is assumed that q and d are vectors of real numbers, and that c contains precomputed collection statistics in addition to the current set of documents. Since the collection may change over time, it may be necessary to change the query representation over time; however, in what follows the training collection is assumed to be static, and successful learning implies that the resulting query generalizes to similar collections.

An IR system can perform several kinds of retrieval tasks. This work is specifically concerned with two retrieval processes: document ranking and document classification. A ranking of documents based on query q is achieved by sorting all documents in a collection by evaluation value. Binary classification is achieved by determining a threshold θ such that for class R, $eval(q, d, c) \geq \theta \rightarrow d \in R$, and

$eval(q, d, c) < \theta \to d \in \bar{R}$, so that R is the set of documents from the collection that are classified as relevant to the query, and $\bar{R}$ is the set classified as non-relevant.

Central to any IR system is a parsing process used for documents and queries, which produces tokens called *terms*. The terms derived from a document are used to build an *inverted list* structure which serves as an index to the collection. The natural-language query is also parsed into a set of terms. Research-based IR systems such as INQUERY, OKAPI [11], and SMART [5], assume that the co-occurrence of a term in a query and a document indicates that the document is relevant to the query to some degree, and that a query with multiple terms requires a mechanism by which to combine the evidence each co-occurrence contributes to the document's degree of relevance to the query. The document representation for such systems is a vector, each element of which is associated with a unique term in the document. The values in the vector are produced by a *term-evaluation function* comprised of a term frequency component, tf, and an inverse document frequency component, idf, which are described in [8, 11]. The tf component causes the term-evaluation value to increase as a query-term's occurrence in the document increases, and the idf component causes the term-evaluation value to decrease as the number of documents in the collection in which the term occurs increases.

3 Query Expansion

Though it is possible to learn weights for terms in the original query, better results are obtained by first expanding the query with additional terms that can contribute to identifying relevant documents, and then learning the weights for the expanded query. The optimal number of terms by which to expand a query is domain-dependent, and query expansion can be performed using several techniques, including thesaurus expansion and statistical methods [12]. The query expansion process performed in this work is a two-step process: *term selection* followed by *weight assignment*. The term selection process ranks all terms found in relevant documents by an information metric described in [8]. The top n terms are used in the expanded query. The experiments in this work used values of 50 and 1000 for n. The most common technique for weight assignment is derived from a closed-form function originally presented by Rocchio in [6], but our experiments show that a single-neuron learning approach is more effective.

3.1 Rocchio Weights

We assume that the terms of the original query are stored in a vector t, and that their associated weights are stored in q. Assuming that the new terms in the expanded query are stored t', the weights for q' can be determined using a method originally developed by Rocchio that has been improved upon in [7, 8]. Using the notation presented above, the weight assignment can be represented in the linear form: $q' = \alpha * f(t) + \beta * r(t', R_q, c) + \gamma * nr(t', \bar{R}_q, c)$, where f is a function operating on the terms in the original query, r is a function operating on the term statistics available from the training set of relevant documents (R_q), and nr is a function operating on the statistics from the non-relevant documents ($\bar{R}_q$). The values for α, β, and γ have been the focus of many IR experiments, and 1.0, 2.0, and 0.5, have been found to work well with various implementations of the functions f, r, and nr [7].

3.2 LMS and EG

In the experiments that follow, LMS and EG were used to learn query term weights. Both algorithms were used in a training process attempting to learn the association between the set of training instances (documents) and their corresponding binary classifications (relevant or non-relevant). A set of weights $\vec{w}$ is updated given an input instance $\vec{x}$ and a target binary classification value y. The algorithms learn the association between $\vec{x}$ and y perfectly if $\vec{w} \cdot \vec{x} = y$, otherwise the value $(y - \vec{w} \cdot \vec{x})$ is the error or *loss* incurred. The task of the learning algorithm is to learn the values of $\vec{w}$ for more than one instance of $\vec{x}$.

The update rule for LMS is $\vec{w}_{t+1} = \vec{w}_t + \vec{r}_t$, where $\vec{r}_t = -2\eta_t(\vec{w}_t \cdot \vec{x}_t - y_t)\vec{x}_t$, where the step-size $\eta_t = \frac{1}{\vec{x}_t \cdot \vec{x}_t}$. The update rule for EG is $\vec{w}_{t+1,i} = \frac{\vec{w}_{t,i} e^{\vec{r}_{t,i}}}{\sum_{j=1}^{N} \vec{w}_{t,j} e^{\vec{r}_{t,j}}}$, where

$\vec{r}_{t,i} = -2\eta_t(\vec{w}_t \cdot \vec{x}_t - y_t)\vec{x}_{t,i}$, and $\eta_t = \frac{2}{3(\max_i(\vec{x}_{t,i}) - \min_i(\vec{x}_{t,i}))}$.

There are several fundamental differences between LMS and EG; the most salient is that EG has a multiplicative exponential update rule, while LMS is additive. A less obvious difference is the derivation of these two update rules. Kivinen and Warmuth [2] show that both rules are *approximately* derivable from an optimization task that minimizes the linear combination of a distance and a loss function: $distance(\vec{w}_{t+1}, \vec{w}_t) + \eta_t loss(y_t, \vec{w}_t \cdot \vec{x}_t)$. But the *distance* component for the derivation leading to the LMS update rule uses the squared Euclidean distance $\|\vec{w}_{t+1} - \vec{w}_t\|_2^2$, while the derivation leading to the EG update rule uses relative entropy or $\sum_{i=1}^{N} \vec{w}_{t+1,i} \ln \frac{\vec{w}_{t+1,i}}{\vec{w}_{t,i}}$. Entropy metrics had previously been used as the *loss* component [4].

One purpose of Kivinen and Warmuth's work was to describe loss bounds for these algorithms; however, they also observed that EG suffers significantly less from irrelevant attributes than does LMS. This hypothesis was tested in the experiments conducted for this work.

4 Experiments

Experiments were conducted on 100 natural-language queries. The queries were manually transformed into INQUERY syntax, expanded using a statistical technique described in [8], and then given a weight assignment as a result of a learning process. One set of experiments expanded each query by 50 terms and another set of experiments expanded each query by 1000 terms. The purpose of the latter was to test the ability of each algorithm to learn in the presence of many irrelevant attributes.

4.1 Data

The queries used are the *description* fields of information requests developed for Text Retrieval Conferences (TREC) [10]. The first set of queries was taken from TREC topics 51-100 and the second set from topics 101-150, for a total of 100 queries. After stopping and stemming, the average number of terms remaining before expansion was 8.34 terms.

Training and testing for all queries was conducted on subsets of the Tipster collection, which currently contains 3.4 gigabytes of text, including 206,201 documents whose relevance to the TREC topics has been evaluated. The collection is partitioned into 3 volumes. The judged documents from volumes 1 and 2 were used for training, while the documents from volume 3 were used for testing. Volumes 1 and 2 contain 741,856 documents from the Associated Press(1988-9), Department of Energy abstract, Federal Register(1988-9), Wall Street Journal(1987-91), and Ziff-Davis Computer-select articles. Volume 3 contains 336,310 documents from Associated Press(1990), San Jose Mercury News(1991), and Ziff-Davis articles.

Only a subset of the data for the TREC-Tipster environment has been judged. Binary judgments are assessed by humans for the top few thousand documents that were retrieved for each query by participating systems from various commercial and research institutions. Based on the judged documents available for volumes 1 and 2, on average 280 relevant documents and 1236 non-relevant documents were used to train each query.

4.2 Training Parameters

Rocchio weights were assigned based on coefficients described in Section 3.1. LMS and EG update rules were applied using 100,000 random presentations of training instances. It was empirically determined that this number of presentations was sufficient to allow both learning algorithms to produce better query weights than the Rocchio assignment based on performance metrics calculated using the training instances.

In reality, of course, the number of documents that will be relevant to a particular query is much smaller than the number of documents that are non-relevant. This property gives rise to the question of what is an appropriate sampling bias of training instances, considering that the ratio of relevant to non-relevant documents approaches 0 in the limit. In the following experiments, LMS benefitted from uniform random sampling from the set of training instances, while EG benefitted from a balanced sampling, that is uniform random sampling from relevant training instances on even iterations and from non-relevant instances on odd iterations.

A *pocketing technique* was applied to the learning algorithms [13]. The purpose of this technique is to find a set of weights that optimize a specific user's utility function. In the following experiments, weights were tested every 1000 iterations using a recall and precision performance metric. If a set of weights produced a new performance-metric maximum, it was saved. The last set saved was assumed to be the result of the algorithm, and was used for testing.

A binary classification value pair (A, B) is supplied as the target for training, where A is the classification value for relevant documents, and B is the classification value for non-relevant documents. Using the standard classification value pair (1, 0), INQUERY's document representation inhibits learning due to the large error caused by these unattainable values. Therefore, testing was done and resulted in the observation that .4 was the lowest attainable evaluation value for a document, and .47 appeared to be a good classification value for relevant documents. The classification value pair used for both the LMS and EG algorithms was thus (.47, .40).

4.3 Evaluation

In the experiments that follow, R-Precision (RP) was used to evaluate ranking performance, and a new metric, Lower Bound Accuracy (LBA) was used to evaluate classification. Both metrics make use of *recall* and *precision*, which are defined as follows: Assume there exists a set of documents sorted by evaluation value and a process that has performed classification, and that a = number of relevant documents classified as relevant, b = number of non-relevant documents classified as relevant, c = number of relevant documents classified as non-relevant, and d = number of non-relevant documents classified as non-relevant; then, $Recall = \frac{a}{a+c}$, and $Precision = \frac{a}{a+b}$ [3].

Precision and *recall* can be calculated at any cut-off point in the sorted list of documents. *R-Precision* is calculated using the top n documents, where n is the number of relevant training documents available for a query.

Lower Bound Accuracy (LBA) is a metric that assumes the minimum of a classifier's accuracy with respect to relevant documents and its accuracy with respect to non-relevant documents. It is defined as $LBA = min(\frac{a}{a+c}, \frac{d}{b+d})$. An LBA value can be interpreted as the lower bound of the percent of instances a classifier will correctly classify, regardless of an imbalance between the actual number of relevant and non-relevant documents. This metric requires a threshold θ. The threshold is taken to be the evaluation value of the document at a cut-off point in the sorted list of training documents where LBA is maximized. Hence, $\theta = max_i(LBA(d_i, R_q, \bar{R}_q))$, where d_i is the ith document in the sorted list.

4.4 Results

Query type	RP	LBA
NL	22.0	88.6
EXP	28.7	92.0
ROC	33.4	94.0
LMS	32.5	89.8
EG	40.3	95.1

Table 1: Query expansion by 50 terms

The following results show the ability of a query weight assignment to generalize. The weights are derived from a subset of the training collection, and the values reported are based on performance on the test collection. The results of the 50-term-expansion experiments are listed in Table 1 [1]. They indicate that the expanded query has an advantage over the original query, and that the EG-trained query generalized better than the other algorithms, while Rocchio appears to be the next best. In terms of ranking, EG gives rise to a 20% improvement over the Rocchio assignment, and realizes 1.2% improvement in terms of classification. This apparently slight improvement in classification in fact implies that EG is correctly classifying at least 3000 documents more than the other approaches.

Table 2 shows a cross-algorithm analysis in which any two algorithms can be compared. The analysis is calculated using both RP and LBA over all queries. An entry for row i column j indicates the number of queries for which the performance of algorithm i was better than algorithm j. Based on sign tests with $\alpha = .01$, the results confirm that EG significantly generalized better than the other algorithms.[2]

Query type	Query counts: RP-LBA				
	NL	EXP	ROC	LMS	EG
NL	-	30 -37	18 - 13	24 - 53	12 - 13
EXP	60 - 62	-	9 - 17	35 - 66	11 - 19
ROC	71 - 86	72 -79	-	53 - 73	17 - 37
LMS	66 - 46	54 -34	38 - 26	-	13 - 15
EG	79 - 85	80 -80	70 - 62	74 - 84	-

Table 2: Cross Algorithm Analysis over 100 queries expanded by 50 terms.

As explained in Section 4.3, the thresholds used to calculate the LBA performance metric are determined by obtaining an evaluation value in the training data corresponding to the cut-off point where LBA was maximized. The threshold analysis in Table 3 shows the best attainable classification performance against performance actually achieved. The results indicate that there is still room for improvement; however, they also indicate that this methodology is acceptable.

The results for queries expanded by 1000 terms are listed in Table 4. Since the average document length in the Tipster collection is 806 terms (non-unique), at least 20% of the terms in the expanded query are generally irrelevant to a particular document. The results indicate that irrelevant attributes prevent all but EG from generalizing well. Comparing the performance of EG and LMS adds evidence to the Kivinen-Warmuth hypothesis that EG yields a smaller *loss* than LMS, given many irrelevant attributes. Juxtaposing the results of the 50-term and 1000-term-expansion experiments suggests that using a statistical filter for selecting the top few terms is better than expanding the query by many terms and having the learning algorithm perform term selection.

5 Conclusion

The experiment results presented here provide evidence that single-neuron learning algorithms can be used to improve retrieval performance in IR systems. Based on performance metrics that test the quality of a classification process and a document ranking process, the weights produced by EG were consistently better than previously available methods.

---

[1] R-Precision (RP) and Lower Bound Accuracy (LBA) performance values are normalized to a 0-100 scale. Values are reported for: NL = original natural language query; EXP = expanded query with weights set to 1.0; ROC = expanded query with weights based on Rocchio assignment; LMS = expanded query with weights based on LMS learning; and EG= expanded query with weights based on EG learning.

[2] Recent experiments using the optimization algorithm DFO (presented in [7]) suggest that certain parameter settings make it competitive with EG.

Query type	Potential LBA	Actual LBA
NL	91.9	88.6
EXP	95.5	92.0
ROC	96.7	94.0
LMS	92.6	89.8
EG	97.1	95.1

Table 3: Threshold Analysis: Query expansion by 50 terms.

Query type	RP	LBA
NL	22.0	88.6
EXP	14.4	76.5
ROC	19.7	82.5
LMS	20.4	86.7
EG	35.0	93.2

Table 4: Query expansion by 1000 terms.

References

[1] B. Widrow and M. Hoff, "Adaptive switching circuits", In 1960 IRE WESCON Convention Record, pp. 96-104, New York, 1960.

[2] J. Kivinen, Manfred Wartmuth, "Exponentiated Gradient Versus Gradient Descent for Linear Predictors", UCSC Tech report: UCSC-CRL-94-16, June 21, 1994.

[3] D. Lewis, R. Schapire, J. Callan, and R. Papka, "Training Algorithms for Linear Text Classifiers", Proceeding of SIGIR 1996.

[4] B.S. Wittner and J.S. Denker, "Strategies for Teaching Layered Networks Classification Tasks", NIPS proceedings, 1987.

[5] G. Salton, "Relevance Feedback and optimization of retrieval effectiveness. In The Smart system - experiments in automatic document processing", 324-336. Englewood Cliffs, NJ: Prentice Hall Inc., 1971.

[6] J.J. Rocchio, "Relevance Feedback in Information Retrieval in The Smart System - Experiments in Automatic document processing", 313-323. Englewood Cliffs, NJ: Prentice Hall Inc., 1971.

[7] C. Buckley and G. Salton, "Optimization of Relevance Feedback Weights", Proceeding of SIGIR 95 Seattle WA, 1995.

[8] J. Allan, L. Ballesteros, J. Callan, W.B. Croft, and Z. Lu, "Recent Experiments with Inquery", TREC-4 Proceedings, 1995.

[9] M. Porter, "An Algorithm for Suffix Stripping", Program, Vol 14(3), pp. 130-137, 1980.

[10] D. Harman, Proceedings of Text REtrievl Conferences (TREC), 1993-5.

[11] S.E. Robertson, W. Walker, S. Jones, M.M. Hancock-Beaulieu, and M.Gatford, "Okapi at TREC-3", TREC-3 Proceedings, 1994.

[12] G. Salton, *Automatic Text Processing*, Addison-Wesley Publishing Co, Massachusetts, 1989.

[13] S.I. Gallant, "Optimal Linear Discrimants", Proceedings of International Conference on Pattern Recognition, 1986.

[14] B.T. Bartell, "Optimizing Ranking Functions: A Connectionist Approach to Adaptive Information Retrieval", Ph.D. Theis, UCSD 1994.

Why did TD-Gammon Work?

Jordan B. Pollack & Alan D. Blair
Computer Science Department
Brandeis University
Waltham, MA 02254
{pollack,blair}@cs.brandeis.edu

Abstract

Although TD-Gammon is one of the major successes in machine learning, it has not led to similar impressive breakthroughs in temporal difference learning for other applications or even other games. We were able to replicate some of the success of TD-Gammon, developing a competitive evaluation function on a 4000 parameter feed-forward neural network, without using back-propagation, reinforcement or temporal difference learning methods. Instead we apply simple hill-climbing in a relative fitness environment. These results and further analysis suggest that the surprising success of Tesauro's program had more to do with the co-evolutionary structure of the learning task and the dynamics of the backgammon game itself.

1 INTRODUCTION

It took great *chutzpah* for Gerald Tesauro to start wasting computer cycles on temporal difference learning in the game of Backgammon (Tesauro, 1992). Letting a machine learning program play itself in the hopes of becoming an expert, indeed! After all, the dream of computers mastering a domain by self-play or "introspection" had been around since the early days of AI, forming part of Samuel's checker player (Samuel, 1959) and used in Donald Michie's MENACE tic-tac-toe learner (Michie, 1961). However such self-conditioning systems, with weak or non-existent internal representations, had generally been fraught with problems of scale and abandoned by the field of AI. Moreover, self-playing learners usually develop eccentric and brittle strategies which allow them to draw each other, yet play poorly against humans and other programs.

Yet Tesauro's 1992 result showed that this self-play approach could be powerful, and after some refinement and millions of iterations of self-play, his TD-Gammon program has become one of the best backgammon players in the world (Tesauro, 1995). His derived weights are viewed by his corporation as significant enough intellectual property to keep as a trade secret, except to leverage sales of their minority operating system (International Business Machines, 1995). Others have replicated this TD result both for research purposes (Boyan, 1992) and commercial purposes.

With respect to the goal of a self-organizing learning machine which starts from a minimal specification and rises to great sophistication, TD-Gammon stands alone. How is its success to be understood, explained, and replicated in other domains? Is TD-Gammon unbridled good news about the reinforcement learning method?

Our hypothesis is that the success of TD-gammon is not due to the back-propagation, reinforcement, or temporal-difference technologies, but to an inherent bias from the dynamics of the game of backgammon, and the co-evolutionary setup of the training, by which the task dynamically changes as the learning progresses. We test this hypothesis by using a much simpler co-evolutionary learning method for backgammon - namely hill-climbing.

2 SETUP

We use a standard feedforward neural network with two layers and the sigmoid function, set up in the same fashion as Tesauro with 4 units to represent the number of each player's pieces on each of the 24 points, plus 2 units each to indicate how many are on the bar and off the board. In addition, we added one more unit which reports whether or not the game has reached the endgame or "race" situation, making a total of 197 input units. These are fully connected to 20 hidden units, which are then connected to one output unit that judges the position. Including bias on the hidden units, this makes a total of 3980 weights. The game is played by generating all legal moves, converting them into the proper network input, and picking the position judged as best by the network. We started with all weights set to zero.

Our initial algorithm was hillclimbing:

1. add gaussian noise to the weights
2. play the network against the mutant for a number of games
3. if the mutant wins more than half the games, select it for the next generation.

The noise was set so each step would have a 0.05 RMS distance (which is the euclidean distance divided by $\sqrt{3980}$).

Surprisingly, this worked reasonably well! The networks so evolved improved rapidly at first, but then sank into mediocrity. The problem we perceived is that comparing two close backgammon players is like tossing a biased coin repeatedly: it may take dozens or even hundreds of games to find out for sure which of them is better. Replacing a well-tested champion is dangerous without enough information to prove the challenger is really a better player and not just a lucky novice. Rather than burden the system with so much computation, we instead introduced the following modifications to the algorithm to avoid this "Buster Douglas Effect":

Firstly, the games are played in pairs, with the order of play reversed and the same random seed used to generate the dice rolls for both games. This washes out some of the unfairness due to the dice rolls when the two networks are very close - in particular, if they were identical, the result would always be one win each. Secondly, when the challenger wins the contest, rather than just replacing the champion by the challenger, we instead make only a small adjustment in that direction:

$$\text{champion} := 0.95*\text{champion} + 0.05*\text{challenger}$$

This idea, similar to the "inertia" term in back-propagation, was introduced on the assumption that small changes in weights would lead to small changes in decision-making by the evaluation function. So, by preserving most of the current champion's decisions, we would be less likely to have a catastrophic replacement of the champion by a lucky novice challenger.

In the initial stages of evolution, two pairs of parallel games were played and the challenger was required to win 3 out of 4 of these games.

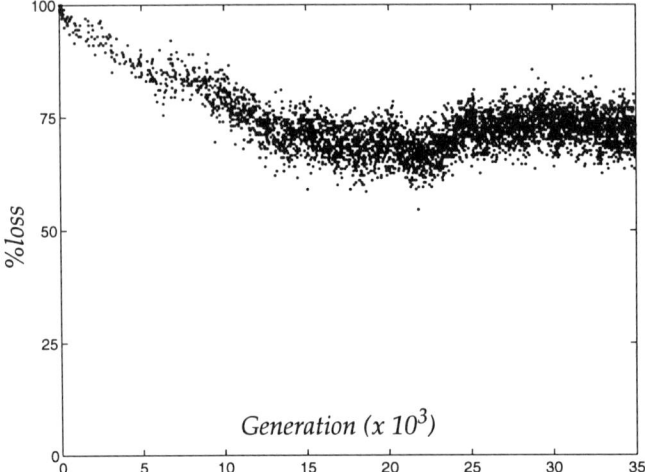

Figure 1. Percentage of losses of our first 35,000 generation players against PUBEVAL. Each match consisted of 200 games.

Figure 1 shows the first 35,000 players rated against PUBEVAL, a strong public-domain player trained by Tesauro using human expert preferences. There are three things to note: (1) the percentage of losses against PUBEVAL falls from 100% to about 67% by 20,000 generations, (2) the frequency of successful challengers increases over time as the player improves, and (3) there are epochs (e.g. starting at 20,000) where the performance against PUBEVAL begins to falter. The first fact shows that our simple self-playing hill-climber is capable of learning. The second fact is quite counter-intuitive - we expected that as the player improved, it would be harder to challenge it! This is true with respect to a uniform sampling of the 4000 dimensional weight space, but not true for a sampling in the neighborhood of a given player: once the player is in a good part of weight space, small changes in weights can lead to mostly similar strategies, ones which make mostly the same moves in the same situations. However, because of the few games we were using to determine relative fitness, this increased frequency of change allows the system to drift, which may account for the subsequent degrading of performance.

To counteract the drift, we decided to change the rules of engagement as the evolution proceeds according to the following "annealing schedule": after 10,000 generations, the number of games that the challenger is required to win was increased from 3 out of 4 to 5 out of 6; after 70,000 generations, it was further increased to 7 out of 8. The numbers 10,000 and 70,000 were chosen on an ad hoc basis from observing the frequency of successful challenges.

After 100,000 games, we have developed a surprisingly strong player, capable of winning 40% of the games against PUBEVAL. The networks were sampled every 100 generations in order to test their performance. Networks at generation 1,000, 10,000 and 100,000 were extracted and used as benchmarks. Figure 2 shows the percentage of losses of the sampled players against the three benchmark networks. Note that the three curves cross the 50% line at 1, 10, and 100, respectively and show a general improvement over time.

The end-game of backgammon, called the "bear-off," can be used as another yardstick of the progress of learning. The bear-off occurs when all of a player's pieces are in the player's home, or first 6 points, and then the dice rolls can be used to remove pieces. We set up a racing board with two pieces on each player's 1 through 7 point and one piece on the 8 point, and played a player against itself 200 games, averaging the number of rolls. We found a monotonic improvement, from 22 to less then 19 rolls, over the 100k generations. PUBEVAL scored 16.6 on this task.

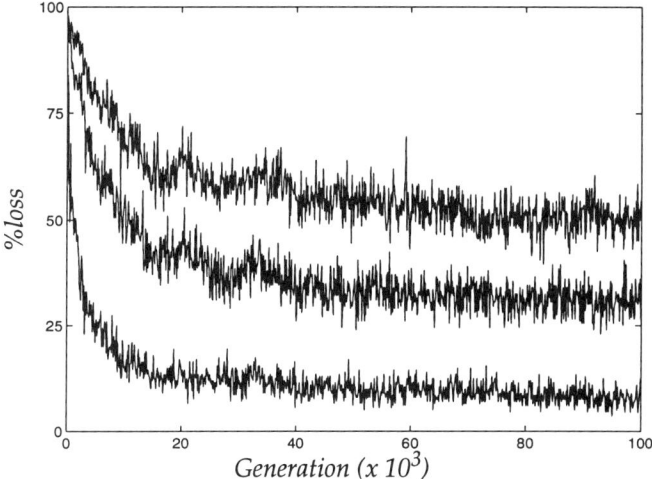

Figure 2. Percentage of losses against benchmark networks at generation 1,000 [lower], 10,000 [middle] and 100,000 [upper].

3 DISCUSSION

3.1 Machine Learning and Evolution

We believe that our evidence of success in learning backgammon using simple hillclimbing indicates that the reinforcement and temporal difference methodology used by Tesauro in TD-gammon was non-essential for its success. Rather, the success came from the setup of co-evolutionary self-play biased by the dynamics of backgammon. Our result is thus similar to the bias found by Mitchell, Crutchfield & Graber in Packard's evolution of cellular automata to the "edge of chaos"(Packard, 1988, Mitchell et al., 1993).

TD-Gammon is a major milestone for a kind of evolutionary machine learning in which the initial specification of model is far simpler than expected because the learning environment is specified implicitly, and emerges as a result of the *co-evolution* between a learning system and its training environment: The learner is embedded in an environment which responds to its own improvements in a never-ending spiral. While this effect has been seen in population models, it is completely unexpected for a "1+1" hillclimbing evolution.

Co-evolution was explored by Hillis (Hillis, 1992) on the sorting problem, by Angeline & Pollack (Angeline and Pollack, 1994) on genetically programmed tic-tac-toe players, on predator/prey games, e.g. (Cliff and Miller, 1995, Reynolds, 1994), and by Juille & Pollack on the intertwined spirals problem (Juille and Pollack, 1995). Rosin & Belew applied competitive fitness to several games (Rosin and Belew, 1995). However, besides Tesauro's TD-Gammon, which has not to date been viewed as an instance of co-evolutionary learning, Sims' artificial robot game (Sims, 1994) is the only other domain as complex as Backgammon to have had substantial success.

3.2 Learnability and Unlearnability

Learnability can be formally defined as a time constraint over a search space. How hard is it to randomly pick 4000 floating-point weights to make a good backgammon evaluator? It is simply impossible. How hard is it to find weights better than the current set? Initially, when all weights are random, it is quite easy. As the playing improves, we would expect it to get harder and harder, perhaps similar to the probability of a tornado constructing a 747 out of a junkyard. However, if we search in the neighborhood of the current weights, we will find many players which make mostly the same moves but which can capitalize on each other's slightly different choices and exposed weaknesses in a tournament.

Although the setting of parameters in our initial runs involved some guesswork, now that we have a large set of "players" to examine, we can try to understand the phenomenon. Taking the 1000th, 10,000th, and 100,000th champions from our run, we sampled random players in their neighborhoods at different RMS distances to find out how likely is it to find a winning challenger. We took 1000 random neighbors at each of 11 different RMS distances, and played them 8 games against the corresponding champion. Figure 3 plots

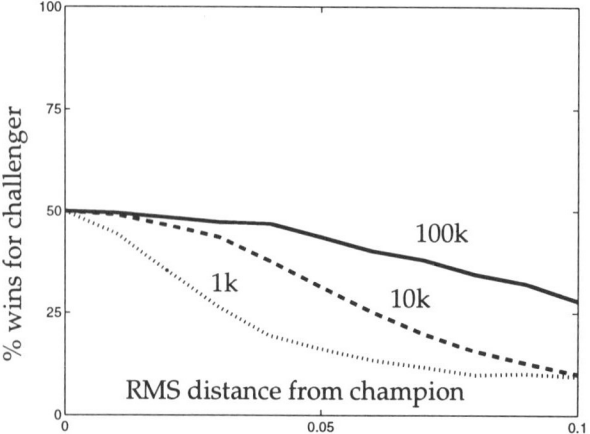

Figure 3. Distance versus probability of random challenger winning against champions at generation 1,000, 10,000 and 100,000.

the average number of games won against the three champions in the range of neighborhoods. This graph demonstrates that as the players improve over time, the probability of finding good challengers in their neighborhood **increases**. This accounts for why the frequency of successful challenges goes up. Each successive challenger is only required to take the small step of changing a few moves of the champion in order to beat it. Therefore, under co-evolution what was apparently unlearnable becomes learnable as we convert from a single question to a continuous stream of questions, each one dependent on the previous answer.

3.3 Avoiding Mediocre Stable States

In general, the problem with learning through self-play is that the player could keep playing the same kinds of games over and over, only exploring some narrow region of the strategy space, missing out on critical areas of the game where it could then be vulnerable to other programs or human experts. Such a learning system might declare success when in reality it has simply converged to a "mediocre stable state" of continual draws or a long term cooperation which merely mimics competition. Such a state can arise in human education systems, where the student gets all the answers right and rewards the teacher with positive feedback for not asking harder questions.

The problem is particularly prevalent in self-play for deterministic games such as chess or tic-tac-toe. We have worked on using a population to get around it (Angeline and Pollack, 1994). Schraudolph et al., 1994 added non-determinism to the game of Go by choosing moves according to the Boltzmann distribution of statistical mechanics. Others, such as Fogel, 1993, expanded exploration by forcing initial moves. Epstein, 1994, has studied a mix of training using self-play, random testing, and playing against an expert in order to better understand this phenomenon.

We are not suggesting that 1+1 hillclimbing is an advanced machine learning technique which others should bring to many tasks. Without internal cognition about an opponent's behavior, co-evolution usually requires a population. Therefore, there must be something about the dynamics of backgammon itself which is helpful because it permitted both TD learning and hill-climbing to succeed where they would clearly fail on other tasks and in other games of this scale. If we can understand why the backgammon domain led to successful acquisition of expert strategies from random initial conditions, we might be able to re-cast other domains in its image.

Tesauro, 1992 pointed out some of the features of Backgammon that make it suitable for approaches involving self-play and random initial conditions. Unlike chess, a draw is impossible and a game played by an untrained network making random moves will eventually terminate (though it may take much longer than a game between competent players). Moreover the randomness of the dice rolls leads self-play into a much larger part of the search space than it would be likely to explore in a deterministic game.

We believe it is not simply the dice rolls which overcome the problems of self-learning. Others have tried to add randomness to deterministic games and have not generally met with success. There is something critical about the dynamics of backgammon which sets its apart from other games with random elements like Monopoly. Namely, that the outcome of the game continues to be uncertain until all contact is broken and one side has a clear advantage. What many observers find exciting about backgammon, and what helps a novice sometimes overcome an expert, is the number of situations where one dice roll, or an improbable sequence, can dramatically reverse which player is expected to win.

A learning system can be viewed as a meta-game between teacher and student, which are identical in a self-play situation. The teacher's goal is to expose the student's mistakes, while the student's goal is to placate the teacher and avoid such exposure. A mediocre stable state for a self-learning system can be seen as an equilibrium situation in this meta-game. A player which learns to repeatedly draw itself will have found a meta-game equilibrium and stop learning. If draws are not allowed, it may still be possible for a self-playing learner to collude with itself - to simulate competition while actually cooperating (Angeline, 1994). For example, if slightly suboptimal moves would allow a player to "throw" a game, a player under self-play could find a meta-game equilibrium by alternately throwing games to itself! Our hypothesis is that the dynamics of backgammon discussed above actively prevent this sort of collusion from forming in the meta-game of self-learning.

4 CONCLUSIONS

Tesauro's 1992 result beat Sun's Gammontool and achieved parity against his own Neurogammon 1.0, trained on expert knowledge. Neither of these is available. Following the 1992 paper on TD-learning, he incorporated a number of hand-crafted expert knowledge features, eventually producing a network which achieved world master level play (Tesauro, 1995). These features included concepts like existence of a prime, probability of blots being hit, and probability of escape from behind the opponent's barrier. Our best players win about 45% against PUBEVAL which was trained using "comparison training"(Tesauro, 1989). Therefore we believe our players achieve approximately the same power as Tesauro's 1992 results, without any advanced learning algorithms. We do not claim that our 100,000 generation player is as good as TD-Gammon, ready to challenge the best humans, just that it is surprisingly good considering its humble origins from hill-climbing with a relative fitness measure. Tuning our parameters or adding more input features would make more powerful players, but that is not the point of this study.

TD-Gammon remains a tremendous success in Machine Learning, but the causes for its success have not been well understood. Replicating some of TD-Gammon's success under a much simpler learning paradigm, we find that the primary cause for success must be the dynamics of backgammon combined with the power of co-evolutionary learning. If we can isolate the features of the backgammon domain which enable evolutionary learning to work so well, it may lead to a better understanding of the conditions necessary, in general, for complex self-organization.

Acknowledgments

This work is supported by ONR grant N00014-96-1-0418 and a Krasnow Foundation Postdoctoral fellowship. Thanks to Gerry Tesauro for providing PUBEVAL and subsequent means to calibrate it, Jack Laurence and Pablo Funes for development of the WWW front end to our evolved player. Interested players can challenge our evolved network using a web browser through our home page at: **http://www.demo.cs.brandeis.edu**

References

Angeline, P. J. (1994). An alternate interpretation of the iterated prisoner's dilemma and the evolution of non-mutual cooperation. In Brooks, R. and Maes, P., editors, *Proceedings 4th Artificial Life Conference*, pages 353–358. MIT Press.

Angeline, P. J. and Pollack, J. B. (1994). Competitive environments evolve better solutions for complex tasks. In Forrest, S., editor, *Genetic Algorithms: Proceedings of the Fifth Inter national Conference*.

Boyan, J. A. (1992). Modular neural networks for learning context-dependent game strategies. Master's thesis, Computer Speech and Language Processing, Cambridge University.

Cliff, D. and Miller, G. (1995). Tracking the red queen: Measurements of adaptive progress in co-evolutionary simulations. In *Third European Conference on Artificial Life*, pages 200–218.

Hillis, D. (1992). Co-evolving parasites improves simulated evolution as an optimization procedure. In C. Langton, C. Taylor, J. F. and Rasmussen, S., editors, *Artificial Life II*. Addison-Wesley, Reading, MA.

International Business Machines (Sept. 12, 1995). IBM's family funpak for os/2 warp hits retail shelves.

Juille, H. and Pollack, J. (1995). Massively parallel genetic programming. In Angeline, P. and Kinnear, K., editors, *Advances in Genetic Programming II*. MIT Press, Cambridge.

Michie, D. (1961). Trial and error. In *Science Survey, part 2*, pages 129–145. Penguin.

Mitchell, M., Hraber, P. T., and Crutchfield, J. P. (1993). Revisiting the edge of chaos: Evolving cellular automata to perform computations. *Complex Systems*, 7.

Packard, N. (1988). Adaptation towards the edge of chaos. In Kelso, J. A. S., Mandell, A. J., and Shlesinger, M. F., editors, *Dynamic patterns in complex systems*, pages 293–301. World Scientific.

Reynolds, C. (1994). Competition, coevolution, and the game of tag. In *Proceedings 4th Artificial Life Conference*. MIT Press.

Rosin, C. D. and Belew, R. K. (1995). Methods for competitive co-evolution: finding opponents worth beating. In *Proceedings of the 6th international conference on Genetic Algorithms*, pages 373–380. Morgan Kaufman.

Samuel, A. L. (1959). some studies of machine learning using the game of checkers. *IBM Joural of Research and Development*.

Sims, K. (1994). Evolving 3d morphology and behavior by competition. In Brooks, R. and Maes, P., editors, *Proceedings 4th Artificial Life Conference*. MIT Press.

Tesauro, G. (1989). Connectionist learning of expert preferences by comparison training. In Touretzky, D., editor, *Advances in Neural Information Processing Systems*, volume 1, pages 99–106, Denver 1988. Morgan Kaufmann, San Mateo.

Tesauro, G. (1992). Practical issues in temporal difference learning. *Machine Learning*, 8:257–277.

Tesauro, G. (1995). Temporal difference learning and td-gammon. *Communications of the ACM*, 38(3):58–68.

Neural Models for Part-Whole Hierarchies

Maximilian Riesenhuber   Peter Dayan
Department of Brain & Cognitive Sciences
Massachusetts Institute of Technology
Cambridge, MA 02139
{max,dayan}@ai.mit.edu

Abstract

We present a connectionist method for representing images that explicitly addresses their hierarchical nature. It blends data from neuroscience about whole-object viewpoint sensitive cells in inferotemporal cortex[8] and attentional basis-field modulation in V4[3] with ideas about hierarchical descriptions based on microfeatures.[5,11] The resulting model makes critical use of bottom-up and top-down pathways for analysis and synthesis.[6] We illustrate the model with a simple example of representing information about faces.

1 Hierarchical Models

Images of objects constitute an important paradigm case of a representational hierarchy, in which 'wholes', such as faces, consist of 'parts', such as eyes, noses and mouths. The representation and manipulation of part-whole hierarchical information in fixed hardware is a heavy millstone around connectionist necks, and has consequently been the inspiration for many interesting proposals, such as Pollack's RAAM.[11]

We turned to the primate visual system for clues. Anterior inferotemporal cortex (IT) appears to construct representations of visually presented objects. Mouths and faces are both objects, and so require fully elaborated representations, presumably at the level of anterior IT, probably using different (or possibly partially overlapping) sets of cells. The natural way to represent the part-whole relationship between mouths and faces is to have a neuronal hierarchy, with connections bottom-up from the mouth units to the face units so that information about the mouth can be used to help recognize or analyze the image of a face, and connections top-down from the face units to the mouth units expressing the generative or synthetic knowledge that if there is a face in a scene, then there is (usually) a mouth too. There is little

---

We thank Larry Abbott, Geoff Hinton, Bruno Olshausen, Tomaso Poggio, Alex Pouget, Emilio Salinas and Pawan Sinha for discussions and comments.

empirical support for or against such a neuronal hierarchy, but it seems extremely unlikely on the grounds that arranging for one with the correct set of levels for all classes of objects seems to be impossible.

There is recent evidence that activities of cells in intermediate areas in the visual processing hierarchy (such as V4) are influenced by the locus of visual attention.[3] This suggests an alternative strategy for representing part-whole information, in which there is an interaction, subject to attentional control, between top-down generative and bottom-up recognition processing. In one version of our example, activating units in IT that represent a particular face leads, through the top-down generative model, to a pattern of activity in lower areas that is closely related to the pattern of activity that would be seen when the entire face is viewed. This activation in the lower areas in turn provides bottom-up input to the recognition system. In the bottom-up direction, the attentional signal controls which aspects of that activation are actually processed, for example, specifying that only the activity reflecting the lower part of the face should be recognized. In this case, the mouth units in IT can then recognize this restricted pattern of activity as being a particular sort of mouth. Therefore, we have provided a way by which the visual system can represent the part-whole relationship between faces and mouths.

This describes just one of many possibilities. For instance, attentional control could be mainly active during the top-down phase instead. Then it would create in V1 (or indeed in intermediate areas) just the activity corresponding to the lower portion of the face in the first place. Also the focus of attention need not be so ineluctably spatial.

The overall scheme is based on an hierarchical top-down synthesis and bottom-up analysis model for visual processing, as in the Helmholtz machine[6] (note that "hierarchy" here refers to a *processing* hierarchy rather than the part-whole hierarchy discussed above) with a synthetic model forming the effective map:

$$\text{'object'} \otimes \text{'attentional eye-position'} \to \text{'image'} \tag{1}$$

(shown in cartoon form in figure 1) where 'image' stands in for the (probabilities over the) activities of units at various levels in the system that would be caused by seeing the aspect of the 'object' selected by placing the focus and scale of attention appropriately. We use this generative model during synthesis in the way described above to traverse the hierarchical description of any particular image. We use the statistical inverse of the synthetic model as the way of analyzing images to determine what objects they depict. This inversion process is clearly also sensitive to the attentional eye-position – it actually determines not only the nature of the object in the scene, but also the way that it is depicted (*ie* its instantiation parameters) as reflected in the attentional eye position.

In particular, the bottom-up analysis model exists in the connections leading to the 2D viewpoint-selective image cells in IT reported by Logothetis *et al*[8] which form population codes for all the represented images (mouths, noses, *etc*). The top-down synthesis model exists in the connections leading in the reverse direction. In generalizations of our scheme, it may, of course, not be necessary to generate an image all the way down in V1.

The map (1) specifies a top-down computational task very like the bottom-up one addressed using a multiplicatively controlled synaptic matrix in the shifter model

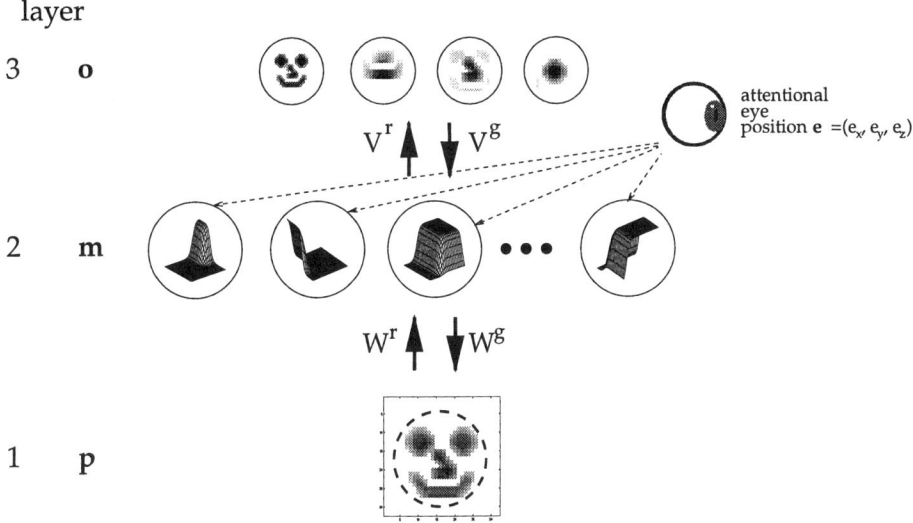

Figure 1: Cartoon of the model. In the top-down, generative, direction, the model generates images of faces, eyes, mouths or noses based on an attentional eye position and a selection of a single top-layer unit; the bottom-up, recognition, direction is the inverse of this map. The response of the neurons in the middle layer is modulated sigmoidally (as illustrated by the graphs shown inside the circles representing the neurons in the middle layer) by the attentional eye position. See section 2 for more details.

of Olshausen et al.[9] Our solution emerges from the control the attentional eye position exerts at various levels of processing, most relevantly modulating activity in V4.[3] Equivalent modulation in the parietal cortex based on actual (rather than attentional) eye position[1] has been characterized by Pouget & Sejnowski[13] and Salinas & Abbott[15] in terms of basis fields. They showed that these basis fields can be used to solve the same tasks as the shifter model but with neuronal rather than synaptic multiplicative modulation. In fact, eye-position modulation almost certainly occurs at many levels in the system, possibly including V1.[12] Our scheme clearly requires that the modulating attentional eye-position must be able to become detached from the spatial eye-position – Connor et al.[3] collected evidence for part of this hypothesis; although the coordinate system(s) of the modulation is not entirely clear from their data.

Bottom-up and top-down mappings are learned taking the eye-position modulation into account. In the experiments below, we used a version of the wake-sleep algorithm,[6] for its conceptual and computational simplicity. This requires learning the bottom-up model from generated imagery (during sleep) and learning the top-down model from assigned explanations (during observation of real input during wake). In the current version, for simplicity, the eye position is set correctly during recognition, but we are also interested in exploring automatic ways of doing this.

2 Results

We have developed a simple model that illustrates the feasibility of the scheme presented above in the context of recognizing and generating cartoon drawings of a face and its parts. Recognition involves taking an image of a face or a part thereof (the mouth, nose or one of the eyes) at an arbitrary position on the retina,

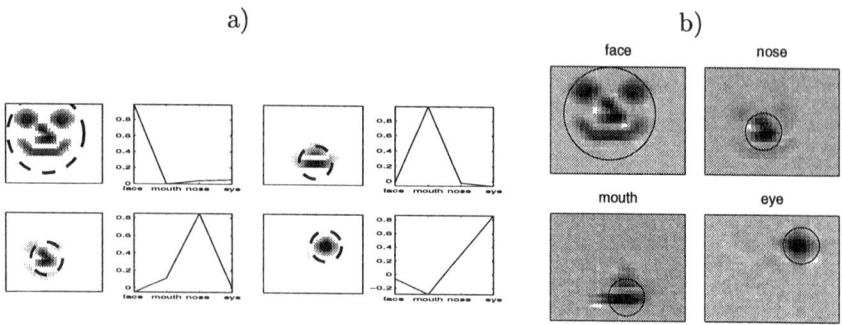

Figure 2: a) Recognition: the left column of each pair shows the stimuli; the right shows the resulting activations in the top layer (ordered as face, mouth, nose and eye). The stimuli are faces at random positions in the retina. Recognition is performed by setting the attentional eye position in the image and setting the attentional scale, which creates a window of attention around the attended to position, shown by a circle of corresponding size and position. b) Generation: each panel shows the output of the generative pathway for a randomly chosen attentional eye position on activating each of the top layer units in turn. The focus of attention is marked by a circle whose size reflects the attentional scale. The name of the object whose neuronal representation in the top layer was activated is shown above each panel.

and setting the appropriate top level unit to 1 (and the remaining units to zero). Generation involves imaging either a whole face or of one of its parts (selected by the active unit in the top layer) at an arbitrary position on the retina.

The model (figure 1) consists of three layers. The lowest layer is a 32 × 32 'retina'. In the recognition direction, the retina feeds into a layer of 500 hidden units. These project to the top layer, which has four neurons. In the generative direction, the connectivity is reversed. The network is fully connected in both directions. The activity of each neuron based on input from the preceding (for recognition) or the following layer (for generation) is a linear function (weight matrices W^r, V^r in the recognition and V^g, W^g in the generative direction). The attentional eye position influences activity through multiplicative modulation of the neuronal responses in the hidden layer. The linear response $r_i = (W^r \mathbf{p})_i$ or $r_i = (V^g \mathbf{o})_i$ of each neuron i in the middle layer based on the bottom-up or top-down connections is multiplied by $\xi_i = \phi_i^x(e_x)\phi_i^y(e_y)\phi_i^s(e_s)$, where $\phi_i^{\{x,y,s\}}$ are the tuning curves in each dimension of the attentional eye position $\mathbf{e} = (e^x, e^y, e^s)$, coding the x- and y- coordinates and the scale of the focus of attention, respectively. Thus, for the activity m_i of hidden neuron i we have $m_i = (W^r \mathbf{p})_i \cdot \xi_i$ in the recognition pathway and $m_i = (V^g \mathbf{o})_i \cdot \xi_i$ in the generative pathway. The tuning curves of the ξ_i are chosen to be sigmoid with random centers c_i and random directions $d_i \in \{-1, 1\}$, eg $\phi_i^s = \sigma(4 * d_i^s * (e^s - c_i^s))$. In other implementations, we have also used Gaussian tuning functions. In fact, the only requirement regarding the shape of the tuning functions is that through a superposition of them one can construct functions that show a peaked dependence on the attentional eye position. In the recognition direction, the attentional eye position also has an influence on the activity in the input layer by defining a 'window of attention',[7] which we implemented using a Gaussian window centered at the attentional eye position with its size given by the attentional scale. This is to allow the system to learn models of parts based on experience with images of whole faces.

To train the model, we employ a variant of the unsupervised wake-sleep algorithm.[6] In this algorithm, the generative pathway is trained during a wake-phase, in which stimuli in the input layer (the retina, in our case) cause activation of the neurons in the network through the recognition pathway, providing an error signal to train the generative pathway using the delta rule. Conversely, in the sleep-phase, random activation of a top layer unit (in conjunction with a randomly chosen attentional eye-position) leads, via the generative connections, to the generation of activation in the middle layer and consequently an image in the input layer that is then used to adapt the recognition weights, again using the delta rule. Although the delta rule in wake-sleep is fine for the recognition direction, it leads to a poor generative model – in our simple case, generation is much more difficult than recognition. As an interim solution, we therefore train the generative weights using back-propagation, which uses the activity in the top layer created by the recognition pathway as the input and the retinal activation pattern as the target signal. Hence, learning is still unsupervised (except that appropriate attentional eye-positions are always set during recognition). We have also experimented with a system in which the weights W^r and W^g are preset and only the weights between layers 2 and 3 are trained. For this model, training could be done with the standard wake-sleep algorithm, *ie* using the local delta-rule for both sets of weights.

Figure 2a shows several examples of the performance of the recognition pathway for the different stimuli after 300,000 iterations. The network is able to recognize the stimuli accurately at different positions in the visual field. Figure 2b shows several examples of the output of the generative model, illustrating its capacity to produce images of faces or their parts at arbitrary locations. By imaging a whole face and then focusing the attention on *eg* an area around its center, which activates the 'nose' unit through the recognition pathway, the relationship that, *eg* a nose is part of a face can be established in a straightforward way.

3 Discussion

Representing hierarchical structure is a key problem for connectionism. Visual images offer a canonical example for which it seems possible to elucidate some of the underlying neural mechanisms. The theory is based on 2D view object selective cells in anterior IT, and attentional eye-position modulation of the firing of cells in V4. These work in the context of analysis by synthesis or recognition and generative models such that the part-whole hierarchy of an object such as a face (which contains eyes, which contain pupils, *etc*) can be traversed in the generative direction by choosing to view the object through a different effective eye-position, and in the recognition direction by allowing the real and the attentional eye-positions to be decoupled to activate the requisite 2D view selective cells.

The scheme is related to Pollack's Recursive Auto-Associative Memory (RAAM) system.[11] RAAM provides a way of representing tree-structured information – for instance to learn an object whose structure is $\{\{A, B\}, \{C, D\}\}$, a standard three-layer auto-associative net would be taught AB, leading to a pattern of hidden unit activations α; then it would learn CD leading to β; and finally $\alpha\beta$ leading to γ, which would itself be the representation of the whole object. The compression operation ($AB \to \alpha$) and its expansion inverse are required as explicit methods for manipulating tree structure.

Our scheme for representing hierarchical information is similar to RAAM, using the notion of an attentional eye-position to perform its compression and expansion operations. However, whereas RAAM normally constructs its own codes for intermediate levels of the trees that it is fed, here, images of faces are as real and as available as those, for instance, of their associated mouths. This not only changes the learning task, but also renders sensible a notion of direct recognition without repeated RAAMification of the parts.

Various aspects of our scheme require comment: the way that eye position affects recognition; the coding of different instances of objects; the use of top-down information during bottom-up recognition; variants of the scheme for objects that are too big or too geometrically challenging to 'fit' in one go into a single image; and hierarchical objects other than images. We are also working on a more probabilistically correct version, taking advantage of the statistical soundness of the Helmholtz machine.

Eye position information is ubiquitous in visual processing areas,[12] including the LGN and V1,[17] as well as the parietal cortex[1] and V4.[3] Further, it can be revealed as having a dramatic effect on perception, as in Ramachandran *et al*'s[14] study on intermittent exotropes. This is a form of squint in which the two eyes are normally aligned, but in which the exotropic eye can deviate (voluntarily or involuntarily) by as much as 60°. The study showed that even if an image is 'burnt' on the retina in this eye as an afterimage, and so is fixed in retinal coordinates, at least one component of the percept *moves* as the eye moves. This argues that information about eye position dramatically effects visual processing in a manner that is consistent with the model presented here of shifts based on modulation. This is also required by Bridgeman *et al*'s[2] theory of perceptual stability across fixations, that essentially builds up an impression of a scene in exactly the form of mapping (1).

In general, there will be many instances for an object, *e.g.,* many different faces. In this general case, the top level would implement a distributed code for the identity and instantiation parameters of the objects. We are currently investigating methods of implementing this form of representation into the model.

A key feature of the model is the interaction of the synthesis and analysis pathways when traversing the part-whole hierarchies. This interaction between the two pathways can also aid the system when performing image analysis by integrating information across the hierarchy. Just as in RAAM, the extra feature required when traversing a hierarchy is short term memory. For RAAM, the memory stores information about the various separate sub-trees that have already been decoded (or encoded). For our system, the memory is required during generative traversal to force 'whole' activity on lower layers to persist even after the activity on upper layers has ceased, to free these upper units to recognize a 'part'. Memory during recognition traversal is necessary in marginal cases to accumulate information across separate 'parts' as well as the 'whole'. This solution to hierarchical representation inevitably gives up the computational simplicity of the naive neuronal hierarchical scheme described in the introduction which does not require any such accumulation.

Knowledge of images that are too large to fit naturally in a single view[4] at a canonical location and scale, or that theoretically cannot fit in a view (like 360° information about a room) can be handled in a straightforward extension of the scheme. All this requires is generalizing further the notion of eye-position. One can explore one's generative model of a room in the same way that one can explore one's generative model of a face.

We have described our scheme from the perspective of images. This is convenient because of the substantial information available about visual processing. However, images are not the only examples of hierarchical structure – this is also very relevant to words, music and also inferential mechanisms. We believe that our mechanisms are also more general – proving this will require the equivalent of the attentional eye-position that lies at the heart of the method.

References

[1] Andersen, R, Essick, GK & Siegel, RM (1985). Encoding of spatial location by posterior parietal neurons. *Science,* **230**, 456-458.

[2] Bridgeman, B, van der Hejiden, AHC & Velichkovsky, BM (1994). A theory of visual stability across saccadic eye movements. *Behavioral and Brain Sciences,* **17**, 247-292.

[3] Connor, CE, Gallant, JL, Preddie, DC & Van Essen, DC (1996). Responses in area V4 depend on the spatial relationship between stimulus and attention. *Journal of Neurophysiology,* **75**, 1306-1308.

[4] Feldman, JA (1985). Four frames suffice: A provisional model of vision and space. *The Behavioral and Brain Sciences,* **8**, 265-289.

[5] Hinton, GE (1981). Implementing semantic networks in parallel hardware. In GE Hinton & JA Anderson, editors, *Parallel Models of Associative Memory.* Hillsdale, NJ: Erlbaum, 161-188.

[6] Hinton, GE, Dayan, P, Frey, BJ & Neal, RM (1995). The wake-sleep algorithm for unsupervised neural networks. *Science,* **268**, 1158-1160.

[7] Koch, C & Ullmann, S (1985). Shifts in selective visual attention: towards the underlying neural circuitry. *Human Neurobiology,* **4**, 219-227.

[8] Logothetis, NK, Pauls, J, & Poggio, T (1995). Shape representation in the inferior temporal cortex of monkeys. *Current Biology,* **5**, 552-563.

[9] Olshausen, BA, Anderson, CH & Van Essen, DC (1993). A neurobiological model of visual attention and invariant pattern recognition based on dynamic routing of information. *Journal of Neuroscience,* **13**, 4700-4719.

[10] Pearl, J (1988). *Probabilistic Reasoning in Intelligent Systems: Networks of Plausible Inference.* San Mateo, CA: Morgan Kaufmann.

[11] Pollack, JB (1990). Recursive distributed representations. *Artificial Intelligence,* **46**, 77-105.

[12] Pouget, A, Fisher, SA & Sejnowski, TJ (1993). Egocentric spatial representation in early vision. *Journal of Cognitive Neuroscience,* **5**, 150-161.

[13] Pouget, A & Sejnowski, TJ (1995). Spatial representations in the parietal cortex may use basis functions. In G Tesauro, DS Touretzky & TK Leen, editors, *Advances in Neural Information Processing Systems 7,* 157-164.

[14] Ramachandran, VS, Cobb, S & Levi, L (1994). The neural locus of binocular rivalry and monocular diplopia in intermittent exotropes. *Neuroreport,* **5**, 1141-1144.

[15] Salinas, E & Abbott LF (1996). Transfer of coded information from sensory to motor networks. *Journal of Neuroscience,* **15**, 6461-6474.

[16] Sung, K & Poggio, T (1995). *Example based learning for view-based human face detection.* AI Memo 1521, CBCL paper 112, Cambridge, MA: MIT.

[17] Trotter, Y, Celebrini, S, Stricanne, B, Thorpe, S & Imbert, M (1992). Modulation of neural stereoscopic processing in primate area V1 by the viewing distance. *Science,* **257**, 1279-1281.

Part II
Neuroscience

Temporal Low-Order Statistics of Natural Sounds

H. Attias* and C.E. Schreiner[†]
Sloan Center for Theoretical Neurobiology and
W.M. Keck Foundation Center for Integrative Neuroscience
University of California at San Francisco
San Francisco, CA 94143-0444

Abstract

In order to process incoming sounds efficiently, it is advantageous for the auditory system to be adapted to the statistical structure of natural auditory scenes. As a first step in investigating the relation between the system and its inputs, we study low-order statistical properties in several sound ensembles using a filter bank analysis. Focusing on the amplitude and phase in different frequency bands, we find simple parametric descriptions for their distribution and power spectrum that are valid for very different types of sounds. In particular, the amplitude distribution has an exponential tail and its power spectrum exhibits a modified power-law behavior, which is manifested by self-similarity and long-range temporal correlations. Furthermore, the statistics for different bands within a given ensemble are virtually identical, suggesting translation invariance along the cochlear axis. These results show that natural sounds are highly redundant, and have possible implications to the neural code used by the auditory system.

1 Introduction

The capacity of the auditory system to represent the auditory scene is restricted by the finite number of cells and by intrinsic noise. This fact limits the ability of the organism to discriminate between different sounds with similar spectro-temporal

---

*Corresponding author. E-mail: hagai@phy.ucsf.edu.
[†]E-mail: chris@phy.ucsf.edu.

characteristics. However, it is possible to enhance the discrimination ability by a suitable choice of the encoding procedure used by the system, namely of the transformation of sounds reaching the cochlea to neural spike trains generated in successive processing stages in response to these sounds. In general, the choice of a good encoding procedure requires knowledge of the statistical structure of the sound ensemble.

For the visual system, several investigations of the statistical properties of image ensembles and their relations to neuronal response properties have recently been performed (Field 1987, Atick and Redlich 1990, Ruderman and Bialek 1994). In particular, receptive fields of retinal ganglion and LGN cells were found to be consistent with an optimal-code prediction formulated within information theory (Atick 1992, Dong and Atick 1995), suggesting that the visual periphery may be designed as to take advantage of simple statistical properties of visual scenes.

In order to investigate whether the auditory system is similarly adapted to the statistical structure of its own inputs, a good characterization of auditory scenes is necessary. In this paper we take a first step in this direction by studying low-order statistical properties of several sound ensembles. The quantities we focus on are the spectro-temporal amplitude and phase defined as follows. For the sound $s(t)$, let $s_\nu(t)$ denote its components at the set of frequencies ν, obtained by filtering it through a bandpass filter bank centered at those frequencies. Then

$$s_\nu(t) = x_\nu(t) cos\left(\nu t + \phi_\nu(t)\right) \qquad (1)$$

where $x_\nu(t) \geq 0$ and $\phi_\nu(t)$ are the spectro-temporal amplitude (STA) and phase (STP), respectively. A complete characterization of a sound ensemble with respect to a given filter bank must be given by the joint distribution of amplitudes and phases at all times, $p(x_{\nu_1}(t_1), \phi_{\nu_1}(t'_1), ..., x_{\nu_n}(t_n), \phi_{\nu_n}(t'_n))$. In this paper, however, we restrict ourselves to second-order statistics in the time domain and examine the distribution and power spectrum of the stochastic processes $x_\nu(t)$ and $\phi_\nu(t)$.

Note that the STA and STP are quantities directly relevant to auditory processing. The different stages of the auditory system are organized in topographic frequency maps, so that cells tuned to the same sound frequency ν are organized in stripes perpendicular to the direction of frequency progression (see, e.g., Pickles 1988). The neuronal responses are thus determined by x_ν and ϕ_ν, and by x_ν alone when phase-locking disappears above 4–5KHz.

2 Methods

Since it is difficult to obtain a reliable sample of an animal's auditory scene over a sufficiently long time, we chose instead to analyze several different sound ensembles, each consisting of a 15min sound of a certain type. We used cat vocalizations, bird songs, wolf cries, environmental sounds, symphonic music, jazz, pop music, and speech. The sounds were obtained from commercially available compact discs and from recordings of animal vocalizations in two laboratories. No attempt has been made to manipulate the recorded sounds in any way (e.g., by removing noise).

Each sound ensemble was loaded into the computer by 30sec segments at a sampling rate of $f_s = 44.1$KHz. After decimating to $f_s/2$, we performed the following frequency-band analysis. Each segment was passed through a bandpass fil-

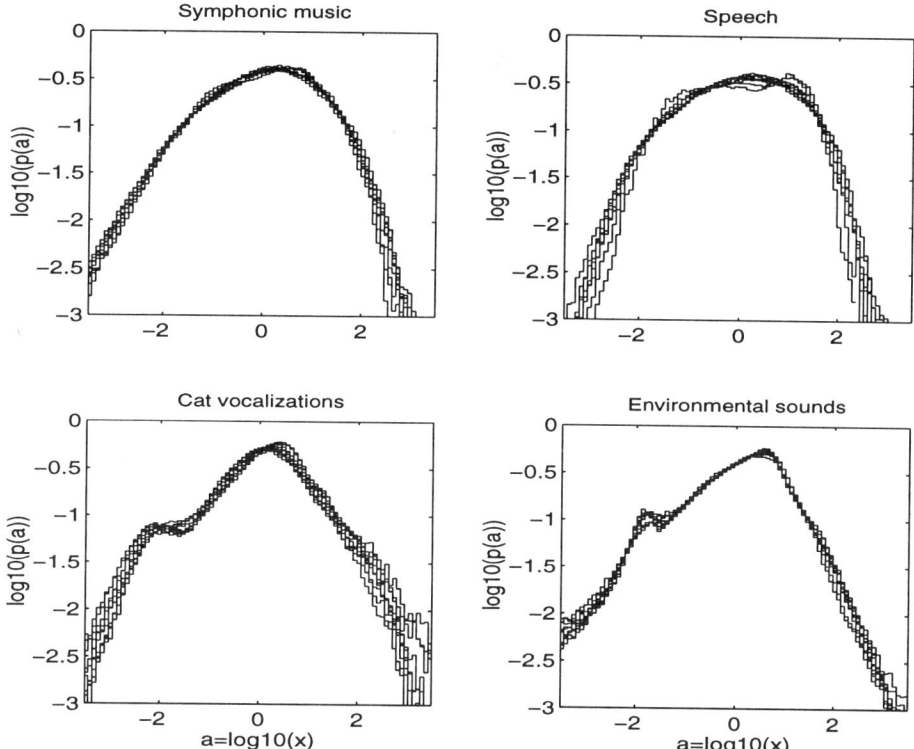

Figure 1: Amplitude probability distribution in different frequency bands for four sound ensembles.

ter bank with impulse responses $h_\nu(t)$ to get the narrow-band component signals $s_\nu(t) = s(t) * h_\nu(t)$. We used square, non-overlapping filters with center frequencies ν logarithmically spaced within the range of $100 - 11025$Hz. The filters were usually 1/8-octave wide, but we experimented with larger bandwidths as well. The amplitude and phase in band ν were then obtained via the Hilbert transform

$$H[s_\nu(t)] = s_\nu(t) + \frac{i}{\pi}\int dt' \frac{s(t')}{t-t'} = x_\nu(t) e^{i(\nu t + \phi_\nu(t))} \,. \qquad (2)$$

The frequency content of x_ν is bounded by 0 and by the bandwidth of h_ν (Flanagan 1980), so keeping the latter below ν guarantees that the low frequencies in s_ν are all contained in x_ν, confirming its interpretation as the amplitude modulator of the carrier $\cos \nu t$ suggested by (1). The phase ϕ_ν, being time-dependent, produces frequency modulation. For a given ν the results were averaged over all segments.

3 Amplitude Distribution

We first examined the STA distribution in different frequency bands ν. Fig. 1 presents historgrams of $p(\log_{10} x_\nu)$ on a logarithmic scale for four different sound ensembles. In order to facilitate a comparison among different bands and ensembles, we normalized the variable to have zero mean and unit variance, $\langle \log_{10} x_\nu(t) \rangle = 0$, $\langle (\log_{10} x_\nu(t))^2 \rangle = 1$, corresponding to a linear gain control.

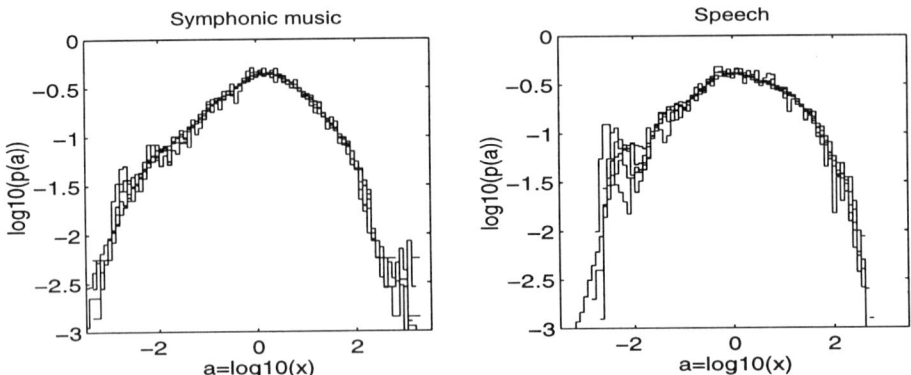

Figure 2: n-point averaged amplitude distributions for $\nu = 800$Hz in two sound ensembles, using $n = 1, 20, 50, 100, 200$. The speech ensemble is different from the one used in Fig. 1.

As shown in the figure, within a given ensemble, the histograms corresponding to different bands lie atop one another. Furthermore, although curves from different ensembles are not identical, we found that they could all be fitted accurately to the same parametric functional form, given by

$$p(x_\nu) \propto \frac{e^{-\gamma x_\nu}}{(b_0^2 + x_\nu^2)^{\beta/2}} \qquad (3)$$

with parameter values roughly in the range of $0.1 \leq \gamma \leq 1$, $0 \leq \beta \leq 2.5$, and $0.1 \leq b_0 \leq 0.6$. In some cases, a mixture of two distributions of the form (3) was necessary, suggesting the presence of two types of sound sources; see, e.g., the slight bimodality in the lower parts of Fig. 1. Details of the fitting procedure will be given in a longer paper. We found the form (3) to be preserved as the filter bandwidths increased.

Whereas this distribution decays exponentially fast at high amplitudes ($p \propto e^{-\gamma x_\nu}/x_\nu^\beta$), it does not vanish at low amplitudes, indicating a finite probability for the occurence of arbitrarily soft sounds. In contrast, the STA of a Gaussian noise signal can be shown to be distributed according to $p \propto x_\nu e^{-\lambda x_\nu^2}$, which vanishes at $x_\nu = 0$ and decays faster than (3) at large x_ν. Hence, the origin of the large dynamic range usually associated with audio signals can be traced to the abundance of soft sounds rather than of loud ones.

4 Amplitude Self-Similarity

An interesting probe of the STA temporal correlations is the property of scale invariance (also called statistical self-similarity). The process $x_\nu(t)$ is scale-invariant when any statistical quantity on a given scale (e.g., at a given temporal resolution, determined by the sampling rate) does not change as that scale is varied. To observe this property we examined the STA distribution $p(x_\nu)$ at different temporal resolutions, by defining the n-point averaged amplitude

$$x_\nu^{(n)}(t) = \frac{1}{n} \sum_{k=0}^{n-1} x_\nu(t + k\Delta) \qquad (4)$$

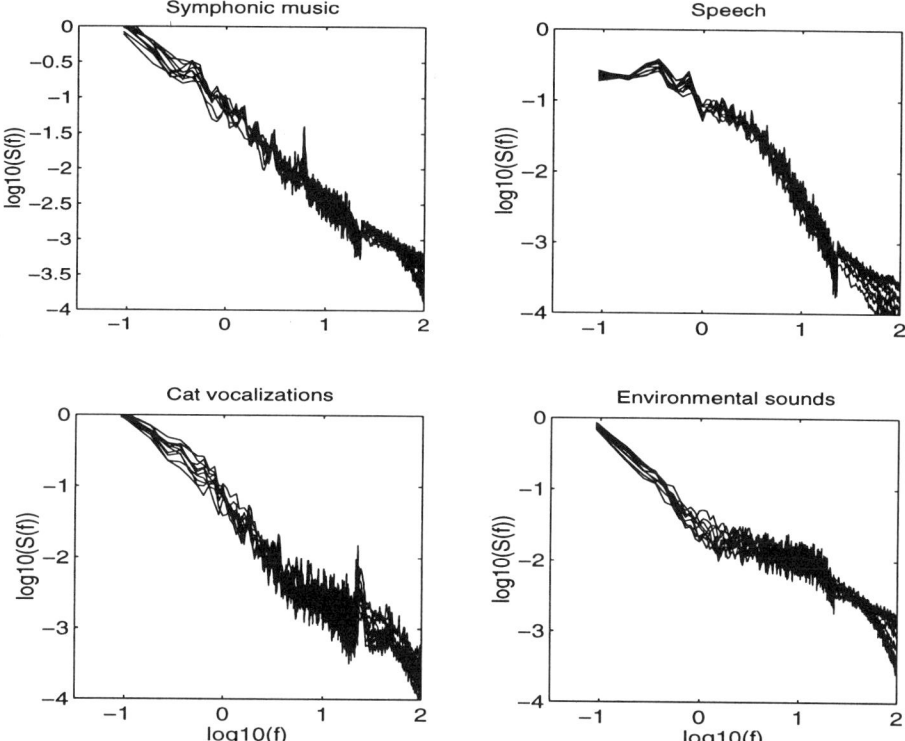

Figure 3: Amplitude power spectrum in different frequency bands for four sound ensembles.

($\Delta = 1/f_s$) and computing its distribution. Fig. 2 displays the histograms of $p(\log_{10} x_\nu^{(n)})$ for the $\nu = 800$Hz frequency band in two sound ensembles on a logarithmic scale, using $n = 1, 20, 50, 100, 200$ which correspond to a temporal resolution range of $0.75 - 150$msec. Remarkably, the histogram remains unmodified even for $n = 200$. Had the $x_\nu(t + k\Delta)$ been statistically independent variables, the central limit theorem would have predicted a Gaussian $p(x_\nu^{(n)})$ for large n. The fact that this non-Gaussian distribution preserves its form as n increases implies the presence of temporal STA correlations over long periods.

Notice the analogy between the invariance of $p(x_\nu)$ under a change in filter bandwidth, reported in the previous section, and under a change in temporal resolution. An x_ν with a broad bandwidth is essentially an average over the x_ν's with narrow bandwidth within the same band, thus bandwidth invariance is a manifestation of STA correlations across frequency bands.

5 Amplitude Power Spectrum

In order to study the temporal amplitude correlations directly, we computed the STA power spectrum $S_\nu(\omega) = \langle |\tilde{x}_\nu(\omega)|^2 \rangle$ in different bands ν, where $\tilde{x}_\nu(\omega)$ is the Fourier transform of the log-amplitude $\log_{10} x_\nu(t)$ obtained by a 512-point FFT. As is well-known, the spectrum $S_\nu(\omega)$ is the Fourier transform of the log-amplitude auto-correlation function $c_\nu(\tau) = \langle \log_{10} x_\nu(t) \log_{10} x_\nu(t + \tau) \rangle$. We used the zero-mean, unit-variance normalization of $\log_{10} x_\nu$, which implies the normalization $\int d\omega S_\nu(\omega) = $ const. of the spectra. Fig. 3 presents S_ν as a function of the modulation frequency $f = \omega/2\pi$ on a logarithmic scale for four different sound ensembles. Notice that, as in the case of the STA distribution, the different curves corresponding to different frequency bands within a given ensemble lie atop one another, including individual peaks; and whereas spectra in different ensembles are not identical, we found a simple parametric description valid for all ensembles which is given by

$$S_\nu(\omega) \propto \frac{1}{(\omega_0^2 + \omega^2)^{\alpha/2}}, \tag{5}$$

with parameter values roughly in the range of $1 \leq \alpha \leq 2.5$ and $10^{-4} \leq \omega_0 \leq 1$. This is a modified power-law form (note that $S_\nu \to C/\omega^\alpha$ at large ω), implying long-rangle temporal correlations in the amplitude: these correlations decrease slowly (as a power law in t) on a time scale of $1/\omega_0$, beyond which they decay exponentially fast. Larger ω_0 contributes more to the flattening of the spectrum at low frequencies (see especially the speech spectra) and corresponds to a shorter correlation time. Again, in some cases a sum of two such forms was necessary, corresponding to a mixture STA distribution as mentioned above; see, e.g., the environmental sound spectra (lower right part of Fig. 3 and Fig. 1).

The form (5) persisted as the filter bandwidth increased. In the limit of allpass filter (not shown) we still observed this form, a fact related to the report of (Voss and Clarke 1975) on $1/f$-like power spectra of sound 'loudness' $s(t)^2$ found in several speech and music ensembles.

6 Phase Distribution and Power Spectrum

Whereas the STA is a non-stationary process which is locally stationary and can thus be studied on the appropriate time scale using our methods, the STP is non-stationary even locally. A more suitable quantity to examine is its rate of change $d\phi_\nu/dt$, called the instantaneous frequency. We studied the statistics of $|d\phi_\nu/dt|$ in different ensembles, and found its distribution to be described accurately by the parametric form (3) with $\gamma = 0$, whereas its power spectrum could be well fitted by the form (5). In addition, those quantities were virtually identical in different bands within a given ensemble. More details on this work will be provided in a longer paper.

7 Implications for Auditory Processing

We have shown that auditory scenes have several robust low-order statistical properties. The STA power spectrum has a modified power-law behavior, which is manifested in self-similarity and temporal correlations over a few hundred milliseconds. The distribution has an exponential tail and features a finite probability for arbitrarily soft sounds. Both the phase and amplitude statistics can be described by simple parametrized functional forms which are valid for very different types of sounds. These results lead to the conclusion that natural sounds are highly redundant, i.e., they occupy a very small subspace in the space of all possible sounds. It would therefore be beneficial for the auditory system to adapt its sound representation to these statistics, thus improving the animal discrimination ability. Whether the auditory system actually follows this design principle is an empirical question which can be attacked by suitable experiments.

Furthermore, since different frequency bands correspond to different spatial locations on the basal membrane (Pickles 1988), the fact that the distributions and spectra in different bands within a given ansemble are identical suggests the existence of translation invariance along the cochlear axis, i.e., all the locations in the cochlea 'see' the same statistics. This is analogous to the translation invariance found in natural images.

Finally, a recent theory for peripheral visual processing (Dong and Atick 1995) proposes that, in order to maximize information transmission into cortex, the LGN performs temporal correlation of retinal images. Within an analogous auditory model, the decorrelation time for sound ensembles reported here implies that the auditory system should process incoming sounds by a few hundred msec-long segments. The ability of cortical neurons to follow in their response modulation rates near and below 10Hz but usually not higher (Schreiner and Urbas 1988) may reflect such a process.

Acknowledgements

We thank B. Bonham, K. Miller, S. Nagarajan, and especially W. Bialek for helpful discussions and suggestions. We also thank F. Theunissen for making his bird song recordings available to us. Supported by The Office of Naval Research (N00014-94-1-0547). H.A. was supported by a Sloan Foundation grant for the Sloan Center for Theoretical Neurobiology.

References

J.J. Atick and N. Redlich (1990), Towards a theory of early visual processing. Neural Comput. **2**, 308-320.

J.J. Atick (1992), Could information theory provide an ecological theory of sensory processing. Network **3**, 213-251.

D.W. Dong and J.J. Atick (1995), Temporal decorrelation: a theory of lagged and non-lagged responses in the lateral geniculate nucleus. Network **6**, 159-178.

D.J. Field (1987), Relations between the statistics of natural images and the response properties of cortical cells. J. Opt. Soc. Am. **4**, 2379-2394.

J.L. Flanagan (1980), Parametric coding of speech spectra. J. Acoust. Soc. Am. **68**, 412-419.

J.O. Pickles (1988), *An introduction to the physiology of hearing* (2nd Ed.). San Diego, CA: Academic Press.

D.L. Ruderman and W. Bialek (1994), Statistics of natural images: scaling in the woods. Phys. Rev. Lett. **73**, 814-817.

C.E. Schreiner and J.V. Urbas, Representation of amplitude modulation in the auditory cortex of the cat. II. Comparison between cortical fields. Hear. Res. **32**, 49-63.

R.F. Voss and J. Clarke (1975), $1/f$ noise in music and speech. Nature **258**, 317-318.

Reconstructing Stimulus Velocity from Neuronal Responses in Area MT

Wyeth Bair, James R. Cavanaugh, J. Anthony Movshon
Howard Hughes Medical Institute, and
Center for Neural Science
New York University
4 Washington Place, Room 809
New York, NY 10003
wyeth@cns.nyu.edu, jamesc@cns.nyu.edu, tony@cns.nyu.edu

Abstract

We employed a white-noise velocity signal to study the dynamics of the response of single neurons in the cortical area MT to visual motion. Responses were quantified using reverse correlation, optimal linear reconstruction filters, and reconstruction signal-to-noise ratio (SNR). The SNR and lower bound estimates of information rate were lower than we expected. Ninety percent of the information was transmitted below 18 Hz, and the highest lower bound on bit rate was 12 bits/s. A simulated opponent motion energy subunit with Poisson spike statistics was able to out-perform the MT neurons. The temporal integration window, measured from the reverse correlation half-width, ranged from 30–90 ms. The window was narrower when a stimulus moved faster, but did not change when temporal frequency was held constant.

1 INTRODUCTION

Area MT neurons can show precise and rapid modulation in response to dynamic noise stimuli (Bair and Koch, 1996); however, computational models of these neurons and their inputs (Adelson and Bergen, 1985; Heeger, 1987; Grzywacz and Yuille, 1990; Emerson et al., 1992; Qian et al., 1994; Nowlan and Sejnowski, 1995) have primarily been compared to electrophysiological results based on time and ensemble averaged responses to deterministic stimuli, e.g., drifting sinusoidal gratings.

Using methods introduced by Bialek et al. (1991) and further analyzed by Gabbiani and Koch (1996) for the estimation of information transmission by a neuron about a white-noise stimulus, we set out to compare the responses of MT neurons for white-noise velocity signals to those of a model based on opponent motion energy sub-units.

The results of two analyses are summarized here. In the first, we compute a lower bound on information transmission using optimal linear reconstruction filters and examine the SNR as a function of temporal frequency. The second analysis examines changes in the reverse correlation (the cross-correlation between the stimulus and the resulting spike trains) as a function of spatial frequency and temporal frequency of the moving stimulus pattern.

2 EXPERIMENTAL METHODS

Spike trains were recorded extracellularly from 26 well-isolated single neurons in area MT of four anesthetized, paralyzed macaque monkeys using methods described in detail elsewhere (Levitt et al., 1994). The size of the receptive fields and the spatial and temporal frequency preferences of the neurons were assessed quantitatively using drifting sinusoidal gratings, after which a white-noise velocity signal, $s(t)$, was used to modulate the position (within a fixed square aperture) of a low-pass filtered 1D Gaussian white-noise (GWN) pattern. The frame rate of the display was 54 Hz or 81 Hz. The spatial noise pattern consisted of 256 discrete intensity values, one per spatial unit. Every 19 ms (or 12 ms at 81 Hz), the pattern shifted, or *jumped*, Δ spatial units along the axis of the neuron's preferred direction, where Δ, the jump size, was chosen according to a Gaussian, binary, or uniform probability distribution. The maximum spatial frequency in the pattern was limited to prevent aliasing.

In the first type of experiment, 10 trials of a 30 s noise sequence, $s(t)$, and 10 trials of its reverse, $-s(t)$, were interleaved. A standard GWN spatial pattern and velocity modulation pattern were used for all cells, but for each cell, the stimulus was scaled for the receptive field size and aligned to the axis of preferred motion. Nine cells were tested with Gaussian noise at 81 Hz, 15 cells with binary noise at 81 Hz and 54 Hz, and 10 cells with uniform noise at 54 Hz.

In another experiment, a sinusoidal spatial pattern (rather than GWN) moved according to a binary white-noise velocity signal. Trials were interleaved with all combinations of four spatial frequencies at octave intervals and four *relative* jump sizes: 1/4, 1/8, 1/16, and 1/32 of each spatial period. Typically 10 trials of length 3 s were run. Four cells were tested at 54 Hz and seven at 81 Hz.

3 ANALYSIS AND MODELING METHODS

We used the linear reconstruction methods introduced by Bialek et al. (1991) and further analyzed by Gabbiani and Koch (1996) to compute an optimal linear estimate of the stimulus, $s(t)$, described above, based on the neuronal response, $x(t)$. A *single* neuronal response was defined as the spike train produced by $s(t)$ minus the spike train produced by $-s(t)$. This overcomes the neuron's limited dynamic range in response to anti-preferred direction motion (Bialek et al., 1991).

The linear filter, $h(t)$, which when convolved with the response yields the minimum mean square error estimate, s_{est}, of the stimulus can be described in terms of its Fourier transform,

$$H(\omega) = \frac{R_{sx}(-\omega)}{R_{xx}(\omega)}, \qquad (1)$$

where $R_{sx}(\omega)$ is the Fourier transform of the cross-correlation $r_{sx}(\tau)$ of the stimulus and the resulting spike train and $R_{xx}(\omega)$ is the power spectrum, i.e., the Fourier transform of the auto-correlation, of the spike train (for details and references, see Bialek et al., 1991; Gabbiani and Koch, 1996). The noise, $n(t)$, is defined as the difference between the stimulus and the reconstruction,

$$n(t) = s_{est}(t) - s(t), \qquad (2)$$

and the SNR is defined as

$$\text{SNR}(\omega) = \frac{R_{ss}(\omega)}{R_{nn}(\omega)}, \qquad (3)$$

where $R_{ss}(\omega)$ is the Fourier power spectrum of the stimulus and $R_{nn}(\omega)$ is the power spectrum of the noise. If the stimulus amplitude distribution is Gaussian, then $\text{SNR}(\omega)$ can be integrated to give a lower bound on the rate of information transmission in bits/s (Gabbiani and Koch, 1996).

The motion energy model consisted of opponent energy sub-units (Adelson and Bergen, 1985) implemented with Gabor functions (Heeger, 1987; Grzywacz and Yuille, 1990) in two spatial dimensions and time. The spatial frequency of the Gabor function was set to match the spatial frequency of the stimulus, and the temporal frequency was set to match that induced by a sequence of jumps equal to the standard deviation (SD) of the amplitude distribution (which is the jump size in the case of a binary distribution). We approximated causality by shifting the output forward in time before computing the optimal linear filter. The model operated on the same stimulus patterns and noise sequences that were used to generate stimuli for the neurons. The time-varying response of the model was broken into two half-wave rectified signals which were interpreted as the firing probabilities of two units, a neuron and an anti-neuron that preferred the opposite direction of motion. From each unit, ten 30 s long spike trains were generated with inhomogeneous Poisson statistics. These 20 model spike trains were used to reconstruct the velocity signal in the same manner as the MT neuron output.

4 RESULTS

Stimulus reconstruction. Optimal linear reconstruction filters, $h(t)$, were computed for 26 MT neurons from responses to 30 s sequences of white-noise motion. A typical $h(t)$, shown in Fig. 1A (large dots), was dominated by a single positive lobe, often preceded by a smaller negative lobe. It was thinner than the reverse correlation $r_{sx}(\tau)$ (Fig. 1A, small dots) from which it was derived due to the division by the low-pass power spectrum of the spikes (see Eqn. 1). Also, $r_{sx}(\tau)$ occasionally had a slower, trailing negative lobe but did not have the preceding negative lobe of $h(t)$. On average, $h(t)$ peaked at -69 ms (SD 17) and was 33 ms (SD 12) wide at half-height. The peak for $r_{sx}(\tau)$ occurred at the same time, but the width was 41 ms (SD 15), ranging from 30–90 ms. The point of half-rise on the right side of the peak was -53 ms (SD 9) for $h(t)$ and -51 ms (SD 9) for $r_{sx}(\tau)$. For all plots, vertical axes for velocity show normalized stimulus velocity, i.e., stimulus velocity was scaled to have unity SD before all computations.

Fig 1C (dots) shows the SNR for the reconstruction using the $h(t)$ in panel A. For 8 cells tested with *Gaussian* velocity noise, the integral of the log of the SNR gives a lower bound for information transmission, which was 6.7 bits/s (SD 2.8), with a high value of 12.3 bits/s. Most of the information was carried below 10 Hz, and 90% of the information was carried below 18.4 Hz (SD 2.1). In Fig. 1D, the failure of the reconstruction (dots) to capture higher frequencies in the stimulus (thick line) is directly visible. Both $h(t)$ and SNR(ω) were similar but on average slightly greater in amplitude for tests using binary and uniform distributed noise. Gaussian noise has many jumps at or near zero which may induce little or no response.

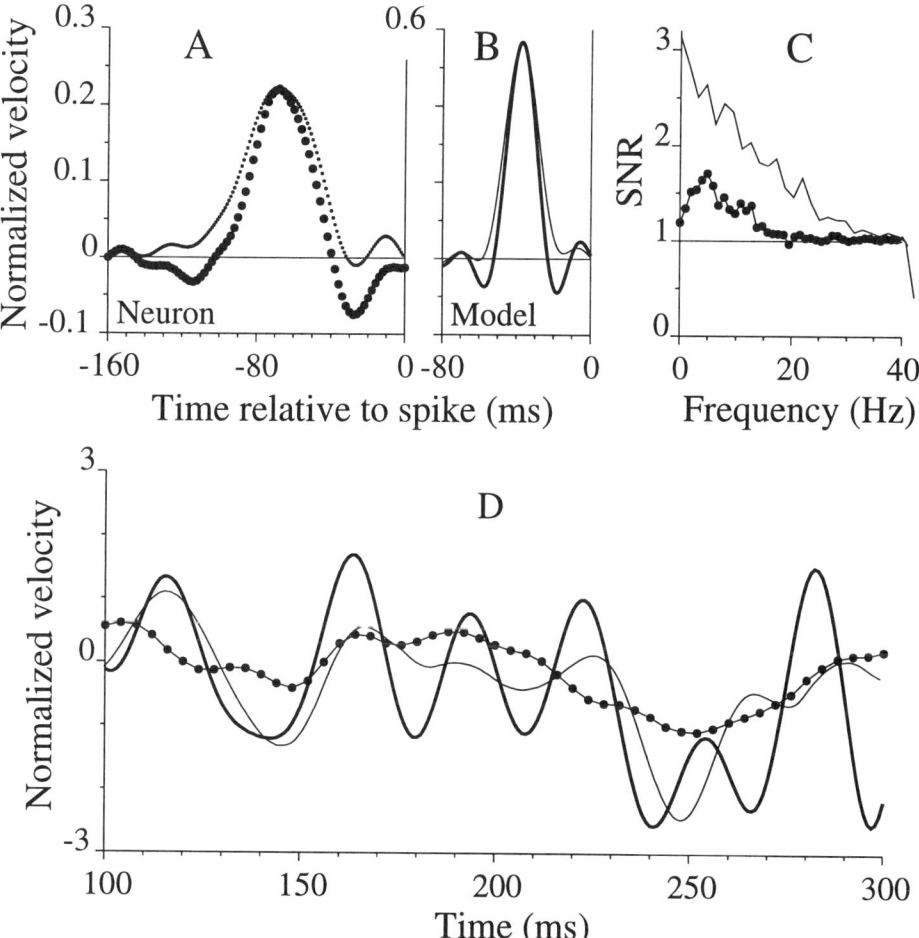

Figure 1: **(A)** Optimal linear filter $h(t)$ (big dots) from Eqn. 1 and cross-correlation $r_{sx}(\tau)$ (small dots) for one MT neuron. **(B)** $h(t)$ (thick line) and $r_{sx}(\tau)$ (thin line) for an opponent motion energy model. **(C)** SNR(ω) for the neuron (dots) and the model (line). **(D)** Reconstruction for the neuron (dots) and model (thin line) of the stimulus velocity (thick line). Velocity was normalized to unity SD. Curves for $r_{sx}(\tau)$ were scaled by 0.5. Note the different vertical scale in B.

An opponent motion energy model using Gabor functions was simulated with spatial SD 0.5°, spatial frequency 0.625 cyc/°, temporal SD 12.5 ms, and temporal frequency 20 Hz. The model was tested with a Gaussian velocity stimulus with SD 32°/s. Because an arbitrary scaling of the spatial parameters in the model does not affect the temporal properties of the information transmission, this was effectively the same stimulus that yielded the neuronal data shown in Fig. 1A. Spike trains were generated from the model at 20 Hz (matched to the neuron) and used to compute $h(t)$ (Fig. 1B, thick line). The model $h(t)$ was narrower than that for the MT neuron, but was similar to $h(t)$ for *V1 neurons* that have been tested (unpublished analysis). This simple model of a putative input sub-unit to MT transmitted 29 bits/s—more than the best MT neurons studied here. The SNR ratio and the reconstruction for the model are shown in Fig. 1C,D (thin lines). The filter $h(t)$ for the model (Fig. 1B thick line) was more symmetric than that for the neuron due to the symmetry of the Gabor function used in the model.

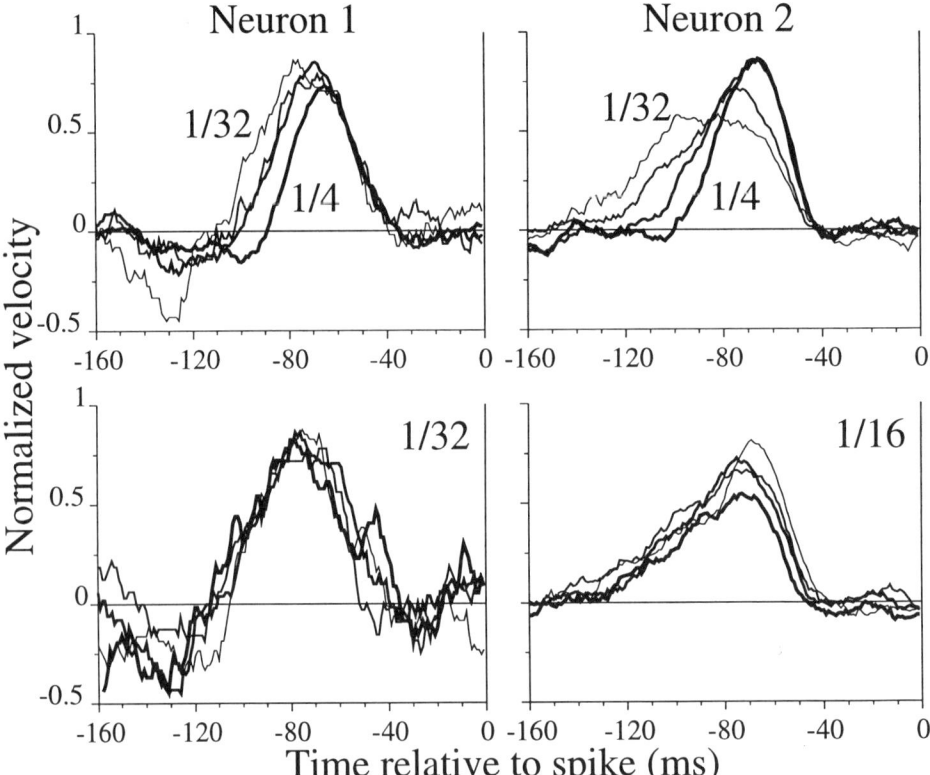

Figure 2: The width of $r_{sx}(\tau)$ changes with temporal frequency, but not spatial frequency. Data from two neurons are shown, one on the left, one on the right. **Top:** $r_{sx}(\tau)$ is shown for binary velocity stimuli with jump sizes 1/4, 1/8, 1/16, and 1/32 (thick to thin lines) of the spatial period (10 trials, 3 s/trial). The left side of the peak shifts leftward as jump size decreases. See text for statistics. **Bottom:** The relative jump size, thus temporal frequency, was constant for the four cases in each panel (1/32 on the left, 1/16 on the right). The peaks do not shift left or right as spatial frequency and jump size change inversely. Thicker lines represent larger jumps and lower spatial frequencies.

Changes in $r_{sx}(\tau)$. We tested 11 neurons with a set of binary white-noise motion stimuli that varied in spatial frequency and jump size. The spatial patterns were sinusoidal gratings. The peaks in $r_{sx}(\tau)$ and $h(t)$ were wider when smaller jumps (slower velocities) were used to move the same spatial pattern. Fig. 2 shows data for two neurons plotted for constant spatial frequency (top) and constant effective temporal frequency, or *contrast frequency* (bottom). Jump sizes were 1/4, 1/8, 1/16, and 1/32 (thick to thin lines, top panels) of the period of the spatial pattern. (Note, a 1/2 period jump would cause an ambiguous motion.) Relative jump size was constant in the bottom panels, but both the spatial period and the velocity increased in octaves from thin to thick lines. One of the plots in the upper panel also appears in the lower panel for each neuron. For 26 conditions in 11 MT neurons (up to 4 spatial frequencies per neuron) the left and right half-rise points of the peak of $r_{sx}(\tau)$ shifted leftward by 19 ms (SD 12) and 4.5 ms (SD 4.0), respectively, as jump size decreased. The width, therefore, increased by 14 ms (SD 12). These changes were statistically significant ($p < 0.001$, t-test). In fact, the left half-rise point moved leftward in all 26 cases, and in no case did the width at half-height decrease. On the other hand, there was no significant change in the peak width or half-rise times when temporal frequency was constant, as demonstrated in the lower panels of Fig. 2.

5 DISCUSSION

From other experiments using frame-based displays to present moving stimuli to MT cells, we know that roughly half of the cells can modulate to a 60 Hz signal in the preferred direction and that some provide reliable bursts of spikes on each frame but do not respond to null direction motion. Therefore, one might expect that these cells could easily be made to transmit nearly 60 bits/s by moving the stimulus randomly in either the preferred or null direction on each video frame. However, the stimuli that we employed here did not result in such high frequency modulation, nor did our best lower bound estimate of information transmission for an MT cell, 12 bits/s, approach the 64 bits/s capacity of the motion sensitive H1 neuron in the fly (Bialek et al., 1991). In recordings from seven V1 neurons (not shown here), two directional complex cells responded to the velocity noise with high temporal precision and fired a burst of spikes on almost every preferred motion frame and no spikes on null motion frames. At 53 frames/s, these cells transmitted over 40 bits/s. We hope that further investigation will reveal whether the lack of high frequency modulation in our MT experiments was due to statistical variation between animals, the structure of the stimulus, or possibly to anesthesia.

In spite of finding less high frequency bandwidth than expected, we were able to document consistent changes, namely narrowing, of the temporal integration window of MT neurons as temporal frequency increased. Similar changes in the time constant of motion processing have been reported in the fly visual system, where it appears that neither velocity nor temporal frequency alone can account for all changes (de Ruyter et al., 1986; Borst & Egelhaaf, 1987). The narrowing of $r_{sx}(\tau)$ with higher temporal frequency does not occur in our simple motion energy model, which lacks adaptive mechanisms, but it could occur in a model which integrated signals from many motion energy units having distributed temporal frequency tuning, even without other sources of adaptation.

We were not able to assess whether changes in the integration window developed quickly at the beginning of individual trials, but an analysis not described here at least indicates that there was very little change in the position and width of $r_{sx}(\tau)$ and $h(t)$ after the first few seconds during the 30 s trials.

Acknowledgements

This work was funded by the Howard Hughes Medical Institute. We thank Fabrizio Gabbiani and Christof Koch for helpful discussion, Lawrence P. O'Keefe for assistance with electrophysiology, and David Tanzer for assistance with software.

References

Adelson EH, Bergen JR (1985) Spatiotemporal energy models for the perception of motion. *J Opt Soc Am A* **2**:284–299.

Bair W, Koch C (1996) Temporal precision of spike trains in extrastriate cortex of the behaving macaque monkey. *Neural Comp* **8**:1185–1202.

Bialek W, Rieke F, de Ruyter van Steveninck RR, Warland D (1991) Reading a neural code. *Science* **252**:1854–1857.

Borst A, Egelhaaf M (1987) Temporal modulation of luminance adapts time constant of fly movement detectors. *Biol Cybern* **56**:209–215.

Emerson RC, Bergen JR, Adelson EH (1992) Directionally selective complex cells and the computation of motion energy in cat visual cortex. *Vision Res* **32**:203–218.

Gabbiani F, Koch C (1996) Coding of time-varying signals in spike trains of integrate-and-fire neurons with random threshold. *Neural Comp* **8**:44–66.

Grzywacz NM, Yuille AL (1990) A model for the estimate of local image velocity by cells in the visual cortex. *Proc R Soc Lond B* **239**:129–161.

Heeger DJ (1987) Model for the extraction of image flow. *J Opt Soc Am A* **4**:1455–1471.

Levitt JB, Kiper DC, Movshon JA (1994) Receptive fields and functional architecture of macaque V2. J.Neurophys. 71:2517–2542.

Nowlan SJ, Sejnowski TJ (1994) Filter selection model for motion segmentation and velocity integration. *J Opt Soc Am A* **11**:3177–3200.

Qian N, Andersen RA, Adelson EH (1994) Transparent motion perception as detection of unbalanced motion signals .3. Modeling. *J Neurosc* **14**:7381–7392.

de Ruyter van Steveninck R, Zaagman WH, Mastebroek HAK (1986) Adaptation of transient responses of a movement-sensitive neuron in the visual-system of the blowfly calliphora-erythrocephala. *Biol Cybern* **54**:223–236.

3D Object Recognition:
A Model of View-Tuned Neurons

Emanuela Bricolo **Tomaso Poggio**
Department of Brain and Cognitive Sciences
Massachusetts Institute of Technology
Cambridge, MA 02139
{emanuela,tp}@ai.mit.edu

Nikos Logothetis
Baylor College of Medicine
Houston, TX 77030
nikos@bcmvision.bcm.tmc.edu

Abstract

In 1990 Poggio and Edelman proposed a view-based model of object recognition that accounts for several psychophysical properties of certain recognition tasks. The model predicted the existence of view-tuned and view-invariant units, that were later found by Logothetis et al. (Logothetis et al., 1995) in IT cortex of monkeys trained with views of specific paperclip objects. The model, however, does not specify the inputs to the view-tuned units and their internal organization. In this paper we propose a model of these view-tuned units that is consistent with physiological data from single cell responses.

1 INTRODUCTION

Recognition of specific objects, such as recognition of a particular face, can be based on representations that are object centered, such as 3D structural models. Alternatively, a 3D object may be represented for the purpose of recognition in terms of a set of views. This latter class of models is biologically attractive because model acquisition – the learning phase – is simpler and more natural.

A simple model for this strategy of object recognition was proposed by Poggio and Edelman (Poggio and Edelman, 1990). They showed that, with few views of an object used as training examples, a classification network, such as a Gaussian radial basis function network, can learn to recognize novel views of that object, in partic-

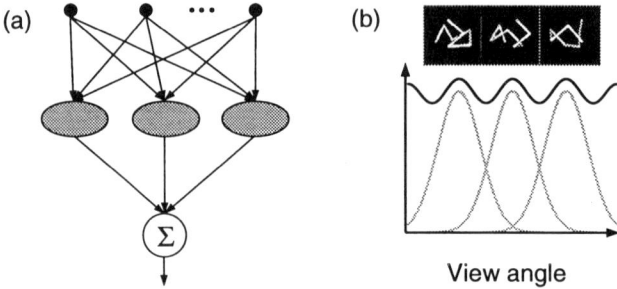

Figure 1: (a) Schematic representation of the architecture of the Poggio-Edelman model. The shaded circles correspond to the view-tuned units, each tuned to a view of the object, while the open circle correspond to the view-invariant, object specific output unit. (b) Tuning curves of the view-tuned (gray) and view-invariant (black) units.

ular views obtained by in depth rotation of the object (translation, rotation in the image plane and scale are probably taken care by object independent mechanisms). The model, sketched in Figure 1, makes several prediction about limited generalization from a single training view and about characteristic generalization patterns between two or more training views (Bülthoff and Edelman, 1992). Psychophysical and neurophysiological results support the main features and predictions of this simple model. For instance, in the case of novel objects, it has been shown that when subjects –both humans and monkeys– are asked to learn an object from a single unoccluded view, their performance decays as they are tested on views farther away from the learned one (Bülthoff and Edelman, 1992; Tarr and Pinker, 1991; Logothetis et al., 1994). Additional work has shown that even when 3D information is provided during training and testing, subjects recognize in a view dependent way and cannot generalize beyond 40 degrees from a single training view (Sinha and Poggio, 1994).

Even more significantly, recent recordings in inferotemporal cortex (IT) of monkeys performing a similar recognition task with paperclip and amoeba-like objects, revealed cells tuned to specific views of the learned object (Logothetis et al., 1995). The tuning, an example of which is shown in Figure 3, was presumably acquired as an effect of the training to views of the particular object. Thus an object can be thought as represented by a set of cells tuned to several of its views, consistently with finding of others (Wachsmuth et al., 1994). This simple model can be extended to deal with symmetric objects (Poggio and Vetter, 1992) as well as objects which are members of a *nice* class (Vetter et al., 1995): in both cases generalization from a single view may be significantly greater than for objects such as the paperclips used in the psychophysical and physiological experiments.

The original model of Poggio and Edelman has a major weakness: it does not specify which features are inputs to the view-tuned units and what is stored as a representation of a view in each unit. The simulation data they presented employed features such as the x,y coordinates of the object vertices in the image plane or the angles between successive segments. This representation, however, is biologically implausible and specific for objects that have easily detectable vertices and measurable angles, like paperclips. In this paper, we suggest a view representation which is more biologically plausible and applies to a wider variety of cases. We will also show that this extension of the Poggio-Edelman model leads to properties that are

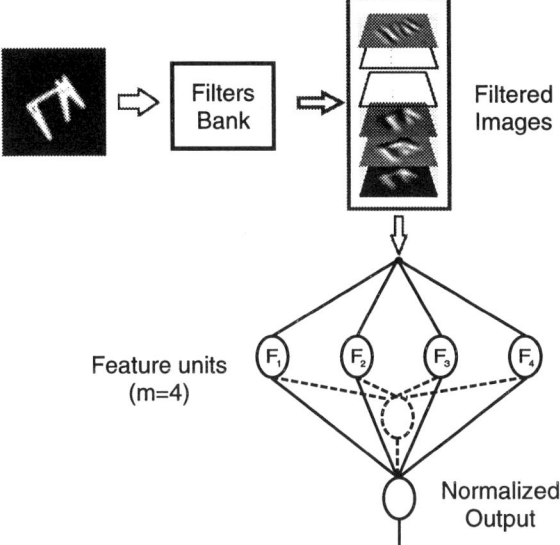

Figure 2: Model overview: during the training phase the images are first filtered through a bank of steerable filters. Then a number of image locations are chosen by an attentional mechanism and the vector of filtered values at these locations is stored in the feature units.

consistent with the cell response to the same objects.

2 A MODEL OF VIEW-TUNED UNITS

Our approach consists in representing a view in terms of a few local features, which can be regarded as local configurations of grey-levels. Suppose one point in the image of the object is chosen. A feature vector is computed by filtering the image with a set of filters with small support centered at the chosen location. The vector of filter responses serves as a description of the local pattern in the image. Four such points were chosen, for example, in the image of Figure 3a, where the white squares indicate the support of the bank of filters that were used. Since the support is local but finite, the value of each filter depends on the pattern contained in the support and not only on the center pixel; since there are several filters one expects that the vector of values may uniquely represent the local feature, for instance a corner of the paperclip.

We used filters that are somewhat similar to oriented receptive fields in V1 (though it is far from being clear whether some V1 cells behave as linear filters). The ten filters we used are the same steerable filters (Freeman and Adelson, 1991) suggested by Ballard and Rao (Rao and Ballard, 1995; Leung et al., 1995). The filters were chosen to be a basis of steerable 2-dimensional filters up to the third order. If G_n represents the nth derivative of a Gaussian in the x direction and we define the rotation operator $(...)^\theta$ as the operator that rotates a function through an angle θ about the origin, the ten basis filters are:

$$G_n^{\theta_k} \quad \begin{array}{l} n = 0, 1, 2, 3 \\ \theta_k = 0, ..., k\pi/(n+1), k = 1, ...n \end{array} \quad (1)$$

Therefore for each one of the chosen locations m in the image we have a 10-value array $\mathbf{T}_m$ given by the output of the filters bank.

$$\mathbf{T}_m = ((I * G_0^0)|_m, (I * G_1^0)|_m, (I * G_1^{\pi/2})|_m, ..., (I * G_3^{3\pi/4})|_m) \qquad (2)$$

The representation of a given view of an object is then the following. First $m = 1, ..., M$ locations are chosen, then for each of these M locations the 10-valued vectors $\mathbf{T}_m$ are computed and stored. These M vectors, with M typically between 1 and 4, form the representation of the view which is learned and commited to memory.

How are the locations chosen? Precise location is not critical. Feature locations can be chosen almost randomly. Of course each specific choice will influence properties of the unit but precise location does not affect the qualitative properties of the model, as verified in simulation experiments. Intuitively, features should be centered at salient locations in the object where there are large changes in contrast and curvature. We have implemented (Riesenhuber and Bricolo, in preparation) a simple attentional mechanism that chooses locations close to edges with various orientations[1]. The locations shown in Figures 3 and 4 were obtained with this unsupervised technique. We emphasize however that all the results and conclusions of this paper do not depend on the specific location of the feature or the precise procedure used to choose them.

We have described so far the learning phase and how views are represented and stored. When a new image $\mathbf{V}$ is presented, recognition takes place in the following way. First the new image is filtered through the bank of filters. Thus at each pixel location i we have the vector of values $\mathbf{f}_i$ provided by the filters. Now consider the first stored vector $\mathbf{T}_1$. The closest $\mathbf{f}_i^*$ is found searching over all i locations and the distance $D_1 = \|\mathbf{T}_1 - \mathbf{f}_i^*\|$ is computed. This process is repeated for the other feature vectors $\mathbf{T}_m$ for $m = 2, ..., M$. Thus for the new image $\mathbf{V}$, M distances D_m are computed; the distance D_m is therefore the distance to the stored feature $\mathbf{T}_m$ of the closest image vector searched over the whole image.

The model uses these M distances as exponents in M Gaussian units. The output of the system is a weighted average of the output of these units with an output non linearity of the sigmoidal type:

$$\mathbf{Y_V} = h\left(\sum_{m=1}^{M} c_m e^{-\frac{D_m^2}{2\sigma^2}}\right) \qquad (3)$$

In the simulations presented in this paper we estimated σ from the distribution of distances over several images; the c_m are $c_m = M^{-1}$, since we have only one training view; h is $h(x) = 1/(1 - e^{-x})$.

In Figure 3b we see the result obtained by simply combining linearly the output of the four feature detectors followed by the sigmoidal non linearity (Figure 4a shows another example). We have also experimented with a multiplicative combination of the output of the feature units. In this case the system performs an AND of the M features. If the response to the distractors is used to set a threshold for

---

[1] A saliency map is at first constructed as the average of the convolutions of the image with four directional filters (first order steerable filters with $\theta = 0, ..., k\pi/(4), k = 1, ...4)$. The locations with higher saliency are extracted one at the time. After each selection, a region around the selected position is inhibited to avoid selecting the same feature over again.

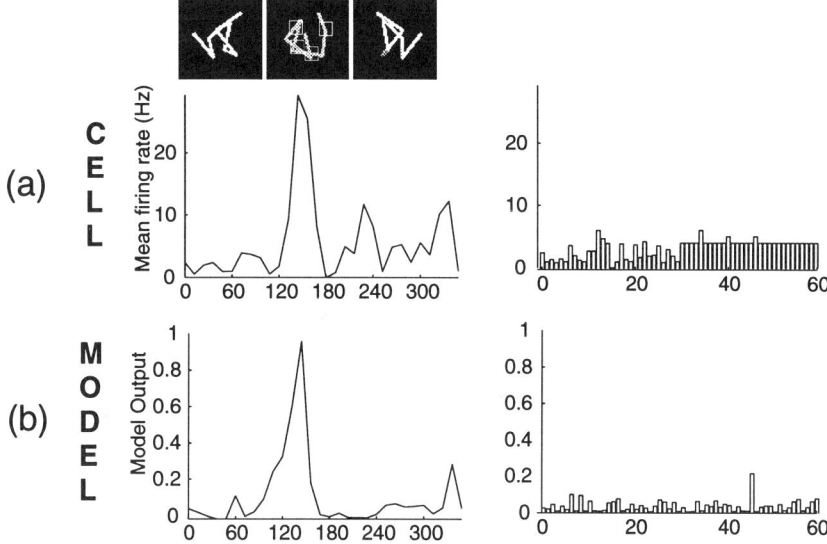

Figure 3: Comparison between a model view-tuned unit and cortical neuron tuned to a view of the same object. (a) Mean spike rate of an inferotemporal cortex cell recorded in response to views of a specific paperclip [left] and to a set of 60 distractor paperclip objects [right],(Logothetis and Pauls, personal communication). (b) Model response for the same set of objects. This is representative for other cells we have simulated, thought there is considerable variability in the cells (and the model) tuning.

classification, then the two versions of the system behave in a similar way. Similar results (not shown) were obtained using other kinds of objects.

3 RESULTS

3.1 COMPARISON BETWEEN VIEW-TUNED UNITS AND CORTICAL NEURONS

Electrophysiological investigations in alert monkeys, trained to recognize wire-like objects presented from any view show that the discharge rate of many IT neurons is a bell-shaped function of orientation centered on a preferred view (Logothetis et al., 1995). The properties of the units here described are comparable to those of the cortical neurons (see Figure 3). The model was tested with the exactly the same objects used in the physiological experiments. As training view for the model we used the view preferred by the cell (the cell became tuned presumably as an effect of training during which the monkey was shown in this particular case several views of this object).

3.2 OCCLUSION EXPERIMENTS

What physiological experiments could lend additional support to our model? A natural question concerns the behavior of the cells when various parts of the object are occluded. The predictions of our model are given in Figure 4 for a specific object and a specific choice of feature units ($m = 4$) and locations.

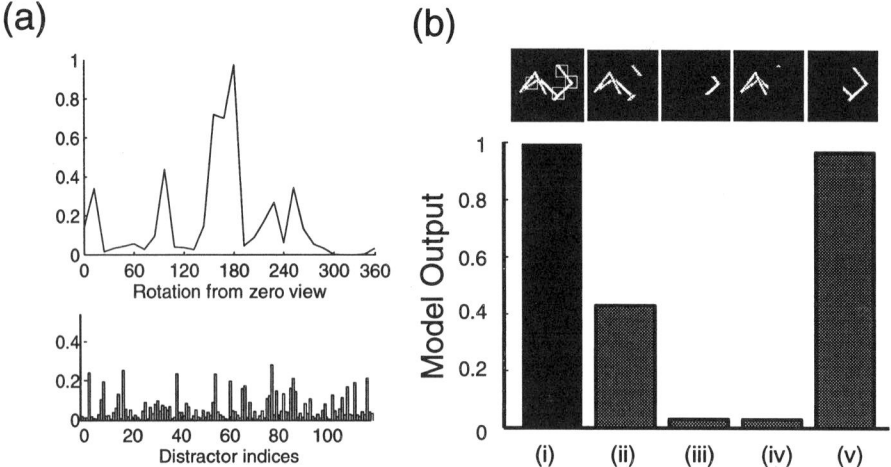

Figure 4: (a) Model behavior in response to a learned object in full view (highlighted on the learned image are the positions of the four features) at different rotations and to 120 other paperclip objects (distractors), (b) Response dependence on occluder characteristics: (i) object in full view at learned location, (ii) object occluded with a small occluder, (iii) occluded region in (ii) presented in isolation, (iv-v) same as (ii-iii) but with a larger occluder.

The simulations show that the behavior depends on the position of key features with respect to the occluder itself. Occluding a part of the object can drastically reduce the response to that specific view (Figure 4b(ii-iv)) because of interference with more than one feature. But since the occluded region does not completely overlap with the occluded features (considering the support of the filters), the presentation of this region alone does not always evoke a significant response (Figure 4b(iii-v)).

4 Discussion

Poggio and Edelman model was designed specifically for paperclip objects and did not explicitly specify how to compute the response for any object and image. In this paper we fill this gap and propose a model of these IT cells that become view tuned as an effect of training. The key aspect of the model is that it relies on a few local features (1-4) that are computed and stored during the training phase. Each feature is represented as the set of responses of oriented filters at one location in the image. During recognition the system computes a robust conjunction of the best matches to the stored features.

Clearly, the version of the model described here does not exploit information about the geometric configuration of the features. This information is available once the features are detected and can be critical to perform more robust recognition. We have devised a model of how to use the relative position of the features $\mathbf{f}_i^*$ in the image. The model can be made translation and scale invariant in a biologically plausible way by using a network of cells with linear receptive fields, similar in spirit to a model proposed for spatial representation in the parietal cortex (Pouget and Sejnowski, 1996). Interestingly enough, this additional information is not needed to account for the selectivity and the generalization properties of the IT cells we have considered so far. The implication is that IT cells may not be sensitive to the overall configuration of the stimulus but to the presence of moderately complex local features (according to our simulations, the number of necessary local features is greater than one for the most selective neurons, such as the one of Figure 3a). Scrambling the image of the object should therefore preserve the selectivity of the neurons, *provided* this can be done without affecting the filtering stage. In practice this may be very difficult. Though our model is still far from being a reasonable neuronal model, it can already be used to make useful predictions for physiological experiments which are presently underway.

References

Bülthoff, H. and Edelman, S. (1992). Psychophisical support for a two-dimensional view interpolation theory of object recognition. *Proceedings of the National Academy of Science. USA*, 89:60–64.

Freeman, W. and Adelson, E. (1991). The design and use of steerable filters. *IEEE transactions on Pattern Analysis and Machine Intelligence*, 13(9):891–906.

Leung, T., Burl, M., and Perona, P. (1995). Finding faces in cluttered scenes using random labelled graph matching. In *Proceedings of the 5th Internatinal Conference on Computer Vision*, Cambridge, Ma.

Logothetis, N., Pauls, J., Bülthoff, H., and Poggio, T. (1994). View dependent object recognition by monkeys. *Current Biology*, 4(5):401–414.

Logothetis, N., Pauls, J., and Poggio, T. (1995). Shape representation in the inferior temporal cortex of monkeys. *Current Biology*, 5(5):552–563.

Poggio, T. and Edelman, S. (1990). A network that learns to recognize three-dimensional objects. *Nature*, 343:263–266.

Poggio, T. and Vetter, T. (1992). Recognition and structure from one 2d model view: observations on prototypes, object classes and symmetries. Technical Report A.I. Memo No.1347, Massachusetts Institute of Technnology, Cambridge, Ma.

Pouget, A. and Sejnowski, T. (1996). Spatial representations in the parietal cortex may use basis functions. In Tesauro, G., Touretzky, D., and Leen, T., editors, *Advances in Neural Information Processing Systems*, volume 7, pages 157–164. MIT Press.

Rao, R. and Ballard, D. (1995). An active vision architecture based on iconic representations. *Artificial Intelligence Journal*, 78:461–505.

Sinha, P. and Poggio, T. (1994). View-based strategies for 3d object recognition. Technical Report A.I. Memo No.1518, Massachusetts Institute of Technnology, Cambridge, Ma.

Tarr, M. and Pinker, S. (1991). Orientation-dependent mechanisms in shape recognition: further issues. *Psychological Science*, 2(3):207–209.

Vetter, T., Hurlbert, A., and Poggio, T. (1995). View-based models of 3d object recognition: Invariance to imaging transformations. *Cerebral Cortex*, 3(261–269).

Wachsmuth, E., Oram, M., and Perrett, D. (1994). Recognition of objects and their component parts: Responses of single units in the temporal cortex of the macaque. *Cerebral Cortex*, 4(5):509–522.

An Hierarchical Model of Visual Rivalry

Peter Dayan
Department of Brain and Cognitive Sciences
E25-210 Massachusetts Institute of Technology
Cambridge, MA 02139
dayan@psyche.mit.edu[1]

Abstract

Binocular rivalry is the alternating percept that can result when the two eyes see different scenes. Recent psychophysical evidence supports an account for one component of binocular rivalry similar to that for other bistable percepts. We test the hypothesis[19,16,18] that alternation can be generated by competition between top-down cortical explanations for the inputs, rather than by direct competition between the inputs. Recent neurophysiological evidence shows that some binocular neurons are modulated with the changing percept; others are not, even if they are selective between the stimuli presented to the eyes. We extend our model to a hierarchy to address these effects.

1 Introduction

Although binocular rivalry leads to distinct perceptual distress, it is revealing about the mechanisms of visual information processing. The first accounts for rivalry argued on the basis of phenomena such as increases in thresholds for test stimuli presented in the suppressed eye[24,8,3] that there was a early competitive process, the outcome of which meant that the system would just ignore input from one eye in favour of the other. Various experiments have suggested that simple input competition cannot be the whole story. For instance, in a case in which rivalry is between a vertical grating in the left eye and a horizontal one in the right, and in which a vertical grating is presented prior to rivalry to cause adaptation, the relative suppression of vertical during rivalry is independent of

---

[1] I am very grateful to Bart Anderson, Adam Elga, Geoff Goodhill, Geoff Hinton, David Leopold, Earl Miller, Read Montague, Bruno Olshausen, Pawan Sinha, Rich Zemel, and particularly Zhaoping Li and Tommi Jaakkola for their comments on earlier drafts and discussions. This work was supported by the NIH.

the eye of origin of the adapting grating.[4] Even more compelling, if the rivalrous stimuli in the two eyes are switched rapidly, the percept switches only slowly – competition is more between coherent percepts than merely inputs. Rivalry is an attractive paradigm for studying models of cortex like the Helmholtz machine[12,7] that construct coherent percepts, and in particular for studying *hierarchical* models, because of electrophysiological data on the behaviour during rivalry of cells at different levels of the visual processing hierarchy.[16]

Leopold & Logothetis[16] trained monkeys to report their percepts during rivalrous and non-rivalrous stimuli whilst recording from neurons V1/2 and V4. Important findings are that striate monocular neurons are unaffected by rivalry; some striate binocular neurons that are selective between the stimuli modulate their activities during rivalry; others do not; some fire more when their preferred stimuli are suppressed; others still are only selective during rivalry. In this paper we consider one form of analysis-by-synthesis model of cortical processing[7] and show how it can exhibit rivalry between explanations in the case that the eyes receive different input. This model can provide an account for many of the behaviours described above.

2 The Model

Figure 1a shows the full generative model. Units in layers $\mathbf{y}$ (modeling V1) and $\mathbf{x}$ and $\mathbf{w}$ (modeling early and late extra-striate areas) are all binocular and jointly explain successively more complex features in the input $\mathbf{z}$ according to a top-down generative model. Apart from the half bars in $\mathbf{y}$, the model is similar to that learned by the Helmholtz machine[12,7] for which increasing complexity in higher layers rather than the increasing input scale is key. In this case, for instance, w_2 specifies the occurrence of vertical bars anywhere in the 8×8 input grids; x_{16} specifies the rightmost vertical bar; and y_{31} and y_{32} the top and bottom half of this vertical bar. These specifications are provided by a top-down generative model in which the activations of units are specified by probabilities such as $\mathcal{P}[y_i = 1|\mathbf{x}] = \sigma\left(b_y + \sum_k x_k J_{\mathbf{xy}}^{ki}\right)$ where the sum k is over all the units in the $\mathbf{x}$ layer, and $\sigma()$ is a robust normal distribution function. We model the percept in terms of the activation in the $\mathbf{w}$ layer.

We model differing input contrasts by representing the input to z_i by d_i, where $\mathcal{P}[z_i = 1] = \sigma(d_i)$ and all the z_i are independent. Recognition is formally the statistical inverse to generation, and should produce distribution $\mathcal{P}[\mathbf{w}, \mathbf{x}, \mathbf{y}|\mathbf{d}]$ over all the choices of the hidden activations. We use a mean field inversion method,[13] using a factorised approximation $\mathcal{Q}[\mathbf{w}, \mathbf{x}, \mathbf{y}; \mu, \xi, \psi] = \mathcal{Q}[\mathbf{w}; \mu]\mathcal{Q}[\mathbf{x}; \xi]\mathcal{Q}[\mathbf{y}; \psi]$, with $\mathcal{Q}[\mathbf{w}; \mu] = \prod_i \sigma(\mu_i)^{w_i}(1 - \sigma(\mu_i))^{1-w_i}$, *etc*, and fitting the parameters μ, ξ, ψ to minimise the approximation cost:

$$\mathcal{F}[\mu, \xi, \psi] = \sum_{\mathbf{z}} \mathcal{P}[\mathbf{z}; \mathbf{d}] \sum_{\mathbf{w}, \mathbf{x}, \mathbf{y}} \mathcal{Q}[\mathbf{w}, \mathbf{x}, \mathbf{y}; \mu, \xi, \psi] \log \frac{\mathcal{Q}[\mathbf{w}, \mathbf{x}, \mathbf{y}; \mu, \xi, \psi]}{\mathcal{P}[\mathbf{w}, \mathbf{x}, \mathbf{y}|\mathbf{z}]}.$$

We report the mean activities of the units in the graphs and use a modified gradient descent method to find appropriate parameters. Figure 1b shows the resulting activities of units in response to binocular horizontal (i) and vertical (ii) bars, and also the two equally likely explanations for rivalrous input (iii and iv). For rivalry,

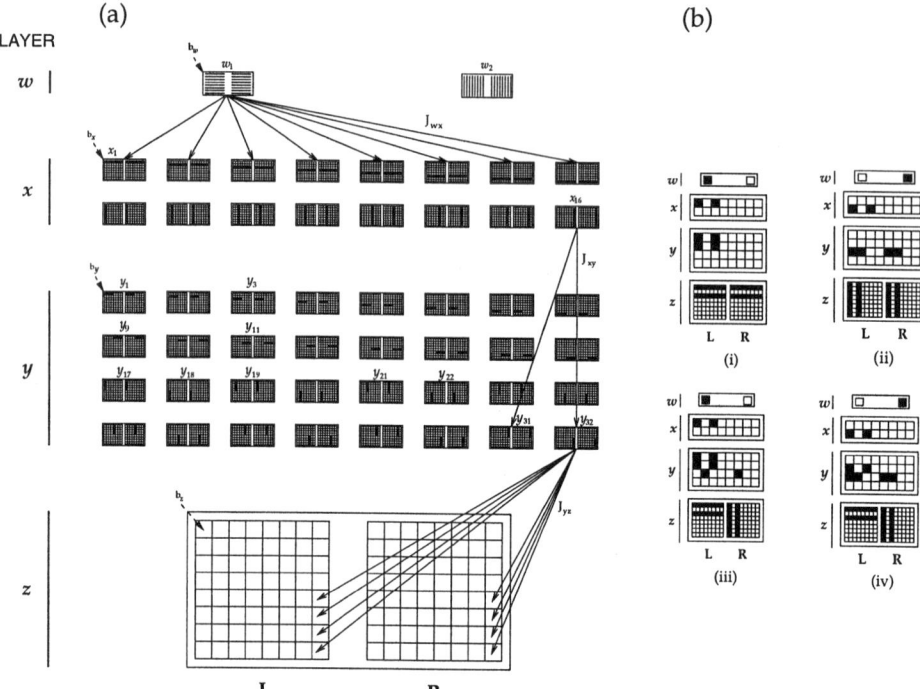

Figure 1: a) Hierarchical generative model for 8 × 8 bar patterns across the two eyes. Units are depicted by their net projective (generative) fields, and characteristic weights are shown. Even though the net projective field of x_1 is the top horizontal bar in both eyes, note that it generates this by increasing the probability that units y_1 and y_9 in the y layer will be active, not by having direct connections to the input z. Unit w_1 connects to $x_1, x_2, \ldots x_8$ through $J_{\mathbf{wx}} = 0.8$; x_{16} connects to y_{31}, y_{32} through $J_{\mathbf{xy}} = 1.0$ and y_{32} connects to the bottom right half vertical bar through $J_{\mathbf{yz}} = 5.8$. Biases are $b_{\mathbf{w}} = -0.75, b_{\mathbf{x}} = -1.5, b_{\mathbf{y}} = -2.7$ and $b_{\mathbf{z}} = -3.3$. b) Recognition activity in the network for four different input patterns. The units are arranged in the same order as (a), and white and black squares imply activities for the units whose means are less than and greater than 0.5. (i) and (ii) represent normal binocular stimulation; (iii) and (iv) show the two alternative stable states during rivalrous stimulation, without the fatigue process.

there is direct competition in the top left hand quadrant of z, which is reflected in the competition between y_1, y_3 and y_{17}, y_{21}. However, the input regions (top right of L and bottom left of R) for which there is no competition, require the constant activity of explanations y_9, y_{11}, y_{18} and y_{22}. Under the generative model, the coactivation of y_1 and y_9 *without* x_1 is quite unlikely ($\mathcal{P}[x_1 = 0 | y_1 = 1, y_3 = 1] = 0.1$), which is why x_1, x_3 and also w_1 become active with y_1 and y_3.

Given just gradient descent for the rivalrous stimulus, the network would just find one of the two equally good (or rather bad) solutions in figure 1b(iii,iv). Alternation ensues when descent is augmented by a fatigue process:

$$\psi_1(t+1) = \psi_1(t) + \delta(-\nabla_{\psi_1} \mathcal{F}[\mu, \xi, \psi] + \alpha(\beta\psi_1(t)) - \psi'_1(t))$$
$$\psi'_1(t+1) = \psi'_1(t) + \delta(\psi_1(t) - \beta\psi'_1(t)),$$

where β is a decay term. In all the simulations, $\alpha = 0.5, \beta = 0.1$ and $\delta = 0.01$.

We adopted various heuristics to simplify the process of using this rather cumbersome mean field model. First, fatigue is only implemented for the units in the y layer, and the ψ follow the equivalent of the dynamical equations above. Although adaptation processes can clearly occur at many levels in the system, and indeed have been used to try to diagnose the mechanisms of rivalry,[15] their exact form is not clear. Bialek & DeWeese[1] argue that the rate of a switching process should be adaptive to the expected rate of change of the associated signal on the basis of prior observations. This is clearly faster nearer to the input.

The second heuristic is that rather than perform gradient descent for the non-fatiguing units, the optimal values of μ and ξ are calculated on each iteration by solving numerically equations such as

$$\nabla_{\xi_i} \mathcal{F}[\mu, \xi, \psi] = 0.$$

The dearth of connections in the network of figure 1a allows μ and ξ to be calculated locally at each unit in an efficient manner. Whether this is reasonable depends on the time constants of settling in the mean field model with respect to the dynamics of switching, and, more particularly on the way that this deterministic model is made appropriately stochastic.

Figure 2a shows the resulting activities during rivalry of units at various levels of the hierarchy including the fatigue process. Broadly, the competing explanations in figure 1b(iii;iv), *ie* horizontal and vertical percepts, alternate, and units without competing inputs, such as y_9, are much less modulated than the others, such as y_1. The activity of y_9 is slightly elevated when horizontal bars are dominant, based on top-down connections. The activities of the units higher up, such as x_1 and w_1, do not decrease to 0 during the suppression period for horizontal bars, leaving weak activity during suppression. Many of the modulating cells in monkeys were not completely silent during their periods of less activity.[16] Figure 2b shows that the hierarchical version of the model also behaves in accordance with experimental results on the effects of varying the input contrast,[17, 10, 22, 16] which suggest that increasing the contrast in both eyes decreases the period of the oscillation (*ie* increases the frequency), and increasing the contrast in just one eye decreases the suppression period for that eye much more than it increases its dominance period.

3 Discussion

Following Logothetis and his colleagues[19, 16, 18] (see also Grossberg[11]) we have suggested an account of rivalry based on competing top-down hierarchical explanations, and have shown how it models various experimental observations on rivalry. Neurons explain inputs in virtue of being capable of generating their activities through a top-down statistical generative model. Competition arises between higher-level explanations of overlapping active regions (*ie* those involving contrast changes) of the input rather than between inputs themselves. Note that alternating the input between the two eyes would have no effect on this behaviour of the model, since *explanations* are competing rather than *inputs*. Of course, the model is greatly simplified – for instance, it only has units that are not modulating with the percept in the earliest binocular layer (layer y), whereas in the monkeys, more than half the cells in V4 were unmodulated during rivalry.[16]

The model's accounts of the neurophysiological findings described in the introduction are: i) monocular cells will generally not be modulated if they are involved in

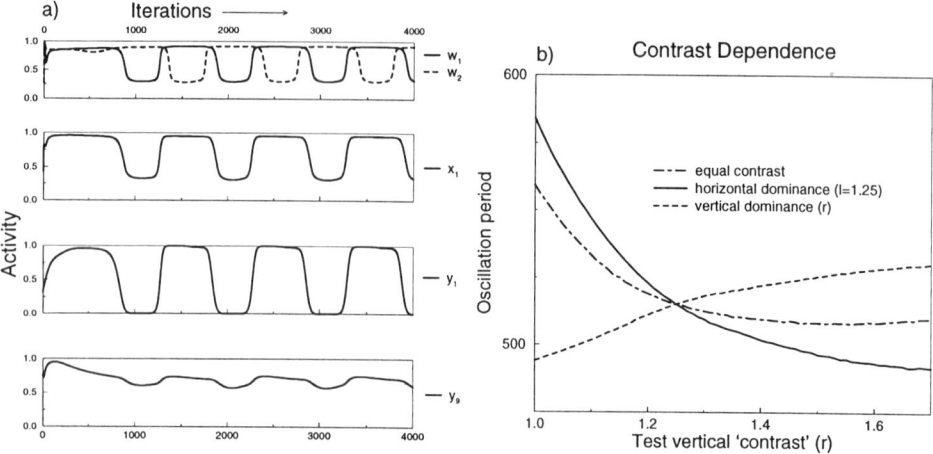

Figure 2: a) Mean activities of units at three levels of the hierarchy in response to rivalrous stimuli with input strengths $l = r = 1.75$. b) Contrast dependence of the oscillation periods for equal input strengths, and when $l = 1.25$ and r is varied.

explaining local correlations in the input from a single eye. This model does not demonstrate this explicitly, but would if, for instance, each of the inputs z_i actually consisted of two units, which are always on or off together. In this case one could get a compact explanation of the joint activities with a set of monocular units which would then not be modulated. ii) Units such as y_9 in the hierarchical model are binocular, are selective between the binocular version of the stimuli, and are barely modulated with the percept. iii) Units such as y_1, x_1 and w_1 are binocular, are selective between the stimuli, and are significantly modulated with the percept.

The final neurophysiological finding is to do with cells that fire when their preferred stimuli are suppressed, or fire selectively between the stimuli *only* during rivalry. There are no units in this model that are selective between the stimuli and are preferentially activated during *suppression* of their preferred stimuli. However, in a model with more complicated stimulus contingencies, they would emerge to account for the parts of the stimulus in the suppressed eye that are *not* accounted for by the explanation of the overlying parts of the dominant explanation, at least provided that this residual between the true monocular stimulus and the current explanation is sufficiently complex as to require explaining itself.

We would expect to find two sets of cells that are activated during the suppressed period by this residual, some of which will form part of the representation of the stimulus when presented binocularly and some of which will not. Those that do not (class A) will only even appear to be selective between the stimuli during rivalry, and will represent parts of the residual that are themselves explained by more overarching explanations for parts of the complete (binocularly presented) stimulus. This suggests the experimental test of presenting binocularly a putative form of the residual (*eg* dotted lines for competing horizontal and vertical gratings). We predict that these cells should be activated.

If there are cells that do participate in the binocular representation, then they will be selective, but will preferentially fire during suppression (class B). Certainly, the residual will have a high correlation with the full suppressed pattern, and so a cell that is selective for part of the residual could have appropriate properties. However, why should such a cell not fire when the full, but currently suppressed, pattern is dominant? In monkeys,[16] there are fewer class B than class A cells (0 versus 3 of 33 cells in V1/2; 6 versus 8 of 68 cells in V4). Under the model, we account for these cells based on a competition between units that represent the residual and those that represent overlapping parts of the complete pattern. In binocular viewing, explanations are generally stronger than during rivalry. So even if both such units participate in representing a binocular stimulus, the cells representing the residual might not reach threshold during the dominance period. However, during suppression, they no longer suffer from competition, and so will be activated. The model's explanation for class B cells seems far less natural than that for class A cells. One experimental test would be to present the preferred pattern binocularly, reduce the contrast, and see if these cells are suppressed more strongly.

The overall model mechanistically has much in common with models which place the competition in rivalry at the level of binocular oriented cells rather than between monocular cells.[11,2] Indeed, the model is based on an explanation-driven account for normal binocular processing, so this is to be expected. The advantage of couching rivalry in terms of explanations is that this provides a natural way of accounting for top-down influences. In fact, one can hope to study top-down control through studying its effects on the behaviour of cells during rivalry.

The model suffers from various lacunæ. Foremost, it is necessary to model the stochasticity of switching between explanations.[9,17] The distributions of dominance times for both humans and monkeys is well characterised by a Γ distribution (Lehky[14] argues that this is descriptive rather than normative), with strong independence between successive dominance periods. Our mean field recognition process is deterministic. The stochastic analogue would be some form of Markov chain Monte-Carlo method such as Gibbs sampling. However, it is not obvious how to incorporate the equivalent of fatigue in a computationally reasonable way. In any case, the nature of neuronal randomness is subject to significant debate at present. Note that the recognition model of a stochastic Helmholtz machine[7,6] would be unsuitable, since it is purely feedforward and does not integrate bottom-up and top-down information.

We have adopted a very simple mean field approach to recognition, giving up neurobiological plausibility for convenience. The determinism of the mean field model in any case rules it out as a complete explanation, but it does at least show clearly the nature of competition between explanations. The architecture of the model is also incomplete. The cortex is replete with what we would model as lateral connections between units within a single layer. We have constructed generative models in which there are no such direct connections, because they significantly complicate the mean field recognition method. It could be that these connections are important for the recognition process,[6] but modeling their effect would require representing them explicitly. This would also allow modeling of the apparent diffusive process by which patches of dominance spread and alter. In a complete model, it would also be necessary to account for competition between eyes in addition to competition between explanations.[24,8,3]

Another gap is some form of contrast gain control.[5] The model is quite sensitive to input contrast. This is obviously important for the effects shown in figures 2, however the range of contrasts over which it works should be larger. It would be particularly revealing to explore the effects of changing the contrast in some parts of images and examine the consequent effects on the spreading of dominance.

References

[1] Bialek, W & DeWeese, M (1995). Random switching and optimal processing in the perception of ambiguous signals. *Physical Review Letters*, **74**, 3077-3080.

[2] Blake, R (1989). A neural theory of binocular rivalry. *Psychological Review*, **96**, 145-167.

[3] Blake, R & Fox, R (1974). Binocular rivalry suppression: Insensitive to spatial frequency and orientation change. *Vision Research*, **14**, 687-692.

[4] Blake, R, Westendorf, DH & Overton, R (1980). What is suppressed during binocular rivalry? *Perception*, **9**, 223-231.

[5] Carandini, M & Heeger, DJ (1994). Summation and division by neurons in primate visual cortex. *Science*, **264**, 1333-1336.

[6] Dayan, P & Hinton, GE (1996). Varieties of Helmholtz machine. *Neural Networks*, **9**, 1385-1403.

[7] Dayan, P, Hinton, GE, Neal, RM & Zemel, RS (1995). The Helmholtz machine. *Neural Computation*, **7**, 889-904.

[8] Fox, R & Check, R (1972). Independence between binocular rivalry suppression duration and magnitude of suppression. *Journal of Experimental Psychology*, **93**, 283-289.

[9] Fox, R & Herrmann, J (1967). Stochastic properties of binocular rivalry alternations. *Perception and Psychophysics*, **2**, 432-436.

[10] Fox, R & Rasche, F (1969). Binocular rivalry and reciprocal inhibition. *Perception and Psychophyics*, **5**, 215-217.

[11] Grossberg, S (1987). Cortical dynamics of three-dimensional form, color and brightness perception: 2. Binocular theory. *Perception & Psychphysics*, **41**, 117-158.

[12] Hinton, GE, Dayan, P, Frey, BJ & Neal, RM (1995). The wake-sleep algorithm for unsupervised neural networks. *Science*, **268**, 1158-1160.

[13] Jaakkola, T, Saul, LK & Jordan, MI (1996). Fast learning by bounding likelihoods in sigmoid type belief networks. *Advances in Neural Information Processing Systems, 8*, forthcoming.

[14] Lehky, SR (1988). An astable multivibrator model of binocular rivalry. *Perception*, **17**, 215-228.

[15] Lehky, SR & Blake, R (1991). Organization of binocular pathways: Modeling and data related to rivalry. *Neural Computation*, **3**, 44-53.

[16] Leopold, DA & Logothetis, NK (1996). Activity changes in early visual cortex reflect monkeys' percepts during binocular rivalry. *Nature*, **379**, 549-554.

[17] Levelt, WJM (1968). *On Binocular Rivalry.* The Hague, Paris: Mouton.

[18] Logothetis, NK, Leopold, DA & Sheinberg, DL (1996). What is rivalling during binocular rivalry. *Nature*, **380**, 621-624.

[19] Logothetis, NK & Schall, JD (1989). Neuronal correlates of subjective visual perception. *Science,*, **245**, 761-763.

[20] Matsuoka, K (1984). The dynamic model of binocular rivalry. *Biological Cybernetics*, **49**, 201-208.

[21] Mueller, TJ (1990). A physiological model of binocular rivalry. *Visual Neuroscience*, **4**, 63-73.

[22] Mueller, TJ & Blake, R (1989). A fresh look at the temporal dynamics of binocular rivalry. *Biological Cybernetics*, **61**, 223-232.

[23] Pearl, J (1988). *Probabilistic Reasoning in Intelligent Systems: Networks of Plausible Inference.* San Mateo, CA: Morgan Kaufmann.

[24] Wales, R & Fox, R (1970). Increment detection thresholds during binocular rivalry suppression. *Perception and Psychophysics*, **8**, 90-94.

[25] Wheatstone, C (1838). Contributions to the theory of vision. I: On some remarkable and hitherto unobserved phenomena of binocular vision. *Philosophical Transactions of the Royal Society of London*, **128**, 371-394.

[26] Wolfe, JM (1986). Stereopsis and binocular rivalry. *Psychological Review*, **93**, 269-282.

Neural network models of chemotaxis in the nematode *Caenorhabditis elegans*

Thomas C. Ferrée, Ben A. Marcotte, Shawn R. Lockery
Institute of Neuroscience, University of Oregon, Eugene, Oregon 97403

Abstract

We train recurrent networks to control chemotaxis in a computer model of the nematode *C. elegans*. The model presented is based closely on the body mechanics, behavioral analyses, neuroanatomy and neurophysiology of *C. elegans*, each imposing constraints relevant for information processing. Simulated worms moving autonomously in simulated chemical environments display a variety of chemotaxis strategies similar to those of biological worms.

1 INTRODUCTION

The nematode *C. elegans* provides a unique opportunity to study the neuronal basis of neural computation in an animal capable of complex goal-oriented behaviors. The adult hermaphrodite is only 1 mm long, and has exactly 302 neurons and 95 muscle cells. The morphology of every cell and the location of most electrical and chemical synapses are known precisely (White et al., 1986), making *C. elegans* especially attractive for study. Whole-cell recordings are now being made on identified neurons in the nerve ring of *C. elegans* to determine electrophysiological properties which underly information processing in this animal (Lockery and Goodman, unpublished). However, the strengths and polarities of synaptic connections are not known, so we use neural network optimization to find sets of synaptic strengths which reproduce actual nematode behavior in a simulated worm.

We focus on chemotaxis, the ability to move up (or down) a gradient of chemical attractants (or repellants). In the laboratory, flat Petri dishes (radius = 4.25 cm) are prepared with a Gaussian-shaped field of attractant at the center, and worms are allowed to move freely about. Worms propel themselves forward by generating an undulatory body wave, which produces sinusoidal movement. In chemotaxis, the nervous system generates motor commands which bias this movement and direct the animal toward higher attractant concentration.

Anatomical constraints pose important problems for *C. elegans* during chemotaxis. In particular, the animal detects the presence of chemicals with a pair of sensory organs (amphids) at the tip of the nose, each containing the processes of multiple chemosensory neurons. During normal locomotion, however, the animal moves on its side so that the two amphids are perpendicular to the Petri dish. *C. elegans* cannot, therefore, sense the gradient directly. One possible strategy for chemotaxis, which has been suggested previously (Ward, 1973), is that the animal computes a temporal derivative of the local concentration during a single head sweep, and combines this with some form of proprioceptive feedback indicating muscle contraction and the direction of head sweep, to compute the spatial gradient for chemotaxis. The existence of this and other strategies is discussed later.

In Section 2, we derive a simple model of the nematode body which produces realistic sinusoidal trajectories in response to motor commands from the nervous system. In Section 3, we give a simple model of the *C. elegans* nervous system based on preliminary physiological data. In Section 4, we use a stochastic optimization algorithm to determine sets of synaptic weights which control chemotaxis, and discuss solutions.

2 BIOMECHANICS OF NEMATODE ORIENTATION

Nematode locomotion has been studied in detail (Niebur and Erdös, 1991; Niebur and Erdös, 1993). These authors derived Newtonian force equations for each muscular segment of the body, which can be solved numerically to generate forward sinusoidal movement. Unfortunately, such a thorough treatment is computationally intensive and not practical to use with network optimization. To simplify the problem we first recognize that chemotaxis is a behavior more of orientation than of locomotion. We therefore derive a set of biomechanical equations which direct the head to generate sinusoidal movement, which can be biased by the network toward higher chemical concentrations.

We focus our attention on the point (x, y) at the tip of the nose, since that is where the animal senses the chemical environment. As shown in Figure 1(a), we assign a velocity vector $\vec{v}$ directed along the midline of the first body segment, *i.e.*, the head. Assuming that the worm moves forward at constant speed v, we can write the velocity vector as

$$\vec{v}(t) \equiv \left(\frac{dx}{dt}, \frac{dy}{dt}\right) = \Big(v\cos\theta(t), v\sin\theta(t)\Big) \tag{1}$$

where x, y and θ are measured relative to fixed coordinates in the Petri dish. Assuming that the worm moves without lateral slipping and that the undulatory wave of muscular contraction initiated in the neck travels posteriorally without modification, then each body segment simply follows the one previous (anterior) to it. In this way, the head directs the movement and the rest of the body simply follows.

Figure 1(b) shows an expanded view of the neck segment. As the worm moves forward, the posterior boundary of that segment assumes the position held by its anterior neighbor at a slightly earlier time. If L is the total body length and N is the number of body segments, then this time delay is $\delta t \simeq L/Nv$. (For $L = 1$ mm, $v = 0.22$ mm/s and $N = 10$ we have $\delta t \simeq 0.45$ s, roughly an order of magnitude smaller than the relevant behavioral time scale: the head-sweep period $T \simeq 4.2$ s.) If we define the neck angle $\alpha(t) \equiv \theta_1(t) - \theta_2(t)$, then the above arguments imply

$$\alpha(t) = \theta_1(t) - \theta_1(t - \delta t) \simeq \frac{d\theta_1}{dt} \delta t \qquad (2)$$

where the second relation is essentially a backward-Euler algorithm for $d\theta_1/dt$. Since $\theta \equiv \theta_1$, we have reached the intuitive result that the neck angle α determines the rate of turning $d\theta/dt$. Note that while θ_1 and θ_2 are defined relative to the fixed laboratory coordinates, their difference α is invariant under rotations of these coordinates, and can therefore be viewed as intrinsic to the body. This allows us to derive an expression for α in terms of muscle cell contraction, or motor neuron depolarization, as follows.

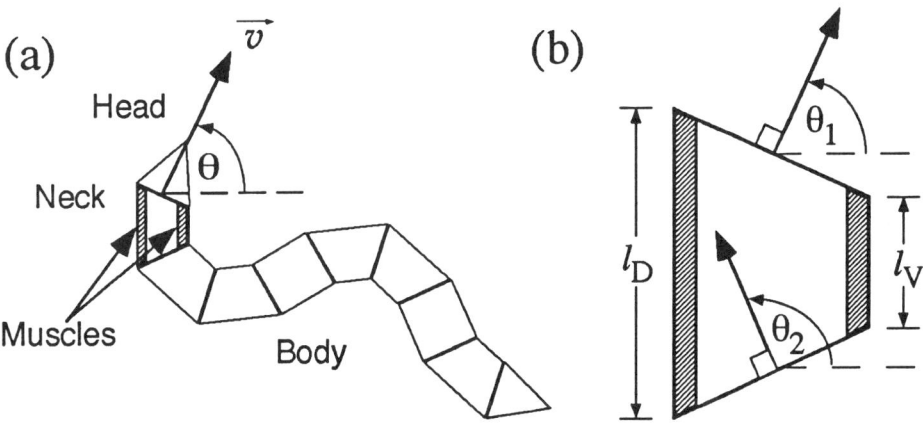

Figure 1: Nematode body mechanics. (a) Segmented model of the nematode body, showing the direction of motion $\vec{v}$. (b) Expanded view of the neck segment, showing dorsal (D) and ventral (V) neck muscles.

Nematodes maintain nearly constant volume during movement. To incorporate this constraint, albeit approximately, we assume that at all times the geometry of each segment is such that $(l_D - l_0) = -(l_V - l_0)$, where $l_0 \equiv L/N$ is the equilibrium length of a relaxed segment. For small angles α, we have $\alpha \simeq (l_V - l_D)/d$, where d is the body diameter. The dashed lines in Figure 1(b) indicate dorsal and ventral muscles, which are believed to develop tension nearly independent of length (Toida et al., 1975). When contracting, these muscles must work against the elasticity of the cuticle, internal fluid pressure, and elasticity and developed tension of the opposing muscles. If these elastic forces act linearly, then $T_D - T_V \simeq k (l_V - l_D)$, where T_D and T_V are dorsal and ventral muscle tensions, and k is an effective force constant. For simplicity, we further assume that each muscle develops tension linearly in response to the voltage of its corresponding motor neuron, i.e., $T_{D,V} = \epsilon V_{D,V}$, where ϵ is a positive constant, and V_D and V_V are dorsal and ventral motor neuron voltages.

Combining these results, we have finally

$$\frac{d\theta}{dt} = \gamma \left(V_D(t) - V_V(t) \right) \qquad (3)$$

where $\gamma = (Nv/L) \cdot (\epsilon/kd)$. With appropriate motor commands, equations (1) and (3) can be integrated numerically to generate sinusoidal worm trajectories like those of biological worms. This model embodies the main anatomical features that are likely to be important in *C. elegans* chemotaxis, yet is sufficiently compact to be embedded in a network optimization procedure.

3 CHEMOTAXIS CONTROL CIRCUIT

C. elegans neurons are tiny and have very simple morpologies: a typical neuron in the head has a spherical soma 1–2 μm in diameter, and a single cylindrical process 60–80 μm in length and 0.1–0.2 μm in diameter. Compartmental models, based on this morphology and preliminary physiological recordings, indicate that *C. elegans* neurons are effectively isopotential (Lockery, 1995). Furthermore, *C. elegans* neurons do not fire classical all-or-none action potentials, but appear to rely primarily on graded signal propagation (Lockery and Goodman, unpublished). Thus, a reasonable starting point for a network model is to represent each neuron by a single isopotential compartment, in which voltage is the state variable, and the membrane conductance in purely ohmic.

Anatomical data indicate that the *C. elegans* nervous system has both electrical and chemical synapses, but the synaptic transfer functions are not known. However, steady-state synaptic transfer functions for chemical synapses have been measured in *Ascaris suum*, a related species of nematode, where it was found that postsynaptic voltage is a graded function of presynaptic voltage, due to tonic neurotransmitter release (Davis and Stretton, 1989). This voltage dependence is sigmoidal, *i.e.*, $V_{\text{post}} \sim \tanh(V_{\text{pre}})$. A simple network model which captures all of these features is

$$\tau \frac{dV_i}{dt} = -V_i + V_{\max} \tanh\left(\beta \sum_{j=1}^{n} w_{ij} (V_j - \bar{V}_j)\right) + V_i^{\text{stim}}(t) \qquad (4)$$

where V_i is the voltage of the ith neuron. Here all voltages are measured relative to a common resting potential, $V_{\max}$ is an arbitrary voltage scale which sets the operational range of the neurons, and β sets the voltage sensitivity of the synaptic transfer function. The weight w_{ij} represents the net strength and polarity of all synaptic connections from neuron j to neuron i, and the constants $\bar{V}_j$ determine the center of each transfer function. The membane time constant τ is assumed to be the same for all cells, and will be discussed further later. Note that in (4), synaptic transmission occurs instantaneously: the time constant τ arises from capacitive current through the cell membrane, and is unrelated to synaptic transmission. Note also that the way in which (4) sums multiple inputs is not unique, *i.e.*, other sigmoidal models which sum inputs differently are equally plausible, since no data on synaptic summation exists for either *C. elegans* or *Ascaris suum*.

The stimulus term $V_i^{\text{stim}}(t)$ is used to introduce chemosensation and sinusoidal locomotion to the network in (4). We use $i = 1$ to label a single chemosensory neuron at the tip of the nose, and $i = n - 1 \equiv D$ and $i = n \equiv V$ to label dorsal and ventral motor neurons. For simplicity we assume that the chemosensory neuron voltage responds linearly to the local chemical concentration:

$$V_1^{\text{stim}}(t) = V_{\text{chem}}\, C(x, y) \qquad (5)$$

where V_{chem} is a positive constant, and the local concentration $C(x,y)$ is always evaluated at the instantaneous nose position.

In the previous section, we emphasized that locomotion is effectively independent of orientation. We therefore assume the existence of a central pattern generator (CPG) which is *outside* the chemotaxis control circuit (4). Thus, in addition to synaptic input from other neurons, each motor neuron receives a sinusoidal stimulus

$$V_{\text{D}}^{\text{stim}}(t) = -V_{\text{V}}^{\text{stim}}(t) = V_{\text{CPG}} \sin(\omega t) \tag{6}$$

where V_{CPG} and $\omega \equiv 2\pi/T$ are positive constants.

4 RESULTS AND DISCUSSION

Equations (1), (3) and (4), together with (5) and (6), comprise a set of $n+3$ first-order nonlinear differential equations, which can be solved numerically given initial conditions and a specification of the chemical environment. We use a fourth-order Runge-Kutta algorithm and find favorable stability and convergence. The necessary body parameters have been measured by observing actual worms (Pierce and Lockery, unpublished): $v = 0.022$ cm/s, $T = 4.2$ s and $\gamma = 0.8/(2V_{\text{CPG}})$. The chemical environment is also chosen to agree roughly with experimental values: $C(x,y) = C_0 \exp(-(x^2+y^2)/\lambda_C^2)$, with $C_0 = 0.052$ μmol/cm^3 and $\lambda_C = 2.3$ cm.

To optimize networks to control chemotaxis, we use a simple simulated annealing algorithm which searches over the (n^2+3)-dimensional space of parameters w_{ij}, β, V_{chem} and V_{CPG}. In the results shown here, we used $n = 12$, and set $\bar{V}_j = 0$. Each set of the resulting parameters represents a different nervous system for the model worm. At the beginning of each run, the worm is initialized by choosing an initial position (x_0, y_0), an initial angle θ_0, and by setting $V_i = 0$. Upon numerically integrating, simulated worms move autonomously in their environment for a predetermined amount of time, typically the real-time equivalent of 10-15 minutes. We quantify the performance, or fitness, of each worm during chemotaxis by computing the average chemical concentration at the tip of its nose over the duration of each run. To avoid lucky scores, the actual score for each worm is obtained by averaging over several initial conditions.

In Figure 2, we show a comparison of tracks produced by (a) biological and (b) simulated worms during chemotaxis. In each case, three worms were placed in a dish with a radial gradient and allowed to move freely for the real-time equivalent of 15 minutes. In (b), the three worms have the same neural parameters (w_{ij}, β, V_{chem}, V_{CPG}), but different initial angles θ_0. In both (a) and (b), all three worms make initial movements, then move toward the center of the dish and remain there. In other optimizations, rather than orbit the center, the simulated worms may approach the center asymptotically from one side, make simple geometric patterns which pass through the center, or exhibit a variety of other distinct strategies for chemotaxis. This is similar to the situation with biological worms, which also have considerable variation in the details of their tracks.

The behavior shown in Figure 2 was produced using $\tau = 500$ ms. However, preliminary electrophysiological recordings from *C. elegans* neurons suggest that the actual value may be as much as an order of magnitude smaller, but not bigger (Lockery and Goodman, unpublished). This presents a potential problem for chemotaxis computation, since shorter time constants require greater sensitivity to small changes in $C(x,y)$ in order to compute a temporal derivative, which is believed to be required. During optimization, we have seen that for a fixed number of neurons n, finding optimal solutions becomes more difficult as τ is decreased. This observation is very difficult to quantify, however, due to the existence of local maxima in the fitness function. Nevertheless, this suggests that additional mechanisms may need to be included to understand neural computation in *C. elegans*. First, time- and voltage-dependent conductances will modify the effective membrane time constant, and may increase the effective time scale for computation by individual neurons. Second, more neurons and synaptic delays will also move the effective neuronal time scale closer to that of the behavior. Either of these will allow comparisons of $C(x,y)$ across greater distances, thereby requiring less sensitivity to compute the gradient, and potentially improving the ability of these networks to control chemotaxis.

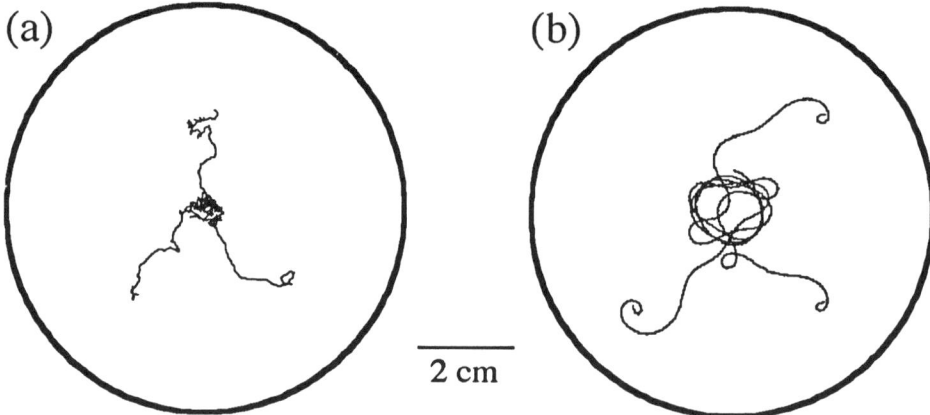

Figure 2: Nematodes performing chemotaxis: (a) biological (Pierce and Lockery, unpublished), and (b) simulated.

We also note, based on a variety of other results, not shown here, that the head-sweep strategy, described in the introduction, is by no means the only strategy for chemotaxis in this system. In particular, we have optimized networks without a CPG, *i.e.*, with $V_{\text{CPG}} = 0$ in (6), and found parameter sets that successfully control chemotaxis. This presents the possibility that even worms with a CPG do not necessarily compute the gradient based on lateral movement of the head, but may instead respond only to changes in concentration along their mean trajectory. Similar results have been reported previously, although based on a somewhat different biomechanical model (Beer and Gallagher, 1992).

Finally, we have also optimized discrete-time networks, obtained by setting $\tau = 0$ in (4) and updating all units synchronously. As is well-known, on relatively short time scales ($\sim T$) such a system tends to "overshoot" at each successive time step, leading to sporadic behavior of the network and the body. Knowing this, it is interesting that simulated worms with such a nervous system are capable of reliable behavior over longer time scales, *i.e.*, they successfully perform chemotaxis.

5 CONCLUSIONS AND FUTURE WORK

The main result of this paper is that a small nervous system, based on graded-potential neurons, is capable of controlling chemotaxis in a worm-like physical body with the dimensions of *C. elegans*. The model presented is based closely on the body mechanics, behavioral analyses, neuroanatomy and neurophysiology of *C. elegans*, and is a reliable starting point for more realistic models to follow. Furthermore, we have established the existence of chemotaxis strategies that had not been anticipated based on behavioral experiments with real worms.

Future work will involve both improvement of the model and analysis of the resulting solutions. Improvements will include introducing voltage- and time-dependent membrane conductances, as this data becomes available, and more realistic models of synaptic transmission. Also, laser ablation experiments have been performed that suggest which interneurons and motor neurons in *C. elegans* may be important for chemotaxis (Bargmann, unpublished), and these data can be used to constrain the synaptic connections during optimization. Analyses will be aimed at determining the role of individual physiological and anatomical features, and how they function together to govern the collective properties of the network as a whole during chemotaxis.

Acknowledgements

The authors would like to thank Miriam Goodman and Jon Pierce for helpful discussions. This work has been supported by NIMH MH11373, NIMH MH51383, NSF IBN 9458102, ONR N00014-94-1-0642, the Sloan Foundation, and The Searle Scholars Program.

References

Beer, R. D. and J. C. Gallagher (1992). Evolving dynamical neural networks for adaptive behavior, *Adaptive Behavior* 1(1):91-122.

Davis, R. E. and A. O. W. Stretton (1989). Signaling properties of *Ascaris* motorneurons: Graded active responses, graded synaptic transmission, and tonic transmitter release, *J. Neurosci.* 9:415-425.

Lockery, S. R. (1995). Signal propagation in the nerve ring of *C. elegans*, *Soc. Neurosci. Abstr.* 569.7:1454.

Niebur, E. and P. Erdös (1991). Theory of the locomotion of nematodes: Dynamics of undulatory progression on a surface, *Biophys. J.* 60:1132-1146.

Niebur, E. and P. Erdös (1993). Theory of the locomotion of nematodes: Control of the somatic motor neurons by interneurons, *Math. Biosci.* 118:51-82.

Toida, N., H. Kuriyama, N. Tashiro and Y. Ito (1975). Obliquely striated muscle, *Physiol. Rev.* 55:700-756.

Ward, S. (1973). Chemotaxis by the nematode *Caenorhabditis elegans*: Identification of attractants and analysis of the response by use of mutants, *Proc. Nat. Acad. Sci. USA* 70:817-821.

White, J. G., E. Southgate, J. N. Thompson and S. Brenner (1986). The structure of the nervous system of *C. elegans*, *Phil. Trans. R. Soc. London* 314:1-340.

Extraction of temporal features in the electrosensory system of weakly electric fish

Fabrizio Gabbiani*
Division of Biology
139-74 Caltech
Pasadena, CA 91125

Walter Metzner
Department of Biology
Univ. of Cal. Riverside
Riverside, CA 92521-0427

Ralf Wessel
Department of Biology
Univ. of Cal. San Diego
La Jolla, CA 92093-0357

Christof Koch
Division of Biology
139-74 Caltech
Pasadena, CA 91125

Abstract

The encoding of random time-varying stimuli in single spike trains of electrosensory neurons in the weakly electric fish *Eigenmannia* was investigated using methods of statistical signal processing. At the first stage of the electrosensory system, spike trains were found to encode faithfully the detailed time-course of random stimuli, while at the second stage neurons responded specifically to features in the temporal waveform of the stimulus. Therefore stimulus information is processed at the second stage of the electrosensory system by extracting temporal features from the faithfully preserved image of the environment sampled at the first stage.

1 INTRODUCTION

The weakly electric fish, *Eigenmannia*, generates a quasi sinusoidal, dipole-like electric field at individually fixed frequencies (250 − 600 Hz) by discharging an electric organ located in its tail (see Bullock and Heilgenberg, 1986 for reviews). The fish sense local changes in the electric field by means of two types of tuberous electroreceptors located on the body surface. T-type electroreceptors fire phase-locked to the zero-crossing of the electric field once per cycle of the electric organ discharge

---

*email: gabbiani@klab.caltech.edu, wmetzner@mail.ucr.edu, rwessel@jeeves.ucsd.edu, koch@klab.caltech.edu.

(EOD) and are thus able to encode phase changes. P-type electroreceptors fire in a more loosely phase-locked manner with a probability smaller than 1 per EOD. Their probability of firing increases with the mean amplitude of the field thereby allowing them to encode amplitude changes (Zakon, 1986).

This information is used by the fish in order to locate objects (electrolocation, Bastian 1986) as well as for communication with conspecifics (Hopkins, 1988). One behavior which has been most thoroughly studied (Heiligenberg, 1991), the jamming avoidance response, occurs when two fish with similar EOD frequency (less than 15 Hz difference) approach close enough to sense each other's field. In order to minimize beat patterns resulting from their summed electric fields, the fish with the higher (resp. lower) EOD raises further (resp. lowers) its own EOD frequency. The resulting frequency difference increase reduces the distortions in the interfering EODs. The fish is known to correlate phase differences computed across body regions with local amplitude increases or decreases in order to determine whether it should raise or lower its own EOD.

At the level of the first central nervous nucleus of the electrosensory pathway, the electrosensory lateral line lobe of the hindbrain (ELL), phase and amplitude information are processed nearly independently of each other (Maler et al., 1981). Amplitude information is encoded in the spike trains of ELL pyramidal cells that receive input from P-receptor afferents and transmit their information to higher order levels of the electrosensory system. Two functional classes of pyramidal cells are distinguished: E-type pyramidal cells respond by raising their firing frequency to increases in the amplitude of an externally applied electric field while I-type pyramidal cells increase their firing frequency when the amplitude decreases (Bastian, 1981).

The aim of this study was to characterize the temporal information processing performed by ELL pyramidal cells on random electric field amplitude modulations and to relate it to the information carried by P-receptor afferents. To this end we recorded the responses of P-receptor afferents and pyramidal cells to random electric field amplitude modulations and analyzed them using two different methods: a signal estimation method characterizing to what extent the neuronal response encodes the detailed time-course of the stimulus and a signal-detection method developed to identify features encoded in spike trains. These two methods as well as the electrophysiology are explained in the next section followed by the result section and a short discussion.

2 METHODS

2.1 ELECTROPHYSIOLOGY

Adult specimens of *Eigenmannia* were immobilized by intramuscular injection of a curare-like drug (Flaxedil). This also strongly attenuated the fish's EODs. The fish were held in place by a foam-lined clamp in an experimental tank and an EOD substitute electric field was established by two electrodes placed in the mouth and near the tail of the fish. The carrier frequency of the electric field, $f_{carrier}$, was chosen equal to the EOD frequency prior to curarization and the voltage generating the stimulus was modulated according to

$$V(t) = A_0(1 + s(t))\cos(2\pi f_{carrier}),$$

where A_0 is the mean amplitude and $s(t)$ is a random, zero-mean modulation having a flat (white) spectrum up to a variable cut-off frequency f_c and a variable standard deviation σ. The modulation $s(t)$ was generated by playing a blank tape on a tape

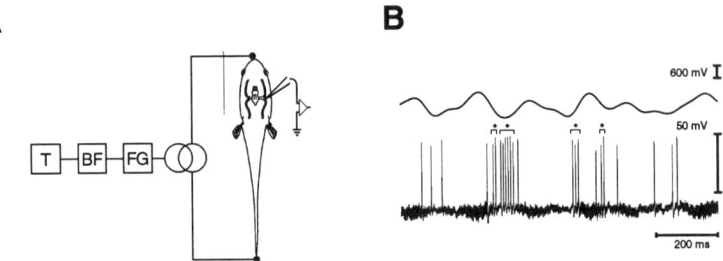

Figure 1: A. Schematic drawing of the experimental set-up. Tape recorder (T), variable cutoff frequency Bessel filter (BF) and function generator (FG). B. Sample amplitude modulation $s(t)$ and intracellular recording from a pyramidal cell (I-type, $f_c = 12$ Hz). Spikes occurring in bursts are marked with an asterisk (see sect. 2.3.2). The intracellular voltage trace reveals a high frequency noise caused by the EOD substitute signal and a high electrode resistance.

recorder, passing the signal through a variable cut-off frequency low-pass filter before multiplying it by the frequency carrier signal in a function generator (fig. 1A).

Extracellular recordings from P-receptor afferents were made by exposing the anterior lateral line nerve. Intracellular recordings from ELL pyramidal cells were obtained by positioning electrodes in the central region of the pyramidal cell layer. Intracellular recording electrodes were filled with neurotracer (neurobiotin) to be used for subsequent intracellular labeling if the recordings were stable long enough. This allowed to verify the cell type and its location within the ELL. In case no intracellular labeling could be made the recording site was verified by setting electrolytic lesions at the conclusion of the experiment. In the subsequent data analysis, data from E- and I-type pyramidal cells and from two different maps (centromedial and lateral, Carr et al., 1982) were pooled. For further experimental details, see Wessel et al. (1996), Metzner and Heiligenberg (1991), Metzner (1993).

2.2 SIGNAL ESTIMATION

The ability of single spike trains to carry detailed time-varying stimulus information was assessed by estimating the stimulus from the spike train. The spike trains, $x(t) = \sum \delta(t - t_i)$, where t_i are the spike occurrence times, were convolved with a filter h (Wiener-Kolmogorov filtering; Poor, 1994; Bialek et al. 1991),

$$s_{est}(t) = \int dt_1 \, h(t_1) x(t - t_1)$$

chosen in order to minimize the mean square error between the true stimulus and the estimated stimulus,

$$\epsilon^2 = \langle (s(t) - s_{est}(t))^2 \rangle.$$

The optimal filter $h(t)$ is determined in Fourier space as the ratio of the Fourier transform of the cross-correlation between stimulus and spike train, $R_{xs}(\tau) = \langle x(t)s(t+\tau) \rangle$ and the Fourier transform of the autocorrelation (power spectrum) of the spike train, $R_{xx}(\tau) = \langle x(t)x(t+\tau) \rangle$. The accuracy at which single spike trains transmit information about the stimulus was characterized in the time domain by the coding fraction, defined as $\gamma = 1 - \epsilon/\sigma$, were σ is the standard deviation of the stimulus. The coding fraction is normalized between 1 when the stimulus is perfectly estimated by the spike train ($\epsilon = 0$) and 0, when the estimation performance of the spike train is at chance level ($\epsilon = \sigma$). Thus, the coding fraction can be compared across experiments. For further details and references on this stimulus estimation method in the context of neuronal sensory processing, see Gabbiani and Koch (1996) and Gabbiani (1996).

2.3 FEATURE EXTRACTION

2.3.1 General procedure

The ability of single spikes to encode the presence of a temporal feature in the stimulus waveform was assessed by adapting a Fisher linear discriminant classification scheme to our data (Anderson, 1984; sect. 6.5). Each random stimulus wave-form and spike response of pyramidal cells (resp. P-receptor afferents) were binned. The bin size Δ was varied between $\Delta_{min} = 0.5$ ms, corresponding to the sampling ratio and Δ_{max}, corresponding to the longest interval leading to a maximum of one spike per bin. The sampling interval yielding the best performance (see below) was finally retained. Typical bin sizes were $\Delta = 7$ ms for pyramidal cells (typical mean firing rate: 30 Hz) and $\Delta = 1$ ms for P-receptor afferents (typical firing rate: 200 Hz). The mean stimulus preceding a spike containing bin ($\mathbf{m_1}$) or no-spike containing bin ($\mathbf{m_0}$) as well as the covariances ($\mathbf{\Sigma_1}, \mathbf{\Sigma_0}$) of these distributions were computed (Anderson, 1984; sect. 3.2). Mean vectors (resp. covariance matrices) had at most 100 (resp. 100 × 100) components. The optimal linear feature vector $\mathbf{f}$ predicting the occurrence or non-occurrence of a spike was found by maximizing the signal-to-noise ratio (see fig. 2A and Poor, 1994; sect. IIIB)

$$\text{SNR}(\mathbf{f}) = \frac{[\mathbf{f} \cdot (\mathbf{m_1} - \mathbf{m_0})]^2}{\mathbf{f} \cdot \frac{1}{2}(\mathbf{\Sigma_0} + \mathbf{\Sigma_1})\mathbf{f}}. \quad (1)$$

The vector $\mathbf{f}$ is solution of $(\mathbf{m_1} - \mathbf{m_0}) = (\mathbf{\Sigma_0} + \mathbf{\Sigma_1})\mathbf{f}$. This equation was solved by diagonalizing $\mathbf{\Sigma_0} + \mathbf{\Sigma_1}$ and retaining the first n largest eigenvalues accounting for 99% of the variance (Jolliffe, 1986; sect. 6.1 and 8.1). The optimal feature vector $\mathbf{f}$ thus obtained corresponded to up- or downstrokes in the stimulus amplitude modulation for E- and I-type pyramidal cells respectively, as expected from their mean response properties to changes in the electric field amplitude (see sect. 1). Similarly, optimal feature vectors for P-receptor afferents corresponded to upstrokes in the electric field amplitude (see sect. 1).

Once $\mathbf{f}$ was determined, we projected the stimuli preceding a spike or no spike onto the optimal feature vector (fig. 2A) and computed the probability of correct classification between the two distributions so obtained by the resubstitution method (Raudys and Jain, 1991). The probability of correct classification (P_{CC}) is obtained by optimizing the value of the threshold used to separate the two distributions in order to maximize

$$P_{CC} = \frac{1}{2}(1 - P_{FA}) + \frac{1}{2}P_{CD}, \quad (2)$$

where the probabilities of false alarm (P_{FA}) and correct detection (P_{CD}) depend on the threshold.

2.3.2 Distinction between isolated spikes and burst-like spike patterns

A large fraction (56% ± 21%, $n = 30$) of spikes generated by pyramidal cells in response to random electric field amplitude modulations occurred in bursts (mean burst length: 18 ± 9 ms, mean number of spikes per burst: 2.9 ± 1.3, n = 30, fig. 1B). In order to verify whether spikes occurring in bursts corresponded to a more reliable encoding of the feature vector, we separated the distribution of stimuli occurring before a spike in two distributions, conditioned on whether the

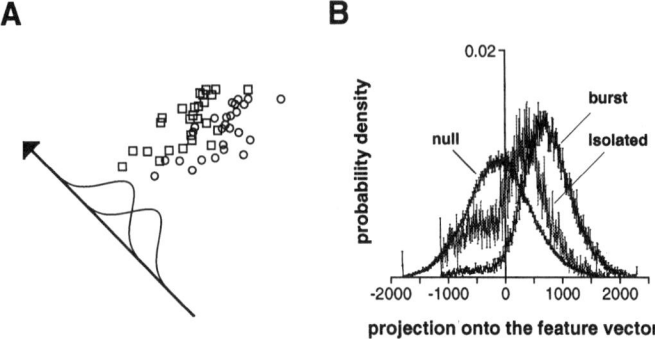

Figure 2: A. 2-dimensional example of two random distributions (circles and squares) as well as the optimal discrimination direction determined by maximizing the signal-to-noise ratio of eq. 1. The 1-dimensional projection of the two distributions onto the optimal direction is also shown (compare with B). B. Example of the distribution of stimuli projected onto the optimal feature vector (same cell as in fig. 1B). Stimuli preceding a bin containing no spike (null), an isolated spike (isolated) and a spike belonging to a burst (burst). Horizontal scale is arbitrary (see eq. 1).

spike belonged to a burst or not. The stimuli were then projected onto the feature vector (fig. 2B), as described in 2.3.1, and the probability of correct classification between the distribution of stimuli occurring before no spike and isolated spike bins was compared to the probability of correct classification between the distribution of stimuli occurring before no spike and burst spike bins (see sect. 3).

3 RESULTS

The results are summarized in fig. 3. Data were analyzed from 30 pyramidal cells (E- and I-type) and 20 P-receptor afferents for a range of stimulus parameters ($f_c = 2 - 40$ Hz, $\sigma = 0.1 - 0.4$, A_0 was varied in order to obtain ± 20 dB changes around the physiological value of the mean electric field amplitude which is of the order of 1 mV/cm). Fig. 3A reports the best probability of correct classification (eq. 2) obtained for each pyramidal cell (white squares) / P-receptor afferent (black dots) as a function of the coding fraction observed in the same experiment (note that for pyramidal cells only burst spikes are shown, see sect. 2.3.2 and fig. 3B). The horizontal axis shows that while the coding fraction of P-receptors afferents can be very high (up to 75% of the detailed stimulus time-course is encoded in a single spike train), pyramidal cells only poorly transmit information on the detailed time-course of the stimulus (less than 20% in most cases). In contrast, the vertical axis shows that pyramidal cells outperform P-receptor afferent in the classification task: it is possible to classify with up to 85% accuracy whether a given stimulus will cause a short burst of spikes or not by comparing it to a single feature vector **f**. This indicates that the presence of an up- or downstroke (the feature vector) is reliably encoded by pyramidal cells. Fig. 3B shows for each experiment on the ordinate the discrimination performance (eq. 2) for stimuli preceding isolated spikes against stimuli preceding no spike. The abscissa plots the discrimination performance (eq. 2) for stimuli preceding spikes occurring in bursts (white squares, fig. 3A) or stimuli preceding all spikes (black squares) against stimuli preceding

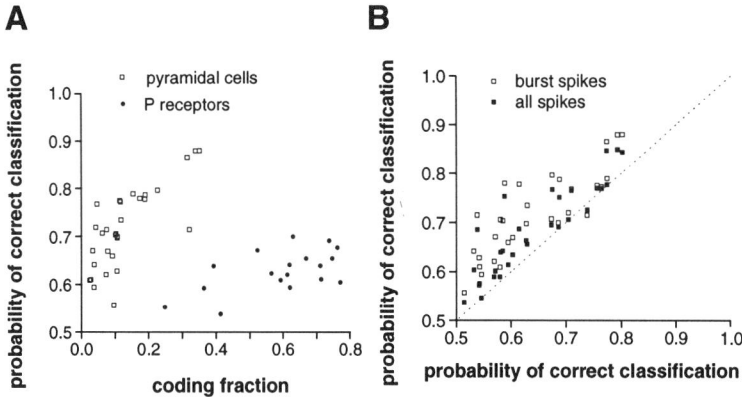

Figure 3: A. Coding fraction and probability of correct classification for pyramidal cells (white squares, burst spikes only) and P-receptor afferents (black circles). B. Probability of correct classification against stimuli preceding no spikes for stimuli preceding burst spikes or all spikes vs. stimuli preceding isolated spikes. Dashed line: identical performance.

no spike. The distribution of stimuli occurring before burst spikes (all spikes) is more easily distinguished from the distribution of stimuli occurring before no spike than the distribution of stimuli preceding isolated spikes. This clearly indicates that spikes occurring in bursts carry more reliable information than isolated spikes.

4 DISCUSSION

We have analyzed the response of P-receptor afferents and pyramidal cells to random electric field amplitude modulations using methods of statistical signal processing. The previously studied mean responses of P-receptor afferents and pyramidal cells to step amplitude changes or sinusoidal modulations of an externally applied electric field left several alternatives open for the encoding and processing of stimulus information in single spike trains. We find that, while P-receptor afferents encode reliably the detailed time-course of the stimulus, pyramidal cells do not. In contrast, pyramidal cells perform better than P-receptor afferents in discriminating the occurrence of up- and downstrokes in the amplitude modulation. The presence of these features is signaled most reliably to higher order stations in the electrosensory system by short bursts of spikes emitted by pyramidal cells in response to the stimulus. This code can be expected to be robust against possible subsequent noise sources, such as synaptic unreliability. The temporal pattern recognition task solved at the level of the ELL is particularly appropriate for computations which have to rely on the temporal resolution of up- and downstrokes, such as those underlying the jamming avoidance response.

Acknowledgments

We thank Jenifer Juranek for computer assistance. Support: UCR and NSF grants, Center of Neuromorphic Systems Engineering as a part of the NSF ERC Program, and California Trade and Commerce Agency, Office of Strategic Technology.

References

Anderson, T.W. (1984) An introduction to Multivariate Statistical Analysis. Wiley, New York.

Bastian, J. (1981) Electrolocation 2. The effects of moving objects and other electrical stimuli on the activities of two categories of posterior lateral line lobe cells in apteronotus albifrons. *J. Comp. Physiol. A*, **144**: 481-494.

Bialek, W., de Ruyter van Steveninck, R.R. & Warland, D. (1991) Reading a neural code. *Science*, **252**: 1854-1857.

Bullock, T.H. & Heiligengerg, W. (1986) Electroreception. Wiley, New York.

Carr, C.C., Maler, L. & Sas, E. (1982). Peripheral Organization and Central Projections of the Electrosensory Nerves in Gymnotiform Fish. *J. Comp. Neurol.*, **211**:139-153.

Gabbiani, F. & Koch, C. (1996) Coding of Time-Varying Signals in Spike Trains of Integrate-and-Fire Neurons with Random Threshold. *Neur. Comput.*, **8**: 44-66.

Gabbiani, F. (1996) Coding of time-varying signals in spike trains of linear and half-wave rectifying neurons. *Network: Comp. Neur. Syst.*, **7**:61-85.

Heiligenberg, W. (1991) Neural Nets in electric fish. MIT Press, Cambridge, MA.

Hopkins, C.D. (1976) Neuroethology of electric communication. *Ann. Rev. Neurosci.*, **11**:497-535.

Jolliffe, I.T. (1986) Principal Component Analysis. Springer-Verlag, New York.

Maler, L., Sas, E.K.B. & Rogers, J. (1981) The cytology of the posterior lateral line lobe of high-frequency weakly electric fish (gymnotidae): Dendritic differentiation and synaptic specificity. *J. Comp. Neurol.*, **255**: 526-537.

Metzner, W. (1993) The jamming avoidance response in Eigenmannia is controlled by two separate motor pathways. *J. Neurosci.*, **13**:1862-1878.

Metzner, W. & Heiligenberg, W. (1991). The coding of signals in the electric communication of the gymnotiform fish Eigenmannia: From electroreceptors to neurons in the torus semicircularis of the midbrain. *J. Comp. Physiol. A*, **169**: 135-150.

Poor, H.V. (1994) An introduction to Signal Detection and Estimation. Springer Verlag, New York.

Raudys, S.J. & Jain, A.K. (1991) Small sample size effects in statistical pattern recognition: Recommendations for practitioners. *IEEE Trans. Patt. Anal. Mach. Intell.*, **13**: 252-264.

Wessel, R., Koch, C. & Gabbiani F. (1996) Coding of Time-Varying Electric Field Amplitude Modulations in a Wave-Type Electric Fish *J. Neurophysiol.* **75**:2280-2293.

Zakon, H. (1986) The electroreceptive periphery. In: Bullock, T.H. & Heiligenberg, W. (eds), Electroreception, pp. 103-156. Wiley, New York.

A neural model of visual contour integration

Zhaoping Li
Computer Science, Hong Kong University of Science and Technology
Clear Water Bay, Hong Kong
zhaoping@uxmail.ust.hk[1]

Abstract

We introduce a neurobiologically plausible model of contour integration from visual inputs of individual oriented edges. The model is composed of interacting excitatory neurons and inhibitory interneurons, receives visual inputs via oriented receptive fields (RFs) like those in V1. The RF centers are distributed in space. At each location, a finite number of cells tuned to orientations spanning 180° compose a model hypercolumn. Cortical interactions modify neural activities produced by visual inputs, selectively amplifying activities for edge elements belonging to smooth input contours. Elements within one contour produce synchronized neural activities. We show analytically and empirically that contour enhancement and neural synchrony increase with contour length, smoothness and closure, as observed experimentally. This model gives testable predictions, and in addition, introduces a feedback mechanism allowing higher visual centers to enhance, suppress, and segment contours.

1. Introduction

The visual system must group local elements in its input into meaningful global features to infer the visual objects in the scene. Sometimes local features group into regions, as in texture segmentation; at other times they group into contours which may represent object boundaries. Although much is known about the processing steps that extract local features such as oriented input edges, it is still unclear how local features are grouped into global ones more meaningful for objects. In this

---

[1] I would very much like to thank Jochen Braun for introducing me to the topic, and Peter Dayan for many helpful conversations and comments on the drafts. This work was supported by the Hong Kong Research Grant Council.

study, we model the neural mechanisms underlying the grouping of edge elements into contours — contour integration.

Recent psychophysical and physiological observations[14, 8] demonstrate a decrease in detection threshold of an edge element, by human observers or a primary cortical cell, if there are aligned neighboring edge elements. Changes in neural responses by visual stimuli presented outside their RFs have been observed physiologically[9, 8]. Human observers easily identify a smooth curve composed of individual, even disconnected, Gabor "edge" elements distributed among many similar elements scattered in the background[4]. Horizontal neural connections observed in the primary visual cortex[5], and the finding that these connections preferably link cells tuned to similar orienations[5], provide a likely neural basis underlying the primitive visual grouping phenomena such as contour integration. These findings suggest that simple and local neural interactions even in V1 could contribute to grouping.

However, it has been difficult to model contour integration using only V1 elements and operation. Most existing models[15, 18] of contour integration lack well-founded biological bases. More neurally based models, e.g., the one by Grossberg and Mingolla[7], require operations beyond V1 or biologically questionable. It is thus desirable to find out whether contour enhancement can indeed occur within V1 or has to be attributed to top-down feedback. We introduce a V1 model of contour integration, using orientation selective cells, local cortical circuits, and horizontal connections. This model captures the essentials of the contour integration behavior. More details of the model can be found in a longer paper[12].

2. The Model

2.1 Model outline

K neuron pairs at each spatial location i model a hypercolumn in V1 (figure 1). Each neuron has a receptive field center i and an optimal orientation $\theta = k\pi/K$ for $k = 1, 2, ...K$. A neuron pair consist of a connected excitatory neuron and inhibitory neuron which are denoted by indice $(i\theta)$ for their receptive field center and preferred orientation, and are referred to as an edge segment. An edge segment receives the visual input via the excitatory cell, whose output quantifies the saliency of the edge segment and projects to higher visual centers. The inhibitory cells are treated as interneurons. When an input image contains an edge at i oriented at θ_o, the edge segment $i\theta$ receives input $I_{i\theta} \propto \phi(\theta - \theta_o)$, where $\phi(\theta) = e^{-|\theta|/(\pi/8)}$ is a cell's orientation tuning curve.

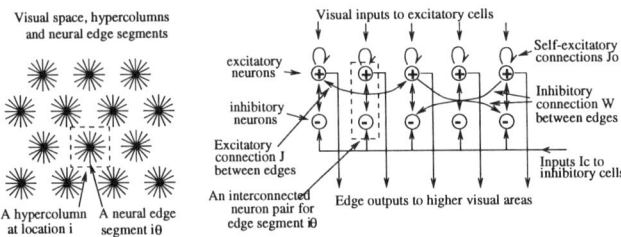

Figure 1: Model visual space, hypercolumn, edge segments, neural elements, visual inputs, and neural connections. The input space is a discrete hexagonal or Manhatten grid.

A Neural Model of Visual Contour Integration

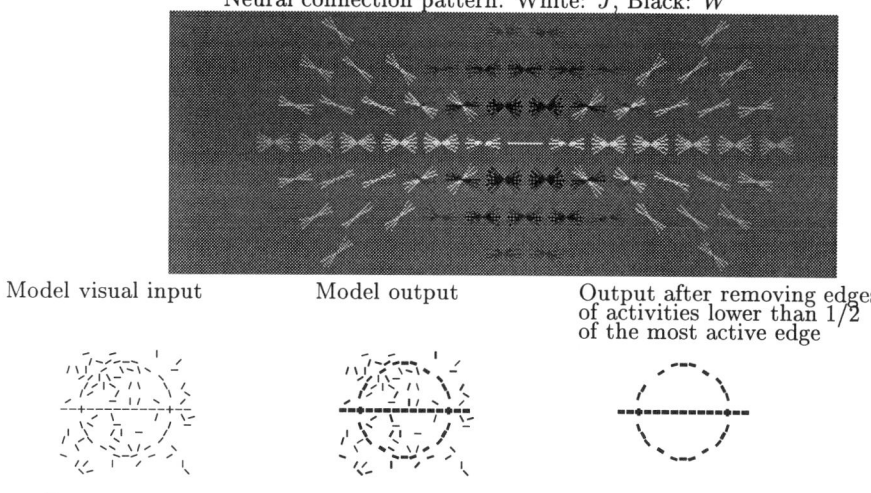

Figure 2: Model neural connections and performance for contour enhancement and noise reduction. The top graph depicts connections $J_{i\theta,j\theta'}$ and $W_{i\theta,j\theta'}$ respectively between the center (white) horizontal edge and other edges. The whiteness and blackness of each edge is proportional to the connection sthength $J_{i\theta,j\theta'}$ and $W_{i\theta,j\theta'}$ respectively. The bottom row plots visual input and the maximum model outputs. The edge thickness in this row is proportional to the value of edge input or activity. The same format applies to the other figures in this paper.

Let $x_{i\theta}$ and $y_{i\theta}$ be the cell membrane potentials for the excitatory and inhibitory cells respectively in the edge segment, then

$$\dot{x}_{i\theta} = -\alpha_x x_{i\theta} - g_y(y_{i\theta}) + J_o g_x(x_{i\theta}) + \sum_{j\theta' \neq i\theta} J_{i\theta j\theta'} g_x(x_{j\theta'}) + I_{i\theta} + I_o \quad (1)$$

$$\dot{y}_{i\theta} = -\alpha_y y_{i\theta} + g_x(x_{i\theta}) + \sum_{j\theta' \neq i\theta} W_{i\theta j\theta'} g_x(x_{j\theta'}) + I_c \quad (2)$$

where $g_x(x_{i\theta})$ and $g_y(y_{i\theta})$ are the firing rates from the excitatory and inhibitory cells respectively, $1/\alpha_x$ and $1/\alpha_y$ are the membrane constants, J_o is the self-excitatory connection weight, $J_{i\theta,j\theta'}$ and $W_{i\theta,j\theta'}$ are synaptic weights between neurons, and I_o and I_c are the background inputs to the excitatory and inhibitory cells. Without loss of generality, we take $\alpha_x = \alpha_y = 1$, $g_x(x)$ as threshold linear with saturation and an unit gain $g'_x(x) = 1$ in the linear range.

The synaptic connections $J_{i\theta,j\theta'}$ and $W_{i\theta,j\theta'}$ are local and translation and rotation invariant (Figure (2)). $J_{i\theta,j\theta'}$ increases with the smoothness (small curvature) of the curve that best connects $(i\theta)$ and $(j\theta')$, and edge elements inhibit each other via $W_{i\theta,j\theta'}$ when they are alternative choices in a smooth curve route. Given an input pattern $I_{i\theta}$, the network approaches a dynamic state after several membrane time constants. As in Figure (2), the neurons with relatively higher final activities are those belonging to smooth curves in the input.

2.2 Model analysis

Ignoring neural connections between edge segments, the neuron in edge segment $i\theta$

has input sensitivity

$$\delta g_x(x_o)/\delta I_{i\theta} = \frac{g'_x(x_o)}{1 + g'_y(y_o)g'_x(x_o) - J_o g'_x(x_o)} \quad (3)$$

$$\delta g_x(x_o)/\delta I_c = -\frac{g'_y(y_o)g'_x(x_o)}{1 + g'_y(y_o)g'_x(x_o) - J_o g'_x(x_o)} \quad (4)$$

where $g_x(x_o)$ and $g_y(y_o)$ are roughly the average neural activities (omitting $i\theta$ for simplicity). Thus the edge activity increases with $I_{i\theta}$ and decreases with I_c (in cases that interest us, $g'_y(y_o)g'_x(x_o) > J_o g'_x(x_o) - 1$). The resulting input-output function given I_c, $g_x(x_o)$ vs. $I_{i\theta}$, corresponds well with physiological data.

By effectively increasing $I_{i\theta}$ or I_c, the edge element $(j\theta')$ can excite or inhibit the element $(i\theta)$ with excitatory-to-excitatory input $J_{i\theta,j\theta'}g_x(x_{j\theta'})$ and excitatory-to-inhibitory input $W_{i\theta j\theta'}g_x(x_{j\theta'})$ respectively. Contour enhancement is so (Fig. 2) achieved. In the simplest example when the visual input has equally spaced equal strength edges from a line and all other edge segments are silent, we can treat the line system as one dimensional, omit θ and take i as locations along the line. A lack of inhibition between line segments gives:

$$\dot{x}_i = -\alpha_x x_i - g_y(y_i) + J_o g_x(x_i) + \sum_{j \neq i} J_{ij} g_x(x_j) + I_o + I_{line-input} \quad (5)$$

$$\dot{y}_i = -\alpha_y y_i + g_x(x_i) + I_c \quad (6)$$

If line is infinite, by symmetry, each edge segment has the same average activity $g_x(x_i) \sim g_x(x_o)$ for all i. This system can then be seen[12] either as a giant edge with self-excitatory connection $(J_o + \sum_{j \neq i} J_{ij})$, or a single edge with extra external input $\Delta I = (\sum_{j \neq i} J_{ij})g_x(x_o)$. Either way, activities $g_x(x_o)$ are enhanced for each edge element in the line (figure 3 and 2).

This analysis is also applicable to constant curvature curves[12]. It can be shown that, in the linear range of $g_x()$, the response ratio between a curve segment and an isolated segment is $(g'_y(y_o) + 1 - J_o)/(g'_y(y_o) + 1 - J_o - \sum_{i \neq j} J_{ij})$. Since $\sum_{i \neq j} J_{ij}$ decreases with increasing curvature, so does the response enhancement. Translation invariance along the curve breaks down in a finite length curve near its two ends, where activity enhancement decays by a decreased excitation from fewer neighboring segments. This suggests that a closed or longer curve has higher saliency than an open or shorter one (figure (3)). This prediction is expected to hold also for curves of non-constant curvature, and should play a significant role in the psychophysical observation[10] showing a decreased detection threshold for closed curves from that of the open ones.

Further analysis[12] shows that the edge segments in a curve normally exhibit neural oscillations around their mean activity levels with near-zero phase delays from each other. The model predicts that, like the contour enhancement, the oscillation is stronger for longer, smoother, and closed curves than open and shorter ones, and tapers off near curve endings where oscillation synchrony also deteriorates (figure (3)).

2.3 Central feedback control for contour enhancement, supression, filling in, and segmentation

A Neural Model of Visual Contour Integration

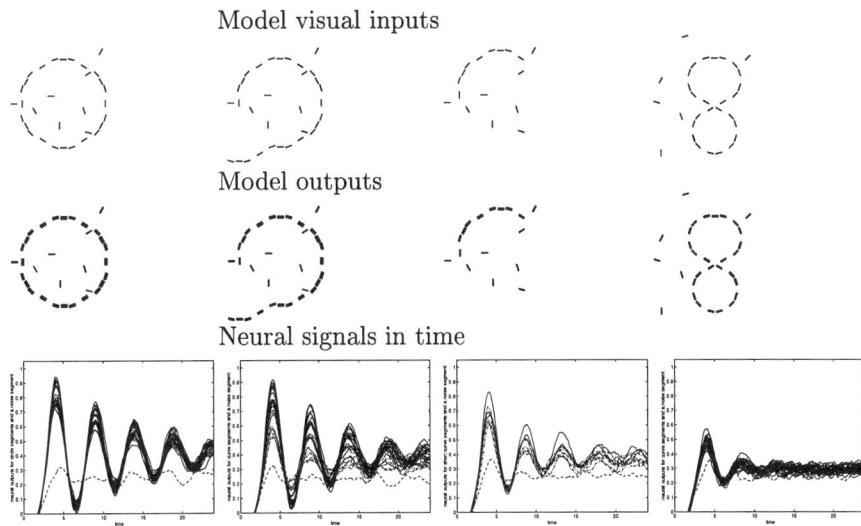

Figure 3: Model performance for input curves and noises. Each column is dedicated to one input condition. The top row is the visual input; the middle row is the maximum neural responses, and the bottom row the segment outputs as a function of time. The neural signals in the bottom row are shown superposed. The solid curves plot outputs for the segments away from the curve endings, the dash-dotted curves for segments near the curve endings, and the dashed curve in each plot, usually the lowest lying one, is an example from a noise segment. Note the decrease in neural signal synchrony between the curve segments, in the oscillation amplitudes, and average neural activities for the curve segments, as the curve becomes open, shorter, and more curled or when the segment is near the curve endings. Because the model employs discrete a grid input space, the figure '8' curve in the right column is almost not a smooth curve, hence the contour is only very weakly enhanced. The enhancement for this curve could be increased by a denser input grid or a multiscale input space.

The model assumes that higher visual centers send inputs I_c to the inhibitory cells, to influence neural activities by equation (4). Take $I_c = I_{c,background} + I_{c,control} \geq 0$, where $I_{c,background}$ is the same for all edge segments and is useful for modulating the overall visual alertness level. By setting $I_{c,control}$ differently for different edge segments, higher centers can selectively suppress or enhance activities for some visual objects (contours) (compare figure 4D,G), and even effectively achieve contour segmentation (figure (4H)) by silencing segments from a given curve. A similar feedback control mechanism was used in an olfactory model for odor sensitivity control and odor segmentation[11]. Nevertheless, the feedback cannot completely substitute for the visual input $I_{i\theta}$. By equation (4), I_c is effective only when $g'_y(y_o)g'_x(x_o) \neq 0$. With insufficient background input I_o, some visual input or excitation from other segments is needed to have $g'_x(x_o) > 0$, even when all the inhibition from I_c is removed by central control. However, a segment with weak visual input or excitation from aligned neighboring segments can increase its activity or become active from subthreshold. Therefore, this model central feedback can enhance a weak contour or fill in an incomplete one (compare figure 4F,I), but can not enhance or "hallucinate" any contour not existing at least partially in the visual input I (figure 4E).

3. Summary and Discussion

We have presented a model which accounts for phenomena of contour enhance-

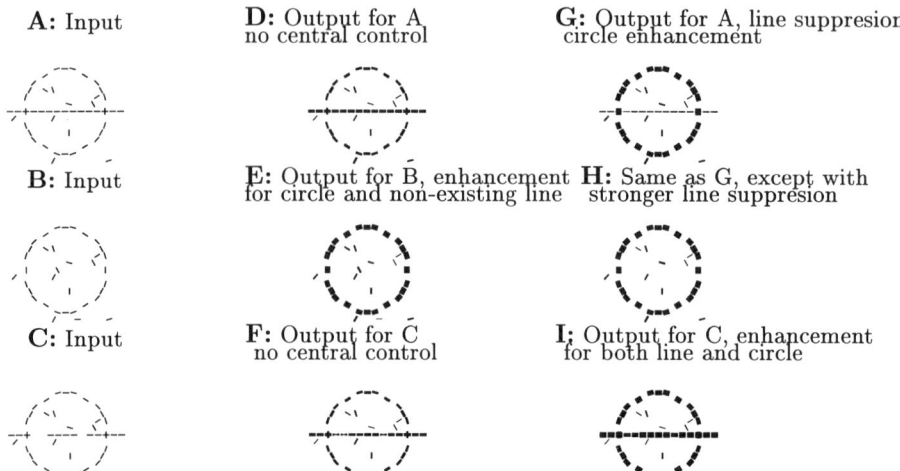

Figure 4: Central feedback control. The visual inputs are in **A**, **B** and **C**. The rest are the model responses under different feedback conditions. **D**: model response for input **A** without central control. **G**: model response for input **A** with line suppression by $I_{c,control} = 0.25 I_{c,background}$ on the line segments, and circle enhancement by $I_{c,control} = -0.29 I_{c,background}$ on the circle elements. **H**: Same as **G** except the line suppression signal $I_{c,control}$ is doubled. **E**: Model response to input **B** with enhancement for the line and the circle by central feedback $I_{c,control} = -0.29 I_{c,background}$. **F**: Response to input **C** with no central control. **I**: Response to input **C** with line and circle enhancement by $I_{c,control} = -0.29 I_{c,background}$. Note how the input gaps are partiallly filled in **F** and almost completely filled in **I**. Note that the apparent gaps in the circle are caused by the underlying discrete grid in the model input space, and hence no gap actually exists, and no filling in is needed, for this circle. Also, with the wrap around boundary condition, the line is actually a closed or infinitely long line, and is thus naturally more salient in this model without feedback.

ment using neurally plausible elements in V1. It is shown analytically and empirically that both the contour enhancement and the neural oscillation amplitudes are stronger for longer, closed, and smaller curvature curves, agreeing with experimental observations[8, 4, 10, 6, 2]. The model predicts that horizontal connections target preferentially excitatory or inhibitory post-synaptic cells when the linked edges are aligned or less aligned (Fig. 2). In addition, we introduce a possible feedback mechanism by which higher visual centers could selectively enhance or suppress contour activities, and achieve contour segmentation. This feedback mechanism has the desirable property that while the higher centers can enhance or complete an existing weak and/or fragmented input contour, they cannot enhance a non-existant contour in the input, thus preventing "hallucination". This property could be exploited by higher visual centers for hypothesis testing and object reconstruction by cooperating with lower visual centers. Analogous computational mechanisms have been used in an olfactory model to achieve odor segmentation and sensitivity modulation[11]. It will be interesting to explore the universality of such computational mechanisms across sensory modalities.

The organization of the model is based on various experimental finding[17, 5, 1, 8, 14]: recurrent excitatory-inhibitory interactions; excitatory and inhibitory linking of edge elements with similar orientation preferences; and neural connection patterns. At the cost of analytical tractability without essential changes in model performance, one can relax the model's idealization of a 1:1 ratio in the excitatory and inhibitory cell numbers, the lack of connections between the inhibitory cells, and the excitatory cells as the exclusive recipients of visual input. While abundant feedback connections are observed from higher visual centers to the primary visual cortex, there is as yet no clear indication of cell types of their targets[3, 16]. It is desirable to find out whether the feedback is indeed directed to the inhibitory cells as predicted.

This model can be extended to stereo, temporal, and chromatic dimensions, by linking edge segments aligned in orientation, depth, motion direction and color. V1 cells have receptive field tuning in all these dimensions, and cortical connections are indeed observed to link cells of similar receptive field properties[5]. This model does not model many other apparently non-contour related visual phenomena such as receptive field adaptations[5]. It is also beyond this model to explain how the higher visual centers decide which segments belong to one contour in order to achieve feedback control, although it has been hypothesized that phase locked neural oscillations and neural correlations can play such a role[13].

References

[1] Douglas R.J. and Martin K. A. "Neocortex" in *Synaptic Organization of the Brain* 3rd Edition, Ed. G. M. Shepherd, Oxford University Press 1990.

[2] Eckhorn R, Bauer, R. Jordan W. Brosch, M. Kruse W., Munk M. and Reitboeck, H. J. 1988. *Biol. Cybern.* 60:121-130.

[3] van Essen D. Peters and E G Jones, Plenum Press, New York, 1985. p. 259-329

[4] Field DJ; Hayes A; Hess RF 1993. *Vision Res.* 1993 Jan; 33(2): 173-93

[5] Gilbert CD *Neuron.* 1992 Jul; 9(1): 1-13

[6] Gray C.M. and Singer W. 1989 *Proc. Natl. Acad. Sci. USA* 86: 1698-1702.

[7] Grossberg S; Mingolla E *Percept Psychophys.* 1985 Aug; 38(2): 141-71

[8] Kapadia MK; Ito M; Gilbert CD; Westheimer G, *Neuron.* 1995 Oct; 15(4): 843-56

[9] Knierim J. J. and van Essen D. C. 1992, *J. Neurophysiol.* 67, 961-980.

[10] Kovacs I; Julesz B *Proc Natl Acad Sci USA.* 1993 Aug 15; 90(16): 7495-7

[11] Li Zhaoping, *Biological Cybernetics*, 62/4 (1990), P. 349-361

[12] Li Zhaoping, "A neural model contour integration in primary visual cortex" manuscript submitted for publication.

[13] von der Malsburg C. 1981 "The correlation theory of brain function." Internal report, Max-Planck-Institute for Biophysical Chemistry, Gottingen, West Germany.

[14] Polat U; Sagi D, 1994 *Vision Res.* 1994 Jan; 34(1): 73-8

[15] Shashua A. and Ullman S. 1988 *Proceedings of the International Conference on Computer Vision.* Tempa, Florida, 482-488.

[16] Valverde F. in *Cerebral Cortex* Eds. A Peters and E G Jones, Plenum Press, New York, 1985. p. 207-258.

[17] White E. L. *Cortical circuits* 46-82, Birkhauser, Boston, 1989

[18] Zucker S. W., David C., Dobbins A, and Iverson L. in *Second international conference on computer vision* pp. 568-577, IEEE computer society press, 1988.

Learning Exact Patterns of Quasi-synchronization among Spiking Neurons from Data on Multi-unit Recordings

Laura Martignon
Max Planck Institute
for Psychological Research
Adaptive Behavior and Cognition
80802 Munich, Germany
laura@mpipf-muenchen.mpg.de

Kathryn Laskey
Dept. of Systems Engineering
and the Krasnow Institute
George Mason University
Fairfax, Va. 22030
klaskey@gmu.edu

Gustavo Deco
Siemens AG
Central Research
Otto Hahn Ring 6
81730 Munich
gustavo.deco@zfe.siemens.de

Eilon Vaadia
Dept. of Physiology
Hadassah Medical School
Hebrew University of Jerusalem
Jerusalem 91010, Israel
eilon@hbf.huji.ac.il

Abstract

This paper develops arguments for a family of temporal log-linear models to represent spatio-temporal correlations among the spiking events in a group of neurons. The models can represent not just pairwise correlations but also correlations of higher order. Methods are discussed for inferring the existence or absence of correlations and estimating their strength.
A frequentist and a Bayesian approach to correlation detection are compared. The frequentist method is based on G^2 statistic with estimates obtained via the Max-Ent principle. In the Bayesian approach a Markov Chain Monte Carlo Model Composition (MC^3) algorithm is applied to search over connectivity structures and Laplace's method is used to approximate their posterior probability. Performance of the methods was tested on synthetic data. The methods were applied to experimental data obtained by the fourth author by means of measurements carried out on behaving Rhesus monkeys at the Hadassah Medical School of the Hebrew University. As conjectured, neural connectivity structures need not be neither hierarchical nor decomposable.

1 INTRODUCTION

Hebb conjectured that information processing in the brain is achieved through the collective action of groups of neurons, which he called *cell assemblies* (Hebb, 1949). His followers were left with a twofold challenge:
- to define cell assemblies in an unambiguous way.
- to conceive and carry out the experiments that demonstrate their existence.

Cell assemblies have been defined in various sometimes conflicting ways, both in terms of anatomy and of shared function. One persistent approach characterizes the cell assembly by near-simultaneity or some other specific timing relation in the firing of the involved neurons. If two neurons converge on a third one, their synaptic influence is much larger for near-coincident firing, due to the spatio-temporal summation in the dendrite (Abeles,1991; Abeles et al. 1993). Thus *syn-firing* is directly available to the brain as a potential code.

The second challenge has led physiologists to develop methods to observe the simultaneous activity of individual neurons to seek evidence for spatio-temporal patterns. It is now possible to obtain multi-unit recordings of up to 100 neurons in awake behaving animals. In the data we analyze, the spiking events (in the 1 msec range) are encoded as sequences of 0's and 1's, and the activity of the whole group is described as a sequence of binary configurations. This paper presents a statistical model in which the parameters represent spatio-temporal firing patterns. We discuss methods for estimating these pararameters and drawing inferences about which interactions are present.

2 PARAMETERS FOR SPATIO-TEMPORAL FIRING PATTERNS

The term spatial correlation has been used to denote synchronous firing of a group of neurons, while the term temporal correlation has been used to indicate chains of firing events at specific temporal intervals. Terms like "couple" or "triplet" have been used to denote spatio-temporal patterns of two or three neurons (Abeles et al., 1993; Grün, 1996) firing simultaneously or in sequence. Establishing the presence of such patterns is not straightforward. For example, three neurons may fire together *more often than expected by chance*[1] without exhibiting an authentic third order interaction. This phenomenon may be due, for instance, to synchronous firing of two couples out of the three neurons. Authentic triplets, and, in general, authentic n-th order correlations, must therefore be distinguished from correlations that can be explained in terms of lower order interactions. In what follows, we present a parameterized model that represents a spatio-temporal correlation by a parameter that depends on the involved neurons and on a set of time intervals, where synchronization is characterized by all time intervals being zero.

Assume that the sequence of configurations $\underline{x}_t = (x_{(1t)}, \cdots, x_{(Nt)})$ of N neurons forms a Markov chain of order r. Let δ be the time step, and denote the conditional distribution for $\underline{x}_t$ given previous configurations by $p(\underline{x}_t | \underline{x}_{(t-\delta)}, \underline{x}_{(t-2\delta)}, \ldots, \underline{x}_{(t-r\delta)})$. We assume that all transition probabilities are strictly positive and expand the logarithm of the conditional distribution as:

---

[1] that is to say, more often than predicted by the null hypothesis of independence.

$$p(\underline{x}_t \mid \underline{x}_{(t-\delta)}, \underline{x}_{(t-2\delta)}, \ldots, \underline{x}_{(t-r\delta)}) = exp\{\theta_0 + \sum_{A \in \Xi} \theta_A X_A\} \quad (1)$$

where each A is a subset of pairs of subscripts of the form $(i, t - s\delta)$ that includes at least one pair of the form (i,t). Here $X_A = \prod_{1 \leq j \leq k} x_{(i_j, t - m_j \delta)}$ denotes the event that all neurons in A are active. The set $\Xi \subseteq 2^\Lambda$ of all subsets for which θ_A is non-zero is called the *interaction structure* for the distribution p. The effect θ_A is called the *interaction strength* for the interaction on subset A. Clearly, $\theta_A = 0$ is equivalent to $A \notin \Xi$ and is taken to indicate absence of an order-$|A|$ interaction among neurons in A. We denote the structure-specific vector of non-zero interaction strengths by $\underline{\theta}_\Xi$. Consider a set Λ of N binary neurons and denote by p the probability distribution on the binary configurations of Λ.

DEFINITION 1: We say that neurons $\{i_1, i_2, \ldots, i_k\}$ exhibit a *spatio-temporal pattern* if there is a set of time intervals $m_1\delta, m_2\delta, \ldots, m_k\delta$ with at least one $m_i = 0$, such that $\theta_A \neq 0$ in Equation (1), where $A = \{(i_1, t - m_1\delta), \ldots, (i_k, t - m_k\delta)\}$.

DEFINITION 2: A subset $\{i_1, i_2, \ldots, i_k\}$ of neurons exhibits a *synchronization* or *spatial correlation* if $\theta_A \neq 0$ for $A = \{(i_1, 0), \ldots, (i_k, 0)\}$.

In the case of absence of any temporal dependencies the configurations are independent and we drop the time index:

$$p(\underline{x}) = exp\{\theta_0 + \sum \theta_A X_A\} \quad (2)$$

where A is any nonempty subset of Λ and $X_A = \prod_{i \in A} x_i$.

Of course (2) is unrealistic. Temporal correlation of some kind is always present, one such example being the refractory period after firing. Nevertheless, (2) may be adequate in cases of weak temporal correlation. Although the models (1) and (2) are statistical not physiological, it is an established conjecture that synaptic connection between two neurons will manifest as a non-zero θ_A for the corresponding set A in the temporal model (1). Another example leading to non-zero θ_A will be simultaneous activation of the neurons in A due to a common input, as illustrated in Figure 1 below. Such a θ_A will appear in model (1) with time intervals equal to 0. An attractive feature of our models is that it is capable of distinguishing between cases a. and b. of Figure 1. This can be seen by extending the model (2) to include the external neurons (H in case a., H,K in case b.) and then marginalizing. An information-theoretic argument supports the choice of $\theta_A \neq 0$ as a natural indicator of an order-$|A|$ interaction among the neurons in A. Assume that we are in the case of no temporal correlation. The absence of interaction of order $|A|$

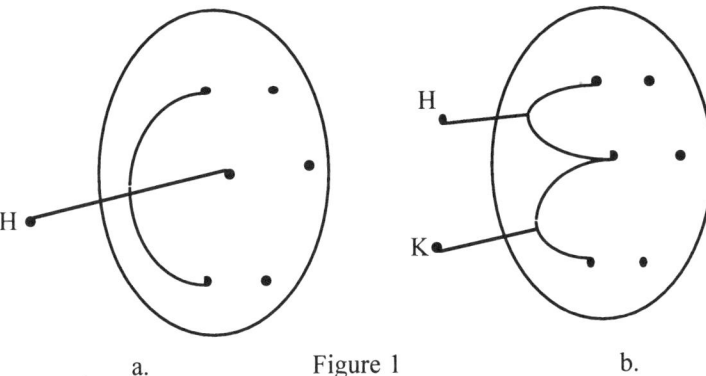

Figure 1

among neurons in A should be taken to mean that the distribution is determined by the marginal distributions on proper subsets of A. A well established criterion for selecting a distribution among those matching the lower order marginals fixed by proper subsets of A, is Max-Ent. According to the Max-Ent principle the distribution that maximizes entropy is the one which is maximally non-committal with regard to missing information. The probability distribution p^* that maximizes entropy among distributions *with the same marginals as the distribution* p *on proper subsets of* A has a log-linear expansion in which only $\theta_B, B \subset A, B \neq A$ can possibly be non-zero.[2]

3 THE FREQUENTIST APPROACH

We treat here the case of no temporal dependencies. The general case is treated in Martignon-Deco,1997; Deco-Martignon,1997. We also assume that our data are stationary. We test the presence of synchronization of neurons in A by the following procedure: we condition on silence of neurons in the complement of A in Λ and call the resulting frequency distribution p. We construct the Max-Ent model determined by the marginals of p on proper subsets of A. The well-known method for constructing this type of Max-Ent models is the I.P.F.P. Algorithm (Bishop et al.,1975). We propose here another simpler and quicker procedure:

If B is a subset of A, denote by χ_B the configuration that has a component 1 for every index in B and 0 elsewhere.

Define $p^*(\chi_B) = p(\chi_B) + (-1)^{|B|} \Delta$, where Δ is to be determined by solving for $\theta^*_A \equiv 0$, where θ^*_A is the coefficient corresponding to A in the log-expansion of p^*. As can be shown (Martignon et al, 1995), θ^*_A can be written as

---

[2] This was observed by J. Good in 1963 (Bishop et al. 1975). It is interesting to note that p^* minimizes the Kullback-Leibler distance from p in the manifold of distributions with a log-linear expansion in which only $\theta_B, B \subset A, B \neq A$ can possibly be non-zero.

$\theta^*_A = \sum_{B \subset A} (-1)^{|A-B|} \ln p^*(\chi_B)$. The distribution p^* maximizes entropy among those with the same marginals of p on proper subsets of A.[3] We use p^* as estimate of p for tests by means of G^2 statistic (Bishop et al., 1975).

4 THE BAYESIAN APPROACH

We treat here the case of no temporal dependencies. The general case is treated in Laskey-Martignon, 1997. Information about $p(x)$ prior to observing any data is represented by a joint probability distribution called the *prior distribution* over Ξ and the θ's. Observations are used to update this probability distribution to obtain a *posterior distribution* over structures and parameters. The posterior probability of a cluster A can be interpreted as the probability that the r nodes in cluster A exhibit a degree-r interaction. The posterior distribution for θ_A represents structure-specific information about the magnitude of the interaction. The mean or mode of the posterior distribution can be used as a point estimate of the interaction strength; the standard deviation of the posterior distribution reflects remaining uncertainty about the interaction strength.

We exhibit a family of log-linear models capable of capturing interactions of all orders. An algorithm is presented for learning both structure and parameters in a unified Bayesian framework. Each model structure specifies a set of clusters of nodes, and structure-specific parameters represent the directions and strengths of interactions among them. The Bayesian learning algorithm gives high posterior probability to models that are consistent with the data. Results include a probability, given the observations, that a set of neurons fires simultaneously, and a posterior probability distribution for the strength of the interaction, conditional on its occurrence.

The prior distribution we used has two components. The first component assigns a prior probability to each structure. In our model, interactions are independent of each other and each interaction has a probability of .1. This reflects the prior expectation that not many interactions are expected to be present. The second component of the prior distribution is the conditional distribution of interaction strengths given the structure. If an interaction is not in the structure, the corresponding strength parameter θ_A is taken to be identically zero given structure Ξ. All interactions belonging to Ξ are taken to be independent and normally distributed with mean zero and standard deviation 2. This reflects the prior expectation that interaction strength magnitudes are rarely larger than 4 in absolute value.

Computing the posterior probability of a structure Ξ requires integrating out of the joint mass-density function of the structure Ξ, the interaction strength θ_A, and the data X. The solution to this integral cannot be obtained in closed form. We use Laplace's method (Kass-Raftery, 1995; Tierney-Kadane, 1986) to estimate the posterior probability of structures. The posterior distribution of θ_A given frequency data also

---

[3] This is due to the fact that there is a unique distribution with the same marginals of p on proper subsets of A such that the coefficient corresponding to A in its log-expansion is zero.

cannot be obtained in closed form. We use the mode of the posterior distribution as a point estimate of θ_A. The standard deviation of θ_A, which indicates how precisely θ_A can be estimated from the given data, is estimated using a normal approximation to the posterior distribution (Laskey-Martignon, 1997). The covariance matrix of the θ_A is estimated as the inverse Fisher information matrix evaluated at the mode of the posterior distribution. The posterior probability of an interaction θ_A is the sum over the posterior probabilities of all structures containing A. We used a Markov chain Monte Carlo Model Composition algorithm (MC^3) to search over structures. This stochastic algorithm converges to a stationary distribution in which structure Ξ is visited with probability equal to its posterior probability. We ran the MC^3 algorithm for 15,000 runs and estimated the posterior probability of a structure as its frequency of occurrence over the 15,000 runs. We estimated interaction strength parameters and standard deviations using only the 100 highest-probability structures. Although the number of possible structures is astronomical, typically most of the posterior probability is contained in relatively few structures. We found this to be the case, which justifies using only the most probable structures to estimate interaction strength parameters.

5 RESULTS

We applied our models to data from an experiment in which spiking events among groups of neurons were analyzed through multi-unit recordings of 6-16 units in the frontal cortex of Rhesus monkeys. The monkeys were trained to localize a source of light and, after a delay, to touch the target from which the light blink was presented. At the beginning of each trial the monkeys touched a "ready-key", then the central ready light was turned on. Later, a visual cue was given in the form of a 200-ms light blink coming from either the left or the right. Then, after a delay of 1 to 32 seconds, the color of the ready light changed from red to orange and the monkeys had to release the ready key and touch the target from which the cue was given. The spiking events (in the 1 millisecond range) of each neuron were encoded as a sequence of zeros and ones, and the activity of the group was described as a sequence of configurations of these binary states. The fourth author provided data corresponding to piecewise stationary segments of the trials, which presented weak temporal correlation, corresponding to intervals of 2000 milliseconds around the ready-signal. He adjoined these 94 segments and formed a data-set of 188,000 msec. The data were then binned in time windows of 40 milliseconds. The criterion we used to fix the binwidth was robustness with regards to variations of the offsets. We selected a subset of eight of the neurons for which data were recorded. We analyzed recordings prior to the ready-signal separately from data recorded after the ready-signal. Each of these data sets is assumed to consist of independent trials from a model of the form (2).

Cluster A	Posterior prob. of A (frequency)	Posterior prob. of A (best 100models)	MAP estimate of θ_A	Standard deviation of θ_A	Significance
6,8	.9	.89	0.47	0.11	4.0853
4,5,6,7	.30	0.32	2.30	0.64	No
2,3,6	.40	0.38	2.30	0.64	2.35
1,3,4	close to prior	close to prior			4.7

Table1: results for pre-ready signal data. Effects with posterior prob. > 0.1

Cluster A	Posterior prob. of A (frequency)	Posterior prob. of A (best 100 models)	MAP estimate of θ_A	Standard deviation of θ_A	Significance
5,6	.79	0.96	1.00	0.27	1.82
4,7	.246	0.18	0.93	0.34	2.68
1,4,5,6	0.18	0.13	1.06	0.36	No
1,3,4,6,7	0.24	0.17	2.69	0.13	No

Table2:results for post-ready signal data. Effects with posterior prob >0.1

Another set of data from 5 simulated neurons was provided by the fourth author for a double-check of the methods. Only second order correlations had been simulated: a synapse lasting 2 msec, an inhibitory common input, and two excitatory common inputs. The Bayesian method was very accurate, detecting exactly the simulated interactions. The frequentist method made one mistake. Other data sets with temporal correlations have also been analyzed. By means of the frequentist approach on shifted data, temporal triplets have been detected and even fourth order correlations. Temporal correlograms are computed for shifts of up to 50 msec (Martignon-Deco, 1997).

References

Hebb, D. (1949) *The Organization of Behavior*. New York: Wiley, 1949.

Abeles, M.(1991)*Corticonics: Neural Circuits of the Cerebral Cortex*. Cambridge: Cambridge University Press, 1991.

Abeles, M., H. Bergman, E. Margalit, and E. Vaadia. (1993) "Spatiotemporal Firing Patterns in the Frontal Cortex of Behaving Monkeys." *Journal of Neurophysiology* 70, 4:, 1629-1638.

Grün S. (1996) *Unitary Joint-Events in Multiple-Neuron Spiking Activity-Detection, Significance and Interpretation*. Verlag Harry Deutsch, Frankfurt.

Martignon L. and Deco G. (1997) "Neurostatistics of Spatio-Temporal Patterns of Neural Activation: the frequentist approach" Technical Report, MPI-ABC no.*3*.

Deco G. and Martignon L. (1997) "Higher-order Phenomena among Spiking Events of Groups of Neurons" Preprint.

Bishop, Y., S. Fienberg, and P. Holland (1975) *Discrete Multivariate Analysis*. Cambridge, MA: MIT Press.

Martignon L,.v.Hasseln H. Grün S, Aertsen A, Palm G.(1995) "Detecting Higher Order Interactions among the Spiking Events of a Group of Neurons" Biol.Cyb. *73*, 69-81.

Kass, . and Raftery A. (1995) "Bayes factors"*Journal of the American Statistical Association 90, no. 430:*, 773-795.

Tierney, L., and J. B. Kadane (1986) "Accurate Approximations for Posterior Moments and Marginal Densities." *Journal of the American Statistical Association 81*, 82-86

Laskey K., and Martignon L.(1997) "Neurostatistics of Spatio-temporal Patterns of Neural Activation: the Bayesian Approach", in preparation

Laskey K., and Martignon, L.(1996) "Bayesian Learning of Log-linear Models for Neural Connectivity" *Proceedings of the XII Conference on Uncertainty in Artificial Intelligence*, Horvitz E. ed., Morgan-Kaufmann, San Mateo.

Complex-Cell Responses Derived from Center-Surround Inputs: The Surprising Power of Intradendritic Computation

Bartlett W. Mel and Daniel L. Ruderman
Department of Biomedical Engineering
University of Southern California
Los Angeles, CA 90089

Kevin A. Archie
Neuroscience Program
University of Southern California
Los Angeles, CA 90089

Abstract

Biophysical modeling studies have previously shown that cortical pyramidal cells driven by strong NMDA-type synaptic currents and/or containing dendritic voltage-dependent Ca^{++} or Na^+ channels, respond more strongly when synapses are activated in several spatially clustered groups of optimal size—in comparison to the same number of synapses activated diffusely about the dendritic arbor [8]. The nonlinear intradendritic interactions giving rise to this "cluster sensitivity" property are akin to a layer of virtual nonlinear "hidden units" in the dendrites, with implications for the cellular basis of learning and memory [7, 6], and for certain classes of nonlinear sensory processing [8]. In the present study, we show that a single neuron, with access only to excitatory inputs from unoriented ON- and OFF-center cells in the LGN, exhibits the principal nonlinear response properties of a "complex" cell in primary visual cortex, namely orientation tuning coupled with translation invariance and contrast insensitivity. We conjecture that this type of intradendritic processing could explain how complex cell responses can persist in the absence of oriented simple cell input [13].

1 INTRODUCTION

Simple and complex cells were first described in visual cortex by Hubel and Wiesel [4]. Simple cell receptive fields could be subdivided into ON and OFF subregions, with spatial summation within a subregion and antagonism between subregions; cells of this type have historically been modeled as linear filters followed by a thresholding nonlinearity (see [13]). In contrast, complex cell receptive fields cannot generally be subdivided into distinct ON and OFF subfields, and as a group exhibit a number of fundamentally nonlinear behaviors, including (1) orientation tuning across a receptive field much wider than an optimal bar, (2) larger responses to thin bars than thick bars—in direct violation of the superposition principle, and (3) sensitivity to both light and dark bars across the receptive field.

The traditional Hubel-Wiesel model for complex cell responses involves a hierarchy, consisting of center-surround inputs that drive simple cells, which in turn provide oriented, phase-dependent input to the complex cell. By pooling over a set of simple cells with different positions and phases, the complex cell could respond selectively to stimulus orientation, while generalizing over stimulus position and contrast. A pure hierarchy involving simple cells is challenged, however, by a variety of more recent experimental results indicating many complex cells receive monosynaptic input from LGN cells [3], or do not depend on simple cell input [10, 5, 1]. It remains unknown how complex cell responses might derive from intracortical network computations that do no depend on simple cells, or whether they could originate directly from intracellular computations.

Previous biophysical modeling studies have indicated that the input-output function of a dendritic tree containing excitatory voltage-dependent membrane mechanisms can be abstracted as low-order polynomial function, i.e. a big sum of little products (see [9] for review). The close match between this type of computation and "energy" models for complex cells [12, 11, 2] suggested that a single-cell origin of complex cell responses was possible.

In the present study, we tested the hypothesis that local nonlinear processing in the dendritic tree of a single neuron, which receives only excitatory synaptic input from unoriented center-surround LGN cells, could in and of itself generate nonlinear complex cell response properties, including orientation selectivity, coupled with position and contrast invariance.

2 METHODS

2.1 BIOPHYSICAL MODELING

Simulations of a layer 5 pyramidal cell from cat visual cortex (fig. 1) were carried out in NEURON[1]. Biophysical parameters and other implementation details were as in [8] and/or shown in Table 2, except dendritic spines were not modeled here. The soma contained modified Hodgkin-Huxley channels with peak somatic conductances of $\bar{g}_{Na}$ and $\bar{g}_{DR}$ 0.20 S/cm^2 and 0.12 S/cm^2, respectively; dendritic membrane was electrically passive. Each synapse included both an NMDA and AMPA-type

---

[1]NEURON simulation environment courtesy Michael Hines and John Moore; synaptic channel implementations courtesy Alan Destexhe and Zach Mainen.

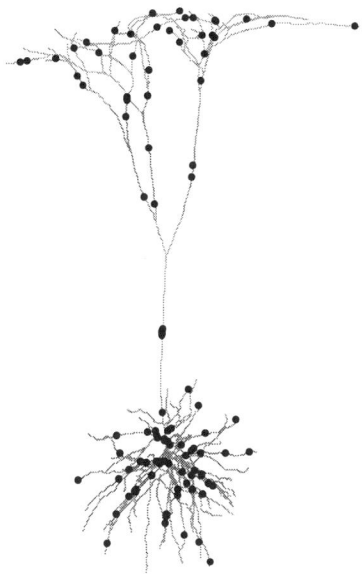

Figure 1: Layer 5 pyramidal neuron used in the simulations, showing 100 synaptic contacts. Morphology courtesy Rodney Douglas and Kevan Martin.

excitatory conductances (see Table 1). Conductances were scaled by an estimate of the local input resistance, to keep local EPSP size approximately uniform across the dendritic tree. Inhibitory synapses were not modeled.

2.2 MAPPING VISUAL STIMULI ONTO THE DENDRITIC TREE

A stimulus image consisted of a 64 × 64 pixel array containing a light or dark bar (pixel value ±1 against a background of 0). Bars of length 45 and width 7 were presented at various orientations and positions within the image. Images were linearly filtered through difference-of-Gaussian receptive fields (center width: 0.6, surround width: 1.2, with no DC response). Filtered images were then mapped onto 64 × 64 arrays of ON-center and OFF-center LGN cells, whose outputs were thresholded at ±0.02 respectively. In a crude model of gain control, only a random subset of 100 of the LGN neurons remained active to drive the modeled cortical cell.

Each LGN neuron gave rise to a single synapse onto the cortical cell's dendritic tree. In a given run, excitatory synapses originating from the 100 active LGN cells were activated asynchronously at 40 Hz, while all other synapses remained silent.

The spatial arrangement of connections from LGN cells onto the pyramidal cell dendrites was generated automatically, such that pairs of LGN cells which are co-active during presentations of optimally oriented bars formed synapses at nearby sites in the dendritic tree. The activity of the LGN cell array to an optimally oriented bar is shown in fig. 3. Frequently co-activated pairs of LGN neurons are hereafter referred to as "friend-pairs", and lie in a geometric arrangement as shown in fig. 4. Correlation-based clustering of friend-pairs was achieved by (1) choosing a random LGN cell and placing it at the next available dendritic site, (2) randomly

Parameter	Value
R_m	$10 \text{k}\Omega \text{cm}^2$
R_a	$200 \Omega \text{cm}$
C_m	$1.0 \mu\text{F}/\text{cm}^2$
V_{rest}	-70 mV
Somatic $\bar{g}_{\text{Na}}$	$0.20 \text{ S}/\text{cm}^2$
Somatic $\bar{g}_{\text{DR}}$	$0.12 \text{ S}/\text{cm}^2$
Synapse count	100
Stimulus frequency	40 Hz
$\tau_{\text{AMPA}}(on, off)$	0.5 ms, 3 ms
$\bar{g}_{\text{AMPA}}$	0.27 nS – 2.95 nS
$\tau_{\text{NMDA}}(on, off)$	0.5 ms, 50 ms
$\bar{g}_{\text{NMDA}}$	0.027 nS – 0.295 nS
E_{syn}	0 mV

Figure 2: Table 1. Simulation Parameters.

choosing one of its friends and placing it at the next available dendritic site, and so on, until until either all of the cell's friends had already been deployed, in which case a new cell was chosen at random to restart the sequence, or all cells had been chosen, meaning that all of the 8192 (= 64 × 64 × 2) LGN synapses had been successfully mapped onto the dendritic tree. In previous modeling work it was shown that this type of clustering of correlated inputs on dendrites is the natural outcome of a balance between activity-independent synapse formation, and activity dependent synapse stabilization [6].

This method guaranteed that an optimally oriented bar stimulus activated a larger number of friend-pairs on average than did bars at non-optimal orientations. This led in turn to relatively clustery distributions of activated synapses in the dendrites in response to optimal bar orientations, in comparison to non-optimal orientations. In previous work, it was shown that synapses activated in clusters about a dendritic arbor could produce significantly larger cell responses than the same number of synapses activated diffusely about the dendritic tree [7, 8].

3 Results

Results for two series of runs are shown in fig. 5. For each bar stimulus, average spike rate was measured over a 250 ms period, beginning with the first spike initiated after stimulus onset (if any). This measure de-emphasized the initial transient climb off the resting potential, and provided a rough steady-state measure of stimulus effectiveness. Spike rates for 30 runs were averaged for each input condition.

Orientation tuning curves for a thin bar (7 × 45 pixels) are shown in fig. 5. The orientation tuning peaks sharply within about 10° of vertical, and then decays slowly for larger angles. Tuning is apparent both for dark and light bars, and remains independent of location within the receptive field.

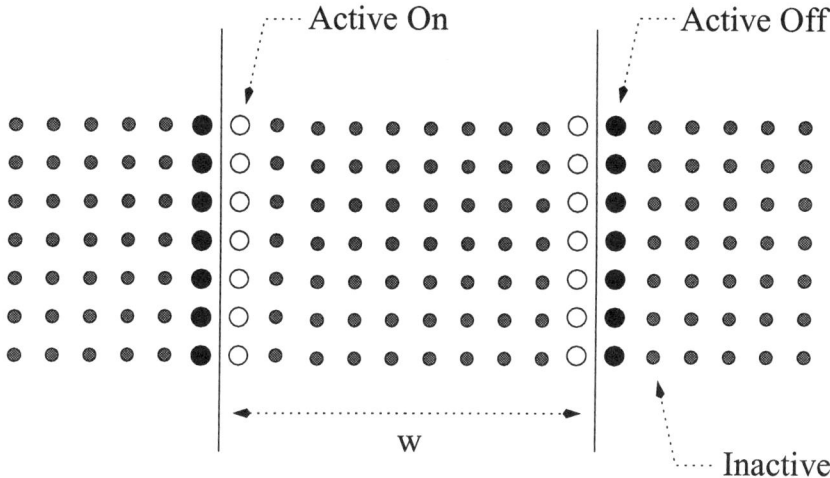

Figure 3: LGN cell activities in response to a vertical light bar of width $w = 10$ presented against a dark background. Large white circles: active on-center cells; large dark circles: active off-center cells; small gray circles: inactive cells. Only a 22×7 section of the array is shown.

4 Discussion

The results of fig. 5 indicate that a pyramidal cell driven exclusively by excitatory inputs from ON- and OFF-center LGN cells, is at a biophysical level *capable* of producing the hallmark nonlinear response property of visual complex cells. Furthermore, the cell's translation-invariant preference for light or dark vertical bars was established by manipulating only the spatial arrangement of connections from LGN cells onto the pyramidal cell dendrites. Since exactly 100 synapses were activated in every tested condition, the significantly larger responses to optimal bar orientations could not be explained by a simple elevation in the total synaptic activity impinging on the neuron in that condition. The origin of the cell's orientation-selective response resulted from nonlinear pooling of a large number of minimally-oriented subunits, i.e. consisting of pairs of ON and OFF cells that were co-consistent with an optimally oriented bar. We have achieved similar results in other experiments with a variety of different friend-neighborhood structures including ones both simpler and more complex than were used here, for LGN arrays with substantially different degrees of receptive field overlap, with random subsampling of the LGN array, with graded LGN activity levels, and for dendritic trees containing active sodium channels in addition to NMDA channels.

Thus far we have not attempted to relate physiologically-measured orientation and width tuning curves, and other detailed aspects of complex cell physiology, to our model cell, as we have been principally interested in establishing whether the most salient nonlinear features of complex cell physiology were biophysically feasible at the single cell level. Detailed comparisons between our results and empirical tuning curves, etc., must be made with caution, since our model cell has been "explanted" from the network in which it normally exists, and is therefore absent the normal recurrent excitatory and inhibitory influences the cortical network provides.

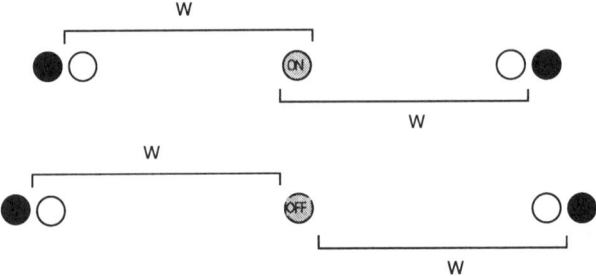

Figure 4: Layout of friends for an ON-center LGN cell for vertically oriented thin bars (top). The linear friendship linkage for a given ideal vertical bar of width w was determined as follows. Suppose an LGN cell is chosen at random, e.g. an ON-center cell at location (i,j) within the cell array. When a vertical bar is presented, LGN cells along the two vertical edges of the bar become active. The ON-center cell at position (i,j) is active to a light bar when it is in a column of cells just inside either edge of the bar. Those cells which are co-active under this circumstance are: (a) other on-center cells in the same vertical column, (b) on-center cells in vertical columns a distance $w-1$ to the right and left (depending on the bar position), (c) off-center cells in columns a distance ± 1 away (due to the negative-going edge adjacent), and (d) off-center cells a distance w to the right and left (due to the opposite edge). As "friend-pairs" we take only those LGN cells a distance $\pm(w-1)$ and $\pm w$ away. Those in the same and neighboring columns are not included. The friends of an off-center cell are shown in the bottom figure. It and its friends are optimally stimulated by bars of width w placed as shown. The width selected for our friend-pairs was $w = 7$, the same width as all bars presented as stimuli.

Experimental validation of these simulation results would imply a significant change in our conception of the role of the single neuron in neocortical processing.

Acknowledgments

This work was funded by grants from the National Science Foundation and the Office of Naval Research.

References

[1] G.M. Ghose, R.D. Freeman, and I. Ohzawa. Local intracortical connections in the cats visual-cortex - postnatal-development and plasticity. *J. Neurophysiol.*, 72:1290–1303, 1994.

[2] D.J. Heeger. Normalization of cell responses in cat striate cortex. *Visual Neurosci.*, 9:181–197, 1992.

[3] K.P. Hoffman and J. Stone. Conduction velocity of afferents to cat visual cortex: a correlation with cortical receptive field properties. *Brain Res.*, 32:460–466, 1971.

[4] D.H. Hubel and T.N. Wiesel. Receptive fields, binocular interaction and functional architecture in the cat's visual cortex. *J. Physiol.*, 160:106–154, 1962.

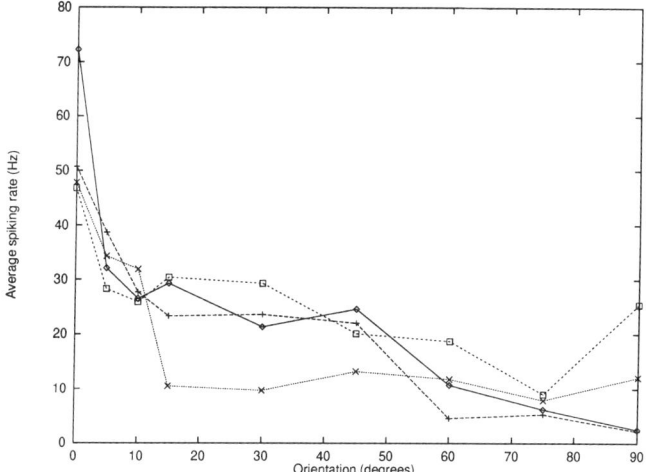

Figure 5: Orientation tuning curves for the model neurons. 'X': light bars centered in the receptive field; diamonds: light bars displaced by 6 pixels horizontally; squares: dark bars centered in the receptive field; '+': dark bars displaced by 6 pixels. Standard errors on the data are about 5 spikes/sec.

[5] J.G. Malpeli, C. Lee, H.D. Schwark, and T.G. Weyand. Cat area 17. I. Pattern of thalamic control of cortical layers. *J. Neurophyiol.*, 46:1102–1119, 1981.

[6] B.W. Mel. The clusteron: Toward a simple abstraction for a complex neuron. In J. Moody, S. Hanson, and R. Lippmann, editors, *Advances in Neural Information Processing Systems, vol. 4*, pages 35–42. Morgan Kaufmann, San Mateo, CA, 1992.

[7] B.W. Mel. NMDA-based pattern discrimination in a modeled cortical neuron. *Neural Computation*, 4:502–516, 1992.

[8] B.W. Mel. Synaptic integration in an excitable dendritic tree. *J. Neurophysiol.*, 70(3):1086–1101, 1993.

[9] B.W. Mel. Information processing in dendritic trees. *Neural Computation*, 6:1031–1085, 1994.

[10] J.A. Movshon. The velocity tuning of single units in cat striate cortex. *J. Physiol. (Lond)*, 249:445–468, 1975.

[11] I. Ohzawa, G.C. DeAngelis, and R.D Freeman. Stereoscopic depth discrimination in the visual cortex: Neurons ideally suited as disparity detectors. *Science*, 279:1037–1041, 1990.

[12] D. Pollen and S. Ronner. Visual cortical neurons as localized spatial frequency filters. *IEEE Trans. Sys. Man Cybern.*, 13:907–916, 1983.

[13] H.R. Wilson, D. Levi, L. Maffei, J. Rovamo, and R. DeValois. The perception of form: retina to striate cortex. In L. Spillman and J.S. Werner, editors, *Visual perception: the neurophysiological foundations*, pages 231–272. Academic Press, San Diego, 1990.

Orientation contrast sensitivity from long-range interactions in visual cortex

Klaus R. Pawelzik, Udo Ernst, Fred Wolf, Theo Geisel
Institut für Theoretische Physik and SFB 185 Nichtlineare Dynamik,
Universität Frankfurt, D-60054 Frankfurt/M., and
MPI für Strömungsforschung, D-37018 Göttingen, Germany
email: {klaus,udo,fred,geisel}@chaos.uni-frankfurt.de

Abstract

Recently Sillito and coworkers (Nature **378**, pp. 492, 1995) demonstrated that stimulation beyond the classical receptive field (cRF) can not only modulate, but radically change a neuron's response to oriented stimuli. They revealed that patch–suppressed cells when stimulated with contrasting orientations inside and outside their cRF can strongly respond to stimuli oriented orthogonal to their nominal preferred orientation. Here we analyze the emergence of such complex response patterns in a simple model of primary visual cortex. We show that the observed sensitivity for orientation contrast can be explained by a delicate interplay between local isotropic interactions and patchy long–range connectivity between distant iso–orientation domains. In particular we demonstrate that the observed properties might arise without specific connections between sites with cross-oriented cRFs.

1 Introduction

Long range horizontal connections form a ubiquitous structural element of intracortical circuitry. In the primary visual cortex long range horizontal connections extend over distances spanning several hypercolumns and preferentially connect cells of similar orientation preference [1, 2, 3, 4]. Recent evidence suggests that their physiological effect depends on the level of postsynaptic depolarization; acting exitatory on weakly activated and inhibitory on strongly activated cells [5, 6]. This differential influence possibly underlies perceptual phenomena as 'pop out' and 'fill in' [9]. Previous modeling studies demonstrated that such differential interactions may arise from a single set of long range excitatory connections terminating both on excitatory and inhibitory neurons in a given target column [7, 8]. By and large these results suggest that long range horizontal connections between columns of like stimulus preference provide a central mechanism for the context dependent regulation of activation in cortical networks.

Recent experiments by Sillito et al. suggest, however, that lateral connections in primary visual cortex can also induce more radical changes in receptive field organization [10]. Most importantly this study shows that patch–suppressed cells can respond selectively to orientation contrast between center and surround of a stimulus even if they are centrally stimulated orthogonal to their preferred orientation. Sillito et al. argued, that these response properties require specific connections between orthogonally tuned columns for which, however, presently there is only weak evidence.

Here we demonstrate that such nonclassical receptive field properties might instead arise as an emergent property of the known intracortical circuitry. We investigate a simple model for intracortical activity dynamics driven by weakly orientation tuned afferent excitation. The cortical actitvity dynamics is based on a continous firing rate description and incorporates both a local center–surround type interaction and long range connections between distant columns of like orientation preference. The connections of distant orientation columns are assumed to act either excitatory or inhibitory depending on the activation of their target neurons. It turns out that this set of interactions not only leads to the emergence of patch–suppressed cells, but also that a large fraction of these cells exhibits a selectivity for orientation contrast very similar to the one observed by Sillito et al. .

2 Model

Our target is the analysis of basic rate modulations emerging from local and long range feedback interactions in a simple model of visual cortex. It is therefore appropriate to consider a simple rate dynamics $\dot{\mathbf{x}} = -c \cdot \mathbf{x} + F(\mathbf{x})$, where $\mathbf{x} = \{x_i, i = 1...N\}$ are the activation levels of N neurons. $F(\mathbf{x}) = g(I_{mex}(\mathbf{x}) + I_{lat}(\mathbf{x}) + I_{ext})$, where $g(I) = c_0 \cdot (I - I_{thres})$ if $I > I_{thres}$, and $g(I) = 0$ otherwise, denotes the firing rate or gain function in dependence of the input I.

The neurons are arranged in a quadratic array representing a small part of the visual cortex. Within this layer, neuron i has a position $\mathbf{r}_i$ and a preferred orientation $\Phi_i \in [0, 180]$. The input to neuron i has three contributions $I_i = I_i^{mex} + I_i^{lat} + I_i^{ext}$. $I_i^{mex} = \epsilon_{mex} \cdot \sum_{j=1}^{N} w_{ij}^{mex} x_j$ is due to a mexican-hat shaped coupling structure with weights w_{ij}^{mex}, $I_{lat} = \epsilon_{lat} \cdot w_L(x_i) \cdot \sum_{j=1}^{N} w_{ij}^{lat} x_j$ denotes input from long-range orientation-specific interactions with weights w_{ij}^{lat}, and the third term models the orientation dependent external input $I_{ext} = \epsilon_{ext} \cdot I_{0,i}^{ext} \cdot (1 + \eta_i)$, where η_i denotes the noise added to the external input. $w_L(x)$ regulates the strength and sign of the long-

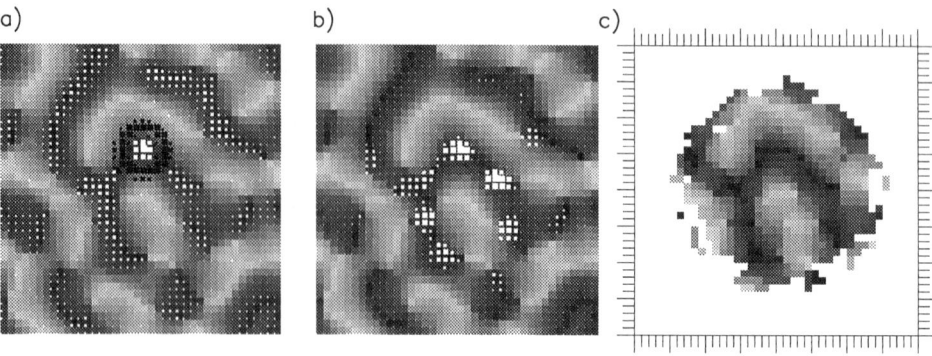

Figure 1: Structure and response properties of the model network. a) Coupling structure from one neuron on a grid of $N = 1600$ elements projected on the orientation preference map which was used for stimulation ($\Phi_i, i = 1...N$). Inhibitory and excitatory couplings are marked with black and white squares, respectively, the sizes of which represent the coupling strength. b) Activation pattern of the network driven by a central stimulus of radius $r_c = 11$ and horizontal orientation. c) Self-consistent orientation map calculated from the activation patterns for all stimulus orientations. Note that this map matches the input orientation preference map shown in a) and b).

range lateral interaction in dependence of the postsynaptic activation, summarizing the behavior of a local circuit in which the inhibitory population has a larger gain.

In particular, $w_l(x)$ can be derived analytically from a simple cortical microcircuit (Fig.2). This circuit consists of an inhibitory and excitatory cell population connected reciprocally. Each population receives lateral input and is driven by the external stimulus I. The effective interaction w_L depends on the lateral input L and external input I. Assuming a piecewise linear gain function for each population, similar as those for the x_i's, the phase-space I-L is partitioned in some regions. Only if both I **and** L are small, w_L is positive; justifying the choice $w_L = x_{sh} - \tanh(0.55 \cdot (x - x_a)/x_b)$ which we used for our simulations.

The weights w_{ij}^{mex} are given by

$$w_{ij}^{mex} = -a_{ex} \cdot |\mathbf{r}_i - \mathbf{r}_j|^2 + b_{ex} \quad \text{for} \quad |\mathbf{r}_i - \mathbf{r}_j| \leq r_{ex}$$
$$w_{ij}^{mex} = a_{in} \cdot |\mathbf{r}_i - \mathbf{r}_j|^2 - b_{in} \quad \text{for} \quad r_{ex} < |\mathbf{r}_i - \mathbf{r}_j| \leq r_{in} \quad (1)$$

and $w_{ij}^{mex} = 0$ otherwise. In this representation of the local interactions weights and scales are independently controllable. In particular if we define

$$a_{ex} = \frac{2}{\pi r_{ex}^4}, \quad a_{in} = \frac{2 \cdot c_{rel}}{\pi (r_{in} + r_{ex})(r_{in} - r_{ex})^3}, \quad b_{ex} = a_{ex} r_{ex}^2, \quad b_{in} = a_{in}(r_{in} - r_{ex})^2 \quad (2)$$

r_{ex} and r_{in} denote the range of the excitatory and inhibitory part of the mexican hat, respectively. Here we used $r_{ex} = 2.5$ and $r_{in} = 4.0$. c_{rel} controls the balances of inhibition and excitation. With constant activation level $x_i = x_0 \; \forall i$ the inhibition is c_{rel} times higher than the excitation and $I_{mex} = \epsilon_{mex} \cdot (1 - c_{rel}) \cdot x_0$.

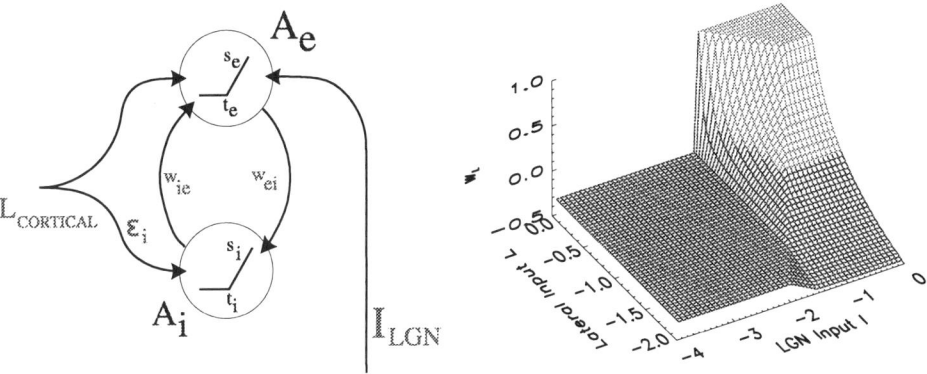

Figure 2: Local cortical circuit (left), consisting of an inhibitory and an excitatory population of neurons interconnected with weights w_{ie}, w_{ei}, and stimulated with lateral input L and external input I. By substituting this circuit with one single excitatory unit, we need a differential instead of a fixed lateral coupling strength (w_L, right), which is positive only for small I and L.

The weights w_{ij}^{lat} are

$$w_{ij}^{lat} = c_{lat} \exp\left(-\frac{|\Phi_i - \Phi_j|^2}{2\sigma_{lat,\Phi}^2}\right) \exp\left(-\frac{|\mathbf{r}_i - \mathbf{r}_j|^2}{2\sigma_{lat,r}^2}\right) \quad \text{if } |\mathbf{r}_i - \mathbf{r}_j| > r_{in} \quad (3)$$

and 0 otherwise. $\sigma_{lat,\phi}$ and $\sigma_{lat,r}$ provide the orientation selectivity and the range of the long-range lateral interaction, respectively. The additional parameter c_{lat} normalizes w_{ij}^{lat} such that $\sum_{j=1}^{N} w_{ij}^{lat} \approx 1$.

[1]

The spatial width and the orientation selectivity of the input fields are modeled by a convolution with a Gaussian kernel before projected onto the cortical layer

$$I_{0,i}^{ext.} = \frac{1}{2\pi\sigma_{recp,r}^2} \sum_{j=1}^{N}\left[\exp\left(\frac{|\mathbf{r}_i - \mathbf{r}_j|^2}{2\sigma_{recp,r}^2}\right) \cdot \exp\left(-\frac{|\Phi_i - \Phi_j|^2}{2\sigma_{recp,\Phi}^2}\right)\right].$$

In our simulations, the orientation preference of a cortical neuron i was given by the orientation preference map displayed in Fig1a.

3 Results

We analyzed stationary states of our model depending on stimulus conditions. The external input, a center stimulus of radius $r_c = 6$ at orientation Φ_c and an annulus

---

[1]The following parameters have been used in our simulations leading to the results shown in Figs.1-4. $\eta_i = 0.1$ (external input noise), $\epsilon_{mex} = 2.2$, $\epsilon_{lat} = 1.5$, $\epsilon_{ext} = 1.3$, $A_{sh} = 0.0$, $A_a = 0.2$, $A_b = 0.05$, $t_e = 0.6$, $s_e = 0.5$, $c_{rel} = 2.0$ (balance between inhibition and excitation), c_{lat} normalizes w_{ij}^{lat} such that $\sum_{j=1}^{N} w_{ij}^{lat} \approx 1$, $\sigma_{lat,\phi} = 20$, $\sigma_{lat,r} = 15$ $\sigma_{recp,r} = 5$, $\sigma_{recp,\Phi} = 40$, $r_{ex} = 2.5$, and $r_{in} = 5.0$.

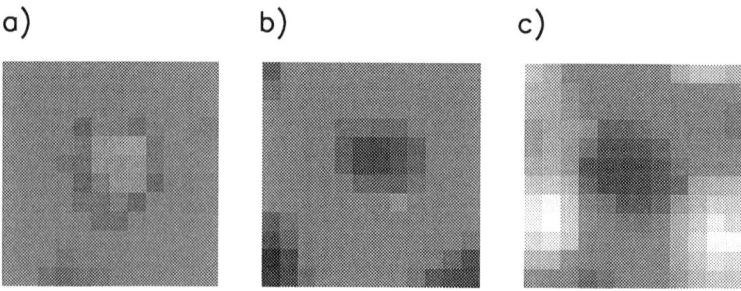

Figure 3: Changes in patterns of activity induced by the additional presentation of a surround stimulus. Grey levels encode increase (darker grey) or decrease (lighter grey) in activation **x**. a) center and surround parallel, b) and c) center and surround orthogonal. While in b), the center is stimulated with the preferred orientation, in c), the center is stimulated with the non-preferred orientation.

of inner radius r_c and outer radius $r_s = 18$ at orientation Φ_s, was projected onto a grid of $N = 40 \times 40$ elements (Fig.1a). Simulations were performed for 20 orientations equally spaced in the interval $[0, 180°]$. When an oriented stimulus was presented to the center we found blob-like activity patterns centered on the corresponding iso–orientation domains (Fig.1b). Simulations utilizing the full set of orientations recovered the input-specificity and demonstrated the self-consistency of the parameter set chosen (Fig.1c). While in this case there were still some deviations, stimulation of the whole field yielded perfect self-consistency (not shown) in the sense of virtually identical afferent and response based orientation preferences.

For combinations of center and surround inputs we observed patch–suppressed regions. These regions exhibited substantial responses for cross–oriented stimuli which often exceeded the response to an optimal center stimulus alone. Figs.3 and 4 summarize these results. Fig.3 shows responses to center–surround combinations compared to activity patterns resulting from center stimulation only. Obviously certain regions within the model were strongly patch–suppressed (Fig.3, light patches for same orientations of center and surround). Interestingly a large fraction of these locations exhibited enhanced activation when center and surround stimulus were orthogonal. Fig.4 displays tuning curves of patch–suppressed cells for variing the orientation of the surround stimulus. Clearly these cells exhibited an enhancement of most responses and a substantial selectivity for orientation contrast. Parameter variation indicated that qualitatively these results do not depend sensitively of the set of parameters chosen.

4 Summary and Discussion

Our model implements only elementary assumptions about intracortical interactions. A local sombrero shaped feedback is well known to induce localized blobs of activity with a stereotyped shape [12]. This effect lies at the basis of many models of visual cortex, as e.g. for the explanation of contrast independence of orientation

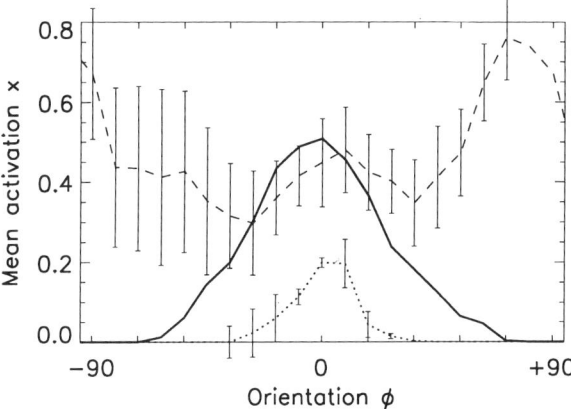

Figure 4: Tuning curves for patch–suppressed cells preferring a horizontal stimulus within their cRF. The bold line shows the orientation tuning curve of the response to an isolated center stimulus. The dashed and dotted lines show the tuning curve when stimulating with a horizontal (dashed) and a vertical (dotted) center stimulus while rotating the surround stimulus. The curves have been averaged over 6 units.

tuning [13, 14]. Long range connections selectively connect columns of similar orientation preference which is consistent with current anatomical knowledge [3, 4]. The differential effect of this set of connections onto the target population was modeled by a continuous sign change of their effective action depending on the level of post-synaptic input or activation. Orientation maps were used to determine the input specificity and we assumed a rather weak selectivity of the afferent connections and a restricted contrast which implies that every stimulus provides some input also to orthogonally tuned cells. This means that long-range excitatory connections, while not effective when only the surround is stimulated, can very well be sufficient for driving cells if the stimulus to the center is orthogonal to their preferred orientation (Contrast sensitivity).

In our model we find a large fraction of cells that exhibit sensitivity for center surround stimuli. It turns out that most of the patch–suppressed cells respond to orientation contrasts, i.e. they are strongly selective for *orientation discontinuities* between center and surround. We also find contrast enhancement, i.e. larger responses to the preferred orientation in the center when stimulated with an orthogonal surround than if stimulated only centrally (Fig.4). The latter constitutes a genuinely emergent property, since no selective cross–oriented connections are present.

This phenomenon can be understood as a desinhibitory effect. Since no cells having long-range connections to the center unit are activated, the additional sub-threshold input from outside the classical receptive field can evoke a larger response (Contrast enhancement). Contrarily, if center and surround are stimulated with the same orientation, all the cells with similar orientation preference become activated such that the long-range connections can strongly inhibit the center unit (Patch suppression). In other words, while the lack of inhibitory influences from the surround should recover the response with an amplitude similar or higher to the local stimulation, the orthogonal surround effectively leads to a desinhibition for some of the cells.

Our results show a surprising agreement with previous findings on non-classical receptive field properties which culminated in the paper by Sillito et al. [10]. Our simple model clearly demonstrates that the known intracortical interactions might lead to surprising effects on receptive fields. While this contribution concentrated on analyzing the origin of selectivities for orientation discontinuities we expect that the pursued level of abstraction has a large potential for analyzing a wide range of non-classical receptive fields. Despite its simplicity we believe that our model captures the main features of rate interactions. More detailed models based on spiking neurons, however, will exhibit additional dynamical effects like correlations and synchrony which will be at the focus of our future research.

Acknowledgement: We acknowledge inspiring discussions with S. Löwel and J. Cowan. This work was supported by the Deutsche Forschungsgemeinschaft.

References

[1] D. Ts'o, C.D. Gilbert, and T.N. Wiesel, J. Neurosci **6**, 1160-1170 (1986).

[2] C.D. Gilbert and T.N. Wiesel, J. Neurosci. **9**, 2432-2442 (1989).

[3] S. Löwel and W. Singer, Science **255**, 209 (1992).

[4] R. Malach, Y. Amir, M. Harel, and A. Grinvald, PNAS **90**, 10469-10473 (1993).

[5] J.A. Hirsch and C.D. Gilbert, J. Neurosci. **6**, 1800-1809 (1991).

[6] M. Weliky, K. Kandler, D. Fitzpatrick, and L.C. Katz, Neuron **15**, 541-552 (1995).

[7] M. Stemmler, M. Usher, and E. Niebur, Science **269**, 1877-1880 (1995).

[8] L.J. Toth, D.C. Sommers, S.C. Rao, E.V. Todorov, D.-S. Kim, S.B. Nelson, A.G. Siapas, and M. Sur, preprint 1995.

[9] U. Polat, D. Sagi, Vision Res. **7**, 993-999 (1993).

[10] A.M. Sillito, K.L. Grieve, H.E. Jones, J. Cudeiro, and J. Davis, Nature **378**, 492-496 (1995).

[11] J.J. Knierim and D.C. van Essen, J. Neurophys. **67**, 961-980 (1992).

[12] H.R. Wilson and J. Cowan, Biol. Cyb. **13**, 55-80 (1973).

[13] R. Ben-Yishai, R.L. Bar-Or, and H. Sompolinsky, Proc. Nat. Acad. Sci. **92**, 3844-3848 (1995).

[14] D. Sommers, S.B. Nelson, and M. Sur, J. Neurosci. **15**, 5448-5465 (1995).

Statistically Efficient Estimation Using Cortical Lateral Connections

Alexandre Pouget
alex@salk.edu

Kechen Zhang
zhang@salk.edu

Abstract

Coarse codes are widely used throughout the brain to encode sensory and motor variables. Methods designed to interpret these codes, such as population vector analysis, are either inefficient, i.e., the variance of the estimate is much larger than the smallest possible variance, or biologically implausible, like maximum likelihood. Moreover, these methods attempt to compute a *scalar* or *vector* estimate of the encoded variable. Neurons are faced with a similar estimation problem. They must read out the responses of the presynaptic neurons, but, by contrast, they typically encode the variable with a further population code rather than as a scalar. We show how a non-linear recurrent network can be used to perform these estimation in an optimal way while keeping the estimate in a coarse code format. This work suggests that lateral connections in the cortex may be involved in cleaning up uncorrelated noise among neurons representing similar variables.

1 Introduction

Most sensory and motor variables in the brain are encoded with coarse codes, i.e., through the activity of large populations of neurons with broad tuning to the variables. For instance, direction of visual motion is believed to be encoded in visual area MT by the responses of a large number of cells with bell-shaped tuning, as illustrated in figure 1-A.

Neurophysiological recordings have shown that, in response to an object moving along a particular direction, the pattern of activity across such a population would look like a noisy hill of activity (figure 1-B). On the basis of this activity, $\vec{A}$, the best that can be done is to recover the conditional probability of the direction of motion, θ, given the activity, $p(\theta|\vec{A})$. A slightly less ambitious goal is to come up with a good "guess", or estimate, $\hat{\theta}$, of the direction, θ, given the activity. Because of the stochastic nature of the noise, the estimator is a random variable, i.e, for

---

[0] AP is at the Institute for Computational and Cognitive Sciences, Georgetown University, Washington, DC 20007 and KZ is at The Salk Institute, La Jolla, CA 92037 . This work was funded by McDonnell-Pew and Howard Hughes Medical Institute.

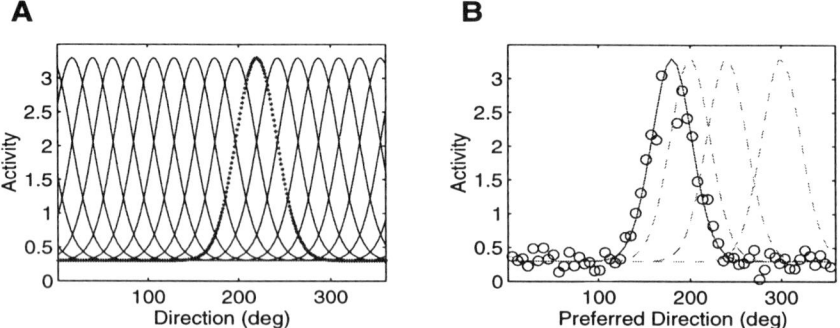

Figure 1: A- Tuning curves for 16 direction tuned neurons. B- Noisy pattern of activity (o) from 64 neurons when presented with a direction of 180°. The ML estimate is found by moving an "expected" hill of activity (dotted line) until the squared distance with the data is minimized (solid line)

the same image, $\hat{\theta}$ will vary from trial to trial. A good estimator should have the smallest possible variance across those trials because the variance determines how well two similar directions can be discriminated using this estimator. The Cramér-Rao bound provides an analytical lower bound for this variance given the noise in the system and the unit tuning curves [5]. Typically, computationally simple estimators, such as optimum linear estimator (OLE), are very inefficient; their variances are several times the bound. By contrast, Bayesian or maximum likelihood (ML) estimators (which are equivalent for the case under consideration in this paper) can reach this bound but require more complex calculations [5].

These decoding technics are valuable for a neurophysiologist interested in reading out the population code but they are not directly relevant for understanding how neural circuits perform estimation. In particular, they all provide the estimate in a format which is incompatible with what we know of sensory representations in the cortex. For example, cells in V4 are estimating orientation from the noisy responses of orientation tuned V1 cells, but, unlike ML or OLE which provide a scalar estimate, V4 neurons retain orientation in a coarse code format, as demonstrated by the fact that V4 cells are just as broadly tuned to orientation as V1 neurons.

Therefore, it seems that a theory of estimation in biological networks should have two critical characteristics: 1- it should preserve the estimate in a coarse code and 2- it should be efficient, i.e., the variance should be close to the Cramér-Rao bound. We explore in this paper various network architectures for performing estimations with coarse code using lateral connections. We start by briefly describing several classical estimators such as OLE or ML. Then, we consider linear and non-linear recurrent networks and compare their performances with the classical estimators.

2 Classical Methods

The simplest estimators are linear of the form $\hat{\theta}_{OLE} = \vec{W}^T \vec{A}$. Better performance can be obtained with a center of mass estimator (COM), $\hat{\theta}_{COM} = \sum_i \theta_i a_i / \sum_i a_i$; however, in the case of a periodic variable, such as direction of motion, the best one-shot method known is the complex estimator (COMP), $\hat{\theta}_{COMP} = phase(z)$ where $z = \sum_{k=1}^{N} a_k e^{i\theta_k}$ [5]. This estimator consists in fitting a cosine through the pattern of activity, like the one shown in figure 1-B, and using the phase of

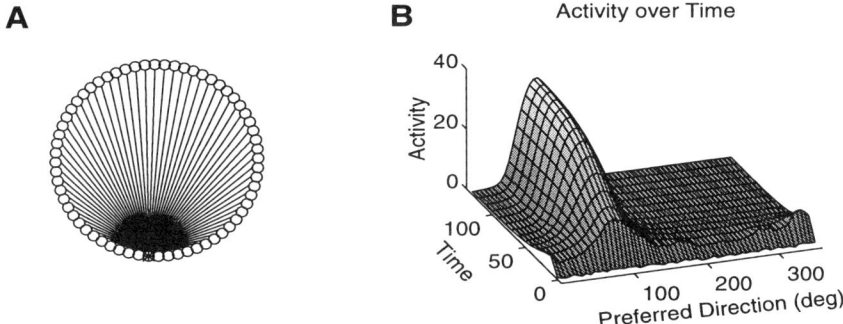

Figure 2: A- Circular network of 64 units. Only the connections originating from one unit are shown. B- Activity over time in the non-linear network when initialized with a random pattern at $t = 0$. The activity of the units are plotted as a function of their position along the circle which is equivalent to their preferred direction of motion with appropriate choice of weights.

the best cosine fit as the estimate of direction. This method is suboptimal if the data were not generated by cosine tuning functions as in the case illustrated in figure 1-A. It is possible to obtain optimum performance by fitting the curve that was actually used to generate the data, i.e, the actual tuning curves of the units. A maximum likelihood estimate, defined as being the direction maximizing $p(\vec{A}|\theta)$, involves exactly this type of curve fitting, a process illustrated in figure 1-B [5]. The estimate is computed by finding first the "expected" hill– the hill that would be obtained in a noise free system– minimizing the distance with the data. In the case of gaussian noise, the appropriate distance measure to minimize is the euclidian squared distance. The final position of the peak of the hill corresponds to the maximum likelihood estimate, $\hat{\theta}_{ML}$.

3 Recurrent Networks

Consider a circular network of 64 units fully connected like the one depicted in figure 2-A. With an appropriate choice of weights and activation function, this network will develop a hill-shaped pattern of activity in response to a transient input as illustrated in figure 2-B. If we initialize this networks with activity patterns $\vec{A} = \{a_i\}$ corresponding to the responses of 64 direction tuned units (figure 1), we can use the final position of the hill across the neuronal array after relaxation as an estimate of the direction, θ. The variance of this estimator will depend on the exact choice of activation function and weights.

3.1 Linear Network

We first consider a network of 64 units whose dynamics is governed by the following difference equation:

$$o_i(t + \delta t) = o_i(t) + \delta t \left(-o_i(t) + \sum_{j=1}^{N} w_{ij} o_j(t) \right) \quad (1)$$

The dynamics of such networks is well understood [3]. If each unit receives the same weight vector $\vec{w}$, then the weight matrix W is symmetric. In this case, the network dynamics amplifies or suppresses the Fourier component of the initial input pattern, $\{a_i\}$, independently by a factors equal to the corresponding component of the Fourier transform, $\vec{\tilde{w}}$, of $\vec{w}$. For example, if the first component of $\vec{\tilde{w}}$ is more than one (resp. less than one) the first Fourier component of the initial pattern of activity will be amplified (resp. suppressed).

Thus, we can choose W such that the network amplifies selectively the first Fourier component of the data while suppressing the others. The network would be unstable but if we stop after a large, yet fixed, number of iterations, the activity pattern would look like a cosine function of direction with a phase corresponding to the phase of the first Fourier components of the data. In other words, the network would end up fitting a cosine function in the data which is equivalent to the COMP method described above. A network for orientation selectivity proposed by Ben-Yishai et al [1] is closely related to this linear network.

Although this method keeps the estimate in a coarse code format, it suffers two problems: it is unclear how it could be extended to non periodic variables, such as disparity, and it is suboptimal since it is equivalent to the COMP estimator.

3.2 Non-Linear Network

We consider next a network of 64 units fully connected whose dynamics is governed by the following difference equations:

$$o_i(t) = g(u_i(t)) = 6.3 \left(\log \left(1 + e^{5+10u_i(t)} \right) \right)^{0.8} \quad (2)$$

$$u_i(t + \delta t) = u_i(t) + \delta t \left(-u_i(t) + \sum_{j=1}^{N} w_{ij} o_j(t) \right) \quad (3)$$

Zhang (1996) has demonstrated that with appropriate symmetric weights, $\{w_{ij}\}$, this network develops a stable hill of activity in response to an arbitrary transient input pattern $\{I_i\}$(figure 2-B). The shape of the hill is fully specified by the weights and activation function whereas, by contrast, the final position of the hill on the neuronal array depends only on the initial input. Therefore, like ML, the network fits an "expected" function through the data. We first present a set of simulations in which we investigated whether ML and the network place the hill at the same location.

Methods: The simulations consisted estimating the value of the direction of a moving bar based on the activity, $\vec{A} = \{a_i\}$, of 64 input units with hill-shaped tuning to direction corrupted by noise. We used circular normal functions like the ones showed in figure 1-A to model the mean activities, $f_i(\theta)$:

$$f_i(\theta) = 3\exp(7(\cos(\theta - \theta_i) - 1)) + 0.3 \quad (4)$$

The value 0.3 corresponds to the mean spontaneous activity of each unit. The peak, θ_i, of the circular normal functions were uniformly spread over the interval $[0°, 360°]$. The activities, $\{a_i\}$, depended on the noise distribution. We used two types of noise, normally distributed with fixed variance, $\sigma_n^2 = 1$ and Poisson distributed:

$$P(a_i = a|\theta) = \frac{1}{\sqrt{2\pi\sigma_n^2}} \exp\left(-\frac{(a - f_i(\theta))^2}{2\sigma_n^2}\right), \quad P(a_i = k|\theta) = \frac{f_i(\theta)^k e^{-f_i(\theta)}}{k!} \quad (5)$$

Our results compare the standard deviation of four estimators, OLE, COM, COMP and ML to the non-linear recurrent network (RN) with *transient* inputs (the input patterns are shown on the first iteration only). In the case of ML, we used the

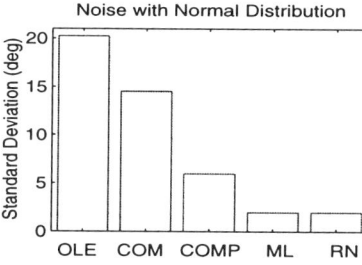 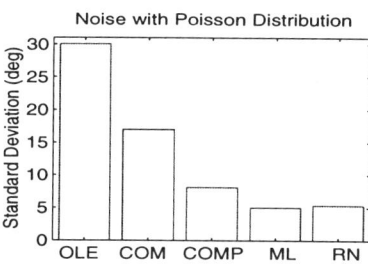

Figure 3: Histogram of the standard deviations of the estimate for all five methods

Cramér-Rao bound to compute the standard deviation as described in Seung and Sompolinsky (1993). The weights in the recurrent network were chosen such that the final pattern of activity in the network have a profile very similar to the tuning function $f_i(\theta)$.

Results: Since the preferred direction of two consecutive units in the network are more than 5° apart, we first wonder whether RN estimates exhibit a bias— a difference between the mean estimate and the true direction— in particular for directions between the peaks of two consecutive units. Our simulations showed no significant bias for any of the orientations tested (not shown). Next, we compared standard deviations of the estimates for all five methods and for the two types of noise. The RN method was found to outperform the OLE, COM and COMP estimators in both cases and to match the Cramér-Rao bound for gaussian noise (figure 3) as suggested by our analysis. For noise with Poisson distribution, the standard deviation for RN was only 0.344° above ML (figure 3).

We also estimated numerically $-\partial\hat{\theta}_{RN}/\partial a_i|_{\theta=170°}$, the derivative of the RN estimate with respect to the *initial* activity of each of 64 units for an orientation of 170°. This derivative in the case of ML matches closely the derivative of the cell tuning curve, $f'(\theta)$. In other words, in ML, units contribute to the estimate according to the amplitude of the derivative of the tuning curve. As shown in figure the same is true for RN, $-\partial\hat{\theta}_{RN}/\partial a_i|_{\theta=170°}$ matches closely the derivative of the units tuning curves. In contrast, the same derivatives for the COMP estimate, (dotted line), or the COM estimate, (dash-dotted line), do not match the profile of $f'(\theta)$. In particular, units with preferred direction far away from 170°, i.e. units whose activity is just noise, end up contributing to the final estimate, hindering the performance of the estimator.

We also looked at the standard deviation of the RN as a function of time, i.e., the number of iterations. Reaching a stable state can take up to several hundred iterations which could make the RN method too slow for any practical purpose. We found however that the standard deviation decreases very rapidly over the first 5-6 iterations and reaches asymptotic values after around 20 iterations (figure 4-B). Therefore, there is no need to wait for a perfectly stable pattern of activity to obtain minimum standard deviation.

Analysis: One way to determine which factors control the final position of the hill is to find a function, called a Lyapunov function, which is minimized over time by the network dynamics. Cohen and Grossberg (1983) have shown that network characterized by the dynamical equation above and in which the input pattern $\{sI_i\}$

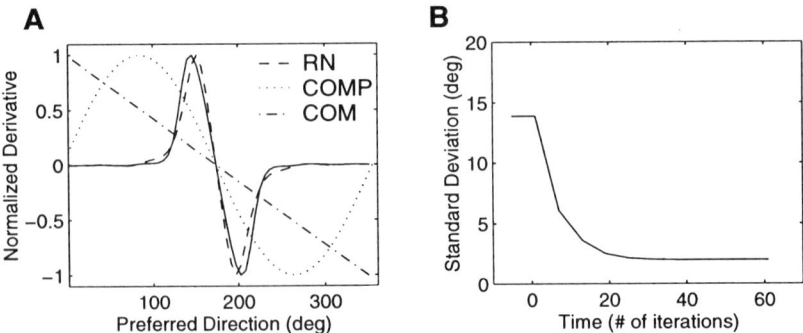

Figure 4: A- Comparison of $g'(\theta)$ (solid line), $-\partial \hat{\theta}/\partial a_i|_{\theta=170°}$ for RN, COMP and COM. All functions have been normalized to one. B- Standard deviation as a function of the number of iterations for RN.

is clamped, minimizes a Lyapunov function of the form:

$$L = -\frac{1}{2}\sum_{i,j} w_{ij} g(u_i) g(u_j) + \sum_i \int_0^{u_i} z g'(z)\, dz - s \sum_i I_i g(u_i). \quad (6)$$

The last term is the dot product between the input pattern, $\{sI_i\}$, and the current activity pattern, $\{g(u_i)\}$, on the neuronal array. Here s is simply a scaling factor for the input pattern. The dynamics of the network will therefore tend to minimize $-\sum_i I_i g(u_i)$, or equivalently, to maximize the overlap between the stable pattern and the input pattern. The other terms however are also dependent on I_i because the shape of the final stable activity profile depends on the input pattern. Therefore the network will settle into a compromise between maximizing overlap and getting the right profile given the clamped input.

We can show however that, for small input (i.e., as the scaling factor $s \to 0$), the dominant term in the Lyapunov function is the dot product. To see this, we consider the Taylor expansion of Lyapunov function L with respect to s. First, let $\{U_i\}$ denote the profile of the stable activity $\{u_i\}$ in the limit of zero input ($s \to 0$), and then write the corresponding value of the Lyapunov function at zero input as L_0. Now keeping only the first-order terms of s in the Taylor expansion, we obtain:

$$L \approx L_0 - s \sum_i I_i g(U_i). \quad (7)$$

This means that the dot product is the only first order term of s, and disturbances to the shape of the final activity profile contribute only to higher order terms of s, which are negligible when s is small. Notice that in the limit of zero input, the shape of the activity profile $\{U_i\}$ is fixed, and the only thing unknown is its peak position. Because L_0 is a constant, the global minimum of the Lyapunov function here should correspond to a peak position which maximizes the dot product. The difference between u_i and U_i is negligible for sufficiently small input because, by definition, $u_i \to U_i$ as $s \to 0$. Consequently, for small input, the network will converge to a solution maximizing primarily $\sum_i I_i g(u_i)$, which is mathematically equivalent to minimizing the square distance between the input and the output pattern.

Therefore, if we use an activity pattern, $\vec{A} = \{a_i\}$, as the input to this network, the stable hill should have its peak at a position very close to the direction corresponding to the maximum likelihood estimate (under the assumption of gaussian noise), provided the network is not attracted into a local minimum of the Liapunov function. This result is valid when using a small *clamped* input but our simulations show that a *transient* input is sufficient to reach the Cramér-Rao bound.

4 Discussion

Our results demonstrate that it is possible to perform efficient unbiased estimation with coarse coding using a neurally plausible architecture. Our model relies on lateral connections to implement a prior expectation on the profile of the activity patterns. As a consequence, units determine their activation according to their own input and the activity of their neighbors. This approach shows that one of the advantages of coarse code is to provide a representation which simplifies the problem of cleaning up uncorrelated noise within a neuronal population.

Unlike OLE, COM and COMP, the RN estimate is not the result of a voting process in which units vote from their preferred direction, θ_i. Instead, units turn out to contribute according to the derivatives of their tuning curves, $f'_i(\theta)$, as in the case of ML. This feature allows the network to ignore background noise, that is to say, responses due to other factors beside the variable of interest. This property also predicts that discrimination of directions around the vertical (90°) would be most affected by shutting off the units tuned at 60° and 120°. This prediction is consistent with psychophysical experiments showing that discrimination around the vertical in human is affected by prior adaptation to orientations displaced from the vertical by ±30° [4].

Our approach can be readily extended to any other periodic sensory or motor variables. For non periodic variables such as the disparity of a line in an image, our network needs to be adapted since it currently relies on circular symmetrical weights. Simply unfolding the network will be sufficient to deal with values around the center of the interval under consideration, but more work is needed to deal with boundary values. We can also generalize this approach to arbitrary mapping between two coarse codes for variables x and y where y is a function of x. Indeed, a coarse code for x provides a set of radial basis functions of x which can be subsequently used to approximate arbitrary functions. It is even conceivable to use a similar approach for one-to-many mappings, a common situation in vision or robotics, by adapting our network such that several hills can coexist simultaneously.

References

[1] R. Ben-Yishai, R. L. Bar-Or, and H. Sompolinsky. *Proc. Natl. Acad. Sci. USA*, 92:3844–3848, 1995.

[2] M. Cohen and S. Grossberg. *IEEE Trans. SMC*, 13:815–826, 1983.

[3] M. Hirsch and S. Smale. *Differential equations, dynamical systems and linear algebra*. Academic Press, New York, 1974.

[4] D. M. Regan and K. I. Beverley. *J. Opt. Soc. Am.*, 2:147–155, 1985.

[5] H. S. Seung and H. Sompolinsky. *Proc. Natl. Acad. Sci. USA*, 90:10749–10753, 1993.

An Architectural Mechanism for Direction-tuned Cortical Simple Cells: The Role of Mutual Inhibition

Silvio P. Sabatini
silvio@dibe.unige.it

Fabio Solari
fabio@dibe.unige.it

Giacomo M. Bisio
bisio@dibe.unige.it

Department of Biophysical and Electronic Engineering
PSPC Research Group
Genova, I-16145, Italy

Abstract

A linear architectural model of cortical simple cells is presented. The model evidences how mutual inhibition, occurring through synaptic coupling functions asymmetrically distributed in space, can be a possible basis for a wide variety of spatio-temporal simple cell response properties, including direction selectivity and velocity tuning. While spatial asymmetries are included explicitly in the structure of the inhibitory interconnections, temporal asymmetries originate from the specific mutual inhibition scheme considered. Extensive simulations supporting the model are reported.

1 INTRODUCTION

One of the most distinctive features of striate cortex neurons is their combined selectivity for stimulus orientation and the direction of motion. The majority of simple cells, indeed, responds better to sinusoidal gratings that are moving in one direction than to the opposite one, exhibiting also a narrower velocity tuning with respect to that of geniculate cells. Recent theoretical and neurophysiological studies [1] [2] pointed out that the initial stage of direction selectivity can be related to the linear space-time receptive field structure of simple cells. A large class of simple cells has a very specific space-time behavior in which the spatial phase of the receptive field changes gradually as a function of time. This results in receptive field profiles that are tilted in the space-time domain. To account for the origin of this particular spatio-temporal inseparability, numerous models have been proposed postulating the existence of structural asymmetries of the geniculo-cortical projections both in the temporal and in the spatial domains (for a review, see [3]

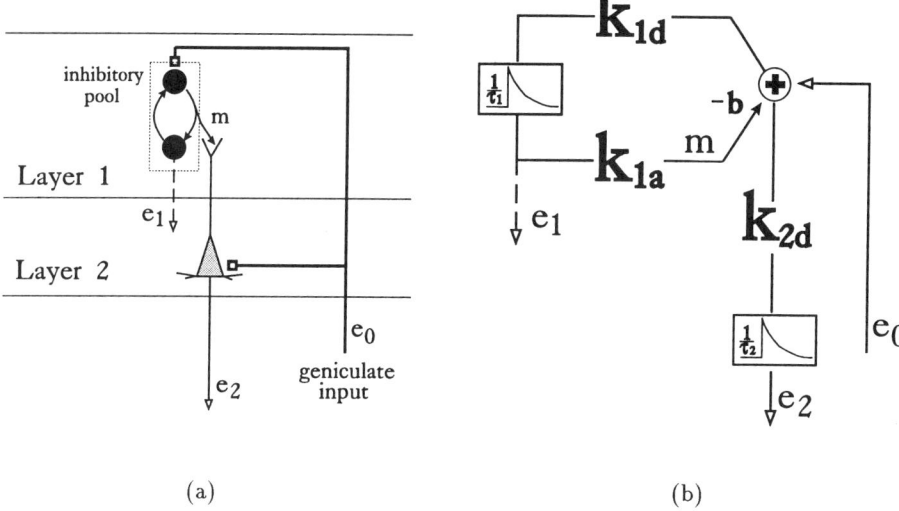

Figure 1: (a) A schematic neural circuitry for the mutual inhibition; (b) equivalent block diagram representation.

[4]). Among them, feed-forward inhibition along the non-preferred direction, and the combination of lagged and non-lagged geniculate inputs to the cortex have been commonly suggested as the major mechanisms.

In this paper, within a linear field theory framework, we propose and analyse an architectural model for dynamic receptive field formation, based on intracortical interactions occurring through asymmetric mutual inhibition schemes.

2 MODELING INTRACORTICAL PROCESSING

The computational characteristics of each neuron are not independent of the ones of other neurons laying in the same layer, rather, they are often the consequence of a collective behavior of neighboring cells. To understand how intracortical circuits may affect the response properties of simple cells one can study their structure and function at many levels of organization, from subcellular, driven primarily by biophysical data, to systemic, driven by functional considerations. In this study, we present a model at the intermediate abstraction level to combine both functional and neurophysiological descriptions into an analytic model of cortical simple cells.

2.1 STRUCTURE OF THE MODEL

Following a linear neural field approach [5] [6], we regard visual cortex as a continuous distribution of neurons and synapses. Accordingly, the geniculo-cortical pathway is modeled by a multi-layer network interconnected through feed-forward and feedback connections, both inter- and intra-layers. Each location on the cortical plane represents a homogeneous population of cells, and connections represent average interactions among populations. Such connections can be modeled by spatial coupling functions which represent the spread of the synaptic influence of a population on its neighbors, as mediated by local axonal and dendritic fields. From an architectural point of view, we assume the superposition of feed-forward (i.e., geniculate) and intracortical contributions which arise from inhibitory pools whose activity is also primed by a geniculate excitatory drive. A schematic diagram showing the "building blocks" of the model is depicted in Fig. 1. The dynamics of each population is modeled as first-order low-pass filters characterized by time constants τ's. For the sake of simplicity, we restrict our analysis to 1-D case, assuming that such direction is orthogonal to the preferred direction of the receptive field [7]. This 1-D model would produce spatio-temporal results that are directly compared with the spatio-temporal plots usually obtained when an optimal stimulus is moved along the direction orthogonal to the preferred direction of the receptive field.

Geniculate contributions $e_0(x,t)$ are modeled directly by a spatiotemporal convolution of the visual input $s(x,t)$ and a separable kernel $h_0(x,t)$ characterized in the spatial domain by a Gaussian shape with spatial extent σ_0 and, in the temporal domain, by a first-order temporal low-pass filter with time constant τ_0. The output $e_1(x,t)$ of the inhibitory neuron population results from the mutual inhibitory scheme through spatially organized pre- and post-synaptic sites, modeled by the kernels $k_{1a}(x-\xi)$ and $k_{1d}(x-\xi)$, respectively:

$$\tau_1 \frac{de_1(x,t)}{dt} = -e_1(x,t) + \int k_{1d}(x-\xi)[e_0(-\xi,t) - bm(-\xi,t)]d\xi \qquad (1)$$

$$m(x,t) = \int k_{1a}(x-\xi)e_1(-\xi)d\xi \qquad (2)$$

where the function $m(x,t)$ describes the spatio-temporal mutual inhibitory interactions, and b is the inhibition strength. The layer 2 cortical excitation $e_2(x,t)$ is the result of feed-forward contributions collected (k_{2d}) from the inhibitory loop, at axonal synaptic sites, and the geniculate input ($e_0(x,t)$). To focus the attention on the inhibitory loop, in the following we assume a one-to-one mapping from layer 1 to layer 2, i.e., $k_{2d}(x-\xi) = \delta(x-\xi)$, consequently:

$$\tau_2 \frac{de_2(x,t)}{dt} = -e_2(x,t) + e_0(x,t) - bm(x,t) \qquad (3)$$

where τ_1 and τ_2 are the time constants associated to layer 1 and layer 2, respectively.

2.2 AVERAGE INTRACORTICAL CONNECTIVITY

When assessing the role of intracortical circuits on the receptive field properties of cortical cells, one important issue concerns the spatial localization of inhibitory and excitatory influences. In a previous work [8] we evidenced how the steady-state solution of Eqs. (1)-(3) can give rise to highly structured Gabor-like receptive field profiles, when inhibition arises from laterally distributed clusters of cells. In this case, the effective intrinsic kernel $k_1(x)$, defined as $k_1(x-\xi) \stackrel{\text{def}}{=} \int \int k_{1a}(-x',-\xi')k_{1d}(x-x',\xi-\xi')dx'd\xi'$, can be modeled as the sum of two Gaussians symmetrically offset with respect to the target cell (see Fig. 2):

$$k_1(x) = \frac{1}{\sqrt{2\pi}} \left(\frac{w_1}{\sigma_1} \exp[-(x-d_1)^2/2\sigma_1^2] + \frac{w_2}{\sigma_2} \exp[-(x+d_2)^2/2\sigma_2^2] \right). \qquad (4)$$

This work is aimed to investigate how spatial asymmetries in the intracortical coupling function lead to non-separable space-time interactions within the resulting discharge field of the simple cells. To this end, we varied systematically the geometrical parameters (σ, w, d) of the inhibitory kernel to consider three different

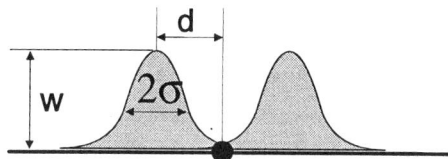

Figure 2: The basic inhibitory kernel used $k_1(x-\xi)$. The cell in the center receives inhibitory contributions from laterally distributed clusters of cells. The asymmetric kernels used in the model derive from this basic kernel by systematic variations of its geometrical parameters (see Table 1).

types of asymmetries: (1) different *spatial spread* of inhibition (i.e., $\sigma_1 \neq \sigma_2$); (2) different *amount* of inhibition ($w_1 \neq w_2$); (3) different *spatial offset* ($d_1 \neq d_2$). A more rigorous treatment should take care also of the continuous distortion of the topographic map [9]. In our analysis this would result in a continuous deformation of the inhibitory kernel, but for the small distances within which inhibition occurs, the approximation of a uniform mapping produces only a negligible error.

Architectural parameters were determined from reliable measured values of receptive fields of simple cells [10] [11]. Concerning the spatial domain, we fixed the size (σ_0) of the initial receptive field (due to geniculate contributions) for an "average" cortical simple cell with a resultant discharge field of $\sim 2°$; and we adjusted, accordingly, the parameters of the inhibitory kernel in order to account for spatial interactions only within the receptive field.

Considering the temporal domain, one should distinguish the time constant τ_1, caused by network interactions, from the time constants τ_0 and τ_2 caused by temporal integration at a single cell membrane. In any case, throughout all simulations, we fixed τ_0 and τ_2 to 20ms, whereas we varied τ_1 in the range 2 - 100ms.

3 RESULTS

Since visual cortex is visuotopically organized, a direct correspondence exists between the spatial organization of intracortical connections and the resulting receptive field topography. Therefore, the dependence of cortical surface activity $e_2(x,t)$ on the visual input $s(x,t)$ can be formulated as $e_2(x,t) = h(x,t) * s(x,t)$, where the symbol $*$ indicates a spatio-temporal convolution, and $h(x,t)$ is the equivalent receptive field interpreted as the spatio-temporal distribution of the signs of all the effects of cortical interactions. In this context, $h(x,t)$ reflects the whole spatio-temporal couplings and not only the direct neuroanatomical connectivity.

To test the efficacy of the various inhibitory schemes, we used a drifting sine wave grating $s(x,t) = C\cos[2\pi(f_x x \pm f_t t)]$ where C is the contrast, f_x and f_t are the spatial and temporal frequency, respectively. The direction selectivity index (DSI) and the optimal velocity (v_{opt}) obtained from the various inhibitory kernels of Fig.2 are summarized in Table 1, for different values of τ_1 and b. The direction selectivity index is defined as $DSI = \frac{R_p - R_{np}}{R_p + R_{np}}$, where R_p is the maximum response amplitude for preferred direction, and R_{np} is the maximum amplitude for non-preferred direction. The optimal velocity is defined as f_t^{opt}/f_x, where f_x is chosen to match the spatial structure of the receptive field, and f_t^{opt} is the frequency which elicits the maximum cell's response. As expected, increasing the parameter b enhances the effects of inhibition, thus resulting in larger DSI and higher optimal velocities. However, for stability reason, b should remain below a theshold value strictly re-

Table 1:

b	$\tau_1 = 2$		$\tau_1 = 10$		$\tau_1 = 20$		$\tau_1 = 100$		
	DSI	v_{opt}	DSI	v_{opt}	DSI	v_{opt}	DSI	v_{opt}	
0.25	0.00	0.00	0.00	0.00	0.00	0.00	0.00	0.00	ASY-1A
0.60	0.00	0.00	0.00	0.00	0.00	0.00	0.00	0.00	
0.80	0.08	1.82	0.24	1.82	0.00	0.00	0.00	0.00	
0.91	0.17	1.82	**0.34**	**1.82**	0.00	0.00	0.00	0.00	
0.50	0.00	0.00	0.00	0.00	0.00	0.00	0.00	0.00	ASY-1B
0.85	0.04	1.82	0.17	1.82	0.25	1.82	0.00	0.00	
1.00	0.06	1.82	0.19	1.82	0.28	1.82	0.00	0.00	
1.30	0.07	1.82	0.28	1.82	**0.37**	**1.82**	0.00	0.00	
0.50	0.00	0.00	0.00	0.00	0.00	0.00	0.00	0.00	ASY-2A
1.00	0.00	0.00	0.00	0.00	0.09	1.82	0.16	1.82	
5.00	0.02	1.82	0.05	1.82	0.09	1.82	**0.39**	**3.64**	
9.00	0.01	1.82	0.03	1.82	0.06	1.82	0.38	3.64	
0.25	0.00	0.00	0.00	0.00	0.00	0.00	0.00	0.00	ASY-2B
0.50	0.06	2.07	0.20	2.07	0.32	2.07	0.00	0.00	
0.60	0.06	2.07	0.39	4.14	0.40	2.07	0.00	0.00	
0.72	0.07	2.00	**0.66**	**6.00**	0.65	4.00	0.00	0.00	
0.25	0.00	0.00	0.00	0.00	0.00	0.00	0.00	0.00	ASY-3A
0.60	0.00	00.0	0.00	0.00	0.00	0.00	0.00	0.00	
0.80	0.08	1.82	0.23	1.82	0.00	0.00	0.00	0.00	
0.88	0.14	1.82	**0.26**	**1.82**	0.00	0.00	0.00	0.00	
0.50	0.00	0.00	0.00	0.00	0.00	0.00	0.00	0.00	ASY-3B
0.85	0.04	1.82	0.16	1.82	0.23	1.82	0.00	0.00	
1.00	0.05	1.82	0.18	1.82	0.26	1.82	0.00	0.00	
1.33	0.06	1.82	0.26	1.82	**0.35**	**1.82**	0.00	0.00	

lated to the inhibitory kernel considered. Moreover, we observe that, except for ASY-2A, the strongest direction selectivity can be obtained when the intracortical time constant τ_1 has values in the range of 10 - 20 ms, i.e., comparable to τ_0 and τ_2. Larger values of τ_1 would result, indeed, in a recrudescence of the velocity low-pass behavior. For each asymmetry, Figs. 3 show the direction tuning curves and the x-t plots, respectively, for the best cases considered (cf. bold-faced values in Table 1). We have evidenced that appreciable DSI can be obtained when inhibition arises from cortical sites at different distance from the target cell (i.e., ASY-2B, $d_1 \neq d_2$). In such conditions we obtained a DSI as high as 0.66 and an optimal velocity up to $\sim 6°/s$, as could be inferred also from the spatio-temporal plot which present a marked motion-type (i.e., oriented) non-separability (see Fig. 3ASY-2B).

4 DISCUSSION AND CONCLUSIONS

As anticipated in the Introduction, direction selectivity mechanisms usually relies upon asymmetric alteration of the spatial and temporal response characteristics of the geniculate input, which are presumably mediated by intracortical circuits. In the architectural model presented in this study, spatial asymmetries were included explicitly in the extension of the inhibitory interconnections, but no explicit asymmetric temporal mechanisms were introduced. It is worth evidencing how temporal asymmetries originate from the specific mutual inhibition scheme considered, which operates, regarding temporal domain, like a quadrature model [12] [13]. This can

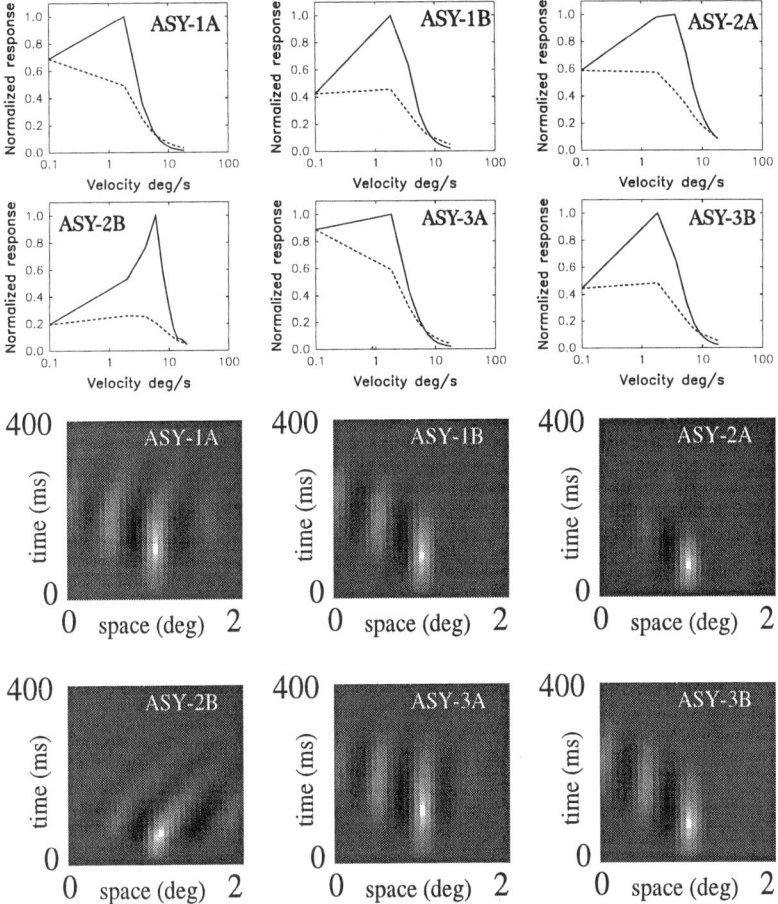

Figure 3: Results from the model related to the bold-typed values indicated in Table 1, for each asymmetry considered. (Top) direction tuning curve; (Bottom) spatio-temporal plots. We can evidence a marked direction tuning for ASY-2B, i.e., when inhibition arises from two differentially offset Gaussians

be inferred by the examination of the equivalent transfer function $H(\omega_x, \omega_t)$ in the Fourier domain:

$$H(\omega_x, \omega_t) = \frac{H_0(\omega_x, \omega_t)}{1 + j\omega_t \tau_2} \left(\frac{1}{1 + j\omega_t \tau_1 + bK_1(\omega_x)} + j\omega_t \tau_1 \frac{1}{1 + j\omega_t \tau_1 + bK_1(\omega_x)} \right) \tag{5}$$

where upper case letters indicate Fourier transforms, and j is the complex variable. The terms in parentheses in Eq. (5) can be interpreted as the sum of temporal components that are approximately arranged in temporal quadrature. Furthermore, one can observe that a direct monosynaptic influence (e_1) from the inhibitory neurons of layer 1 to the excitatory cells of layer 2, would result in the cancellation of the quadrature component in Eq. (5).

Further improvement of the model should take into account also transmission delays between spatially separated interacting cells, theshold non-linearities, and ON-OFF interactions.

Acknowledgements

This research was partially supported by CEC-Esprit CORMORANT 8503, and by MURST 40%-60%.

References

[1] R.C. Reid, R.E. Soodak, and R.M. Shapley. Directional selectivity and spatiotemporal structure of receptive fields of simple cells in cat striate cortex. *J. Neurophysiol.*, 66:505–529, 1991.

[2] D.B. Hamilton, D.G. Albrecht, and W.S. Geisler. Visual cortical receptive fields in monkey and cat: spatial and temporal phase transfer function. *Vision Res.*, 29(10):1285–1308, 1989.

[3] K. Nakayama. Biological image motion processing: a review. *Vision Res.*, 25:625–660, 1985.

[4] E.C. Hildreth and C. Koch. The analysis of visual motion: From computational theory to neuronal mechanisms. *Ann. Rev. Neurosci.*, 10:477–533, 1987.

[5] G. Krone, H. Mallot, G. Palm, and A. Schüz. Spatiotemporal receptive fields: A dynamical model derived from cortical architectonics. *Proc. R. Soc. London Biol*, 226:421–444, 1986.

[6] H.R. Wilson and J.D. Cowan. A mathematical theory of the functional dynamics of cortical and thalamic nervous tissue. *Kibernetik*, 13:55–80, 1973.

[7] G.C. De Angelis, I. Ohzawa, and R.D. Freeman. Spatiotemporal organization of simple-cell receptive fields in the cat's striate cortex.I. General characteristics and postnatal development. *J. Neurophysiol.*, 69:1091–1117, 1993.

[8] S.P. Sabatini, L. Raffo, and G.M. Bisio. Functional periodic intracortical couplings induced by structured lateral inhibition in a linear cortical network. *Neural Computation*, 9(3):525–531, 1997.

[9] H.A. Mallot, W. von Seelen, and F. Giannakopoulos. Neural mapping and space variant image processing. *Neural Networks*, 3:245–263, 1990.

[10] K. Albus. A quantitative study of the projection area of the central and the paracentral visual field in area 17 of the cat. *Exp. Brain Res.*, 24:159–202, 1975.

[11] J. Jones and L. Palmer. The two-dimensional spatial structure of simple receptive fields in cat striate cortex. *J. Neurophysiol.*, 58:1187–1211, 1987.

[12] A.B. Watson and A.J. Ahumada. Model of human visual-motion sensing. *J. Opt. Soc. Amer.*, 2:322–341, 1985.

[13] E.H. Adelson and J.R. Bergen. Spatiotemporal energy models for the perception of motion. *J. Opt. Soc. Amer.*, 2:284–321, 1985.

Cholinergic Modulation Preserves Spike Timing Under Physiologically Realistic Fluctuating Input

Akaysha C. Tang
The Salk Institute
Howard Hughes Medical Institute
Computational Neurobiology Laboratory
La Jolla, CA 92037

Andreas M. Bartels
Zoological Institute
University of Zürich
Zürich
Switzerland

Terrence J. Sejnowski
The Salk Institute
Howard Hughes Medical Institute
Computational Neurobiology Laboratory
La Jolla, CA 92037

Abstract

Neuromodulation can change not only the mean firing rate of a neuron, but also its pattern of firing. Therefore, a reliable neural coding scheme, whether a rate coding or a spike time based coding, must be robust in a dynamic neuromodulatory environment. The common observation that cholinergic modulation leads to a reduction in spike frequency adaptation implies a modification of spike timing, which would make a neural code based on precise spike timing difficult to maintain. In this paper, the effects of cholinergic modulation were studied to test the hypothesis that precise spike timing can serve as a reliable neural code. Using the whole cell patch-clamp technique in rat neocortical slice preparation and compartmental modeling techniques, we show that cholinergic modulation, surprisingly, preserved spike timing in response to a fluctuating inputs that resembles *in vivo* conditions. This result suggests that in vivo spike timing may be much more resistant to changes in neuromodulator concentrations than previous physiological studies have implied.

1 Introduction

Recently, there has been a vigorous debate concerning the nature of neural coding (Rieke et al. 1996; Stevens and Zador 1995; Shadlen and Newsome 1994). The prevailing view has been that the mean firing rate conveys all information about the sensory stimulus in a spike train and the precise timing of the individual spikes is noise. This belief is, in part, based on a lack of correlation between the precise timing of the spikes and the sensory qualities of the stimulus under study, particularly, on a lack of spike timing repeatability when identical stimulation is delivered. This view has been challenged by a number of recent studies, in which highly repeatable temporal patterns of spikes can be observed both *in vivo* (Bair and Koch 1996; Abeles et al. 1993) and *in vitro* (Mainen and Sejnowski 1994). Furthermore, application of information theory to the coding problem in the frog and house fly (Bialek et al. 1991; Bialek and Rieke 1992) suggested that additional information could be extracted from spike timing. In the absence of direct evidence for a timing code in the cerebral cortex, the role of spike timing in neural coding remains controversial.

1.1 A necessary condition for a spike timing code

If spike timing is important in defining a stimulus, precisely timed spikes must be maintained under a range of physiological conditions. One important aspect of a neuron's environment is the presence of various neuromodulators. Due to their widespread projections in the nervous system, major neuromodulators, such as acetylcholine (ACh) and norepinephrine (NA), can have a profound influence on the firing properties of most neurons. If a change in concentration of a neuromodulator completely alters the temporal structure of the spike train, it would be unlikely that spike timing could serve as a reliable neural code. A major effect of cholinergic modulation on cortical neurons is a reduction in spike frequency adaptation, which is characterized by a shortening of inter-spike-intervals and an increase in neuronal excitability (McCormick 1993; Nicoll 1988). One obvious consequence of this cholinergic effect is a modification of spike timing (Fig. 1A). This modification of spike timing due to a change in neuromodulator concentration would seem to preclude the possibility of a neural code based on precise spike timing.

1.2 Re-examination of the cholinergic modulation of spike timing

Despite its popularity, the square pulse stimulus used in most eletrophysiological studies is rarely encountered by a cortical neuron under physiological conditions. The corresponding behavior of the neuron at the input/output level may have limited relevance to the behavior of the neuron under its natural condition, which is characterized *in vivo* by highly fluctuating synaptic inputs. In this paper, we re-examine the effect of cholinergic modulation on spike timing under two contrasting stimulus conditions: the physiologically unrealistic square pulse input versus the more plausible fluctuating input. We report that under physiologically more realistic fluctuating inputs, effects of cholinergic modulation preserved the timing of each individual spike (Fig. 1B). This result is consistent with the hypothesis that spike timing may be relevant to information encoding.

2 Methods

2.1 Experimental

Using the whole cell patch-clamp technique, we made somatic recordings from layer 2/3 neocortical neurons in the rat visual cortex. Coronal slices of 400 μm were prepared from 14 to 18 days old Long Evans rats (for details see (Mainen and Sejnowski 1994). Spike trains elicited by current injection of 900 ms were recorded for the square pulse inputs and fluctuating inputs with equal mean synaptic inputs, in the absence and presence of a cholinergic agonist carbachol. The fluctuating inputs were constructed from Gaussian noise and convolved with an alpha function with a time constant of 3 ms, reflecting the time course of the synaptic events. The amplitude of fluctuation was such that the subthreshold membrane potential fluctuation observed in our experiments were comparable to that in whole-cell patch clamp study in vivo (Ferster and Jagadeesh 1992). The cholinergic agonist carbachol at concentrations of 5, 7.5, 15, 30 μM was delivered through bath perfusion (perfusion time: between 1 and 6 min). For each cell, three sets of blocks were recorded before, during and after carbachol perfusion at a given concentration. Each block contained 20 trials of stimulation under identical experimental conditions.

2.2 Simulation

We used a compartmental model of a neocortical neuron to explore the contribution of three potassium conductances affected by cholinergic modulation (Madison et al. 1987). Simulations were performed in a reduced 9 compartment model, based on a layer 2 pyramidal cell reconstruction using the NEURON program. The model had five conductances: g_{Na}, g_{K_v}, g_{K_M}, g_{Ca}, $g_{K(Ca)}$. Membrane resistivity was $40 K\Omega cm^2$, capacitance was $1\mu F/\mu m^2$, and axial resistance was $200\Omega cm$. Intrinsic noise was simulated by injecting a randomly fluctuating current to fit the spike jitter observed experimentally. Different potassium conductances were manipulated as independent variables and the spike timing displacement was measured for multiple levels of conductance change corresponding to multiple concentrations of carbachol.

2.3 Data analysis

For both experimental and simulation data, first derivatives were used to detect spikes and to determine the timing for spike initiation. Raster plots of the spike trains were derived from the series of membrane potentials for each trial, and a smoothed histogram was then constructed to reflect the instantaneous firing rate for each block of trials under identical stimulation and pharmacological conditions. An event was then defined as a period of increase in instantaneous firing rate that is greater than a threshold level (set at 3 times of the mean firing rate within the block of trials) (Mainen and Sejnowski 1994).

The effect of carbachol on spike timing under fluctuating inputs was quantified by defining the displacement in spike timing for each event, d_i, as the time difference between the nearest peaks of the events under carbachol and control condition. The weight for each event, w_i, is determined by the peak of the event. The higher the peak, the less the spike jitter. The mean displacement is

$$D = \sum d_i w_i / \sum w_i, \qquad (1)$$

where i= 1, 2, ...nth event in the control condition.

3 Results

3.1 Experimental

The effects of carbachol on spike timing under the square pulse and fluctuating inputs are shown in Fig. 1A and B respectively. In the absence of carbachol, a square pulse input produced a spike train with clear spike frequency adaptation (Fig. 1A1). Similar to previous reports from the literature, addition of carbachol to the perfusion medium reduced spike frequency adaptation (Fig. 1A2). This reduction in spike frequency adaptation is reflected in the shortening of inter-spike-intervals and an increase in the firing frequency. Most importantly, spike timing was altered by carbachol perfusion. When a fluctuating current was injected, the strong spike frequency adaptation observed under a square pulse input was no longer apparent (Fig. 1B1). Unlike the results under the square pulse condition, addition of carbachol to the bath medium preserved the timing of the spikes (Fig. 1B2). An increased excitability was achieved with the insertion of additional spikes between the existing spikes.

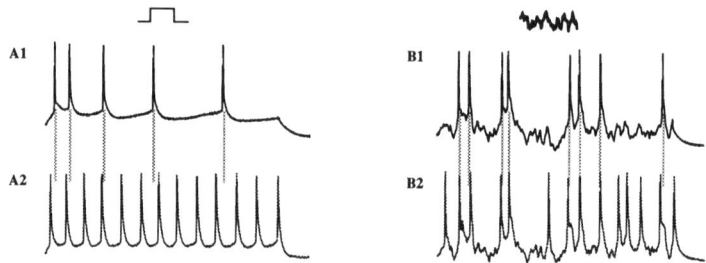

Figure 1: Response of a cortical neuron to square pulse current injection (A) and a fluctuating input (B). The membrane potential during the 1024 ms sampling period is plotted as a function of time for the two types of inputs (onset: 5 ms; duration: 900 ms). The grey lines show where the spikes occurred in the upper traces.

Preservation of spike timing under carbachol was examined at concentrations of 5, 7.5, 15, and 30μM, here shown in one cell (Fig. 2, 5μM). The smoothed histograms (as described in section 2.3) were plotted for blocks of 20 identical trials under the same fluctuating input. The alignment of the events between the control and carbachol indicates that spike timing was well preserved. The table gives the mean spike displacement, D, for a range of carbachol concentrations. The spike jitter within the control and carbachol conditions was approximately 1 ms, and was not changed significantly by carbachol (control: 0.96 ± 0.3; carbachol: 0.94 ± 0.42 ms.)

3.2 Simulation

The model captured the basic characteristics of experimental data. In response to fluctuating inputs, the model neurons showed reduced spike frequency adaptation and preservation of spike timing. The *in vitro* experiment were limited to only two levels of stimulus fluctuation. To show that reduced adaptation in response

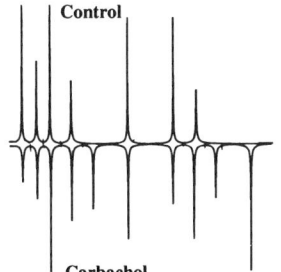

Cholinergic Modification of Spike Timing

D (ms)	N	Carbachol (microM)
2.76 ± 0.38	15	5–7.5
3.33	1	15
9.3	2	30

Figure 2: Preservation of spike timing for a range of carbachol concentrations. Left: the top portion is the histogram for the control condition; the bottom is the histogram for the carbachol condition shown inverted. The alignment of the events between the control and carbachol indicates preserved timing. Right: statistics of spike displacement.

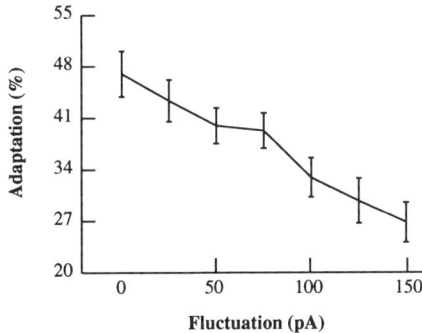

Figure 3: Reduced adaptation as a function of increasing stimulus fluctuation. Adaptation measured as a normalized spike count difference between the first and second halves of the 900 ms stimulation: (C2-C1)/C1.

to fluctuating inputs is a general phenomenon, in the model neuron we measured adaptation for multiple levels of stimulus fluctuation. As shown in Fig. 3, spike frequency adaptation decreased as a function of increasing stimulus fluctuation over a range of fluctuation amplitude. The effects cholinergic modulation on spike timing were studied under simulated cholinergic modulation. Similar to the experimental finding, increased neuronal excitability to fluctuating inputs was accompanied by insertion of additional spikes (Fig. 4 left) and spike timing was preserved simultaneously (Fig. 4 right).

In real neurons, the total effects of cholinergic modulation depends on its effects on at least three potassium conductances. Using the model, we examined the effects of manipulating each of the three potassium conductances on spike displacement and spike jitter. We found that (1) spike displacement due to reduction in potassium conductances were all very small, on the order of a few milliseconds (Fig. 5 top row); (2) Compared to the conductances underlying I_M and I_{leak}, spike displacement was most sensitive to changes in the conductance underlying I_{AHP} (Fig. 5 top row), whose reduction alone led to the best reproduction of the experimental data; (3) spike jitters of approximately 1 ms were independent of the values of the three

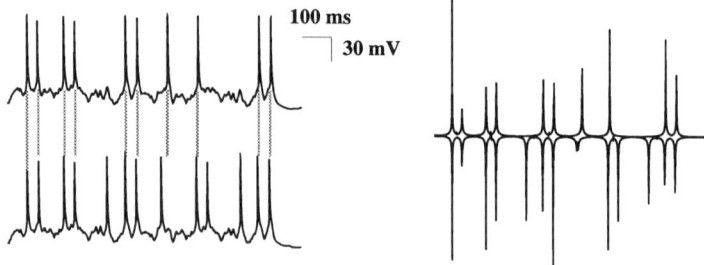

Figure 4: Preservation of spike timing in the model neocortical neuron. Left: Responses of the model neuron to fluctuating input. Top: replicating data from the control condition. Bottom: reproducing the carbachol effect by blocking the adaptation current, I_{AHP}. Right: histogram display of preservation of spike timing in a block of 20 trials.

potassium conductances (Fig. 5 bottom row). These results make predictions for new experiments where each individual current is blocked selectively.

4 Conclusions

The results showed that under the physiologically realistic fluctuating input, the effects of cholinergic modulation on spike timing are rather different from that observed when unphysiological square pulse inputs were used. Instead of moving the spikes forward in time by shortening the inter-spike-intervals, cholinergic modulation preserved spike timing. This preservation of spike timing was achieved simultaneously with an increase in neuronal excitability.

According to the classical view of neuromodulation, one would have expected that a spike timing based neural code would be difficult to maintain across a range of neuromodulator concentrations. The fact that spike timing was rather resistant to changes in the neuromodulatory environment raises the possibility that spike timing may serve some function in the cortex.

The differential effect of cholinergic modulation on spike timing observed under the square pulse and fluctuating inputs also calls for caution in generalizing an observation from one set of parameter values to another, especially when generalizing from *in vitro* to *in vivo*. This concern for external validity is particularly important for computational neuroscientists whose work involves integrating phenomena from the cellular, systems and finally, to behavioral levels.

Acknowledgments

Supported by the Howard Hughes Medical Institute. We are grateful to Zachary Mainen, Barak Pearlmutter, Raphael Ritz, Anthony Zador, David Horn, Chuck Stevens, William Bialek, and Christof Koch for helpful discussions.

References

Abeles, M., Bergman, H., Margalit, E., and Vaadia, E. (1993). Spatiotemporal

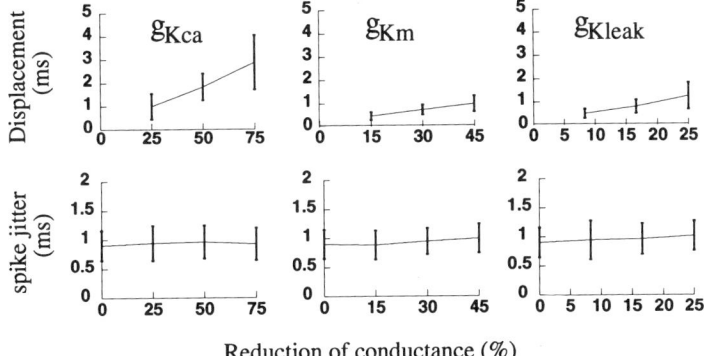

Figure 5: Effects of individual conductance changes on spike timing. Top: spike displacement as a function of changing conductances. Bottom: spike jitter as a function of changing conductances. Each conductance was reduced from its control value which was determined by fitting experimentally observed spike trains. The range of change for the leak conductance was constrained by the experimentally observed resting membrane potential changes (avg. 5 mV.)

firing patterns in the frontal cortex of behaving monkeys. *J. Neurophysiol.*, 70, 1629–1638.

Bair, W. and Koch, C. (1996). Temporal precision of spike trains in extrastriate cortex of the behaving Macaque monkey. *Neural Computation*, 8(6), 1184–1202.

Bialek, W. and Rieke, F. (1992). Reliability and information transmission in spiking neurons. *Trends Neurosci.*, 15, 428–434.

Bialek, W., Rieke, F., de Ruyter van Stevenick, R. R., and Warland, D. (1991). Reading a neural code. *Science*, 252, 1854–7.

Ferster, D. and Jagadeesh, B. (1992). EPSP-IPSP interactions in cat visual cortex studied with *in vivo* whole-cell patch recording. *J. Neurosci.*, 12(4), 1262–1274.

Madison, D. V., Lancaster, B., and Nicoll, R. A. (1987). Voltage clamp analysis of cholinergic action in the hippocampus. *J. Neurosci.*, 7(3), 733–741.

Mainen, Z. F. and Sejnowski, T. J. (1994). Reliability of spike timing in neocortical neurons. *Science*, 268, 1503–6.

McCormick, D. A. (1993). Actions of acetylecholine in the cerebral cortex and thalamus and implications for function.. *Prog. Brain Res.*, 98, 303–308.

Nicoll, R. (1988). The coupling of neurotransmitter receptors to ion channels in the brain. *Science*, 241, 545–550.

Rieke, F., Warland, D., de Ruyter van Steveninck, R., and Bialek, W. (1996). *Spikes: Exploring the Neural Code.* MIT Press.

Shadlen, M. N. and Newsome, W. T. (1994). Noise, neural codes and cortical organization. *Current Opinion in Neurobiology*, 4, 569–579.

Stevens, C. and Zador, A. (1995). The enigma of the brain. *Current Biology*, 5, 1–2.

A Model of Recurrent Interactions in Primary Visual Cortex

Emanuel Todorov, Athanassios Siapas and David Somers
Dept. of Brain and Cognitive Sciences
E25-526, MIT, Cambridge, MA 02139
Email: {emo,thanos,somers}@ai.mit.edu

Abstract

A general feature of the cerebral cortex is its massive interconnectivity - it has been estimated anatomically [19] that cortical neurons receive upwards of 5,000 synapses, the majority of which originate from other nearby cortical neurons. Numerous experiments in primary visual cortex (V1) have revealed strongly nonlinear interactions between stimulus elements which activate classical and non-classical receptive field regions. Recurrent cortical connections likely contribute substantially to these effects. However, most theories of visual processing have either assumed a feedforward processing scheme [7], or have used recurrent interactions to account for isolated effects only [1, 16, 18]. Since nonlinear systems cannot in general be taken apart and analyzed in pieces, it is not clear what one learns by building a recurrent model that only accounts for one, or very few phenomena. Here we develop a relatively simple model of recurrent interactions in V1, that reflects major anatomical and physiological features of intracortical connectivity, and *simultaneously* accounts for a wide range of phenomena observed physiologically. All phenomena we address are strongly nonlinear, and cannot be explained by linear feedforward models.

1 The Model

We analyze the mean firing rates observed in oriented V1 cells in response to stimuli consisting of an inner circular grating and an outer annular grating. Mean responses of individual cells are modeled by single-valued "cellular" response functions, whose arguments are the mean firing rates of the cell's inputs and their maximal synaptic conductances.

1.1 Neuronal model

Each neuron is modeled as a single voltage compartment in which the membrane potential V is given by:

$$C_m \frac{dV(t)}{dt} = g_{\text{ex}}(t)(E_{\text{ex}} - V(t)) + g_{\text{inh}}(t)(E_{\text{inh}} - V(t)) + \\ g_{\text{leak}}(E_{\text{leak}} - V(t)) + g_{\text{ahp}}(t)(E_{\text{ahp}} - V(t))$$

where C_m is the membrane capacitance, E_x is the reversal potential for current x, and g_x is the conductance for that current. If the voltage exceeds a threshold V_θ, a spike is generated, and afterhyperpolarizing currents are activated. The conductances for excitatory and inhibitory currents are modeled as sums of α-functions, and the *ahp* conductance is modeled as a decaying exponential. The model consists of two distinct cell types, excitatory and inhibitory, with realistic cellular parameters [13], similar to the ones used in [17]. To compute the response functions for the two cell types, we simulated one cell of each type, receiving excitatory and inhibitory Poisson inputs. The synaptic strengths were held constant, while the rates of the excitatory and inhibitory inputs were varied independently.

Although the driving forces for excitation and inhibition vary, we found that single cell responses can be accurately modeled if incoming excitation and inhibition are combined linearly, and the net input is passed through a response function that is approximately threshold-linear, with some smoothing around threshold. This is consistent with the results of intracellular experiments that show linear synaptic interactions in visual cortex[5]. Note that the cellular functions are not sigmoids, and thus saturating responses could be achieved only through network interactions.

1.2 Cortical connectivity

The visual cortex shares with many other cortical areas a similar pattern of intra-areal connections [12]. Excitatory cells make dense local projections, as well as long-range horizontal projections that usually contact cells with similar response properties. Inhibitory cells make only local projections, which are spread further in space than the local excitatory connections [10]. We assume that cells with similar response properties have a higher probability of connection, and that probability falls down with distance in "feature" space. For simplicity, we consider only two feature dimensions: orientation and RF center in visual space. Since we are dealing with stimuli with radial symmetry, one spatial dimension is sufficient. The extension to more dimensions, i.e. another spatial dimension, direction selectivity, ocularity, etc., is straightforward.

We assume that the feature space is filled uniformly with excitatory and inhibitory cells. Rather than modeling individual cells, we model a grid of locations, and for each location we compute the mean firing rate of cells present there. The connectivity is defined by two projection kernels K_{ex}, K_{in} (one for each presynaptic cell type) and weights $W_{ee}, W_{ei}, W_{ie}, W_{ii}$, corresponding to the number and strength of synapses made onto excitatory/inhibitory cells. The excitatory projection has sharper tuning in orientation space, and bigger spread in visual space (Figure 1).

1.3 Visual stimuli and thalamocortical input

The visual stimulus is defined by five parameters: diameter d of the inner grating (the outer is assumed infinite), log contrast c_1, c_2, and orientation θ_1, θ_2 of each grating. The two gratings are always centered in the spatial center of the model.

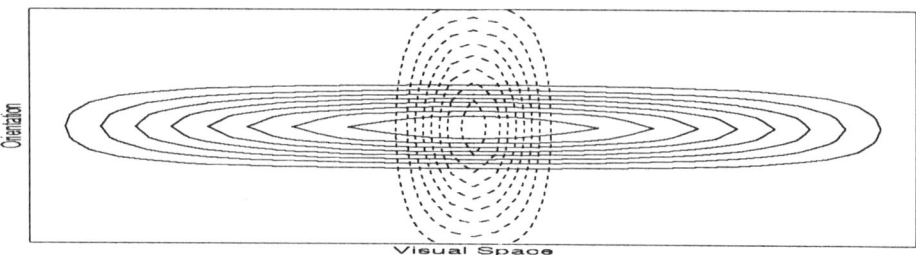

Figure 1: Excitatory (solid) and Inhibitory (dashed) connectivity kernels.

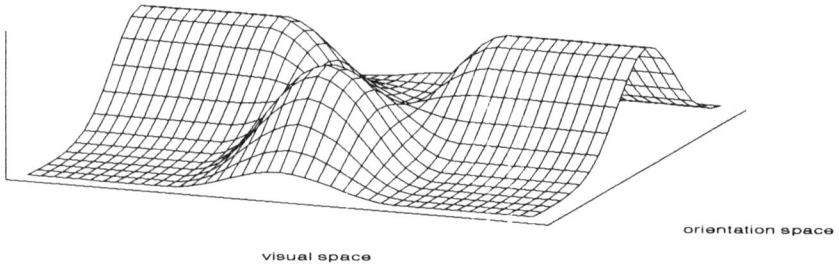

Figure 2: LGN input for a stimulus with high contrast, orthogonal orientations of center and surround gratings.

Each cortical cell receives LGN input which is the product of log contrast, orientation tuning, and convolution of the stimulus with a spatial receptive field. The LGN input computed in this way is multiplied by LGN_{ex}, LGN_{in} and sent to the cortical cells. Figure 2 shows an example of what the LGN input looks like.

2 Results

For given input LGN input, we computed the steady-state activity in cortex iteratively (about 30 iteration were required). Since we studied the model for gradually changing stimulus parameters, it was possible to use the solution for one set of parameters as an initial guess for the next solution, which resulted in significant speedup. The results presented here are for the excitatory population, since i) it provides the output of the cortex; ii) contains four times more cells than the inhibitory population, and therefore is more likely to be recorded from. All results were obtained for the same set of parameters.

2.1 Classical RF effects

First we simulate responses to a central grating ($1 deg$ diameter) for increasing log-contrast levels. It has been repeatedly observed that although LGN firing increases linearly with stimulus log-contrast, the contrast response functions observed in V1 saturate, and may even supersaturate or decline[11, 2]. The most complete and recent model of that phenomena [6, 3] assumes shunting inhibition, which contradicts recent intracellular observations [4, 5]. Furthermore, that model cannot explain supersaturation. Our model achieves saturation (Figure 3A) for high contrast levels,

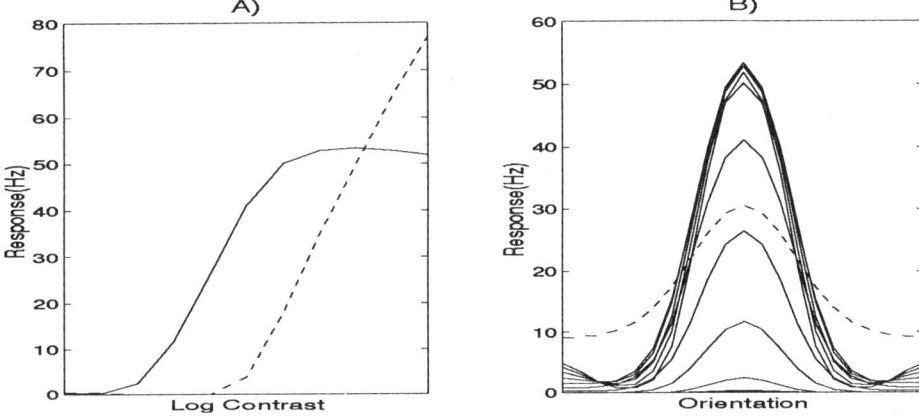

Figure 3: Classical RF effects. A) Contrast response function for excitatory (solid) and inhibitory (dashed) cells. B) Orientation tuning for different contrast levels (solid); scaled LGN input (dashed).

and can easily achieve supersaturation for different parameter setting. Instead of using shunting (divisive) inhibition, we suggest that inhibitory neurons have higher contrast thresholds than excitatory neurons, i.e. the direct LGN input to inhibitory cells is weaker. Note that we only need a subpopulation of inhibitory neurons with that property; the rest can have the same response threshold as the excitatory population.

Another well-known property of V1 neurons is that their orientation tuning is roughly contrast-invariant[14]. The LGN input tuning is invariant, therefore this property is easily obtained in models where V1 responses are almost linear, rather than saturating [1, 16]. Achieving both contrast-invariant tuning and contrast saturation for the entire population (while singe cell feedforward response functions are non-saturating) is non-trivial. The problem is that invariant tuning requires the responses at all orientations saturate simultaneously. This is the case in our model (Figure 3B) - we found that the tuning (half width at half amplitude) varied within a $5deg$ range as contrast increased.

2.2 Extraclassical RF effects

Next we consider stimuli which include both a center and a surround grating. In the first set of simulations we held the diameter constant (at $1deg$) and varied stimulus contrast and orientation. It has been observed [9, 15] that a high contrast iso–orientation surround stimulus facilitates responses to a low contrast, but suppresses responses to a high contrast center stimulus. This behavior is captured very well by our model (Figure 4A). The strong response to the surround stimulus alone is partially due to direct thalamic input (i.e. the thalamocortical projective field is larger than the classical receptive field of a V1 cell). The response to an orthogonal surround is between the center and iso–orientation surround responses, as observed in [9].

Many neurons in V1 respond optimally to a center grating with a certain diameter, but their response decreases as the diameter increases (end-stopping). End-stopping in the model is shown in Figure 4B - responses to increasing grating diameter reach a peak and then decrease. In experiments it has been observed that the

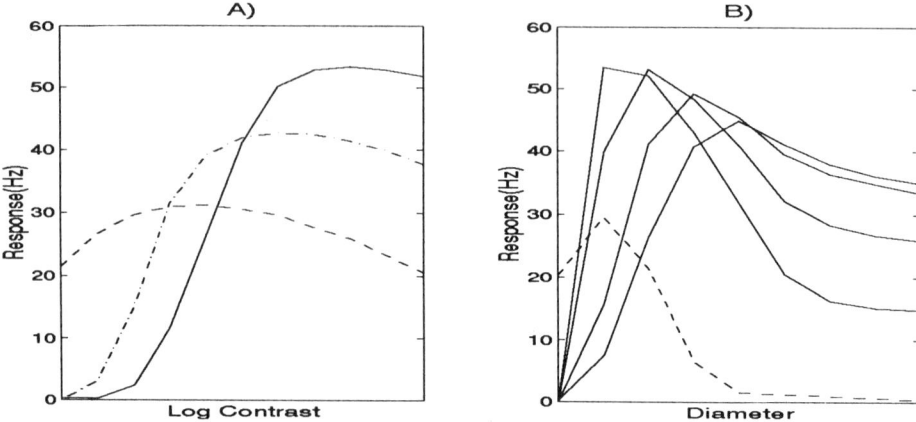

Figure 4: Extraclassical RF effects. A) Contrast response functions for center (solid), center + iso–orientation surround (dashed), center + orthogonal surround (dash-dot). B) Length tuning for 4 center log contrast levels (1, .75, .5, .4), response to surround of high contrast (dashed).

border between the excitatory and inhibitory regions shifts outward (rightward) as stimulus contrast levels decline[8]. Our model also achieves this effect (for other parameter settings it can shift more downward than rightward). Note also that a center grating with maximal contrast reaches its peak response for a diameter value which is 3 times smaller than the diameter for which responses to a surround grating disappear. This is interesting because both the peak response to a central grating, and the first response to a surround grating can be used to define the extent of the classical RF - in this case clearly leading to very different definitions. This effect (shown in Figure 4B) has also been recently observed in V1 [15].

3 Population Modeling and Variability

So far we have analyzed the population firing rates in the model, and compared them to physiological observations. Unfortunately, in many cases the limited sample size, or the variability in a given physiological experiment does not allow an accurate estimate of what the population response might be. In such cases researchers only describe individual cells, which are not necessarily representative. How can findings reported in this way be captured in a population model? The parameters of the model could be modified in order capture the behavior of individual cells on the population level; or, further subdivisions into neuronal subpopulations may be introduced explicitly. The approach we prefer is to increase the variance of the number of connections made across individual cells, while maintaining the same mean values. We consider variations in the amount of excitatory and inhibitory synapses that a particular cell receives from other cortical neurons. Note that the presynaptic origin of these inputs is still the "average" cortical cell , and is not chosen from a subpopulation with special response properties.

The two examples we show have recently been reported in [15]. If we increase the cortical input (excitation by 100%, inhibition by 30%), we obtain a completely patch-suppressed cell, i.e. it does not respond to a center + iso–orientation surround stimulus - Figure 5A. Figure 5B shows that this cell is an "orientation contrast detector", i.e. it responds well to $0deg$ center + $90deg$ surround, and to $90deg$

center + $0deg$ surround. Interestingly, the cells with that property reported in [15] were all patch-suppressed. Note also that our cell has a supersaturating center response - we found that it always accompanies patch suppression in the model.

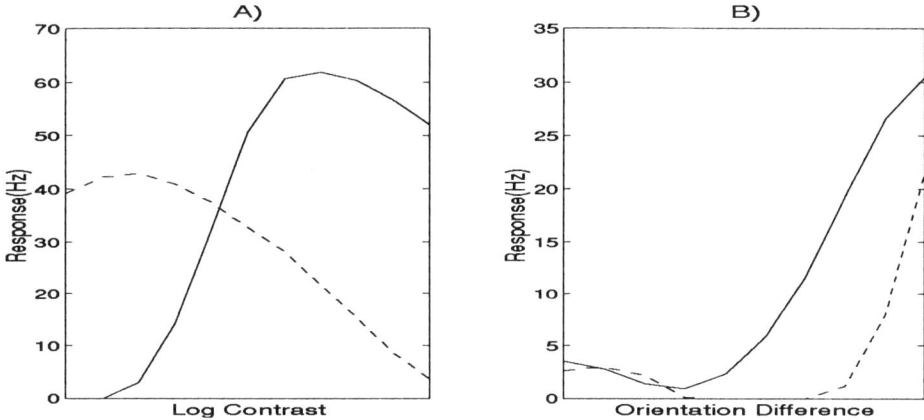

Figure 5: Orientation discontinuity detection for a strongly patch-suppressed cell. A) Contrast response functions for center (solid) and center + iso-orientation surround (dashed). B) Cell's response for $0deg$ center, $0-90deg$ surround (solid) and $90deg$ center, $90-0deg$ surround.

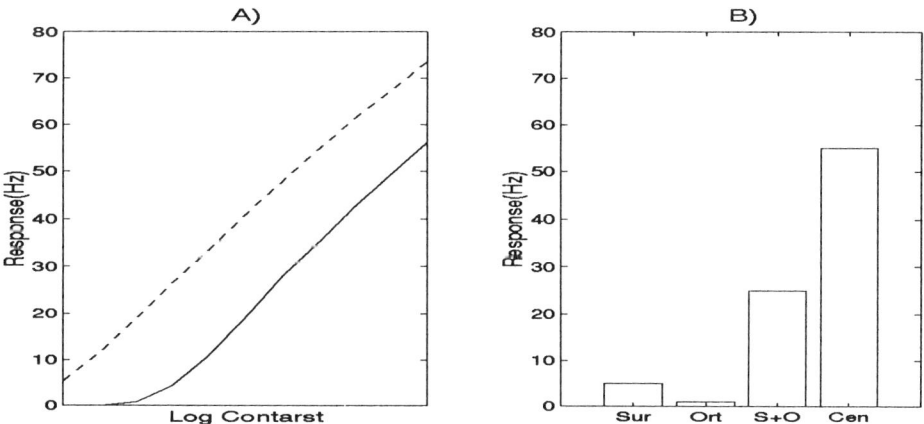

Figure 6: Nonlinear summation for a non patch-suppressed cell. A) Contrast response functions for center (solid) and center + iso-orientation surround (dashed). B) Cell's response for iso-orientation surround, orthogonal center, surround + center, center only.

The second example is a cell receiving 15% of the average cortical input. Not surprisingly, its contrast response function does not saturate - Figure 6A. However, this cell exhibits an interesting nonlinear property - it respond well to a combination of an iso-orientation surround + orthogonal center, but does not respond to either stimulus alone (Figure 6B). It is not clear from [15] whether the cells with this property had saturating contrast response functions.

4 Conclusion

We presented a model of recurrent computation in primary visual cortex that relies on a limited set of physiologically plausible mechanisms. In particular, we used the different cellular properties of excitatory and inhibitory neurons and the non-isotropic shape of lateral connections (Figure 1). Due to space limitations, we only presented simulation results, rather than analyzing the effects of specific parameters. A preliminary version of such analysis is given in [17] for local effects, and will be developed elsewhere for lateral interaction effects.

Our goal here was to propose a framework for studying recurrent computation in V1, that is relatively simple, yet rich enough to simultaneously account for a wide range of physiological observations. Such a framework is needed if we are to analyse systematically the fundamental role of recurrent interactions in neocortex.

References

[1] Ben-Yishai, R., Lev Bar-Or, R. & Sompolinsky, H. *Proc. Natl. Acad. Sci. U.S.A.* **92**, 3844-3848 (1995).

[2] Bonds, A.B. *Visual Neurosci.* **6**, 239-255 (1991).

[3] Carandini, M. & Heeger, D.J. *Science,* **264**, 1333-1336 (1994).

[4] Douglas R.J., Martin K.C., Whitteridge D. An intracellular analysis of the visual responses on neurones in cat visual cortex. *J Physiology* **44**, 659-696, 1991.

[5] Ferster,D & Jagadeesh, B. *J. Neurosci.* **12**, 1262-1274(1992).

[6] Heeger, D.J. *Visual Neurosci.* **70**, 181-197 (1992).

[7] Hubel, D.H. & Wiesel, T.N. *J. Neurophysiol.* **148**, 574-591 (1959).

[8] Jagadeesh, B. & Ferster, D. *Soc Neursci Abstr.* **16** 130.11. (1990).

[9] Knierim, J.J. & Van Essen, D.C. *J. Neurophysiol.* **67**, 961-980 (1992).

[10] Kisvarday, Z.F., Martin, K.A.C., Freund, T.F., Magloczky, Z.F., Whitteridge, D., and Somogyi, D. *Exp. Brain Res.* **64**, 541-552.

[11] Li, C.Y. & Creutzfeldt, O.D. *Pflugers Arch.* **401**, 304-314 (1984).

[12] Lund J.S., Yoshioka T., Levitt, J.B. *Cereb. Cortex* **3**, 148-162.

[13] McCormick, D.A., Connors, B.W., Lighthall, J.W. & Prince, D.A. *J. Neurophysiol.* **54**, 782-806 (1985).

[14] Sclar, G. & Freeman, R.D. *Exp. Brain Res.* **46**, 457-461.

[15] Sillito, A.M., Grieve, K.L., Jones, H.E., Cudeiro, J., & Davis, J. *Nature*, Nov 1995.

[16] Somers, D.C., Nelson, S.B. & Sur, M. *J. Neurosci.* **15**, 5448-5465 (1995).

[17] Siapas A, Todorov E, Somers D. Computing the mean firing rates of ensembles of realistic neurons. *Soc Neuroscience Abstract*, 1995.

[18] Stemmler, M., Usher, M. & Niebur, E *Science* **269**, 1877-1880, (1995).

[19] White, E.L. *Cortical Circuits* 46-82 (Birkhauser, Boston, 1989).

PART III
THEORY

Neural Learning in Structured Parameter Spaces
— Natural Riemannian Gradient

Shun-ichi Amari
RIKEN Frontier Research Program, RIKEN,
Hirosawa 2-1, Wako-shi 351-01, Japan
amari@zoo.riken.go.jp

Abstract

The parameter space of neural networks has a Riemannian metric structure. The natural Riemannian gradient should be used instead of the conventional gradient, since the former denotes the true steepest descent direction of a loss function in the Riemannian space. The behavior of the stochastic gradient learning algorithm is much more effective if the natural gradient is used. The present paper studies the information-geometrical structure of perceptrons and other networks, and prove that the on-line learning method based on the natural gradient is asymptotically as efficient as the optimal batch algorithm. Adaptive modification of the learning constant is proposed and analyzed in terms of the Riemannian measure and is shown to be efficient. The natural gradient is finally applied to blind separation of mixtured independent signal sources.

1 Introduction

Neural learning takes place in the parameter space of modifiable synaptic weights of a neural network. The role of each parameter is different in the neural network so that the parameter space is structured in this sense. The Riemannian structure which represents a local distance measure is introduced in the parameter space by information geometry (Amari, 1985).

On-line learning is mostly based on the stochastic gradient descent method, where the current weight vector is modified in the gradient direction of a loss function. However, the ordinary gradient does not represent the steepest direction of a loss function in the Riemannian space. A geometrical modification is necessary, and it is called the natural Riemannian gradient. The present paper studies the remarkable effects of using the natural Riemannian gradient in neural learning.

We first studies the asymptotic behavior of on-line learning (Opper, NIPS'95 Workshop). Batch learning uses all the examples at any time to obtain the optimal weight vector, whereas on-line learning uses an example once when it is observed. Hence, in general, the target weight vector is estimated more accurately in the case of batch learning. However, we prove that, when the Riemannian gradient is used, on-line learning is asymptotically as efficient as optimal batch learning.

On-line learning is useful when the target vector fluctuates slowly (Amari, 1967). In this case, we need to modify a learning constant η_t depending on how far the current weight vector is located from the target function. We show an algorithm adaptive changes in the learning constant based on the Riemannian criterion and prove that it gives asymptotically optimal behavior. This is a generalization of the idea of Sompolinsky et al. [1995].

We then answer the question what is the Riemannian structure to be introduced in the parameter space of synaptic weights. We answer this problem from the point of view of information geometry (Amari [1985, 1995], Amari et al [1992]). The explicit form of the Riemannian metric and its inverse matrix are given in the case of simple perceptrons.

We finally show how the Riemannian gradient is applied to blind separation of mixtured independent signal sources. Here, the mixing matrix is unknown so that the parameter space is the space of matrices. The Riemannian structure is introduced in it. The natural Riemannian gradient is computationally much simpler and more effective than the conventional gradient.

2 Stochastic Gradient Descent and On-Line Learning

Let us consider a neural network which is specified by a vector parameter $\boldsymbol{w} = (w_1, \cdots w_n) \in \boldsymbol{R}^n$. The parameter $\boldsymbol{w}$ is composed of modifiable connection weights and thresholds. Let us denote by $l(\boldsymbol{x}, \boldsymbol{w})$ a loss when input signal $\boldsymbol{x}$ is processed by a network having parameter $\boldsymbol{w}$. In the case of multilayer perceptrons, a desired output or teacher signal $\boldsymbol{y}$ is associated with $\boldsymbol{x}$, and a typical loss is given

$$l(\boldsymbol{x}, \boldsymbol{y}, \boldsymbol{w}) = \frac{1}{2} \parallel \boldsymbol{y} - \boldsymbol{f}(\boldsymbol{x}, \boldsymbol{w}) \parallel^2, \qquad (1)$$

where $\boldsymbol{z} = \boldsymbol{f}(\boldsymbol{x}, \boldsymbol{w})$ is the output from the network.

When input $\boldsymbol{x}$, or input-output training pair $(\boldsymbol{x}, \boldsymbol{y})$, is generated from a fixed probability distribution, the expected loss $L(\boldsymbol{w})$ of the network specified by $\boldsymbol{w}$ is

$$L(\boldsymbol{w}) = \mathrm{E}[l(\boldsymbol{x}, \boldsymbol{y}; \boldsymbol{w})], \qquad (2)$$

where E denotes the expectation. A neural network is trained by using training examples $(\boldsymbol{x}_1, \boldsymbol{y}_1), (\boldsymbol{x}_2, \boldsymbol{y}_2), \cdots$ to obtain the optimal network parameter $\boldsymbol{w}^*$ that minimizes $L(\boldsymbol{w})$. If $L(\boldsymbol{w})$ is known, the gradient method is described by

$$\boldsymbol{w}_{t+1} = \boldsymbol{w}_t - \eta_t \nabla L(\boldsymbol{w}_t), \qquad t = 1, 2, \cdots$$

where η_t is a learning constant depending on t and $\nabla L = \partial L / \partial \boldsymbol{w}$. Usually $L(\boldsymbol{w})$ is unknown. The stochastic gradient learning method

$$\boldsymbol{w}_{t+1} = \boldsymbol{w}_t - \eta_t \nabla l(\boldsymbol{x}_{t+1}, \boldsymbol{y}_{t+1}; \boldsymbol{w}_t) \qquad (3)$$

was proposed by an old paper (Amari [1967]). This method has become popular since Rumelhart et al. [1986] rediscovered it. It is expected that, when η_t converges to 0 in a certain manner, the above $\boldsymbol{w}_t$ converges to $\boldsymbol{w}^*$. The dynamical behavior of

(3) was studied by Amari [1967], Heskes and Kappen [1992] and many others when η_t is a constant.

It was also shown in Amari [1967] that

$$w_{t+1} = w_t - \eta_t G^{-1}\nabla l(x_{t+1}, y_{t+1}, w_t) \tag{4}$$

works well for any positive-definite matrix, in particular for the metric G. Geometrically speaking $\partial l/\partial w$ is a covariant vector while $\Delta w_t = w_{t+1} - w_t$ is a contravariant vector. Therefore, it is natural to use a (contravariant) metric tensor G^{-1} to convert the covariant gradient into the contravariant form

$$\tilde{\nabla} l = G^{-1}\frac{\partial l}{\partial w} = \left(\sum_j g^{ij}\frac{\partial}{\partial w_j}(w)\right), \tag{5}$$

where $G^{-1} = (g^{ij})$ is the inverse matrix of $G = (g_{ij})$. The present paper studies how the matrix tensor matrix G should be defined in neural learning and how effective is the new gradient learning rule

$$w_{t+1} = w_t - \eta_t \tilde{\nabla} l(x_t, y_t, w_t). \tag{6}$$

3 Gradient in Riemannian spaces

Let $S = \{w\}$ be the parameter space and let $l(w)$ be a function defined on S. When S is a Euclidean space and w is an orthonormal coordinate system, the squared length of a small incremental vector dw connecting w and $w + dw$ is given by

$$|dw|^2 = \sum_{i=1}^n (dw_i)^2. \tag{7}$$

However, when the coordinate system is non-orthonormal or the space S is Riemannian, the squared length is given by a quadratic form

$$|dw|^2 = \sum_{i,j} g_{ij}(w) dw_i dw_j = w'Gw. \tag{8}$$

Here, the matrix $G = (g_{ij})$ depends in general on w and is called the metric tensor. It reduces to the identity matrix I in the Euclidean orthonormal case. It will be shown soon that the parameter space S of neural networks has Riemannian structure (see Amari et al. [1992], Amari [1995], etc.).

The steepest descent direction of a function $l(w)$ at w is defined by a vector dw that minimize $l(w+dw)$ under the constraint $|dw|^2 = \varepsilon^2$ (see eq.8) for a sufficiently small constant ε.

Lemma 1. The steepest descent direction of $l(w)$ in a Riemannian space is given by

$$-\tilde{\nabla} l(w) = -G^{-1}(w)\nabla l(w).$$

We call

$$\tilde{\nabla} l(w) = G^{-1}(w)\nabla l(w)$$

the natural gradient of $l(w)$ in the Riemannian space. It shows the steepest descent direction of l, and is nothing but the contravariant form of ∇l in the tensor notation. When the space is Euclidean and the coordinate system is orthonormal, G is the unit matrix I so that $\tilde{\nabla} l = \nabla l$.

4 Natural gradient gives efficient on-line learning

Let us begin with the simplest case of noisy multilayer analog perceptrons. Given input x, the network emits output $z = f(x, w) + n$, where f is a differentiable deterministic function of the multilayer perceptron with parameter w and n is a noise subject to the normal distribution $N(0, I)$. The probability density of an input-output pair (x, z) is given by

$$p(x, z; w) = q(x)p(z|x; w),$$

where $q(x)$ is the probability distribution of input x, and

$$p(z|x; w) = \frac{1}{\sqrt{2\pi}} \exp\left\{-\frac{1}{2} \| z - f(x, w) \|^2\right\}.$$

The squared error loss function (1) can be written as

$$l(x, z, w) = -\log p(x, z; w) + \log q(x) - \log \sqrt{2\pi}.$$

Hence, minimizing the loss is equivalent to maximizing the likelihood function $p(x, z; w)$.

Let $D_T = \{(x_1, z_1), \cdots, (x_T, z_T)\}$ be T independent input-output examples generated by the network having the parameter w^*. Then, maximum likelihood estimator $\hat{w}_T$ minimizes the log loss $l(x, z; w) = -\log p(x, z; w)$ over the training data D_T, that is, it minimizes the training error

$$E_{\text{train}}(w) = \frac{1}{T} \sum_{t=1}^{T} l(x_t, z_t; w). \tag{9}$$

The maximum likelihood estimator is efficient (or Fisher-efficient), implying that it is the best consistent estimator satisfying the Cramér-Rao bound asymptotically,

$$\lim_{T \to \infty} T E[(\hat{w}_T - w^*)(\hat{w}_T - w^*)'] = G^{-1}, \tag{10}$$

where G^{-1} is the inverse of the Fisher information matrix $G = (g_{ij})$ defined by

$$g_{ij} = E\left[\frac{\partial \log p(x, z; w)}{\partial w_i} \frac{\partial \log p(x, z; w)}{\partial w_j}\right] \tag{11}$$

in the component form. Information geometry (Amari, 1985) proves that the Fisher information G is the only invariant metric to be introduced in the space $S = \{w\}$ of the parameters of probability distributions.

Examples $(x_1, z_1), (x_2, z_2) \cdots$ are given one at a time in the case of on-line learning. Let $\tilde{w}_t$ be the estimated value at time t. At the next time $t+1$, the estimator $\tilde{w}_t$ is modified to give a new estimator $\tilde{w}_{t+1}$ based on the observation (x_{t+1}, z_{t+1}). The old observations $(x_1, z_1), \cdots, (x_t, z_t)$ cannot be reused to obtain $\tilde{w}_{t+1}$, so that the learning rule is written as $\tilde{w}_{t+1} = m(x_{t+1}, z_{t+1}, \tilde{w}_t)$. The process $\{\tilde{w}_t\}$ is hence Markovian. Whatever a learning rule m we choose, the behavior of the estimator $\tilde{w}_t$ is never better than that of the optimal batch estimator $\hat{w}_t$ because of this restriction. The conventional on-line learning rule is given by the following gradient form $\tilde{w}_{t+1} = \tilde{w}_t - \eta_t \nabla l(x_{t+1}, z_{t+1}; \tilde{w}_t)$. When η_t satisfies a certain condition, say $\eta_t = c/t$, the stochastic approximation guarantees that $\tilde{w}_t$ is a consistent estimator converging to w^*. However, it is not efficient in general.

There arises a question if there exists an on-line learning rule that gives an efficient estimator. If it exists, the asymptotic behavior of on-line learning is equivalent to that of the batch estimation method. The present paper answers the question by giving an efficient on-line learning rule

$$\tilde{w}_{t+1} = \tilde{w}_t - \frac{1}{t}\tilde{\nabla}l(x_{t+1}, z_{t+1}; \tilde{w}_t). \tag{12}$$

Theorem 1. The natural gradient on-line learning rule gives an Fisher-efficient estimator, that is,

$$\tilde{V}_t = E[(\tilde{w}_t - w^*)(\tilde{w}_t - w^*)'] \approx \frac{1}{t}G^{-1}(w^*). \tag{13}$$

5 Adaptive modification of learning constant

We have proved that $\eta_t = 1/t$ with the coefficient matrix G^{-1} is the asymptotically best choice for on-line learning. However, when the target parameter w^* is not fixed but fluctuating or changes suddenly, this choice is not good, because the learning system cannot follow the change if η_t is too small. It was proposed in Amari [1967] to choose η_t adaptively such that η_t becomes larger when the current target w^* is far from w_t and becomes small when it is close to w_t adaptively. However, no definite scheme was analyzed there. Sompolinsky et al. [1995] proposed an excellent scheme of an adaptive choice of η_t for a deterministic dichotomy neural networks. We extend their idea to be applicable to stochastic cases, where the Riemannian structure plays a role.

We assume that $l(x, z; w)$ is differentiable with respect to w. (The non-differentiable case is usually more difficult to analyze. Sompolinsky et al [1995] treated this case.) We moreover treat the realizable teacher so that $L(w^*) = 0$.

We propose the following learning scheme:

$$\hat{w}_{t+1} = \hat{w}_t - \eta_t \tilde{\nabla}l(x_{t+1}, z_{t+1}; \hat{w}_t) \tag{14}$$

$$\eta_{t+1} = \eta_t + \alpha\eta_t[\beta l(x_{t+1}, z_{t+1}; \hat{w}_t) - \eta_t], \tag{15}$$

where α and β are constants. We try to analyze the dynamical behavior of learning by using the continuous version of the algorithm,

$$\frac{d}{dt}\hat{w}_t = -\eta_t \tilde{\nabla}l(x_t, z_t; \hat{w}_t), \tag{16}$$

$$\frac{d}{dt}\eta_t = \alpha\eta_t[\beta l(x_t, z_t; \hat{w}_t) - \eta_t]. \tag{17}$$

In order to show the dynamical behavior of $(\hat{w}_t, \eta_t)$, we use the averaged version of the above equation with respect to the current input-output pair (x_t, z_t). We introduce the squared error variable

$$e_t = \frac{1}{2}(w_t - w^*)'G^*(w_t - w^*). \tag{18}$$

By using the average and continuous time version

$$\dot{w}_t = -\eta_t G^{-1}(w_t)\left\langle \frac{\partial}{\partial w}l(x_t, z_t; w_t)\right\rangle,$$

$$\dot{\eta}_t = \alpha\eta_t\{\beta\langle l(x_t, z_t; w_t)\rangle - \eta_t\},$$

where $\dot{}$ denotes d/dt and $\langle\,\rangle$ the average over the current (x, z), we have

$$\dot{e}_t = -2\eta_t e_t, \tag{19}$$

$$\dot{\eta}_t = \alpha\beta\eta_t e_t - \alpha\eta_t^2. \tag{20}$$

The behavior of the above equation is interesting : The origin (0,0) is its attractor. However, the basin of attraction has a fractal boundary. Anyway, starting from an adequate initial value, it has the solution of the form

$$e_t \approx \frac{1}{\beta}\left(\frac{1}{2} - \frac{1}{\alpha}\right)\frac{1}{t}, \tag{21}$$

$$\eta_t \approx \frac{1}{2t}. \tag{22}$$

This proves the $1/t$ convergence rate of the generalization error, that is optimal in order for any estimator $\hat{\boldsymbol{w}}_t$ converging to $\boldsymbol{w}^*$.

6 Riemannian structures of simple perceptrons

We first study the parameter space S of simple perceptrons to obtain an explicit form of the metric G and its inverse G^{-1}. This suggests how to calculate the metric in the parameter space of multilayer perceptrons.

Let us consider a simple perceptron with input $\boldsymbol{x}$ and output z. Let $\boldsymbol{w}$ be its connection weight vector. For the analog stochastic perceptron, its input-output behavior is described by $z = f(\boldsymbol{w}'\boldsymbol{x}) + n$, where n denotes a random noise subject to the normal distribution $N(0, \sigma^2)$ and f is the hyperbolic tangent,

$$f(u) = \frac{1 - e^{-u}}{1 + e^{-u}}.$$

In order to calculate the metric G explicitly, let $\boldsymbol{e_w}$ be the unit column vector in the direction of $\boldsymbol{w}$ in the Euclidean space $\boldsymbol{R}^n$,

$$\boldsymbol{e_w} = \frac{\boldsymbol{w}}{\|\boldsymbol{w}\|},$$

where $\|\boldsymbol{w}\|$ is the Euclidean norm. We then have the following theorem.

Theorem 2. The Fisher metric G and its inverse G^{-1} are given by

$$G(\boldsymbol{w}) = c_1(w)I + \{c_2(w) - c_1(w)\}\boldsymbol{e_w}\boldsymbol{e}'_{\boldsymbol{w}}, \tag{23}$$

$$G^{-1}(\boldsymbol{w}) = \frac{1}{c_1(w)}I + \left(\frac{1}{c_2(w)} - \frac{1}{c_1(w)}\right)\boldsymbol{e_w}\boldsymbol{e}'_{\boldsymbol{w}}. \tag{24}$$

where $w = |\boldsymbol{w}|$ (Euclidean norm) and $c_1(w)$ and $c_2(w)$ are given by

$$c_1(w) = \frac{1}{4\sqrt{2\pi}\sigma^2}\int\{f^2(w\varepsilon) - 1\}^2 \exp\left\{-\frac{1}{2}\varepsilon^2\right\}d\varepsilon, \tag{25}$$

$$c_2(w) = \frac{1}{4\sqrt{2\pi}\sigma^2}\int\{f^2(w\varepsilon) - 1\}^2\varepsilon^2 \exp\left\{-\frac{1}{2}\varepsilon^2\right\}d\varepsilon. \tag{26}$$

Theorem 3. The Jeffrey prior is given by

$$\sqrt{|G(\boldsymbol{w})|} = \frac{1}{V_n}\sqrt{c_2(w)\{c_1(w)\}^{n-1}}. \tag{27}$$

7 The natural gradient for blind separation of mixtured signals

Let $\boldsymbol{s} = (s_1, \cdots, s_n)$ be n source signals which are n independent random variables. We assume that their n mixtures $\boldsymbol{x} = (x_1, \cdots, x_n)$,

$$\boldsymbol{x} = A\boldsymbol{s} \tag{28}$$

are observed. Here, A is a matrix. When s is time serieses, we observe $x(1), \cdots, x(t)$. The problem of blind separation is to estimate $W = A^{-1}$ adaptively from $x(t)$, $t = 1, 2, 3, \cdots$ without knowing $s(t)$ nor A. We can then recover original s by

$$y = \hat{W}x \qquad (29)$$

when $\hat{W} = A^{-1}$. Let $W \in Gl(n)$, that is a nonsingular $n \times n$-matrix, and $\phi(W)$ be a scalar function. This is given by a measure of independence such as $\phi(W) = KL[\tilde{p}(y); p(y)]$, which is represented by the expectation of a loss function. We define the natural gradient of $\phi(W)$.

Now we return to our manifold $Gl(n)$ of matrices. It has the Lie group structure : Any $A \in Gl(n)$ maps $Gl(n)$ to $Gl(n)$ by $W \to WA$. We impose that the Riemannian structure should be invariant by this operation A.

We can then prove that the natural gradient in this case is

$$\tilde{\nabla}\phi = \nabla\phi W'W. \qquad (30)$$

The natural gradient works surprisingly well for adaptive blind signal separation Amari et al. [1995], Cardoso and Laheld [1996].

References

[1] S. Amari. Theory of adaptive pattern classifiers, *IEEE Trans.*, **EC-16**, No.3, 299–307, 1967.

[2] S. Amari. *Differential-Geometrical Methods in Statistics, Lecture Notes in Statistics*, vol.**28**, Springer, 1985.

[3] S. Amari. Information geometry of the EM and em algorithms for neural networks, *Neural Networks*, **8**, No.9, 1379–1408, 1995.

[4] S. Amari, A. Cichocki and H.H. Yang. A new learning algorithm for blind signal separation, in *NIPS'95*, vol.**8**, 1996, MIT Press, Cambridge, Mass.

[5] S. Amari, K. Kurata, H. Nagaoka. Information geometry of Boltzmann machines, *IEEE Trans. on Neural Networks*, **3**, 260–271, 1992.

[6] J. F. Cardoso and Beate Laheld. Equivariant adaptive source separation, to appear *IEEE Trans. on Signal Processing*, 1996.

[7] T. M. Heskes and B. Kappen. Learning processes in neural networks, *Physical Review A*, **440**, 2718–2726, 1991.

[8] D. Rumelhart, G.E. Hinton and R. J. Williams. Learning internal representation, in *Parallel Distributed Processing: Explorations in the Microstructure of Cognition*, **1**, *Foundations*, MIT Press, Cambridge, MA, 1986.

[9] H. Sompolinsky, N. Barkai and H. S. Seung. On-line learning of dichotomies: algorithms and learning curves, *Neural Networks: The statistical Mechanics Perspective*, Proceedings of the CTP-PBSRI Joint Workshop on Theoretical Physics, J.-H. Oh et al eds, 105–130, 1995.

For valid generalization, the size of the weights is more important than the size of the network

Peter L. Bartlett
Department of Systems Engineering
Research School of Information Sciences and Engineering
Australian National University
Canberra, 0200 Australia
Peter.Bartlett@anu.edu.au

Abstract

This paper shows that if a large neural network is used for a pattern classification problem, and the learning algorithm finds a network with small weights that has small squared error on the training patterns, then the generalization performance depends on the size of the weights rather than the number of weights. More specifically, consider an ℓ-layer feed-forward network of sigmoid units, in which the sum of the magnitudes of the weights associated with each unit is bounded by A. The misclassification probability converges to an error estimate (that is closely related to squared error on the training set) at rate $O((cA)^{\ell(\ell+1)/2}\sqrt{(\log n)/m})$ ignoring log factors, where m is the number of training patterns, n is the input dimension, and c is a constant. This may explain the generalization performance of neural networks, particularly when the number of training examples is considerably smaller than the number of weights. It also supports heuristics (such as weight decay and early stopping) that attempt to keep the weights small during training.

1 Introduction

Results from statistical learning theory give bounds on the number of training examples that are necessary for satisfactory generalization performance in classification problems, in terms of the Vapnik-Chervonenkis dimension of the class of functions used by the learning system (see, for example, [13, 5]). Baum and Haussler [4] used these results to give sample size bounds for multi-layer threshold networks that grow at least as quickly as the number of weights (see also [7]). However, for pattern classification applications the VC-bounds seem loose; neural networks often perform successfully with training sets that are considerably smaller than the number of weights. This paper shows that for classification problems on which neural networks perform well, if the weights are not too big, the size of the weights determines the generalization performance.

In contrast with the function classes and algorithms considered in the VC-theory, neural networks used for binary classification problems have real-valued outputs, and learning algorithms typically attempt to minimize the squared error of the network output over a training set. As well as encouraging the correct classification, this tends to push the output away from zero and towards the target values of $\{-1, 1\}$. It is easy to see that if the total squared error of a hypothesis on m examples is no more than $m\epsilon$, then on no more than $m\epsilon/(1-\alpha)^2$ of these examples can the hypothesis have either the incorrect sign or magnitude less than α.

The next section gives misclassification probability bounds for hypotheses that are "distinctly correct" in this way on most examples. These bounds are in terms of a scale-sensitive version of the VC-dimension, called the fat-shattering dimension. Section 3 gives bounds on this dimension for feedforward sigmoid networks, which imply the main results. The proofs are sketched in Section 4. Full proofs can be found in the full version [2].

2 Notation and bounds on misclassification probability

Denote the space of input patterns by X. The space of labels is $\{-1, 1\}$. We assume that there is a probability distribution P on the product space $X \times \{-1, 1\}$, that reflects both the relative frequency of different input patterns and the relative frequency of an expert's classification of those patterns. The learning algorithm uses a class of real-valued functions, called the hypothesis class H. An hypothesis h is correct on an example (x, y) if $\text{sgn}(h(x)) = y$, where $\text{sgn}(\alpha) : \mathbb{R} \to \{-1, 1\}$ takes value 1 iff $\alpha \geq 0$, so the misclassification probability (or error) of h is defined as

$$\text{er}_P(h) = P\{(x, y) \in X \times \{-1, 1\} : \text{sgn}(h(x)) \neq y\}.$$

The crucial quantity determining misclassification probability is the fat-shattering dimension of the hypothesis class H. We say that a sequence $x_1, \ldots, x_d$ of d points from X is shattered by H if functions in H can give all classifications of the sequence. That is, for all $b = (b_1, \ldots, b_m) \in \{-1, 1\}^m$ there is an h in H satisfying $\text{sgn}(h(x_i)) = b_i$. The VC-dimension of H is defined as the size of the largest shattered sequence.[1]

For a given scale parameter $\gamma > 0$, we say that a sequence $x_1, \ldots, x_d$ of d points from X is γ-shattered by H if there is a sequence $r_1, \ldots, r_d$ of real values such that for all $b = (b_1, \ldots, b_m) \in \{-1, 1\}^m$ there is an h in H satisfying $(h(x_i) - r_i)b_i \geq \gamma$. The fat-shattering dimension of H at γ, denoted $\text{fat}_H(\gamma)$, is the size of the largest γ-shattered sequence. This dimension reflects the complexity of the functions in the class H, when examined at scale γ. Notice that $\text{fat}_H(\gamma)$ is a nonincreasing function of γ. The following theorem gives generalization error bounds in terms of $\text{fat}_H(\gamma)$. A related result, that applies to the case of no errors on the training set, will appear in [12].

Theorem 1 *Define the input space X, hypothesis class H, and probability distribution P on $X \times \{-1, 1\}$ as above. Let $0 < \delta < 1/2$, and $0 < \gamma < 1$. Then, with probability $1 - \delta$ over the training sequence $(x_1, y_1), \ldots, (x_m, y_m)$ of m labelled*

---
[1]In fact, according to the usual definition, this is the VC-dimension of the class of thresholded versions of functions in H.

examples, every hypothesis h in H satisfies

$$\text{er}_P(h) < \frac{1}{m}|\{i : |h(x_i)| < \gamma \text{ or } \text{sgn}(h(x_i)) \neq y_i\}| + \epsilon(\gamma, m, \delta),$$

where

$$\epsilon^2(\gamma, m, \delta) = \frac{2}{m}\left(d\ln(50em/d)\log_2(1250m) + \ln(4/\delta)\right), \qquad (1)$$

and $d = \text{fat}_H(\gamma/16)$.

2.1 Comments

It is informative to compare this result with the standard VC-bound. In that case, the bound on misclassification probability is

$$\text{er}_P(h) < \frac{1}{m}|\{i : \text{sgn}(h(x_i)) \neq y_i\}| + \left(\frac{c}{m}(d\log(m/d) + \log(1/\delta))\right)^{1/2},$$

where $d = \text{VCdim}(H)$ and c is a constant. We shall see in the next section that there are function classes H for which VCdim(H) is infinite but $\text{fat}_H(\gamma)$ is finite for all $\gamma > 0$; an example is the class of functions computed by any two-layer neural network with an arbitrary number of parameters but constraints on the size of the parameters. It is known that if the learning algorithm and error estimates are constrained to make use of the sample only by considering the proportion of training examples that hypotheses misclassify, there are distributions P for which the second term in the VC-bound above cannot be improved by more than log factors. Theorem 1 shows that it can be improved if the learning algorithm makes use of the sample by considering the proportion of training examples that are correctly classified and have $|h(x_i)| < \gamma$. It is possible to give a lower bound (see the full paper [2]) which, for the function classes considered here, shows that Theorem 1 also cannot be improved by more than log factors.

The idea of using the magnitudes of the values of $h(x_i)$ to give a more precise estimate of the generalization performance was first proposed by Vapnik in [13] (and was further developed by Vapnik and co-workers). There it was used only for the case of linear hypothesis classes. Results in [13] give bounds on misclassification probability for a test sample, in terms of values of h on the training and test data. This result is extended in [11], to give bounds on misclassification probability (that is, for unseen data) in terms of the values of h on the training examples. This is further extended in [12] to more general function classes, to give error bounds that are applicable when there is a hypothesis with no errors on the training examples. Lugosi and Pintér [9] have also obtained bounds on misclassification probability in terms of similar properties of the class of functions containing the true regression function (conditional expectation of y given x). However, their results do not extend to the case when the true regression function is not in the class of real-valued functions used by the estimator.

It seems unnatural that the quantity γ is specified in advance in Theorem 1, since it depends on the examples. The full paper [2] gives a similar result in which the statement is made uniform over all values of this quantity.

3 The fat-shattering dimension of neural networks

Bounds on the VC-dimension of various neural network classes have been established (see [10] for a review), but these are all at least linear in the number of parameters. In this section, we give bounds on the fat-shattering dimension for several neural network classes.

We assume that the input space X is some subset of $\mathbb{R}^n$. Define a sigmoid unit as a function from $\mathbb{R}^k$ to $\mathbb{R}$, parametrized by a vector of weights $w \in \mathbb{R}^k$. The unit computes $x \mapsto \sigma(x \cdot w)$, where σ is a fixed bounded function satisfying a Lipchitz condition. (For simplicity, we ignore the offset parameter. It is equivalent to including an extra input with a constant value.) A multi-layer feed-forward sigmoid network of depth ℓ is a network of sigmoid units with a single output unit, which can be arranged in a layered structure with ℓ layers, so that the output of a unit passes only to the inputs of units in later layers. We will consider networks in which the weights are bounded. The relevant norm is the ℓ_1 norm: for a vector $w \in \mathbb{R}^k$, define $\|w\|_1 = \sum_{i=1}^k |w_i|$. The following result gives a bound on the fat-shattering dimension of a (bounded) linear combination of real-valued functions, in terms of the fat-shattering dimension of the basis function class. We can apply this result in a recursive fashion to give bounds for single output feed-forward networks.

Theorem 2 *Let F be a class of functions that map from X to $[-M/2, M/2]$, such that $0 \in F$ and, for all f in F, $-f \in F$. For $A > 0$, define the class H of weight-bounded linear combinations of functions from F as*

$$H = \left\{ \sum_{i=1}^k w_i f_i : k \in \mathbb{N}, f_i \in F, \|w\|_1 \leq A \right\}.$$

Suppose $\gamma > 0$ is such that $d = \text{fat}_F(\gamma/(32A)) \geq 1$. Then $\text{fat}_H(\gamma) \leq (cM^2 A^2 d/\gamma^2) \log^2(MAd/\gamma)$, for some constant c.

Gurvits and Koiran [6] have shown that the fat-shattering dimension of the class of two-layer networks with bounded output weights and linear threshold hidden units is $O\left((A^2 n^2/\gamma^2) \log(n/\gamma)\right)$, when $X = \mathbb{R}^n$. As a special case, Theorem 2 improves this result.

Notice that the fat-shattering dimension of a function class is not changed by more than a constant factor if we compose the functions with a fixed function satisfying a Lipschitz condition (like the standard sigmoid function). Also, for $X = \mathbb{R}^n$ and $H = \{x \mapsto x_i\}$ we have $\text{fat}_H(\gamma) \leq \log n$ for all γ. Finally, for $H = \{x \mapsto w \cdot x : w \in \mathbb{R}^n\}$ we have $\text{fat}_H(\gamma) \leq n$ for all γ. These observations, together with Theorem 2, give the following corollary. The $\tilde{O}(\cdot)$ notation suppresses log factors. (Formally, $f = \tilde{O}(g)$ if $f = o(g^{1+\alpha})$ for all $\alpha > 0$.)

Corollary 3 *If $X \subseteq \mathbb{R}^n$ and H is the class of two-layer sigmoid networks with the weights in the output unit satisfying $\|w\|_1 \leq A$, then $\text{fat}_H(\gamma) = \tilde{O}\left(A^2 n/\gamma^2\right)$.*

If $X = \{x \in \mathbb{R}^n : \|x\|_\infty \leq B\}$ and the hidden unit weights are also bounded, then $\text{fat}_H(\gamma) = \tilde{O}\left(B^2 A^6 (\log n)/\gamma^4\right)$.

Applying Theorem 2 to this result gives the following result for deeper networks. Notice that there is no constraint on the number of hidden units in any layer, only on the total magnitude of the weights associated with a processing unit.

Corollary 4 *For some constant c, if $X \subseteq \mathbb{R}^n$ and H is the class of depth ℓ sigmoid networks in which the weight vector w associated with each unit beyond the first layer satisfies $\|w\|_1 \leq A$, then $\text{fat}_H(\gamma) = \tilde{O}\left(n(cA)^{\ell(\ell-1)}/\gamma^{2(\ell-1)}\right)$.*

If $X = \{x \in \mathbb{R}^n : \|x\|_\infty \leq B\}$ and the weights in the first layer units also satisfy $\|w\|_1 \leq A$, then $\text{fat}_H(\gamma) = \tilde{O}\left(B^2 (cA)^{\ell(\ell+1)}/\gamma^{2\ell} \log n\right)$.

In the first part of this corollary, the network has fat-shattering dimension similar to the VC-dimension of a linear network. This formalizes the intuition that when the weights are small, the network operates in the "linear part" of the sigmoid, and so behaves like a linear network.

3.1 Comments

Consider a depth ℓ sigmoid network with bounded weights. The last corollary and Theorem 1 imply that if the training sample size grows roughly as $B^2 A^{\ell^2}/\epsilon^2$, then the misclassification probability of a network is within ϵ of the proportion of training examples that the network classifies as "distinctly correct."

These results give a plausible explanation for the generalization performance of neural networks. If, in applications, networks with many units have small weights and small squared error on the training examples, then the VC-dimension (and hence number of parameters) is not as important as the magnitude of the weights for generalization performance.

It is possible to give a version of Theorem 1 in which the probability bound is uniform over all values of a complexity parameter indexing the function classes (using the same technique mentioned at the end of Section 2.1). For the case of sigmoid network classes, indexed by a weight bound, minimizing the resulting bound on misclassification probability is equivalent to minimizing the sum of a sample error term and a penalty term involving the weight bound. This supports the use of two popular heuristic techniques, weight decay and early stopping (see, for example, [8]), which aim to minimize squared error while maintaining small weights.

These techniques give bounds on the fat-shattering dimension and hence generalization performance for any function class that can be expressed as a bounded number of compositions of either bounded-weight linear combinations or scalar Lipschitz functions with functions in a class that has finite fat-shattering dimension. This includes, for example, radial basis function networks.

4 Proofs

4.1 Proof sketch of Theorem 1

For $A \subseteq S$, where (S, ρ) is a pseudometric space, a set $T \subseteq S$ is an ϵ-cover of A if for all a in A there is a t in T with $\rho(t, a) < \epsilon$. We define $\mathcal{N}(A, \epsilon, \rho)$ as the size of the smallest ϵ-cover of A. For $x = (x_1, \ldots, x_m) \in X^m$, define the pseudometric $d_{\ell_\infty(x)}$ on the set S of functions defined on X by $d_{\ell_\infty(x)}(f, g) = \max_i |f(x_i) - g(x_i)|$. For a set A of functions, denote $\max_{x \in X^m} \mathcal{N}(A, \epsilon, d_{\ell_\infty(x)})$ by $\mathcal{N}_\infty(A, \epsilon, m)$. Alon et al. [1] have obtained the following bound on $\mathcal{N}_\infty$ in terms of the fat-shattering dimension.

Lemma 5 *For a class F of functions that map from $\{1, \ldots, n\}$ to $\{1, \ldots, b\}$ with $\text{fat}_F(1) \leq d$, $\log_2 \mathcal{N}_\infty(F, 2, n) < 1 + \log_2(nb^2) \log_2 \left(\sum_{i=0}^d \binom{n}{i} b^i \right)$, provided that $n \geq 1 + \log_2 \left(\sum_{i=0}^d \binom{n}{i} b^i \right)$.*

For $\gamma > 0$ define $\pi_\gamma : \mathbb{R} \to [-\gamma, \gamma]$ as the piecewise-linear squashing function satisfying $\pi_\gamma(\alpha) = \gamma$ if $\alpha \geq \gamma$, $\pi_\gamma(\alpha) = -\gamma$ if $\alpha \leq -\gamma$, and $\pi_\gamma(\alpha) = \alpha$ otherwise. For a class H of real-valued functions, define $\pi_\gamma(H)$ as the set of compositions of π_γ with functions in H.

Lemma 6 *For $X, H, P, \delta,$ and γ as in Theorem 1,*

$$P^m \left\{ z : \exists h \in H, \text{er}_P(h) \geq \left(\frac{2}{m} \ln \left(\frac{2\mathcal{N}_\infty(\pi_\gamma(H), \gamma/2, 2m)}{\delta} \right) \right)^{1/2} + \frac{1}{m} |\{i : |h(x_i)| < \gamma \text{ or } \text{sgn}(h(x_i)) \neq y_i\}| \right\} < \delta.$$

The proof of the lemma relies on the observation that

$$P^m \left\{ z : \exists h \in H, \text{er}_P(h) \geq \epsilon + \frac{1}{m} |\{i : |h(x_i)| < \gamma \text{ or } \text{sgn}(h(x_i)) \neq y_i\}| \right\}$$
$$\leq P^m \left\{ z : \exists h \in H, P\left(|\pi_\gamma(h(x)) - \gamma y| \geq \gamma\right) \geq \epsilon + \frac{1}{m} |\{i : \pi_\gamma(h(x_i)) \neq \gamma y_i\}| \right\}.$$

We then use a standard symmetrization argument and the permutation argument introduced by Vapnik and Chervonenkis to bound this probability by the probability under a random permutation of a double-length sample that a related property holds. For any fixed sample, we can then use Pollard's approach of approximating the hypothesis class using a $(\gamma/2)$-cover, except that in this case the appropriate cover is with respect to the ℓ_∞ pseudometric. Applying Hoeffding's inequality gives the lemma.

To prove Theorem 1, we need to bound the covering numbers in terms of the fat-shattering dimension. It is easy to apply Lemma 5 to a quantized version of the function class to get such a bound, taking advantage of the range constraint imposed by the squashing function π_γ.

4.2 Proof sketch of Theorem 2

For $x = (x_1, \ldots, x_m) \in X^m$, define the pseudometric $d_{\ell_1(x)}$ on the class of functions defined on X by $d_{\ell_1(x)}(f,g) = \frac{1}{m} \sum_{i=1}^m |f(x_i) - g(x_i)|$. Similarly, define $d_{\ell_2(x)}(f,g) = \left(\frac{1}{m} \sum_{i=1}^m (f(x_i) - g(x_i))^2\right)^{1/2}$. If A is a set of functions defined on X, denote $\max_{x \in X^m} \mathcal{N}(A, \gamma, d_{\ell_1(x)})$ by $\mathcal{N}_1(A, \gamma, m)$, and similarly for $\mathcal{N}_2(A, \gamma, m)$.

The idea of the proof of Theorem 2 is to first derive a general upper bound on an ℓ_1 covering number of the class H, and then apply the following result (which is implicit in the proof of Theorem 2 in [3]) to give a bound on the fat-shattering dimension.

Lemma 7 *For a class F of $[0,1]$-valued functions on X satisfying $\text{fat}_F(4\gamma) \geq d$, we have $\log_2 \mathcal{N}_1(F, \gamma, d) \geq d/32$.*

To derive an upper bound on $\mathcal{N}_1(\gamma, H, m)$, we start with the bound that Lemma 5 implies on the ℓ_∞ covering number $\mathcal{N}_\infty(F, \gamma, m)$ for the class F of hidden unit functions. Since $d_{\ell_2}(f,g) \leq d_{\ell_\infty}(f,g)$, this implies the following bound on the ℓ_2 covering number for F (provided m satisfies the condition required by Lemma 5, and it turns out that the theorem is trivial otherwise).

$$\log_2 \mathcal{N}_2(F, \gamma, m) < 1 + d \log_2 \left(\frac{4emM}{d\gamma}\right) \log_2 \left(\frac{9mM^2}{\gamma^2}\right). \quad (2)$$

Next, we use the following result on approximation in ℓ_2, which A. Barron attributes to Maurey.

Lemma 8 (Maurey) *Suppose G is a Hilbert space and $F \subseteq G$ has $\|f\| \leq b$ for all f in F. Let f be an element from the convex closure of F. Then for all $k \geq 1$ and all $c > b^2 - \|f\|^2$, there are functions $\{f_1, \ldots, f_k\} \subseteq F$ such that $\left\| f - \frac{1}{k} \sum_{i=1}^k f_i \right\|^2 \leq \frac{c}{k}$.*

This implies that any element of H can be approximated to a particular accuracy (with respect to ℓ_2) using a fixed linear combination of a small number of elements of F. It follows that we can construct an ℓ_2 cover of H from the ℓ_2 cover of F; using Lemma 8 and Inequality 2 shows that

$$\log_2 \mathcal{N}_2(H, \gamma, m) < \frac{2M^2 A^2}{\gamma^2} \left(1 + d \log_2 \left(\frac{8emMA}{d\gamma}\right) \log_2 \left(\frac{36mM^2 A^2}{\gamma^2}\right)\right).$$

Now, Jensen's inequality implies that $d_{l_1(x)}(f,g) \leq d_{l_2(x)}(f,g)$, which gives a bound on $\mathcal{N}_1(H, \gamma, m)$. Comparing with the lower bound given by Lemma 7 and solving for m gives the result. A more refined analysis for the neural network case involves bounding $\mathcal{N}_2$ for successive layers, and solving to give a bound on the fat-shattering dimension of the network.

Acknowledgements

Thanks to Andrew Barron, Jonathan Baxter, Mike Jordan, Adam Kowalczyk, Wee Sun Lee, Phil Long, John Shawe-Taylor, and Robert Slaviero for helpful discussions and comments.

References

[1] N. Alon, S. Ben-David, N. Cesa-Bianchi, and D. Haussler. Scale-sensitive dimensions, uniform convergence, and learnability. In *Proceedings of the 1993 IEEE Symposium on Foundations of Computer Science*. IEEE Press, 1993.

[2] P. L. Bartlett. The sample complexity of pattern classification with neural networks: the size of the weights is more important than the size of the network. Technical report, Department of Systems Engineering, Australian National University, 1996. (available by anonymous ftp from syseng.anu.edu.au:pub/peter/TR96d.ps).

[3] P. L. Bartlett, S. R. Kulkarni, and S. E. Posner. Covering numbers for real-valued function classes. Technical report, Australian National University and Princeton University, 1996.

[4] E. Baum and D. Haussler. What size net gives valid generalization? *Neural Computation*, 1(1):151–160, 1989.

[5] A. Blumer, A. Ehrenfeucht, D. Haussler, and M. K. Warmuth. Learnability and the Vapnik-Chervonenkis dimension. *J. ACM*, 36(4):929–965, 1989.

[6] L. Gurvits and P. Koiran. Approximation and learning of convex superpositions. In *Computational Learning Theory: EUROCOLT'95*, 1995.

[7] D. Haussler. Decision theoretic generalizations of the PAC model for neural net and other learning applications. *Inform. Comput.*, 100(1):78–150, 1992.

[8] J. Hertz, A. Krogh, and R. G. Palmer. *Introduction to the Theory of Neural Computation*. Addison-Wesley, 1991.

[9] G. Lugosi and M. Pintér. A data-dependent skeleton estimate for learning. In *Proc. 9th Annu. Conference on Comput. Learning Theory*. ACM Press, New York, NY, 1996.

[10] W. Maass. Vapnik-Chervonenkis dimension of neural nets. In M. A. Arbib, editor, *The Handbook of Brain Theory and Neural Networks*, pages 1000–1003. MIT Press, Cambridge, 1995.

[11] J. Shawe-Taylor, P. L. Bartlett, R. C. Williamson, and M. Anthony. A framework for structural risk minimisation. In *Proc. 9th Annu. Conference on Comput. Learning Theory*. ACM Press, New York, NY, 1996.

[12] J. Shawe-Taylor, P. L. Bartlett, R. C. Williamson, and M. Anthony. Structural risk minimization over data-dependent hierarchies. Technical report, 1996.

[13] V. N. Vapnik. *Estimation of Dependences Based on Empirical Data*. Springer-Verlag, New York, 1982.

Dynamics of Training

Siegfried Bös[*]
Lab for Information Representation
RIKEN, Hirosawa 2–1, Wako–shi
Saitama 351–01, Japan

Manfred Opper
Theoretical Physics III
University of Würzburg
97074 Würzburg, Germany

Abstract

A new method to calculate the full training process of a neural network is introduced. No sophisticated methods like the replica trick are used. The results are directly related to the actual number of training steps. Some results are presented here, like the maximal learning rate, an exact description of early stopping, and the necessary number of training steps. Further problems can be addressed with this approach.

1 INTRODUCTION

Training guided by empirical risk minimization does not always minimize the expected risk. This phenomenon is called overfitting and is one of the major problems in neural network learning. In a previous work [Bös 1995] we developed an approximate description of the training process using statistical mechanics. To solve this problem exactly, we introduce a new description which is directly dependent on the actual training steps. As a first result we get analytical curves for empirical risk and expected risk as functions of the training time, like the ones shown in Fig. 1.

To make the method tractable we restrict ourselves to a quite simple neural network model, which nevertheless demonstrates some typical behavior of neural nets. The model is a single layer perceptron, which has one N–dim. layer of adjustable weights $\vec{W}$ between input $\vec{x}$ and output z. The outputs are linear, i.e.

$$z = h = \frac{1}{\sqrt{N}} \sum_{i=1}^{N} W_i x_i \,. \qquad (1)$$

We are interested in supervised learning, where examples x_i^μ ($\mu = 1, ..., P$) are given for which the correct output z_* is known. To define the task more clearly and to monitor the training process, we assume that the examples are provided by another network, the so called *teacher* network. The teacher is not restricted to linear outputs, it can have a nonlinear output function $g_*(h_*)$.

---

[*]email: boes@zoo.riken.go.jp and opper@physik.uni-wuerzburg.de

Learning by examples attempts to minimize the error averaged over all examples, i.e. $E_T := 1/2 <(z_*^\mu - z^\mu)^2>_{\{\vec{x}^\mu\}}$, which is called *training error* or empirical risk. In fact what we are interested in is a minimal error averaged over all possible inputs $\vec{x}$, i.e $E_G := 1/2 <(z_* - z)^2>_{\{\vec{x} \in \text{Input}\}}$, called *generalization error* or expected risk.

It can be shown [see Bös 1995] that for random inputs, i.e. all components x_i are independent and have zero means and unit variance, the generalization error can be described by the order parameters R and Q,

$$E_G(t) = \frac{1}{2}[G - 2H\,R(t) + Q(t)] \quad \text{with} <\ldots>_h = \int_{-\infty}^{\infty} \frac{dh}{\sqrt{2\pi}} e^{-\frac{h^2}{2}} \ldots, \qquad (2)$$

with the two parameters $G = <[g_*(h)]^2>_h$ and $H = <g_*(h)\,h>_h$. The order parameters are defined as:

$$R(t) = <\frac{1}{N}\sum_{i=1}^{N} W_i^* W_i(t)>_{\{W_i^*\}}, \quad Q(t) = <\frac{1}{N}\sum_{i=1}^{N}(W_i(t))^2>_{\{W_i^*\}}. \qquad (3)$$

As a novelty in this paper we average the order parameters not as usual in statistical mechanics over many example realizations $\{x_i^\mu\}$, but over many teacher realizations $\{W_i^*\}$, where we use a spherical distribution. This corresponds to a Bayesian average over the unknown teacher. A study of the static properties of this model was done by Saad [1996]. Further comments about the averages can be found in the appendix.

In the next section we introduce our new method briefly. Readers, who do not wish to go into technical details in first reading, can turn directly to the results (15) and (16). The remainder of the section can be read later, as a proof. In the third section results will be presented and discussed. Finally, we conclude the paper with a summary and a perspective on further problems.

2 DYNAMICAL APPROACH

Basically we exploit the gradient descent learning rule, using the linear student, i.e $g'(h) = 1$ and $z^\mu = h^\mu = \frac{1}{\sqrt{N}}\vec{W}\vec{x}^\mu$,

$$W_i(t+1) = W_i(t) - \eta\frac{\partial(PE_T)}{\partial W_i} = W_i(t) + \frac{\eta}{\sqrt{N}}\sum_{\mu=1}^{P}(z_*^\mu - z^\mu)x_i^\mu, \qquad (4)$$

For $P < N$, the weights are linear combinations of the example inputs x_i^μ, if $W_i(0) = 0$,

$$W_i(t) =: \frac{1}{\sqrt{N}}\sum_{\mu=1}^{P}\sigma_\mu(t)\,x_i^\mu. \qquad (5)$$

After some algebra a recursion for $\sigma_\mu(t)$ can be found, i.e.

$$\sigma_\mu(t+1) = \sum_{\nu=1}^{P}\left[\delta_{\mu\nu} - \eta\left(\frac{1}{N}\sum_{i=1}^{N}x_i^\mu x_i^\nu\right)\right]\sigma_\nu(t) + \eta z_*^\mu, \qquad (6)$$

where the term in the round brackets defines the *overlap matrix* $\mathbf{C}_{\mu\nu}$. From the geometric series we know the solution of this recursion, and therefore for the weights

$$W_i(t) = \frac{\eta}{\sqrt{N}}\sum_{\mu,\nu=1}^{P} z_*^\mu \left[\frac{\mathbf{E} - (\mathbf{E} - \eta\,\mathbf{C})^t}{\mathbf{E} - (\mathbf{E} - \eta\,\mathbf{C})}\right]_{\mu\nu} x_i^\nu. \qquad (7)$$

Dynamics of Training

It fulfills the initial conditions $W_i(0) = 0$ and $W_i(1) = \eta \sum_{\mu=1}^{P} z_*^{\mu} x_i^{\mu}$ (Hebbian), and yields after infinite time steps the so called *Pseudo-inverse* weights, i.e.

$$W_i(\infty) = \frac{1}{\sqrt{N}} \sum_{\mu,\nu=1}^{P} z_*^{\mu} (\mathbf{C}^{-1})_{\mu\nu} x_i^{\nu}. \tag{8}$$

This is valid as long as the examples are linearly independent, i.e. $P < N$. Remarks about the other case $(P > N)$ will follow later.

With the expression (7) we can calculate the behavior of the order parameters for the whole training process. For $R(t)$ we get

$$\begin{aligned} R(t) &= \frac{1}{N} \sum_{\mu,\nu=1}^{P} \left[\frac{\mathbf{E} - (\mathbf{E} - \eta\mathbf{C})^t}{\mathbf{C}} \right]_{\mu\nu} < z_*^{\mu} \left(\frac{1}{\sqrt{N}} \sum_{i=1}^{N} W_i^* x_i^{\nu} \right) >_{\{W_i^*\}} \\ &= \alpha H \left(1 - \frac{1}{P} \sum_{\mu=1}^{P} \left[(\mathbf{E} - \eta\mathbf{C})^t \right]_{\mu\mu} \right). \end{aligned} \tag{9}$$

For the average we have used expression (21) from the appendix. Similarly we get for the other order parameter,

$$\begin{aligned} Q(t) &= \frac{1}{N} \sum_{\mu,\nu,\tau,\sigma=1}^{P} \left[\frac{\mathbf{E} - (\mathbf{E} - \eta\mathbf{C})^t}{\mathbf{C}} \right]_{\mu\nu} \left[\frac{\mathbf{E} - (\mathbf{E} - \eta\mathbf{C})^t}{\mathbf{C}} \right]_{\tau\sigma} \\ &\quad \times < z_*^{\mu} z_*^{\tau} \left(\frac{1}{N} \sum_{i=1}^{N} x_i^{\nu} x_i^{\sigma} \right) >_{\{W_i^*\}} \\ &= \frac{\alpha(G - H^2)}{P} \sum_{\mu=1}^{P} \left[\mathbf{C}^{-1} \left(\mathbf{E} - (\mathbf{E} - \eta\mathbf{C})^t \right)^2 \right]_{\mu\mu} \\ &\quad + \frac{\alpha H^2}{P} \sum_{\mu=1}^{P} \left[\left(\mathbf{E} - (\mathbf{E} - \eta\mathbf{C})^t \right)^2 \right]_{\mu\mu}. \end{aligned} \tag{10}$$

Again we have applied an identity (20) from the appendix and we did some matrix algebra. Note, up to this point the order parameters were calculated without any assumption about the statistics of the inputs. The results hold, even without the thermodynamic limit.

The trace can be calculated by an integration over the eigenvalues, thus we attain integrals of the following form,

$$\frac{1}{P} \sum_{\mu=1}^{P} \left[(\mathbf{E} - \eta\mathbf{C})^l \mathbf{C}^m \right]_{\mu\mu} = \int_{\xi_{\min}}^{\xi_{\max}} d\xi \, \rho(\xi) (1 - \eta\xi)^l \xi^m =: I_m^l(t, \alpha, \eta), \tag{11}$$

with $l = \{0, t, 2t\}$ and $m = \{-1, 0, 1\}$.

These integrals can be calculated once we know the density of the eigenvalues $\rho(\xi)$. The determination of this density can be found in recent literature calculated by Opper [1989] using replicas, by Krogh [1992] using perturbation theory and by Sollich [1994] with matrix identities. We should note, that the thermodynamic limit and the special assumptions about the inputs enter the calculation here. All authors found

$$\rho(\xi) = \frac{1}{2\pi\alpha\xi} \sqrt{(\xi_{\max} - \xi)(\xi - \xi_{\min})}, \tag{12}$$

for $\alpha < 1$. The maximal and the minimal eigenvalues are $\xi_{\text{max,min}} := (1 \pm \sqrt{\alpha})^2$. So all that remains now is a numerical integration.

Similarly we can calculate the behavior of the training error from

$$E_T(t) = < \frac{1}{2P} \sum_{\mu=1}^{P} (z_*^\mu - h^\mu)^2 >_{\{W_i^*\}} . \quad (13)$$

For the overdetermined case ($P > N$) we can find a recursion analog to (6),

$$W_i(t+1) = \sum_{j=1}^{N} \left[\delta_{ij} - \left(\frac{1}{N} \sum_{\mu=1}^{P} x_i^\mu x_j^\mu \right) \right] W_j(t) + \frac{\eta}{\sqrt{N}} \sum_{\mu=1}^{P} z_*^\mu x_i^\mu . \quad (14)$$

The term in the round brackets defines now the matrix $\mathbf{B}_{ij}$. The calculation is therefore quite similar to above with the matrix $\mathbf{B}$ playing the role of matrix $\mathbf{C}$. The density of the eigenvalues $\rho(\lambda)$ for matrix $\mathbf{B}$ is the one from above (12) multiplied by α.

Altogether, we find the following results in the case of $\alpha < 1$,

$$E_G(t, \alpha, \eta) = \frac{G}{2} + \frac{G - H^2}{2} \alpha \left(\frac{1}{1-\alpha} - 2I_{-1}^t + I_{-1}^{2t} \right) - \frac{H^2}{2} \alpha \left(1 - I_0^{2t} \right) ,$$

$$E_T(t, \alpha, \eta) = \frac{G - H^2}{2} I_0^{2t} + \frac{H^2}{2} I_1^{2t} , \quad (15)$$

and in the case of $\alpha > 1$,

$$E_G(t, \alpha, \eta) = \frac{G - H^2}{2} \left(1 + \frac{1}{\alpha - 1} - 2I_{-1}^t + I_{-1}^{2t} \right) + \frac{H^2}{2} I_0^{2t} ,$$

$$E_T(t, \alpha, \eta) = \frac{G - H^2}{2} \left(1 - \frac{1}{\alpha} + \frac{I_0^{2t}}{\alpha} \right) + \frac{H^2}{2} \frac{I_1^{2t}}{\alpha} . \quad (16)$$

If $t \to \infty$ all the time–dependent integrals I_k^t and I_k^{2t} vanish. The remaining first two terms describe, in the limit $\alpha \to \infty$, the optimal convergence rate of the errors. In the next section we discuss the implications of this result.

3 RESULTS

First we illustrate how well the theoretical results describe the training process. If we compare the theory with simulations, we find a very good correspondence, see Fig. 1.

Trying other values for the learning rate we can see that there is a maximal learning rate. It is twice the inverse of the maximal eigenvalue of the matrix $\mathbf{B}$, i.e.

$$\eta_{\text{max}} = \frac{2}{\xi_{\text{max}}} = \frac{2}{(1 + \sqrt{\alpha})^2} . \quad (17)$$

This is consistent with a more general result, that the maximal learning is twice the inverse of the maximal eigenvalue of the Hessian. In the case of the linear perceptron the matrix $\mathbf{B}$ is identical to the Hessian.

As our approach is directly related to the actual number of training steps we can examine how training time varies in different training scenarios. Training can be stopped if the training error reaches a certain minimal value, i.e if $E_T(t) \leq E_T^{\text{min}} + \epsilon$. Or, in cross-validated early stopping, we will terminate training if the generalization error starts to increase, i.e. if $E_G(t+1) > E_G(t)$.

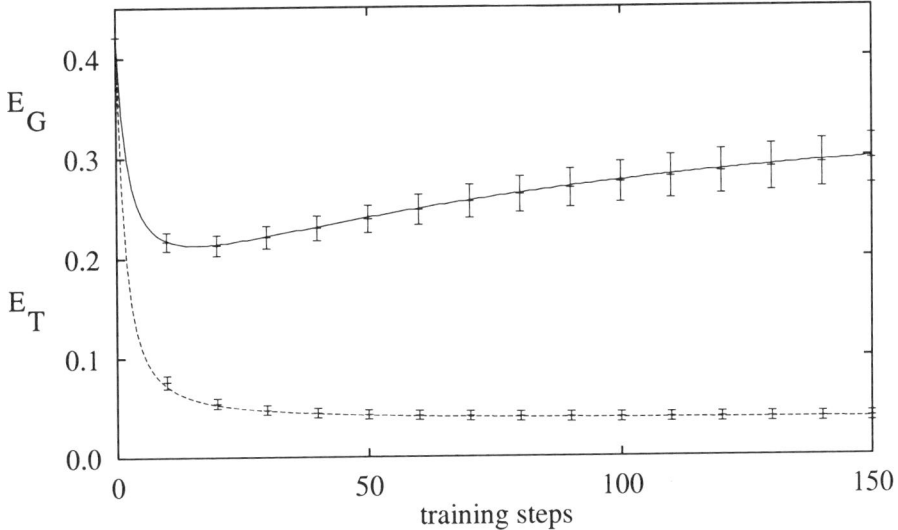

Figure 1: Behavior of the generalization error E_G (upper line) and the training error E_T (lower line) during the training process. As the loading rate $\alpha = P/N = 1.5$ is near the storage capacity ($\alpha = 1$) of the net overfitting occurs. The theory describes the results of the simulations very well. Parameters: learning rate $\eta = 0.1$, system size $N = 200$, and $g_*(h) = \tanh(\gamma h)$ with gain $\gamma = 5$.

Fig. 2 shows that in exhaustive training the training time diverges for α near 1, in the region where also the overfitting occurs. In the same region early stopping shows only a slight increase in training time.

Furthermore, we can guess from Fig. 2 that asymptotically only a few training steps are necessary to fulfill the stopping criteria. This has to be specified more precisely. First we study the behavior of E_G after only one training step, i.e. $t = 1$. Since we interested in the limit of many examples ($\alpha \to \infty$) we choose the learning rate as a fraction of the maximal learning rate (17), i.e. $\eta = \eta_0/\xi_{\max}$. Then we can calculate the behavior of $E_G(t = 1, \alpha, \xi_{\max}^{-1})$ analytically. We find that only in the case of $\eta_0 = 1$, the generalization error can reach its asymptotic minimum $E_{\inf}$. The rate of the convergence is α^{-1} like in the optimal case, but the prefactor is different.

However, already for $t = 2$ we find,

$$\bar{E}_G\left(t = 2, \alpha, \eta = \xi_{\max}^{-1}\right) := E_G - E_{\inf} = \frac{G - H^2}{2} \frac{1}{\alpha - 1} + \mathcal{O}\left(\frac{1}{\alpha^2}\right). \quad (18)$$

If α is large, so that we can neglect the α^{-2} term, then two batch training steps are already enough to get the optimal convergence rate. These results are illustrated in Fig. 3.

4 SUMMARY

In this paper we have calculated the behavior of the learning and the training error during the whole training process. The novel approach relates the errors directly to the actual number of training steps. It was shown how good this theory describes the training process. Several results have been presented, such as the maximal learning rate and the training time in different scenarios, like early stopping. If the learning rate is chosen appropriately, then only two batch training steps are necessary to reach the optimal convergence rate for sufficiently large α.

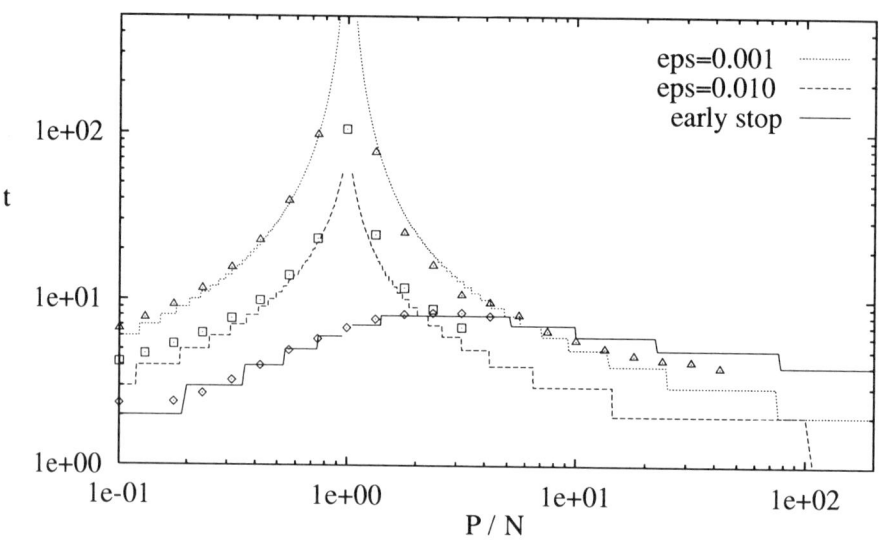

Figure 2: Number of necessary training steps to fulfill certain stopping criteria. The upper lines show the result if training is stopped when the training error is lower than $E_T^{\min}+\epsilon$, with $\epsilon = 0.001$ (dotted line) and $\epsilon = 0.01$ (dashed line). The solid line is the early stopping result where training is stopped, when the generalization error started to increase, $E_G(t+1) > E_G(t)$. Simulation results are indicated by marks. Parameters: learning rate $\eta = 0.01$, system size $N = 200$, and $g_*(h) = \tanh(\gamma h)$ with gain $\gamma = 5$.

Further problems, like the dynamical description of weight decay, and the relation of the dynamical approach to the thermodynamic description of the training process [see Bös, 1995] can not be discussed here due to lack of space. These problems are examined in an extended version of this work [Bös and Opper 1996]. It would be very interesting if this method could be extended towards other, more realistic models.

A APPENDIX

Here we add some identities which are necessary for the averages over the teacher weight distributions, eqs. (9) and (10). In the statistical mechanics approach one assumes that the distribution of the local fields h is Gaussian. This becomes true, if one averages over random inputs x_i, with first moments zero and one, which is the usual approach [see Bös 1995 and ref.]. In principle it is also possible to average over many tasks, i.e many teacher realizations $\vec{W}^*$, which is done here. The Gaussian local fields h_*^μ fulfill,

$$< h_*^\mu >= 0, \quad < h_*^\mu h_*^\nu >= C_{\mu\nu}. \tag{19}$$

This implies

$$< z_*^\mu z_*^\nu >_{\{W_i^*\}} = \int_{-\infty}^{\infty} D\tilde{h}_*^\mu \int_{-\infty}^{\infty} D\tilde{h}_*^\nu \, g_*(\sqrt{1-(C_{\mu\nu})^2}\,\tilde{h}_*^\mu + C_{\mu\nu}\tilde{h}_*^\nu) \, g_*(\tilde{h}_*^\nu)$$

$$= \delta_{\mu\nu} G + (C_{\mu\nu} - \delta_{\mu\nu}) H^2. \tag{20}$$

In the second identity we first calculated the diagonal term and for the non-diagonal term we made an expansion assuming small correlations. Similarly the following

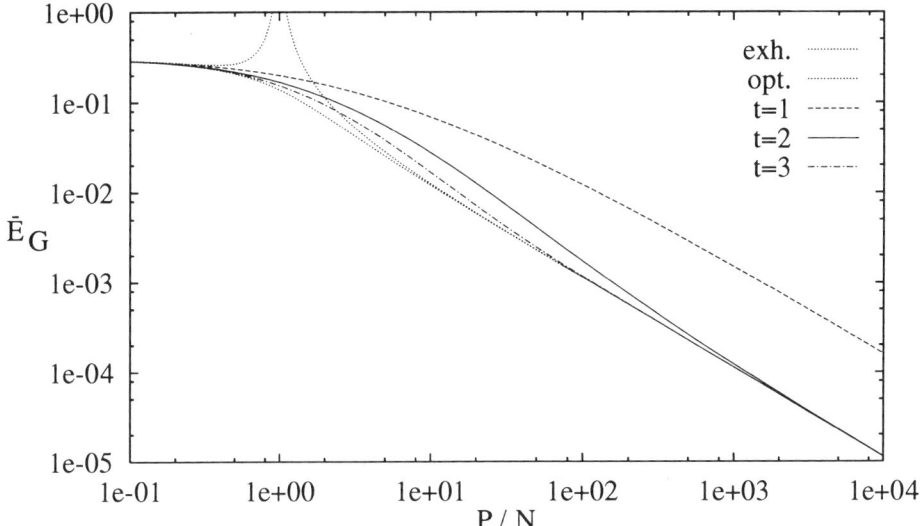

Figure 3: Behavior of $\bar{E}_G = E_G - E_{\text{inf}}$ after t training steps. Results for $t = 1$, 2 and 3 are given. For large enough α it is already after $t = 2$ training steps possible to reach the optimal convergence (solid line). If $t = 3$ the optimal result is reached even faster. Parameters: learning rate $\eta = \xi_{\max}^{-1}$ and $g_*(h) = \tanh(\gamma h)$ with gain $\gamma = 5$.

identity can be proved,

$$< z_*^\mu h_*^\nu >_{\{W_i^*\}} = \delta_{\mu\nu} H + (C_{\mu\nu} - \delta_{\mu\nu}) H. \tag{21}$$

Acknowledgment: We thank Shun-ichi Amari for many discussions and E. Helle, A. Stevenin–Barbier for proofreading and valuable comments.

References

Bös S. (1995), 'Avoiding overfitting by finite temperature learning and cross-validation', in *Int. Conference on Artificial Neural Networks 95 (ICANN'95)*, edited by EC2 & Cie, Vol.2, p.111–116.

Bös S., and Opper M. (1996), 'An exact description of early stopping and weight decay', submitted.

Kinzel W., and Opper M. (1995), 'Dynamics of learning', in *Models of Neural Networks I*, edited by E. Domany, J. L. van Hemmen and K. Schulten, Springer, p.157–179.

Krogh A. (1992), 'Learning with noise in a linear perceptron', *J. Phys. A* **25**, p.1135–1147.

Opper M. (1989), 'Learning in neural networks: Solvable dynamics', *Europhys. Lett.* **8**, p.389–392.

Saad D. (1996), 'General Gaussian priors for improved generalization', submitted to *Neural Networks*.

Sollich P. (1995), 'Learning in large linear perceptrons and why the thermodynamic limit is relevant to the real world', in *NIPS 7*, p.207–214.

Multilayer neural networks: one or two hidden layers?

G. Brightwell
Dept of Mathematics
LSE, Houghton Street
London WC2A 2AE, U.K.

C. Kenyon, H. Paugam-Moisy
LIP, URA 1398 CNRS
ENS Lyon, 46 allée d'Italie
F69364 Lyon cedex, FRANCE

Abstract

We study the number of hidden layers required by a multilayer neural network with threshold units to compute a function f from $\mathcal{R}^d$ to $\{0, 1\}$. In dimension $d = 2$, Gibson characterized the functions computable with just one hidden layer, under the assumption that there is no "multiple intersection point" and that f is only defined on a compact set. We consider the restriction of f to the neighborhood of a multiple intersection point or of infinity, and give necessary and sufficient conditions for it to be locally computable with one hidden layer. We show that adding these conditions to Gibson's assumptions is not sufficient to ensure global computability with one hidden layer, by exhibiting a new non-local configuration, the "critical cycle", which implies that f is not computable with one hidden layer.

1 INTRODUCTION

The number of hidden layers is a crucial parameter for the architecture of multilayer neural networks. Early research, in the 60's, addressed the problem of exactly realizing Boolean functions with binary networks or binary multilayer networks. On the one hand, more recent work focused on approximately realizing real functions with multilayer neural networks with one hidden layer [6, 7, 11] or with two hidden units [2]. On the other hand, some authors [1, 12] were interested in finding bounds on the architecture of multilayer networks for exact realization of a finite set of points. Another approach is to search the minimal architecture of multilayer networks for exactly realizing real functions, from $\mathcal{R}^d$ to $\{0, 1\}$. Our work, of the latter kind, is a continuation of the effort of [4, 5, 8, 9] towards characterizing the real dichotomies which can be exactly realized with a single hidden layer neural network composed of threshold units.

1.1 NOTATIONS AND BACKGROUND

A finite set of hyperplanes $\{H_i\}_{1 \leq i \leq h}$ defines a partition of the d-dimensional space into convex polyhedral open regions, the union of the H_i's being neglected as a subset of measure zero. A *polyhedral dichotomy* is a function $f : \mathcal{R}^d \to \{0,1\}$, obtained by associating a class, equal to 0 or to 1, to each of those regions. Thus both $f^{-1}(0)$ and $f^{-1}(1)$ are unions of a finite number of convex polyhedral open regions. The h hyperplanes which define the regions are called the *essential hyperplanes* of f. A point P is an *essential point* if it is the intersection of some set of essential hyperplanes.

In this paper, all *multilayer networks* are supposed to be feedforward neural networks of threshold units, fully interconnected from one layer to the next, without skipping interconnections. A network is said to *realize* a function $f : \mathcal{R}^d \to \{0,1\}$ if, for an input vector x, the network output is equal to $f(x)$, almost everywhere in $\mathcal{R}^d$. The functions realized by our multilayer networks are the polyhedral dichotomies.

By definition of threshold units, each unit of the first hidden layer computes a binary function y_j of the real inputs $(x_1, \ldots, x_d)$. Therefore, subsequent layers compute a Boolean function. Since any Boolean function can be written in DNF-form, two hidden layers are sufficient for a multilayer network to realize any polyhedral dichotomy. Two hidden layers are sometimes also necessary, e.g. for realizing the "four-quadrant" dichotomy which generalizes the XOR function [4].

For all j, the jth unit of the first hidden layer can be seen as separating the space by the hyperplane $H_j : \sum_{i=1}^{d} w_{ij} x_i = \theta_j$. Hence the first hidden layer necessarily contains at least one hidden unit for each essential hyperplane of f. Thus each region R can be labelled by a binary number $y = (y_1, \ldots, y_h)$ (see [5]). The jth digit y_j will be denoted by $H_j(R)$.

Usually there are fewer than 2^h regions and not all possible labels actually exist. The *Boolean family* $\mathcal{B}_f$ of a polyhedral dichotomy f is defined to be the set of all Boolean functions on h variables which are equal to f on all the existing labels.

1.2 PREVIOUS RESULTS

It is straightforward that all polyhedral dichotomies which have at least one linearly separable function in their Boolean family can be realized by a one-hidden-layer network. However the converse is far from true. A counter-example was produced in [5]: adding extra hyperplanes (i.e. extra units on the first hidden layer) can eliminate the need for a second hidden layer. Hence the problem of finding a minimal architecture for realizing dichotomies cannot be reduced to the neural computation of Boolean functions. Finding a generic description of all the polyhedral dichotomies which can be realized exactly by a one-hidden-layer network is still an open problem. This paper is a new step towards its resolution.

One approach consists of finding geometric configurations which imply that a function is not realizable with a single hidden layer. There are three known such geometric configurations: the XOR-situation, the XOR-bow-tie and the XOR-at-infinity (see Figure 1).

A polyhedral dichotomy is said to be *in an XOR-situation* iff one of its essential hyperplanes H is *inconsistent*, i.e. if there are four regions B, B', W, W' such that B and B' are in class 1, W and W' are in class 0, B and W' are on one side of H, B' and W are on the other side of H, and B and W are adjacent along H, as well as B' and W'.

Given a point P, two regions containing P in their closure are called *opposite with respect to P* if they are in different halfspaces w.r.t. all essential hyperplanes going through P. A polyhedral dichotomy is said to be *in an XOR-bow-tie* iff there exist four distinct regions B, B', W, W', such that B and B', both in class 1 (resp. W and W', both in class 0), are opposite with respect to point P.

The third configuration is the *XOR-at-infinity*, which is analogous to the XOR-bow-tie at a point ∞ added to $\mathcal{R}^d$. There exist four distinct unbounded regions B, B' (in class 1), W, W' (in class 0) such that, for every essential hyperplane H, either all of them are on the same side of H (e.g. the horizontal line), or B and B' are on opposite sides of H, and W and W' are on opposite sides of H (see [3]).

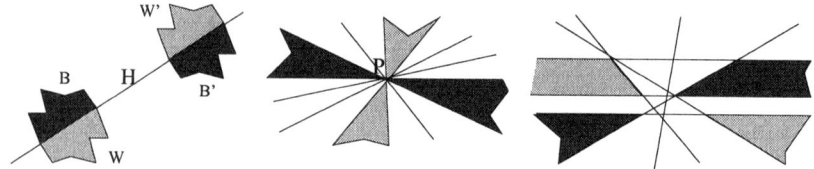

figure 1: Geometrical representation of XOR-situation, XOR-bow-tie and XOR-at-infinity in the plane (black regions are in class 1, grey regions are in class 0).

Theorem 1 *If a polyhedral dichotomy f, from $\mathcal{R}^d$ to $\{0, 1\}$, can be realized by a one-hidden-layer network, then it cannot be in an XOR-situation, nor in an XOR-bow-tie, nor in an XOR-at-infinity.*

The proof can be found in [5] for the XOR-situation, in [13] for the XOR-bow-tie, and in [5] for the XOR-at-infinity.

Another research direction, implying a function is realizable by a single hidden layer network, is based on the universal approximator property of one-hidden-layer networks, applied to intermediate functions obtained constructively adding extra hyperplanes to the essential hyperplanes of f. This direction was explored by Gibson [9], but there are virtually no results known beyond two dimensions. Gibson's result can be reformulated as follows:

Theorem 2 *If a polyhedral dichotomy f is defined on a compact subset of $\mathcal{R}^2$, if f is not in an XOR-situation, and if no three essential hyperplanes (lines) intersect, then f is realizable with a single hidden layer network.*

Unfortunately Gibson's proof is not constructive, and extending it to remove some of the assumptions or to go to higher dimensions seems challenging. Both XOR-bow-tie and XOR-at-infinity are excluded by his assumptions of compactness and no multiple intersections. In the next section, we explore the two cases which are excluded by Gibson's assumptions. We prove that, in $\mathcal{R}^2$, the XOR-bow-tie and the XOR-at-infinity are the only restrictions to local realizability.

2 LOCAL REALIZATION IN $\mathcal{R}^2$

2.1 MULTIPLE INTERSECTION

Theorem 3 *Let f be a polyhedral dichotomy on $\mathcal{R}^2$ and let P be a point of multiple intersection. Let C_P be a neighborhood of P which does not intersect any essential hyperplane other than those going through P. The restriction of f to C_P is realizable by a one-hidden-layer network iff f is not in an XOR-bow-tie at P.*

The proof is in three steps: first, we reorder the hyperplanes in the neighborhood of P, so as to get a nice looking system of inequalities; second, we apply Farkas' lemma; third, we show how an XOR-bow-tie can be deduced.

Proof: Let P be the intersection of $k \geq 3$ essential hyperplanes of f. All the hyperplanes which intersect at P can be renumbered and re-oriented so that the intersecting hyperplanes are totally ordered. Thus the label of the regions which have the point P in their closure is very regular. If one drops all the digits corresponding to the essential hyperplanes of f which do not contain P, the remaining part of the region labels are exactly like those of Figure 2.

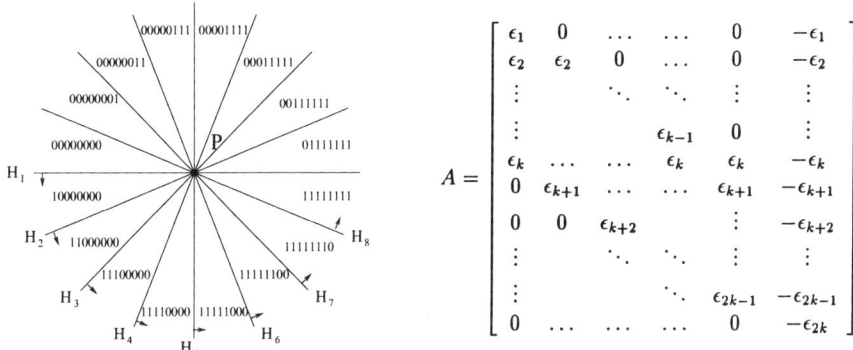

Figure 2: Labels of the regions in the neighborhood of P, and matrix A.

The problem of finding a one-hidden-layer network which realizes f can be rewritten as a system of inequalities. The unknown variables are the weights w_i and threshold θ of the output unit. Let $(\mathcal{S})$ denote the subsystem of inequalities obtained from the $2k$ regions which have the point P in their closure. The regular numbering of these $2k$ regions allows us to write the system as follows

$$(\mathcal{S}) \begin{cases} 1 \leq i \leq k & \begin{cases} \sum_{m=1}^{i} w_m < \theta & \text{if class 0} \\ \sum_{m=1}^{i} w_m > \theta & \text{if class 1} \end{cases} \\ k+1 \leq i \leq 2k & \begin{cases} \sum_{m=i-k+1}^{k} w_m < \theta & \text{if class 0} \\ \sum_{m=i-k+1}^{k} w_m > \theta & \text{if class 1} \end{cases} \end{cases}$$

The system $(\mathcal{S})$ can be rewritten in the matrix form $Ax \leq b$, where

$$x^\top = [w_1, w_2, \ldots, w_k, \theta] \text{ and } b^\top = [b_1, b_2, \ldots, b_k, b_{k+1}, \ldots, b_{2k}]$$

where $b_i = -\epsilon$, for all i, and ϵ is an arbitrary small positive number. Matrix A can be seen in figure 2, where $\epsilon_j = +1$ or -1 depending on whether region j is in class 0 or 1. The next step is to apply Farkas lemma, or an equivalent version [10], which gives a necessary and sufficient condition for finding a solution of $Ax \leq b$.

Lemma 1 (Farkas lemma) *There exists a vector $x \in \mathcal{R}^n$ such that $Ax \leq b$ iff there does not exist a vector $y \in \mathcal{R}^m$ such that $y^\top A = 0$, $y \geq 0$ and $y^\top b < 0$.*

Assume that $Ax \leq b$ is not solvable. Then, by Lemma 1 for $n = k+1$ and $m = 2k$, a vector y can be found such that $y \geq 0$. Since in addition $y^\top b = -\epsilon \sum_{j=1}^{2k} y_j$, the condition $y^\top b < 0$ implies $(\exists j_1)\, y_{j_1} > 0$. But $y^\top A = 0$ is equivalent to the system

($\mathcal{E}$) of $k+1$ equations

$$(\mathcal{E})\begin{cases} 1 \leq i \leq k & \sum_{m=i}^{i+k-1} y_{m/class\ 0} = \sum_{m=i}^{i+k-1} y_{m/class\ 1} \\ i = k+1 & \sum_{m=1}^{2k} y_{m/class\ 0} = \sum_{m=1}^{2k} y_{m/class\ 1} \end{cases}$$

Since $(\exists j_1)$ $y_{j_1} > 0$, the last equation (E_{k+1}) of system $(\mathcal{E})$ implies that $(\exists j_2 \ / \ \text{class}(\text{region } j_1) \neq \text{class}(\text{region } j_2))$ $y_{j_2} > 0$. Without loss of generality, assume that j_1 and j_2 are less than k and that region j_1 is in class 0 and region j_2 is in class 1. Comparing two successive equations of $(\mathcal{E})$, for $i < k$, we can write

$$(\forall \lambda \in \{0,1\}) \ \sum_{(E_{i+1})} y_{m/class\ \lambda} = \sum_{(E_i)} y_{m/class\ \lambda} - y_{i/class\ \lambda} + y_{i+k/class\ \lambda}$$

Since $y_{j_1} > 0$ and region j_1 is in class 0, the transition from E_{j_1} to E_{j_1+1} implies that $y_{j_1+k} = y_{j_1} > 0$ and region $j_1 + k$, which is opposite to region j_1, is also in class 0. Similarly, the transition from E_{j_2} to E_{j_2+1} implies that both opposite regions $j_2 + k$ and j_2 are in class 1. These conditions are necessary for the system $(\mathcal{E})$ to have a non-negative solution and they correspond exactly to the definition of an XOR-bow-tie at point P. The converse comes from theorem 1. ■

2.2 UNBOUNDED REGIONS

If no two essential hyperplanes are parallel, the case of unbounded regions is exactly the same as a multiple intersection. All the unbounded regions can be labelled as on figure 2. The same argument holds for proving that, if the local system $(\mathcal{S})$ $Ax \leq b$ is not solvable, then there exists an XOR-at-infinity. The case of parallel hyperplanes is more intricate because matrix A is more complex. The proof requires a heavy case-by-case analysis and cannot be given in full in this paper (see [3]).

Theorem 4 *Let f be a polyhedral dichotomy on $\mathcal{R}^2$. Let C_∞ be the complementary region of the convex hull of the essential points of f. The restriction of f to C_∞ is realizable by a one-hidden-layer network iff f is not in an XOR-at-infinity.*

From theorems 3 and 4 we can deduce that a polyhedral dichotomy is locally realizable in $\mathcal{R}^2$ by a one-hidden-layer network iff f has no XOR-bow-tie and no XOR-at-infinity. Unfortunately this result cannot be extended to the global realization of f in $\mathcal{R}^2$ because more intricate distant configurations can involve contradictions in the complete system of inequalities. The object of the next section is to point out such a situation by producing a new geometric configuration, called a *critical cycle*, which implies that f cannot be realized with one hidden layer.

3 CRITICAL CYCLES

In contrast to section 2, the results of this section hold for any dimension $d \geq 2$.

We first need some definitions. Consider a pair of regions $\{T, T'\}$ in the same class and which both contain an essential point P in their closure. This pair is called *critical* with respect to P and H if there is an essential hyperplane H going through P such that T' is adjacent along H to the region opposite to T. Note that T and T' are both on the same side of H.

We define a graph G whose nodes correspond to the critical pairs of regions of f. There is a red edge between $\{T, T'\}$ and $\{U, U'\}$ if the pairs, in different classes, are both critical with respect to the same point (e.g., $\{B_P, B'_P\}$ and $\{W_P, W'_P\}$ in figure 3). There is a green edge between $\{T, T'\}$ and $\{U, U'\}$ if the pairs are both critical with respect to the same hyperplane H, and either the two pairs are on the same side of H, but in different classes (e.g., $\{W_P, W_P'\}$ and $\{B_Q, B_Q'\}$), or they are on different sides of H, but in the same class (e.g., $\{B_P, B_P'\}$ and $\{B_R, B_R'\}$).

Definition 1 *A critical cycle is a cycle in graph G, with alternating colors.*

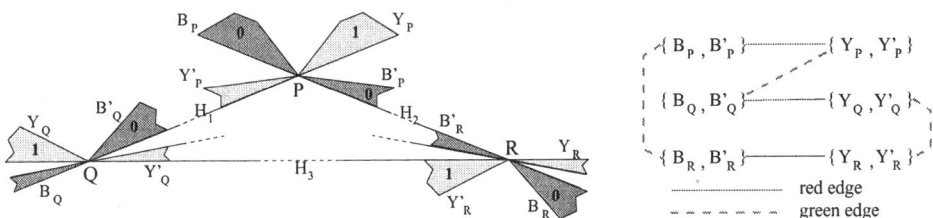

Figure 3: Geometrical configuration and graph of a critical cycle, in the plane. Note that one can augment the figure in such a way that there is no XOR-situation, no XOR-bow-tie, and no XOR-at-infinity.

Theorem 5 *If a polyhedral dichotomy f, from $\mathcal{R}^d$ to $\{0,1\}$, can be realized by a one-hidden-layer network, then it cannot have a critical cycle.*

Proof: For the sake of simplicity, we will restrict ourselves to doing the proof for a case similar to the example figure 3, with notation as given in that figure, but without any restriction on the dimension d of f. Assume, for a contradiction, that f has a critical cycle and can be realized by a one-hidden-layer network. Consider the sets of regions $\{B_P, B_P', B_Q, B_Q', B_R, B_R'\}$ and $\{W_P, W_P', W_Q, W_Q', W_R, W_R'\}$. Consider the regions defined by all the hyperplanes associated to the hidden layer units (in general, these hyperplanes are a large superset of the essential hyperplanes). There is a region $b_P \subseteq B_P$, whose border contains P and a $(d-1)$-dimensional subset of H_1. Similarly we can define $b_P', \ldots, b_R', w_P, \ldots, w_R'$. Let $\mathcal{B}$ be the set of such regions which are in class 1 and $\mathcal{W}$ be the set of such regions in class 0.

Let H be the hyperplane associated to one of the hidden units. For T a region, let $H(T)$ be the digit label of T w.r.t. H, i.e. $H(T) = 1$ or 0 according to whether T is above or below H (cf. section 1.1). We do a case-by-case analysis.

If H does not go through P, then $H(b_P) = H(b_P') = H(w_P) = H(w_P')$; similar equalities hold for lines not going through Q or R. If H goes through P but is not equal to H_1 or to H_2, then, from the viewpoint of H, things are as if b_P' was opposite to b_P, and w_P' was opposite to w_P, so the two regions of each pair are on different sides of H, and so $H(b_P) + H(b_P') = H(w_P) + H(w_P') = 1$; similar equalities hold for hyperplanes going through Q or R. If $H = H_1$, then we use the fact that there is a green edge between $\{W_P, W_P'\}$ and $\{B_Q, B_Q'\}$, meaning in the case of the figure that all four regions are on the same side of H_1 but in different classes. Then $H(b_P) + H(b_P') + H(b_Q) + H(b_Q') = H(w_P) + H(w_P') + H(w_Q) + H(w_Q')$. In fact, this equality would also hold in the other case, as can easily be checked. Thus for all H, we have $\sum_{b \in \mathcal{B}} H(b) = \sum_{w \in \mathcal{W}} H(w)$. But such an equality is impossible: since each b is in class 1 and each w is in class 0, this implies a contradiction in the system of inequalities and f cannot be realized by a one-hidden-layer network.

Obviously there can exist cycles of length longer than 3, but the extension of the proof is straightforward. ∎

4 CONCLUSION AND PERSPECTIVES

This paper makes partial progress towards characterizing functions which can be realized by a one-hidden-layer network, with a particular focus on dimension 2. Higher dimensions are more challenging, and it is difficult to even propose a conjecture: new cases of inconsistency emerge in subspaces of intermediate dimension. Gibson gives an example of an inconsistent line (dimension 1) resulting of its intersection with two hyperplanes (dimension 2) which are not inconsistent in $\mathcal{R}^3$.

The principle of using Farkas lemma for proving local realizability still holds but the matrix A becomes more and more complex. In $\mathcal{R}^d$, even for $d = 3$, the labelling of the regions, for instance around a point P of multiple intersection, can become very complex.

In conclusion, it seems that neither the topological method of Gibson, nor our algebraic point of view, can easily be extended to higher dimensions. Nevertheless, we conjecture that in dimension 2, a function can be realized by a one-hidden-layer network iff it does not have any of the four forbidden types of configurations: XOR-situation, XOR-bow-tie, XOR-at-infinity, and critical cycle.

Acknowledgements

This work was supported by European Esprit III Project n^0 8556, NeuroCOLT.

References

[1] E. B. Baum. On the capabilities of multilayer perceptrons. *Journal of Complexity*, 4:193–215, 1988.

[2] E. K. Blum and L. K. Li. Approximation theory and feedforward networks. *Neural Networks*, 4(4):511–516, 1991.

[3] G. Brightwell, C. Kenyon, and H. Paugam-Moisy. Multilayer neural networks: one or two hidden layers? Research Report 96-37, LIP, ENS Lyon, 1996.

[4] M. Cosnard, P. Koiran, and H. Paugam-Moisy. Complexity issues in neural network computations. In I. Simon, editor, *Proc. of LATIN'92*, volume 583 of *LNCS*, pages 530–544. Springer Verlag, 1992.

[5] M. Cosnard, P. Koiran, and H. Paugam-Moisy. A step towards the frontier between one-hidden-layer and two-hidden layer neural networks. In I. Simon, editor, *Proc. of IJCNN'93-Nagoya*, volume 3, pages 2292–2295. Springer Verlag, 1993.

[6] G. Cybenko. Approximation by superpositions of a sigmoidal function. *Math. Control, Signal Systems*, 2:303–314, October 1988.

[7] K. Funahashi. On the approximate realization of continuous mappings by neural networks. *Neural Networks*, 2(3):183–192, 1989.

[8] G. J. Gibson. A combinatorial approach to understanding perceptron decision regions. *IEEE Trans. Neural Networks*, 4:989–992, 1993.

[9] G. J. Gibson. Exact classification with two-layer neural nets. *Journal of Computer and System Science*, 52(2):349–356, 1996.

[10] M. Grötschel, L. Lovsz, and A. Schrijver. *Geometric Algorithms and Combinatorial Optimization*. Springer-Verlag, Berlin, Heidelberg, 1988.

[11] K. Hornik, M. Stinchcombe, and H. White. Multilayer feedforward networks are universal approximators. *Neural Networks*, 2(5):359–366, 1989.

[12] S.-C. Huang and Y.-F. Huang. Bounds on the number of hidden neurones in multilayer perceptrons. *IEEE Trans. Neural Networks*, 2:47–55, 1991.

[13] P. J. Zweitering. *The complexity of multi-layered perceptrons*. PhD thesis, Technische Universiteit Eindhoven, 1994.

Support Vector Regression Machines

Harris Drucker*   Chris J.C. Burges**   Linda Kaufman**
Alex Smola**   Vladimir Vapnik [+]

*Bell Labs and Monmouth University
Department of Electronic Engineering
West Long Branch, NJ 07764
**Bell Labs   [+]AT&T Labs

Abstract

A new regression technique based on Vapnik's concept of support vectors is introduced. We compare support vector regression (SVR) with a committee regression technique (bagging) based on regression trees and ridge regression done in feature space. On the basis of these experiments, it is expected that SVR will have advantages in high dimensionality space because SVR optimization does not depend on the dimensionality of the input space.

1. Introduction

In the following, lower case bold characters represent vectors and upper case bold characters represent matrices. Superscript "t" represents the transpose of a vector. y represents either a vector (in bold) or a single observance of the dependent variable in the presence of noise. $y^{(p)}$ indicates a predicted value due to the input vector $x^{(p)}$ not seen in the training set.

Suppose we have an unknown function $G(x)$ (the "truth") which is a function of a vector x (termed *input space*). The vector $x^t = [x_1, x_2, ..., x_d]$ has d components where d is termed the dimensionality of the input space. $F(x, w)$ is a family of functions parameterized by w. $\hat{w}$ is that value of w that minimizes a measure of error between $G(x)$ and $F(x, \hat{w})$. Our objective is to estimate w with $\hat{w}$ by observing the N training instances v_j, $j=1,\cdots,N$. We will develop two approximations for the truth $G(x)$. The first one is $F_1(x, \hat{w})$ which we term a feature space representation. One (of many) such feature vectors is:

$$z^t = [x_1^2, \cdots, x_d^2, x_1 x_2, \cdots, x_i x_j, \cdots, x_{d-1} x_d, x_1, \cdots, x_d, 1]$$

which is a quadratic function of the input space components. Using the feature space representation, then $F_1(x, \hat{w}) = z^t \hat{w}$, that is, $F_1(x, \hat{w})$ is linear in *feature space* although it is quadratic in input space. In general, for a p'th order polynomial and d'th dimensional input space, the feature dimensionality f of $\hat{w}$ is

$$f = \sum_{i=d-1}^{p+d-1} C_{d-1}^i$$

where $C_k^n = \dfrac{n!}{k!(n-k)!}$.

The second representation is a support vector regression (SVR) representation that was developed by Vladimir Vapnik (1995):

$$F_2(x,\hat{w}) = \sum_{i=1}^{N} (\alpha_i^* - \alpha_i)(v_i^t x + 1)^p + b$$

F_2 is an expansion explicitly using the training examples. The rationale for calling it a support vector representation will be clear later as will the necessity for having both an α^* and an α rather than just one multiplicative constant. In this case we must choose the 2N + 1 values of α_i α_i^* and b. If we expand the term raised to the p'th power, we find f coefficients that multiply the various powers and cross product terms of the components of x. So, in this sense F_1 looks very similar to F_2 in that they have the same number of terms. However F_1 has f free coefficients while F_2 has 2N+1 coefficients that must be determined from the N training vectors.

We let α represent the 2N values of α_i and α_i^*. The optimum values for the components of $\hat{w}$ or α depend on our definition of the loss function and the objective function. Here the primal objective function is:

$$U \sum_{j=1}^{N} L[y_j - F(v_j, \hat{w})] + ||\hat{w}||^2$$

where L is a general loss function (to be defined later) and F could be F_1 or F_2, y_j is the observation of $G(x)$ in the presence of noise, and the last term is a regularizer. The regularization constant is U which in typical developments multiplies the regularizer but is placed in front of the first term for reasons discussed later.

If the loss function is quadratic, i.e., we $L[\cdot]=[\cdot]^2$, and we let $F=F_1$, i.e., the feature space representation, the objective function may be minimized by using linear algebra techniques since the feature space representation is linear in that space. This is termed ridge regression (Miller, 1990). In particular let V be a matrix whose i'th row is the i'th training vector represented in feature space (including the constant term "1" which represents a bias). V is a matrix where the number of rows is the number of examples (N) and the number of columns is the dimensionality of feature space f. Let E be the $f x f$ diagonal matrix whose elements are 1/U. y is the Nx1 column vector of observations of the dependent variable. We then solve the following matrix formulation for $\hat{w}$ using a linear technique (Strang, 1986) with a linear algebra package (e.g., MATLAB):

$$V^t y = [V^t V + E] \hat{w}$$

The rationale for the regularization term is to trade off mean square error (the first term) in the objective function against the size of the $\hat{w}$ vector. If U is large, then essentially we are minimizing the mean square error on the training set which may give poor generalization to a test set. We find a good value of U by varying U to find the best performance on a validation set and then applying that U to the test set.

Let us now define a different type of loss function termed an ε-insensitive loss (Vapnik, 1995):

$$L = \begin{cases} 0 & \text{if } |y_i - F_2(x_i, \hat{w})| < \varepsilon \\ |y_i - F_2(x_i, \hat{w})| - \varepsilon & \text{otherwise} \end{cases}$$

This defines an ε tube (Figure 1) so that if the predicted value is within the tube the loss is zero, while if the predicted point is outside the tube, the loss is the magnitude of the difference between the predicted value and the radius ε of the tube.

Specifically, we minimize:

$$U(\sum_{i=1}^{N} \xi_i^* + \sum_{i=1}^{N} \xi_i) + \frac{1}{2}(w^t w)$$

where ξ_i or ξ_i^* is zero if the sample point is inside the tube. If the observed point is "above" the tube, ξ_i is the positive difference between the observed value and ε and α_i will be nonzero. Similarly, ξ_i^* will be nonzero if the observed point is below the tube and in this case α_i^* will be nonzero. Since an observed point can not be simultaneously on both sides of the tube, either α_i or α_i^* will be nonzero, unless the point is within the tube, in which case, both constants will be zero. If U is large, more emphasis is placed on the error while if U is small, more emphasis is placed on the norm of the weights leading to (hopefully) a better generalization. The constraints are: (for all i, i=1,N)

$$y_i - (w^t v_i) - b \leq \varepsilon + \xi_i$$
$$(w^t v_i) + b - y_i \leq \varepsilon + \xi_i^*$$
$$\xi_i^* \geq 0$$
$$\xi_i \geq 0$$

The corresponding Lagrangian is:

$$L = \frac{1}{2}(w^t w) + U(\sum_{i=1}^{N} \xi_i^* + \sum_{i=1}^{N} \xi_i) - \sum_{i=1}^{N} \alpha_i^* [y_i - (w^t v_i) - b + \varepsilon + \xi_i^*]$$
$$- \sum_{i=1}^{N} \alpha_i [(w^t v_i) + b - y_i + \varepsilon + \xi_i] - \sum_{i=1}^{N} (\gamma_i^* \xi_i^* + \gamma_i \xi_i)$$

where the γ_i and α_i are Lagrange multipliers.

We find a saddle point of L (Vapnik, 1995) by differentiating with respect to w_i, b, and ξ which results in the equivalent maximization of the (dual space) objective function:

$$W(\alpha, \alpha^*) = -\varepsilon \sum_{i=1}^{N} (\alpha_i^* + \alpha_i) + \sum_{i=1}^{N} y_i(\alpha_i^* - \alpha_i) - \frac{1}{2} \sum_{i,j=1}^{N} (\alpha_i^* - \alpha_i)(\alpha_j^* - \alpha_j)(v_i^t v_j + 1)^p$$

with the constraints:

$$0 \leq \alpha_i \leq U \quad 0 \leq \alpha_i^* \leq U \quad i=1,...,N$$
$$\sum_{i=1}^{N} \alpha_i^* = \sum_{i=1}^{N} \alpha_i$$

We must find N Largrange multiplier pairs (α_i, α_i^*). We can also prove that the product of α_i and α_i^* is zero which means that at least one of these two terms is zero. A v_i corresponding to a non-zero α_i or α_i^* is termed a support vector. There can be at most N support vectors. Suppose now, we have a new vector $x^{(p)}$, then the corresponding prediction of $y^{(p)}$ is:

$$y^{(p)} = \sum_{i=1}^{N}(\alpha_i^* - \alpha_i)(v_i^t x^{(p)} + 1)^p + b$$

Maximizing W is a quadratic programming problem but the above expression for W is not in standard form for use in quadratic programming packages (which usually does minimization). If we let

$$\beta_i = \alpha_i^* \quad \beta_{i+N} = \alpha_i \quad i=1,...,N$$

then we minimize:

$$f(\beta) = \frac{1}{2}\beta^t Q \beta + c^t \beta$$

subject to the constraints

$$\sum_{i=1}^{N}\beta_i = \sum_{N+1}^{2N}\beta_i \quad \text{and} \quad 0 \leq \beta_i \leq U \quad i=1,\cdots,2N$$

where

$$c^t = [\varepsilon-y_1, \varepsilon-y_2, \cdots, \varepsilon-y_N, \varepsilon+y_1, \varepsilon+y_2, \cdots, \varepsilon+y_N]$$

$$Q = \begin{bmatrix} D & -D \\ -D & D \end{bmatrix}$$

$$d_{ij} = (v_i^t v_j + 1)^p \quad i,j = 1, \cdots, N$$

We use an active set method (Bunch and Kaufman, 1980) to solve this quadratic programming problem.

2. Nonlinear Experiments

We tried three artificial functions from (Friedman, 1991) and a problem (Boston Housing) from the UCI database. Because the first three problems are artificial, we know both the observed values and the truths. Boston Housing has 506 cases with the dependent variable being the median price of housing in the Boston area. There are twelve continuous predictor variables. This data was obtaining from the UCI database (anonymous ftp at ftp.ics.uci.edu in directory /pub/machine-learning-databases) In this case, we have no "truth", only the observations.

In addition to the input space representation and the SVR representation, we also tried bagging. Bagging is a technique that combines regressors, in this case regression trees (Breiman, 1994). We used this technique because we had a local version available. In the case of regression trees, the validation set was used to prune the trees.

Suppose we have test points with input vectors $x_i^{(p)}$ $i=1,M$ and make a prediction $y_i^{(p)}$ using any procedure discussed here. Suppose y_i is the actually observed value, which is the truth $G(x)$ plus noise. We define the prediction error (PE) and the modeling error (ME):

$$ME = \frac{1}{M}\sum_{i=1}^{M}(y_i^{(p)} - G(x_i))^2$$

$$PE = \frac{1}{M}\sum_{i=1}^{M}(y_i^{(p)} - y_i)^2$$

For the three Friedman functions we calculated both the prediction error and modeling error. For Boston Housing, since the "truth" was not known, we calculated the prediction error only. For the three Friedman functions, we generated (for each experiment) 200 training set examples and 40 validation set examples. The validation set examples were used to find the optimum regularization constant in the feature space representation. The following procedure was followed. Train on the 200 members of the training set with a choice of regularization constant and obtain the prediction error on the validation set. Now repeat with a different regularization constant until a minimum of prediction error occurs on the validation set. Now, use that regularizer constant that minimizes the validation set prediction error and test on a 1000 example test set. This experiment was repeated for 100 different training sets of size 200 and validation sets of size 40 but one test set of size 1000. Different size polynomials were tried (maximum power 3). Second order polynomials fared best. For Friedman function #1, the dimensionality of feature space is 66 while for the last two problems, the dimensionality of feature space was 15 (for $d=2$). Thus the size of the feature space is smaller than that of the number of examples and we would expect that a feature space representation should do well.

A similar procedure was followed for the SVR representation except the regularizer constant U, ε and power p were varied to find the minimum validation prediction error. In the majority of cases p=2 was the optimum choice of power.

For the Boston Housing data, we picked randomly from the 506 cases using a training set of size 401, a validation set of size 80 and a test set of size 25. This was repeated 100 times. The optimum power as picked by the validations set varied between p=4 and p=5.

3. Results of experiments

The first experiments we tried were bagging regression trees versus support regression (Table I).

Table I. Modeling error and prediction error
on the three Friedman problems (100 trials).

	bagging ME	SVR ME	bagging PE	SVR PE	# trials better
#1	2.26	.67	3.36	1.75	100
#2	10,185	4,944	66,077	60,424	92
#3	.0302	.0261	.0677	.0692	46

Rather than report the standard error, we did a comparison for each training set. That is, for the first experiment we tried both SVR and bagging on the same training, validation, and test set. If SVR had a better modeling error on the test set, it counted as a win. Thus for Friedman #1, SVR was always better than bagging on the 100 trials. There is no clear winner for Friedman function #3.

Subsequent to our comparison of bagging to SVR, we attempted working directly in feature space. That is, we used F_1 as our approximating function with square loss and a second degree polynomial. The results of this ridge regression (Table II) are better than SVR. In retrospect, this is not surprising since the dimensionality of feature space is small ($f=66$ for Friedman #1 and $f=15$ for the two remaining functions) in relation to the number of training examples (200). This was due to the fact that the best approximating polynomial is second order. The other advantages of the feature space representation in this particular case are that both PE and ME are mean squared error and the loss function is mean squared error also.

Table II. Modeling error for SVR and
feature space polynomial approximation.

	SVR	feature space
#1	.67	.61
#2	4,944	3051
#3	.0261	.0176

We now ask the question whether U and ε are important in SVR by comparing the results in Table I with the results obtaining by setting ε to zero and U to 100,000 making the regularizer insignificant (Table III). On Friedman #2 (and less so on Friedman #3), the proper choice of ε and U are important.

Table III. Comparing the results above with those obtained by setting
ε to zero and U to 100,000 (labeled suboptimum).

	optimum ME	suboptimum ME
#1	.67	.70
#2	4,944	34,506
#3	.0261	.0395

For the case of Boston Housing, the prediction error using bagging was 12.4 while for SVR we obtained 7.2 and SVR was better than bagging on 71 out of 100 trials. The optimum power seems to be about five. We never were able to get the feature representation to work well because the number of coefficients to be determined (6885) was much larger than the number of training examples (401).

4 Conclusions

Support vector regression was compared to bagging and a feature space representation on four nonlinear problems. On three of these problems a feature space representation was best, bagging was worst, and SVR came in second. On the fourth problem, Boston Housing, SVR was best and we were unable to construct a feature space representation because of the high dimensionality required of the feature space. On linear problems, forward subset selection seems to be the method of choice for the two linear problems we tried at varying signal to noise ratios.

In retrospect, the problems we decided to test on were too simple. SVR probably has greatest use when the dimensionality of the input space and the order of the approximation creates a dimensionality of a feature space representation much larger than that of the number of examples. This was not the case for the problems we considered. We thus need real life examples that fulfill these requirements.

5. Acknowledgements

This project was supported by ARPA contract number N00014-94-C-1086.

6. References

Leo Breiman, "Bagging Predictors", Technical Report 421, September 1994, Department of Statistics, University of California Berkeley, CA Also at anonymous ftp site: ftp.stat.berkeley.edu/pub/tech-reports/421.ps.Z.

Jame R. Bunch and Linda C. Kaufman, " A Computational Method of the Indefinite Quadratic Programming Problem", *Linear Algebra and Its Applications*, Elsevier-North Holland, 1980.

Jerry Friedman, "Multivariate Adaptive Regression Splines", *Annal of Statistics*, vol 19, No. 1, pp. 1-141

Alan J. Miller, *Subset Selection in Regression*, Chapman and Hall, 1990.

Gilbert Strang, *Introduction to Applied Mathematics*, Wellesley Cambridge Press, 1986.

Vladimir N. Vapnik, *The Nature of Statistical Learning Theory*, Springer, 1995.

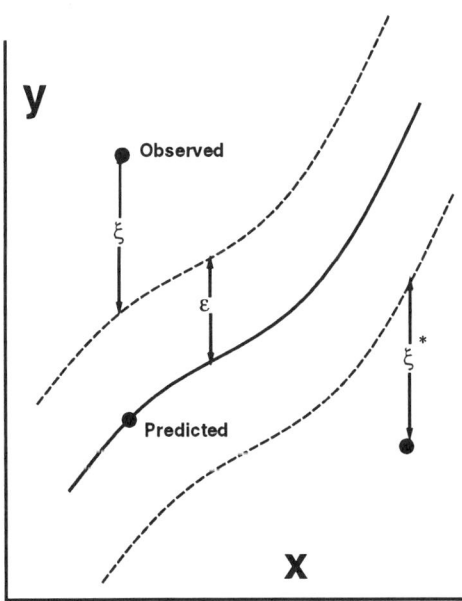

Figure 1: The parameters for the support vector regression.

Size of multilayer networks for exact learning: analytic approach

André Elisseeff
Dept Mathématiques et Informatique
École Normale Supérieure de Lyon
46 allée d'Italie
F69364 Lyon cedex 07, FRANCE

Hélène Paugam-Moisy
LIP, URA 1398 CNRS
École Normale Supérieure de Lyon
46 allée d'Italie
F69364 Lyon cedex 07, FRANCE

Abstract

This article presents a new result about the size of a multilayer neural network computing real outputs for exact learning of a finite set of real samples. The architecture of the network is feedforward, with one hidden layer and several outputs. Starting from a fixed training set, we consider the network as a function of its weights. We derive, for a wide family of transfer functions, a lower and an upper bound on the number of hidden units for exact learning, given the size of the dataset and the dimensions of the input and output spaces.

1 RELATED WORKS

The context of our work is rather similar to the well-known results of Baum et al. [1, 2, 3, 5, 10], but we consider both real inputs and outputs, instead of the dichotomies usually addressed. We are interested in learning exactly all the examples of a fixed database, hence our work is different from stating that multilayer networks are universal approximators [6, 8, 9]. Since we consider real outputs and not only dichotomies, it is not straightforward to compare our results to the recent works about the VC-dimension of multilayer networks [11, 12, 13]. Our study is more closely related to several works of Sontag [14, 15], but with different hypotheses on the transfer functions of the units. Finally, our approach is based on geometrical considerations and is close to the model of Coetzee and Stonick [4].

First we define the model of network and the notations and second we develop our analytic approach and prove the fundamental theorem. In the last section, we discuss our point of view and propose some practical consequences of the result.

2 THE NETWORK AS A FUNCTION OF ITS WEIGHTS

General concepts on neural networks are presented in matrix and vector notations, in a geometrical perspective. All vectors are written in bold and considered as column vectors, whereas matrices are denoted with upper-case script.

2.1 THE NETWORK ARCHITECTURE AND NOTATIONS

Consider a multilayer network with N_I input units, N_H hidden units and N_S output units. The inputs and outputs are real-valued. The hidden units compute a non-linear function f which will be specified later on. The output units are assumed to be linear. A learning set of N_P examples is given and fixed. For all $p \in \{1..N_P\}$, the pth example is defined by its input vector $\boldsymbol{d}_p \in \Re^{N_I}$ and the corresponding desired output vector $\boldsymbol{t}_p \in \Re^{N_S}$. The learning set can be represented as an *input matrix*, with both row and column notations, as follows

$$\mathcal{D} = \begin{bmatrix} d_{11} & d_{12} & \ldots & d_{1N_I} \\ \vdots & \vdots & & \vdots \\ d_{N_P 1} & d_{N_P 2} & \ldots & d_{N_P N_I} \end{bmatrix} = \begin{bmatrix} \boldsymbol{d}_1^T \\ \vdots \\ \boldsymbol{d}_{N_P}^T \end{bmatrix} = [\boldsymbol{\delta}_1, \ldots, \boldsymbol{\delta}_{N_I}]$$

Similarly, the *target matrix* is $\mathcal{T} = \begin{bmatrix} \boldsymbol{t}_1^T, \ldots, \boldsymbol{t}_{N_P}^T \end{bmatrix}^T$, with independent row vectors.

2.2 THE NETWORK AS A FUNCTION g OF ITS WEIGHTS

For all $h \in \{1..N_H\}$, $\boldsymbol{w}_h^1 = (w_{h1}^1, \ldots, w_{hN_I}^1)^T \in \Re^{N_I}$ is the vector of the weights between all the input units and the hth hidden unit. The *input weight matrix* W^1 is defined as $W^1 = \begin{bmatrix} \boldsymbol{w}_1^1, \ldots, \boldsymbol{w}_{N_H}^1 \end{bmatrix}$. Similarly, a vector $\boldsymbol{w}_s^2 = (w_{s1}^2, \ldots, w_{sN_H}^2)^T \in \Re^{N_H}$ represents the weights between all the hidden units and the sth output unit, for all $s \in \{1..N_S\}$. Thus the *output weight matrix* W^2 is defined as $W^2 = \begin{bmatrix} \boldsymbol{w}_1^2, \ldots, \boldsymbol{w}_{N_S}^2 \end{bmatrix}$. For an input matrix $\mathcal{D}$, the network computes an *output matrix*

$$\mathcal{Z}(\mathcal{D}) = \begin{bmatrix} z_1(\boldsymbol{d}_1) & \ldots & z_{N_S}(\boldsymbol{d}_1) \\ \vdots & & \vdots \\ z_1(\boldsymbol{d}_{N_P}) & \ldots & z_{N_S}(\boldsymbol{d}_{N_P}) \end{bmatrix} = \begin{bmatrix} \boldsymbol{z}(\boldsymbol{d}_1)^T \\ \vdots \\ \boldsymbol{z}(\boldsymbol{d}_{N_P})^T \end{bmatrix} = [\boldsymbol{\zeta}_1(\mathcal{D}), \ldots, \boldsymbol{\zeta}_{N_S}(\mathcal{D})]$$

where each output vector $\boldsymbol{z}(\boldsymbol{d}_p)$ must be equal to the target $\boldsymbol{t}_p$ for exact learning. The network computation can be detailed as follows, for all $s \in \{1..N_S\}$

$$\begin{aligned} z_s(\boldsymbol{d}_p) &= \sum_{h=1}^{N_H} w_{sh}^2 . f(\sum_{i=1}^{N_I} d_{pi} . w_{hi}^1) \\ &= \sum_{h=1}^{N_H} w_{sh}^2 . f(\boldsymbol{d}_p^T . \boldsymbol{w}_h^1) \end{aligned}$$

Hence, for the whole learning set, the sth output component is

$$\boldsymbol{\zeta}_s(\mathcal{D}) = \sum_{h=1}^{N_H} w_{sh}^2 . \begin{bmatrix} f(\boldsymbol{d}_1^T . \boldsymbol{w}_h^1) \\ \vdots \\ f(\boldsymbol{d}_{N_P}^T . \boldsymbol{w}_h^1) \end{bmatrix}$$

(1) $$\boldsymbol{\zeta}_s(\mathcal{D}) = \sum_{h=1}^{N_H} w_{sh}^2 . F(\mathcal{D} . \boldsymbol{w}_h^1)$$

In equation (1), F is a vector operator which transforms a n vector v into a n vector $F(v)$ according to the relation $[F(v)]_i = f([v]_i)$, $i \in \{1..n\}$. The same notation F will be used for the matrix operator. Finally, the expression of the output matrix can be deduced from equation (1) as follows

$$\mathcal{Z}(\mathcal{D}) = [F(\mathcal{D}.w_1^1), \ldots, F(\mathcal{D}.w_{N_H}^1)] \cdot [w_1^2, \ldots, w_{N_S}^2]$$
(2) $$\mathcal{Z}(\mathcal{D}) = F(\mathcal{D}.W^1).W^2$$

From equation (2), the network output matrix appears as a simple function of the input matrix and the network weights. Unlike Coetzee and Stonick, we will consider that the input matrix $\mathcal{D}$ is not a variable of the problem. Thus we express the network output matrix $\mathcal{Z}(\mathcal{D})$ as a function of its weights. Let g be this function

$$g : \mathcal{R}^{N_I \times N_H + N_H \times N_S} \longrightarrow \mathcal{R}^{N_P \times N_S}$$
$$W = (W^1, W^2) \longrightarrow F(\mathcal{D}.W^1).W^2$$

The g function clearly depends on the input matrix and could have been denoted by $g_\mathcal{D}$ but this index will be dropped for clarity.

3 FUNDAMENTAL RESULT

3.1 PROPERTY OF FUNCTION g

Learning is said to be exact on $\mathcal{D}$ if and only if there exists a network such that its output matrix $\mathcal{Z}(\mathcal{D})$ is equal to the target matrix $\mathcal{T}$. If g is a diffeomorphic function from $R^{N_I \times N_H + N_H \times N_S}$ onto $R^{N_P \times N_S}$ then the network can learn any target in $R^{N_P \times N_S}$ exactly. We prove that it is sufficient for the network function g to be a local diffeomorphism. Suppose there exist a set of weights X, an open subset $U \subset \mathcal{R}^{N_I N_H + N_H N_S}$ including X and an open subset $V \subset \mathcal{R}^{N_P N_S}$ including $g(X)$ such that g is diffeomorphic from U to V. Since V is an open neighborhood of $g(X)$, there exist a real λ and a point y in V such that $\mathcal{T} = \lambda(y - g(X))$. Since g is diffeomorphic from U to V, there exists a set of weights Y in U such that $y = g(Y)$, hence $\mathcal{T} = \lambda(g(Y) - g(X))$. The output units of the network compute a linear transfer function, hence the linear combination of $g(X)$ and $g(Y)$ can be integrated in the output weights and a network with twice $N_I N_H + N_H N_S$ weights can learn $(\mathcal{D}, \mathcal{T})$ exactly (see Figure 1).

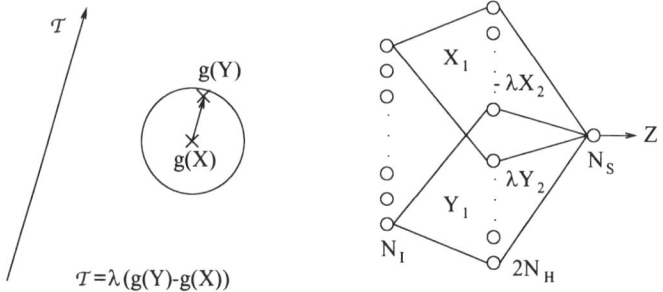

Figure 1: A network for exact learning of a target $\mathcal{T}$ (unique output for clarity)

For g a local diffeomorphism, it is sufficient to find a set of weights X such that the Jacobian of g in X is non-zero and to apply the theorem of local inversion. This analysis is developed in next sections and requires some assumptions on the transfer function f of the hidden units. A function which verifies such an hypothesis $\mathcal{H}$ will be called a $\mathcal{H}$-function and is defined below.

3.2 DEFINITION AND THEOREM

Definition 1 *Consider a function $f : \mathcal{R} \to \mathcal{R}$ which is $\mathcal{C}^1(\mathcal{R})$ (i.e. with continuous derivative) and which has finite limits in $-\infty$ and $+\infty$. Such a function is called a $\mathcal{H}$-function iff it verifies the following property*

$$(\mathcal{H}) \quad (\forall a \in \mathcal{R} / \mid a \mid > 1) \quad \lim_{x \to \pm\infty} \mid \frac{f'(ax)}{f'(x)} \mid = 0$$

From this hypothesis on the transfer function of all the hidden units, the fundamental result can be stated as follows

Theorem 1 *Exact learning of a set of N_P examples, in general position, from $\mathcal{R}^{N_I}$ to $\mathcal{R}^{N_S}$, can be realized by a network with linear output units and a transfer function which is a $\mathcal{H}$-function, if the size N_H of its hidden layer verifies the following bounds*

Lower Bound $\quad N_H = \lceil \frac{N_P N_S}{N_I + N_S} \rceil \quad$ *hidden units are necessary*

Upper Bound $\quad N_H = 2 \lceil \frac{N_P}{N_I + N_S} \rceil N_S \quad$ *hidden units are sufficient*

The proof of the lower bound is straightforward, since a condition for g to be diffeomorphic from $R^{N_I \times N_H + N_H \times N_S}$ onto $R^{N_P \times N_S}$ is the equality of its input and output space dimensions $N_I N_H + N_H N_S = N_P N_S$.

3.3 SKETCH OF THE PROOF FOR THE UPPER BOUND

The g function is an expression of the network as a function of its weights, for a given input matrix: $g(W^1, W^2) = F(\mathcal{D}.W^1).W^2$ and g can be decomposed according to its vectorial components on the learning set (which are themselves vectors of size N_S). For all $p \in \{1..N_P\}$

$$g_p(W^1, W^2) = \mathbf{z}(\mathbf{d}_p) = \left[\sum_{h=1}^{N_H} w_{1h}^2 \, f(\mathbf{d}_p^T.\mathbf{w}_h^1), \ldots, \sum_{h=1}^{N_H} w_{N_S h}^2 \, f(\mathbf{d}_p^T.\mathbf{w}_h^1) \right]^T$$

The derivatives of g w.r.t. the input weight matrix W^1 are, for all $i \in \{1..N_I\}$, for all $h \in \{1..N_H\}$

$$\frac{\partial g_p}{\partial w_{hi}^1} = \left[w_{1h}^2 \, f'(\mathbf{d}_p^T.\mathbf{w}_h^1) d_{pi}, \ldots, w_{N_S h}^2 \, f'(\mathbf{d}_p^T.\mathbf{w}_h^1) d_{pi} \right]^T$$

For the output weight matrix W^2, the derivatives of g are, for all $h \in \{1..N_H\}$, for all $s \in \{1..N_S\}$

$$\frac{\partial g_p}{\partial w_{sh}^2} = [\ \underbrace{0, \ldots, 0}_{s-1}, f(\mathbf{d}_p^T.\mathbf{w}_h^1), \underbrace{0, \ldots, 0}_{N_S - s}\ ]^T$$

The Jacobian matrix $\mathcal{M}_J(g)$ of g, the size of which is $N_I N_H + N_H N_S$ columns and $N_S N_P$ rows, is thus composed of a block-diagonal part (derivatives w.r.t. W^2) and several other blocks (derivatives w.r.t. W^1). Hence the Jacobian $J(g)$ can be rewritten $J(g) = \mid J_1, J_2, \ldots, J_{N_H} \mid$, after permutations of rows and columns, and using the Hadamard and Kronecker product notations, each J_h being equal to

$$(3) \quad J_h = \left[F(\mathcal{D}.\mathbf{w}_h^1) \otimes I_{N_S}, \left[F'(\mathcal{D}.\mathbf{w}_h^1) \circ \delta_1 \ldots F'(\mathcal{D}.\mathbf{w}_h^1) \circ \delta_{N_I} \right] \otimes \left[w_{1h}^2 \ldots w_{N_S h}^2 \right] \right]$$

where I_{N_S} is for the identity matrix in dimension N_S.

Our purpose is to prove that there exists a point $X = (W^1, W^2)$ such that the Jacobian $J(g)$ is non-zero at X, i.e. such that the column vectors of the Jacobian matrix $\mathcal{M}_J(g)$ are linearly independent at X. The proof can be divided in two steps. First we address the case of a single output unit. Afterwards, this proof can be used to extend the result to several output units. Since the complete development of both proofs require a lot of calculations, we only present their sketchs below. More details can be found in [7].

3.3.1 Case of a single output unit

The proof is based on a linear arrangement of the projections of the column vectors of J_h onto a subspace. This subspace is orthogonal to all the J_i for $i < h$. We build a vector $\boldsymbol{w}_h^1$ and a scalar w_{1h}^2 such that the projected column vectors are an independent family, hence they are independent with the J_i for $i < h$. Such a construction is recursively applied until $h = N_H$. We derive then vectors $\boldsymbol{w}_1^1, \ldots, \boldsymbol{w}_{N_H}^1$ and $\boldsymbol{w}_1^2$ such that $J(g)$ is non-zero. The assumption on $\mathcal{H}$-fonctions is essential for proving that the projected column vectors of J_h are independent.

3.3.2 Case of multiple output units

In order to extend the result from a single output to s output units, the usual idea consists in considering as many subnetworks as the number of output units. From this point of view, the bound on the hidden units would be $N_H = 2\frac{N_P N_S}{N_I + 1}$ which differs from the result stated in theorem 1. A new direct proof can be developed (see [7]) and get a better bound: the denominator is increased to $N_I + N_S$.

4 DISCUSSION

The definition of a $\mathcal{H}$-function includes both sigmoids and gaussian functions which are commonly used for multilayer perceptrons and RBF networks, but is not valid for threshold functions. Figure 2 shows the difference between a sigmoid, which is a $\mathcal{H}$-function, and a saturation which is not a $\mathcal{H}$-function. Figures (a) and (b) represent the span of the output space by the network when the weights are varying, i.e. the image of g. For clarity, the network is reduced to 1 hidden unit, 1 input unit, 1 output unit and 2 input patterns. For a $\mathcal{H}$-function, a ball can be extracted from the output space $\mathcal{R}^2$, onto which the g function is a diffeomorphism. For the saturation, the image of g is reduced to two lines, hence g cannot be onto on a ball of $\mathcal{R}^2$. The assumption of the activation function is thus necessary to prove that the jacobian is non-zero.

Our bound on the number of hidden units is very similar to Baum's results for dichotomies and functions from real inputs to binary outputs [1]. Hence the present result can be seen as an extension of Baum's results to the case of real outputs, and for a wide family of transfer functions, different from the threshold functions addressed by Baum and Haussler in [2]. An early result on sigmoid networks has been stated by Sontag [14]: for a single output and at least two input units, the number of examples must be twice the number of hidden units. Our upper bound on the number of hidden units is strictly lower than that (as soon as the number of input units is more than two). A counterpart of considering real data is that our results bear little relation to the VC-dimension point of view.

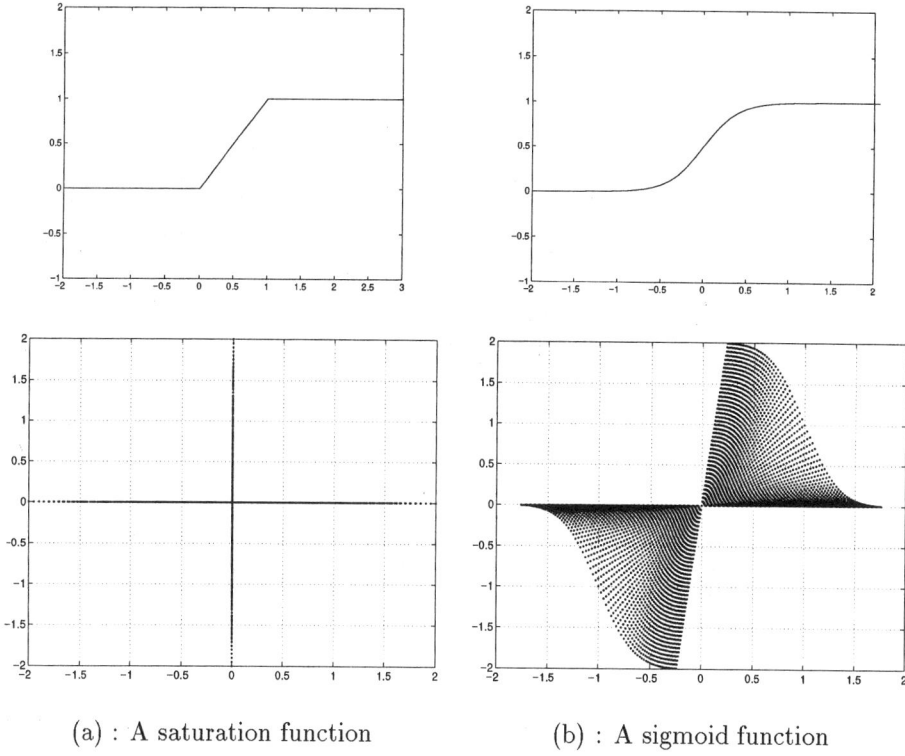

(a) : A saturation function   (b) : A sigmoid function

Figure 2: Positions of output vectors, for given data, when varying network weights

5 CONCLUSION

In this paper, we show that a number of hidden units $N_H = 2 \lceil N_P N_S/(N_I+N_S) \rceil$ is sufficient for a network of $\mathcal{H}$-functions to exactly learn a given set of N_P examples in general position. We now discuss some of the practical consequences of this result.

According to this formula, the size of the hidden layer required for exact learning may grow very high if the size of the learning set is large. However, without *a priori* knowledge on the degree of redundancy in the learning set, exact learning is not the right goal in practical cases. Exact learning usually implies overfitting, especially if the examples are very noisy. Nevertheless, a right point of view could be to previously reduce the dimension and the size of the learning set by feature extraction or data analysis as pre-processing. Afterwards, our theoretical result could be a precious indication for scaling a network to perform exact learning on this representative learning set, with a good compromise between bias and variance.

Our bound is more optimistic than the rule-of-thumb $N_P = 10w$ derived from the theory of PAC-learning. In our architecture, the number of weights is $w = 2N_P N_S$. However the proof is not constructive enough to be derived as a learning algorithm, especially the existence of $g(Y)$ in the neighborhood of $g(X)$ where g is a local diffeomorphism (cf. figure 1). From this construction we can only conclude that $N_H = \lceil N_P N_S/(N_I+N_S) \rceil$ is necessary and $N_H = 2 \lceil N_P N_S/(N_I+N_S) \rceil$ is sufficient to realize exact learning of N_P examples, from $\mathcal{R}^{N_I}$ to $\mathcal{R}^{N_S}$.

The opportunity of using multilayer networks as auto-associative networks and for data compression can be discussed at the light of this results. Assume that $N_S = N_I$ and the expression of the number of hidden units is reduced to $N_H = N_P$ or at least $N_H = N_P/2$. Since $N_P \geq N_I + N_S$, the number of hidden units must verify $N_H \geq N_I$. Therefore, an architecture of "diabolo" network seems to be precluded for exact learning of auto-associations. A consequence may be that exact retrieval from data compression is hopeless by using internal representations of a hidden layer smaller than the data dimension.

Acknowledgements

This work was supported by European Esprit III Project n^0 8556, NeuroCOLT Working Group. We thank C.S. Poon and J.V. Shah for fruitful discussions.

References

[1] E. B. Baum. On the capabilities of multilayer perceptrons. *J. of Complexity*, 4:193–215, 1988.

[2] E. B. Baum and D. Haussler. What size net gives valid generalization ? *Neural Computation*, 1:151–160, 1989.

[3] E. K. Blum and L. K. Li. Approximation theory and feedforward networks. *Neural Networks*, 4(4):511–516, 1991.

[4] F. M. Coetzee and V. L. Stonick. Topology and geometry of single hidden layer network, least squares weight solutions. *Neural Computation*, 7:672–705, 1995.

[5] M. Cosnard, P. Koiran, and H. Paugam-Moisy. Bounds on the number of units for computing arbitrary dichotomies by multilayer perceptrons. *J. of Complexity*, 10:57–63, 1994.

[6] G. Cybenko. Approximation by superpositions of a sigmoidal function. *Math. Control, Signal Systems*, 2:303–314, October 1988.

[7] A. Elisseeff and H. Paugam-Moisy. Size of multilayer networks for exact learning: analytic approach. Rapport de recherche 96-16, LIP, July 1996.

[8] K. Funahashi. On the approximate realization of continuous mappings by neural networks. *Neural Networks*, 2(3):183–192, 1989.

[9] K. Hornik, M. Stinchcombe, and H. White. Multilayer feedforward networks are universal approximators. *Neural Networks*, 2(5):359–366, 1989.

[10] S.-C. Huang and Y.-F. Huang. Bounds on the number of hidden neurons in multilayer perceptrons. *IEEE Trans. Neural Networks*, 2:47–55, 1991.

[11] M. Karpinski and A. Macintyre. Polynomial bounds for vc dimension of sigmoidal neural networks. In *27th ACM Symposium on Theory of Computing*, pages 200–208, 1995.

[12] P. Koiran and E. D. Sontag. Neural networks with quadratic vc dimension. In *Neural Information Processing Systems (NIPS*95)*, 1995. to appear.

[13] W. Maass. Bounds for the computational power and learning complexity of analog neural networks. In *25th ACM Symposium on Theory of Computing*, pages 335–344, 1993.

[14] E. D. Sontag. Feedforward nets for interpolation and classification. *J. Comp. Syst. Sci.*, 45:20–48, 1992.

[15] E. D. Sontag. Shattering all sets of k points in "general position" requires $(k-1)/2$ parameters. Technical Report Report 96-01, Rutgers Center for Systems and Control (SYCON), February 1996.

The effect of correlated input data on the dynamics of learning

Søren Halkjær and Ole Winther

CONNECT, The Niels Bohr Institute
Blegdamsvej 17
2100 Copenhagen, Denmark
halkjaer,winther@connect.nbi.dk

Abstract

The convergence properties of the gradient descent algorithm in the case of the linear perceptron may be obtained from the response function. We derive a general expression for the response function and apply it to the case of data with simple input correlations. It is found that correlations severely may slow down learning. This explains the success of PCA as a method for reducing training time. Motivated by this finding we furthermore propose to transform the input data by removing the mean across input variables as well as examples to decrease correlations. Numerical findings for a medical classification problem are in fine agreement with the theoretical results.

1 INTRODUCTION

Learning and generalization are important areas of research within the field of neural networks. Although good generalization is the ultimate goal in feed-forward networks (perceptrons), it is of practical importance to understand the mechanism which control the amount of time required for learning, i. e. the dynamics of learning. This is of course particularly important in the case of a large data set. An exact analysis of this mechanism is possible for the linear perceptron and as usual it is hoped that the results to some extend may be carried over to explain the behaviour of non-linear perceptrons.

We consider N dimensional input vectors $\mathbf{x} \in \mathcal{R}^N$ and scalar output y. The linear perceptron is parametrized by the weight vector $\mathbf{w} \in \mathcal{R}^N$

$$y(\mathbf{x}) = \frac{1}{\sqrt{N}} \mathbf{w}^T \mathbf{x} \qquad (1)$$

Let the training set be $\{(\mathbf{x}^\mu, y^\mu), \mu = 1, \ldots, p\}$ and the training error be the usual squared error, $E(\mathbf{w}) = \frac{1}{2} \sum_\mu (y^\mu - y(\mathbf{x}^\mu))^2$. We will use the well-known gradient descent algorithm[1] $\mathbf{w}(k+1) = \mathbf{w}(k) - \eta \nabla E(\mathbf{w}(k))$ to estimate the minimum points $\mathbf{w}^*$ of E. Here η denotes the learning parameter. Collecting the input examples in the $N \times p$ matrix $\mathbf{X}$ and the corresponding output in $\mathbf{y}$, the error function is written $E(\mathbf{w}) = \frac{1}{2}(\mathbf{w}^T \mathbf{R} \mathbf{w} - 2 \mathbf{q}^T \mathbf{w} + c)$, where $\mathbf{R} \equiv \frac{1}{N} \sum_\mu \mathbf{x}^\mu (\mathbf{x}^\mu)^T$, $\mathbf{q} = \frac{1}{\sqrt{N}} \mathbf{X} \mathbf{y}$ and $c = \mathbf{y}^T \mathbf{y}$. As in (Le Cun et al., 1991) the convergence properties of the minimum points $\mathbf{w}^*$ are examined in the coordinate system where $\mathbf{R}$ is diagonal. Let $\mathbf{U}$ denote the matrix whose columns are the eigenvectors of $\mathbf{R}$ and $\Delta = \mathrm{diag}(\lambda_1, \ldots, \lambda_N)$ the diagonal matrix containing the eigenvalues of $\mathbf{R}$. The new coordinates then become $\mathbf{v} = \mathbf{U}^T(\mathbf{w} - \mathbf{w}^*)$ with corresponding error function[2]

$$E(\mathbf{v}) = \frac{1}{2} \mathbf{v}^T \Delta \mathbf{v} + E_0 = \frac{1}{2} \sum_i \lambda_i v_i^2 + E_0 \qquad (2)$$

where $E_0 = E(\mathbf{w}^*)$. Gradient descent now leads to the decoupled equations

$$v_i(k+1) = (1 - \eta \lambda_i) v_i(k) = (1 - \eta \lambda_i)^k v_i(0) \qquad (3)$$

with $i = 1, \ldots, N$. Clearly, $\mathbf{v} \to \mathbf{0}$ requires $|1 - \eta \lambda_i| < 1$ for all i, so that η must be chosen in the interval $0 < \eta < 2/\lambda_{max}$. In the extreme case $\lambda_i = \lambda$ we will have convergence in one step for $\eta = 1/\lambda$. However, in the usual case of unequal λ_i the convergence for large k will be exponential $v_i(k) = \exp(-\eta \lambda_i k) v_i(0)$. $(\eta \lambda_i)^{-1}$ therefore defines the time constant of the i'th equation giving a slowest time constant $(\eta \lambda_{min})^{-1}$. A popular choice for the learning parameter is $\eta = 1/\lambda_{max}$ resulting in a slowest time constant $\lambda_{max}/\lambda_{min}$ called the learning time τ in the following. The convergence properties of the gradient descent algorithm is thus characterized by τ. In the case of a singular matrix $\mathbf{R}$, one or more of the eigenvalues will be zero, and there will be no convergence along the corresponding eigendirections. This has however no influence on the error according to (2). Thus, λ_{min} will in the following denote the smallest non-zero eigenvalue.

We will in the article calculate the eigenvalue spectrum of $\mathbf{R}$ in order to obtain the learning time of the gradient descent algorithm. This may be done by introducing the response function

$$G_\mathbf{L} \equiv G(\mathbf{L}, \mathbf{H}) = \frac{1}{N} \mathrm{Tr} \mathbf{L} \frac{1}{1 - \mathbf{R} \mathbf{H}} \equiv \left\langle \mathbf{L} \frac{1}{1 - \mathbf{R} \mathbf{H}} \right\rangle \qquad (4)$$

where $\mathbf{L}, \mathbf{H}$ are arbitrary $N \times N$ matrices. Using a standard representation of the Dirac δ-function (Krogh, 1992) we may write the eigenvalue spectrum of $\mathbf{R}$ as

$$\rho(\lambda) = \frac{1}{N} \sum_i \delta(\lambda - \lambda_i) = -\frac{1}{\pi} \mathrm{Im}\, G(\lambda^{-1}, \lambda^{-1}) \qquad (5)$$

---

[1] The Newton-Raphson method, $\mathbf{w}(k+1) = \mathbf{w}(k) - \nabla E(\mathbf{w}(k))(\nabla^2 E(\mathbf{w}(k)))^{-1}$ is of course much more effective in the linear case since it gives convergence in one step. This method however requires an inversion of the Hessian matrix.

[2] Note that this analysis is valid for any part of an error surface in which a quadratic approximation is valid. In the general case $\mathbf{R}$ should be exchanged with the Hessian $\nabla \nabla E(\mathbf{w}^*)$.

where λ has an infinitesimal imaginary part which is set equal to zero at the end of the calculation.

In the 'thermodynamic limit' $N \to \infty$ keeping $\alpha = \frac{P}{N}$ constant and finite, G (and thus the eigenvalue spectrum) is a self-averaging quantity (Sollich, 1996) i. e. $G - \overline{G} = \mathcal{O}(N^{-1})$, where $\overline{G}$ is defined as the response function averaged over the input distribution. Previously $\overline{G}$ has been calculated for independent input variables (Hertz et al., 1989; Sollich, 1996). In section 2 we derive an implicit equation for the averaged response function for arbitrary correlations using random matrix techniques (Brody et al., 1981). This equation is solved showing that simple input correlations may slow down learning significantly. Based on this finding we propose in section 3 data transformations for improving the learning speed and test the transformation numerically on a medical classification problem in section 4. We conclude in section 5 with a discussion of the results.

2 THE RESPONSE FUNCTION

The method for deriving the averaged response function is based on the fact that the response function (4) may be written as a geometrical series $G_\mathbf{L} = \sum_{r=0}^{\infty} \langle \mathbf{L}(\mathbf{RH})^r \rangle$. We will assume that the input examples $\mathbf{x}^\mu$ are drawn independently from a Gaussian distribution with means m_i and correlations $\overline{x_i x_j} - m_i m_j = C_{ij}$, i. e. $\overline{\mathbf{x}^\mu (\mathbf{x}^\nu)^T} = \delta_{\mu\nu} \mathbf{Z}$ and $\overline{\mathbf{R}} = \alpha \mathbf{Z}$ where $\mathbf{Z} \equiv \mathbf{C} + \mathbf{m}\mathbf{m}^T$. The Gaussian distribution has the property that the average of products of x's can be calculated by making all possible pair correlations, e.g. $\overline{x_i x_j x_k x_l} = Z_{ij} Z_{kl} + Z_{ik} Z_{jl} + Z_{il} Z_{jk}$. To take the average of $\langle \mathbf{L}(\mathbf{RH})^r \rangle$, we must therefore make all possible pairs of the $\mathbf{x}$'s and exchange each pair $x_i x_j$ with Z_{ij}. This combinatorial problem will be solved below in a recursive fashion leading to an implicit equation for $\overline{G}_L$. Using underbraces to indicate pairings of $\mathbf{x}$'s, we get for $r \geq 2$

$$
\begin{aligned}
\overline{\langle \mathbf{L}(\mathbf{RH})^r \rangle} &= \frac{1}{N} \sum_\mu \overline{\left\langle \mathbf{L} \underbrace{\mathbf{x}^\mu (\mathbf{x}^\mu)^T}_{} \mathbf{H}(\mathbf{RH})^{r-1} \right\rangle} \\
&\quad + \frac{1}{N^2} \sum_{s=0}^{r-2} \sum_{\mu,\nu} \overline{\left\langle \mathbf{L}\mathbf{x}^\mu \underbrace{(\mathbf{x}^\mu)^T \mathbf{H}(\mathbf{RH})^s \mathbf{x}^\nu}_{} (\mathbf{x}^\nu)^T \mathbf{H}(\mathbf{RII})^{r-s-2} \right\rangle} \\
&= \alpha \overline{\langle \mathbf{LZH}(\mathbf{RH})^{r-1} \rangle} + \sum_{s=0}^{r-2} \overline{\langle \mathbf{L}(\mathbf{RH})^{r-s-1} \rangle}\, \overline{\langle \mathbf{ZH}(\mathbf{RH})^s \rangle} \quad (6)
\end{aligned}
$$

Resumming this we get the response function

$$\overline{G}_\mathbf{L} = \langle \mathbf{L} \rangle + \alpha \sum_{r=0}^{\infty} \overline{\langle \mathbf{LZH}(\mathbf{RH})^r \rangle} + \sum_{r=0}^{\infty} \sum_{s=0}^{r-2} \overline{\langle \mathbf{L}(\mathbf{RH})^{r-s-1} \rangle}\, \overline{\langle \mathbf{ZH}(\mathbf{RH})^s \rangle} \quad (7)$$

Exchanging the order of summation in the last term we can write everything in terms of the response function

$$
\begin{aligned}
\overline{G}_\mathbf{L} &= \langle \mathbf{L} \rangle + \alpha \overline{G}_\mathbf{LZH} + \sum_{s=0}^{\infty} \sum_{r=s+1}^{\infty} \overline{\langle \mathbf{L}(\mathbf{RH})^{r-s} \rangle}\, \overline{\langle \mathbf{ZH}(\mathbf{RH})^s \rangle} \\
&= \langle \mathbf{L} \rangle + \alpha \overline{G}_\mathbf{LZH} + (\overline{G}_\mathbf{L} - \langle \mathbf{L} \rangle)\overline{G}_\mathbf{CH}
\end{aligned}
$$

$$= \langle \mathbf{L} \rangle + \frac{\alpha \overline{G}_{\mathbf{LZH}}}{1 - \overline{G}_{\mathbf{ZH}}} \qquad (8)$$

Using (8) recursively setting $\mathbf{L}$ equal to $\mathbf{LZH}$, $\mathbf{L(ZH)}^2$ etc. one obtains

$$\overline{G}_{\mathbf{L}} = \sum_{r=0}^{\infty} \left\langle \mathbf{L} \left(\frac{\alpha \mathbf{ZH}}{1 - \overline{G}_{\mathbf{ZH}}} \right)^r \right\rangle = \left\langle \mathbf{L} \frac{1}{1 - \frac{\alpha \mathbf{ZH}}{1 - \overline{G}_{\mathbf{ZH}}}} \right\rangle \qquad (9)$$

This is our main result for the response function. To get the response function $\overline{G}_{\frac{1}{\lambda}} = G(\lambda^{-1}, \lambda^{-1})$ requires two steps, first set $\mathbf{L} = \mathbf{ZH}$ and solve for $\overline{G}_{\mathbf{ZH}}$ and then solve for $\overline{G}_{\frac{1}{\lambda}}$. If $\mathbf{Z}$ has a particularly simple form (9) may be solved analytically, but in general it must be solved numerically.

In the following we will calculate the eigenvalue spectrum for a correlation matrix on the form $\mathbf{C} = \mathbf{nn}^T + r\mathbf{I}$ and general mean $\mathbf{m}$. To ensure that $\mathbf{C}$ is positive semi definite $r \geq 0$ and $|\mathbf{n}|^2 + r \geq 0$ where $|\mathbf{n}|^2 \equiv \mathbf{n} \cdot \mathbf{n}$. The eigenvalues of $\mathbf{Z} = \mathbf{nn}^T + \mathbf{mm}^T + r\mathbf{I}$ are straight forwardly shown to be $a_1 = r$ (with multiplicity $N - 2$), $a_2 = r + \left[|\mathbf{n}|^2 + |\mathbf{m}|^2 - \sqrt{D}\right]/2$ and $a_3 = r + \left[|\mathbf{n}|^2 + |\mathbf{m}|^2 + \sqrt{D}\right]/2$ with $D = (|\mathbf{n}|^2 - |\mathbf{m}|^2)^2 + 4(\mathbf{n} \cdot \mathbf{m})^2$. Carrying out the trace in eq. (9) we get

$$\overline{G}_{\frac{1}{\lambda}} = \frac{N-2}{N} \frac{1}{\lambda - \frac{\alpha a_1}{1 - \overline{G}_{\mathbf{ZH}}}} + \frac{1}{N} \frac{1}{\lambda - \frac{\alpha a_2}{1 - \overline{G}_{\mathbf{ZH}}}} + \frac{1}{N} \frac{1}{\lambda - \frac{\alpha a_3}{1 - \overline{G}_{\mathbf{ZH}}}} \qquad (10)$$

This expression suggests that we may solve $\overline{G}_{\frac{1}{\lambda}}$ in powers of $1/N$ (see e.g. (Sollich, 1996)). However for purposes of the discussion of learning times the only $\frac{1}{N}$-term that will be of importance is the last term above. We therefore only need to solve for $\overline{G}_{\mathbf{ZH}}$ (setting $\mathbf{L} = \mathbf{ZH}$ in (9)) to leading order

$$\overline{G}_{\mathbf{ZH}} = \frac{\lambda + a_1(1-\alpha) - \sqrt{(\lambda + a_1(1-\alpha)^2) - 4\lambda a_1}}{2\lambda} \qquad (11)$$

Note that $\overline{G}_{\mathbf{ZH}}$ will vanish for large λ implying that the last term in (10) to leading order is singular for $\lambda = \alpha a_3$. Inserting the result in (10) gives

$$\overline{G}_{\frac{1}{\lambda}} = \frac{1}{2\lambda a_2} \left[\lambda + a_2(1-\alpha) - \sqrt{(\lambda + a_2(1-\alpha))^2 - 4\lambda a_2} \right] + \frac{1}{N} \frac{1}{\lambda - \alpha a_1} \qquad (12)$$

According to (5) the eigenvalue spectrum is determined by the imaginary part and poles of $\overline{G}_{\frac{1}{\lambda}}$. $\overline{G}_{\frac{1}{\lambda}}$ has an imaginary part for $\lambda_- < \lambda < \lambda_+$ where $\lambda_\pm = a_1(1 \pm \sqrt{\alpha})^2$ and the poles $\lambda = 0$, $\lambda = \alpha a_3$. The poles contribute each with a δ-function such that the eigenvalue spectrum up to corrections of order $\frac{1}{N}$ becomes

$$\overline{\rho}(\lambda) = (1-\alpha)\Theta(1-\alpha)\delta(\lambda) + \frac{1}{N}\delta(\lambda - \alpha a_3) + \frac{1}{2\pi\lambda a_1}\sqrt{(\lambda_+ - \lambda)(\lambda - \lambda_-)} \qquad (13)$$

where $\Theta(x) = 1$ for $x > 0$ and 0 otherwise. The first term expresses the trivial fact that for $p < N$ the whole input space is not spanned and $\mathbf{R}$ will have a fraction of $1 - \alpha$ zero-eigenvalues. The continuous spectrum (the root term) only contributes for $\lambda_- < \lambda < \lambda_+$. Numerical simulations has been performed to test the validity of the spectrum (13) (Halkjær, 1996). They are in good agreement with predicted results indicating that finite size effects are unimportant. The continuous spectrum in (13) has also been calculated using the replica method (Halkjær, 1996).

From the spectrum the learning time τ may be read of directly

$$\tau = \max\left(\frac{\lambda_+}{\lambda_-}, \frac{\alpha a_3}{\lambda_-}\right) = \max\left(\left(\frac{1+\sqrt{\alpha}}{1-\sqrt{\alpha}}\right)^2, \frac{\alpha a_3}{a_1\left(1-\sqrt{\alpha}\right)^2}\right) \qquad (14)$$

To illustrate how input correlations and bias may affect learning time consider simple correlations $C_{ij} = \delta_{ij}v(1-c) + vc$ and $m_i = m$. With this special choice $\tau = \frac{\alpha N(m^2 + vc)}{v(1-c)\left(1-\sqrt{\alpha}\right)^2}$. For $m^2 + cv > 0$, i.e. for non-zero mean or positive correlations, the convergence time will blow up by a factor proportional to N. The input bias effect has previously been observed by (Le Cun et al., Wendemuth et al.). In the next section we will consider transformations to remove the large eigenvalue and thus to speed up learning.

3 DATA TRANSFORMATIONS FOR INCREASING LEARNING SPEED

In this section we consider two data transformations for minimizing the learning time τ of a data set, based on the results obtained in the previous sections.

The PCA transformation (Jackson, 1991) is a data transformation often used in data analysis. Let $\mathbf{U}$ be the matrix whose columns are the eigenvectors of the sample covariance matrix and let $\mathbf{x}^{mean}$ denote the sample average vector (see below). It is easy to check that the transformed data set

$$\tilde{\mathbf{x}}^\mu = \mathbf{U}^T(\mathbf{x}^\mu - \mathbf{x}^{mean}) \qquad (15)$$

have uncorrelated (zero-mean) variables. However, the new PCA variables will often have a large spread in variances which might result in slow convergence. A simple rescaling of the new variables will remove this problem, such that according to (14) a PCA transformed data set with rescaled variables will have optimal convergence properties.

The other transformation, which we will call *double centering*, is based on the removal of the observation means and the variable means. However, whereas the PCA transformation doesn't care about the initial distribution, this transformation is optimal for a data set generated from the matrix $Z_{ij} = \delta_{ij}v(1-c) + vc + m_i m_j$ studied earlier. Define $x_i^{mean} = \frac{1}{p}\sum_\mu x_i^\mu$ (mean of the i'th variable), $x_{mean}^\mu = \frac{1}{N}\sum_i x_i^\mu$ (mean of the μ'th example) and $x_{mean}^{mean} = \frac{1}{pN}\sum_{\mu i} x_i^\mu$ (grand mean). Consider first the transformed data set

$$\tilde{x}_i^\mu = x_i - x_i^{mean} - x_{mean}^\mu + x_{mean}^{mean}$$

The new variables are readily seen to have zero mean, variance $\tilde{v} = v(1-c) - \frac{v}{N}(1-c)$ and correlation $\tilde{c} = \frac{-1}{N-1}$. Since $\tilde{v}(1-\tilde{c}) = v(1-c)$ we immediately get from (13) that the continuous eigenvalue spectrum is unchanged by this transformation. Furthermore the 'large' eigenvalue αa_1 is equal to zero and therefore uninteresting. Thus the learning time becomes $\tau = (1+\sqrt{\alpha})^2/(1-\sqrt{\alpha})^2$. This transformation however removes perhaps important information from the data set, namely the observation means. Motivated by these findings, we create a new data set $\{\tilde{\mathbf{x}}^\mu\}$ where this information is added as an extra component

$$\tilde{\mathbf{x}}^\mu = (\tilde{x}_1^\mu, \ldots, \tilde{x}_N^\mu, x_{mean}^\mu - x_{mean}^{mean}) \qquad (16)$$

Table 1: Required number of iterations and corresponding learning times for different data transformations. 'Raw' is the original data set, 'Var. cent.' indicates the variable centered ($m_i = 0$) data set, 'Doub. cent.' denotes (16), while the two last columns concerns the PCA transformed data set (15) without and with rescaled variables.

	Raw	Var. cent.	Doub. cent.	PCA	PCA (res.)
Iterations	∞	300	50	630	7
τ	161190	3330	237	3330	1

The matrix $\tilde{\mathbf{R}}$ resulting from this data set is identical to the above case except that a column and a row have been added. We therefore conclude that the eigenvalue spectrum of this data set consists of a continuous spectrum equal to the above and a single eigenvalue which is found to be $\lambda = \frac{1}{N}v(1-c) + cv$. For $c \neq 0$ we will therefore have a learning time τ of order one indicating fast convergence. For independent variables ($c = 0$) the transformation results in a learning time of order N but in this case a simple removal of the variable means will be optimal. After training, when an $(N+1)$-dim parameter set $\tilde{\mathbf{w}}$ has been obtained, it is possible to transform back to the original data set using the parameter transformation $w_l = \tilde{w}_l + \frac{1}{N}\tilde{w}_{N+1} - \frac{1}{N}\sum_{i=1}^{N}\tilde{w}_i$.

4 NUMERICAL INVESTIGATIONS

The suggested transformations for improving the convergence properties have been tested on a medical classification problem. The data set consisted of 40 regional values of cerebral glucose metabolism from 85 patients, 48 HIV-negatives and 37 HIV-positives. A simple perceptron with sigmoidal tanh output was trained using gradient descent on the entropic error function to diagnose the 85 patients correctly. The choice of an entropic error function was due to it's superior convergence properties compared to the quadratic error function considered in the analysis. The learning was stopped once the perceptron was able to diagnose all patients correctly. Table 1 shows the average number of required iterations for each of the transformed data sets (see legend) as well as the ratio $\tau = \lambda_{max}/\lambda_{min}$ for the corresponding matrix $\mathbf{R}$. The 'raw' data set could not be learned within the allowed 1000 iterations which is indicated by an ∞. Overall, there's fine agreement between the order of calculated learning times and the corresponding order of required number of iterations. Note especially the superiority of the PCA transformation with rescaled variables.

5 CONCLUSION

For linear networks the convergence properties of the gradient descent algorithm may be derived from the eigenvalue spectrum of the covariance matrix of the input data. The convergence time is controlled by the ratio between the largest and smallest (non-zero) eigenvalue. In this paper we have calculated the eigenvalue spectrum of a covariance matrix for correlated and biased inputs. It turns out that correlation and bias give rise to an eigenvalue of order the input dimension as well as a continuous spectrum of order one. This explains why a PCA transformation (with a variable rescaling) may increase learning speed significantly. We have proposed to center (setting equal to zero) the empirical mean both for each variable and each observation in order to remove the large eigenvalue. We add an additional component containing the observation mean to the input vector in order have this information in the training set. At the end of training it is possible to transform the solution back to the original representation. Numerical investigations are in fine agreement with the theoretical analysis for improving the convergence properties.

6 ACKNOWLEDGMENTS

We would like to thank Sara A. Solla and Lars Kai Hansen for valuable comments and discussions. Furthermore we wish to thank Ido Kanter for providing us with notes on some of his previous work. This work has been supported by the Danish National Councils for the Natural and Technical Sciences through the Danish Computational Neural Network Center CONNECT.

REFERENCES

Brody, T. A., Flores J., French J. B., Mello, P. A., Pendey, A., & Wong, S. S. (1981) Random-matrix physics. *Rev. Mod. Phys.* 53:385.

Halkjær, S. (1996) *Dynamics of learning in neural networks: application to the diagnosis of HIV and Alzheimer patients.* Master's thesis, University of Copenhagen.

Hertz, J. A., Krogh, A. & Thorbergsson G. I. (1989) Phase transitions in simple learning. *J. Phys. A* 22:2133-2150.

Jackson, J. E. (1991) *A User's Guide to Principal Components.* John Wiley & Sons.

Krogh, A. (1992) Learning with noise in a linear perceptron *J. Phys A* 25:1119-1133.

Le Cun, Y., Kanter, I. & Solla, S.A. (1991) Second Order Properties of Error Surfaces : Learning Time and Generalization. *NIPS*, 3:918-924.

Sollich, P. (1996) Learning in large linear perceptrons and why the thermodynamic limit is relevant to the real world. *NIPS*, 7:207-214

Wendemuth, A., Opper, M. & Kinzel W. (1993) The effect of correlations in neural networks, *J. Phys. A* 26:3165.

Practical confidence and prediction intervals

Tom Heskes
RWCP Novel Functions SNN Laboratory,[*] University of Nijmegen
Geert Grooteplein 21, 6525 EZ Nijmegen, The Netherlands
tom@mbfys.kun.nl

Abstract

We propose a new method to compute prediction intervals. Especially for small data sets the width of a prediction interval does not only depend on the variance of the target distribution, but also on the accuracy of our estimator of the mean of the target, i.e., on the width of the confidence interval. The confidence interval follows from the variation in an ensemble of neural networks, each of them trained and stopped on bootstrap replicates of the original data set. A second improvement is the use of the residuals on validation patterns instead of on training patterns for estimation of the variance of the target distribution. As illustrated on a synthetic example, our method is better than existing methods with regard to extrapolation and interpolation in data regimes with a limited amount of data, and yields prediction intervals which actual confidence levels are closer to the desired confidence levels.

1 STATISTICAL INTERVALS

In this paper we will consider feedforward neural networks for regression tasks: estimating an underlying mathematical function between input and output variables based on a finite number of data points possibly corrupted by noise. We are given a set of p_{data} pairs $\{\vec{x}^\mu, t^\mu\}$ which are assumed to be generated according to

$$t(\vec{x}) = f(\vec{x}) + \xi(\vec{x}), \tag{1}$$

where $\xi(\vec{x})$ denotes noise with zero mean. Straightforwardly trained on such a regression task, the output of a network $o(\vec{x})$ given a new input vector $\vec{x}$ can be

---

[*]RWCP: Real World Computing Partnership; SNN: Foundation for Neural Networks.

interpreted as an estimate of the regression $f(\vec{x})$, i.e., of the mean of the target distribution given input $\vec{x}$. Sometimes this is all we are interested in: a reliable estimate of the regression $f(\vec{x})$. In many applications, however, it is important to quantify the accuracy of our statements. For regression problems we can distinguish two different aspects: the accuracy of our estimate of the true regression and the accuracy of our estimate with respect to the observed output. Confidence intervals deal with the first aspect, i.e., consider the distribution of the quantity $f(\vec{x}) - o(\vec{x})$, prediction intervals with the latter, i.e., treat the quantity $t(\vec{x}) - o(\vec{x})$. We see from

$$t(\vec{x}) - o(\vec{x}) = [f(\vec{x}) - o(\vec{x})] + \xi(\vec{x}), \tag{2}$$

that a prediction interval necessarily encloses the corresponding confidence interval.

In [7] a method somewhat similar to ours is introduced to estimate both the mean and the variance of the target probability distribution. It is based on the assumption that there is a sufficiently large data set, i.e., that their is no risk of overfitting and that the neural network finds the correct regression. In practical applications with limited data sets such assumptions are too strict. In this paper we will propose a new method which estimates the inaccuracy of the estimator through bootstrap resampling and corrects for the tendency to overfit by considering the residuals on validation patterns rather than those on training patterns.

2 BOOTSTRAPPING AND EARLY STOPPING

Bootstrapping [3] is based on the idea that the available data set is nothing but a particular realization of some unknown probability distribution. Instead of sampling over the "true" probability distribution, which is obviously impossible, one defines an empirical distribution. With so-called naive bootstrapping the empirical distribution is a sum of delta peaks on the available data points, each with probability content $1/p_{\text{data}}$. A bootstrap sample is a collection of p_{data} patterns drawn with replacement from this empirical probability distribution. This bootstrap sample is nothing but our training set and all patterns that do not occur in the training set are by definition part of the validation set. For large p_{data}, the probability that a pattern becomes part of the validation set is $(1 - 1/p_{\text{data}})^{p_{\text{data}}} \approx 1/e \approx 0.37$.

When training a neural network on a particular bootstrap sample, the weights are adjusted in order to minimize the error on the training data. Training is stopped when the error on the validation data starts to increase. This so-called early stopping procedure is a popular strategy to prevent overfitting in neural networks and can be viewed as an alternative to regularization techniques such as weight decay. In this context bootstrapping is just a procedure to generate subdivisions in training and validation set similar to k-fold cross-validation or subsampling.

On each of the n_{run} bootstrap replicates we train and stop a single neural network. The output of network i on input vector $\vec{x}^\mu$ is written $o_i(\vec{x}^\mu) \equiv o_i^\mu$. As "the" estimate of our ensemble of networks for the regression $f(\vec{x})$ we take the average output[1]

$$m(\vec{x}) \equiv \frac{1}{n_{\text{run}}} \sum_{i=1}^{n_{\text{run}}} o_i(\vec{x}).$$

---

[1] This is a so-called "bagged" estimator [2]. In [5] it is shown that a proper balancing of the network outputs can yield even better results.

3 CONFIDENCE INTERVALS

Confidence intervals provide a way to quantify our confidence in the estimate $m(\vec{x})$ of the regression $f(\vec{x})$, i.e., we have to consider the probability distribution $P(f(\vec{x})|m(\vec{x}))$ that the true regression is $f(\vec{x})$ given our estimate $m(\vec{x})$. Our line of reasoning goes as follows (see also [8]).

We assume that our ensemble of neural networks yields a more or less unbiased estimate for $f(\vec{x})$, i.e., the distribution $P(f(\vec{x})|m(\vec{x}))$ is centered around $m(\vec{x})$. The truth is that neural networks are biased estimators. For example, neural networks trained on a finite number of examples will always have a tendency (as almost any other model) to oversmooth a sharp peak in the data. This introduces a bias, which, to arrive at asymptotically correct confidence intervals, should be taken into account. However, if it would be possible to compute such a bias correction, one should do it in the first place to arrive at a better estimator. Our working hypothesis here is that the bias component of the confidence intervals is negligible in comparison with the variance component.

There do exist methods that claim to give confidence intervals that are "second-order correct", i.e., up to and including terms of order $1/p_{\text{data}}^{3/2}$ (see e.g. the discussion after [3]). Since we do not know how to handle the bias component anyways, such precise confidence intervals, which require a tremendous amount of bootstrap samples, are too ambitious for our purposes. First-order correct intervals up to and including terms of order $1/p_{\text{data}}$ are always symmetric and can be derived by assuming a Gaussian distribution $P(f(\vec{x})|m(\vec{x}))$.

The variance of this distribution can be estimated from the variance in the outputs of the n_{run} networks:

$$\sigma^2(\vec{x}) \equiv \frac{1}{n_{\text{run}} - 1} \sum_{i=1}^{n_{\text{run}}} [o_i(\vec{x}) - m(\vec{x})]^2 \,. \tag{3}$$

This is the crux of the bootstrap method (see e.g. [3]). Since the distribution of $P(f(\vec{x})|m(\vec{x}))$ is a Gaussian, so is the "inverse" distribution $P(m(\vec{x})|f(\vec{x}))$ to find the regression $m(\vec{x})$ by randomly drawing data sets consisting of p_{data} data points according to the prescription (1). Not knowing the true distribution of inputs and corresponding targets[2], the best we can do is to define the empirical distribution as explained before and estimate $P(m(\vec{x})|f(\vec{x}))$ from the distribution $P(o(\vec{x})|m(\vec{x}))$. This then yields the estimate (3).

So, following this bootstrap procedure we arrive at the confidence intervals

$$m(\vec{x}) - c_{\text{confidence}}\sigma(\vec{x}) \leq f(\vec{x}) \leq m(\vec{x}) + c_{\text{confidence}}\sigma(\vec{x}) \,,$$

where $c_{\text{confidence}}$ depends on the desired confidence level $1-\alpha$. The factors $c_{\text{confidence}}$ can be taken from a table with the percentage points of the Student's t-distribution with number of degrees of freedom equal to the number of bootstrap runs n_{run}. A more direct alternative is to choose $c_{\text{confidence}}$ such that for no more than $100\alpha\%$ of all $n_{\text{run}} \times p_{\text{data}}$ network predictions $|o_i^\mu - m^\mu| \geq c_{\text{confidence}}\, \sigma^\mu$.

---

[2] In this paper we assume that both the inputs and the outputs are stochastic. For the case of deterministic input variables other bootstrapping techniques (see e.g. [4]) are more appropriate, since the statistical intervals resulting from naive bootstrapping may be too conservative.

4 PREDICTION INTERVALS

Confidence intervals deal with the accuracy of our prediction of the regression, i.e., of the mean of the target probability distribution. Prediction intervals consider the accuracy with which we can predict the targets themselves, i.e., they are based on estimates of the distribution $P(t(\vec{x})|m(\vec{x}))$. We propose the following method.

The two noise components $f(\vec{x}) - m(\vec{x})$ and $\xi(\vec{x})$ in (2) are independent. The variance of the first component has been estimated in our bootstrap procedure to arrive at confidence intervals. The remaining task is to estimate the noise inherent to the regression problem. We assume that this noise is more or less Gaussian such that it again suffices to compute its variance which may however depend on the input $\vec{x}$. In mathematical symbols,

$$s^2(\vec{x}) \equiv \langle [t(\vec{x}) - m(\vec{x})]^2 \rangle = \langle [f(\vec{x}) - m(\vec{x})]^2 \rangle + \langle \xi^2(\vec{x}) \rangle = \sigma^2(\vec{x}) + \chi^2(\vec{x}) .$$

Of course, we are interested in prediction intervals for new points $\vec{x}$ for which we do not know the targets t. Suppose that we had left aside a set of test patterns $\{\vec{x}^\nu, t^\nu\}$ that we had never used for training nor for validating our neural networks. Then we could try and estimate a model $\chi^2(\vec{x})$ to fit the remaining residuals

$$r^2(\vec{x}^\nu) \equiv \max\left([t^\nu - m(\vec{x}^\nu)]^2 - \sigma^2(\vec{x}^\nu), 0\right) , \qquad (4)$$

using minus the loglikelihood as the error measure:

$$L \equiv -\sum_\nu \log\left[\frac{1}{\sqrt{2\pi\chi^2(\vec{x}^\nu)}} \exp\left(-\frac{r^2(\vec{x}^\nu)}{2\chi^2(\vec{x}^\nu)}\right)\right] . \qquad (5)$$

Of course, leaving out these test patterns is a waste of data and luckily our bootstrap procedure offers an alternative. Each pattern is in about 37% of all bootstrap runs not part of the training set. Let us write $q_i^\mu = 1$ if pattern μ is in the validation set of run i and $q_i^\mu = 0$ otherwise. If we, for each pattern μ, use the average

$$m_{\text{validation}}(\vec{x}^\mu) = \sum_{i=1}^{n_{\text{run}}} q_i^\mu o_i^\mu \bigg/ \sum_{\mu=1}^{n_{\text{run}}} q_i^\mu ,$$

instead of the average $m(\vec{x}^\mu)$ we get as close as possible to an unbiased estimate for the residual on independent test patterns as we can, without wasting any training data. So, summarizing, we suggest to find a function $\chi(\vec{x})$ that minimizes the error (5), yet not by leaving out test patterns, which would be a waste of data, nor by straightforwardly using the training data, which would underestimate the error, but by exploiting the information about the residuals on the validation patterns.

Once we have found the function $\chi(\vec{x})$, we can compute for any $\vec{x}$ both the mean $m(\vec{x})$ and the deviation $s(\vec{x})$ which are combined in the prediction interval

$$m(\vec{x}) - c_{\text{prediction}} s(\vec{x}) \leq t(\vec{x}) \leq m(\vec{x}) + c_{\text{prediction}} s(\vec{x}) .$$

Again, the factor $c_{\text{prediction}}$ can be found in a Student's t-table or chosen such that for no more than $100\alpha\%$ of all p_{data} patterns $|t^\mu - m_{\text{validation}}(\vec{x}^\mu)| \geq c_{\text{prediction}} s(\vec{x}^\mu)$.

The function $\chi^2(\vec{x})$ may be modelled by a separate neural network, similar to the method proposed in [7] with an exponential instead of a linear transfer function for the output unit to ensure that the variance is always positive.

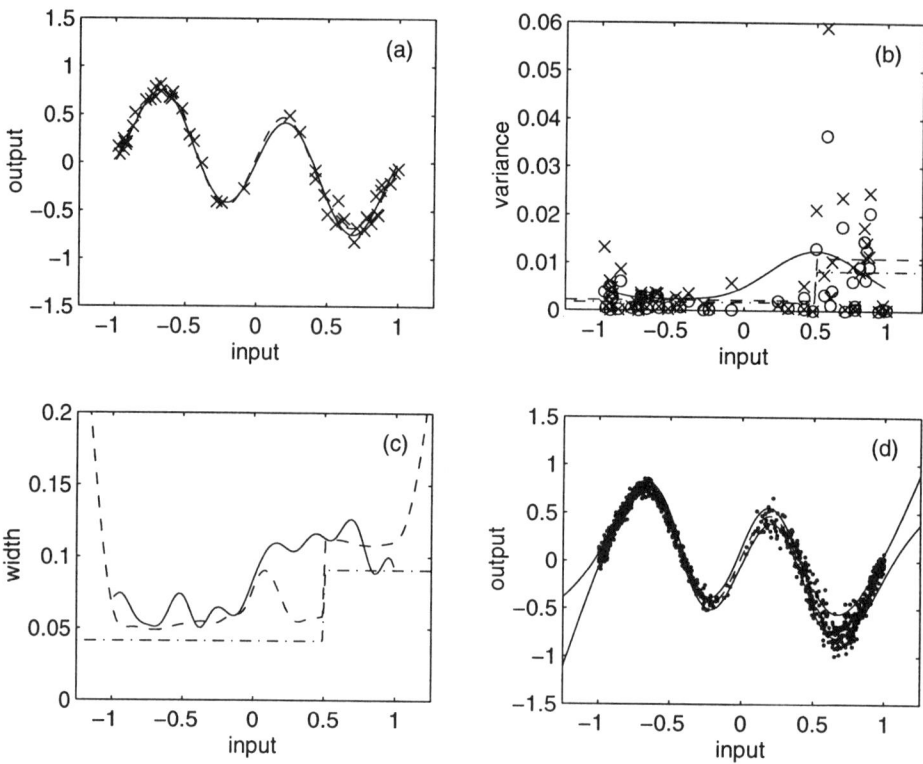

Figure 1: Prediction intervals for a synthetic problem. (a) Training set (crosses), true regression (solid line), and network prediction (dashed line). (b) Validation residuals (crosses), training residuals (circles), true variance (solid line), estimated variance based on validation residuals (dashed line) and based on training residuals (dash-dotted line). (c) Width of standard error bars for the more advanced method (dashed line), the simpler procedure (dash-dotted line) and what it should be (solid line). (d) Prediction intervals (solid line), network prediction (dashed line), and 1000 test points (dots).

5 ILLUSTRATION

We consider a synthetic problem similar to the one used in [7]. With this example we will demonstrate the desirability to incorporate the inaccuracy of the regression estimator in the prediction intervals. Inputs x are drawn from the interval $[-1, 1]$ with probability density $\rho(x) = |x|$, i.e., more examples are drawn at the boundary than in the middle. Targets t are generated according to

$$t = \sin(\pi x)\cos(5\pi x/4) + \xi(x) \quad \text{with} \quad \langle \xi^2(x) \rangle = 0.005 + 0.005\left[1 + \sin(\pi x)\right]^2 .$$

The regression is the solid line in Figure 1(a), the variance of the target distribution the solid line in Figure 1(b). Following this prescription we obtain a training set of $p_{\text{data}} = 50$ data points [the crosses in Figure 1(a)] on which we train an ensemble of $n_{\text{run}} = 25$ networks, each having 8 hidden units with tanh-transfer function and one linear output unit. The average network output $m(x)$ is the dashed line in Figure 1(a) and (d). In the following we compare two methods to arrive at prediction intervals: the more advanced method described in Section 4, i.e., taking into account the uncertainty of the estimator and correcting for the tendency to overfit on the training data, and a simpler procedure similar to [7] which disregards both effects.

We compute the (squared) "validation residuals" $(m^\mu_{\text{validation}} - t^\mu)^2$ [crosses in Figure 1(b)], based on runs in which pattern μ was part of the validation set, and the "training residuals" $(m^\mu_{\text{train}} - t^\mu)^2$ (circles), based on runs in which pattern μ was part of the training set. The validation residuals are most of the time somewhat larger than the training residuals.

For our more advanced method we substract the uncertainty of our model from the validation residuals as in (4). The other procedure simply keeps the training residuals to estimate the variance of the target distribution. It is obvious that the distribution of residuals in Figure 1(b) does not allow for a complex model. Here we take a feedforward network with one hidden unit:

$$\chi^2(x) = \exp\left[v_1 \tanh(v_3 x + v_2) + v_0\right].$$

The parameters $\{v_0, v_1, v_2, v_3\}$ are found through minimization of the error (5). Both for the advanced method (dashed line) and for the simpler procedure (dash-dotted line) the variance of the target distribution is estimated to be a step function. The former, being based on the validation residuals minus the uncertainty of the estimator, is slightly more conservative than the latter, being based on the training residuals. Both estimates are pretty far from the truth (solid line), especially for $0 < x < 0.5$, yet considering such a limited amount of noisy residuals we can hardly expect anything better.

Figure 1(c) considers the width of standard error bars, i.e., of prediction intervals for error level $\alpha \approx 0.32$. For the simpler procedure the width of the prediction interval [dash-dotted line in Figure 1(c)] follows directly from the estimate of the variance of the target distribution. Our more advanced method adds the uncertainty of the estimator to arrive at the dashed line. The correct width of the prediction interval, i.e., the width that would include 68% of all targets for a particular input, is given by the solid line. The prediction intervals obtained through the more advanced procedure are displayed in Figure 1(d) together with a set of 1000 test points visualizing the probability distribution of inputs and corresponding targets.

The method proposed in Section 4 has several advantages. The prediction intervals of the advanced method include 65% of the test points in Figure 1(d), pretty close to the desired confidence level of 68%. The simpler procedure is too liberal with an actual confidence level of only 58%. This difference is mainly due to the use of validation residuals instead of training residuals. Incorporation of the uncertainty of the estimator is important in regions of input space with just a few training data. In this example the density of training data affects both extrapolation and interpolation. For $|x| > 1$ the prediction intervals obtained with the advanced method become wider and wider whereas those obtained through the simpler procedure remain more or less constant. The bump in the prediction interval (dashed line) near the origin is a result of the relatively large variance in the network predictions in this region. It shows that our method also incorporates the effect that the density of training data has on the accuracy of interpolation.

6 CONCLUSION AND DISCUSSION

We have presented a novel method to compute prediction intervals for applications with a limited amount of data. The uncertainty of the estimator itself has been taken into account by the computation of the confidence intervals. This explains the qualitative improvement over existing methods in regimes with a low density of training data. Usage of the residuals on validation instead of on training patterns yields prediction intervals with a better coverage. The price we have to pay is in the computation time: we have to train an ensemble of networks on about 20 to 50 different bootstrap replicates [3, 8]. There are other good reasons for resampling: averaging over networks improves the generalization performance and early stopping is a natural strategy to prevent overfitting. It would be interesting to see how our "frequentist" method compares with Bayesian alternatives (see e.g. [1, 6]).

Prediction intervals can also be used for the detection of outliers. With regard to the training set it is straightforward to point out the targets that are not enclosed by a prediction interval of error level say $\alpha = 0.05$. A wide prediction interval for a new test pattern indicates that this test pattern lies in a region of input space with a low density of training data making any prediction completely unreliable.

A weak point in our method is the assumption of unbiasedness in the computation of the confidence intervals. This assumption makes the confidence intervals in general too liberal. However, as discussed in [8], such bootstrap methods tend to perform better than other alternatives based on the computation of the Hessian matrix, partly because they incorporate the variability due to the random initialization. Furthermore, when we model the prediction interval as a function of the input $\vec{x}$ we will, to some extent, repair this deficiency. But still, incorporating even a somewhat inaccurate confidence interval ensures that we can never severely overestimate our accuracy in regions of input space where we have never been before.

References

[1] C. Bishop and C. Qazaz. Regression with input-dependent noise: a Bayesian treatment. *These proceedings*, 1997.

[2] L. Breiman. Bagging predictors. *Machine Learning*, 24:123–140, 1996.

[3] B. Efron and R. Tibshirani. *An Introduction to the Bootstrap*. Chapman & Hall, London, 1993.

[4] W. Härdle. *Applied Nonparametric Regression*. Cambridge University Press, 1991.

[5] T. Heskes. Balancing between bagging and bumping. *These proceedings*, 1997.

[6] D. MacKay. A practical Bayesian framework for backpropagation. *Neural Computation*, 4:448–472, 1992.

[7] D. Nix and A. Weigend. Estimating the mean and variance of the target probability distribution. In *Proceedings of the IJCNN '94*, pages 55–60. IEEE, 1994.

[8] R. Tibshirani. A comparison of some error estimates for neural network models. *Neural Computation*, 8:152–163, 1996.

Statistical Mechanics of the Mixture of Experts

Kukjin Kang and Jong-Hoon Oh
Department of Physics
Pohang University of Science and Technology
Hyoja San 31, Pohang, Kyongbuk 790-784, Korea
E-mail: `kkj,jhoh@galaxy.postech.ac.kr`

Abstract

We study generalization capability of the mixture of experts learning from examples generated by another network with the same architecture. When the number of examples is smaller than a critical value, the network shows a symmetric phase where the role of the experts is not specialized. Upon crossing the critical point, the system undergoes a continuous phase transition to a symmetry breaking phase where the gating network partitions the input space effectively and each expert is assigned to an appropriate subspace. We also find that the mixture of experts with multiple level of hierarchy shows multiple phase transitions.

1 Introduction

Recently there has been considerable interest among neural network community in techniques that integrate the collective predictions of a set of networks[1, 2, 3, 4]. The mixture of experts [1, 2] is a well known example which implements the philosophy of divide-and-conquer elegantly. Whereas this model are gaining more popularity in various applications, there have been little efforts to evaluate generalization capability of these modular approaches theoretically. Here we present the first analytic study of generalization in the mixture of experts from the statistical physics perspective. Use of statistical mechanics formulation have been focused on the study of feedforward neural network architectures close to the multilayer perceptron[5, 6], together with the VC theory[8]. We expect that the statistical mechanics approach can also be effectively used to evaluate more advanced architectures including mixture models.

In this letter we study generalization in the mixture of experts[1] and its variety with two-level hierarchy[2]. The network is trained by examples given by a teacher network with the same architecture. We find an interesting phase transition driven by symmetry breaking among the experts. This phase transition is closely related to the 'division-and-conquer' mechanism which this mixture model was originally designed to accomplish.

2 Statistical Mechanics Formulation for the Mixture of Experts

The mixture of experts[2] is a tree consisted of expert networks and gating networks which assign weights to the outputs of the experts. The expert networks sit at the leaves of the tree and the gating networks sit at its branching points of the tree. For the sake of simplicity, we consider a network with one gating network and two experts. Each expert produces its output μ_j as a generalized linear function of the N dimensional input $\mathbf{x}$:

$$\mu_j = f(\mathbf{W}_j \cdot \mathbf{x}), \qquad j = 1, 2, \tag{1}$$

where $\mathbf{W}_j$ is a weight vector of the j th expert with spherical constraint[5]. We consider a transfer function $f(x) = \text{sgn}(x)$ which produces binary outputs. The principle of divide-and-conquer is implemented by assigning each expert to a subspace of the input space with different local rules. A gating network makes partitions in the input space and assigns each expert a weighting factor:

$$g_j(\mathbf{x}) = \Theta(\mathbf{V}_j \cdot \mathbf{x}), \tag{2}$$

where the gating function $\Theta(x)$ is the Heaviside step function. For two experts, this gating function defines a sharp boundary between the two subspace which is perpendicular to the vector $\mathbf{V}_1 = -\mathbf{V}_2 = \mathbf{V}$, whereas the softmax function used in the original literature [2] yield a soft boundary. Now the weighted output from the mixture of expert is written:

$$\mu(\mathbf{V}, \mathbf{W}; \mathbf{x}) = \sum_{j=1}^{2} g_j(\mathbf{x}) \mu_j(\mathbf{x}). \tag{3}$$

The whole network as well as the individual experts generates binary outputs. Therefore, it can learn only dichotomy rules. The training examples are generated by a teacher with the same architecture as:

$$\sigma(\mathbf{x}_\mu) = \sum_{j=1}^{2} \Theta(\mathbf{V}_j^0 \cdot \mathbf{x}) \text{sgn}(\mathbf{W}_j^0 \cdot \mathbf{x}), \tag{4}$$

where V_j^0 and W_j^0 are the weights of the jth gating network and the expert of the teacher.

The learning of the mixture of experts is usually interpreted probabilistically, hence the learning algorithm is considered as a maximum likelihood estimation. Learning algorithms originated from statistical methods such as the EM algorithm are often used. Here we consider Gibbs algorithm with noise level T $(= 1/\beta)$ that leads to a Gibbs distribution of the weights after a long time:

$$P(\mathbf{V}, \mathbf{W}_j) = \frac{1}{Z} e^{-\beta E(\mathbf{V}, \mathbf{W}_j)}, \tag{5}$$

where $Z = \int d\mathbf{V} d\mathbf{W} \exp(-\beta E(\mathbf{V}, \mathbf{W}_j))$ is the partition function. Training both the experts and the gating network is necessary for a good generalization performance. The energy E of the system is defined as a sum of errors over P examples:

$$E(\mathbf{V}, \mathbf{W}_j) = \sum_{l=1}^{P} \epsilon(\mathbf{V}, \mathbf{W}_j; \mathbf{x}^l), \tag{6}$$

$$\epsilon(\mathbf{V}, \mathbf{W}_j; \mathbf{x}^l) = \Theta(-\mu(\mathbf{V}, \mathbf{W}_j; \mathbf{x}^l)\sigma(\mathbf{V}^0, \mathbf{W}_j^0; \mathbf{x}^l)). \tag{7}$$

The performance of the network is measured by the generalization function $\epsilon(\mathbf{V}, \mathbf{W}_j) = \int d\mathbf{x}\, \epsilon(\mathbf{V}, \mathbf{W}_j; \mathbf{x})$, where $\int d\mathbf{x}$ represents an average over the whole input space. The generalization error ϵ_g is defined by $\epsilon_g = \langle\!\langle \langle \epsilon(\mathbf{W}) \rangle_T \rangle\!\rangle$ where $\langle\!\langle \cdots \rangle\!\rangle$ denotes the quenched average over the examples and $\langle \cdots \rangle_T$ denotes the thermal average over the probability distribution of Eq. (5).

Since the replica calculation turns out to be intractable, we use the annealed approximation:

$$\langle\!\langle \log Z \rangle\!\rangle \simeq \log \langle\!\langle Z \rangle\!\rangle . \tag{8}$$

The annealed approximation is exact only in the high temperature limit, but it is known that the approximation usually gives qualitatively good results for the case of learning realizable rules[5, 6].

3 Generalization Curve and the Phase Transition

The generalization function $\epsilon(\mathbf{V}, \mathbf{W}_j)$ is can be written as a function of overlaps between the weight vectors of the teacher and the student:

$$\epsilon(\mathbf{V}, \mathbf{W}_j) = \sum_{i=1}^{2} \sum_{j=1}^{2} P_{ij} \epsilon_{ij} \tag{9}$$

where

$$P_{ij} = \frac{1}{2}\left(1 - \frac{1}{\pi}\cos^{-1} R_{ij}^V\right) \tag{10}$$

$$\epsilon_{ij} = \frac{1}{\pi}\cos^{-1} R_{ij}, \tag{11}$$

and

$$R_{ij}^V = \frac{1}{N}\mathbf{V}_i \cdot \mathbf{V}_j^0, \qquad (12)$$

$$R_{ij} = \frac{1}{N}\mathbf{W}_i \cdot \mathbf{W}_j^0. \qquad (13)$$

is the overlap order parameters. Here, P_{ij} is a probability that the i th expert of the student learns from examples generated by the j th expert of the teacher. It is a volume fraction in the input space where $\mathbf{V}_i \cdot \mathbf{x}$ and $\mathbf{V}_j^0 \cdot \mathbf{x}$ are both positive. For that particular examples, the ith expert of the student gives wrong answer with probability ϵ_{ij} with respect to the j th expert of the teacher. We assume that the weight vectors of the teacher, $\mathbf{V}_0, \mathbf{W}_1^0$ and $\mathbf{W}_2^0$, are orthogonal to each other, then the overlap order parameters other than the ones shown above vanish. We use the symmetry properties of the network such as $R_V = R_{11}^V = R_{22}^V = -R_{12}^V$, $R = R_{11} = R_{22}$, and $r = R_{12} = R_{21}$.

The free energy also can be written as a function of three order parameters R_V, R, and r. Now we consider a thermodynamic limit where the dimension of the input space N and the number of examples P goes to infinity, keeping the ratio $\alpha = P/N$ finite. By minimizing the free energy with respect to the order parameters, we find the most probable values of the order parameters as well as the generalization error.

Fig 1.(a) plots the overlap order parameters R_V, R and r versus α at temperature $T = 5$. Examining the plot, we find an interesting phase transition driven by symmetry breaking among the experts. Below the phase transition point $\alpha_c = 51.5$, the overlap between the gating networks of the teacher and the student is zero ($R_V = 0$) and the overlaps between the experts are symmetric ($R = r$). In the symmetric phase, the gating network does not have enough examples to learn proper partitioning, so its performance is not much better than a random partitioning. Consequently each expert of the student can not specialize for the subspaces with a particular local rule given by an expert of the teacher. Each expert has to learn multiple linear rules with linear structure, which leads to a poor generalization performance. Unless more than a critical amount of examples is provided, the divide-and-conquer strategy does not work.

Upon crossing the critical point α_c, the system undergoes a continuous phase transition to the symmetry breaking phase. The order parameter R_V, related to the goodness of partition, begins to increase abruptly and approaches 1 with increasing α. The gating network now provides a better partition which is close to that of the teacher. The plot of order parameter R and r, which is overlap between experts of teacher and student, branches at α_c and approaches 1 and 0 respectively. It means that each expert specializes its role by making appropriate pair with a particular expert of the teacher. Fig. 1(b) plots the generalization curve (ϵ_g versus α) in the same scale. Though the generalization curve is continuous, the slope of the curve changes discontinuously at the transition point so that the generalization curve has

Statistical Mechanics of the Mixture of Experts

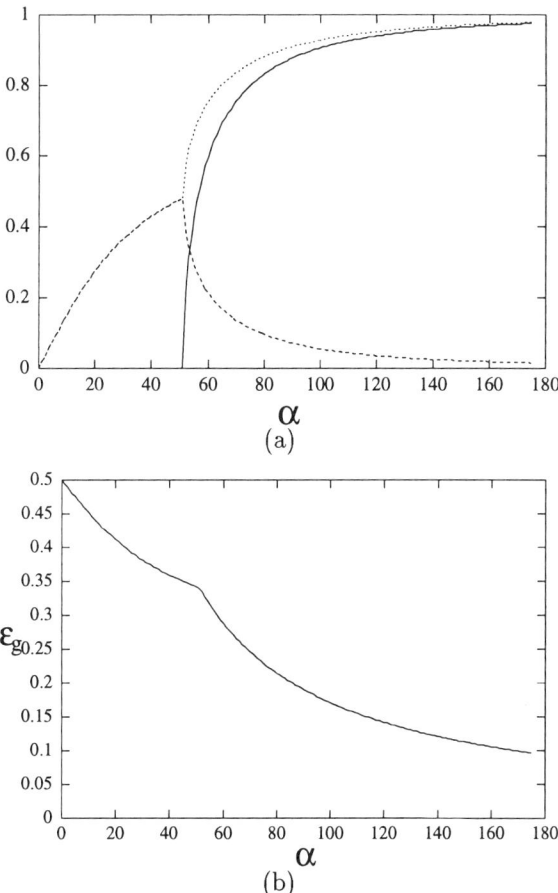

Figure 1: (a) The overlap order parameters R_V, R, r versus α at $T = 5$. For $\alpha < \alpha_c = 51.5$, we find $R_V = 0$ (solid line that follows x axis), and $R = r$ (dashed line). At the transition point, R_V begins to increase abruptly, R (dotted line) and r (dashed line) branches, which approach 1 and 0 respectively. (b) The generalization curve (ϵ_g versus α) for the mixture of experts in the same scale. A cusp at the transition point α_c is shown.

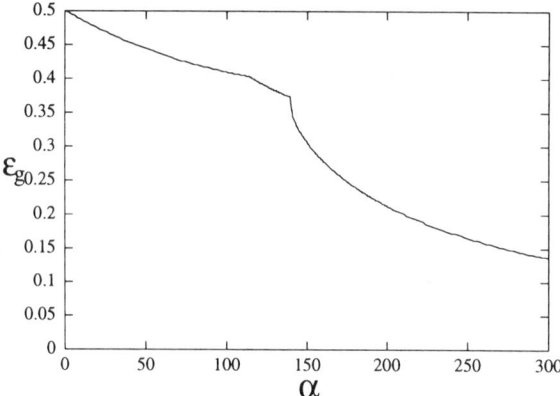

Figure 2: A typical generalization error curve for HME network with continuous weight. $T = 5$.

a cusp. The asymptotic behavior of ϵ_g at large α is given by:

$$\epsilon \simeq \frac{3}{1 - e^{-\beta}} \frac{1}{\alpha}, \qquad (14)$$

where the $1/\alpha$ decay is often observed in learning of other feedforward networks.

4 The Mixture of Experts with Two-Level Hierarchy

We also study generalization in the hierarchical mixture of experts [2]. Consider a two-level hierarchical mixture of experts consisted of three gating networks and four experts. At the top level the tree is divided into two branch, and they are in turn divided into two branches at the lower level. The experts sit at the four leaves of the tree, and the three gating networks sit at the top and lower-level branching points. The network also learns from the training examples drawn from a teacher network with the same architecture.

FIG 2. (b) shows corresponding learning curve which has two cusps related to the phase transitions. For $\alpha < \alpha_{c1}$, the system is in the fully symmetric phase. The gating networks do not provide correct partition for the experts at both levels of hierarchy and the experts cannot specialize at all. All the overlaps with the weights of the teacher experts have the same value. The first phase transition at the smaller α_{c1} is related to the symmetry breaking by the top-level gating network. For $\alpha_{c1} < \alpha < \alpha_{c2}$, the top-level gating network partition the input space into two parts, but the lower-level gating network is not functioning properly. The overlap between the gating networks at the lower level of the tree and that of the teacher is still zero. The experts partially specialize into two groups. Specialization among the same group is not accomplished yet. The overlap order parameter R_{ij} can have two distinct values. The bigger one is the overlap with the two experts of the teacher for which the group is specializing, and the smaller is with the experts of the teacher which belong to the other group. At the second transition point α_{c2}, the symmetry related to the lower-level hierarchy breaks. For $\alpha > \alpha_{c2}$, all the gating networks work properly and the input space is divided into four. Each expert makes appropriate pair with an expert of the teacher. Now the overlap order parameters can have three distinct values. The largest is the overlap with matching expert of teacher. The next largest is the overlap with the neighboring teacher expert in the tree hierarchy. The smallest is with the experts of the other group. The two phase transition result in the two cusps of the learning curve.

5 Conclusion

Whereas the phase transition of the mixture of experts can be interpreted as a symmetry breaking phenomenon which is similar to the one already observed in the committee machine and the multi-layer-perceptron[6, 7], the transition is novel in that it is continuous. This means that symmetry breaking is easier for the mixture of experts than in the multi-layer perceptron. This can be a big advantage in learning of highly nonlinear rules as we do not have to worry about the existence of local minima. We find that the hierarchical mixture of experts can have multiple phase transitions which are related to symmetry breaking at different levels. Note that symmetry breaking comes first from the higher-level branch, which is desirable property of the model.

We thank M. I. Jordan, L. K. Saul, H. Sompolinsky, H. S. Seung, H. Yoon and C. Kwon for useful discussions and comments. This work was partially supported by the Basic Science Special Program of the POSTECH Basic Science Research Institute.

References

[1] R. A. Jacobs, M. I Jordan, S. J. Nolwan, and G. E. Hinton, Neural Computation **3**, 79 (1991).

[2] M. I. Jordan, and R. A. Jacobs, Neural Computation **6**, 181 (1994).

[3] M.P. Perrone and L. N. Cooper, Neural Networks for Speech and Image Processing, R. J. Mammone. Ed., Chapman-Hill, London, 1993.

[4] D. Wolpert, Neural Networks, **5**, 241 (1992).

[5] H. S. Seung, H. Sompolinsky, and N. Tishby, Phys. Rev. A **45**, 6056 (1992).

[6] K. Kang, J.-H. Oh, C. Kwon and Y. Park, Phys. Rev. E **48**, 4805 (1993); K. Kang, J.-H. Oh, C. Kwon and Y. Park, Phys. Rev. E **54**, 1816 (1996).

[7] E. Baum and D. Haussler, Neural Computation **1**, 151 (1989).

MLP can provably generalise much better than VC-bounds indicate.

A. Kowalczyk and H. Ferrá
Telstra Research Laboratories
770 Blackburn Road, Clayton, Vic. 3168, Australia
({a.kowalczyk, h.ferra}@trl.oz.au)

Abstract

Results of a study of the worst case learning curves for a particular class of probability distribution on input space to MLP with hard threshold hidden units are presented. It is shown in particular, that in the thermodynamic limit for scaling by the number of connections to the first hidden layer, although the true learning curve behaves as $\approx \alpha^{-1}$ for $\alpha \approx 1$, its VC-dimension based bound is trivial ($\equiv 1$) and its VC-entropy bound is trivial for $\alpha \leq 6.2$. It is also shown that bounds following the true learning curve can be derived from a formalism based on the density of error patterns.

1 Introduction

The VC-formalism and its extensions link the generalisation capabilities of a binary valued neural network with its *counting function*[1], e.g. via upper bounds implied by VC-dimension or VC-entropy on this function [17, 18]. For linear perceptrons the counting function is constant for almost every selection of a fixed number of input samples [2], and essentially equal to its upper bound determined by VC-dimension and Sauer's Lemma. However, in the case for *multilayer perceptrons* (MLP) the counting function depends essentially on the selected input samples. For instance, it has been shown recently that for MLP with sigmoidal units although the largest number of input samples which can be shattered, i.e. VC-dimension, equals $\Omega(w^2)$ [6], there is always a non-zero probability of finding a $(2w+2)$-element input sample which cannot be shattered, where w is the number of weights in the network [16]. In the case of MLP using Heaviside rather than sigmoidal activations (McCulloch-Pitts neurons), a similar claim can be made: VC-dimension is $\Omega(w_1 log_2 \mathcal{H}_1)$ [13, 15],

---
[1]Known also as *the partition function* in computational learning theory.

where w_1 is the number of weights to the first hidden layer of $\mathcal{H}_1$ units, but there is a non-zero probability of finding a sample of size $w_1 + 2$ which cannot be shattered [7, 8]. The results on these "hard to shatter samples" for the two MLP types differ significantly in terms of techniques used for derivation. For the sigmoidal case the result is "existential" (based on recent advances in "model theory") while in the Heaviside case the proofs are constructive, defining a class of probability distributions from which "hard to shatter" samples can be drawn randomly; the results in this case are also more explicit in that a form for the counting function may be given [7, 8].

Can the existence of such hard to shatter samples be essential for generalisation capabilities of MLP? Can they be an essential factor for improvement of theoretical models of generalisation? In this paper we show that at least for the McCulloch-Pitts case with specific (continuous) probability distributions on the input space the answer is "yes". We estimate "directly" the real learning curve in this case and show that its bounds based on VC-dimension or VC-entropy are loose at low learning sample regimes (for training samples having less than $12 \times w_1$ examples) even for the linear perceptron. We also show that a modification to the VC-formalism given in [9, 10] provides a significantly better bound. This latter part is a more rigorous and formal extension and re-interpretation of some results in [11, 12]. All the results are presented in the thermodynamic limit, i.e. for MLP with $w_1 \to \infty$ and training sample size increasing proportionally, which simplifies their mathematical form.

2 Overview of the formalism

On a sample space X we consider a class H of binary functions $h : X \to \{0,1\}$ which we shall call *a hypothesis space*. Further we assume that there are given a probability distribution μ on X and a *target concept* $t : X \to \{0,1\}$. The quadruple $\mathcal{L} = (X, \mu, H, t)$ will be called *a learning system*.

In the usual way, with each hypothesis $h \in H$ we associate *the generalization error* $\epsilon_h \stackrel{def}{=} \mathbf{E}_X[|t(x) - h(x)|]$ and *the training error* $\epsilon_{h,\vec{x}} \stackrel{def}{=} \frac{1}{m}\sum_{i=1}^{m}|t(x_i) - h(x_i)|$ for any *training m-sample* $\vec{x} = (x_1, ..., x_m) \in X^m$.

Given a *learning threshold* $0 \leq \lambda \leq 1$, let us introduce an auxiliary random variable $\epsilon_\lambda^{\max}(\vec{x}) \stackrel{def}{=} \max\{\epsilon_h \; ; \; h \in H \; \& \; \epsilon_{h,\vec{x}} \leq \lambda\}$ for $\vec{x} \in X^m$, giving the worst generalization error of all hypotheses with training error $\leq \lambda$ on the m-sample $\vec{x} \in X^m$.[2] The basic objects of interest in this paper are *the learning curve*[3] defined as

$$\epsilon_\lambda^{wc}(m) \stackrel{def}{=} \mathbf{E}_{X^m}[\epsilon_\lambda^{\max}(\vec{x})].$$

2.1 Thermodynamic limit

Now we introduce the thermodynamic limit of the learning curve. The underlying idea of such asymptotic analysis is to capture the essential features of learning

---

[2]In this paper $\max(S)$, where $S \subset \mathbf{R}$, denotes the maximal element in the closure of S, or ∞ if no such element exists. Similarly, we understand $\min(S)$.

[3]Note that our learning curve is determined by the worst generalisation error of acceptable hypotheses and in this respect differs from "average generalisation error" learning curves considered elsewhere, e.g. [3, 5].

systems of very large size. Mathematically it turns out that in the thermodynamic limit the functional forms of learning curves simplify significantly and analytic characterizations of these are possible.

We are given a sequence of learning systems, or shortly, $\mathcal{L}_N = (X_N, \mu_N, H_N, t_N)$, $N = 1, 2, ...$ and *a scaling* $N \mapsto \tau_N \in \mathbf{R}^+$, with the property $\tau_N \to \infty$; the scaling can be thought of as a measure of the size (complexity) of a learning system, e.g. VC-dimension of H_N. *The thermodynamic limit* of *scaled learning curves* is defined for $\alpha > 0$ as follows [4]

$$\epsilon^{wc}_{\lambda\infty}(\alpha) \stackrel{def}{=} \limsup_{N \to \infty} \epsilon^{wc}_{\lambda,N}(\lfloor \alpha \tau_N \rfloor), \qquad (1)$$

Here, and below, the additional subscript N refers to the N-th learning system.

2.2 Error pattern density formalism

This subsection briefly presents a thermodynamic version of a modified VC formalism discussed previously in [9]; more details and proofs can be found in [10]. The main innovation of this approach comes from splitting error patterns into error shells and using estimates on the size of these error shells rather than the total number of error patterns. We shall see on examples discussed in the following section that this improves results significantly.

The space $\{0,1\}^m$ of all binary m-vectors naturally splits into $m+1$ *error pattern shells* $\mathcal{E}^m_i$, $i = 0, 1, ..., m$, with the i-th shell composed of all vectors with exactly i entries equal to 1. For each $h \in H$ and $\vec{x} = (x_1, ..., x_m) \in X^m$, let $\vec{v}_h(\vec{x}) \in \{0,1\}^m$ denote a vector (*error pattern*) having 1 in the j-th position if and only if $h(x_j) \neq t(x_j)$. As the i-th error shell has $\binom{m}{i}$ elements, *the average error pattern density* falling into this error shell is

$$\Delta^m_i \stackrel{def}{=} \binom{m}{i}^{-1} \mathbf{E}_{X^m}[\#(\{\vec{v}_h(\vec{x}) ; h \in H\} \cap \mathcal{E}^m_i)] \qquad (i = 0, 1, ..., m), \qquad (2)$$

where $\#$ denotes the cardinality of a set[5].

Theorem 1 *Given a sequence of learning systems* $\mathcal{L}_N = (X_N, \mu_N, H_N, t_N)$, *a scaling* τ_N *and a function* $\varphi : \mathbf{R}^+ \times (0,1) \to \mathbf{R}^+$ *such that*

$$\ln\left(\Delta^m_{i,N}\right) \leq -\tau_N \varphi\left(\frac{m}{\tau_N}, \frac{i}{m}\right) + o(\tau_N), \qquad (3)$$

for all $m, N = 1, 2, ..., 0 \leq i \leq m$.

Then

$$\epsilon^{wc}_{\lambda\infty}(\alpha) \leq \epsilon_{\lambda\beta}(\alpha), \qquad (4)$$

---

[4]We recall that $\lfloor x \rfloor$ denotes the largest integer $\leq x$ and $\limsup_{N \to \infty} x_N$ is defined as $\lim_{N \to \infty}$ of the monotonic sequence $N \mapsto \max\{x_1, x_2, ..., x_N\}$. Note that in contrast to the ordinary limit, lim sup always exists.

[5]Note the difference to the concept of error shells used in [4] which are partitions of the finite hypothesis space H according to the generalisation error values. Both formalisms are related though, and the central result in [4], Theorem 4, can be derived from our Theorem 1 below.

for any $0 \leq \lambda \leq 1$ and $\alpha, \beta > 0$, where

$$\epsilon_{\lambda\beta}(\alpha) \stackrel{def}{=} \max\left\{ \epsilon \in (0,1) \; ; \; \exists_{\substack{0 \leq y \leq \lambda \\ \epsilon \leq x \leq 1}} \alpha(\mathcal{H}(y) + \beta\mathcal{H}(x)) - \varphi\left(\alpha + \alpha\beta, \frac{y + \beta x}{1 + \beta}\right) \geq 0 \right\}$$

and $\mathcal{H}(y) \stackrel{def}{=} -y \ln y - (1-y)\ln(1-y)$ denotes the entropy function.

3 Main results : applications of the formalism

3.1 VC-bounds

We consider a learning sequence $\mathcal{L}_N = (X_N, \mu_N, H_N, t_N)$, $t_N \in H_N$ (realisable case) and the scaling of this sequence by VC-dimension [17], i.e. we assume $\tau_N = d_{VC}(H_N) \to \infty$. The following bounds for the N-th learning system can be derived for $\lambda = 0$ (consistent learning case) [1, 17]:

$$\epsilon_{0,N}^{wc}(m) \leq \int_0^1 \min\left(1, 2^{2-m\epsilon/2}\left(\frac{2em}{d_{VC}(H_N)}\right)^{d_{VC}(H_N)}\right) d\epsilon. \quad (5)$$

In the thermodynamic limit, i.e. as $N \to \infty$, we get for any $\alpha > 1/e$

$$\epsilon_{0\infty}^{wc}(\alpha) \leq \min\left(1, \frac{2\log_2(2e\alpha)}{\alpha}\right), \quad (6)$$

Note that this bound is independent of probability distributions μ_N.

3.2 Piecewise constant functions

Let $PC(d)$ denote the class of piecewise constant binary functions on the unit segment $[0,1)$ with up to $d \geq 0$ discontinuities and with their values defined as 1 at all these discontinuity points. We consider here the learning sequence $\mathcal{L}_N = ([0,1), \mu_N, PC(d_N), t_N)$ where μ_N is any continuous probability distributions on $[0,1)$, d_N is a monotonic sequence of positive integers diverging to ∞ and targets $t_N \in PC(d_{t_N})$ are such that the limit $\delta_t \stackrel{def}{=} \lim_{N\to\infty} \frac{d_N}{d_{t_N}}$ exists. (Without loss of generality we can assume that all μ_N are the uniform distribution on $[0,1)$.)

For this learning sequence the following can be established.

Claim 1. The following function defined for $\alpha > 1$ and $0 \leq x \leq 1$ as

$$\varphi(\alpha, x) \stackrel{def}{=} -\alpha(1-x)\mathcal{H}\left(\frac{1+\delta_t}{2\alpha(1-x)}\right) - \alpha x \mathcal{H}\left(\frac{1+\delta_t}{2\alpha x}\right) + \alpha \mathcal{H}(x) \quad \text{for } 2\alpha x(1-x) > 1,$$

and as 0, otherwise, satisfies assumption (3) with respect to the scaling $\tau_N \stackrel{def}{=} d_N$.

Claim 2. The following two sided bound on the learning curve holds:

$$\frac{1}{2\alpha^-}(1 + \ln(2\alpha^-)) \leq \epsilon_{\lambda\infty}^{wc}(\alpha) \leq \frac{1}{2\alpha^+}(1 + \ln(2\alpha^+)) \quad (7)$$

for $\alpha > 1$, $0 \leq \lambda \leq 1$ and $0 \leq \delta_t \leq \alpha\lambda/2$, where $\alpha^- \stackrel{def}{=} \frac{\alpha}{1-\delta_t+\alpha\lambda/2}$, $\alpha^+ \stackrel{def}{=} \frac{\alpha}{1+\delta_t+\alpha\lambda}$.

We outline the main steps of proof of these two claims now.

For Claim 1 we start with a combinatorial argument establishing that in the particular case of constant target

$$\Delta_{i,N}^m = \begin{cases} \binom{m-1}{i-1}^{-1} \sum_{j=0}^{d_N/2} \binom{m-i-1}{j-1}\binom{i-1}{j} & \text{for } d + d_t < \min(2i, 2(m-i)), \\ 1 & \text{otherwise.} \end{cases}$$

Next we observe that that the above sum equals

$$e^{o(d_N)} \times \max_{0 \leq j \leq d_N/2} (\binom{m-i}{j}\binom{i}{j}) = e^{\max_{0 \leq x \leq i/m} \alpha(1-x)\mathcal{H}\left(\frac{1}{2\alpha(1-x)}\right) + \alpha x \mathcal{H}\left(\frac{1}{2\alpha x}\right) + o(d_N)}.$$

This easily gives Claim 1 for constant target ($\delta_t = 0$). Now we observe that this particular case gives an upper bound for the general case (of non-constant target) if we use the "effective" number of discontinuities $d_N + d_{t_N}$ instead of d_N.

For Claim 2 we start with the estimate [12, 11]

$$\frac{\lfloor d_N/2 \rfloor}{m+1}\left(1 + \sum_{j=\lfloor d_N/2 \rfloor+1}^{m+1} \frac{1}{j}\right) \leq \epsilon_0^{wc}(m) \leq \frac{\lfloor d_N/2 \rfloor + 1}{m+1}\left(1 + \sum_{j=\lfloor d_N/2 \rfloor+2}^{m+1} \frac{1}{j}\right).$$

derived from the Mauldon result [14] for the constant target $t_N = \text{const}$, $m \geq d_N$. This implies immediately the expression

$$\epsilon_{0\infty}^{wc}(\alpha) = \frac{1}{2\alpha}\left(1 + \ln(2\alpha)\right). \tag{8}$$

for the constant target, which extends to the estimate (7) with a straightforward lower and upper bound on the "effective" number of discontinuities in the case of a non-constant target.

3.3 Link to multilayer perceptron

Let $MLP^n(w_1)$ denote the class of function from $\mathbf{R}^n$ to $\{0,1\}$ which can be implemented by a multilayer perceptron (feedforward neural network) with ≥ 1 number of hidden layers, with w_1 connections to the first hidden layer and the first hidden layer composed entirely of fully connected, linear threshold logic units (i.e. units able to implement any mapping of the form $(x_1, .., x_n) \mapsto \theta(a_0 + \sum_{i=1}^n a_i x_i)$ for $a_i \in \mathbf{R}$). It can be shown from the properties of Vandermonde determinant (c.f. [7, 8]) that if $f : [0, 1) \to \mathbf{R}^n$ is a mapping with coordinates composed of linearly independent polynomials (generic situation) of degree $\leq n$, then

$$PC(w_1) = f^* MLP^n(w_1) \stackrel{def}{=} \{h \circ f \,;\, h \in MLP^n(w_1)\}. \tag{9}$$

This implies immediately that all results for learning the class of PC functions in Section 5.2 are applicable (with obvious modifications) to this class of multilayer perceptrons with probability distribution concentrated on the 1-dimensional curves of the form $f([0, 1))$ with f as above.

However, we can go a step further. We can extend such a distribution to a continuous distribution on $\mathbf{R}^n$ with support "sufficiently close" to the curve $f([0, 1))$,

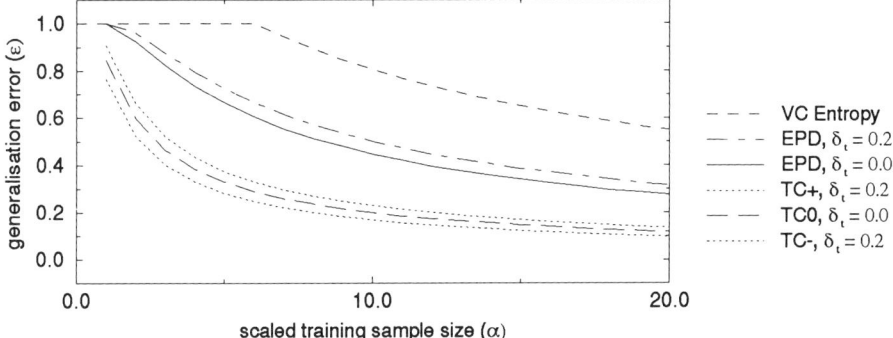

Figure 1: Plots of different estimates for thermodynamic limit of learning curves for the sequence of multilayer perceptrons as in Claim 3 for consistent learning ($\lambda = 0$). Estimates on true learning curve from (7) are for $\delta_t = 0$ ('TC0') and $\delta_t = 0.2$ ('TC+' and 'TC−' for the upper and lower bound, respectively). Two upper bounds of the form (4) from the modified VC-formalism for φ as in Claim 1 and $\beta = 1$ are plotted for $\delta_t = 0.0$ and $\delta_t = 0.2$ (marked EPD). For comparison, we plot also the bound (10) based on the VC-entropy; VC bound (5) being trivial for this scaling, $\equiv 1$, c.f. Corollary 2, is not shown.

with changes to the error pattern densities $\Delta_{i,N}^m$, the learning curves, etc., as small as desired. This observation implies the following result:

Claim 3 *For any sequence of multilayer perceptrons, $MLP^{n_N}(w_{1N})$, $w_{1N} \to \infty$, there exists a sequence of continuous probability distributions μ_N on $\mathbf{R}^{n_N}$ with properties as follows. For any sequence of targets $t_N \in MLP^{n_N}(w_{1t_N})$, both Claim 1 and Claim 2 of Section 3.2 hold for the learning sequence $\left(\mathbf{R}^{n_N}, \mu_N, MLP^{n_N}(w_{1N}), t_N\right)$ with scaling $\tau_N \stackrel{def}{=} n_{1N}$ and $\delta_t = \lim_{N \to \infty} w_{1t_N}/w_{1N}$. In particular bound (4) on the learning curve holds for φ as in Claim 1.*

Corollary 2 *If additionally the number of units in first hidden layer $\mathcal{H}_{1N} \to \infty$, then the thermodynamic limit of VC-bound (5) with respect to the scaling $\tau_N = w_{1N}$ is trivial, i.e. $= 1$ for all $\alpha > 0$.*

Proof. The bound (5) is trivial for $m \leq 12 d_N$, where $d_N \stackrel{def}{=} d_{VC}(MLP^{n_N}(w_{1t_N}))$. As $d_N = \Omega(w_{1N} \log_2(\mathcal{H}_{1N}))$ [13, 15] for any *continuous* probability on the input space, this bound is trivial for any $\alpha = \frac{m}{w_{1N}} \leq 12 \frac{d_N}{w_{1N}} \to \infty$ if $N \to \infty$. □

There is a possibility that VC dimension based bounds are applicable but fail to capture the true behavior because of their independence from the distribution. One option to remedy the situation is to try a distribution-specific estimate such as VC entropy (i.e. the expectation of the logarithm of the counting function $\Pi_N(x_1, ..., x_m)$ which is the number of dichotomies realised by the perceptron for the m-tuple of input points [18]). However, in our case, $\Pi_N(x_1, ..., x_m)$ has the lower bound $2 \sum_{i=0}^{\min(w_{1N}/2, m-1)} \binom{m}{i}$, for $x_1, ..., x_m$ in general position, which is virtually the expression from Sauer's lemma with VC-dimension replaced by $w_{1N}/2$. Thus using

VC entropy instead of VC dimension (and Sauer's Lemma) we cannot hope for a better result than bounds of the form (5) with $w_{1N}/2$ replacing VC-dimension resulting in the bound

$$\epsilon_0^{wc}(\alpha) \leq \min(1, \alpha^{-1}\log_2(4e\alpha)) \qquad (\alpha > 1/e) \tag{10}$$

in the thermodynamic limit with respect to the scaling $\tau_N = w_{1N}$. (Note that more "optimistic" VC entropy based bounds can be obtained if prior distribution on hypothesis space is given and taken into account [3].)

The plots of learning curves are shown in Figure 1.

Acknowledgement. The permission of Director of Telstra Research Laboratories to publish this paper is gratefully acknowledged.

References

[1] A. Blumer, A. Ehrenfeucht, D. Haussler, and M.K. Warmuth. Learnability and the Vapnik-Chervonenkis dimensions. *Journal of the ACM*, **36**:929–965, (Oct. 1989).

[2] T.M. Cover. Geometrical and statistical properties of linear inequalities with applications to pattern recognition. *IEEE Trans. Elec. Comp.*, **EC-14**:326-334, 1965.

[3] D. Hausler, M. Kearns, and R. Shapire. Bounds on the Sample Complexity of Bayesian Learning Using Information Theory and VC Dimension. *Machine Learning*, **14**:83–113, (1994).

[4] D. Haussler, M. Kearns, H.S. Seung, and N. Tishby. Rigorous learning curve bounds from statistical mechanics. In *Proc. COLT'94*, pages 76–87, 1994.

[5] S.B. Holden and M. Niranjan. On the Practical Applicability of VC Dimension Bounds. *Neural Computation*, **7**:1265–1288, 1995).

[6] P. Koiran and E.D. Sontag. Neural networks with quadratic VC-dimension. In *Proc. NIPS 8*, pages 197–203, The MIT Press, Cambridge, Ma., 1996. .

[7] A. Kowalczyk. Counting function theorem for multi-layer networks. In *Proc. NIPS 6*, pages 375–382. Morgan Kaufman Publishers, Inc., 1994.

[8] A. Kowalczyk. Estimates of storage capacity of multi-layer perceptron with threshold logic hidden units. Neural networks, to appear.

[9] A. Kowalczyk and H. Ferra. Generalisation in feedforward networks. Proc. NIPS 6, pages 215–222, The MIT Press, Cambridge, Ma., 1994.

[10] A. Kowalczyk. An asymptotic version of EPD-bounds on generalisation in learning systems. 1996. Preprint.

[11] A. Kowalczyk, J. Szymanski, and R.C. Williamson. Learning curves from a modified VC-formalism: a case study. In *Proc. of ICNN'95* , 2939–2943, IEEE, 1995.

[12] A. Kowalczyk, J. Szymański, P.L. Bartlett, and R.C. Williamson. Examples of learning curves from a modified VC-formalism. Proc. NIPS 8, pages 344–350, The MIT Press, 1996.

[13] W. Maas. Neural Nets with superlinear VC-dimesnion. *Neural Computation*, **6**:877–884, 1994.

[14] J.G. Mauldon. Random division of an interval. *Proc. Cambridge Phil. Soc.*, **47**:331–336, 1951.

[15] A. Sakurai. Tighter bounds of the VC-dimension of three-layer networks. In *Proc. of the 1993 World Congress on Neural Networks*, 1993.

[16] E. Sontag. Shattering all sets of k points in "general position" requires $(k-1)/2$ parameters. Report 96-01, Rutgers Center for Systems and Control, 1996.

[17] V. Vapnik. *Estimation of Dependences Based on Empirical Data*. Springer-Verlag, 1982.

[18] V. Vapnik. *The Nature of Statistical Learning Theory*. Springer-Verlag, 1995.

Radial Basis Function Networks and Complexity Regularization in Function Learning

Adam Krzyżak
Department of Computer Science
Concordia University
Montreal, Canada
krzyzak@cs.concordia.ca

Tamás Linder
Dept. of Math. & Comp. Sci.
Technical University of Budapest
Budapest, Hungary
linder@inf.bme.hu

Abstract

In this paper we apply the method of complexity regularization to derive estimation bounds for nonlinear function estimation using a single hidden layer radial basis function network. Our approach differs from the previous complexity regularization neural network function learning schemes in that we operate with random covering numbers and l_1 metric entropy, making it possible to consider much broader families of activation functions, namely functions of bounded variation. Some constraints previously imposed on the network parameters are also eliminated this way. The network is trained by means of complexity regularization involving empirical risk minimization. Bounds on the expected risk in terms of the sample size are obtained for a large class of loss functions. Rates of convergence to the optimal loss are also derived.

1 INTRODUCTION

Artificial neural networks have been found effective in learning input-output mappings from noisy examples. In this learning problem an unknown target function is to be inferred from a set of independent observations drawn according to some unknown probability distribution from the input-output space $\mathbb{R}^d \times \mathbb{R}$. Using this data set the learner tries to determine a function which fits the data in the sense of minimizing some given empirical loss function. The target function may or may not be in the class of functions which are realizable by the learner. In the case when the class of realizable functions consists of some class of artificial neural networks, the above problem has been extensively studied from different viewpoints.

In recent years a special class of artificial neural networks, the radial basis function (RBF) networks have received considerable attention. RBF networks have been shown to be the solution of the regularization problem in function estimation with certain standard smoothness functionals used as stabilizers (see [5], and the references therein). Universal convergence of RBF nets in function estimation and classification has been proven by Krzyżak et al. [6]. Convergence rates of RBF approximation schemes have been shown to be comparable with those for sigmoidal nets by Girosi and Anzellotti [4]. In a recent paper Niyogi and Girosi [9] studied the tradeoff between approximation and estimation errors and provided an extensive review of the problem.

In this paper we consider one hidden layer RBF networks. We look at the problem of choosing the size of the hidden layer as a function of the available training data by means of complexity regularization. Complexity regularization approach has been applied to model selection by Barron [1], [2] resulting in near optimal choice of sigmoidal network parameters. Our approach here differs from Barron's in that we are using l_1 metric entropy instead of the supremum norm. This allows us to consider a more general class of activation function, namely the functions of bounded variation, rather than a restricted class of activation functions satisfying a Lipschitz condition. For example, activations with jump discontinuities are allowed. In our complexity regularization approach we are able to choose the network parameters more freely, and no discretization of these parameters is required. For RBF regression estimation with squared error loss, we considerably improve the convergence rate result obtained by Niyogi and Girosi [9].

In Section 2 the problem is formulated and two results on the estimation error of complexity regularized RBF nets are presented: one for general loss functions (Theorem 1) and a sharpened version of the first one for the squared loss (Theorem 2). Approximation bounds are combined with the obtained estimation results in Section 3 yielding convergence rates for function learning with RBF nets.

2 PROBLEM FORMULATION

The task is to predict the value of a real random variable Y upon the observation of an $\mathbb{R}^d$ valued random vector X. The accuracy of the predictor $f : \mathbb{R}^d \to \mathbb{R}$ is measured by the expected risk

$$J(f) = \mathbf{E}L(f(X), Y),$$

where $L : \mathbb{R} \times \mathbb{R} \to \mathbb{R}^+$ is a nonnegative loss function. It will be assumed that there exists a minimizing predictor f^* such that

$$J(f^*) = \inf_f J(f).$$

A good predictor f_n is to be determined based on the data $(X_1, Y_1), \ldots, (X_n, Y_n)$ which are i.i.d. copies of (X, Y). The goal is to make the expected risk $\mathbf{E}J(f_n)$ as small as possible, while f_n is chosen from among a given class $\mathcal{F}$ of candidate functions.

In this paper the set of candidate functions $\mathcal{F}$ will be the set of single-layer feedforward neural networks with radial basis function activation units and we let $\mathcal{F} = \cup_{k=1}^{\infty} \mathcal{F}_k$, where $\mathcal{F}_k$ is the family of networks with k hidden nodes whose weight parameters satisfy certain constraints. In particular, for radial basis functions characterized by a kernel $K : \mathbb{R}^+ \to \mathbb{R}$, $\mathcal{F}_k$ is the family of networks

$$f(x) = \sum_{i=1}^{k} w_i K\left([x - c_i]^t A_i [x - c_i]\right) + w_0,$$

where $w_0, w_1 \ldots, w_k$ are real numbers called weights, $c_1, \ldots, c_k \in \mathbb{R}^d$, A_i are nonnegative definite $d \times d$ matrices, and x^t denotes the transpose of the column vector x.

The complexity regularization principle for the learning problem was introduced by Vapnik [10] and fully developed by Barron [1], [2] (see also Lugosi and Zeger [8]). It enables the learning algorithm to choose the candidate class $\mathcal{F}_k$ automatically, from which is picks

Radial Basis Function Networks and Complexity Regularization

the estimate function by minimizing the empirical error over the training data. Complexity regularization penalizes the large candidate classes, which are bound to have small approximation error, in favor of the smaller ones, thus balancing the estimation and approximation errors.

Let $\mathcal{F}$ be a subset of a space $\mathcal{X}$ of real functions over some set, and let ρ be a pseudometric on $\mathcal{X}$. For $\epsilon > 0$ the *covering number* $N(\epsilon, \mathcal{F}, \rho)$ is defined to be the minimal number of closed ϵ balls whose union cover $\mathcal{F}$. In other words, $N(\epsilon, \mathcal{F}, \rho)$ is the least integer such that there exist $f_1, \ldots, f_N$ with $N = N(\epsilon, \mathcal{F}, \rho)$ satisfying

$$\sup_{f \in \mathcal{F}} \min_{1 \le i \le N} \rho(f, f_i) \le \epsilon.$$

In our case, $\mathcal{F}$ is a family of real functions on $\mathbb{R}^m$, and for any two functions f and g, ρ is given by

$$\rho(f, g) = \frac{1}{n} \sum_{i=1}^{n} |f(z_i) - g(z_i)|,$$

where $z_1, \ldots, z_n$ are n given points in $\mathbb{R}^m$. In this case we will use the notation $N(\epsilon, \mathcal{F}, \rho) = N(\epsilon, \mathcal{F}, z_1^n)$, emphasizing the dependence of the metric ρ on $z_1^n = (z_1, \ldots, z_n)$. Let us define the families of functions $\mathcal{H}_k$, $k = 1, 2, \ldots$ by

$$\mathcal{H}_k = \{L(f(\cdot), \cdot) : f \in \mathcal{F}_k\}.$$

Thus each member of $\mathcal{H}_k$ maps $\mathbb{R}^{d+1}$ into $\mathbb{R}$. It will be assumed that for each k we are given a finite, almost sure uniform upper bound on the random covering numbers $N(\epsilon, \mathcal{H}_k, Z_1^n)$, where $Z_1^n = ((X_1, Y_1), \ldots, (X_n, Y_n))$. We may assume without loss of generality that $N(\epsilon, \mathcal{H}_k)$ is monotone decreasing in ϵ. Finally, assume that $L(f(X), Y)$ is uniformly almost surely bounded by a constant B, i.e.,

$$\mathbf{P}\{L(f(X), Y) \le B\} = 1, \quad f \in \mathcal{F}_k, \quad k = 1, 2, \ldots \tag{1}$$

The complexity penalty of the kth class for n training samples is a nonnegative number Δ_{kn} satisfying

$$\Delta_{kn} \ge \sqrt{128 B^2 \frac{\log N(\Delta_{kn}/8, \mathcal{H}_k) + c_k}{n}}, \tag{2}$$

where the nonnegative constants c_k satisfy $\sum_{k=1}^{\infty} e^{-c_k} \le 1$. Note that since $N(\epsilon, \mathcal{H}_k)$ is nonincreasing in ϵ, it is possible to choose such Δ_{kn} for all k and n. The resulting complexity penalty optimizes the upper bound on the estimation error in the proof of Theorem 1 below. We can now define our estimate. Let

$$f_{kn} = \arg\min_{f \in \mathcal{F}_k} J_n(f) = \arg\min_{f \in \mathcal{F}_k} \frac{1}{n} \sum_{i=1}^{n} L(f(X_i), Y_i),$$

that is, f_{kn} minimizes over $\mathcal{F}_k$ the empirical risk for n training samples. The penalized empirical risk is defined for each $f \in \mathcal{F}_k$ as

$$\widehat{J}_n(f) = J_n(f) + \Delta_{kn}.$$

The estimate f_n is then defined as the f_{kn} minimizing the penalized empirical risk over all classes:

$$f_n = \arg\min_{f_{kn}: k \ge 1} \widehat{J}_n(f_{kn}). \tag{3}$$

We have the following theorem for the expected estimation error of the above complexity regularization scheme.

Theorem 1 *For any n and k the complexity regularization estimate* (3) *satisfies*

$$\mathbf{E}J(f_n) - J(f^*) \leq \min_{k \geq 1}\left(R_{kn} + \inf_{f \in \mathcal{F}_k} J(f) - J(f^*)\right),$$

where

$$R_{kn} = \min_{u \geq 4\Delta_{kn}}\left(u + 9Be^{-nu^2/(512B^2)}\right).$$

Assuming without loss of generality that $\log N(\epsilon, \mathcal{H}_k) \geq 1$, it is easy to see that the choice

$$\Delta_{kn} = \sqrt{128B^2 \frac{\log N(B/\sqrt{n}, \mathcal{H}_k) + c_k}{n}} \tag{4}$$

satisfies (2).

2.1 SQUARED ERROR LOSS

For the special case when

$$L(x, y) = (x - y)^2$$

we can obtain a better upper bound. The estimate will be the same as before, but instead of (2), the complexity penalty Δ_{kn} now has to satisfy

$$\Delta_{kn} \geq C_1 \frac{\log N(\Delta_{kn}/C_2, \mathcal{F}_k) + c_k}{n}, \tag{5}$$

where $C_1 = 3499C^4$, $C_2 = 256C^3$, and $C = \max\{B, 1\}$. Here $N(\epsilon, \mathcal{F}_k)$ is a uniform upper bound on the random l_1 covering numbers $N(\epsilon, \mathcal{F}_k, X_1^n)$. Assume that the class $\mathcal{F} = \cup_k \mathcal{F}_k$ is convex, and let $\overline{\mathcal{F}}$ be the closure of $\mathcal{F}$ in $L^2(\mu)$, where μ denotes the distribution of X. Then there is a unique $\bar{f} \in \overline{\mathcal{F}}$ whose squared loss $J(\bar{f})$ achieves $\inf_{f \in \mathcal{F}} J(f)$. We have the following bound on the difference $\mathbf{E}J(f_n) - J(\bar{f})$.

Theorem 2 *Assume that $\mathcal{F} = \cup_k \mathcal{F}_k$ is a convex set of functions, and consider the squared error loss. Suppose that $|f(x)| \leq B$ for all $x \in \mathbb{R}^d$ and $f \in \mathcal{F}$, and $\mathbf{P}(|Y| > B) = 0$. Then complexity regularization estimate with complexity penalty satisfying* (5) *gives*

$$\mathbf{E}J(f_n) - J(\bar{f}) \leq 2\min_{k \geq 1}\left(\Delta_{kn} + \inf_{f \in \mathcal{F}_k} J(f) - J(\bar{f})\right) + \frac{C_1}{2n}.$$

The proof of this result uses an idea of Barron [1] and a Bernstein-type uniform probability inequality recently obtained by Lee *et al.* [7].

3 RBF NETWORKS

We will consider radial basis function (RBF) networks with one hidden layer. Such a network is characterized by a kernel $K : \mathbb{R}^+ \to \mathbb{R}$. An RBF net of k nodes is of the form

$$f(x) = \sum_{i=1}^{k} w_i K\left([x - c_i]^t A_i [x - c_i]\right) + w_0, \tag{6}$$

where $w_0, w_1, \ldots, w_k$ are real numbers called weights, $c_1, \ldots, c_k \in \mathbb{R}^d$, and the A_i are nonnegative definite $d \times d$ matrices. The kth candidate class $\mathcal{F}_k$ for the function estimation task is defined as the class of networks with k nodes which satisfy the weight condition $\sum_{i=0}^{k}|w_i| \leq b$ for a fixed $b > 0$:

$$\mathcal{F}_k = \left\{\sum_{i=1}^{k} w_i K\left([x - c_i]^t A_i [x - c_i]\right) + w_0 : \sum_{i=0}^{k}|w_i| \leq b\right\}. \tag{7}$$

Let $L(x,y) = |x-y|^p$, and
$$J(f) = \mathbf{E}|f(X) - Y|^p, \tag{8}$$

where $1 \le p < \infty$. Let μ denote the probability measure induced by X. Define $\overline{\mathcal{F}}$ to be the closure in $L^p(\mu)$ of the convex hull of the functions $\widehat{b}K([x-c]^t A[x-c])$ and the constant function $h(x) = 1$, $x \in \mathbb{R}^d$, where $|\widehat{b}| \le b$, $c \in \mathbb{R}^d$, and A varies over all nonnegative $d \times d$ matrices. That is, $\overline{\mathcal{F}}$ is the closure of $\mathcal{F} = \cup_k \mathcal{F}_k$, where $\mathcal{F}_k$ is given in (7). Let $g \in \overline{\mathcal{F}}$ be arbitrary. If we assume that $|K|$ is uniformly bounded, then by Corollary 1 of Darken et al. [3], we have for $1 \le p \le 2$ that

$$\inf_{f \in \mathcal{F}_k} \|f - g\|_{L^p(\mu)} = O(1/\sqrt{k}), \tag{9}$$

where $\|f - g\|_{L^p(\mu)}$ denotes the $L^p(\mu)$ norm $\left(\int |f - f^*|^p d\mu\right)^{1/p}$, and $\mathcal{F}_k$ is given in (7). The approximation error $\inf_{f \in \mathcal{F}_k} J(f) - J(f^*)$ can be dealt with using this result if the optimal f^* happens to be in $\overline{\mathcal{F}}$. In this case, we obtain

$$\inf_{f \in \mathcal{F}_k} J(f) - J(f^*) = O(1/\sqrt{k})$$

for all $1 \le p \le 2$. Values of p close to 1 are of great importance for robust neural network regression.

When the kernel K has a bounded total variation, it can be shown that $N(\epsilon, \mathcal{H}_k) \le (A_1/\epsilon)^{A_2 k}$, where the constants A_1, A_2 depend on $\sup_x |K(x)|$, the total variation V of K, the dimension d, and on the the constant b in the definition (7) of $\mathcal{F}_k$. Then, if $1 \le p \le 2$, the following consequence of Theorem 1 can be proved for L^p regression estimation.

Theorem 3 *Let the kernel K be of bounded variation and assume that $|Y|$ is bounded. Then for $1 \le p \le 2$ the error (8) of the complexity regularized estimate satisfies*

$$\mathbf{E}J(f_n) - J(f^*) \le \min_{k \ge 1} \left[O\left(\sqrt{\frac{k \log n}{n}}\right) + O\left(\sqrt{\frac{1}{k}}\right) \right]$$
$$= O\left(\left(\frac{\log n}{n}\right)^{1/4}\right).$$

For $p = 1$, i.e., for L^1 regression estimation, this rate is known to be optimal within the logarithmic factor.

For squared error loss $J(f) = \mathbf{E}(f(X) - Y)^2$ we have $f^*(x) = \mathbf{E}(Y|X=x)$. If $f^* \in \overline{\mathcal{F}}$, then by (9) we obtain

$$\inf_{f \in \mathcal{F}_k} J(f) - J(f^*) = O(1/k). \tag{10}$$

It is easy to check that the class $\cup_k \mathcal{F}_k$ is convex if the $\mathcal{F}_k$ are the collections of RBF nets defined in (7). The next result shows that we can get rid of the square root in Theorem 3.

Theorem 4 *Assume that K is of bounded variation. Suppose furthermore that $|Y|$ is a bounded random variable, and let $L(x,y) = (x-y)^2$. Then the complexity regularization RBF squared regression estimate satisfies*

$$\mathbf{E}J(f_n) - \inf_{f \in \mathcal{F}} J(f) \le 2 \min_{k \ge 1} \left(\inf_{f \in \mathcal{F}_k} J(f) - \inf_{f \in \mathcal{F}} J(f) + O\left(\frac{k \log n}{n}\right) \right) + O\left(\frac{1}{n}\right).$$

If $f^* \in \overline{\mathcal{F}}$, this result and (10) give

$$\mathbf{E}J(f_n) - J(f^*) \leq \min_{k \geq 1}\left[O\left(\frac{k\log n}{n}\right) + O\left(\frac{1}{k}\right)\right]$$
$$= O\left(\left(\frac{\log n}{n}\right)^{1/2}\right). \qquad (11)$$

This result sharpens and extends Theorem 3.1 of Niyogi and Girosi [9] where the weaker $O\left(\sqrt{\frac{k\log n}{n}}\right) + O\left(\frac{1}{k}\right)$ convergence rate was obtained (in a PAC-like formulation) for the squared loss of Gaussian RBF network regression estimation. The rate in (11) varies linearly with dimension. Our result is valid for a very large class of RBF schemes, including the Gaussian RBF networks considered in [9]. Besides having improved on the convergence rate, our result has the advantage of allowing kernels which are not continuous, such as the window kernel.

The above convergence rate results hold in the case when there exists an f^* minimizing the risk which is a member of the $L^p(\mu)$ closure of $\mathcal{F} = \cup \mathcal{F}_k$, where $\mathcal{F}_k$ is given in (7). In other words, f^* should be such that for all $\epsilon > 0$ there exists a k and a member f of $\mathcal{F}_k$ with $\|f - f^*\|_{L^p(\mu)} < \epsilon$. The precise characterization of $\overline{\mathcal{F}}$ seems to be difficult. However, based on the work of Girosi and Anzellotti [4] we can describe a large class of functions that is *contained* in $\overline{\mathcal{F}}$.

Let $H(x,t)$ be a real and bounded function of two variables $x \in \mathbb{R}^d$ and $t \in \mathbb{R}^n$. Suppose that λ is a signed measure on $\mathbb{R}^n$ with finite total variation $\|\lambda\|$. If $g(x)$ is defined as

$$g(x) = \int_{\mathbb{R}^n} H(x,t)\lambda(dt),$$

then $g \in L^p(\mu)$ for any probability measure μ on $\mathbb{R}^d$. One can reasonably expect that g can be approximated well by functions $f(x)$ of the form

$$f(x) = \sum_{i=1}^k w_i H(x, t_i),$$

where $t_1, \ldots, t_k \in \mathbb{R}^n$ and $\sum_{i=1}^k |w_i| \leq \|\lambda\|$. The case $m = d$ and $H(x,t) = G(x-t)$ is investigated in [4], where a detailed description of function spaces arising from the different choices of the basis function G is given. Niyogi and Girosi [9] extends this approach to approximation by convex combinations of translates and dilates of a Gaussian function. In general, we can prove the following

Lemma 1 *Let*

$$g(x) = \int_{\mathbb{R}^n} H(x,t)\lambda(dt), \qquad (12)$$

where $H(x,t)$ and λ are as above. Define for each $k \geq 1$ the class of functions

$$\mathcal{G}_k = \left\{f(x) = \sum_{i=1}^k w_i H(x, t_i) : \sum_{i=0}^k |w_i| \leq \|\lambda\|\right\}.$$

Then for any probability measure μ on $\mathbb{R}^d$ and for any $1 \leq p < \infty$, the function g can be approximated in $L^p(\mu)$ arbitrarily closely by members of $\mathcal{G} = \cup \mathcal{G}_k$, i.e.,

$$\inf_{f \in \mathcal{G}_k} \|f - g\|_{L^p(\mu)} \to 0 \quad as \quad k \to \infty.$$

To prove this lemma one need only slightly adapt the proof of Theorem 8.2 in [4], or in a more elementary way following the lines of the probabilistic proof of Theorem 1 of [6]. To apply the lemma for RBF networks considered in this paper, let $n = d^2 + d$, $t = (A, c)$, and $H(x, t) = K\left([x-c]^t A[x-c]\right)$. Then we obtain that $\overline{\mathcal{F}}$ contains all the functions g with the integral representation

$$g(x) = \int_{\mathbb{R}^{d^2+d}} K\left([x-c]^t A[x-c]\right) \lambda(dc\,dA),$$

for which $\|\lambda\| \leq b$, where b is the constraint on the weights as in (7).

Acknowledgements

This work was supported in part by NSERC grant OGP000270, Canadian National Networks of Centers of Excellence grant 293 and OTKA grant F014174.

References

[1] A. R. Barron. Complexity regularization with application to artificial neural networks. In G. Roussas, editor, *Nonparametric Functional Estimation and Related Topics*, pages 561–576. NATO ASI Series, Kluwer Academic Publishers, Dordrecht, 1991.

[2] A. R. Barron. Approximation and estimation bounds for artificial neural networks. *Machine Learning*, 14:115–133, 1994.

[3] C. Darken, M. Donahue, L. Gurvits, and E. Sontag. Rate of approximation results motivated by robust neural network learning. In *Proc. Sixth Annual Workshop on Computational Learning Theory*, pages 303–309. Morgan Kauffman, 1993.

[4] F. Girosi and G. Anzellotti. Rates of convergence for radial basis functions and neural networks. In R. J. Mammone, editor, *Artificial Neural Networks for Speech and Vision*, pages 97–113. Chapman & Hall, London, 1993.

[5] F. Girosi, M. Jones, and T. Poggio. Regularization theory and neural network architectures. *Neural Computation*, 7:219–267, 1995.

[6] A. Krzyżak, T. Linder, and G. Lugosi. Nonparametric estimation and classification using radial basis function nets and empirical risk minimization. *IEEE Transactions on Neural Networks*, 7(2):475–487, March 1996.

[7] W. S. Lee, P. L. Bartlett, and R. C. Williamson. Efficient agnostic learning of neural networks with bounded fan-in. to be published in *IEEE Transactions on Information Theory*, 1995.

[8] G. Lugosi and K. Zeger. Concept learning using complexity regularization. *IEEE Transactions on Information Theory*, 42:48–54, 1996.

[9] P. Niyogi and F. Girosi. On the relationship between generalization error, hypothesis complexity, and sample complexity for radial basis functions. *Neural Computation*, 8:819–842, 1996.

[10] V. N. Vapnik. *Estimation of Dependencies Based on Empirical Data*. Springer-Verlag, New York, 1982.

An Apobayesian Relative of Winnow

Nick Littlestone
NEC Research Institute
4 Independence Way
Princeton, NJ 08540

Chris Mesterharm
NEC Research Institute
4 Independence Way
Princeton, NJ 08540

Abstract

We study a mistake-driven variant of an on-line Bayesian learning algorithm (similar to one studied by Cesa-Bianchi, Helmbold, and Panizza [CHP96]). This variant only updates its state (learns) on trials in which it makes a mistake. The algorithm makes binary classifications using a linear-threshold classifier and runs in time linear in the number of attributes seen by the learner. We have been able to show, theoretically and in simulations, that this algorithm performs well under assumptions quite different from those embodied in the prior of the original Bayesian algorithm. It can handle situations that we do not know how to handle in linear time with Bayesian algorithms. We expect our techniques to be useful in deriving and analyzing other apobayesian algorithms.

1 Introduction

We consider two styles of on-line learning. In both cases, learning proceeds in a sequence of trials. In each trial, a learner observes an *instance* to be classified, makes a *prediction* of its classification, and then observes a *label* that gives the correct classification. One style of on-line learning that we consider is Bayesian. The learner uses probabilistic assumptions about the world (embodied in a prior over some model class) and data observed in past trials to construct a probabilistic model (embodied in a posterior distribution over the model class). The learner uses this model to make a prediction in the current trial. When the learner is told the correct classification of the instance, the learner uses this information to update the model, generating a new posterior to be used in the next trial.

In the other style of learning that we consider, the attention is on the correctness of the predictions rather than on the model of the world. The internal state of the learner is only changed when the learner makes a mistake (when the prediction fails to match the label). We call such an algorithm *mistake-driven*. (Such algorithms are often called *conservative* in the computational learning theory literature.) There is a simple way to derive a mistake-driven algorithm from any on-line learning algorithm (we restrict our attention in this paper to deterministic algorithms). The derived algorithm is just like the original algorithm, except that before every trial, it makes a record of its entire state, and after every trial in which its prediction is correct, it resets its state to match the recorded state, entirely forgetting the intervening trial. (Typically this is actually implemented not by making such a record, but by merely omitting the step that updates the state.) For example, if some algorithm keeps track of the number of trials it has seen, then the mistake-driven version of this algorithm will end up keeping track of the number of mistakes it has made. Whether the original or mistake-driven algorithm will do better depends on the task and on how the algorithms are evaluated.

We will start with a Bayesian learning algorithm that we call *SBSB* and use this procedure to derive a mistake-driven variant, *SASB*. Note that the variant cannot be expected to be a Bayesian learning algorithm (at least in the ordinary sense) since a Bayesian algorithm would make a prediction that minimizes the Bayes risk based on all the available data, and the mistake-driven variant has forgotten quite a bit. We call such algorithms *apobayesian* learning algorithms. This name is intended to suggest that they are derived from Bayesian learning algorithms, but are not themselves Bayesian. Our algorithm *SASB* is very close to an algorithm of [CHP96]. We study its application to different tasks than they do, analyzing its performance when it is applied to linearly separable data as described below.

In this paper instances will be chosen from the instance space $\mathbf{X} = \{0,1\}^n$ for some n. Thus instances are composed of n boolean attributes. We consider only two category classifications tasks, with predictions and labels chosen from $\mathbf{Y} = \{0,1\}$.

We obtain a bound on the number of mistakes *SASB* makes that is comparable to bounds for various Winnow family algorithms given in [Lit88,Lit89]. As for those algorithms, the bound holds under the assumption that the points labeled 1 are linearly separable from the points labeled 0, and the bound depends on the size δ of the gap between the two classes. (See Section 3 for a definition of δ.) The mistake bound for *SASB* is $O(\frac{1}{\delta^2} \log \frac{n}{\delta})$. While this bound has an extra factor of $\log \frac{1}{\delta}$ not present in the bounds for the Winnow algorithms, SASB has the advantage of not needing any parameters. The Winnow family algorithms have parameters, and the algorithms' mistake bounds depend on setting the parameters to values that depend on δ. (Often, the value of δ will not be known by the learner.) We expect the techniques used to obtain this bound to be useful in analyzing other apobayesian learning algorithms.

A number of authors have done related research regarding worst-case on-line loss bounds including [Fre96,KW95,Vov90]. Simulation experiments involving a Bayesian algorithm and a mistake-driven variant are described in [Lit95]. That paper provides useful background for this paper. Note that our present analysis techniques do not apply to the apobayesian algorithm studied there. The closest of the original Winnow family algorithms to *SASB* appears to be the Weighted Majority algorithm [LW94], which was analyzed for a case similar to that considered in this paper in [Lit89]. One should get a roughly correct impression of *SASB* if one thinks of it as a version of the Weighted Majority algorithm that learns its parameters.

In the next section we describe the Bayesian algorithm that we start with. In Section 3 we discuss its mistake-driven apobayesian variant. Section 4 mentions some simulation experiments using these algorithms, and Section 5 is the conclusion.

2 A Bayesian Learning Algorithm

To describe the Bayesian learning algorithm we must specify a family of distributions over $\mathbf{X} \times \mathbf{Y}$ and a prior over this family of distributions. We parameterize the distributions with parameters $(\theta_1, \ldots, \theta_{n+1})$ chosen from $\Theta = [0,1]^{n+1}$. The parameter θ_{n+1} gives the probability that the label is 1, and the parameter θ_i gives the probability that the ith attribute matches the label. Note that the probability that the ith attribute is 1 given that the label is 1 equals the probability that the ith attribute is 0 given that the label is 0. We speak of this linkage between the probabilities for the two classes as a symmetry condition. With this linkage, the observation of a point from either class will affect the posterior distribution for both classes. It is perhaps more typical to choose priors that allow the two classes to be treated separately, so that the posterior for each class (giving the probability of elements of $\mathbf{X}$ conditioned on the label) depends only on the prior and on observations from that class. The symmetry condition that we impose appears to be important to the success of our analysis of the apobayesian variant of this algorithm. (Though we impose this condition to *derive* the algorithm, it turns out that the apobayesian variant can actually handle tasks where this condition is not satisfied.)

We choose a prior on Θ that gives probability 1 to the set of all elements $\boldsymbol{\theta} = (\theta_1, \ldots, \theta_{n+1}) \in \Theta$ for which at most one of $\theta_1, \ldots, \theta_n$ does not equal $\frac{1}{2}$. The prior is uniform on this set. Note that for any $\boldsymbol{\theta}$ in this set only a single attribute has a probability other than $\frac{1}{2}$ of matching the label, and thus only a single attribute is relevant. Concentrating on this set turns out to lead to an apobayesian algorithm that can, in fact, handle more than one relevant attribute and that performs particularly well when only a small fraction of the attributes are relevant.

This prior is related to to the familiar Naive Bayes model, which also assumes that the attributes are conditionally independent given the labels. However, in the typical Naive Bayes model there is no restriction to a single relevant attribute and the symmetry condition linking the two classes is not imposed.

Our prior leads to the following algorithm. (The name *SBSB* stands for "**S**ymmetric **B**ayesian Algorithm with **S**ingly-variant prior for **B**ernoulli distribution.")

Algorithm *SBSB* Algorithm *SBSB* maintains counts s_i of the number of times each attribute matches the label, a count M of the number of times the label is 1, and a count t of the number of trials.

Initialization $s_i \leftarrow 0$ for $i = 1, \ldots, n$ $M \leftarrow 0$ $t \leftarrow 0$

Prediction Predict 1 given instance $(x_1, \ldots, x_n)$ if and only if
$$(M+1) \sum_{i=1}^{n} \frac{x_i(s_i+1) + (1-x_i)(t-s_i+1)}{\binom{t}{s_i}} > (t-M+1) \sum_{i=1}^{n} \frac{(1-x_i)(s_i+1) + x_i(t-s_i+1)}{\binom{t}{s_i}}$$

Update $M \leftarrow M + y$, $t \leftarrow t+1$, and for each i, if $x_i = y$ then $s_i \leftarrow s_i + 1$

3 An Apobayesian Algorithm

We construct an apobayesian algorithm by converting algorithm *SBSB* into a mistake-driven algorithm using the standard conversion given in the introduction. We call the resulting learning algorithm *SASB*; we have replaced "Bayesian" with "Apobayesian" in the acronym.

In the previous section we made assumptions made about the generation of the instances and labels that led to *SBSB* and thence to *SASB*. These assumptions have served their purpose and we now abandon them. In analyzing the apobayesian algorithm we do not assume that the instances and labels are generated by some stochastic process. Instead we assume that the instance-label pairs in all of the trials are linearly-separable, that is, that there exist some $w_1, \ldots, w_n$, and c such that for every instance-label pair $(\mathbf{x}, y)$ we have $\sum_{i=1}^n w_i x_i \geq c$ when $y = 1$ and $\sum_{i=1}^n w_i x_i \leq c$ when $y = 0$. We actually make a somewhat stronger assumption, given in the following theorem, which gives our bound for the apobayesian algorithm.

Theorem 1 *Suppose that $\gamma_i \geq 0$ and $\overline{\gamma}_i \geq 0$ for $i = 1, \ldots, n$, and that $\sum_{i=1}^n \gamma_i + \overline{\gamma}_i = 1$. Suppose that $0 \leq b_0 < b_1 \leq 1$ and let $\delta = b_1 - b_0$. Suppose that algorithm SASB is run on a sequence of trials such that the instance $\mathbf{x}$ and label y in each trial satisfy $\sum_{i=1}^n \gamma_i x_i + \overline{\gamma}_i (1 - x_i) \leq b_0$ if $y = 0$ and $\sum_{i=1}^n \gamma_i x_i + \overline{\gamma}_i (1 - x_i) \geq b_1$ if $y = 1$. Then the number of mistakes made by SASB will be bounded by $\frac{16}{\delta^2} \log \frac{8n}{\delta}$.*

We have space to say only a little about how the derivation of this bound proceeds. Details are given in [Lit96].

In analyzing *SASB* we work with an abstract description of the associated algorithm *SBSB*. This algorithm starts with a prior on Θ as described above. We represent this with a density ρ_0. Then after each trial it calculates a new posterior density $\rho_t(\boldsymbol{\theta}) = \frac{\rho_{t-1}(\boldsymbol{\theta}) P(\mathbf{x}, y | \boldsymbol{\theta})}{\int \rho_{t-1}(\boldsymbol{\theta}) P(\mathbf{x}, y | \boldsymbol{\theta})}$, where ρ_t is the density after trial t and $P(\mathbf{x}, y | \boldsymbol{\theta})$ is the conditional probability of the instance $\mathbf{x}$ and label y observed in trial t given $\boldsymbol{\theta}$. Thus we can think of the algorithm as maintaining a current distribution on Θ that is initially the prior. *SASB* is similar, but it leaves the current distribution unchanged when a mistake is not made. For there to exist a finite mistake bound there must exist some possible choice for the current distribution for which *SASB* would make perfect predictions, should it ever arrive at that distribution. We call any such distribution leading to perfect predictions a possible *target distribution*. It turns out that the separability condition given in Theorem 1 guarantees that a suitable target distribution exists. The analysis proceeds by showing that for an appropriate choice of a target density $\tilde{\rho}$ the relative entropy of the current distribution with respect to the target distribution, $\int \tilde{\rho}(\boldsymbol{\theta}) \log(\tilde{\rho}(\boldsymbol{\theta})/\rho_t(\boldsymbol{\theta}))$, decreases by at least some amount $R > 0$ whenever a mistake is made. Since the relative entropy is never negative, the number of mistakes is bounded by the initial relative entropy divided by R. This form of analysis is very similar to the analysis of the various members of the Winnow family in [Lit89,Lit91].

The same technique can be applied to other apobayesian algorithms. The abstract update of ρ_t given above is quite general. The success of the analysis depends on conditions on ρ_0 and $P(\mathbf{x}, y | \boldsymbol{\theta})$ that we do not have space here to discuss.

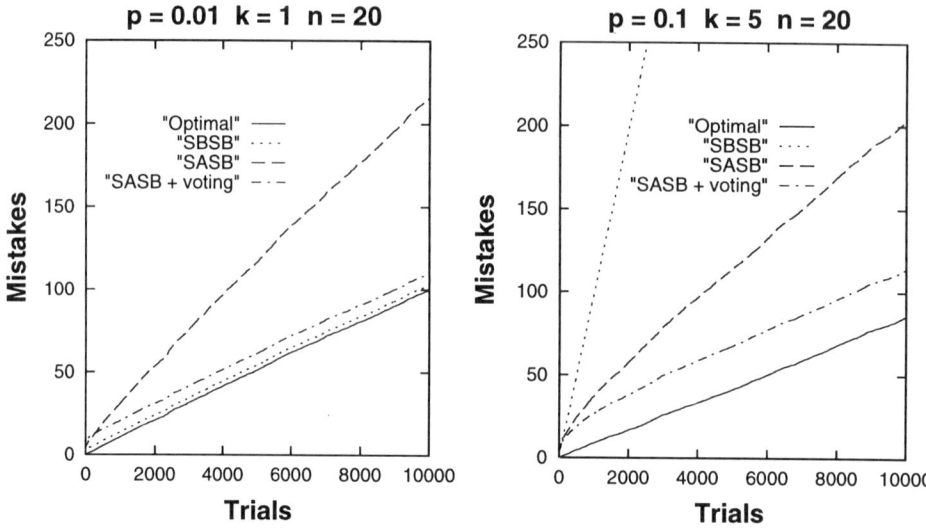

Figure 1: Comparison of *SASB* with *SBSB*

4 Simulation Experiments

The bound of the previous section was for perfectly linearly-separable data. We have also done some simulation experiments exploring the performance of *SASB* on non-separable data and comparing it with *SBSB* and with various other mistake-driven algorithms. A sample comparison of *SASB* with *SBSB* is shown in Figure 1. In each experimental run we generated 10000 trials with the instances and labels chosen randomly according to a distribution specified by $\theta_1 = \ldots = \theta_k = 1 - p$, $\theta_{k+1} = \ldots = \theta_{n+1} = .5$ where $\theta_1, \ldots, \theta_{n+1}$ are interpreted as specified in Section 2, n is the number of attributes, and n, p, and k are as specified at the top of each plot. The line labeled "optimal" shows the performance obtained by an optimal predictor that knows the distribution used to generate the data ahead of time, and thus does not need to do any learning. The lines labeled "SBSB" and "SASB" show the performance of the corresponding learning algorithms. The lines labeled "SASB + voting" show the performance of *SASB* with the addition of a voting procedure described in [Lit95]. This procedure improves the asymptotic mistake rate of the algorithms. Each line on the graph is the average of 30 runs. Each line plots the cumulative number of mistakes made by the algorithm from the beginning of the run as a function of the number of trials.

In the left hand plot, there is only 1 relevant attribute. This is exactly the case that *SBSB* is intended for, and it does better than *SASB*. In right hand plot, there are 5 relevant attributes; *SBSB* appears unable to take advantage of the extra information present in the extra relevant attributes, but *SASB* successfully does.

Comparison of *SASB* and previous Winnow family algorithms is still in progress, and we defer presenting details until a clearer picture has been obtained. *SASB* and the Weighted Majority algorithm often perform similarly in simulations. Typically, as one would expect, the Weighted Majority algorithm does somewhat better than

$SASB$ when its parameters are chosen optimally for the particular learning task, and worse for bad choices of parameters.

5 Conclusion

Our mistake bounds and simulations suggest that $SASB$ may be a useful alternative to the existing algorithms in the Winnow family. Based on the analysis style and the bounds, $SASB$ should perhaps itself be considered a Winnow family algorithm. Further experiments are in progress comparing $SASB$ with Winnow family algorithms run with a variety of parameter settings.

Perhaps of even greater interest is the potential application of our analytic techniques to a variety of other apobayesian algorithms (though as we have observed earlier, the techniques do not appear to apply to all such algorithms). We have already obtained some preliminary results regarding an interpretation of the Perceptron algorithm as an apobayesian algorithm. We are interested in looking for entirely new algorithms that can be derived in this way and also in better understanding the scope of applicability of our techniques. All of the analyses that we have looked at depend on symmetry conditions relating the probabilities for the two classes. It would be of interest to see what can be said when such symmetry conditions do not hold. In simulation experiments [Lit95], a mistake-driven variant of the standard Naive Bayes algorithm often does very well, despite the absence of such symmetry in the prior that it is based on.

Our simulation experiments and also the analysis of the related algorithm Winnow [Lit91] suggest that $SASB$ can be expected to handle some instance-label pairs inside of the separating gap or on the wrong side, especially if they are not too far on the wrong side. In particular it appears to be able to handle data generated according to the distributions on which $SBSB$ is based, which do not in general yield perfectly separable data.

It is of interest to compare the capabilities of the original Bayesian algorithm with the derived apobayesian algorithm. When the data is stochastically generated in a manner consistent with the assumptions behind the original algorithm, the original Bayesian algorithm can be expected to do better (see, for example, Figure 1). On the other hand, the apobayesian algorithm can handle data beyond the capabilities of the original Bayesian algorithm. For example, in the case we consider, the apobayesian algorithm can take advantage of the presence of more than one relevant attribute, even though the prior behind the original Bayesian algorithm assumes a single relevant attribute. Furthermore, as for all of the Winnow family algorithms, the mistake bound for the apobayesian algorithm does not depend on details of the behavior of the irrelevant attributes (including redundant attributes).

Instead of using the apobayesian variant, one might try to construct a Bayesian learning algorithm for a prior that reflects the actual dependencies among the attributes and the labels. However, it may not be clear what the appropriate prior is. It may be particularly unclear how to model the behavior of the irrelevant attributes. Furthermore, such a Bayesian algorithm may end up being computationally expensive. For example, attempting to keep track of correlations among all pairs of attributes may lead to an algorithm that needs time and space quadratic in the number of attributes. On the other hand, if we start with a Bayesian algorithm that uses time and space linear in the number of attributes we can obtain an apobayesian algorithm that still uses linear time and space but that can handle situations beyond the capabilities of the original Bayesian algorithm.

Acknowledgments This paper has benefited from discussions with Adam Grove.

References

[CHP96] Nicolo Cesa-Bianchi, David P. Helmbold, and Sandra Panizza. On bayes methods for on-line boolean prediction. In *Proceedings of the Ninth Annual Conference on Computational Learning Theory*, pages 314–324, 1996.

[Fre96] Yoav Freund. Predicting a binary sequence almost as well as the optimal biased coin. In *Proceedings of the Ninth Annual Conference on Computational Learning Theory*, pages 89–98, 1996.

[KW95] J. Kivinen and M. K. Warmuth. Additive versus exponentiated gradient updates for linear prediction. In *Proc. 27th ACM Symp. on Theory of Computing*, pages 209–218, 1995.

[Lit88] N. Littlestone. Learning quickly when irrelevant attributes abound: A new linear-threshold algorithm. *Machine Learning*, 2:285–318, 1988.

[Lit89] N. Littlestone. *Mistake Bounds and Logarithmic Linear-threshold Learning Algorithms*. PhD thesis, Tech. Rept. UCSC-CRL-89-11, Univ. of Calif., Santa Cruz, 1989.

[Lit91] N. Littlestone. Redundant noisy attributes, attribute errors, and linear-threshold learning using Winnow. In *Proc. 4th Annu. Workshop on Comput. Learning Theory*, pages 147–156. Morgan Kaufmann, San Mateo, CA, 1991.

[Lit95] N. Littlestone. Comparing several linear-threshold learning algorithms on tasks involving superfluous attributes. In *Proceedings of the XII International conference on Machine Learning*, pages 353–361, 1995.

[Lit96] N. Littlestone. Mistake-driven bayes sports: Bounds for symmetric apobayesian learning algorithms. Technical report, NEC Research Institute, Princeton, NJ, 1996.

[LW94] N. Littlestone and M. K. Warmuth. The weighted majority algorithm. *Information and Computation*, 108:212–261, 1994.

[Vov90] Volodimir G. Vovk. Aggregating strategies. In *Proceedings of the 1990 Workshop on Computational Learning Theory*, pages 371–383, 1990.

Noisy Spiking Neurons with Temporal Coding have more Computational Power than Sigmoidal Neurons

Wolfgang Maass
Institute for Theoretical Computer Science
Technische Universitaet Graz, Klosterwiesgasse 32/2
A-8010 Graz, Austria, e-mail: maass@igi.tu-graz.ac.at

Abstract

We exhibit a novel way of simulating sigmoidal neural nets by networks of noisy spiking neurons in temporal coding. Furthermore it is shown that networks of noisy spiking neurons with temporal coding have a strictly larger computational power than sigmoidal neural nets with the same number of units.

1 Introduction and Definitions

We consider a formal model SNN for a spiking neuron network that is basically a reformulation of the spike response model (and of the leaky integrate and fire model) without using δ-functions (see [Maass, 1996a] or [Maass, 1996b] for further background).

An SNN consists of a finite set V of *spiking neurons*, a set $E \subseteq V \times V$ of *synapses*, a *weight* $w_{u,v} \geq 0$ and a *response function* $\varepsilon_{u,v} : \mathbf{R}^+ \to \mathbf{R}$ for each synapse $\langle u, v \rangle \in E$ (where $\mathbf{R}^+ := \{x \in \mathbf{R} : x \geq 0\}$) , and a *threshold function* $\Theta_v : \mathbf{R}^+ \to \mathbf{R}^+$ for each neuron $v \in V$.

If $F_u \subseteq \mathbf{R}^+$ is the set of *firing times* of a neuron u, then the *potential* at the trigger zone of neuron v at time t is given by

$$P_v(t) := \sum_{u : \langle u,v \rangle \in E} \sum_{s \in F_u : s < t} w_{u,v} \cdot \varepsilon_{u,v}(t - s) .$$

In a noise-free model a neuron v fires at time t as soon as $P_v(t)$ reaches $\Theta_v(t - t')$, where t' is the time of the most recent firing of v. One says then that neuron v sends out an "action potential" or "spike" at time t.

For some specified subset $V_{in} \subseteq V$ of *input neurons* one assumes that the firing times ("spike trains") F_u for neurons $u \in V_{in}$ are not defined by the preceding convention, but are given from the outside. The firing times F_v for all other neurons $v \in V$ are determined by the previously described rule, and the output of the network is given in the form of the spike trains F_v for a specified set of *output neurons* $V_{out} \subseteq V$.

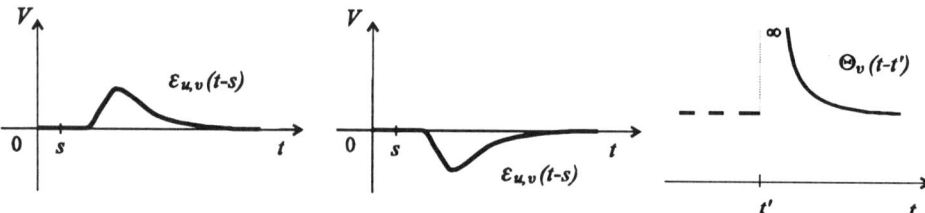

Figure 1: *Typical shapes of response functions $\varepsilon_{u,v}$ (EPSP and IPSP) and threshold functions Θ_v for biological neurons.*

We will assume in our subsequent constructions that all response functions $\varepsilon_{u,v}$ and threshold functions Θ_v in an SNN are "stereotyped", i.e. that the response functions differ apart from their "sign" (EPSP or IPSP) only in their delay $d_{u,v}$ (where $d_{u,v} := \inf\{t \geq 0 : \varepsilon_{u,v}(t) \neq 0\}$), and that the threshold functions Θ_v only differ by an additive constant (i.e. for all u and v there exists a constant $c_{u,v}$ such that $\Theta_u(t) = \Theta_v(t) + c_{u,v}$ for all $t \geq 0$). We refer to a term of the form $w_{u,v} \cdot \varepsilon_{u,v}(t-s)$ as an <u>e</u>xcitatory respectively <u>i</u>nhibitory <u>p</u>ost<u>s</u>ynaptic <u>p</u>otential (abbreviated: EPSP respectively IPSP).

Since biological neurons do not always fire in a reliable manner one also considers the related model of *noisy spiking neurons*, where $P_v(t)$ is replaced by $P_v^{noisy}(t) := P_v(t) + \alpha_v(t)$ and $\Theta_v(t-t')$ is replaced by $\Theta_v^{noisy}(t-t') := \Theta_v(t-t') + \beta_v(t-t')$. $\alpha_v(t)$ and $\beta_v(t-t')$ are allowed to be arbitrary functions with bounded absolute value (hence they can also represent "systematic noise").

Furthermore one allows that the current value of the difference $D(t) := P_v^{noisy}(t) - \Theta_v^{noisy}(t-t')$ does not determine directly the firing time of neuron v, but only its current *firing probability*. We assume that the firing probability approaches 1 if $D \to \infty$, and 0 if $D \to -\infty$. We refer to spiking neurons with these two types of noise as "noisy spiking neurons".

We will explore in this article the power of *analog* computations with noisy spiking neurons, and we refer to [Maass, 1996a] for results about *digital* computations in this model. Details to the results in this article appear in [Maass, 1996b] and [Maass, 1997].

2 Fast Simulation of Sigmoidal Neural Nets with Noisy Spiking Neurons in Temporal Coding

So far one has only considered simulations of sigmoidal neural nets by spiking neurons where each analog variable in the sigmoidal neural net is represented by the *firing rate* of a spiking neuron. However this "firing rate interpretation" is inconsistent with a number of empirical results about computations in biological neural systems. For example [Thorpe & Imbert, 1989] have demonstrated that visual pattern analysis and pattern classification can be carried out by humans in just 150 ms, in spite of the fact that it involves a minimum of 10 synaptic stages from the retina to the temporal lobe. [de Ruyter van Steveninck & Bialek, 1988] have found that a blowfly can produce flight torques within 30 ms of a visual stimulus by a neural system with several synaptic stages. However the firing rates of neurons involved in all these computations are usually below 100 Hz, and interspike intervals tend to be quite irregular. Hence one cannot interpret these analog computations with spiking neurons on the basis of an encoding of analog variables by firing rates.

On the other hand experimental evidence has accumulated during the last few years which indicates that many biological neural systems use the *timing* of action potentials to encode information (see e.g. [Bialek & Rieke, 1992], [Bair & Koch, 1996]).

We will now describe a new way of simulating sigmoidal neural nets by networks of spiking neurons that is based on *temporal coding*. The *key mechanism* for this alternative simulation is based on the well known fact that EPSP's and IPSP's are able to *shift* the firing time of a spiking neuron. This mechanism can be demonstrated very clearly in our formal model if one assumes that EPSP's rise (and IPSP's fall) *linearly* during a certain initial time period. Hence we assume in the following that there exists some constant $\Delta > 0$ such that each response function $\varepsilon_{u,v}(x)$ is of the form $\alpha_{u,v} \cdot (x - d_{u,v})$ with $\alpha_{u,v} \in \{-1, 1\}$ for $x \in [d_{u,v}, d_{u,v} + \Delta]$, and $\varepsilon_{u,v}(x) = 0$ for $x \in [0, d_{u,v}]$.

Consider a spiking neuron v that receives postsynaptic potentials from n presynaptic neurons $a_1, \ldots, a_n$. For simplicity we assume that interspike intervals are so large that the firing time t_v of neuron v depends just on a single firing time t_{a_i} of each neuron a_i, and Θ_v has returned to its "resting value" $\Theta_v(0)$ before v fires again. Then if the next firing of v occurs at a time when the postsynaptic potentials described by $w_{a_i,v} \cdot \varepsilon_{a_i,v}(t - t_{a_i})$ are all in their initial *linear* phase, its firing time t_v is determined in the noise-free model for $w_i := w_{a_i,v} \cdot \alpha_{a_i,v}$ by the equation $\sum_{i=1}^{n} w_i \cdot (t_v - t_{a_i} - d_{a_i,v}) = \Theta_v(0)$, or equivalently

$$t_v = \frac{\Theta_v(0)}{\sum_{i=1}^{n} w_i} + \frac{\sum_{i=1}^{n} w_i \cdot (t_{a_i} + d_{a_i,v})}{\sum_{i=1}^{n} w_i} \tag{1}$$

This equation reveals the somewhat surprising fact that (for a certain range of their parameters) spiking neurons can compute a *weighted sum* in terms of *firing times*, i.e. *temporal coding*. One should also note that in the case where all delays $d_{a_i,v}$ have the same value, the "weights" w_i of this weighted sum are encoded in the "strengths" $w_{a_i,v}$ of the synapses and their "sign" $\alpha_{a_i,v}$, as in the "firing rate interpretation". Finally according to (1) the coefficients of the presynaptic firing times t_{a_i} are automatically *normalized*, which appears to be of biological interest.

In the simplest scheme for temporal coding (which is closely related to that in [Hopfield, 1995]) an analog variable $x \in [0, 1]$ is encoded by the firing time $T - \gamma \cdot x$ of a neuron, where T is assumed to be independent of x (in a biological context T might be time-locked to the onset of a stimulus, or to some oscillation) and γ is some constant that is determined in the proof of Theorem 2.1 (e.g. $\gamma = \Delta/2$ in the noise-free case). In contrast to [Hopfield, 1995] we assume that both the inputs *and the outputs* of computations are encoded in this fashion. This has the advantage that one can *compose* computational modules.

We will first focus in Theorem 2.1 on the simulation of sigmoidal neural nets that employ the piecewise linear "linear saturated" activation function $\pi : \mathbf{R} \to [0,1]$ defined by $\pi(y) = 0$ if $y < 0$, $\pi(y) = y$ if $0 \leq y \leq 1$, and $\pi(y) = 1$ if $y > 1$. The Theorem 3.1 in the next section will imply that one can simulate with spiking neurons also sigmoidal neural nets that employ *arbitrary* continuous activation functions. Apart from the previously mentioned assumptions we will assume for the proofs of Theorem 2.1 and 3.1 that any EPSP satisfies $\varepsilon_{u,v}(x) = 0$ for all sufficiently large x, and $\varepsilon_{u,v}(x) \geq \varepsilon_{u,v}(d_{u,v} + \Delta)$ for all $x \in [d_{u,v} + \Delta, d_{u,v} + \Delta + \gamma]$. We assume that each IPSP is continuous, and has value 0 except for some interval of $\mathbf{R}$. Furthermore we assume for each EPSP and IPSP that $|\varepsilon_{u,v}(x)|$ grows at most linearly during the interval $[d_{u,v} + \Delta, d_{u,v} + \Delta + \gamma]$. In addition we assume that $\Theta_v(x) = \Theta_v(0)$ for sufficiently large x, and that $\Theta_v(x)$ is sufficiently large for $0 < x \leq \gamma$.

Theorem 2.1 *For any given $\varepsilon, \delta > 0$ one can simulate any given feedforward sigmoidal neural net N with activation function π by a network $\mathcal{N}_{N,\varepsilon,\delta}$ of noisy spiking neurons in temporal coding. More precisely, for any network input $x_1, \ldots, x_m \in [0,1]$ the output of $\mathcal{N}_{N,\varepsilon,\delta}$ differs with probability $\geq 1 - \delta$ by at most ε from that of N. Furthermore the computation time of $\mathcal{N}_{N,\varepsilon,\delta}$ depends neither on the number of gates in N nor on the parameters ε, δ, but only on the number of <u>layers</u> of the sigmoidal neural network N.*

We refer to [Maass, 1997] for details of the somewhat complicated proof. One employs the mechanism described by (1) to simulate through the firing time of a spiking neuron v a sigmoidal gate with activation function π for those gate-inputs where π operates in its linearly rising range. With the help of an auxiliary spiking neuron that fires at time T one can avoid the automatic "normalization" of the weights w_i that is provided by (1), and thereby compute a weighted sum with *arbitrary* given weights. In order to simulate in temporal coding the behaviour of the gate in the input range where π is "saturated" (i.e. constant), it suffices to employ some auxiliary spiking neurons which make sure that v fires exactly once during the relevant time window (and not shortly before that).

Since inputs and outputs of the resulting modules for each single gate of N are all given in temporal coding, one can compose these modules to simulate the multi-layer sigmoidal neural net N. With a bit of additional work one can ensure that this construction also works with *noisy* spiking neurons. ∎

3 Universal Approximation Property of Networks of Noisy Spiking Neurons with Temporal Coding

It is known [Leshno et al., 1993] that feedforward sigmoidal neural nets whose gates employ the activation function π can approximate with a single hidden layer for any $n, k \in \mathbf{N}$ any given continuous function $F : [0,1]^n \to [0,1]^k$ within any $\varepsilon > 0$ with regard to the L_∞-norm (i.e. uniform convergence). Hence we can derive the following result from Theorem 2.1:

Theorem 3.1 *Any given continuous function $F : [0,1]^n \to [0,1]^k$ can be approximated within any given $\varepsilon > 0$ with arbitrarily high reliability in temporal coding by* a network of noisy spiking neurons (SNN) with a single hidden layer (and hence within 15 ms for biologically realistic values of their time-constants). ■

Because of its generality this Theorem implies the same result also for *more general schemes of coding analog variables by the firing times of neurons*, besides the particular one that we have considered so far. In fact it implies that the same result holds for any other coding scheme C that is "continuously related" to the previously considered one in the sense that the transformation between firing times that encode an analog variable x in the here considered coding scheme and in the coding scheme C can be described by uniformly continuous functions in both directions.

4 Spiking Neurons have more Computational Power than Sigmoidal Neurons

We consider the *"element distinctness function"* $ED_n : (\mathbf{R}^+)^n \to \{0,1\}$ defined by

$$ED_n(s_1,\ldots,s_n) = \begin{cases} 1, & \text{if } s_i = s_j \text{ for some } i \neq j \\ 0, & \text{if } |s_i - s_j| \geq 1 \text{ for all } i,j \text{ with } i \neq j \\ \text{arbitrary}, & \text{else .} \end{cases}$$

If one encodes the value of input variable s_i by a firing of input neuron a_i at time $T_{in} - c \cdot s_i$, then for sufficiently large values of the constant $c > 0$ *a single noisy spiking neuron v can compute ED_n* with arbitrarily high reliability. This holds for any reasonable type of response functions, e.g. the ones shown in Fig. 1. The binary output of this computation is assumed to be encoded by the firing/non-firing of v. Hair-trigger situations are avoided since no assumptions have to be made about the firing or non-firing of v if EPSP's arrive with a temporal distance *between* 0 and c.

On the other hand the following result shows that a fairly large *sigmoidal* neural net is needed to compute the same function. Its proof provides the first application for Sontag's recent results about a new type of "dimension" d of a neural network N, where d is chosen maximal so that *every* subset of d inputs is shattered by N. Furthermore it expands a method due to [Koiran, 1995] for using the VC-dimension to prove lower bounds on network size.

Theorem 4.1 *Any sigmoidal neural net N that computes ED_n has at least $\frac{n-4}{2} - 1$ hidden units.*

Proof: Let N be an arbitrary sigmoidal neural net with k gates that computes ED_n. Consider *any* set $S \subseteq \mathbf{R}^+$ of size $n - 1$. Let $\lambda > 0$ be sufficiently large so that the numbers in $\lambda \cdot S$ have pairwise distance ≥ 2. Let A be a set of $n - 1$ numbers $> \max(\lambda \cdot S) + 2$ with pairwise distance ≥ 2.

By assumption N can decide for n arbitrary inputs from $\lambda \cdot S \cup A$ whether they are all different. Let N_λ be a variation of N where all weights on edges from the first input variable are multiplied with λ. Then N_λ can compute any function from

S into $\{0, 1\}$ after one has assigned a suitable fixed set of $n-1$ pairwise different numbers from $\lambda \cdot S \cup A$ to the last $n-1$ input variables.

Thus if one considers as *programmable* parameters of $\mathcal{N}$ the factor λ in the weights on edges from the first input variable and the $\leq k$ thresholds of gates that are connected to some of the other $n-1$ input variables, then $\mathcal{N}$ shatters S with these $k+1$ programmable parameters.

Since $S \subseteq \mathbf{R}^+$ of size $n-1$ was chosen *arbitrarily*, we can now apply the result from [Sontag, 1996], which yields an upper bound of $2w + 1$ for the maximal number d such that *every* set of d different inputs can be shattered by a sigmoidal neural net with w programmable parameters (note that this parameter d is in general much smaller than the VC-dimension of the neural net). For $w := k+1$ this implies in our case that $n - 1 \leq 2(k + 1) + 1$, hence $k \geq (n - 4)/2$. Thus $\mathcal{N}$ has at least $(n-4)/2$ computation nodes, and therefore at least $(n-4)/2 - 1$ hidden units. One should point out that due to the generality of Sontag's result this lower bound is valid for all common activation functions of sigmoidal gates, and even if $\mathcal{N}$ employs heaviside gates besides sigmoidal gates. ∎

Theorem 4.1 yields a lower bound of 4997 for the number of hidden units in any sigmoidal neural net that computes ED_n for $n = 10\,000$, where 10 000 is a common estimate for the number of inputs (i.e. synapses) of a biological neuron.

Finally we would like to point out that to the best of our knowledge Theorem 4.1 provides the largest known lower bound for *any* concrete function with n inputs on a sigmoidal neural net. The largest previously known lower bound for sigmoidal neural nets was $\Omega(n^{1/4})$, due to [Koiran, 1995].

5 Conclusions

Theorems 2.1 and 3.1 provide a model for analog computations in network of spiking neurons that is consistent with experimental results on the maximal computation speed of biological neural systems. As explained after Theorem 3.1, this result holds for a large variety of possible schemes for encoding analog variables by firing times.

These theoretical results hold *rigorously* only for a rather small time window of length γ for temporal coding. However a closer inspection of the construction shows that the actual shape of EPSP's and IPSP's in biological neurons provides an automatic adjustment of extreme values of the inputs t_{a_i} towards their average, which allows them to carry out rather similar computations for a substantially larger window size. It also appears to be of interest from the biological point of view that the synaptic weights play for temporal coding in our construction basically the same role as for rate coding, and hence the *same* network is in principle able to compute closely related analog functions in *both* coding schemes.

We have focused in our constructions on feedforward nets, but our method can for example also be used to simulate a Hopfield net with graded response by a network of noisy spiking neurons in temporal coding. A stable state of the Hopfield net corresponds then to a firing pattern of the simulating SNN where all neurons fire at the same frequency, with the *"pattern"* of the stable state encoded in their phase differences.

The theoretical results in this article may also provide additional goals and directions for a new computer technology based on *artificial* spiking neurons.

Acknowledgement

I would like to thank David Haussler, Pascal Koiran, and Eduardo Sontag for helpful communications.

References

[Bair & Koch, 1996] W. Bair, C. Koch, "Temporal precision of spike trains in extrastriate cortex of the behaving macaque monkey", *Neural Computation*, vol. 8, pp 1185–1202, 1996.

[Bialek & Rieke, 1992] W. Bialek, and F. Rieke, "Reliability and information transmission in spiking neurons", *Trends in Neuroscience*, vol. 15, pp 428–434, 1992.

[Hopfield, 1995] J. J. Hopfield, "Pattern recognition computation using action potential timing for stimulus representations", *Nature*, vol. 376, pp 33–36, 1995.

[Koiran, 1995] P. Koiran, "VC-dimension in circuit complexity", *Proc. of the 11th IEEE Conference on Computational Complexity*, pp 81–85, 1996.

[Leshno et al., 1993] M. Leshno, V. Y. Lin, A. Pinkus, and S. Schocken, "Multilayer feedforward networks with a nonpolynomial activation function can approximate any function", *Neural Networks*, vol. 6, pp 861–867, 1993.

[Maass, 1996a] W. Maass, "On the computational power of noisy spiking neurons", *Advances in Neural Information Processing Systems*, vol. 8, pp 211-217, MIT Press, Cambridge, 1996.

[Maass, 1996b] W. Maass, "Networks of spiking neurons: the third generation of neural network models", FTP-host: archive.cis.ohio-state.edu, FTP-filename: /pub/neuroprose/maass.third-generation.ps.Z, *Neural Networks*, to appear.

[Maass, 1997] W. Maass, "Fast sigmoidal networks via spiking neurons", to appear in Neural Computation. FTP-host: archive.cis.ohio-state.edu FTP-filename: /pub/neuroprose/maass.sigmoidal-spiking.ps.Z, *Neural Computation*, to appear in vol. 9, 1997.

[de Ruyter van Steveninck & Bialek, 1988] R. de Ruyter van Steveninck, and W. Bialek, "Real-time performance of a movement sensitive neuron in the blowfly visual system", *Proc. Roy. Soc. B*, vol. 234, pp 379–414, 1988.

[Sontag, 1996] E. D. Sontag, "Shattering all sets of k points in 'general position' requires $(k-1)/2$ parameters", http://www.math.rutgers.edu/~sontag/ , follow links to FTP archive.

[Thorpe & Imbert, 1989] S. T. Thorpe, and M. Imbert, "Biological constraints on connectionist modelling", In: *Connectionism in Perspective*, R. Pfeifer, Z. Schreter, F. Fogelman-Soulié, and L. Steels, eds., Elsevier, North-Holland, 1989.

On the Effect of Analog Noise in Discrete-Time Analog Computations

Wolfgang Maass
Institute for Theoretical Computer Science
Technische Universität Graz*

Pekka Orponen
Department of Mathematics
University of Jyväskylä[†]

Abstract

We introduce a model for noise-robust analog computations with discrete time that is flexible enough to cover the most important concrete cases, such as computations in noisy analog neural nets and networks of noisy spiking neurons. We show that the presence of arbitrarily small amounts of analog noise reduces the power of analog computational models to that of finite automata, and we also prove a new type of upper bound for the VC-dimension of computational models with analog noise.

1 Introduction

Analog noise is a serious issue in practical analog computation. However there exists no formal model for reliable computations by noisy analog systems which allows us to address this issue in an adequate manner. The investigation of noise-tolerant *digital* computations in the presence of stochastic failures of gates or wires had been initiated by [von Neumann, 1956]. We refer to [Cowan, 1966] and [Pippenger, 1989] for a small sample of the numerous results that have been achieved in this direction. In all these articles one considers computations which produce a correct output not with perfect reliability, but with probability $\geq \frac{1}{2} + \rho$ (for some parameter $\rho \in (0, \frac{1}{2}]$). The same framework (with stochastic failures of gates or wires) has been applied to analog neural nets in [Siegelmann, 1994].

The abovementioned approaches are insufficient for the investigation of noise in analog computations, because in analog computations one has to be concerned not only with occasional total failures of gates or wires, but also with "imprecision", i.e. with omnipresent smaller (and occasionally larger) perturbations of analog outputs

---

* Klosterwiesgasse 32/2, A-8010 Graz, Austria. E-mail: maass@igi.tu-graz.ac.at.
[†] P. O. Box 35, FIN-40351 Jyväskylä, Finland. E-mail: orponen@math.jyu.fi. Part of this work was done while this author was at the University of Helsinki, and during visits to the Technische Universität Graz and the University of Chile in Santiago.

of internal computational units. These perturbations may for example be given by Gaussian distributions. Therefore we introduce and investigate in this article a notion of noise-robust computation by noisy analog systems where we assume that the values of intermediate analog values are moved according to some quite arbitrary probability distribution. We consider – as in the traditional framework for noisy *digital* computations – arbitrary computations whose output is correct with some given probability $\geq \frac{1}{2} + \rho$ (for $\rho \in (0, \frac{1}{2}])$. We will restrict our attention to analog computation with *digital* output. Since we impose no restriction (such as continuity) on the type of operations that can be performed by computational units in an analog computational system, an output unit of such system can convert an analog value into a binary output via "thresholding".

Our model and our Theorem 3.1 are somewhat related to the analysis of probabilistic finite automata in [Rabin, 1963]. However there the finiteness of the state space simplifies the setup considerably. [Casey, 1996] addresses the special case of analog computations on recurrent neural nets (for those types of analog noise that can move an internal state at most over a distance ε) whose digital output is *perfectly reliable* (i.e. $\rho = 1/2$ in the preceding notation).[1]

The restriction to perfect reliability in [Casey, 1996] has immediate consequences for the types of analog noise processes that can be considered, and for the types of mathematical arguments that are needed for their investigation. In a computational model with perfect reliability of the output it cannot happen that an intermediate state $\underline{s}$ occurs at some step t both in a computation for an input $\underline{x}$ that leads to output "0" , and at step t in a computation for the same input "$\underline{x}$" that leads to output "1" . Hence an analysis of perfectly reliable computations can focus on *partitions* of intermediate states $\underline{s}$ according to the computations and the computation steps where they may occur.

Apparently many important concrete cases of noisy analog computations require a different type of analysis. Consider for example the special case of a sigmoidal neural net (with thresholding at the output), where for each input the output of an internal noisy sigmoidal gate is distributed according to some Gaussian distribution (perhaps restricted to the range of all possible output values which this sigmoidal gate can actually produce). In this case an intermediate state $\underline{s}$ of the computational system is a vector of values which have been produced by these Gaussian distributions. Obviously each such intermediate state $\underline{s}$ can occur at any fixed step t in *any* computation (in particular in computations with different network output for the same network input). Hence perfect reliability of the network output is unattainable in this case. For an investigation of the actual computational power of a sigmoidal neural net with Gaussian noise one has to drop the requirement of perfect reliability of the output, and one has to analyze how *probable* it is that a particular network output is given, and how *probable* it is that a certain intermediate state is assumed. Hence one has to analyze for each network input and each step t the different

---
[1] There are relatively few examples for nontrivial computations on common digital or analog computational models that can achieve *perfect reliability* of the output in spite of noisy internal components. Most constructions of noise-robust computational models rely on the *replication* of noisy computational units (see [von Neumann, 1956], [Cowan, 1966]). The idea of this method is that the average of the outputs of k identical noisy computational units (with stochastically independent noise processes) is with high probability close to the expected value of their output, if k is sufficiently large. However for *any* value of k there exists in general a small but nonzero probability that this average deviates strongly from its expected value. In addition, if one assumes that the computational unit that produces the output of the computations is also noisy, one cannot expect that the reliability of the output of the computation is larger than the reliability of this last computational unit. Consequently there exist many methods for *reducing* the error-probability of the output *to a small value*, but these methods cannot achieve error probability 0 at the output.

probability distributions over intermediate states $\underline{s}$ that are induced by computations of the noisy analog computational system. In fact, one may view the set of these probability distributions over intermediate states $\underline{s}$ as a generalized set of "states" of a noisy analog computational system. In general the mathematical structure of this generalized set of "states" is substantially more complex than that of the original set of intermediate states $\underline{s}$. We have introduced in [Maass, Orponen, 1996] some basic methods for analyzing this generalized set of "states", and the proofs of the main results in this article rely on this analysis.

The preceding remarks may illustrate that if one drops the assumption of perfect reliability of the output, it becomes more difficult to prove *upper* bounds for the power of noisy analog computations. We prove such upper bounds even for the case of *stochastic dependencies* among noises for different internal units, and for the case of *nonlinear dependencies* of the noise on the current internal state. Our results also cover noisy computations in hybrid analog/digital computational models, such as for example a neural net combined with a binary register, or a network of noisy spiking neurons where a neuron may temporarily assume the discrete state "not-firing". Obviously it becomes quite difficult to analyze the computational effect of such complex (but practically occuring) types of noise without a rigorous mathematical framework. We introduce in section 2 a mathematical framework that is general enough to subsume all these cases. The traditional case of noisy *digital* computations is captured as a special case of our definition.

One goal of our investigation of the effect of analog noise is to find out *which* features of analog noise have the most detrimental effect on the computational power of an analog computational system. This turns out to be a nontrivial question.[2] As a first step towards characterizing those aspects and parameters of analog noise that have a strong impact on the computational power of a noisy analog system, the proof of Theorem 3.1 (see [Maass, Orponen, 1996]) provides an explicit bound on the number of states of any finite automaton that can be implemented by an analog computational system with a given type of analog noise. It is quite surprising to see on which specific parameters of the analog noise the bound depends. Similarly the proofs of Theorem 3.4 and Theorem 3.5 provide explicit (although very large) upper bounds for the VC-dimension of noisy analog neural nets with batch input, which depend on specific parameters of the analog noise.

2 Preliminaries: Definitions and Examples

An *analog discrete-time computational system* (briefly: *computational system*) M is defined in a general way as a 5-tuple $\langle \Omega, p^0, F, \Sigma, s \rangle$, where Ω, the set of *states*, is a bounded subset of $\mathbf{R}^d$, $p^0 \in \Omega$ is a distinguished *initial state*, $F \subseteq \Omega$ is the set of *accepting states*, Σ is the *input domain*, and $s : \Omega \times \Sigma \to \Omega$ is the *transition function*. To avoid unnecessary pathologies, we impose the conditions that Ω and F are Borel subsets of $\mathbf{R}^d$, and for each $a \in \Sigma$, $s(p, a)$ is a measurable function of p. We also assume that Σ contains a distinguished null value ⊔, which may be used to pad the actual input to arbitrary length. The nonnull input domain is denoted by $\Sigma_0 = \Sigma - \{⊔\}$.

---

[2] For example, one might think that analog noise which is likely to move an internal state over a *large* distance is more harmful than another type of analog noise which keeps an internal state within its *neighborhood*. However this intuition is deceptive. Consider the extreme case of analog noise in a sigmoidal neural net which moves a gate output $x \in [-1, 1]$ to a value in the ε-neighborhood of $-x$. This type of noise moves some values x over large distances, but it appears to be less harmful for noise-robust computing than noise which moves x to an arbitrary value in the 10ε-neighborhood of x.

The intended noise-free dynamics of such a system M is as follows. The system starts its computation in state p^0, and on each single computation step on input element $a \in \Sigma_0$ moves from its current state p to its next state $s(p, a)$. After the actual input sequence has been exhausted, M may still continue to make pure computation steps. Each pure computation step leads it from a state p to the state $s(p, \sqcup)$. The system accepts its input if it enters a state in the class F at some point after the input has finished.

For instance, the *recurrent analog neural net* model of [Siegelmann, Sontag, 1991] (also known as the *"Brain State in a Box"* model) is obtained from this general framework as follows. For a network $\mathcal{N}$ with d neurons and activation values between -1 and 1, the state space is $\Omega = [-1, 1]^d$. The input domain may be chosen as either $\Sigma = \mathbf{R}$ or $\Sigma = \{-1, 0, 1\}$ (for "online" input) or $\Sigma = \mathbf{R}^n$ (for "batch" input).

Feedforward analog neural nets may also be modeled in the same manner, except that in this case one may wish to select as the state set $\Omega := ([-1, 1] \cup \{dormant\})^d$, where *dormant* is a distinguished value not in $[-1, 1]$. This special value is used to indicate the state of a unit whose inputs have not all yet been available at the beginning of a given computation step (e.g. for units on the l-th layer of a net at computation steps $t < l$).

The completely different model of a *network of m stochastic spiking neurons* (see e.g. [Maass, 1997]) is also a special case of our general framework.[3]

Let us then consider the *effect of noise in a computational system* M. Let $Z(p, B)$ be a function that for each state $p \in \Omega$ and Borel set $B \subseteq \Omega$ indicates the probability of noise moving state p to some state in B. The function Z is called the *noise process affecting* M, and it should satisfy the mild conditions of being a *stochastic kernel*, i.e., for each $p \in \Omega$, $Z(p, \cdot)$ should be a probability distribution, and for each Borel set B, $Z(\cdot, B)$ should be a measurable function.

We assume that there is some measure μ over Ω so that $Z(p, \cdot)$ is absolutely continuous with respect to μ for each $p \in \Omega$, i.e. $\mu(B) = 0$ implies $Z(p, B) = 0$ for every measurable $B \subseteq \Omega$. By the Radon–Nikodym theorem, Z then possesses a *density kernel* with respect to μ, i.e. there exists a function $z(\cdot, \cdot)$ such that for any state $p \in \Omega$ and Borel set $B \subseteq \Omega$, $Z(p, B) = \int_{q \in B} z(p, q) \, d\mu$.

We assume that this function $z(\cdot, \cdot)$ has values in $[0, \infty)$ and is measurable. (Actually, in view of our other conditions this can be assumed without loss of generality.)

The dynamics of a computational system M affected by a noise process Z is now defined as follows.[4] If the system starts in a state p, the distribution of states q obtained after a single computation step on input $a \in \Sigma$ is given by the density kernel $\pi_a(p, q) = z(s(p, a), q)$. Note that as a composition of two measurable func-

---

[3]In this case one wants to set $\Omega_{sp} := (\bigcup_{j=1}^{l} [0, T)^j \cup \{not\text{-}firing\})^m$, where $T > 0$ is a sufficiently large constant so that it suffices to consider only the firing history of the network during a preceding time interval of length T in order to determine whether a neuron fires (e.g. $T = 30$ ms for a biological neural system). If one partitions the time axis into discrete time windows $[0, T), [T, 2T), \ldots$, then in the noise-free case the firing events during each time window are completely determined by those in the preceding one. A component $p_i \in [0, T)^j$ of a state in this set Ω_{sp} indicates that the corresponding neuron i has fired exactly j times during the considered time interval, and it also specifies the j firing times of this neuron during this interval. Due to refractory effects one can choose $l < \infty$ for biological neural systems, e.g. $l = 15$ for $T = 30$ ms. With some straightforward formal operations one can also write this state set Ω_{sp} as a bounded subset of $\mathbf{R}^d$ for $d := l \cdot m$.

[4]We would like to thank Peter Auer for helpful conversations on this topic.

tions, π_a is again a measurable function. The long-term dynamics of the system is given by a Markov process, where the distribution $\pi_{xa}(p,q)$ of states after $|xa|$ computation steps with input $xa \in \Sigma^*$ starting in state p is defined recursively by $\pi_{xa}(p,q) = \int_{r \in \Omega} \pi_x(p,r) \cdot \pi_a(r,q) \, d\mu$.

Let us denote by $\pi_x(q)$ the distribution $\pi_x(p^0,q)$, i.e. the distribution of states of M after it has processed string x, starting from the initial state p^0. Let $\rho > 0$ be the required reliability level. In the most basic version the system M accepts (rejects) some input $x \in \Sigma_0^*$ if $\int_F \pi_x(q) \, d\mu \geq \frac{1}{2} + \rho$ (respectively $\leq \frac{1}{2} - \rho$). In less trivial cases the system may also perform pure computation steps after it has read all of the input. Thus, we define more generally that the system M *recognizes a set* $L \subseteq \Sigma_0^*$ *with reliability* ρ if for any $x \in \Sigma_0^*$:

$$x \in L \iff \int_F \pi_{xu}(q) \, d\mu \geq \frac{1}{2} + \rho \text{ for some } u \in \{\sqcup\}^*$$

$$x \notin L \iff \int_F \pi_{xu}(q) \, d\mu \leq \frac{1}{2} - \rho \text{ for all } u \in \{\sqcup\}^*.$$

This covers also the case of batch input, where $|x| = 1$ and Σ_0 is typically quite large (e.g. $\Sigma_0 = \mathbf{R}^n$).

3 Results

The proofs of Theorems 3.1, 3.4, 3.5 require a mild continuity assumption for the density functions $z(r, \cdot)$, which is satisfied in all concrete cases that we have examined. We do *not* require any *global* continuity property over Ω for the density functions $z(r, \cdot)$ because there are important special cases (see [Maass, Orponen, 1996]), where the state space Ω is a disjoint union of subspaces $\Omega_1, \ldots, \Omega_k$ with different measures on each subspace. We only assume that for some arbitrary partition of Ω into Borel sets $\Omega_1, \ldots, \Omega_k$ the density functions $z(r, \cdot)$ are uniformly continuous over each Ω_j, with moduli of continuity that can be bounded independently of r. In other words, we require that $z(\cdot, \cdot)$ satisfies the following condition:

We call a function $\pi(\cdot, \cdot)$ from Ω^2 into $\mathbf{R}$ *piecewise uniformly continuous* if for every $\varepsilon > 0$ there is a $\delta > 0$ such that for every $r \in \Omega$, and for all $p, q \in \Omega_j$, $j = 1, \ldots, k$:

$$\| p - q \| \leq \delta \quad \text{implies} \quad |\pi(r,p) - \pi(r,q)| \leq \varepsilon. \qquad (1)$$

If $z(\cdot, \cdot)$ satisfies this condition, we say that the resulting noise process Z is *piecewise uniformly continuous*.

Theorem 3.1 *Let $L \subseteq \Sigma_0^*$ be a set of sequences over an arbitrary input domain Σ_0. Assume that some computational system M, affected by a piecewise uniformly continuous noise process Z, recognizes L with reliability ρ, for some arbitrary $\rho > 0$. Then L is regular.*

The *proof* of Theorem 3.1 relies on an analysis of the space of probability density functions over the state set Ω. An upper bound on the number of states of a deterministic finite automaton that simulates M can be given in terms of the number k of components Ω_j of the state set Ω, the dimension and diameter of Ω, a bound on the values of the noise density function z, and the value of δ for $\varepsilon = \rho/4\mu(\Omega)$ in condition (1). For details we refer to [Maass, Orponen, 1996].[5] ∎

---

[5]A corresponding result is claimed in Corollary 3.1 of [Casey, 1996] for the special case

Remark 3.2 *In stark contrast to the results of [Siegelmann, Sontag, 1991] and [Maass, 1996] for the noise-free case, the preceding Theorem implies that both recurrent analog neural nets and recurrent networks of spiking neurons with online input from Σ_0^* can only recognize regular languages in the presence of any reasonable type of analog noise, even if their computation time is unlimited and if they employ arbitrary real-valued parameters.*

Let us say that a noise process Z defined on a set $\Omega \subseteq \mathbf{R}^d$ is *bounded by η* if it can move a state p only to other states q that have a distance $\leq \eta$ from p in the L_1-norm over $\mathbf{R}^d$, i.e. if its density kernel z has the property that for any $p = \langle p_1, \ldots, p_d \rangle$ and $q = \langle q_1, \ldots, q_d \rangle \in \Omega$, $z(p,q) > 0$ implies that $|q_i - p_i| \leq \eta$ for $i = 1, \ldots, d$. Obviously η-bounded noise processes are a very special class. However they provide an example which shows that the general upper bound of Theorem 3.1 is a sense optimal:

Theorem 3.3 *For every regular language $L \subseteq \{-1,1\}^*$ there is a constant $\eta > 0$ such that L can be recognized with perfect reliability (i.e. $\rho = \frac{1}{2}$) by a recurrent analog neural net in spite of any noise process Z bounded by η.* ∎

We now consider the effect of analog noise on discrete time analog computations with *batch-input*. The *proofs* of Theorems 3.4 and 3.5 are quite complex (see [Maass, Orponen, 1996]).

Theorem 3.4 *There exists a finite upper bound for the VC-dimension of layered feedforward sigmoidal neural nets and feedforward networks of spiking neurons with piecewise uniformly continuous analog noise (for arbitrary real-valued inputs, Boolean output computed with some arbitrary reliability $\rho > 0$, and arbitrary real-valued "programmable parameters") which does <u>not</u> depend on the size or structure of the network beyond its first hidden layer.* ∎

Theorem 3.5 *There exists a finite upper bound for the VC-dimension of recurrent sigmoidal neural nets and networks of spiking neurons with piecewise uniformly continuous analog noise (for arbitrary real valued inputs, Boolean output computed with some arbitrary reliability $\rho > 0$, and arbitrary real valued "programmable parameters") which does <u>not</u> depend on the computation time of the network, even if the computation time is allowed to vary for different inputs.* ∎

4 Conclusions

We have introduced a new framework for the analysis of analog noise in discrete-time analog computations that is better suited for "real-world" applications and

---

of recurrent neural nets with bounded noise and $\rho = 1/2$, i.e. for certain computations with *perfect reliability*. This case may not require the consideration of probability density functions. However it turns out that the proof for this special case in [Casey, 1996] is wrong. The proof of Corollary 3.1 in [Casey, 1996] relies on the argument that a compact set "can contain only a finite number of disjoint sets with nonempty interior". This argument is wrong, as the counterexample of the intervals $[1/(2i+1), 1/2i]$ for $i = 1, 2, \ldots$ shows. These infinitely many disjoint intervals are all contained in the compact set $[0,1]$. In addition, there is an independent problem with the *structure* of the proof of Corollary 3.1 in [Casey, 1996]. It is derived as a consequence of the proof of Theorem 3.1 in [Casey, 1996]. However that proof relies on the *assumption* that the recurrent neural net accepts a regular language. Hence the proof via probability density functions in [Maass, Orponen, 1996] provides the first valid proof for the claim of Corollary 3.1 in [Casey, 1996].

more flexible than previous models. In contrast to preceding models it also covers important concrete cases such as analog neural nets with a Gaussian distribution of noise on analog gate outputs, noisy computations with less than perfect reliability, and computations in networks of noisy spiking neurons.

Furthermore we have introduced adequate mathematical tools for analyzing the effect of analog noise in this new framework. These tools differ quite strongly from those that have previously been used for the investigation of noisy computations. We show that they provide new bounds for the computational power and VC-dimension of analog neural nets and networks of spiking neurons in the presence of analog noise.

Finally we would like to point out that our model for noisy analog computations can also be applied to completely different types of models for discrete time analog computation than neural nets, such as arithmetical circuits, the random access machine (RAM) with analog inputs, the parallel random access machine (PRAM) with analog inputs, various computational discrete-time dynamical systems and (with some minor adjustments) also the BSS model [Blum, Shub, Smale, 1989]. Our framework provides for each of these models an adequate definition of noise-robust computation in the presence of analog noise, and our results provide upper bounds for their computational power and VC-dimension in terms of characteristica of their analog noise.

References

[Blum, Shub, Smale, 1989] L. Blum, M. Shub, S. Smale, On a theory of computation over the real numbers: NP-completeness, recursive functions and universal machines. *Bulletin of the Amer. Math. Soc. 21* (1989), 1–46.

[Casey, 1996] M. Casey, The dynamics of discrete-time computation, with application to recurrent neural networks and finite state machine extraction. *Neural Computation 8* (1996), 1135–1178.

[Cowan, 1966] J. D. Cowan, Synthesis of reliable automata from unreliable components. *Automata Theory* (E. R. Caianiello, ed.), 131–145. Academic Press, New York, 1966.

[Maass, 1996] W. Maass, Lower bounds for the computational power of networks of spiking neurons. *Neural Computation 8* (1996), 1–40.

[Maass, 1997] W. Maass, Fast sigmoidal networks via spiking neurons, to appear in *Neural Computation 9*, 1997. FTP-host: archive.cis.ohio-state.edu, FTP-filename: /pub/neuroprose /maass.sigmoidal-spiking.ps.Z.

[Maass, Orponen, 1996] W. Maass, P. Orponen, On the effect of analog noise in discrete-time analog computations (journal version), submitted for publication; see http://www.math.jyu.fi/~orponen/papers/noisyac.ps.

[Pippenger, 1989] N. Pippenger, Invariance of complexity measures for networks with unreliable gates. *J. Assoc. Comput. Mach. 36* (1989), 531–539.

[Rabin, 1963] M. Rabin, Probabilistic automata. *Information and Control 6* (1963), 230–245.

[Siegelmann, 1994] H. T. Siegelmann, On the computational power of probabilistic and faulty networks. *Proc. 21st International Colloquium on Automata, Languages, and Programming*, 23–34. Lecture Notes in Computer Science 820, Springer-Verlag, Berlin, 1994.

[Siegelmann, Sontag, 1991] H. T. Siegelmann, E. D. Sontag, Turing computability with neural nets. *Appl. Math. Letters 4(6)* (1991), 77–80.

[von Neumann, 1956] J. von Neumann, Probabilistic logics and the synthesis of reliable organisms from unreliable components. *Automata Studies* (C. E. Shannon, J. E. McCarthy, eds.), 329–378. Annals of Mathematics Studies 34, Princeton University Press, Princeton, NJ, 1956.

A mean field algorithm for Bayes learning in large feed-forward neural networks

Manfred Opper
Institut für Theoretische Physik
Julius-Maximilians-Universität, Am Hubland
D-97074 Würzburg, Germany
opper@physik.Uni-Wuerzburg.de

Ole Winther
CONNECT
The Niels Bohr Institute
Blegdamsvej 17
2100 Copenhagen, Denmark
winther@connect.nbi.dk

Abstract

We present an algorithm which is expected to realise Bayes optimal predictions in large feed-forward networks. It is based on mean field methods developed within statistical mechanics of disordered systems. We give a derivation for the single layer perceptron and show that the algorithm also provides a leave-one-out cross-validation test of the predictions. Simulations show excellent agreement with theoretical results of statistical mechanics.

1 INTRODUCTION

Bayes methods have become popular as a consistent framework for regularization and model selection in the field of neural networks (see e.g. [MacKay,1992]). In the Bayes approach to statistical inference [Berger,1985] one assumes that the prior uncertainty about parameters of an unknown data generating mechanism can be encoded in a probability distribution, the so called *prior*. Using the prior and the likelihood of the data given the parameters, the *posterior* distribution of the parameters can be derived from Bayes rule. From this posterior, various estimates for functions of the parameter, like predictions about unseen data, can be calculated. However, in general, those predictions cannot be realised by specific parameter values, but only by an ensemble average over parameters according to the posterior probability.

Hence, exact implementations of Bayes method for neural networks require averages over network parameters which in general can be performed by time consuming

Monte Carlo procedures. There are however useful approximate approaches for calculating posterior averages which are based on the assumption of a Gaussian form of the posterior distribution [MacKay,1992]. Under regularity conditions on the likelihood, this approximation becomes asymptotically exact when the number of data is large compared to the number of parameters. This Gaussian ansatz for the posterior may not be justified when the number of examples is small or comparable to the number of network weights. A second cause for its failure would be a situation where discrete classification labels are produced from a probability distribution which is a nonsmooth function of the parameters. This would include the case of a network with *threshold* units learning a *noise free* binary classification problem.

In this contribution we present an alternative approximate realization of Bayes method for neural networks, which is not based on asymptotic posterior normality. The posterior averages are performed using mean field techniques known from the statistical mechanics of disordered systems. Those are expected to become exact in the limit of a large number of network parameters under additional assumptions on the statistics of the input data. Our analysis follows the approach of [Thouless, Anderson& Palmer,1977] (TAP) as adapted to the simple perceptron by [Mézard,1989].

The basic set up of the Bayes method is as follows: We have a training set consisting of m input-output pairs $D_m = \{(\mathbf{s}^\mu, \sigma^\mu), m = 1, \ldots, \mu\}$, where the outputs are generated independently from a conditional probability distribution $P(\sigma^\mu|\mathbf{w}, \mathbf{s}^\mu)$. This probability is assumed to describe the output σ^μ to an input $\mathbf{s}^\mu$ of a neural network with weights $\mathbf{w}$ subject to a suitable noise process. If we assume that the unknown parameters $\mathbf{w}$ are randomly distributed with a prior distribution $p(\mathbf{w})$, then according to Bayes theorem our knowledge about $\mathbf{w}$ after seeing m examples is expressed through the posterior distribution

$$p(\mathbf{w}|D_m) = Z^{-1} p(\mathbf{w}) \prod_{\mu=1}^{m} P(\sigma^\mu|\mathbf{w}, \mathbf{s}^\mu) \qquad (1)$$

where $Z = \int d\mathbf{w} p(\mathbf{w}) \prod_{\mu=1}^{m} P(\sigma^\mu|\mathbf{w}, \mathbf{s}^\mu)$ is called the partition function in statistical mechanics and the *evidence* in Bayesian terminology. Taking the average with respect to the posterior eq. (1), which in the following will be denoted by angle brackets, gives Bayes estimates for various quantities. For example the optimal predictive probability for an output σ to a new input $\mathbf{s}$ is given by $\hat{P}^{\text{Bayes}}(\sigma|\mathbf{s}) = \langle P(\sigma|\mathbf{w}, \mathbf{s}) \rangle$.

In section 2 exact equations for the posterior averaged weights $\langle \mathbf{w} \rangle$ are derived for arbitrary networks. In 3 we specialize these equations to a perceptron and develop a mean field ansatz in section 4. The resulting system of mean field equations equations is presented in section 5. In section 6 we consider Bayes optimal predictions and a leave-one-out estimator for the generalization error. We conclude in section 7 with a discussion of our results.

2 A RESULT FOR POSTERIOR AVERAGES FROM GAUSSIAN PRIORS

In this section we will derive an interesting equation for the posterior mean of the weights for arbitrary networks when the prior is Gaussian. This average of the weights can be calculated for the distribution (1) by using the following simple and well known result for averages over Gaussian distributions.

Let v be a Gaussian random variable with zero means. Then for any function $f(v)$, we have
$$\langle v f(v)\rangle_G = \langle v^2 \rangle_G \cdot \langle \frac{df(v)}{dv}\rangle_G. \tag{2}$$
Here $\langle \ldots \rangle_G$ denotes the average over the Gaussian distribution of v. The relation is easily proved from an integration by parts.

In the following we will specialize to an isotropic Gaussian prior $p(\mathbf{w}) = \frac{1}{\sqrt{2\pi}^N} e^{-\frac{1}{2}\mathbf{w}\cdot\mathbf{w}}$. In [Opper & Winter,1996] anisotropic priors are treated as well. Applying (2) to each component of $\mathbf{w}$ and the function $\prod_{\mu=1}^m P(\sigma^\mu|\mathbf{w},\mathbf{s}^\mu)$, we get the following equations

$$\langle \mathbf{w} \rangle = Z^{-1} \int d\mathbf{w}\ \mathbf{w} p(\mathbf{w}) \prod_{\nu=1}^m P(\sigma^\nu|\mathbf{w},\mathbf{s}^\nu)$$

$$= Z^{-1} \sum_{\mu=1}^m \int d\mathbf{w} p(\mathbf{w}) \prod_{\nu\neq\mu}^m P(\sigma^\nu|\mathbf{w},\mathbf{s}^\nu) \nabla_\mathbf{w} P(\sigma^\mu|\mathbf{w},\mathbf{s}^\mu) \tag{3}$$

$$= \sum_{\mu=1}^m \frac{\langle \nabla_\mathbf{w} P(\sigma^\mu|\mathbf{w},\mathbf{s}^\mu)\rangle_\mu}{\langle P(\sigma^\mu|\mathbf{w},\mathbf{s}^\mu)\rangle_\mu}.$$

Here $\langle \ldots \rangle_\mu = \frac{\int d\mathbf{w} p(\mathbf{w}) \ldots \prod_{\nu\neq\mu} P(\sigma^\nu|\mathbf{w},\mathbf{s}^\nu)}{\int d\mathbf{w} p(\mathbf{w}) \prod_{\nu\neq\mu} P(\sigma^\nu|\mathbf{w},\mathbf{s}^\nu)}$ is a *reduced* average over a posterior where the μ-th example is kept out of the training set and $\nabla_\mathbf{w}$ denotes the gradient with respect to $\mathbf{w}$.

3 THE PERCEPTRON

In the following, we will utilize the fact that for neural networks, the probability (1) depends only on the so called internal fields $\Delta = \frac{1}{\sqrt{N}}\mathbf{w}\cdot\mathbf{s}$.

A simple but nontrivial example is the perceptron with N dimensional input vector $\mathbf{s}$ and output $\sigma(\mathbf{w},\mathbf{s}) = \text{sign}(\Delta)$. We will generalize the noise free model by considering label noise in which the output is flipped, i.e. $\sigma\Delta < 0$ with a probability $(1+e^\beta)^{-1}$. (For simplicity, we will assume that β is known such that no prior on β is needed.) The conditional probability may thus be written as

$$P(\sigma^\mu\Delta^\mu) \equiv P(\sigma^\mu|\mathbf{w},\mathbf{s}^\mu) = \frac{e^{-\beta\Theta(-\sigma^\mu\Delta^\mu)}}{1+e^{-\beta}}, \tag{4}$$

where $\Theta(x) = 1$ for $x > 0$ and 0 otherwise. Obviously, this a nonsmooth function of the weights $\mathbf{w}$, for which the posterior will not become Gaussian asymptotically.

For this case (3) reads

$$\langle \mathbf{w} \rangle = \frac{1}{\sqrt{N}}\sum_{\mu=1}^m \frac{\langle P'(\sigma^\mu\Delta^\mu)\rangle_\mu}{\langle P(\sigma^\mu\Delta^\mu)\rangle_\mu}\ \sigma^\mu\mathbf{s}^\mu = \tag{5}$$

$$\frac{1}{\sqrt{N}}\sum_{\mu=1}^m \frac{\int d\Delta f_\mu(\Delta) P'(\sigma^\mu\Delta)}{\int d\Delta f_\mu(\Delta) P(\sigma^\mu\Delta)}\ \sigma^\mu\mathbf{s}^\mu$$

$f_\mu(\Delta)$ is the density of $\frac{1}{\sqrt{N}}\mathbf{w} \cdot \mathbf{s}^\mu$, when the weights $\mathbf{w}$ are randomly drawn from a posterior, where example $(\mathbf{s}^\mu, \sigma^\mu)$ was kept out of the training set. This result states that the weights are linear combinations of the input vectors. It gives an example of the ability of Bayes method to regularize a network model: the effective number of parameters will never exceed the number of data points.

4 MEAN FIELD APPROXIMATION

Sofar, no approximations have been made to obtain eqs. (3,5). In general $f_\mu(\Delta)$ depends on the entire set of data D_m and can not be calculated easily. Hence, we look for a useful approximation to these densities.

We split the internal field into its average and fluctuating parts, i.e. we set $\Delta^\mu = \langle \Delta^\mu \rangle_\mu + v^\mu$, with $v^\mu = \frac{1}{\sqrt{N}}(\mathbf{w} - \langle \mathbf{w} \rangle_\mu)\mathbf{s}^\mu$. Our mean field approximation is based on the assumption of a central limit theorem for the fluctuating part of the internal field, v^μ which enters in the reduced average of eq. (5). This means, we assume that the *non-Gaussian fluctuations* of w_i around $\langle w_i \rangle_\mu$, when mulitplied by s_i^μ will sum up to make v^μ a Gaussian random variable. The important point is here that for the reduced average, the w_i are not correlated to the s_i^μ! [1]

We expect that this Gaussian approximation is reasonable, when N, the number of network weights is sufficiently large.Following ideas of [Mézard, Parisi & Virasoro,1987] and [Mézard,1989], who obtained mean field equations for a variety of disordered systems in statistical mechanics, one can argue that in many cases this assumption may be exactly fulfilled in the 'thermodynamic limit' $m, N \to \infty$ with $\alpha = \frac{m}{N}$ fixed. According to this ansatz, we get

$$f_\mu(\Delta) \simeq \frac{\exp\left[-\frac{(\Delta - \langle \Delta^\mu \rangle_\mu)^2}{2\lambda^\mu}\right]}{\sqrt{2\pi\lambda^\mu}}$$

in terms of the second moment of v^μ $\lambda^\mu \equiv \frac{1}{N} \sum_{i,j} s_i^\mu s_j^\mu (\langle w_i w_j \rangle_\mu - \langle w_i \rangle_\mu \langle w_j \rangle_\mu)$.

To evaluate (5) we need to calculate the mean $\langle \Delta^\mu \rangle_\mu$ and the variance λ^μ. The first problem is treated easily within the Gaussian approximation.

$$\begin{aligned}\langle \Delta_k^\mu \rangle_\mu &= \langle \Delta^\mu \rangle - \langle v^\mu \rangle \\ &= \langle \Delta^\mu \rangle - \frac{\langle v^\mu P(\sigma^\mu \Delta^\mu) \rangle_\mu}{\langle P(\sigma^\mu \Delta^\mu) \rangle_\mu} \\ &= \langle \Delta^\mu \rangle - \lambda^\mu \frac{\langle P'(\sigma^\mu \Delta^\mu) \rangle_\mu}{\langle P(\sigma^\mu \Delta^\mu) \rangle_\mu} \sigma^\mu \end{aligned} \qquad (6)$$

In the third line (2) has been used again for the Gaussian random variable v^μ.

Sofar, the calculation of the variance λ^μ for *general inputs* is an open problem. However, we can make a further reasonable ansatz, when the distribution of the inputs is known. The following approximation for λ^μ is expected to become exact in the thermodynamic limit if the inputs of the training set are drawn independently

---

[1] Note that the fluctuations of the internal field with respect to the *full* posterior mean (which depends on the input $\mathbf{s}^\mu$) is *non* Gaussian, because the different terms in the sum become slightly correlated.

from a distribution, where all components s_i are uncorrelated and normalized i.e. $\overline{s_i} = 0$ and $\overline{s_i s_j} = \delta_{ij}$. The bars denote expectation over the distribution of inputs. For the generalisation to a correlated input distribution see [Opper& Winther,1996]. Our basic mean field assumption is that the fluctuations of the λ^μ with the data set can be neglected so that we can replace them by their averages $\overline{\lambda^\mu}$. Since the reduced posterior averages are not correlated with the data s_i^μ, we obtain $\lambda^\mu \simeq \frac{1}{N}\sum_i(\langle w_i^2\rangle_\mu - \langle w_i\rangle_\mu^2)$. Finally, we replace the reduced average by the expectation over the full posterior, neglecting terms of order $1/N$. Using $\sum_i \langle w_i^2 \rangle = N$, which follows from our choice of the Gaussian prior, we get $\lambda^\mu \simeq \lambda = 1 - \frac{1}{N}\sum_i \langle w_i \rangle^2$. This depends only on known quantities.

5 MEAN FIELD EQUATIONS FOR THE PERCEPTRON

(5) and (6) give a selfconsistent set of equations for the variable $x^\mu \equiv \frac{\langle P'(\sigma^\mu \Delta^\mu)\rangle_\mu}{\langle P(\sigma^\mu \Delta^\mu)\rangle_\mu}$. We finally get

$$\langle \mathbf{w} \rangle = \frac{1}{\sqrt{N}} \sum_{\mu=1}^{m} x^\mu \sigma^\mu \mathbf{s}^\mu \quad (7)$$

with

$$x^\mu = \frac{(1-e^{-\beta})e^{-z^{\mu 2}/2}}{\sqrt{2\pi\lambda}[e^{-\beta} + (1-e^{-\beta})H(-\sigma^\mu z^\mu)]} \quad (8)$$

$$z^\mu = \frac{\frac{1}{\sqrt{N}}\langle \mathbf{w} \rangle \cdot \mathbf{s}^\mu - \lambda \sigma^\mu x^\mu}{\sqrt{\lambda}}. \quad (9)$$

$$H(t) = \int_t^\infty dx e^{-x^2/2}/\sqrt{2\pi}$$

$$\lambda = 1 - \frac{1}{N}\sum_i \langle w_i \rangle^2.$$

These mean field equations can be solved by iteration. It is useful to start with a small number of data and then to increase the number of data in steps of 1 - 10. Numerical work show that the algorithm works well even for small systems sizes, $N \simeq 15$.

6 BAYES PREDICTIONS AND LEAVE-ONE-OUT

After solving the mean field equations we can make optimal Bayesian classifications for new data $\mathbf{s}$ by chosing the output label with the largest predictive probability. In case of output noise this reduces to $\sigma^{\text{Bayes}}(\mathbf{s}) = \text{sign}\langle \sigma(\mathbf{w}, \mathbf{s})\rangle$ Since the posterior distribution is independent of the new input vector we can apply the Gaussian assumption again to the internal field, Δ. and obtain $\sigma^{\text{Bayes}}(\mathbf{s}) = \sigma(\langle \mathbf{w}\rangle, \mathbf{s})$, i.e for the simple perceptron the averaged weights implement the Bayesian prediction. This will not be the case for multi-layer neural networks.

We can also get an estimate for the generalization error which occurs on the prediction of new data. The generalization error for the Bayes prediction is defined by $\epsilon^{\text{Bayes}} = \langle \Theta\left(-\sigma(\mathbf{s})\langle\sigma(\mathbf{w},\mathbf{s})\rangle\right)\rangle_\mathbf{s}$, where $\sigma(\mathbf{s})$ is the true output and $\langle\ldots\rangle_\mathbf{s}$ denotes average over the input distribution. To obtain the *leave-one-out estimator* of ϵ one

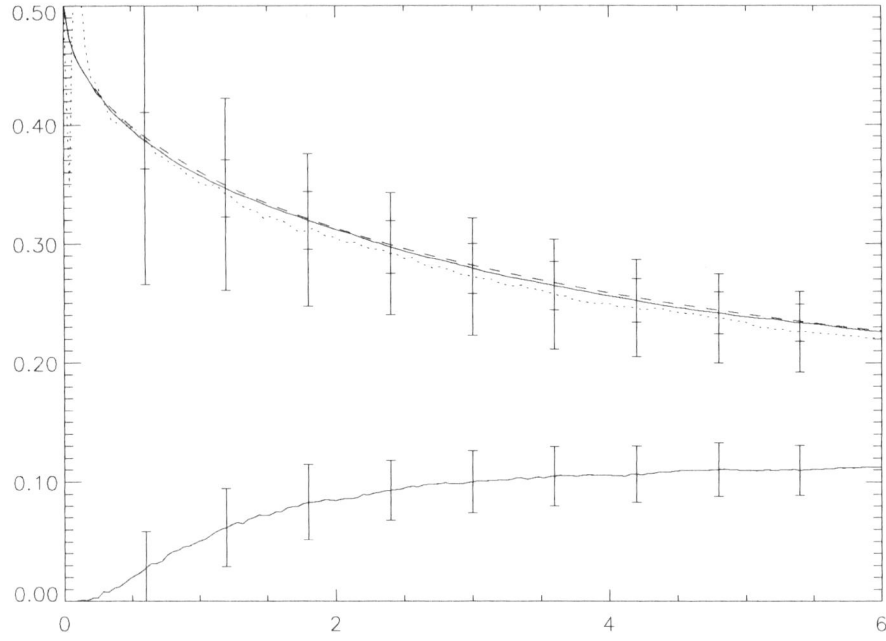

Figure 1: Error vs. $\alpha = m/N$ for the simple perceptron with output noise $\beta = 0.5$ and $N = 50$ averaged over 200 runs. The full lines are the simulation results (upper curve shows prediction error and the lower curve shows training error). The dashed line is the theoretical result for $N \to \infty$ obtained from statistical mechanics [Opper & Haussler,1991]. The dotted line with larger error bars is the moving control estimate.

removes the μ-th example from the training set and trains the network using only the remaining $m - 1$ examples. The μ'th example is used for testing. Repeating this procedure for all μ an unbiased estimate for the Bayes generalization error with $m-1$ training data is obtained as the mean value $\epsilon_{\text{MC}}^{\text{Bayes}} = \frac{1}{m} \sum_\mu \Theta\left(-\sigma^\mu \langle \sigma(\mathbf{w}, \mathbf{s}^\mu) \rangle_\mu\right)$ which is exactly the type of reduced averages which are calculated within our approach. Figure 1 shows a result of simulations of our algorithm when the inputs are uncorrelated and the outputs are generated from a teacher perceptron with fixed noise rate β.

7 CONCLUSION

In this paper we have presented a mean field algorithm which is expected to implement a Bayesian optimal classification well in the limit of large networks. We have explained the method for the single layer perceptron. An extension to a simple multilayer network, the so called committee machine with a tree architecture is discussed in [Opper& Winther,1996]. The algorithm is based on a Gaussian assumption for the distribution of the internal fields, which seems reasonable for large networks. The main problem sofar is the restriction to ideal situations such as a known distribution of inputs which is not a realistic assumption for real world data. However, this assumption only entered in the calculation of the variance of the Gaussian field. More theoretical work is necessary to find an approximation to the variance which is valid in more general cases. A promising approach is a derivation of the mean field equations directly from an approximation to the free energy $-\ln(Z)$. Besides a deeper understanding this would also give us the possibility to use the method with the so called evidence framework, where the partition function (evidence) can be used to estimate unknown (hyper-) parameters of the model class [Berger,1985]. It will further be important to extend the algorithm to fully connected architectures. In that case it might be necessary to make further approximations in the mean field method.

ACKNOWLEDGMENTS

This research is supported by a Heisenberg fellowship of the *Deutsche Forschungsgemeinschaft* and by the Danish Research Councils for the Natural and Technical Sciences through the Danish Computational Neural Network Center (CONNECT).

REFERENCES

Berger, J. O. (1985) *Statistical Decision theory and Bayesian Analysis*, Springer-Verlag, New York.

MacKay, D. J. (1992) *A practical Bayesian framework for backpropagation networks*, Neural Comp. **4** 448.

Mézard, M., Parisi G. & Virasoro M. A. (1987) *Spin Glass Theory and Beyond*, Lecture Notes in Physics, 9, World Scientific, .

Mézard, M. (1989) *The space of interactions in neural networks: Gardner's calculation with the cavity method* J. Phys. A **22**, 2181 .

Opper, M. & Haussler, D. (1991) in *IVth Annual Workshop on Computational Learning Theory (COLT91)*, Morgan Kaufmann.

Opper M. & Winther O (1996) *A mean field approach to Bayes learning in feedforward neural networks*, Phys. Rev. Lett. **76** 1964.

Thouless, D.J., Anderson, P. W. & Palmer, R.G. (1977), *Solution of 'Solvable model of a spin glass'* Phil. Mag. **35**, 593.

Removing Noise in On-Line Search using Adaptive Batch Sizes

Genevieve B. Orr
Department of Computer Science
Willamette University
900 State Street
Salem, Oregon 97301
gorr@willamette.edu

Abstract

Stochastic (on-line) learning can be faster than batch learning. However, at late times, the learning rate must be annealed to remove the noise present in the stochastic weight updates. In this annealing phase, the convergence rate (in mean square) is at best proportional to $1/\tau$ where τ is the number of input presentations. An alternative is to increase the batch size to remove the noise. In this paper we explore convergence for LMS using 1) small but fixed batch sizes and 2) an adaptive batch size. We show that the best adaptive batch schedule is exponential and has a rate of convergence which is the same as for annealing, i.e., at best proportional to $1/\tau$.

1 Introduction

Stochastic (on-line) learning can speed learning over its batch training particularly when data sets are large and contain redundant information [Møl93]. However, at late times in learning, noise present in the weight updates prevents complete convergence from taking place. To reduce the noise, the learning rate is slowly decreased (annealed) at late times. The optimal annealing schedule is asymptotically proportional to $\frac{1}{t}$ where t is the iteration [Gol87, LO93, Orr95]. This results in a rate of convergence (in mean square) that is also proportional to $\frac{1}{t}$.

An alternative method of reducing the noise is to simply switch to (noiseless) batch mode when the noise regime is reached. However, since batch mode can be slow, a better idea is to slowly increase the batch size starting with 1 (pure stochastic) and slowly increasing it only "as needed" until it reaches the training set size (pure batch). In this paper we 1) investigate the convergence behavior of LMS when using small fixed batch sizes, 2) determine the best schedule when using an adaptive batch size at each iteration, 3) analyze the convergence behavior of the adaptive batch algorithm, and 4) compare this convergence rate to the alternative method of annealing the learning rate.

Other authors have approached the problem of redundant data by also proposing techniques for training on subsets of the data. For example, Pluto [PW93] uses active data selection to choose a concise subset for training. This subset is slowly added to over time as needed. Moller [Møl93] proposes combining scaled conjugate gradient descent (SCG) with what he refers to as blocksize updating. His algorithm uses an iterative approach and assumes that the block size does not vary rapidly during training. In this paper, we take the simpler approach of just choosing exemplars *at random* at each iteration. Given this, we then analyze in detail the convergence behavior. Our results are more of theoretical than practical interest since the equations we derive are complex functions of quantities such as the Hessian that are impractical to compute.

2 Fixed Batch Size

In this section we examine the convergence behavior for LMS using a fixed batch size. We assume that we are given a large but finite sized training set $T \equiv \{z_i \equiv (x_i, d_i)\}_{i=1}^{N}$ where $x_i \in \mathcal{R}^m$ is the ith input and $d_i \in \mathcal{R}$ is the corresponding target. We further assume that the targets are generated using a signal plus noise model so that we can write

$$d_i = w_*^T x_i + \epsilon_i \tag{1}$$

where $\omega_* \in \mathcal{R}^m$ is the optimal weight vector and the ϵ_i is zero mean noise. Since the training set is assumed to be large we take the average of ϵ_i and $x_i \epsilon_i$ over the training set to be approximately zero. Note that we consider only the problem of optimization of the ω *over the training set* and do not address the issue of obtaining good generalization over the distribution from which the training set was drawn.

At each iteration, we assume that exactly n samples are randomly drawn *without replacement* from T where $1 \leq n \leq N$. We denote this batch of size n drawn at time t by $B_n(t) \equiv \{z_{k_i}\}_{i=1}^{n}$. When $n = 1$ we have pure on-line training and when $n = N$ we have pure batch. We choose to sample without replacement so that as the batch size is increased, we have a smooth transition from on line to batch.

For LMS, the squared error at iteration t *for a batch* of size n is

$$\mathcal{E}_{B_n(t)} \equiv \frac{1}{n} \sum_{z_i \in B_n(t)} \mathcal{E}(z_i) \quad \text{where} \quad \mathcal{E}(z_i) = \frac{1}{2}(d_i - \omega_t^T x_i)^2 \tag{2}$$

and where $\omega_t \in \mathcal{R}^m$ is the current weight in the network. The update weight equation is then $\omega_{t+1} = \omega_t - \mu \frac{\partial \mathcal{E}_{B_n}}{\partial \omega_t}$ where μ is the fixed learning rate. Rewriting this in terms of the weight error $v \equiv \omega - \omega_*$ and defining $g_{B_n,t} \equiv \partial \mathcal{E}_{B_n(t)} / \partial v_t$ we obtain

$$v_{t+1} = v_t + \frac{\mu}{n} \sum_{z_i \in B_n} (\epsilon_i - v_t^T x_i) x_i = v_t - \mu g_{B_n,t}. \tag{3}$$

Convergence (in mean square) to ω_* can be characterized by the rate of change of the average squared norm of the weight error $E[v^2]$ where $v^2 \equiv v^T v$. From (3) we obtain an expression for v_{t+1}^2 in terms of v_t,

$$v_{t+1}^2 = v_t^2 - 2\mu v_t^T g_{B_n,t} + \mu^2 g_{B_n,t}^2. \tag{4}$$

To compute the expected value of v_{t+1}^2 conditioned on v_t we can average the right side of (4) over all possible ways that the batch $B_n(t)$ can be chosen from the N training examples. In appendix A, we show that

$$\langle g_{B_n,t}\rangle_B = \langle g_{i,t}\rangle_N \tag{5}$$

$$\langle g_{B_n,t}^2\rangle_B = \frac{N-n}{n(N-1)}\langle g_{i,t}^2\rangle_N + \frac{(n-1)N}{(N-1)n}\langle g_{i,t}\rangle_N^2 \tag{6}$$

where $\langle\cdot\rangle_N$ denotes average over all examples *in the training set*, $\langle\cdot\rangle_B$ denotes average *over the possible batches* drawn at time t, and $g_{i,t} \equiv \partial\mathcal{E}(z_i)/\partial v_t$. The averages over the entire training set are

$$\langle g_{i,t}\rangle_N = \frac{1}{N}\sum_{i=1}^N \frac{\partial\mathcal{E}(z_i)}{\partial v_t} = -\sum_{i=1}^N \epsilon_i x_i - v_t^T x_i x_i = Rv_t \tag{7}$$

$$\langle g_{i,t}^2\rangle_N = \frac{1}{N}\sum_{i=1}^N (\epsilon_i x_i - v_t^T x_i x_i)^T (\epsilon_i x_i - v_t^T x_i x_i) = \sigma_\epsilon^2(\text{Tr } R) + v_t^T S v_t \tag{8}$$

where $R \equiv \langle xx^T\rangle_N$, $S \equiv \langle xx^T xx^T\rangle_N$[1], $\sigma_\epsilon^2 \equiv \langle\epsilon^2\rangle$ and $(\text{Tr } R)$ is the trace of R. These equations together with (5) and (6) in (4) gives the expected value of v_{t+1} conditioned on v_t

$$\langle v_{t+1}^2|v_t\rangle = v_t^T\left\{I - 2\mu R + \mu^2\left(\frac{N(n-1)}{(N-1)n}R^2 + \frac{N-n}{(N-1)n}S\right)\right\}v_t + \frac{\mu^2\sigma_\epsilon^2(\text{Tr } R)(N-n)}{n(N-1)}. \tag{9}$$

Note that this reduces to the standard stochastic and batch update equations when $n = 1$ and $n = N$, respectively.

2.0.1 Special Cases: 1-D solution and Spherically Symmetric

In 1-dimension we can average over v_t in (9) to give

$$\langle v_{t+1}^2\rangle = \alpha\langle v_t^2\rangle + \beta \tag{10}$$

where

$$\alpha = 1 - 2\mu R + \mu^2\left(\frac{N(n-1)}{(N-1)n}R^2 + \frac{N-n}{(N-1)n}S\right), \quad \beta = \frac{\mu^2\sigma_\epsilon^2 R(N-n)}{n(N-1)} \tag{11}$$

and where R and S simplify to $R = \langle x^2\rangle_N$, $S = \langle x^4\rangle_N$. This is a difference equation which can be solved exactly to give

$$\langle v_t^2\rangle = \alpha^{t-t_0}\langle v_0^2\rangle + \frac{1-\alpha^{t-t_0}}{1-\alpha}\beta \tag{12}$$

where $\langle v_0^2\rangle$ is the expected squared weight error at the initial time t_0.

Figure 1a compares equation (12) with simulations of 1-D LMS with gaussian inputs for $N = 1000$ and batch sizes $n =$10, 100, and 500. As can be seen, the agreement is good. Note that $\langle v^2\rangle$ decreases exponentially until flattening out. The equilibrium value can be computed from (12) by setting $t = \infty$ (assuming $|\alpha| < 1$) to give

$$\langle v^2\rangle_\infty = \frac{\beta}{1-\alpha} = \frac{\mu\sigma_\epsilon^2 R(N-n)}{2Rn(N-1) - \mu(N(n-1)R^2 + (N-n)S)}. \tag{13}$$

Note that $\langle v^2\rangle_\infty$ decreases as n increases and is zero only if $n = N$.

---

[1]For real zero mean gaussian inputs, we can apply the gaussian moment factoring theorem [Hay91] which states that $\langle x_i x_j x_k x_l\rangle_N = R_{ij}R_{kl} + R_{ik}R_{jl} + R_{il}R_{jk}$ where the subscripts on x denote components of x. From this, we find that $S = (\text{Trace }R)R + 2R^2$.

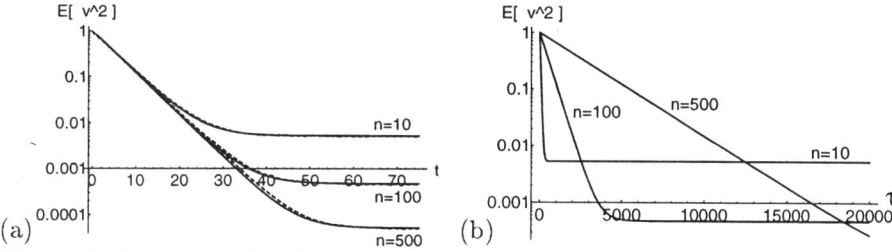

Figure 1: Simulations(solid) vs Theoretical (dashed) predictions of the squared weight error of 1-D LMS a) as function of the number of t, the batch updates (iterations), and b) as function of the number of input presentations, τ. Training set size is $N = 1000$ and batch sizes are $n = 10$, 100, and 500. Inputs were gaussian with $R = 1$, $\sigma_\epsilon = 1$ and $\mu = .1$. Simulations used 10000 networks

Equation (9) can also be solved exactly in multiple dimensions in the rather restrictive case where we assume that the inputs are spherically symmetric gaussians with $R = aI$ where a is a constant, I is the identity matrix, and m is the dimension. The update equation and solution are the same as (10) and (12), respectively, but where α and β are now

$$\alpha = 1 - 2\mu a + \mu^2 a^2 \left(\frac{N(n-1)}{(N-1)n} + \frac{N-n}{(N-1)n}(m+2) \right), \beta = \frac{\mu^2 \sigma_\epsilon^2 ma(N-n)}{n(N-1)}. \quad (14)$$

3 Adaptive Batch Size

The time it takes to compute the weight update in one iteration is roughly proportional to the number of input presentations, i.e the batch size. To make the comparison of convergence rates for different batch sizes meaningful, we must compute the change in squared weight error as a function of the number of input presentations, τ, rather than iteration number t.

For fixed batch size, $\tau = nt$. Figure 1b displays our 1-D LMS simulations plotted as a function of τ. As can be seen, training with a large batch size is slow but results in a lower equilibrium value than obtained with a small batch size. This suggests that we could obtain the fastest decrease of $\langle v^2 \rangle$ overall by varying the batch size at each iteration. The batch size to choose for the current $\langle v^2 \rangle$ would be the *smallest* n that has yet to reach equilibrium, i.e. for which $\langle v^2 \rangle > \langle v^2 \rangle_\infty$.

To determine the best batch size, we take the greedy approach by demanding that *at each iteration* the batch size is chosen so as to reduce the weight error at the next iteration by the greatest amount per input presentation. This is equivalent to asking what value of n maximizes $h \equiv (\langle v_t^2 \rangle - \langle v_{t+1}^2 \rangle)/n$? Once we determine n we then express it as a function of τ.

We treat the 1-D case, although the analysis would be similar for the spherically symmetric case. From (10) we have $h = \frac{1}{n}\left((\alpha - 1)\langle v_t^2 \rangle + \beta\right)$. Differentiating h with respect to n and solving yields the batch size that decreases the weight error the most to be

$$n_t = \min\left(N, \frac{2\mu N((S - R^2)\langle v_t^2 \rangle + \sigma_\epsilon^2 R)}{(2R(N-1) + \mu(S - NR^2))\langle v_t^2 \rangle + \mu\sigma_\epsilon^2 R}\right). \quad (15)$$

We have n_t exactly equal to N when the current value of $\langle v_t^2 \rangle$ satisfies

$$\langle v_t^2 \rangle < \gamma_c \equiv \frac{\mu \sigma_\epsilon^2 R}{2R(N-1) - \mu(R^2(N-2) - S)} \quad (n_t = N). \quad (16)$$

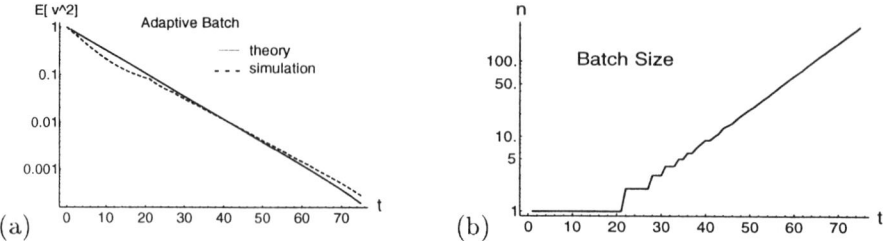

Figure 2: 1-D LMS: a) Comparison of the simulated and theoretically predicted (equation (18)) squared weight error as a function of t with $N = 1000$, $R = 1$, $\sigma_\epsilon = 1$, $\mu = .1$, and 10000 networks. b) Corresponding batch sizes used in the simulations.

Thus, after $\langle v_t^2 \rangle$ has decreased to γ_c, training will proceed as pure batch. When $\langle v_t^2 \rangle > \gamma_c$, we have $n_t < N$ and we can put (15) into (10) to obtain

$$\langle v_{t+1}^2 \rangle = \left(1 - \mu R + \mu^2 \frac{(NR^2 - S)}{2(N-1)}\right) \langle v_t^2 \rangle - \frac{\mu^2 \sigma_\epsilon^2 R}{2(N-1)}. \tag{17}$$

Solving (17) we get

$$\langle v_t^2 \rangle = \alpha_1^{t-t_0} \langle v_0^2 \rangle + \frac{1 - \alpha_1^{t-t_0}}{1 - \alpha_1} \beta_1 \tag{18}$$

where α_1, and β_1 are constants

$$\alpha_1 = 1 - \mu R + \mu^2 \frac{(S - NR^2)}{2(N-1)}, \qquad \beta_1 = -\mu^2 \frac{\sigma_\epsilon^2 R}{2(N-1)}. \tag{19}$$

Figure 2a compares equation (18) with 1-D LMS simulations. The adaptive batch size was chosen by rounding (15) to the nearest integer. Early in training, the predicted n_t is always smaller than 1 but the simulation always rounds up to 1 (can't have n=0). Figure 2b displays the batch sizes that were used in the simulations. A logarithmic scale is used to show that the batch size increases exponentially in t. We next examine the batch size as a function of τ.

3.1 Convergence Rate per Input Presentation

When we use (15) to choose the batch size, the number of input presentations will vary at each iteration. Thus, τ is not simply a multiple of t. Instead, we have

$$\tau(t) = \tau_0 + \sum_{i=t_0}^{t} n_i \tag{20}$$

where τ_0 is the number of inputs that have been presented by t_0. This can be evaluated when N is very large. In this case, equations (18) and (15) reduce to

$$\langle v_t^2 \rangle = \langle v_0^2 \rangle \alpha_3^{t-t_0} \quad \text{where} \quad \alpha_3 \equiv 1 - \mu R + \frac{1}{2}\mu^2 R^2 \tag{21}$$

$$n_t = \frac{2\mu((S - R^2)\langle v_t^2 \rangle + \sigma_\epsilon^2 R)}{(2R - \mu R^2)\langle v_t^2 \rangle} = \frac{2\mu(S - R^2)}{2R - \mu R^2} + \frac{2\mu\sigma_\epsilon^2}{(2 - \mu R)\langle v_0^2 \rangle \alpha_3^{t-t_0}}. \tag{22}$$

Putting (22) into (20), and summing gives gives

$$\Delta\tau(t) = \frac{2\mu(S - R^2)}{(2 - \mu R)R}\Delta t + \frac{2\mu\sigma_\epsilon^2}{(2 - \mu R)\langle v_0^2 \rangle} \frac{\alpha_3^{-\Delta t} - \alpha_3}{1 - \alpha_3} \tag{23}$$

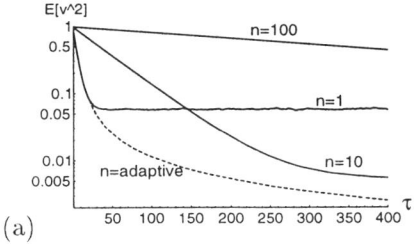 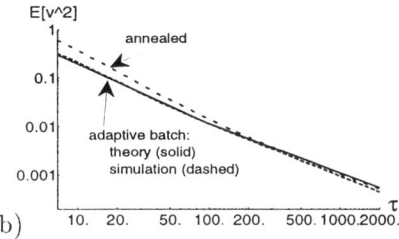

Figure 3: 1-D LMS: a) Simulations of the squared weight error as a function of τ, the number of input presentations for $N = 1000$, $R = 1$, $\sigma_\epsilon = 1$, $\mu = .1$, and 10000 networks. Batch sizes are $n = 1, 10, 100$, and n_t (see (15)). b) Comparison of simulation (dashed) and theory (see (24)) using adaptive batch size. Simulation (long dash) using an annealed learning rate with $n = 1$ and $\mu = R^{-1}$ is also shown.

where $\Delta t \equiv t - t_0$ and $\Delta \tau \equiv \tau - \tau_0$. Assuming that $|\alpha_3| < 1$, the term with $\alpha_3^{-\Delta t}$ will dominate at late times. Dropping the other terms and solving for α_3^t gives

$$\langle v_t^2 \rangle = \langle v_t^2 \rangle \alpha_3^{\Delta t} \approx \frac{4\sigma_\epsilon^2}{(2 - \mu R)^2 R (\tau - \tau_0)}. \tag{24}$$

Thus, when using an adaptive batch size, $\langle v^2 \rangle$ converges at late times as $\frac{1}{\tau}$. Figure 3a compares simulations of $\langle v^2 \rangle$ with adaptive and constant batch sizes. As can be seen, the adaptive n curve follows the $n = 1$ curve until just before the $n = 1$ curve starts to flatten out. Figure 3b compares (24) with the simulation. Curves are plotted on a log-log plot to illustrate the $1/\tau$ relationship at late times (straight line with slope of -1).

4 Learning Rate Annealing vs Increasing Batch Size

With online learning ($n = 1$), we can reduce the noise at late times by annealing the learning rate using a μ/t schedule. During this phase, $\langle v^2 \rangle$ decreases at a rate of $1/\tau$ if $\mu > R^{-1}/2$ [LO93] and slower otherwise. In this paper, we have presented an alternative method for reducing the noise by increasing the batch size exponentially in t. Here, $\langle v^2 \rangle$ also decreases at rate of $1/\tau$ so that, from this perspective, an adaptive batch size is equivalent to annealing the learning rate. This is confirmed in Figure 3b which compares using an adaptive batch size with annealing.

An advantage of the adaptive batch size comes when n reaches N. At this point n remains constant so that $\langle v^2 \rangle$ decreases exponentially in τ. However, with annealing, the convergence rate of $\langle v^2 \rangle$ always remains proportional to $1/\tau$. A disadvantage, though, occurs in multiple dimensions with nonspherical R where the best choice of n_t would likely be different along different directions in the weight space. Though it is possible to have a different learning rate along different directions, it is not possible to have different batch sizes.

5 Appendix A

In this appendix we use simple counting arguments to derive the two results in equations (5) and (6). We first note that there are $M \equiv \binom{N}{n}$ ways of choosing n examples out of a total of N examples. Thus, (5) can be rewritten as

$$\langle g_{B_n,t} \rangle_B = \frac{1}{M} \sum_{i=1}^{M} g_{B_n^{(i)},t} = \frac{1}{M} \sum_{i=1}^{M} \frac{1}{n} \sum_{z_j \in B_n^{(i)}} g_{j,t}. \tag{25}$$

where $B_n^{(i)}$ is the ith batch ($i = 1, \ldots, M$), and $g_{j,t} \equiv \partial \mathcal{E}(z_j)/\partial v_t$ for $j = 1, \ldots, N$. If we were to expand (25) we would find that there are exactly nM terms. From symmetry and since there are only N unique $g_{j,t}$, we conclude that each $g_{j,t}$ occurs exactly $\frac{nM}{N}$ times. The above expression can then be written as

$$\langle g_{B_n,t} \rangle_B = \frac{1}{nM} \frac{nM}{N} \sum_{j=1}^{N} g_{j,t} = \frac{1}{N} \sum_{j=1}^{N} g_{j,t} = \langle g_{i,t} \rangle_N. \tag{26}$$

Thus, we have equation (5). The second equation (6) is

$$\langle g_{B_n,t}^2 \rangle_B = \frac{1}{M} \sum_{i=1}^{M} g_{B_n,t}^T g_{B_n,t} = \frac{1}{M} \sum_{i=1}^{M} \left(\frac{1}{n} \sum_{z_j \in B_n^{(i)}} g_{j,t}^T \right) \left(\frac{1}{n} \sum_{z_k \in B_n^{(i)}} g_{k,t} \right)$$

$$= \frac{1}{n^2 M} \sum_{i=1}^{M} \sum_{z_j, z_k \in B_n^{(i)}} g_{j,t}^T g_{k,t} = \frac{1}{n^2 M} \sum_{i=1}^{M} \left(\sum_{z_j \in B_n^{(i)}} g_{j,t}^2 + \sum_{\substack{z_j, z_k \in B_n^{(i)} \\ j \neq k}} g_{j,t}^T g_{k,t} \right). \tag{27}$$

By the same argument to derive (5), the first term on the right $(1/n)\langle g_{i,t}^2 \rangle_N$. In the second term, there are a total $n(n-1)M$ terms in the sum, of which only $N(N-1)$ are unique. Thus, a given $g_{j,t}^T g_{k,t}$ occurs exactly $n(n-1)M/(N(N-1))$ times so that

$$\frac{1}{n^2 M} \sum_{i=1}^{M} \sum_{\substack{z_j, z_k \in B_n^{(i)}, j \neq k}} g_{j,t} g_{k,t} = \frac{1}{n^2 M} \frac{n(n-1)M}{N(N-1)} \sum_{j,k=1, j \neq k}^{N} g_{j,t} g_{k,t}$$

$$= \frac{N(n-1)}{n(N-1)} \left(\frac{1}{N^2} \cdot \left(\sum_{j,k=1, j \neq k}^{N} g_{j,t} g_{k,t} + \sum_{j=1}^{N} g_{j,t}^2 \right) - \frac{1}{N} \left(\frac{1}{N} \sum_{j=1}^{N} g_{j,t}^2 \right) \right)$$

$$= \frac{N(n-1)}{n(N-1)} \langle g_{i,t} \rangle_N^2 - \frac{(n-1)}{n(N-1)} \langle g_{i,t}^2 \rangle_N. \tag{28}$$

Putting the simplified first term together and (28) both into (27) we obtain our second result in equation (6).

References

[Gol87] Larry Goldstein. Mean square optimality in the continuous time Robbins Monro procedure. Technical Report DRB-306, Dept. of Mathematics, University of Southern California, LA, 1987.

[Hay91] Simon Haykin. *Adaptive Filter Theory*. Prentice Hall, New Jersey, 1991.

[LO93] Todd K. Leen and Genevieve B. Orr. Momentum and optimal stochastic search. In *Advances in Neural Information Processing Systems, vol. 6*, 1993. to appear.

[Møl93] Martin Møller. Supervised learning on large redundant training sets. *International Journal of Neural Systems*, 4(1):15–25, 1993.

[Orr95] Genevieve B. Orr. *Dynamics and Algorithms for Stochastic learning*. PhD thesis, Oregon Graduate Institute, 1995.

[PW93] Mark Plutowski and Halbert White. Selecting concise training sets from clean data. *IEEE Transactions on Neural Networks*, 4:305–318, 1993.

Are Hopfield Networks Faster Than Conventional Computers?

Ian Parberry[*] and Hung-Li Tseng[†]
Department of Computer Sciences
University of North Texas
P.O. Box 13886
Denton, TX 76203-6886

Abstract

It is shown that conventional computers can be exponentially faster than planar Hopfield networks: although there are planar Hopfield networks that take exponential time to converge, a stable state of an arbitrary planar Hopfield network can be found by a conventional computer in polynomial time. The theory of $\mathcal{PLS}$-completeness gives strong evidence that such a separation is unlikely for nonplanar Hopfield networks, and it is demonstrated that this is also the case for several restricted classes of nonplanar Hopfield networks, including those who interconnection graphs are the class of bipartite graphs, graphs of degree 3, the dual of the knight's graph, the 8-neighbor mesh, the hypercube, the butterfly, the cube-connected cycles, and the shuffle-exchange graph.

1 Introduction

Are Hopfield networks faster than conventional computers? This apparently straightforward question is complicated by the fact that conventional computers are universal computational devices, that is, they are capable of simulating any discrete computational device including Hopfield networks. Thus, a conventional computer could in a sense cheat by imitating the fastest Hopfield network possible.

---

[*]Email: ian@cs.unt.edu. URL: http://hercule.csci.unt.edu/ian.
[†]Email: htseng@ponder.csci.unt.edu.

But the question remains, is it faster for a computer to imitate a Hopfield network, or to use other computational methods? Although the answer is likely to be different for different benchmark problems, and even for different computer architectures, we can make our results meaningful in the long term by measuring *scalability*, that is, how the running time of Hopfield networks and conventional computers increases with the size of any benchmark problem to be solved.

Stated more technically, we are interested in the computational complexity of the *stable state problem* for Hopfield networks, which is defined succinctly as follows: given a Hopfield network, determine a stable configuration. As previously stated, this stable configuration can be determined by imitation, or by other means. The following results are known about the scalability of Hopfield network imitation. Any imitative algorithm for the stable state problem must take exponential time on *some* Hopfield networks, since there exist Hopfield networks that require exponential time to converge (Haken and Luby [4], Goles and Martinez [2]). It is unlikely that even non-imitative algorithms can solve the stable state problem in polynomial time, since the latter is $\mathcal{PLS}$-complete (Papadimitriou, Schäffer, and Yannakakis [9]). However, the stable state problem is more difficult for some classes of Hopfield networks than others. Hopfield networks will converge in polynomial time if their weights are bounded in magnitude by a polynomial of the number of nodes (for an expository proof see Parberry [11, Corollary 8.3.4]). In contrast, the stable state problem for Hopfield networks whose interconnection graph is bipartite is $\mathcal{PLS}$-complete (this can be proved easily by adapting techniques from Bruck and Goodman [1]) which is strong evidence that it too requires superpolynomial time to solve even with a nonimitative algorithm.

We show in this paper that although there exist planar Hopfield networks that take exponential time to converge in the worst case, the stable state problem for planar Hopfield networks can be solved in polynomial time by a non-imitative algorithm. This demonstrates that imitating planar Hopfield networks is exponentially slower than using non-imitative algorithmic techniques. In contrast, we discover that the stable state problem remains $\mathcal{PLS}$-complete for many simple classes of nonplanar Hopfield network, including bipartite networks, networks of degree 3, and some networks that are popular in neurocomputing and parallel computing.

The main part of this manuscript is divided into four sections. Section 2 contains some background definitions and references. Section 3 contains our results about planar Hopfield networks. Section 4 describes our $\mathcal{PLS}$-completeness results, based on a pivotal lemma about a nonstandard type of graph embedding.

2 Background

This section contains some background which are included for completeness but may be skipped on a first reading. It is divided into two subsections, the first on Hopfield networks, and the second on $\mathcal{PLS}$-completeness.

2.1 Hopfield Networks

A *Hopfield network* [6] is a discrete neural network model with symmetric connections. Each processor in the network computes a hard binary weighted threshold

function. Only one processor is permitted to change state at any given time. That
processor becomes active if its excitation level exceeds its threshold, and inactive
otherwise. A Hopfield network is said to be in a *stable state* if the states of all of
its processors are consistent with their respective excitation levels. It is well-known
that all Hopfield networks converge to a stable state. The proof defines a measure
called *energy*, and demonstrates that energy is positive but decreases with every
computation step. Essentially then, a Hopfield network finds a local minimum in
some energy landscape.

2.2 $\mathcal{PLS}$-completeness

While the theory of $\mathcal{NP}$-completeness measures the complexity of global optimization, the theory of $\mathcal{PLS}$-completeness developed by Johnson, Papadimitriou, and Yannakakis [7] measures the complexity of local optimization. It is similar to the theory of $\mathcal{NP}$-completeness in that it identifies a set of difficult problems known collectively as $\mathcal{PLS}$-*complete* problems. These are difficult in the sense that if a fast algorithm can be developed for any $\mathcal{PLS}$-complete problem, then it can be used to give fast algorithms for a substantial number of other local optimization problems including many important problems for which no fast algorithms are currently known. Recently, Papadimitriou, Schäffer, and Yannakakis [9] proved that the problem of finding stable states in Hopfield networks is $\mathcal{PLS}$-complete.

3 Planar Hopfield Networks

A planar Hopfield network is one whose interconnection graph is planar, that is, can be drawn on the Euclidean plane without crossing edges. Haken and Luby [4] describe a planar Hopfield network that provably takes exponential time to converge, and hence any imitative algorithm for the stable state problem must take exponential time on *some* Hopfield network. Yet there exists a nonimitative algorithm for the stable state problem that runs in polynomial time on *all* Hopfield networks:

Theorem 3.1 *The stable state problem for Hopfield networks with planar interconnection pattern can be solved in polynomial time.*

PROOF: (Sketch.) The proof follows from the fact that the maximal cut in a planar graph can be found in polynomial time (see, for example, Hadlock [3]), combined with results of Papadimitriou, Schäffer, and Yannakakis [9]. □

4 $\mathcal{PLS}$-completeness Results

Our $\mathcal{PLS}$-completeness results are a straightforward consequence of a new result that characterizes the difficulty of the stable state problem of an arbitrary class of Hopfield networks based on a graph-theoretic property of their interconnection patterns. Let $G = (V, E)$ and $H = (V', E')$ be graphs. An *embedding* of G into H is a function $f: V \to 2^{V'}$ such that the following properties hold. (1) For all $v \in V$, the subgraph of H induced by $f(v)$ is connected. (2) For all $(u, v) \in E$, there exists a path (which we will denote $f(u, v)$) in H from a member of $f(u)$ to a member of $f(v)$. (3) Each vertex $w \in H$ is used at most once, either as a member of $f(v)$

for some $v \in V$, or as an internal vertex in a path $f(u, v)$ for some $u, v \in V$. The graph G is called the *guest* graph, and H is called the *host* graph. Our definition of embedding is different from the standard notion of embedding (see, for example, Hong, Mehlhorn, and Rosenberg [5]) in that we allow the image of a single guest vertex to be a *set* of host vertices, and we insist in properties (2) and (3) that the images of guest edges be distinct paths. The latter property is crucial to our results, and forms the major difficulty in the proofs.

Let S, T be sets of graphs. S is said to be *polynomial-time embeddable* into T, written $S \leq_e T$, if there exists polynomials $p_1(n), p_2(n)$ and a function f with the following properties: (1) f can be computed in time $p_1(n)$, and (2) for every $G \in S$ with n vertices, there exists $H \in T$ with at most $p_2(n)$ vertices such that G can be embedded into H by f. A set S of graphs is said to be *pliable* if the set of all graphs is polynomial-time embeddable into S.

Lemma 4.1 *If S is pliable, then the problem of finding a stable state in Hopfield networks with interconnection graphs in S is $\mathcal{PLS}$-complete.*

PROOF: (Sketch.) Let S be a set of graphs with the property that the set of all graphs is polynomial-time embeddable into S. By the results of Papadimitriou, Schäffer, and Yannakakis [9], it is enough to show that the max-cut problem for graphs in S is $\mathcal{PLS}$-complete.

Let G be an arbitrary labeled graph. Suppose G is embedded into $H \in S$ under the polynomial-time embedding. For each edge e in G of cost c, select one edge from the path connecting the vertices in $f(e)$ and assign it cost c. We call this special edge $f'(e)$. Assign all other edges in the path cost $-\infty$. For all $v \in V$, assign the edges linking the vertices in $f(v)$ a cost of $-\infty$. Assign all other edges of H a cost of zero.

It can be shown that every cut in G induces a cut of the same cost in H, as follows. Suppose $C \subseteq E$ is a cut in G, that is, a set of edges that if removed from G, disconnects it into two components containing vertices V_1 and V_2 respectively. Then, removing vertices $f'(C)$ and all zero-cost edges from H will disconnect it into two components containing vertices $f(V_1)$ and $f(V_2)$ respectively. Furthermore, each cut of positive cost in H induces a cut of the same cost in G, since a positive cost cut in H cannot contain any edges of cost $-\infty$, and hence must consist only of $f'(e)$ for some edges $e \in E$. Therefore, every max-cost cut in H induces in polynomial time a max-cost cut in G. □

We can now present our $\mathcal{PLS}$-completeness results. A graph has *degree* 3 if all vertices are connected to at most 3 other vertices each.

Theorem 4.2 *The problem of finding stable states in Hopfield networks of degree 3 is $\mathcal{PLS}$-complete.*

PROOF: (Sketch.) By Lemma 4.1, it suffices to prove that the set of degree-3 graphs is pliable. Suppose $G = (V, E)$ is an arbitrary graph. Replace each degree-k vertex $x \in V$ by a path consisting of k vertices, and attach each edge incident with v by a new edge incident with one of the vertices in the path. Figure 1 shows an example of this embedding. □

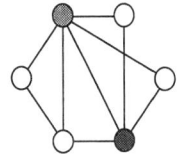 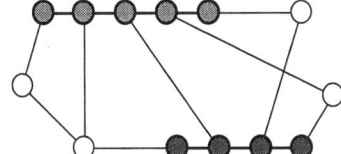

Figure 1: A guest graph of degree 5 (left), and the corresponding host of degree 3 (right). Shading indicates the high-degree nodes that were embedded into paths. All other nodes were embedded into single nodes.

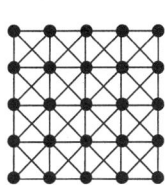 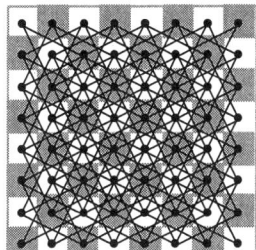

Figure 2: An 8-neighbor mesh with 25 vertices (left), and the 8 × 8 knight's graph superimposed on an 8 × 8 board (right).

The *8-neighbor mesh* is the degree-8 graph $G = (V, E)$ defined as follows: $V = \{1, 2, \ldots, m\} \times \{1, 2, \ldots, n\}$, and vertex (u, v) is connected to vertices $(u, v \pm 1)$, $(u \pm 1, v)$, $(u \pm 1, v \pm 1)$. Figure 2 shows an 8-neighbor mesh with 25 vertices.

Theorem 4.3 *The problem of finding stable states in Hopfield networks on the 8-neighbor mesh is $\mathcal{PLS}$-complete.*

PROOF: (Sketch.) By Lemma 4.1, it suffices to prove that the 8-neighbor mesh is pliable. An arbitrary graph can be embedded on an 8-neighbor mesh by mapping each node to a set of consecutive nodes in the bottom row of the grid, and mapping edges to disjoint rectilinear paths which use the diagonal edges of the grid for crossovers. □

The *knight's graph* for an $n \times n$ chessboard is the graph $G = (V, E)$ where $V = \{(i, j) \mid 1 \leq i, j \leq n\}$, and $E = \{((i, j), (k, \ell)) \mid \{|i - k|, |j - \ell|\} = \{1, 2\}\}$. That is, there is a vertex for every square of the board and an edge between two vertices exactly when there is a knight's move from one to the other. For example, Figure 2 shows the knight's graph for the 8 × 8 chessboard. Takefuji and Lee [15] (see also Parberry [12]) use the dual of the knight's graph for a Hopfield-style network to solve the knight's tour problem. That is, they have a vertex v_e for each edge e of the knight's graph, and an edge between two vertices v_d and v_e when d and e share a common vertex in the knight's graph.

Theorem 4.4 *The problem of finding stable states in Hopfield networks on the dual of the knight's graph is $\mathcal{PLS}$-complete.*

PROOF: (Sketch.) By Lemma 4.1, it suffices to prove that the dual of the knight's graph is pliable. It can be shown that the knight's graph is pliable using the technique of Theorem 4.3. It can also be proved that if a set S of graphs is pliable, then the set consisting of the duals of graphs in S is also pliable. □

The *hypercube* is the graph with 2^d nodes for some d, labelled with the binary representations of the d-bit natural numbers, in which two nodes are connected by an edge iff their labels differ in exactly one bit. The hypercube is an important graph for parallel computation (see, for example, Leighton [8], and Parberry [10]).

Theorem 4.5 *The problem of finding stable states in Hopfield networks on the hypercube is $\mathcal{PLS}$-complete.*

PROOF: (Sketch.) By Lemma 4.1, it suffices to prove that the hypercube is pliable. Since the "$\leq_e$" relation is transitive, it further suffices by Theorem 4.2 to show that the set of degree-3 graphs is polynomial-time embeddable into the hypercube. To embed a degree-3 graph G into the hypercube, first break it into a degree-1 graph G_1 and a degree-2 graph G_2. Since G_2 consists of cycles, paths, and disconnected vertices, it can easily be embedded into a hypercube (since a hypercube is rich in cycles). G_1 can be viewed as a permutation of vertices in G and can hence be realized using a hypercube implementation of Waksman's permutation network [16]. □

We conclude by stating $\mathcal{PLS}$-completeness results for three more graphs that are important in the parallel computing literature the *butterfly* (see, for example, Leighton [8]), the *cube-connected cycles* (Preparata and Vuillemin [13]), and the *shuffle-exchange* (Stone [14]). The proofs use Lemma 4.1 and Theorem 4.5, and are omitted for conciseness.

Theorem 4.6 *The problem of finding stable states in Hopfield networks on the butterfly, the cube-connected cycles, and the shuffle-exchange is $\mathcal{PLS}$-complete.*

Conclusion

Are Hopfield networks faster than conventional computers? The answer seems to be that it depends on the interconnection graph of the Hopfield network. Conventional nonimitative algorithms can be exponentially faster than planar Hopfield networks. The theory of $\mathcal{PLS}$-completeness shows us that such an exponential separation result is unlikely not only for nonplanar graphs, but even for simple nonplanar graphs such as bipartite graphs, graphs of degree 3, the dual of the knight's graph, the 8-neighbor mesh, the hypercube, the butterfly, the cube-connected cycles, and the shuffle-exchange graph.

Acknowledgements

The research described in this paper was supported by the National Science Foundation under grant number CCR–9302917, and by the Air Force Office of Scientific

Research, Air Force Systems Command, USAF, under grant number F49620-93-1-0100.

References

[1] J. Bruck and J. W. Goodman. A generalized convergence theorem for neural networks. *IEEE Transactions on Information Theory*, 34(5):1089–1092, 1988.

[2] E. Goles and S. Martinez. Exponential transient classes of symmetric neural networks for synchronous and sequential updating. *Complex Systems*, 3:589–597, 1989.

[3] F. Hadlock. Finding a maximum cut of a planar graph in polynomial time. *SIAM Journal on Computing*, 4(3):221–225, 1975.

[4] A. Haken and M. Luby. Steepest descent can take exponential time for symmetric conenction networks. *Complex Systems*, 2:191–196, 1988.

[5] J.-W. Hong, K. Mehlhorn, and A.L. Rosenberg. Cost tradeoffs in graph embeddings. *Journal of the ACM*, 30:709–728, 1983.

[6] J. J. Hopfield. Neural networks and physical systems with emergent collective computational abilities. *Proc. National Academy of Sciences*, 79:2554–2558, April 1982.

[7] D. S. Johnson, C. H. Papadimitriou, and M. Yannakakis. How easy is local search? In *26th Annual Symposium on Foundations of Computer Science*, pages 39–42. IEEE Computer Society Press, 1985.

[8] F. T. Leighton. *Introduction to Parallel Algorithms and Architectures: Arrays · Trees · Hypercubes*. Morgan Kaufmann, 1992.

[9] C. H. Papadimitriou, A. A. Schäffer, and M. Yannakakis. On the complexity of local search. In *Proceedings of the Twenty Second Annual ACM Symposium on Theory of Computing*, pages 439–445. ACM Press, 1990.

[10] I. Parberry. *Parallel Complexity Theory*. Research Notes in Theoretical Computer Science. Pitman Publishing, London, 1987.

[11] I. Parberry. *Circuit Complexity and Neural Networks*. MIT Press, 1994.

[12] I. Parberry. Scalability of a neural network for the knight's tour problem. *Neurocomputing*, 12:19–34, 1996.

[13] F. P. Preparata and J. Vuillemin. The cube-connected cycles: A versatile network for parallel computation. *Communications of the ACM*, 24(5):300–309, 1981.

[14] H. S. Stone. Parallel processing with the perfect shuffle. *IEEE Transactions on Computers*, C-20(2):153–161, 1971.

[15] Y. Takefuji and K. C. Lee. Neural network computing for knight's tour problems. *Neurocomputing*, 4(5):249–254, 1992.

[16] A. Waksman. A permutation network. *Journal of the ACM*, 15(1):159–163, January 1968.

Hebb Learning of Features based on their Information Content

Ferdinand Peper
Communications Research Laboratory
588-2, Iwaoka, Iwaoka-cho
Nishi-ku, Kobe 651-24
Japan
peper@crl.go.jp

Hideki Noda
Kyushu Institute of Technology
Dept. Electr., Electro., and Comp. Eng.
1-1 Sensui-cho, Tobata-ku
Kita-Kyushu 804, Japan
noda@kawa.comp.kyutech.ac.jp

Abstract

This paper investigates the stationary points of a Hebb learning rule with a sigmoid nonlinearity in it. We show mathematically that when the input has a low information content, as measured by the input's variance, this learning rule suppresses learning, that is, forces the weight vector to converge to the zero vector. When the information content exceeds a certain value, the rule will automatically begin to learn a feature in the input. Our analysis suggests that under certain conditions it is the first principal component that is learned. The weight vector length remains bounded, provided the variance of the input is finite. Simulations confirm the theoretical results derived.

1 Introduction

Hebb learning, one of the main mechanisms of synaptic strengthening, is induced by cooccurrent activity of pre- and post-synaptic neurons. It is used in artificial neural networks like perceptrons, associative memories, and unsupervised learning neural networks. Unsupervised Hebb learning typically employs rules of the form:

$$\mu \dot{\mathbf{w}}(t) = \mathbf{x}(t)y(t) - \mathbf{d}(\mathbf{x}(t), y(t), \mathbf{w}(t)), \tag{1}$$

where $\mathbf{w}$ is the vector of a neuron's synaptic weights, $\mathbf{x}$ is a stochastic input vector, y is the output expressed as a function of $\mathbf{x}^T\mathbf{w}$, and the vector function $\mathbf{d}$ is a forgetting term forcing the weights to decay when there is little input. The integration constant μ determines the learning speed and will be assumed 1 for convenience.

The dynamics of rule (1) determines which features are learned, and, with it, the rule's stationary points and the boundedness of the weight vector. In some cases, weight vectors grow to zero or grow unbounded. Either is biologically implausible. Suppression and unbounded growth of weights is related to the characteristics of the input $\mathbf{x}$ and to the choice for $\mathbf{d}$. Understanding this relation is important to enable a system, that employs Hebb learning, to learn the right features and avoid implausible weight vectors.

Unbounded or zero length of weight vectors is avoided in [5] by keeping the total synaptic strength $\sum_i w_i$ constant. Other studies, like [7], conserve the sum-squared synaptic strength. Another way to keep the weight vector length bounded is to limit the range of each of the individual weights [4]. The effect of these constraints on the learning dynamics of a linear Hebb rule is studied in [6].

This paper constrains the weight vector length by a nonlinearity in a Hebb rule. It uses a rule of the form (1) with $y = S(\mathbf{x}^T\mathbf{w} - h)$ and $\mathbf{d}(\mathbf{x}, y, \mathbf{w}) = c.\mathbf{w}$, the function S being a smooth sigmoid, h being a constant, and c being a positive constant (see [1] for a similar rule). We prove that the weight vector $\mathbf{w}$ assumes a bounded nonzero solution if the largest eigenvalue λ_1 of the input covariance matrix satisfies $\lambda_1 > c/S'(-h)$. Furthermore, if $\lambda_1 \leq c/S'(-h)$ the weight vector converges to the vector $\mathbf{0}$. Since λ_1 equals the variance of the input's first principal component, that is, λ_1 is a measure for the amount of information in the input, learning is enabled by a high information content and suppressed by a low information content.

The next section describes the Hebb neuron and its input in more detail. After characterizing the stationary points of the Hebb learning rule in section 3, we analyze their stability in section 4. Simulations in section 5 confirm that convergence towards a nonzero bounded solution occurs only when the information content of the input is sufficiently high. We finish this paper with a discussion.

2 The Hebb Neuron and its Input

Assume that the n-dimensional input vectors $\mathbf{x}$ presented to the neuron are generated by a stationary white stochastic process with mean $\mathbf{0}$. The process's covariance matrix $\Sigma = \mathrm{E}[\mathbf{x}\mathbf{x}^T]$ has eigenvalues $\lambda_1, ..., \lambda_n$ (in order of decreasing size) and corresponding eigenvectors $\mathbf{u}_1, ..., \mathbf{u}_n$. Furthermore, $\mathrm{E}[\|\mathbf{x}\|^2]$ is finite. This implies that the eigenvalues are finite because $\mathrm{E}[\|\mathbf{x}\|^2] = \mathrm{E}[\mathrm{tr}[\mathbf{x}\mathbf{x}^T]] = \mathrm{tr}[\mathrm{E}[\mathbf{x}\mathbf{x}^T]] = \sum_{i=1}^{n} \lambda_i$. It is assumed that the probability density function of $\mathbf{x}$ is continuous. Given an input $\mathbf{x}$ and a synaptic weight vector $\mathbf{w}$, the neuron produces an output $y = S(\mathbf{x}^T\mathbf{w} - h)$, where $S: \mathbb{R} \to \mathbb{R}$ is a function that satisfies the conditions:

C1. S is smooth, i.e., S is continuous and differentiable and S' is continuous.

C2. S is sublinear, i.e., $\lim_{z \to \infty} S(z)/z = \lim_{z \to -\infty} S(z)/z = 0$.

C3. S is monotonically nondecreasing.

C4. S' has one maximum, which is at the point $z = -h$.

Typically, these conditions are satisfied by smooth sigmoidal functions. This includes sigmoids with infinite saturation values, like $S(z) = \mathrm{sign}(z)|z|^{1/2}$ (see [9]). The point at which a sigmoid achieves maximal steepness (condition C4) is called its *base*. Though the step function is discontinuous at its base, thus violating condition C1, the results in this paper apply to the step function too, because it is the limit of a sequence of continuous sigmoids, and the input density function is continuous and thus Lebesgue-integrable. The learning rule of the neuron is given by

$$\dot{\mathbf{w}} = \mathbf{x}y - c\mathbf{w}, \qquad (2)$$

c being a positive constant. Use of a linear $S(z) = az$ in this rule gives unstable dynamics: if $a > c/\lambda_1$, then the length of the weight vector $\mathbf{w}$ grows out of bound though ultimately $\mathbf{w}$ becomes collinear with $\mathbf{u}_1$. It is proven in the next section that a sublinear S prevents unbounded growth of $\mathbf{w}$.

3 Stationary Points of the Learning Rule

To get insight into what stationary points the weight vector **w** ultimately converges to, we average the stochastic equation (2) over the input patterns and obtain

$$\langle \dot{\mathbf{w}} \rangle = \mathrm{E}\left[\mathbf{x} S\left(\mathbf{x}^T \langle \mathbf{w} \rangle - h \right) \right] - c \langle \mathbf{w} \rangle, \tag{3}$$

where $\langle \mathbf{w} \rangle$ is the averaged weight vector and the expectation is taken over **x**, as with all expectations in this paper. Since the solutions of (2) correspond with the solutions of (3) under conditions described in [2], the averaged $\langle \mathbf{w} \rangle$ will be referred to as **w**. Learning in accordance to (2) can then be interpreted [1] as a gradient descent process on an averaged energy function J associated with (3):

$$J(\mathbf{w}) = -\mathrm{E}\left[T\left(\mathbf{x}^T \mathbf{w} - h \right) \right] + \frac{1}{2} c \mathbf{w}^T \mathbf{w} \quad \text{with} \quad T(z) = \int_{-\infty}^{z} S(v) dv.$$

To characterize the solutions of (3) we use the following lemma.

Lemma 1. Given a unit-length vector **u**, the function $f_{\mathbf{u}} : \mathbb{R} \to \mathbb{R}$ is defined by

$$f_{\mathbf{u}}(z) = \frac{1}{c} \mathrm{E}\left[\mathbf{u}^T \mathbf{x} S\left(z \mathbf{x}^T \mathbf{u} - h \right) \right]$$

and the constant $\lambda_{\mathbf{u}}$ by $\lambda_{\mathbf{u}} = \mathrm{E}[\mathbf{u}^T \mathbf{x} \mathbf{x}^T \mathbf{u}]$. The fixed points of $f_{\mathbf{u}}$ are as follows.

1. If $\lambda_{\mathbf{u}} S'(-h) \leq c$ then $f_{\mathbf{u}}$ has one fixed point, i.e., $z = 0$.

2. If $\lambda_{\mathbf{u}} S'(-h) > c$ then $f_{\mathbf{u}}$ has three fixed points, i.e., $z = 0$, $z = \alpha_{\mathbf{u}}^+$, and $z = \alpha_{\mathbf{u}}^-$, where $\alpha_{\mathbf{u}}^+$ ($\alpha_{\mathbf{u}}^-$) is a positive (negative) value depending on **u**.

Proof:(Sketch; for a detailed proof see [11]). Function $f_{\mathbf{u}}$ is a smooth sigmoid, since conditions C1 to C4 carry over from S to $f_{\mathbf{u}}$. The steepness of $f_{\mathbf{u}}$ in its base at $z = 0$ depends on vector **u**. If $\lambda_{\mathbf{u}} S'(-h) \leq c$, function $f_{\mathbf{u}}$ intersects the line $h(z) = z$ only at the origin, giving $z = 0$ as the only fixed point. If $\lambda_{\mathbf{u}} S'(-h) > c$, the steepness of $f_{\mathbf{u}}$ is so large as to yield two more intersections: $z = \alpha_{\mathbf{u}}^+$ and $z = \alpha_{\mathbf{u}}^-$. □

Thus characterizing the fixed points of $f_{\mathbf{u}}$, the lemma allows us to find the fixed points of a vector function $\mathbf{g} : \mathbb{R}^n \to \mathbb{R}^n$ that is closely related to (3). Defining

$$\mathbf{g}(\mathbf{w}) = \frac{1}{c} \mathrm{E}\left[\mathbf{x} S\left(\mathbf{x}^T \mathbf{w} - h \right) \right],$$

we find that a fixed point $z = \alpha_{\mathbf{u}}$ of $f_{\mathbf{u}}$ corresponds to the fixed point $\mathbf{w} = \alpha_{\mathbf{u}} \mathbf{u}$ of **g**. Then, since (3) can be written as $\dot{\mathbf{w}} = c.\mathbf{g}(\mathbf{w}) - c.\mathbf{w}$, its stationary points are the fixed points of **g**, that is, $\mathbf{w} = \mathbf{0}$ is a stationary point and for each **u** for which $\lambda_{\mathbf{u}} S'(-h) > c$ there exists one bounded stationary point associated with $\alpha_{\mathbf{u}}^+$ and one associated with $\alpha_{\mathbf{u}}^-$. Consequently, if $\lambda_1 \leq c/S'(-h)$ then the only fixed point of **g** is $\mathbf{w} = \mathbf{0}$, because $\lambda_1 \geq \lambda_{\mathbf{u}}$ for all **u**.

What is the implication of this result? The relation $\lambda_1 \leq c/S'(-h)$ indicates a low information content of the input, because λ_1—equaling the variance of the input's first principal component—is a measure for the input's information content. A low information content thus results in a zero **w**, suppressing learning. Section 4 shows that a high information content results in a nonzero **w**. The turnover point of what is considered high/low information is adjusted by changing the steepness of the sigmoid in its base or changing constant c in the forgetting term.

To show the boundedness of **w**, we consider an arbitrary point P: $\mathbf{w} = \beta \mathbf{u}$ sufficiently far away from the origin O (but at finite distance) and calculate the component of $\dot{\mathbf{w}}$ along the line OP as well as the components orthogonal to OP. Vector **u** has unit length, and β may be assumed positive since its sign can be absorbed by **u**. Then, the component along OP is given by the projection of $\dot{\mathbf{w}}$ on **u**:

$$\mathbf{u}^T \dot{\mathbf{w}} \Big|_{\mathbf{w}=\beta\mathbf{u}} = \mathbf{u}^T c\mathbf{g}(\beta\mathbf{u}) - \mathbf{u}^T c\beta\mathbf{u} = -c\left[\beta - f_\mathbf{u}(\beta)\right].$$

This is negative for all β exceeding the fixed points of $f_\mathbf{u}$ because of the sigmoidal shape of $f_\mathbf{u}$. So, for any point P in $\mathbb{R}^n$ lying far enough from O the vector component of $\dot{\mathbf{w}}$ in P along the line OP is directed towards O and not away from it. This component decreases as we move away from O, because the value of $[\beta - f_\mathbf{u}(\beta)]$ increases as β increases ($f_\mathbf{u}$ is sublinear). Orthogonal to this is a component given by the projection of $\dot{\mathbf{w}}$ on a unit-length vector **v** that is orthogonal to **u**:

$$\mathbf{v}^T \dot{\mathbf{w}} \Big|_{\mathbf{w}=\beta\mathbf{u}} = \mathbf{v}^T c\mathbf{g}(\beta\mathbf{u}) - \mathbf{v}^T c\beta\mathbf{u} = c\mathbf{v}^T \mathbf{g}(\beta\mathbf{u}).$$

This component increases as we move away from O; however, it changes at a slower pace than the component along OP, witness the quotient of both components:

$$\lim_{\beta \to \infty} \frac{\mathbf{v}^T \dot{\mathbf{w}}}{\mathbf{u}^T \dot{\mathbf{w}}} \Big|_{\mathbf{w}=\beta\mathbf{u}} = \lim_{\beta \to \infty} \frac{c\mathbf{v}^T \mathbf{g}(\beta\mathbf{u})}{-c[\beta - f_\mathbf{u}(\beta)]} = \lim_{\beta \to \infty} \frac{\mathbf{v}^T \mathbf{g}(\beta\mathbf{u})/\beta}{f_\mathbf{u}(\beta)/\beta - 1} = 0.$$

Vector $\dot{\mathbf{w}}$ thus becomes increasingly dominated by the component along OP as β increases. So, the origin acts as an attractor if we are sufficiently far away from it, implying that **w** remains bounded during learning.

4 Stability of the Stationary Points

To investigate the stability of the stationary points, we use the Hessian of the averaged energy function J described in the last section. The Hessian at point **w** equals: $H(\mathbf{w}) = cI - \mathrm{E}\left[\mathbf{xx}^T S'\left(\mathbf{x}^T \mathbf{w} - h\right)\right]$. A stationary point $\mathbf{w} = \hat{\mathbf{w}}$ is stable iff $H(\hat{\mathbf{w}})$ is a positive definite matrix. The latter is satisfied if for every unit-length vector **v**,

$$\mathbf{v}^T \mathrm{E}\left[\mathbf{xx}^T S'\left(\mathbf{x}^T \hat{\mathbf{w}} - h\right)\right] \mathbf{v} < c, \tag{4}$$

that is, if all eigenvalues of the matrix $\mathrm{E}[\mathbf{xx}^T S'(\mathbf{x}^T\hat{\mathbf{w}} - h)]$ are less than c. First consider the stationary point $\mathbf{w} = \mathbf{0}$. The eigenvalues of $\mathrm{E}[\mathbf{xx}^T S'(-h)]$ in decreasing order are $\lambda_1 S'(-h), ..., \lambda_n S'(-h)$. The Hessian $H(\mathbf{0})$ is thus positive definite iff $\lambda_1 S'(-h) < c$. In this case $\mathbf{w} = \mathbf{0}$ is stable. It is also stable in the case $\lambda_1 = c/S'(-h)$, because then (4) holds for all $\mathbf{v} \neq \mathbf{u}_1$, preventing growth of **w** in directions other than $\mathbf{u}_1$. Moreover, **w** will not grow in the direction of $\mathbf{u}_1$, because $|f_{\mathbf{u}_1}(\beta)| < |\beta|$ for all $\beta \neq 0$. Combined with the results of the last section this implies:

Corollary 1. If $\lambda_1 \leq c/S'(-h)$ then the averaged learning equation (3) will have as its only stationary point $\mathbf{w} = \mathbf{0}$, and this point is stable. If $\lambda_1 > c/S'(-h)$ the stationary point $\mathbf{w} = \mathbf{0}$ is not stable, and there will be other stationary points.

We now investigate the other stationary points. Let $\mathbf{w} = \alpha_\mathbf{u}\mathbf{u}$ be such a point, $\mathbf{u}$ being a unit-length vector and $\alpha_\mathbf{u}$ a nonzero constant. To check whether the Hessian $H(\alpha_\mathbf{u}\mathbf{u})$ is positive definite, we apply the relation $\mathrm{E}[XY] = \mathrm{E}[X]\mathrm{E}[Y] + \mathrm{Cov}[X,Y]$ to the expression $\mathrm{E}\left[\mathbf{u}^T\mathbf{x}\mathbf{x}^T\mathbf{u}\,S'(\alpha_\mathbf{u}\mathbf{x}^T\mathbf{u} - h)\right]$ and obtain after rewriting:

$$\mathrm{E}\left[S'(\alpha_\mathbf{u}\mathbf{x}^T\mathbf{u} - h)\right] = \frac{1}{\lambda_\mathbf{u}}\mathrm{E}\left[\mathbf{u}^T\mathbf{x}\mathbf{x}^T\mathbf{u}\,S'(\alpha_\mathbf{u}\mathbf{x}^T\mathbf{u} - h)\right] - \frac{1}{\lambda_\mathbf{u}}\mathrm{Cov}\left[\mathbf{u}^T\mathbf{x}\mathbf{x}^T\mathbf{u}, S'(\alpha_\mathbf{u}\mathbf{x}^T\mathbf{u} - h)\right].$$

The sigmoidal shape of the function $f_\mathbf{u}$ implies that $f_\mathbf{u}$ is less steep than the line $h(z) = z$ at the intersection at $z = \alpha_\mathbf{u}$, that is, $f'_\mathbf{u}(\alpha_\mathbf{u}) < 1$. It then follows that $\mathrm{E}\left[\mathbf{u}^T\mathbf{x}\mathbf{x}^T\mathbf{u}\,S'(\alpha_\mathbf{u}\mathbf{x}^T\mathbf{u} - h)\right] = cf'_\mathbf{u}(\alpha_\mathbf{u}) < c$, giving:

$$\mathrm{E}\left[S'(\alpha_\mathbf{u}\mathbf{x}^T\mathbf{u} - h)\right] < \frac{1}{\lambda_\mathbf{u}}\left\{c - \mathrm{Cov}\left[\mathbf{u}^T\mathbf{x}\mathbf{x}^T\mathbf{u}, S'(\alpha_\mathbf{u}\mathbf{x}^T\mathbf{u} - h)\right]\right\}.$$

Then, $\mathbf{v}^T\mathrm{E}\left[\mathbf{x}\mathbf{x}^T S'(\alpha_\mathbf{u}\mathbf{x}^T\mathbf{u} - h)\right]\mathbf{v} =$
$\lambda_\mathbf{v}\mathrm{E}\left[S'(\alpha_\mathbf{u}\mathbf{x}^T\mathbf{u} - h)\right] + \mathrm{Cov}\left[\mathbf{v}^T\mathbf{x}\mathbf{x}^T\mathbf{v}, S'(\alpha_\mathbf{u}\mathbf{x}^T\mathbf{u} - h)\right] <$
$\frac{\lambda_\mathbf{v}}{\lambda_\mathbf{u}}c - \frac{\lambda_\mathbf{v}}{\lambda_\mathbf{u}}\mathrm{Cov}\left[\mathbf{u}^T\mathbf{x}\mathbf{x}^T\mathbf{u}, S'(\alpha_\mathbf{u}\mathbf{x}^T\mathbf{u} - h)\right] + \mathrm{Cov}\left[\mathbf{v}^T\mathbf{x}\mathbf{x}^T\mathbf{v}, S'(\alpha_\mathbf{u}\mathbf{x}^T\mathbf{u} - h)\right].$

The probability distribution of $\mathbf{x}$ unspecified, it is hard to evaluate this upper bound. For certain distributions the upper bound is minimized when $\lambda_\mathbf{u}$ is maximized, that is, when $\mathbf{u} = \mathbf{u}_1$ and $\lambda_\mathbf{u} = \lambda_1$, implying the Hebb neuron to be a nonlinear principal component analyzer. Distributions that are symmetric with respect to the eigenvectors of Σ are probably examples of such distributions, as suggested by [11, 12]. For other distributions vector $\mathbf{w}$ may assume a solution not collinear with $\mathbf{u}_1$ or may periodically traverse (part of) the nonzero fixed-point set of $\mathbf{g}$.

5 Simulations

We carry out simulations to test whether learning behaves in accordance with corollary 1. The following difference equation is used as the learning rule:

$$\Delta\mathbf{w} = \gamma\left[\mathbf{x}\cdot\tanh\left(a\mathbf{x}^T\mathbf{w}\right) - \mathbf{w}\right], \qquad (5)$$

where γ is the learning rate and a a constant. The use of a difference Δ in (5) rather than the differential in (2) is computationally easier, and gives identical results if γ decreases over training time in accordance with conditions described in [3]. We use $\gamma(t) = 1/(0.01t + 20)$. It satisfies these conditions and gives fast convergence without disrupting stability [10]. Its precise choice is not very critical here, though.

The neuron is trained on multivariate normally distributed random input samples of dimension 6 with mean $\mathbf{0}$ and a covariance matrix Σ that has the eigenvalues 4.00, 2.25, 1.00, 0.09, 0.04, and 0.01. The degree to which the weight vector and Σ's first eigenvector $\mathbf{u}_1$ are collinear is measured by the match coefficient [10], defined by: $m = \cos^2\angle(\mathbf{u}_1, \mathbf{w})$. In every experiment the neuron is trained for 10000 iterations by (5) with the value of parameter a set to 0.20, 0.25, and 0.30, respectively. This corresponds to the situations in which $\lambda_1 < c/S'(-h)$, $\lambda_1 = c/S'(-h)$, and $\lambda_1 > c/S'(-h)$, respectively, since $c = 1$ and the steepness of the sigmoid $S(z) = \tanh(az)$

in its base $z = -h = 0$ is $S'(0) = a$. We perform each experiment 2000 times, which allows us to obtain the match coefficients beyond iteration 100 within ±0.02 with a confidence coefficient of 95% (and a smaller confidence coefficient on the first 100 iterations). The random initialization of the weight vector—its initial elements are uniformly distributed in the interval $(-1, 1)$—is different in each experiment.

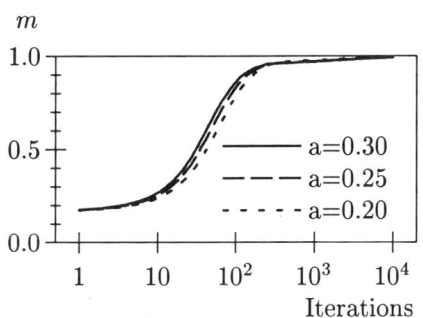
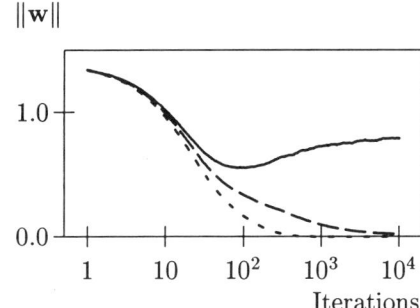

Figure 1: Match coefficients averaged over 2000 experiments for parameter values $a = 0.20, 0.25$, and 0.30.

Figure 2: Lengths of the weight vector averaged over 2000 experiments. The curve types are similar to those in Fig. 1.

Fig. 1 shows that for all tested values of parameter a the weight vector gradually becomes collinear with $\mathbf{u}_1$ over 10000 iterations. The length of the weight vector converges to 0 when $a = 0.20$ or $a = 0.25$ (see Fig. 2). In the case $a = 0.30$, corresponding to $\lambda_1 > c/S'(-h)$, the length converges to a nonzero bounded value. In conclusion, convergence is as predicted by corollary 1: the weight vector converges to $\mathbf{0}$ if the information content in the input is too low for climbing the slope of the sigmoid in its base, and otherwise the weight vector becomes nonzero.

6 Discussion

Learning by the Hebb rule discussed in this paper is enabled if the input's information content as measured by the variance is sufficiently high, and only then. The results, though valid for a single neuron, have implications for systems consisting of multiple neurons connected by inhibitory connections. A neuron in such a system would have as output $y = S(\mathbf{x}^T\mathbf{w} - h - \mathbf{v}^T\mathbf{y}')$, where the inhibitory signal $\mathbf{v}^T\mathbf{y}'$ would consist of the vector of output signals $\mathbf{y}'$ of the other neurons, weighted by the vector $\mathbf{v}$ (see also [1]). Function $f_\mathbf{u}$ in lemma 1 would, when extended to contain the signal $\mathbf{v}^T\mathbf{y}'$, still pass through the origin because of the zero-meanness of the input, but would have a reduced steepness at the origin caused by the shift in S's argument away from the base. The reduced steepness would make an intersection of $f_\mathbf{u}$ with the line $h(z) = z$ in a point other than the origin less likely. Consequently, an inhibitory signal would bias the neuron towards suppressing its weights. In a system of neurons this would reduce the emergence of neurons with correlated outputs, because of the mutual presence of their outputs in each other's inhibitory signals. The neurons, then, would extract different features, while suppressing information-poor features.

In conclusion, the Hebb learning rule in this paper combines well with inhibitory connections, and can potentially be used to build a system of nonredundant feature extractors, each of which is optimized to extract only information-rich features.

Moreover, the suppression of weights with a low information content suggests a straightforward way [8] to adaptively control the number of neurons, thus minimizing the necessary neural resources.

Acknowledgments

We thank Dr. Mahdad N. Shirazi at Communications Research Laboratory (CRL) for the helpful discussions, Prof. Dr. S.-I. Amari for his encouragement, and Dr. Hidefumi Sawai at CRL for providing financial support to present this paper at NIPS'96 from the Council for the Promotion of Advanced Information and Communications Technology. This work was financed by the Japan Ministry of Posts and Telecommunications as part of their Frontier Research Project in Telecommunications.

References

[1] S.-I. Amari, "Mathematical Foundations of Neurocomputing," *Proceedings of the IEEE*, vol. 78, no. 9, pp. 1443-1463, 1990.

[2] S. Geman, "Some Averaging and Stability Results for Random Differential Equations," *SIAM J. Appl. Math.*, vol. 36, no. 1, pp. 86-105, 1979.

[3] H.J. Kushner and D.S. Clark, "Stochastic Approximation Methods for Constrained and Unconstrained Systems," *Applied Mathematical Sciences*, vol. 26, New York: Springer-Verlag, 1978.

[4] R. Linsker, "Self-Organization in a Perceptual Network," *Computer*, vol. 21, pp. 105-117, 1988.

[5] C. von der Malsburg, "Self-Organization of Orientation Sensitive Cells in the Striate Cortex," *Kybernetik*, vol. 14, pp. 85-100, 1973.

[6] K.D. Miller and D.J.C. MacKay, "The Role of Constraints in Hebbian Learning," *Neural Computation*, vol. 6, pp. 100-126, 1994.

[7] E. Oja, "A simplified neuron model as a principal component analyzer," *Journal of Mathematics and Biology*, vol. 15, pp. 267-273, 1982.

[8] F. Peper and H. Noda, "A Mechanism for the Development of Feature Detecting Neurons," *Proc. Second New-Zealand Int. Two-Stream Conf. on Artificial Neural Networks and Expert Systems, ANNES'95*, Dunedin, New-Zealand, pp. 59-62, 20-23 Nov. 1995.

[9] F. Peper and H. Noda, "A Class of Simple Nonlinear 1-unit PCA Neural Networks," *1995 IEEE Int. Conf. on Neural Networks, ICNN'95*, Perth, Australia, pp. 285-289, 27 Nov.-1 Dec. 1995.

[10] F. Peper and H. Noda, "A Symmetric Linear Neural Network that Learns Principal Components and their Variances," *IEEE Trans. on Neural Networks*, vol. 7, pp. 1042-1047, 1996.

[11] F. Peper and H. Noda, "Stationary Points of a Hebb Learning Rule for a Nonlinear Neural Network," *Proc. 1996 Int. Symp. Nonlinear Theory and Appl. (NOLTA'96)*, Kochi, Japan, pp. 241-244, 7-9 Oct 1996.

[12] F. Peper and M.N. Shirazi, "On the Eigenstructure of Nonlinearized Covariance Matrices," *Proc. 1996 Int. Symp. Nonlinear Theory and Appl. (NOLTA'96)*, Kochi, Japan, pp. 491-493, 7-9 Oct 1996.

The Generalisation Cost of RAMnets

Richard Rohwer and Michał Morciniec
rohwerrj@cs.aston.ac.uk   morcinim@cs.aston.ac.uk
Neural Computing Research Group
Aston University
Aston Triangle, Birmingham B4 7ET, UK.

Abstract

Given unlimited computational resources, it is best to use a criterion of minimal expected generalisation error to select a model and determine its parameters. However, it may be worthwhile to sacrifice some generalisation performance for higher learning speed. A method for quantifying sub-optimality is set out here, so that this choice can be made intelligently. Furthermore, the method is applicable to a broad class of models, including the ultra-fast memory-based methods such as RAMnets. This brings the added benefit of providing, for the first time, the means to analyse the generalisation properties of such models in a Bayesian framework.

1 Introduction

In order to quantitatively predict the performance of methods such as the ultra-fast RAMnet, which are not trained by minimising a cost function, we develop a Bayesian formalism for estimating the generalisation cost of a wide class of algorithms.

We consider the noisy interpolation problem, in which each output data point y^i results from adding noise to the result $y = f(x)$ of applying unknown function f to input data point x, which is generated from a distribution $P(x)$. We follow a similar approach to (Zhu & Rohwer, to appear 1996) in using a Gaussian process to define a prior over the space of functions, so that the expected generalisation cost under the posterior can be determined. The optimal model is defined in terms of the restriction of this posterior to the subspace defined by the model. The optimum is easily determined for linear models over a set of basis functions. We go on to compute the generalisation cost (with an error bar) for all models of this class, which we demonstrate to include the RAMnets.

Section 2 gives a brief overview of RAMnets. Sections 3 and 4 supply the formalism for computing expected generalisation costs under Gaussian process priors. Numerical experiments with this formalism are presented in Section 5. Finally, we discuss the current limitations of this technique and future research directions in Section 6.

2 RAMnets

The RAMnet, or n-tuple network is a very fast 1-pass learning system that often gives excellent results competitive with slower methods such as Radial Basis Function networks or Multi-layer Perceptrons (Rohwer & Morciniec, 1996). Although a semi-quantitative theory explains how these systems generalise, no formal framework has previously been given to precisely predict the accuracy of n-tuple networks.

Essentially, a RAMnet defines a set of "features" which can be regarded as Boolean functions of the input variables. Let the $a^{\underline{th}}$ feature of x be given by a $\{0,1\}$-valued function $\phi_a(x)$. We will focus on the n-tuple regression network (Allinson & Kołcz, 1995), which outputs

$$y = \overset{m}{\mathbf{f}}(x) = \frac{\sum_a \phi_a(x) \sum_i y^i \phi_a(x^i)}{\sum_a \phi_a(x) \sum_i \phi_a(x^i)} = \frac{\sum_i y^i U(x, x^i)}{\sum_i U(x, x^i)} \quad (1)$$

in response to input x, if trained on the set of N samples $\{\mathbf{x}_{(N)}\mathbf{y}_{(N)}\} = \{(x^i, y^i)\}_{i=1}^N$. Here $U(x, x') = \sum_a \phi_a(x)\phi_a(x')$ can be seen to play the role of a smoothing kernel, provided that it turns out to have a suitable shape. It is well-know that it does, for appropriate choices of feature sets. The strength of this method is that the sums over training data can be done in one pass, producing a table containing two totals for each feature. Only this table is required for recognition.

It is interesting to note that there is a familiar way to expand a kernel into the form $U(x, x') = \sum_a \phi_a(x)\phi_a(x')$, at least when $U(x, x') = U(x - x')$, if the range of ϕ is not restricted to $\{0,1\}$: an eigenfunction expansion[1]. Indeed, principal component analysis[2] applied to a Gaussian with variance $\mathbf{V}$ shows that the smallest feature set for a given generalisation cost consists of the (real-valued) projections onto the leading eigenfunctions of $\mathbf{V}$. Be that as it may, the treatment here applies to arbitrary feature sets.

3 Bayesian inference with Gaussian priors

Gaussian processes provide a diverse set of priors over function spaces. To avoid mathematical details of peripheral interest, let us approximate the infinite-dimensional space of functions by a finite-dimensional space of discretised functions, so that function f is replaced by high-dimensional vector $\mathbf{f}$, and $f(x)$ is replaced by $\mathbf{f}_x$, with $f(x) \approx \mathbf{f}_x$ within a volume Δx around x. We develop the case of scalar functions f, but the generalisation to vector-valued functions is straightforward.

---

[1] In physics, this is essentially the mode function expansion of U^{-1}, the differential operator with Green's function U.

[2] V^{-1} needs to be a compact operator for this to work in the infinite-dimensional limit.

The Generalisation Cost of RAMnets

We assume a Gaussian prior on $\mathbf{f}$, with zero mean and covariance $\mathbf{V}/\alpha$:

$$P(\mathbf{f}) = (1/Z_\alpha)e^{-\frac{\alpha}{2}\mathbf{f}^T\mathbf{V}^{-1}\mathbf{f}} \quad (2)$$

where $Z_\alpha = \det(\frac{2\pi}{\alpha}\mathbf{V})^{\frac{1}{2}}$. The overall scale of variation of $\mathbf{f}$ is controlled by α. Illustrative samples of the functions generated from various choices of covariance are given in (Zhu & Rohwer, to appear 1996). With q_x/β denoting the (possibly position-dependent) variance of the Gaussian output noise, the likelihood of outputs $\mathbf{y}_{(N)}$ given function $\mathbf{f}$ and inputs $\mathbf{x}_{(N)}$ is

$$P(\mathbf{y}_{(N)}|\mathbf{x}_{(N)},\mathbf{f}) = (1/Z_\beta)\exp-\frac{\beta}{2}\sum_i(\mathbf{f}_{x^i} - y^i)q_{x^i}^{-1}(\mathbf{f}_{x^i} - y^i) \quad (3)$$

where $Z_\beta^2 = \prod_i \frac{2\pi}{\beta} q_{x^i} = \det\left[\frac{2\pi}{\beta}\mathbf{Q}\right]$ with $\mathbf{Q}_{ij} = q_{x^i}\delta_{ij}$.

Because $\mathbf{f}$ and $\mathbf{x}_{(N)}$ are independent the joint distribution is

$$P(\mathbf{y}_{(N)},\mathbf{f}|\mathbf{x}_{(N)}) = P(\mathbf{y}_{(N)}|\mathbf{f},\mathbf{x}_{(N)})P(\mathbf{f}) = (e^{\frac{1}{2}\mathbf{b}^T\mathbf{A}\mathbf{b}+c})/(Z_\alpha Z_\beta)e^{-\frac{1}{2}(\mathbf{f}-\mathbf{Ab})^T\mathbf{A}^{-1}(\mathbf{f}-\mathbf{Ab})} \quad (4)$$

where δ_{x,x^i} is understood to be 1 whenever x^i is in the same cell of the discretisation as x, and $\mathbf{A}_{xx'}^{-1} = \alpha\mathbf{V}_{xx'}^{-1} + \beta\sum_i q_{x^i}^{-1}\delta_{x,x^i}\delta_{x',x^i}$, $\mathbf{b}_x = \beta\sum_i y^i q_{x^i}^{-1}\delta_{x,x^i}$, and $c = -\frac{1}{2}\beta\sum_i y^i q_{x^i}^{-1}y^i$. One can readily verify that

$$\mathbf{A}_{xx'} = (1/\alpha)\mathbf{V}_{xx'} + \sum_{tu}\mathbf{V}_{xx^t}\mathbf{K}_{tu}\mathbf{V}_{x^u x'} \quad (5)$$

where $\mathbf{K}$ is the $N \times N$ matrix defined by

$$\mathbf{K}_{tu}^{-1} = -(\alpha^2/\beta)q_{x^t}\delta_{t,u} - \alpha\mathbf{V}_{x^t x^u}. \quad (6)$$

The posterior is readily determined to be

$$P(\mathbf{f}|\mathbf{x}_{(N)},\mathbf{y}_{(N)}) = \frac{P(\mathbf{y}_{(N)},\mathbf{f}|\mathbf{x}_{(N)})}{P(\mathbf{y}_{(N)}|\mathbf{x}_{(N)})} = \det[2\pi\mathbf{A}]^{-\frac{1}{2}}e^{-\frac{1}{2}(\mathbf{f}-\overset{*}{\mathbf{f}})^T\mathbf{A}^{-1}(\mathbf{f}-\overset{*}{\mathbf{f}})}. \quad (7)$$

where $\overset{*}{\mathbf{f}} = \mathbf{Ab}$ is the posterior mean estimate of the true function $\mathbf{f}$.

4 Calculation of the expected cost and its variance

Let us define the cost of associating an output $\overset{m}{\mathbf{f}}_x$ of the model with an input x that actually produced an output y as

$$C(\overset{m}{\mathbf{f}}_x, y) = \tfrac{1}{2}(\overset{m}{\mathbf{f}}_x - y)^2 r_x$$

where r_x is a position dependent cost weight.

The average of this cost defines a cost functional, given input data $\mathbf{x}_{(N)}$:

$$C(\overset{m}{\mathbf{f}}, \mathbf{f}|\mathbf{x}_{(N)}) = \int C(\overset{m}{\mathbf{f}_x}, y) P(x|\mathbf{x}_{(N)}) P(y|x, \mathbf{f}) dx dy. \tag{8}$$

This form is obtained by noting that the function $\mathbf{f}$ carries no information about the input point x, and the input data $\mathbf{x}_{(N)}$ supplies no information about y beyond that supplied by $\mathbf{f}$. The distributions in (8) are unchanged by further conditioning on $\mathbf{y}_{(N)}$, so we could write $C(\overset{m}{\mathbf{f}}, \mathbf{f}|\mathbf{x}_{(N)}) = C(\overset{m}{\mathbf{f}}, \mathbf{f}|\mathbf{x}_{(N)}, \mathbf{y}_{(N)})$. This cost functional therefore has the posterior expectation value

$$\langle C|\mathbf{x}_{(N)}, \mathbf{y}_{(N)} \rangle = \int C(\overset{m}{\mathbf{f}_x}, y|\mathbf{x}_{(N)}) P(x, y, \mathbf{f}|\mathbf{x}_{(N)}, \mathbf{y}_{(N)}) dx dy d\mathbf{f} \tag{9}$$

and variance

$$\mathrm{var}\left[C(\overset{m}{\mathbf{f}}, \mathbf{f}|\mathbf{x}_{(N)})\right] = \int C(\overset{m}{\mathbf{f}}, \mathbf{f}|\mathbf{x}_{(N)})^2 P(\mathbf{f}|\mathbf{x}_{(N)}, \mathbf{y}_{(N)}) d\mathbf{f} - \langle C|\mathbf{x}_{(N)}, \mathbf{y}_{(N)} \rangle^2. \tag{10}$$

Plugging in the distributions (2) (applied to a single sample), (3) and (7) leads to:

$$\langle C|\mathbf{x}_{(N)}, \mathbf{y}_{(N)} \rangle = \tfrac{1}{2}\mathrm{tr}[\mathbf{AR}] + \tfrac{1}{2}(\overset{*}{\mathbf{f}} - \overset{m}{\mathbf{f}})^{\mathrm{T}} \mathbf{R}(\overset{*}{\mathbf{f}} - \overset{m}{\mathbf{f}}) + \frac{\mathrm{tr}[\mathbf{QR}]}{2\beta} \tag{11}$$

where the diagonal matrices $\mathbf{R}$ and $\mathbf{Q}$ have the elements $\mathbf{R}_{xx'} = P(x|X) r_x \Delta x \delta_{x,x'}$ and $\mathbf{Q}_{xx'} = q_x \delta_{xx'}$.

Similar calculations lead to the expression for the variance

$$\mathrm{var}\left[C(\overset{m}{\mathbf{f}}, \mathbf{f}|\mathbf{x}_{(N)}, \mathbf{y}_{(N)})\right] = \tfrac{1}{2}\mathrm{tr}[\mathbf{ARAR}] + \mathrm{tr}[\mathbf{ARRFF}]. \tag{12}$$

where the elements of $\mathbf{F}$ are $\mathbf{F}_{xx'} = (\overset{m}{\mathbf{f}_x} - \overset{*}{\mathbf{f}_x}) \delta_{x,x'}$.

Note that the RAMnet (1) has the form $\overset{m}{\mathbf{f}_x} = \sum_i \mathbf{J}_{xx^i} y^i$ linear in the output data $\mathbf{y}_{(N)}$, with $\mathbf{J}_{xx^i} = U(x, x^i)/\sum_j U(x, x_j)$. Let us take $\mathbf{V}$ to have the form $\mathbf{V}(x, x') = p(x) G(x - x') p(x')$, combining translation-invariant and non-invariant factors in a plausible way. Then with the sums over x replaced by integrals, (11) becomes explicitly

$$\begin{aligned}
2\langle C|\mathbf{x}_{(N)}, \mathbf{y}_{(N)} \rangle &= \frac{1}{\beta} \int dx P(x|\mathbf{x}_{(N)}) q_x r_x + \frac{1}{\alpha} \int P(x|\mathbf{x}_{(N)}) r_x p_x^2 \mathbf{G}_{xx} \\
&+ \frac{1}{\alpha} \sum_{tu} p_{x^t} \mathbf{K}_{tu} p_{x^u} \int dx P(x|\mathbf{x}_{(N)}) r_x p_x^2 \mathbf{G}_{x^u x} \mathbf{G}_{xx^t} \\
&+ \alpha^2 \sum_{tuvs} y^u \mathbf{K}_{ut} p_{x^t} \int dx P(x|\mathbf{x}_{(N)}) r_x p_x^2 \mathbf{G}_{x^t x} \mathbf{G}_{xx^s} p_{x^s} \mathbf{K}_{sv} y^v \\
&+ 2\alpha \sum_{tuv} y^u \mathbf{K}_{ut} p_{x^t} \int dx P(x|\mathbf{x}_{(N)}) r_x p_x \mathbf{G}_{x^t x} \mathbf{J}_{xx^v} y^v \\
&+ \sum_{uv} y^u \int dx P(x|\mathbf{x}_{(N)}) r_x \mathbf{J}_{x^u x} \mathbf{J}_{xx^v} y^v. \tag{13}
\end{aligned}$$

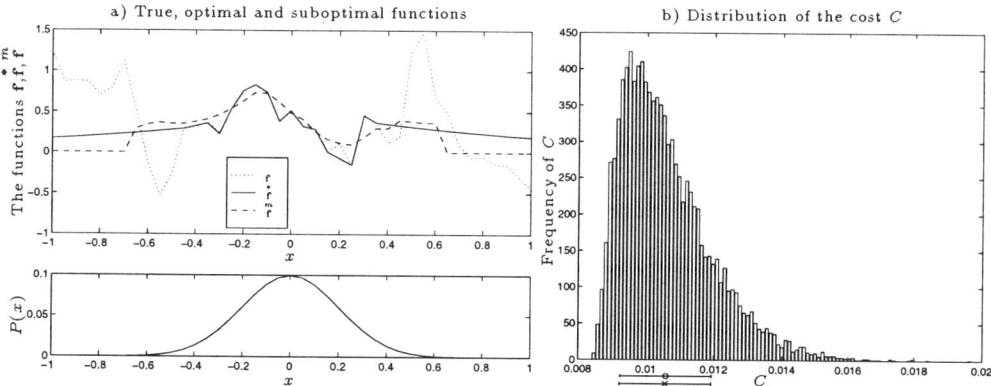

Figure 1: **a)** The lower figure shows the input distribution. The upper figure shows the true function **f** generated from a Gaussian prior with covariance matrix **V** (dotted line), the optimal function $\overset{*}{\mathbf{f}} = \mathbf{Ab}$ (solid line) and the suboptimal solution $\overset{m}{\mathbf{f}}$ (dashed line). **b)** The distribution of the cost function obtained by generating functions from the posterior Gaussian with covariance matrix **A** and calculating the cost according to equation 14. The mean and one standard deviation calculated analytically and numerically are shown by the lower and upper error bars respectively.

Taking $P(x|\mathbf{x}_{(N)})$ to be Gaussian (the maximum likelihood estimate would be reasonable) and p, r, and q uniform, the first four integrals are straightforward. The latter two involve the model **J**, and were evaluated numerically in the work reported below.

5 Numerical results

We present one numerical example to illustrate the formalism, and another to illustrate its application.

For the first illustration, let the input and output variables be one dimensional real numbers. Let the input distribution $P(x)$ be a Gaussian with mean $\mu_x = 0$ and standard deviation $\sigma_x = 0.2$. Nearly all inputs then fall within the range $[-1, 1]$, which we uniformly quantise into 41 bins. The true function **f** is generated from a Gaussian distribution with $\mu_\mathbf{f} = 0$ and 41×41 covariance matrix **V** with elements $\mathbf{V}_{xx'} = e^{-|x-x'|}$. 50 training inputs x were generated from the input distribution and assigned corresponding outputs $y = \mathbf{f}_x + \epsilon$, where ϵ is Gaussian noise with zero mean and standard deviation $\sqrt{q_x/\beta} \equiv 0.01$. The cost weight $r_x \equiv 1$.

The inputs were thermometer coded[3] over 256 bits, from which 100 subsets of 30 bits were randomly selected. Each of the 100×2^{30} patterns formed over these bits defines a RAMnet feature which evaluates to 1 when that pattern is present in the input x. (Only those features which actually appear in the data need to be tabulated.) The 50 training data points were used in this way to train an n-tuple

---
[3] The first $256(x+1)/2$ bits are set to 1, and the remaining bits to 0.

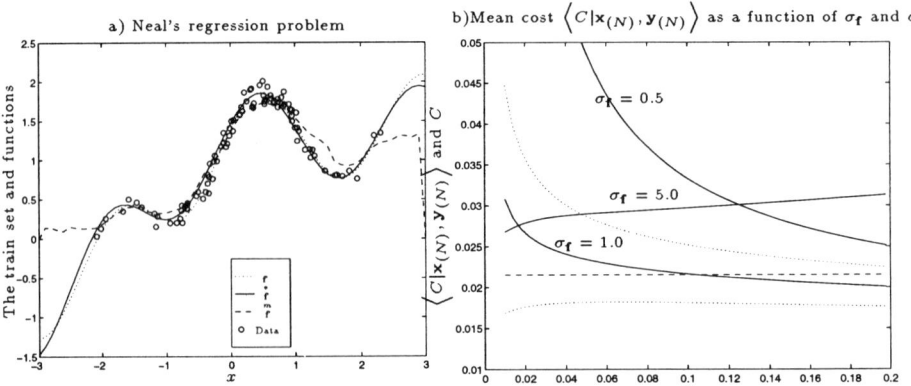

Figure 2: **a)** Neal's Regression problem. The true function **f** is indicated by a dotted line, the optimal function $\overset{*}{\mathbf{f}}$ is denoted by a solid line and the suboptimal solution $\overset{m}{\mathbf{f}}$ is indicated by a dashed line. Circles indicate the training data. **b)** Dependence of the cost prediction on the values of parameters α and $\sigma_{\mathbf{f}}$. The cost evaluated from the test set is plotted as a dashed line, predicted cost is shown as a solid line with one standard deviation indicated by a dotted line.

regression network. The input distribution and functions $\mathbf{f}, \overset{m}{\mathbf{f}}, \overset{*}{\mathbf{f}}$ are plotted in figure 1a.

A Gaussian distribution with mean $\overset{*}{\mathbf{f}}$ and posterior covariance matrix $\mathbf{A}$ was then used to generate 10^4 functions. For each such function **fp**, the generalisation cost

$$C = \tfrac{1}{2} \sum_x P\left(x|\mathbf{x}_{(N)}\right) (\mathbf{fp}_x - \overset{m}{\mathbf{f}}_x)^2. \tag{14}$$

was computed. A histogram of these costs appears in figure 1b, together with the theoretical and numerically computed average generalisation cost and its variance. Good agreement is evident.

Another one-dimensional problem illustrates the use of this formalism for predicting the generalisation performance of a RAMnet when the prior over functions can only be guessed. The true function, taken from (Neal, 1995) is given by

$$\mathbf{f}_x = 0.3 + 0.4x + 0.5\sin(2.7x) + 1.1/(1 + x^2) + \epsilon \tag{15}$$

where the Gaussian noise variable ϵ has mean $\mu_\epsilon = 0$ and standard deviation $\sqrt{q_x/\beta} \equiv 0.1$. The cost weight $r_x \equiv 1$. The training and test set each comprised 100 data-points. The inputs were generated by the standard normal distribution ($\mu_x = 0$, $\sigma_x = 1$) and converted into the binary strings using a thermometer code. The input range $[-3, 3]$ was quantised into 61 uniform bins.

The training set and the functions $\mathbf{f}, \overset{m}{\mathbf{f}}, \overset{*}{\mathbf{f}}$ are shown on figure 2a for $\alpha = 0.1$. The function space covariance matrix was defined to have the Gaussian form $\mathbf{V}_{xx'} = e^{-\frac{1}{2}\frac{(x-x')^2}{\sigma_{\mathbf{f}}^2}}$ where $\sigma_{\mathbf{f}} = 1.0$.

$\sigma_{\mathbf{f}}$ is the correlation length of the functions, which is of order 1, judging from figure 2a. The overall scale of variation is $1/\sqrt{\alpha}$, which appears to be about 3, so α should be about 1/9. Figure 2b shows the expected cost as a function of α for various choices of $\sigma_{\mathbf{f}}$, with error bars on the $\sigma_{\mathbf{f}} = 1.0$ curve. The actual cost computed from the test set according to $C = \frac{1}{2}\sum_{i}^{m}(y^i - \mathbf{f}_x)^2$ is plotted with a dashed line. There is good agreement around the sensible values of α and $\sigma_{\mathbf{f}}$.

6 Conclusions

This paper demonstrates that unusual models, such as the ultra-fast RAMnets which are not trained by directly optimising a cost function, can be analysed in a Bayesian framework to determine their generalisation cost. Because the formalism is constructed in terms of distributions over function space rather than distributions over model parameters, it can be used for model comparison, and in particular to select RAMnet parameters.

The main drawback with this technique, as it stands, is the need to numerically integrate two expressions which involve the model. This difficulty intensifies rapidly as the input dimension increases. Therefore, it is now a research priority to search for RAMnet feature sets which allow these integrals to be performed analytically.

It would also be interesting to average the expected costs over the training data, producing an expected generalisation cost for an algorithm. The $\mathbf{y}_{(N)}$ integral is straightforward, but the $\mathbf{x}_{(N)}$ integral is difficult. However, similar integrals have been carried out in the thermodynamic limit (high input dimension) (Sollich, 1994), so the investigation of these techniques in the current setting is another promising research direction.

7 Acknowledgements

We would like to thank the Aston Neural Computing Group, and especially Huaiyu Zhu, Chris Williams, and David Saad for helpful discussions.

References

Allinson, N.M., & Kołcz, A. 1995. *N-tuple Regression Network*. to be published in Neural Networks.

Neal, R. 1995. *Introductory documentation for software implementing Bayesian learning for neural networks using Markov chain Monte Carlo techniques*. Tech. rept. Dept of Computer Science, University of Toronto.

Rohwer, R., & Morciniec, M. 1996. A theoretical and experimental account of the n-tuple classifier performance. *Neural Computation*, **8**(3), 657–670.

Sollich, Peter. 1994. Finite-size effects in learning and generalization in linear perceptrons. *J. Phys. A*, **27**, 7771–7784.

Zhu, H., & Rohwer, R. to appear 1996. Bayesian regression filters and the issue of priors. *Neural Computing and Applications*. ftp://cs.aston.ac.uk/neural/zhuh/reg_fil_prior.ps.Z.

Learning with Noise and Regularizers in Multilayer Neural Networks

David Saad
Dept. of Comp. Sci. & App. Math.
Aston University
Birmingham B4 7ET, UK
D.Saad@aston.ac.uk

Sara A. Solla
AT&T Research Labs
Holmdel, NJ 07733, USA
solla@research.att.com

Abstract

We study the effect of noise and regularization in an on-line gradient-descent learning scenario for a general two-layer student network with an arbitrary number of hidden units. Training examples are randomly drawn input vectors labeled by a two-layer teacher network with an arbitrary number of hidden units; the examples are corrupted by Gaussian noise affecting either the output or the model itself. We examine the effect of both types of noise and that of weight-decay regularization on the dynamical evolution of the order parameters and the generalization error in various phases of the learning process.

1 Introduction

One of the most powerful and commonly used methods for training large layered neural networks is that of on-line learning, whereby the internal network parameters $\{\mathbf{J}\}$ are modified after the presentation of each training example so as to minimize the corresponding error. The goal is to bring the map $f_{\mathbf{J}}$ implemented by the network as close as possible to a desired map $\tilde{f}$ that generates the examples. Here we focus on the learning of continuous maps via gradient descent on a differentiable error function.

Recent work [1]-[4] has provided a powerful tool for the analysis of gradient-descent learning in a very general learning scenario [5]: that of a *student* network with N input units, K hidden units, and a single linear output unit, trained to implement a continuous map from an N-dimensional input space $\boldsymbol{\xi}$ onto a scalar ζ. Examples of the target task $\tilde{f}$ are in the form of input-output pairs $(\boldsymbol{\xi}^\mu, \zeta^\mu)$. The output labels ζ^μ to independently drawn inputs $\boldsymbol{\xi}^\mu$ are provided by a *teacher* network of similar architecture, except that its number M of hidden units is not necessarily equal to K.

Here we consider the possibility of a noise process ρ^μ that corrupts the teacher output. Learning from corrupt examples is a realistic and frequently encountered scenario. Previous analysis of this case have been based on various approaches: Bayesian [6], equilibrium statistical physics [7], and nonequilibrium techniques for analyzing learning dynamics [8]. Here we adapt our previously formulated techniques [2] to investigate the effect of different noise mechanisms on the dynamical evolution of the learning process and the resulting generalization ability.

2 The model

We focus on a *soft committee machine* [1], for which all hidden-to-output weights are positive and of unit strength. Consider the student network: hidden unit i receives information from input unit r through the weight J_{ir}, and its activation under presentation of an input pattern $\boldsymbol{\xi} = (\xi_1, \ldots, \xi_N)$ is $x_i = \mathbf{J}_i \cdot \boldsymbol{\xi}$, with $\mathbf{J}_i = (J_{i1}, \ldots, J_{iN})$ defined as the vector of incoming weights onto the i-th hidden unit. The output of the student network is $\sigma(\mathbf{J}, \boldsymbol{\xi}) = \sum_{i=1}^{K} g\left(\mathbf{J}_i \cdot \boldsymbol{\xi}\right)$, where g is the activation function of the hidden units, taken here to be the error function $g(x) \equiv \mathrm{erf}(x/\sqrt{2})$, and $\mathbf{J} \equiv \{\mathbf{J}_i\}_{1 \le i \le K}$ is the set of input-to-hidden adaptive weights.

The components of the input vectors $\boldsymbol{\xi}^\mu$ are uncorrelated random variables with zero mean and unit variance. Output labels ζ^μ are provided by a teacher network of similar architecture: hidden unit n in the teacher network receives input information through the weight vector $\mathbf{B}_n = (B_{n1}, \ldots, B_{nN})$, and its activation under presentation of the input pattern $\boldsymbol{\xi}^\mu$ is $y_n^\mu = \mathbf{B}_n \cdot \boldsymbol{\xi}^\mu$. In the noiseless case the teacher output is given by $\zeta_0^\mu = \sum_{n=1}^{M} g\left(\mathbf{B}_n \cdot \boldsymbol{\xi}^\mu\right)$. Here we concentrate on the architecturally matched case $M = K$, and consider two types of Gaussian noise: additive output noise that results in $\zeta^\mu = \rho^\mu + \sum_{n=1}^{K} g\left(\mathbf{B}_n \cdot \boldsymbol{\xi}^\mu\right)$, and model noise introduced as fluctuations in the activations y_n^μ of the hidden units, $\zeta^\mu = \sum_{n=1}^{K} g\left(\rho_n^\mu + \mathbf{B}_n \cdot \boldsymbol{\xi}^\mu\right)$. The random variables ρ^μ and ρ_n^μ are taken to be Gaussian with zero mean and variance σ^2.

The error made by a student with weights $\mathbf{J}$ on a given input $\boldsymbol{\xi}$ is given by the quadratic deviation

$$\epsilon(\mathbf{J}, \boldsymbol{\xi}) \equiv \frac{1}{2}\left[\, \sigma(\mathbf{J}, \boldsymbol{\xi}) - \zeta_0 \,\right]^2 = \frac{1}{2}\left[\sum_{i=1}^{K} g(x_i) - \sum_{n=1}^{K} g(y_n)\right]^2, \quad (1)$$

measured with respect to the noiseless teacher (it is also possible to measure performance as deviations with respect to the actual output ζ provided by the noisy teacher). Performance on a typical input defines the generalization error $\epsilon_g(\mathbf{J}) \equiv \,<\epsilon(\mathbf{J}, \boldsymbol{\xi})>_{\{\xi\}}$, through an average over all possible input vectors $\boldsymbol{\xi}$ to be performed implicitly through averages over the activations $\mathbf{x} = (x_1, \ldots, x_K)$ and $\mathbf{y} = (y_1, \ldots, y_K)$. These averages can be performed analytically [2] and result in a compact expression for ϵ_g in terms of *order parameters*: $Q_{ik} \equiv \mathbf{J}_i \cdot \mathbf{J}_k$, $R_{in} \equiv \mathbf{J}_i \cdot \mathbf{B}_n$, and $T_{nm} \equiv \mathbf{B}_n \cdot \mathbf{B}_m$, which represent student-student, student-teacher, and teacher-teacher overlaps, respectively. The parameters T_{nm} are characteristic of the task to be learned and remain fixed during training, while the overlaps Q_{ik} among student hidden units and R_{in} between a student and a teacher hidden units are determined by the student weights $\mathbf{J}$ and evolve during training.

A gradient descent rule on the error made with respect to the actual output provided by the noisy teacher results in $\mathbf{J}_i^{\mu+1} = \mathbf{J}_i^\mu + \frac{\eta}{N} \delta_i^\mu \boldsymbol{\xi}^\mu$ for the update of the student weights, where the learning rate η has been scaled with the input size N, and δ_i^μ depends on the type of noise. The time evolution of the overlaps R_{in} and Q_{ik} can be written in terms of similar difference equations. We consider the large N limit, and introduce a normalized number of examples $\alpha = \mu/N$ to be interpreted as a continuous time variable in the $N \to \infty$ limit. The time evolution of R_{in} and Q_{ik} is thus described in terms of first-order differential equations.

3 Output noise

The resulting equations of motion for the student-teacher and student-student overlaps are given in this case by:

$$\frac{dR_{in}}{d\alpha} = \eta <\delta_i\, y_n>, \tag{2}$$

$$\frac{dQ_{ik}}{d\alpha} = \eta <\delta_i\, x_k> + \eta <\delta_k\, x_i> + \eta^2 <\delta_i\, \delta_k> + \eta^2 \sigma^2 <g'(x_i)\, g'(x_k)>,$$

where each term is to be averaged over all possible ways in which an example $\boldsymbol{\xi}$ could be chosen at a given time step. These averages have been performed using the techniques developed for the investigation of the noiseless case [2]; the only difference due to the presence of additive output noise is the need to evaluate the fourth term in the equation of motion for Q_{ik}, proportional to both η^2 and σ^2.

We focus on isotropic uncorrelated teacher vectors: $T_{nm} = T\, \delta_{nm}$, and choose $T = 1$ in our numerical examples. The time evolution of the overlaps R_{in} and Q_{ik} follows from integrating the equations of motion (2) from initial conditions determined by a random initialization of the student vectors $\{\mathbf{J}_i\}_{1 \leq i \leq K}$. Random initial norms Q_{ii} for the student vectors are taken here from a uniform distribution in the $[0, 0.5]$ interval. Overlaps Q_{ik} between independently chosen student vectors $\mathbf{J}_i$ and $\mathbf{J}_k$, or R_{in} between $\mathbf{J}_i$ and an unknown teacher vector $\mathbf{B}_n$, are small numbers of order $1/\sqrt{N}$ for $N \gg K$, and taken here from a uniform distribution in the $[0, 10^{-12}]$ interval.

We show in Figures 1.a and 1.b the evolution of the overlaps for a noise variance $\sigma^2 = 0.3$ and learning rate $\eta = 0.2$. The example corresponds to $M = K = 3$. The qualitative behavior is similar to the one observed for $M = K$ in the noiseless case extensively analyzed in [2]. A very short transient is followed by a long plateau characterized by lack of differentiation among student vectors: all student vectors have the same norm $Q_{ii} = Q$, the overlap between any two different student vectors takes a unique value $Q_{ik} = C$ for $i \neq k$, and the overlap R_{in} between an arbitrary student vector i and a teacher vector n is independent of i (as student vectors are indistinguishable in this regime) and of n (as the teacher is isotropic), resulting in $R_{in} = R$. This phase is characterized by an unstable symmetric solution; the perturbation introduced through the nonsymmetric initialization of the norms Q_{ii} and overlaps R_{in} eventually takes over in a transition that signals the onset of specialization.

This process is driven by a breaking of the uniform symmetry of the matrix of student-teacher overlaps: each student vector acquires an increasingly dominant overlap R with a specific teacher vector which it begins to imitate, and a gradually decreasing secondary overlap S with the remaining teacher vectors. In the example of Figure 1.b the assignment corresponds to $i = 1 \to n = 1$, $i = 2 \to n = 3$, and $i = 3 \to n = 2$. A relabeling of the student hidden units allows us to identify R with the diagonal elements and S with the off-diagonal elements of the matrix of student-teacher overlaps.

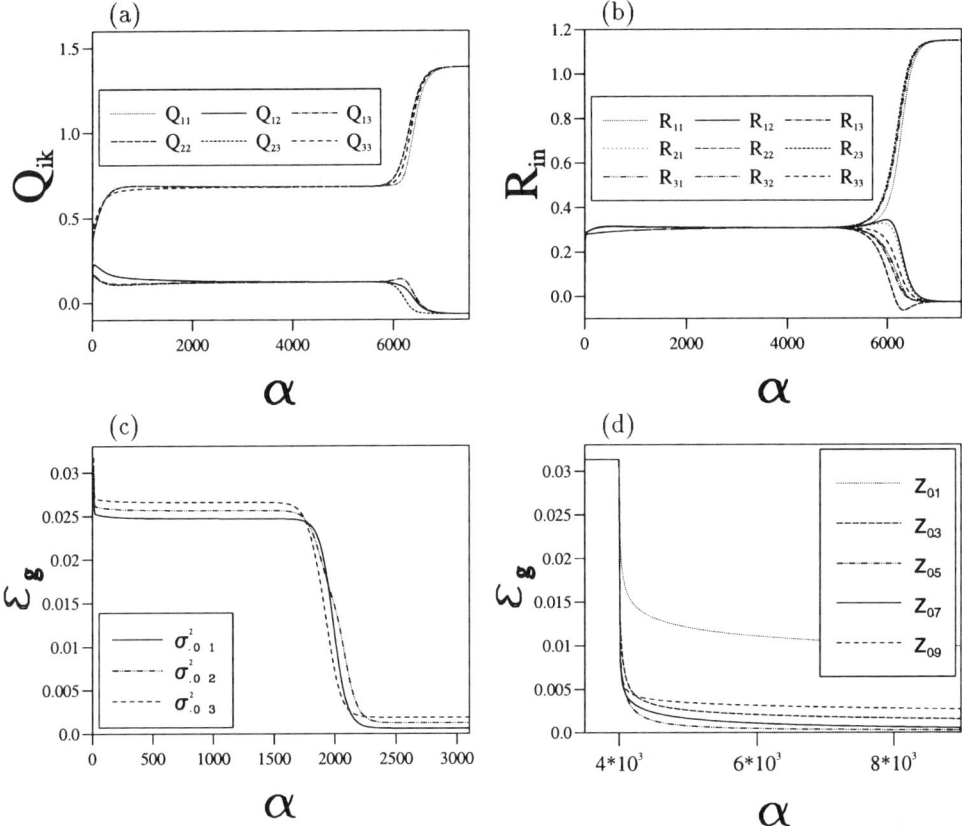

Figure 1: Dependence of the overlaps and the generalization error on the normalized number of examples α for a three-node student learning corrupted examples generated by an isotropic three-node teacher. (a) student-student overlaps Q_{ik} and (b) student-teacher overlaps R_{in} for $\sigma^2 = 0.3$. The generalization error is shown in (c) for different values of the noise variance σ^2, and in (d) for different powers of the polynomial learning rate decay, focusing on $\alpha > \alpha_0$ (asymptotic regime).

Asymptotically the secondary overlaps S decay to zero, while $R_{in} \to \sqrt{Q_{ii}}$ indicates full alignment for $T_{nn} = 1$. As specialization proceeds, the student weight vectors grow in length and become increasingly uncorrelated. It is interesting to observe that in the presence of noise the student vectors grow asymptotically longer than the teacher vectors: $Q_{ii} \to Q_\infty > 1$, and acquire a small negative correlation with each other. Another detectable difference in the presence of noise is a larger gap between the values of Q and C in the symmetric phase. Larger norms for the student vectors result in larger generalization errors: as shown in Figure 1.c, the generalization error increases monotonically with increasing noise level, both in the symmetric and asymptotic regimes.

For an isotropic teacher, the teacher-student and student-student overlaps can thus be fully characterized by four parameters: $Q_{ik} = Q\delta_{ik} + C(1-\delta_{ik})$ and $R_{in} = R\delta_{in} + S(1-\delta_{in})$. In the symmetric phase the additional constraint $R = S$ reflects the lack of differentiation among student vectors and reduces the number of parameters to three.

The symmetric phase is characterized by a fixed point solution to the equations of motion (2) whose coordinates can be obtained analytically in the small noise approximation: $R^* = 1/\sqrt{K(2K-1)} + \eta\,\sigma^2\,r_s$, $Q^* = 1/(2K-1) + \eta\,\sigma^2\,q_s$, and $C^* = 1/(2K-1) + \eta\,\sigma^2\,c_s$, with r_s, q_s, and c_s given by relatively simple functions of K. The generalization error in this regime is given by:

$$\epsilon_g^* = \frac{K}{\pi}\left(\frac{\pi}{6} - K\arcsin\left(\frac{1}{2K}\right)\right) + \frac{\sigma^2\eta}{2\pi}\frac{(2K-1)^{3/2}}{(2K+1)^{1/2}}\;; \qquad (3)$$

note its increase over the corresponding noiseless value, recovered for $\sigma^2 = 0$.

The asymptotic phase is characterized by a fixed point solution with $R^* \neq S^*$. The coordinates of the asymptotic fixed point can also be obtained analytically in the small noise approximation: $R^* = 1 + \eta\,\sigma^2\,r_a$, $S^* = -\eta\,\sigma^2\,s_a$, $Q^* = 1 + \eta\,\sigma^2\,q_a$, and $C^* = -\eta\,\sigma^2\,c_a$, with r_a, s_a, q_a, and c_a given by rational functions of K with corrections of order η. The asymptotic generalization error is given by

$$\epsilon_g^* = \frac{\sqrt{3}}{6\pi}\,\eta\,\sigma^2 K\;. \qquad (4)$$

Explicit expressions for the coefficients $r_s, q_s, c_s, r_a, s_a, q_a$, and c_a will not be given here for lack of space; suffice it to say that the fixed point coordinates predicted on the basis of the small noise approximation are found to be in excellent agreement with the values obtained from the numerical integration of the equations of motion for $\sigma^2 \leq 0.3$.

It is worth noting in Figure 1.c that in the small noise regime the length of the symmetric plateau decreases with increasing noise. This effect can be investigated analytically by linearizing the equations of motion around the symmetric fixed point and identifying the positive eigenvalue responsible for the escape from the symmetric phase. This calculation has been carried out in the small noise approximation, to obtain $\lambda = (2/\pi)K(2K-1)^{-1/2}(2K+1)^{-3/2} + \lambda_\sigma \sigma^2 \eta$, where λ_σ is positive and increases monotonically with K for $K > 1$. A faster escape from the symmetric plateau is explained by this increase of the positive eigenvalue. The calculation is valid for $\sigma^2\eta \ll 1$; we observe experimentally that the trend is reversed as σ^2 increases. A small level of noise assists in the process of differentiation among student vectors, while larger levels of noise tend to keep student vectors equally ignorant about the task to be learned.

The asymptotic value (4) for the generalization error indicates that learning at finite η will result in asymptotically suboptimal performance for $\sigma^2 > 0$. A monotonic decrease of the learning rate is necessary to achieve optimal asymptotic performance with $\epsilon_g^* = 0$. Learning at small η results in long trapping times in the symmetric phase; we therefore suggest starting the training process with a relatively large value of η and switching to a decaying learning rate at $\alpha = \alpha_0$, after specialization begins. We propose $\eta = \eta_0$ for $\alpha \leq \alpha_0$ and $\eta = \eta_0/(\alpha - \alpha_0)^z$ for $\alpha > \alpha_0$. Convergence to the asymptotic solution requires $z \leq 1$. The value $z = 1$ corresponds to the fastest decay for $\eta(\alpha)$; the question of interest is to determine the value of z which results in fastest decay for $\epsilon_g(\alpha)$. Results shown in Figure 1.d for $\alpha > \alpha_0 = 4000$ correspond to $M = K = 3$, $\eta_0 = 0.7$, and $\sigma^2 = 0.1$. Our numerical results indicate optimal decay of $\epsilon_g(\alpha)$ for $z = 1/2$. A rigorous justification of this result remains to be found.

4 Model noise

The resulting equations of motion for the student-teacher and student-student overlaps can also be obtained analytically in this case; they exhibit a structure remark-

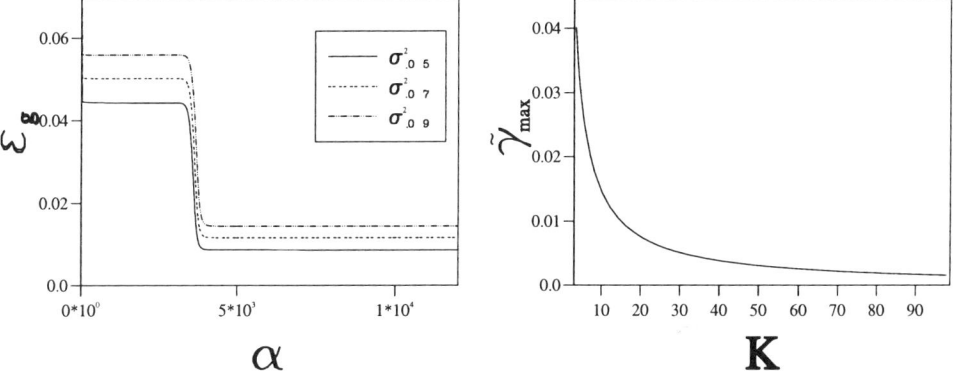

Figure 2: Left - The generalization error for different values of the noise variance σ^2; training examples are corrupted by model noise. Right - $\tilde{\gamma}_{max}$ as a function of K.

ably similar to those for the noiseless case reported in [2], except for some changes in the relevant covariance matrices.

A numerical investigation of the dynamical evolution of the overlaps and generalization error reveals qualitative and quantitative differences with the case of additive output noise: 1) The sensitivity to noise is much higher for model noise than for output noise. 2) The application of independent noise to the individual teacher hidden units results in an effective anisotropic teacher and causes fluctuations in the symmetric phase; the various student hidden units acquire some degree of differentiation and the symmetric phase can no longer be fully characterized by unique values of Q and C. 3) The noise level does not affect the length of the symmetric phase.

The effect of model noise on the generalization error is illustrated in Figure 2 for $M = K = 3$, $\eta = 0.2$, and various noise levels. The generalization error increases monotonically with increasing noise level, both in the symmetric and asymptotic regimes, but there is no modification in the length of the symmetric phase. The dynamical evolution of the overlaps, not shown here for the case of model noise, exhibits qualitative features quite similar to those discussed in the case of additive output noise: we observe again a noise-induced widening of the gap between Q and C in the symmetric phase, while the asymptotic phase exhibits an enhancement of the norm of the student vectors and a small degree of negative correlation between them.

Approximate analytic expressions based on a small noise expansion have been obtained for the coordinates of the fixed point solutions which describe the symmetric and asymptotic phases. In the case of model noise the expansions for the symmetric solution are independent of η and depend only on σ^2 and K. The coordinates of the asymptotic fixed point can be expressed as: $R^* = 1 + \sigma^2 \, r_a$, $S^* = -\sigma^2 \, s_a$, $Q^* = 1 + \sigma^2 \, q_a$, $C^* = -\sigma^2 \, c_a$, with coefficients r_a, s_a, q_a, and c_a given by rational functions of K with corrections of order η. The important difference with the output noise case is that the asymptotic fixed point is shifted from its noiseless position even for $\eta = 0$. It is therefore not possible to achieve optimal asymptotic performance even if a decaying learning rate is utilized. The asymptotic generalization error is given by

$$\epsilon_g^* = \frac{\sqrt{3}}{12\pi} \sigma^2 K + \eta \, \sigma^2 K \, \epsilon_a(K, \eta) \,. \tag{5}$$

Note that the asymptotic generalization error remains finite even as $\eta \to 0$.

5 Regularizers

A method frequently used in real world training scenarios to overcome the effects of noise and parameter redundancy ($K > M$) is the use of regularizers such as weight decay (for a review see [6]).

Weight-decay regularization is easily incorporated within the framework of on-line learning; it leads to a rule for the update of the student weights of the form $\mathbf{J}_i^{\mu+1} = \mathbf{J}_i^{\mu} + \frac{\eta}{N} \delta_i^{\mu} \boldsymbol{\xi}^{\mu} - \frac{\gamma}{N} \mathbf{J}_i^{\mu}$. The corresponding equations of motion for the dynamical evolution of the teacher-student and student-student overlaps can again be obtained analytically and integrated numerically from random initial conditions.

The picture that emerges is basically similar to that described for the noisy case: the dynamical evolution of the learning process goes through the same stages, although specific values for the order parameters and generalization error at the symmetric phase and in the asymptotic regime are changed as a consequence of the modification in the dynamics.

Our numerical investigations have revealed no scenario, either when training from noisy data or in the presence of redundant parameters, where weight decay improves the system performance or speeds up the training process. This lack of effect is probably a generic feature of on-line learning, due to the absence of an additive, stationary error surface defined over a finite and fixed training set. In off-line (batch) learning, regularization leads to improved performance through the modification of such error surface. These observations are consistent with the absence of 'overfitting' phenomena in on-line learning. One of the effects that arises when weight-decay regularization is introduced in on-line learning is a prolongation of the symmetric phase, due to a decrease in the positive eingenvalue that controls the onset of specialization. This positive eigenvalue, which signals the instability of the symmetric fixed point, decreases monotonically with increasing regularization strength γ, and crosses zero at $\gamma_{max} = \eta \, \tilde{\gamma}_{max}$. The dependence of $\tilde{\gamma}_{max}$ on K is shown in Figure 2; for $\gamma > \gamma_{max}$ the symmetric fixed point is stable and the system remains trapped there for ever.

The work reported here focuses on an architecturally matched scenario, with $M = K$. Over-realizable cases with $K > M$ show a rich behavior that is rather less amenable to generic analysis. It will be of interest to examine the effects of different types of noise and regularizers in this regime.

Acknowledgement: D.S. acknowledges support from EPSRC grant GR/L19232.

References

[1] M. Biehl and H. Schwarze, *J. Phys. A* **28**, 643 (1995).

[2] D. Saad and S.A. Solla, *Phys. Rev. E* **52**, 4225 (1995).

[3] D. Saad and S.A. Solla, preprint (1996).

[4] P. Riegler and M. Biehl, *J. Phys. A* **28**, L507 (1995).

[5] G. Cybenko, *Math. Control Signals and Systems* **2**, 303 (1989).

[6] C.M. Bishop, *Neural networks for pattern recognition*, (Oxford University Press, Oxford, 1995).

[7] T.L.H. Watkin, A. Rau, and M. Biehl, *Rev. Mod. Phys.* **65**, 499 (1993).

[8] K.R. Müller, M. Finke, N. Murata, K. Schulten, and S. Amari, *Neural Computation* **8**, 1085 (1996).

A variational principle for model-based morphing

Lawrence K. Saul* and Michael I. Jordan
Center for Biological and Computational Learning
Massachusetts Institute of Technology
79 Amherst Street, E10-034D
Cambridge, MA 02139

Abstract

Given a multidimensional data set and a model of its density, we consider how to define the optimal interpolation between two points. This is done by assigning a cost to each path through space, based on two competing goals—one to interpolate through regions of high density, the other to minimize arc length. From this path functional, we derive the Euler-Lagrange equations for extremal motion; given two points, the desired interpolation is found by solving a boundary value problem. We show that this interpolation can be done efficiently, in high dimensions, for Gaussian, Dirichlet, and mixture models.

1 Introduction

The problem of non-linear interpolation arises frequently in image, speech, and signal processing. Consider the following two examples: (i) given two profiles of the same face, connect them by a smooth animation of intermediate poses[1]; (ii) given a telephone signal masked by intermittent noise, fill in the missing speech. Both these examples may be viewed as instances of the same abstract problem. In qualitative terms, we can state the problem as follows[2]: given a multidimensional data set, and two points from this set, find a smooth adjoining path that is consistent with available models of the data. We will refer to this as the problem of *model-based morphing*.

In this paper, we examine this problem it arises from statistical models of multidimensional data. Specifically, our focus is on models that have been derived from

---
*Current address: AT&T Labs, 600 Mountain Ave 2D-439, Murray Hill, NJ 07974

some form of density estimation. Though there exists a large body of work on the use of statistical models for regression and classification, there has been comparatively little work on the other types of operations that these models support. Non-linear morphing is an example of such an operation, one that has important applications to video email[3], low-bandwidth teleconferencing[4], and audiovisual speech recognition[2].

A common way to describe multidimensional data is some form of mixture modeling. Mixture models represent the data as a collection of two or more clusters; thus, they are well-suited to handling complicated (multimodal) data sets. Roughly speaking, for these models the problem of interpolation can be divided into two tasks—how to interpolate between points in the same cluster, and how to interpolate between points in different clusters. Our paper will therefore be organized along these lines.

Previous studies of morphing have exploited the properties of radial basis function networks[1] and locally linear models[2]. We have been influenced by both these works, especially in the abstract formulation of the problem. New features of our approach include: the fundamental role played by the density, the treatment of non-Gaussian models, the use of a continuous variational principle, and the description of the interpolant by a differential equation.

2 Intracluster interpolation

Let $Q = \{\mathbf{q}^{(1)}, \mathbf{q}^{(2)}, \ldots, \mathbf{q}^{|Q|}\}$ denote a set of multidimensional data points, and let $P(\mathbf{q})$ denote a model of the distribution from which these points were generated. Given two points, our problem is to find a smooth adjoining path that respects the statistical model of the data. In particular, the desired interpolant should not pass through regions of space that the modeled density $P(\mathbf{q})$ assigns low probability.

2.1 Clusters and metrics

To develop these ideas further, we begin by considering a special class of models—namely, those that represent clusters. We say that $P(\mathbf{q})$ models a *data cluster* if $P(\mathbf{q})$ has a unique (global) maximum; in turn, we identify the location of this maximum, $\mathbf{q}^*$, as the *prototype*.

Let us now consider the geometry of the space inhabited by the data. To endow this space with a geometric structure, we must define a metric, $g_{\alpha\beta}(\mathbf{q})$, that provides a measure of the distance between two nearby points:

$$\mathcal{D}[\mathbf{q}, \mathbf{q} + \mathbf{dq}] = \left[\sum_{\alpha\beta} g_{\alpha\beta}(\mathbf{q}) \, dq_\alpha dq_\beta \right]^{\frac{1}{2}} + O\left(|\mathbf{dq}|^2 \right). \quad (1)$$

Intuitively speaking, the metric should reflect the fact that as one moves away from the center of the cluster, the density of the data dies off more quickly in some directions than in others. A natural choice for the metric, one that meets the above criteria, is the negative Hessian of the log-likelihood:

$$g_{\alpha\beta}(\mathbf{q}) = -\frac{\partial^2}{\partial q_\alpha \partial q_\beta} \left[\ln P(\mathbf{q}) \right]. \quad (2)$$

A Variational Principle for Model-based Morphing

This metric is positive-definite if $\ln P(\mathbf{q})$ is concave; this will be true for all the examples we discuss.

2.2 From densities to paths

The problem of model-based interpolation is to balance two competing goals—one to interpolate through regions of high density, the other to avoid excessive deformations. Using the metric in eq. (1), we can now assign a cost (or penalty) to each path based on these competing goals.

Consider the path parameterized by $\mathbf{q}(t)$. We begin by dividing the path into segments, each of which is traversed in some small time interval, dt. We assign a value to each segment by

$$\phi(t) = \left\{ \left[\frac{P(\mathbf{q}(t))}{P(\mathbf{q}^*)}\right] e^{-\ell} \right\}^{\mathcal{D}[\mathbf{q}(t),\mathbf{q}(t+dt)]}, \tag{3}$$

where $\ell \geq 0$. For reasons that will become clear shortly, we refer to ℓ as the *line tension*. The value assigned to each segment depends on two terms: a ratio of probabilities, $P(\mathbf{q}(t))/P(\mathbf{q}^*)$, which favors points near the prototype, and the constant multiplier, $e^{-\ell}$. Both these terms are upper bounded by unity, and hence so is their product. The value of the segment also decays with its length, as a result of the exponent, $\mathcal{D}[\mathbf{q}(t), \mathbf{q}(t+dt)]$.

We derive a path functional by piecing these segments together, multiplying their individual contributions, and taking the continuum limit. A value for the entire path is obtained from the product:

$$e^{-\mathcal{S}} = \prod_t \phi(t). \tag{4}$$

Taking the logarithm of both sides, and considering the limit $dt \to 0$, we obtain the path functional

$$\mathcal{S}[\mathbf{q}(t)] = \int \left\{ -\ln\left[\frac{P(\mathbf{q}(t))}{P(\mathbf{q}^*)}\right] + \ell \right\} \left[\sum_{\alpha\beta} g_{\alpha\beta}(\mathbf{q})\, \dot{q}_\alpha \dot{q}_\beta\right]^{\frac{1}{2}} dt, \tag{5}$$

where $\dot{\mathbf{q}} \equiv \frac{d}{dt}[\mathbf{q}]$ is the tangent vector to the path at time t. The terms in this functional balance the two competing goals for non-linear interpolation. The first favors paths that interpolate through regions of high density, while the second favors paths with small arc lengths; both are computed under the metric induced by the modeled density. The line tension ℓ determines the cost per unit arc length and modulates the competition between the two terms. Note that the value of the functional does not depend on the rate at which the path is traversed.

To minimize this functional, we use the following result from the calculus of variations. Let $\mathcal{L}(\mathbf{q}, \dot{\mathbf{q}})$ denote the integrand of eq. (5), such that $\mathcal{S}[\mathbf{q}(t)] = \int dt\, \mathcal{L}(\mathbf{q}, \dot{\mathbf{q}})$. Then the path which minimizes this functional obeys the Euler-Lagrange equations[5]:

$$\frac{d}{dt}\left(\frac{\partial \mathcal{L}}{\partial \dot{\mathbf{q}}}\right) = \frac{\partial \mathcal{L}}{\partial \mathbf{q}}. \tag{6}$$

We define the model-based interpolant between two points as the path which minimizes this functional; it is found by solving the associated boundary value problem. The function $\mathcal{L}(\mathbf{q}, \dot{\mathbf{q}})$ is known as the *Lagrangian*. In the next sections, we present eq. (5) for two distributions of interest—the multivariate Gaussian and the Dirichlet.

2.3 Gaussian cloud

The simplest model of multidimensional data is the multivariate Gaussian. In this case, the data is modeled by

$$P(\mathbf{x}) = \frac{|\mathbf{M}|^{1/2}}{(2\pi)^{N/2}} \exp\left\{-\frac{1}{2}[\mathbf{x}^T \mathbf{M} \mathbf{x}]\right\}, \tag{7}$$

where $\mathbf{M}$ is the inverse covariance matrix and N is the dimensionality. Without loss of generality, we have chosen the coordinate system so that the mean of the data coincides with the origin. For the Gaussian, the mean also defines the location of the prototype; moreover, from eq. (2), the metric induced by this model is just the inverse covariance matrix. From eq. (5), we obtain the path functional:

$$\mathcal{S}[\mathbf{x}(t)] = \int \left\{\frac{1}{2}[\mathbf{x}^T \mathbf{M} \mathbf{x}] + \ell\right\} [\dot{\mathbf{x}}^T \mathbf{M} \dot{\mathbf{x}}]^{\frac{1}{2}} dt, \tag{8}$$

To find a model-based interpolant, we seek the path that minimizes this functional. Because the functional is parameterization-invariant, it suffices to consider paths that are traversed at a constant (unit) rate: $\dot{\mathbf{x}}^T \mathbf{M} \dot{\mathbf{x}} = 1$. From eq. (6), we find that the optimal path with this parameterization satisfies:

$$\left\{\frac{1}{2}[\mathbf{x}^T \mathbf{M} \mathbf{x}] + \ell\right\} \ddot{\mathbf{x}} + [\mathbf{x}^T \mathbf{M} \dot{\mathbf{x}}] \dot{\mathbf{x}} = \mathbf{x}. \tag{9}$$

This is a set of coupled non-linear equations for the components of $\mathbf{x}(t)$. However, note that at any moment in time, the acceleration, $\ddot{\mathbf{x}}$, can be expressed as a linear combination of the position, $\mathbf{x}$, and the velocity, $\dot{\mathbf{x}}$. It follows that the motion of $\mathbf{x}$ lies in a plane; in particular, it lies in the plane spanned by the initial conditions, $\mathbf{x}$ and $\dot{\mathbf{x}}$, at time $t = 0$. This enables one to solve the boundary value problem efficiently, even in very high dimensions.

Figure 1a shows some solutions to this boundary value problem for different values of the line tension, ℓ. Note how the paths bend toward the origin, with the degree of curvature determined by the line tension, ℓ.

2.4 Dirichlet simplex

For many types of data, the multivariate Gaussian distribution is not the most appropriate model. Suppose that the data points are vectors of positive numbers whose elements sum to one. In particular, we say that $\mathbf{w}$ is a *probability vector* if $\mathbf{w} = (w_1, w_2, \ldots, w_N) \in \mathcal{R}^N$, $w_\alpha > 0$ for all α, and $\sum_\alpha w_\alpha = 1$. Clearly, the multivariate Gaussian is not suited to data of this form, since no matter what the mean and covariance matrix, it cannot assign zero probability to vectors outside the simplex. Instead, a more natural model is the Dirichlet distribution:

$$P(\mathbf{w}) = \Gamma(\theta) \prod_\alpha \frac{w_\alpha^{\theta_\alpha - 1}}{\Gamma(\theta_\alpha)}, \tag{10}$$

where $\theta_\alpha > 0$ for all α, and $\theta \equiv \sum_\alpha \theta_\alpha$. Here, $\Gamma(\cdot)$ is the gamma function, and θ_α are parameters that determine the statistics of $P(\mathbf{w})$. Note that $P(\mathbf{w}) = 0$ for vectors that are not probability vectors; in particular, the simplex constraints on $\mathbf{w}$ are implicit assumptions of the model.

We can rewrite the Dirichlet distribution in a more revealing form as follows. First, let $\mathbf{w}^*$ denote the probability vector with elements $w_\alpha^* = \theta_\alpha/\theta$. Then, making a change of variables from $\mathbf{w}$ to $\ln \mathbf{w}$, we have:

$$P(\ln \mathbf{w}) = \frac{1}{Z_\theta} \exp\left\{-\theta \left[\mathrm{KL}\left(\mathbf{w}^*||\mathbf{w}\right)\right]\right\}, \tag{11}$$

where Z_θ is a normalization factor that depends on θ_α (but not $\mathbf{w}$), and the quantity in the exponent is θ times the Kullback-Leibler (KL) divergence,

$$\mathrm{KL}\left(\mathbf{w}^*||\mathbf{w}\right) = \sum_\alpha w_\alpha^* \ln\left[\frac{w_\alpha^*}{w_\alpha}\right]. \tag{12}$$

The KL divergence measures the mismatch between $\mathbf{w}$ and $\mathbf{w}^*$, with $\mathrm{KL}(\mathbf{w}^*||\mathbf{w}) = 0$ if and only if $\mathbf{w} = \mathbf{w}^*$. Since $\mathrm{KL}(\mathbf{w}^*||\mathbf{w})$ has no other minima besides the one at $\mathbf{w}^*$, we shall say that $P(\ln \mathbf{w})$ models a data cluster *in the variable* $\ln \mathbf{w}$.

The metric induced by this modeled density is computed by following the prescription of eq. (2). For two nearby points inside the simplex, $\mathbf{w}$ and $\mathbf{w} + d\mathbf{w}$, the result of this prescription is that the squared distance is given by

$$ds^2 = \theta \sum_\alpha \frac{dw_\alpha^2}{w_\alpha}. \tag{13}$$

Up to a multiplicative factor of 2θ, eq. (13) measures the infinitesimal KL divergence between $\mathbf{w}$ and $\mathbf{w} + d\mathbf{w}$. This is a natural metric for vectors whose elements can be interpreted as probabilities.

The functional for non-linear interpolation is found by substituting the modeled density and the induced metric into eq. (5). For the Dirichlet distribution, this gives:

$$\mathcal{S}[\mathbf{w}(t)] = \int \left\{\theta\left[\mathrm{KL}\left(\mathbf{w}^*||\mathbf{w}\right)\right] + \ell\right\} \left[\theta \sum_\alpha \frac{\dot{w}_\alpha^2}{w_\alpha}\right]^{\frac{1}{2}} dt. \tag{14}$$

Our problem is to find the path that minimizes this functional. Because the functional is parameterization-invariant, it again suffices to consider paths that are traversed at a constant rate, or $\sum_\alpha \dot{w}_\alpha^2/w_\alpha = 1$. In addition to this, however, we must also enforce the constraint that $\mathbf{w}$ remains inside the simplex; this is done by introducing a Lagrange multiplier. Following this procedure, we find that the optimal path is described by:

$$\left[\theta\,\mathrm{KL}(\mathbf{w}^*||\mathbf{w}) + \ell\right]\left\{\ddot{w}_\alpha - \frac{\dot{w}_\alpha^2}{2w_\alpha} + \frac{w_\alpha}{2}\right\} - \theta\left[\sum_\beta \frac{w_\beta^*}{w_\beta}\dot{w}_\beta\right]\dot{w}_\alpha = \theta(w_\alpha - w_\alpha^*). \tag{15}$$

Given two endpoints, this differential equation defines a boundary value problem for the optimal path. Unlike before, however, in this case the motion of $\mathbf{w}$ is not confined to a plane. Hence, the boundary value problem for eq. (15) does not collapse to one dimension, as does its Gaussian counterpart, eq. (9).

To remedy this situation, we have developed an efficient approximation that finds a near-optimal interpolant, in lieu of the optimal one. This is done in two steps: first, by solving eq. (15) exactly in the limit $\ell \to \infty$; second, by using this limiting solution, $\mathbf{w}^\infty(t)$, to find the lowest-cost path that can be expressed as the convex combination:

$$\mathbf{w}(t) = m(t)\mathbf{w}^* + [1 - m(t)]\,\mathbf{w}^\infty(t). \tag{16}$$

The lowest-cost path of this form is found by substituting eq. (16) into the Dirichlet functional, eq. (14), and solving the Euler-Lagrange equations for $m(t)$. The motivation for eq. (16) is that for finite ℓ, we expect the optimal interpolant to deviate from $\mathbf{w}^\infty(t)$ and bend toward the prototype at $\mathbf{w}^*$. In practice, this approximation works very well, and by collapsing the boundary value problem to one dimension, it allows cheap computation of the Dirichlet interpolants. Some paths from eq. (16), as well as the $\ell \to \infty$ paths on which they are based, are shown in figure 1b. These paths were computed for the twelve dimensional simplex ($N = 12$), then projected onto the $w_1 w_2$-plane.

3 Intercluster interpolation

The Gaussian and Dirichlet distributions of the previous section are clearly inadequate for modeling for multimodal data sets. In this section, we extend the variational principle to mixture models, which describe the data as a collection of $k \geq 2$ clusters. In particular, suppose the data is modeled by

$$P(\mathbf{q}) = \sum_{z=1}^{k} \pi_z P(\mathbf{q}|z). \tag{17}$$

Here, we have assumed that the conditional densities $P(\mathbf{q}|z)$ model data clusters as defined in section 2.1, and the coefficients $\pi_z = P(z)$ define prior probabilities for the latent variable, $z \in \{1, 2, \ldots, k\}$.

The crucial step for mixture models is to develop the appropriate generalization of eq. (5). To this end, let $\mathcal{L}_z(\mathbf{q}, \dot{\mathbf{q}})$ denote the Lagrangian derived from the conditional density, $P(\mathbf{q}|z)$, and ℓ_z the line tension[1] that appears in this Lagrangian. We now combine these Lagrangians into a single functional:

$$\mathcal{S}[\mathbf{q}(t), z(t)] = \int dt\; \mathcal{L}_{z(t)}(\mathbf{q}, \dot{\mathbf{q}}). \tag{18}$$

Note that eq. (18) is a functional of two arguments, not one. For mixture models, which define a joint density $P(\mathbf{q}, z) = \pi_z P(\mathbf{q}|z)$, our goal is to find the optimal path in the joint space $\mathbf{q} \otimes z$. Here, $z(t)$ is a piecewise-constant function of time that assigns a discrete label to each point along the path; in other words, it provides a temporal segmentation of the path, $q(t)$. The purpose of $z(t)$ in eq. (18) is to select which Lagrangian is used to compute the contribution from the interval $[t, t+dt]$.

---

[1] To respect the weighting of the mixture components in eq. (17), we set the line tensions according to $\ell_z = \ell - \ln \pi_z$. Thus, components with higher weights have lower line tensions.

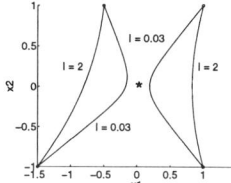 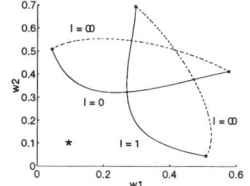 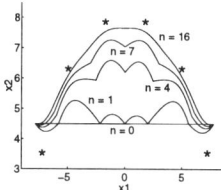

Figure 1: Model-based morphs for (a) Gaussian distribution; (b) Dirichlet distribution; (c) mixture of Gaussians. The prototypes are shown as asterisks; ℓ denotes the line tension. Figure 1c shows the convergence of the iterative algorithm; n denotes the number of iterations.

As before, we define the model-based interpolant as the path $\mathbf{q}(t)$ that minimizes eq. (18). In this case, however, both $\mathbf{q}(t)$ and $z(t)$ must be simultaneously optimized to recover this path. We have implemented an iterative scheme to perform this optimization, one that alternately (i) estimates the segmentation $z(t)$, (ii) computes the model-based interpolant within each cluster based on this segmentation, and (iii) reestimates the points (along the cluster boundaries) where $z(t)$ changes value. In short, the strategy is to optimize $z(t)$ for fixed $\mathbf{q}(t)$, then optimize $\mathbf{q}(t)$ for fixed $z(t)$.

Figure 1c shows how this algorithm operates on a simple mixture of Gaussians. In this example, the covariance matrices were set equal to the identity matrix, and the means of the Gaussians were distributed along a circle in the $x_1 x_2$-plane. Note that with each iteration, the interpolant converges more closely to the path that traverses this circle. The effect is similar to the manifold-snake algorithm of Bregler and Omohundro[2].

4 Discussion

In this paper we have proposed a variational principle for model-based interpolation. Our framework handles Gaussian, Dirichlet, and mixture models, and the resulting algorithms scale well to high dimensions. Future work will concentrate on the application to real images.

References

[1] T. Poggio and F. Girosi. Networks for approximation and learning. *Proc. of IEEE*, vol 78:9 (1990).

[2] C. Bregler and S. Omohundro. Nonlinear image interpolation using manifold learning. In G. Tesauro, D. Touretzky, and T. Leen (eds.). *Advances in Neural Information Processing Systems 7*, 973–980. MIT Press, Cambridge, MA (1995).

[3] T. Ezzat. Example based analysis and synthesis for images of faces. *MIT EECS M.S. thesis* (1996).

[4] D. Beymer, A. Shashua, and T. Poggio. Example based image analysis and synthesis. *AI Memo 1161*, MIT (1993).

[5] H. Goldstein. *Classical Mechanics*. Addison-Wesley, London (1980).

Online learning from finite training sets: An analytical case study

Peter Sollich*
Department of Physics
University of Edinburgh
Edinburgh EH9 3JZ, U.K.
P.Sollich@ed.ac.uk

David Barber[†]
Neural Computing Research Group
Department of Applied Mathematics
Aston University
Birmingham B4 7ET, U.K.
D.Barber@aston.ac.uk

Abstract

We analyse online learning from *finite* training sets at *non-infinitesimal* learning rates η. By an extension of statistical mechanics methods, we obtain exact results for the time-dependent generalization error of a linear network with a large number of weights N. We find, for example, that for small training sets of size $p \approx N$, larger learning rates can be used without compromising asymptotic generalization performance or convergence speed. Encouragingly, for optimal settings of η (and, less importantly, weight decay λ) at given final learning time, the generalization performance of online learning is essentially as good as that of offline learning.

1 INTRODUCTION

The analysis of online (gradient descent) learning, which is one of the most common approaches to supervised learning found in the neural networks community, has recently been the focus of much attention [1]. The characteristic feature of online learning is that the weights of a network ('student') are updated each time a new training example is presented, such that the error on this example is reduced. In offline learning, on the other hand, the total error on all examples in the training set is accumulated before a gradient descent weight update is made. Online and

---

* Royal Society Dorothy Hodgkin Research Fellow
[†] Supported by EPSRC grant GR/J75425: Novel Developments in Learning Theory for Neural Networks

offline learning are equivalent only in the limiting case where the learning rate $\eta \to 0$ (see, e.g., [2]). The main quantity of interest is normally the evolution of the generalization error: How well does the student approximate the input-output mapping ('teacher') underlying the training examples after a given number of weight updates?

Most analytical treatments of online learning assume either that the size of the training set is infinite, or that the learning rate η is vanishingly small. Both of these restrictions are undesirable: In practice, most training sets are finite, and non-infinitesimal values of η are needed to ensure that the learning process converges after a reasonable number of updates. General results have been derived for the difference between online and offline learning to first order in η, which apply to training sets of any size (see, e.g., [2]). These results, however, do not directly address the question of generalization performance. The most explicit analysis of the time evolution of the generalization error for finite training sets was provided by Krogh and Hertz [3] for a scenario very similar to the one we consider below. Their $\eta \to 0$ (i.e., offline) calculation will serve as a baseline for our work. For finite η, progress has been made in particular for so-called soft committee machine network architectures [4, 5], but only for the case of infinite training sets.

Our aim in this paper is to analyse a simple model system in order to assess how the combination of non-infinitesimal learning rates η and finite training sets (containing α examples per weight) affects online learning. In particular, we will consider the dependence of the asymptotic generalization error on η and α, the effect of finite α on both the critical learning rate and the learning rate yielding optimal convergence speed, and optimal values of η and weight decay λ. We also compare the performance of online and offline learning and discuss the extent to which infinite training set analyses are applicable for finite α.

2 MODEL AND OUTLINE OF CALCULATION

We consider online training of a linear student network with input-output relation

$$y = \mathbf{w}^T \mathbf{x}/\sqrt{N}.$$

Here $\mathbf{x}$ is an N-dimensional vector of real-valued inputs, y the single real output and $\mathbf{w}$ the weight vector of the network. 'T' denotes the transpose of a vector and the factor $1/\sqrt{N}$ is introduced for convenience. Whenever a training example $(\mathbf{x}, y)$ is presented to the network, its weight vector is updated along the gradient of the squared error on this example, i.e.,

$$\Delta \mathbf{w} = -\eta \, \nabla_\mathbf{w} \tfrac{1}{2}(y - \mathbf{w}^T\mathbf{x}/\sqrt{N})^2 = \eta \, (y\mathbf{x}/\sqrt{N} - \tfrac{1}{N}\mathbf{x}\mathbf{x}^T\mathbf{w})$$

where η is the learning rate. We are interested in online learning from finite training sets, where for each update an example is randomly chosen from a given set $\{(\mathbf{x}^\mu, y^\mu), \mu = 1 \ldots p\}$ of p training examples. (The case of cyclical presentation of examples [6] is left for future study.) If example μ is chosen for update n, the weight vector is changed to

$$\mathbf{w}_{n+1} = \{1 - \eta \, \tfrac{1}{N}[\mathbf{x}^\mu(\mathbf{x}^\mu)^T + \gamma]\}\mathbf{w}_n + \eta \, y^\mu \mathbf{x}^\mu/\sqrt{N} \qquad (1)$$

Here we have also included a weight decay γ. We will normally parameterize the strength of the weight decay in terms of $\lambda = \gamma \alpha$ (where $\alpha = p/N$ is the number of examples per weight), which plays the same role as the weight decay commonly used in offline learning [3]. For simplicity, all student weights are assumed to be initially zero, i.e., $\mathbf{w}_{n=0} = \mathbf{0}$.

The main quantity of interest is the evolution of the *generalization error* of the student. We assume that the training examples are generated by a linear 'teacher', i.e., $y^\mu = \mathbf{w}_*^T \mathbf{x}^\mu / \sqrt{N} + \xi^\mu$, where ξ^μ is zero mean additive noise of variance σ^2. The teacher weight vector is taken to be normalized to $\mathbf{w}_*^2 = N$ for simplicity, and the input vectors are assumed to be sampled randomly from an isotropic distribution over the hypersphere $\mathbf{x}^2 = N$. The generalization error, defined as the average of the squared error between student and teacher outputs for random inputs, is then

$$\epsilon_g = \tfrac{1}{2N}(\mathbf{w}_n - \mathbf{w}_*)^2 = \tfrac{1}{2N}\mathbf{v}_n^2 \quad \text{where} \quad \mathbf{v}_n = \mathbf{w}_n - \mathbf{w}_*.$$

In order to make the scenario analytically tractable, we focus on the limit $N \to \infty$ of a large number of input components and weights, taken at constant number of examples per weight $\alpha = p/N$ and updates per weight ('learning time') $t = n/N$. In this limit, the generalization error $\epsilon_g(t)$ becomes self-averaging and can be calculated by averaging both over the random selection of examples from a given training set and over all training sets. Our results can be straightforwardly extended to the case of perceptron teachers with a nonlinear transfer function, as in [7].

The usual statistical mechanical approach to the online learning problem expresses the generalization error in terms of 'order parameters' like $R = \tfrac{1}{N}\mathbf{w}_n^T \mathbf{w}_*$ whose (self-averaging) time evolution is determined from appropriately averaged update equations. This method works because for *infinite* training sets, the average order parameter updates can again be expressed in terms of the order parameters alone. For *finite* training sets, on the other hand, the updates involve new order parameters such as $R_1 = \tfrac{1}{N}\mathbf{w}_n^T \mathbf{A} \mathbf{w}_*$, where $\mathbf{A}$ is the correlation matrix of the training inputs, $\mathbf{A} = \tfrac{1}{N}\sum_{\mu=1}^p \mathbf{x}^\mu (\mathbf{x}^\mu)^T$. Their time evolution is in turn determined by order parameters involving higher powers of $\mathbf{A}$, yielding an infinite hierarchy of order parameters. We solve this problem by considering instead *order parameter* (generating) *functions* [8] such as a generalized form of the generalization error $\epsilon(t;h) = \tfrac{1}{2N}\mathbf{v}_n^T \exp(h\mathbf{A})\mathbf{v}_n$. This allows powers of $\mathbf{A}$ to be obtained by differentiation with respect to h, resulting in a closed system of (partial differential) equations for $\epsilon(t;h)$ and $R(t;h) = \tfrac{1}{N}\mathbf{w}_n^T \exp(h\mathbf{A})\mathbf{w}_*$.

The resulting equations and details of their solution will be given in a future publication. The final solution is most easily expressed in terms of the Laplace transform of the generalization error

$$\hat{\epsilon}_g(z) = \frac{\eta}{\alpha}\int_0^\infty dt\, \epsilon_g(t) e^{-z(\eta/\alpha)t} = \frac{\epsilon_1(z) + \eta\epsilon_2(z) + \eta^2 \epsilon_3(z)}{1 - \eta\epsilon_4(z)} \qquad (2)$$

The functions $\epsilon_i(z)$ ($i = 1\ldots 4$) can be expressed in closed form in terms of α, σ^2 and λ (and, of course, z). The Laplace transform (2) yields directly the asymptotic value of the generalization error, $\epsilon_\infty = \epsilon_g(t \to \infty) = \lim_{z \to 0} z\hat{\epsilon}_g(z)$, which can be calculated analytically. For finite learning times t, $\epsilon_g(t)$ is obtained by numerical inversion of the Laplace transform.

3 RESULTS AND DISCUSSION

We now discuss the consequences of our main result (2), focusing first on the asymptotic generalization error ϵ_∞, then the convergence speed for large learning times,

Online Learning from Finite Training Sets: An Analytical Case Study

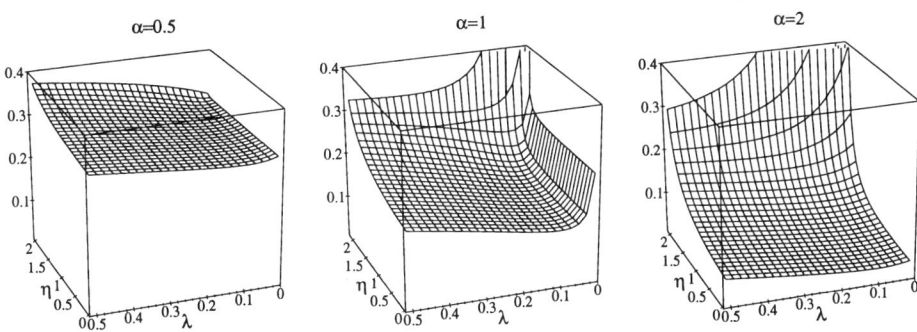

Figure 1: Asymptotic generalization error ϵ_∞ vs η and λ. α as shown, $\sigma^2 = 0.1$.

and finally the behaviour at small t. For numerical evaluations, we generally take $\sigma^2 = 0.1$, corresponding to a sizable noise-to-signal ratio of $\sqrt{0.1} \approx 0.32$.

The asymptotic generalization error ϵ_∞ is shown in Fig. 1 as a function of η and λ for $\alpha = 0.5, 1, 2$. We observe that it is minimal for $\lambda = \sigma^2$ and $\eta = 0$, as expected from corresponding results for offline learning [3][1]. We also read off that for fixed λ, ϵ_∞ is an increasing function of η: The larger η, the more the weight updates tend to overshoot the minimum of the (total, i.e., offline) training error. This causes a diffusive motion of the weights around their average asymptotic values [2] which increases ϵ_∞. In the absence of weight decay ($\lambda = 0$) and for $\alpha < 1$, however, ϵ_∞ is independent of η. In this case the training data can be fitted perfectly; every term in the total sum-of-squares training error is then zero and online learning does not lead to weight diffusion because all individual updates vanish. In general, the relative increase $\epsilon_\infty(\eta)/\epsilon_\infty(\eta=0) - 1$ due to nonzero η depends significantly on α. For $\eta = 1$ and $\alpha = 0.5$, for example, this increase is smaller than 6% for all λ (at $\sigma^2 = 0.1$), and for $\alpha = 1$ it is at most 13%. This means that in cases where training data is limited ($p \approx N$), η can be chosen fairly large in order to optimize learning speed, without seriously affecting the asymptotic generalization error. In the large α limit, on the other hand, one finds $\epsilon_\infty = (\sigma^2/2)[1/\alpha + \eta/(2-\eta)]$. The relative increase over the value at $\eta = 0$ therefore grows linearly with α; already for $\alpha = 2$, increases of around 50% can occur for $\eta = 1$.

Fig. 1 also shows that ϵ_∞ diverges as η approaches a critical learning rate η_c: As $\eta \to \eta_c$, the 'overshoot' of the weight update steps becomes so large that the weights eventually diverge. From the Laplace transform (2), one finds that η_c is determined by $\eta_c \epsilon_4(z=0) = 1$; it is a function of α and λ only. As shown in Fig. 2b-d, η_c increases with λ. This is reasonable, as the weight decay reduces the length of the weight vector at each update, counteracting potential weight divergences. In the small and large α limit, one has $\eta_c = 2(1+\lambda)$ and $\eta_c = 2(1+\lambda/\alpha)$, respectively. For constant λ, η_c therefore decreases[2] with α (Fig. 2b-d).

We now turn to the large t behaviour of the generalization error $\epsilon_g(t)$. For small η, the most slowly decaying contribution (or 'mode') to $\epsilon_g(t)$ varies as $\exp(-ct)$, its

---

[1]The optimal value of the *unscaled* weight decay decreases with α as $\gamma = \sigma^2/\alpha$, because for large training sets there is less need to counteract noise in the training data by using a large weight decay.

[2]Conversely, for constant γ, η_c *increases* with α from $2(1+\gamma\alpha)$ to $2(1+\gamma)$: For large α, the weight decay is applied more often between repeat presentations of a training example that would otherwise cause the weights to diverge.

decay constant $c = \eta[\lambda+(\sqrt{\alpha}-1)^2]/\alpha$ scaling linearly with η, the size of the weight updates, as expected (Fig. 2a). For small α, the condition $ct \gg 1$ for $\epsilon_g(t)$ to have reached its asymptotic value ϵ_∞ is $\eta(1+\lambda)(t/\alpha) \gg 1$ and scales with t/α, which is the number of times each training example has been used. For large α, on the other hand, the condition becomes $\eta t \gg 1$: The size of the training set drops out since convergence occurs before repetitions of training examples become significant.

For larger η, the picture changes due to a new 'slow mode' (arising from the denominator of (2)). Interestingly, this mode exists only for η above a finite threshold $\eta_{\min} = 2/(\alpha^{1/2}+\alpha^{-1/2}-1)$. For finite α, it could therefore not have been predicted from a small η expansion of $\epsilon_g(t)$. Its decay constant c_{slow} decreases to zero as $\eta \to \eta_c$, and crosses that of the normal mode at $\eta_x(\alpha, \lambda)$ (Fig. 2a). For $\eta > \eta_x$, the slow mode therefore determines the convergence speed for large t, and fastest convergence is obtained for $\eta = \eta_x$. However, it may still be advantageous to use lower values of η in order to lower the asymptotic generalization error (see below); values of $\eta > \eta_x$ would deteriorate both convergence speed and asymptotic performance. Fig. 2b-d shows the dependence of $\eta_{\min}$, η_x and η_c on α and λ. For λ not too large, η_x has a maximum at $\alpha \approx 1$ (where $\eta_x \approx \eta_c$), while decaying as $\eta_x = 1+2\alpha^{-1/2} \approx \frac{1}{2}\eta_c$ for larger α. This is because for $\alpha \approx 1$ the (total training) error surface is very anisotropic around its minimum in weight space [9]. The steepest directions determine η_c and convergence along them would be fastest for $\eta = \frac{1}{2}\eta_c$ (as in the isotropic case). However, the overall convergence speed is determined by the shallow directions, which require maximal $\eta \approx \eta_c$ for fastest convergence.

Consider now the small t behaviour of $\epsilon_g(t)$. Fig. 3 illustrates the dependence of $\epsilon_g(t)$ on η; comparison with simulation results for $N = 50$ clearly confirms our calculations and demonstrates that finite N effects are not significant even for such fairly small N. For $\alpha = 0.7$ (Fig. 3a), we see that nonzero η acts as effective update noise, eliminating the minimum in $\epsilon_g(t)$ which corresponds to over-training [3]. ϵ_∞ is also seen to be essentially independent of η as predicted for the small value of $\lambda = 10^{-4}$ chosen. For $\alpha = 5$, Fig. 3b clearly shows the increase of ϵ_∞ with η. It also illustrates how convergence first speeds up as η is increased from zero and then slows down again as $\eta_c \approx 2$ is approached.

Above, we discussed optimal settings of η and λ for minimal asymptotic generalization error ϵ_∞. Fig. 4 shows what happens if we minimize $\epsilon_g(t)$ instead for a given *final learning time* t, corresponding to a fixed amount of computational effort for training the network. As t increases, the optimal η decreases towards zero as required by the tradeoff between asymptotic performance and convergence

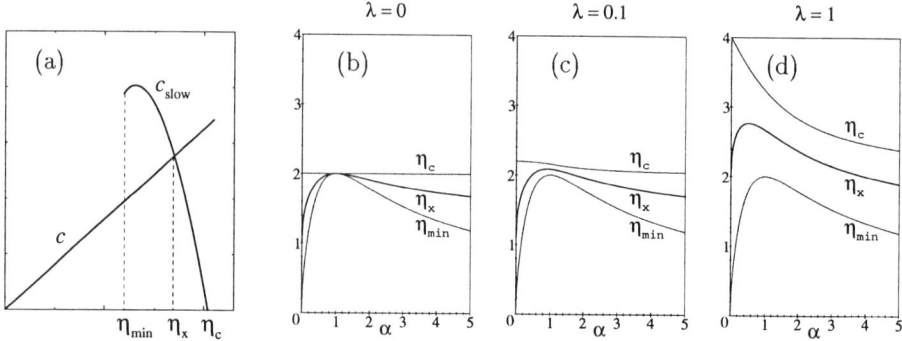

Figure 2: Definitions of $\eta_{\min}$, η_x and η_c, and their dependence on α (for λ as shown).

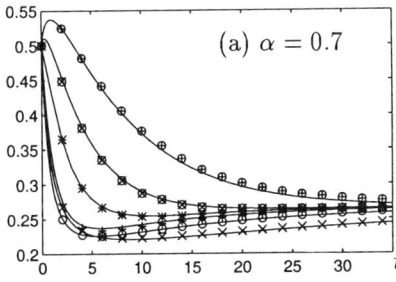
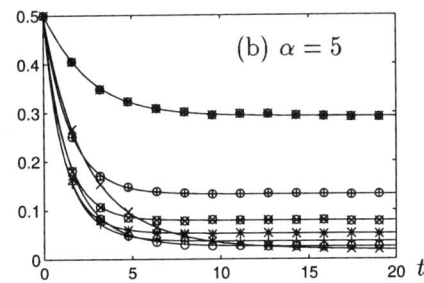

Figure 3: ϵ_g vs t for different η. Simulations for $N = 50$ are shown by symbols (standard errors less than symbol sizes). $\lambda=10^{-4}$, $\sigma^2=0.1$, α as shown. The learning rate η increases from below (at large t) over the range (a) $0.5\ldots 1.95$, (b) $0.5\ldots 1.75$.

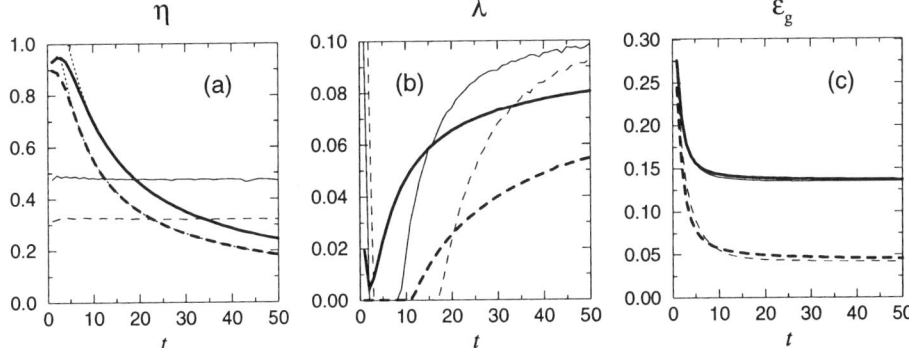

Figure 4: Optimal η and λ vs given final learning time t, and resulting ϵ_g. Solid/dashed lines: $\alpha=1$ / $\alpha=2$; bold/thin lines: online/offline learning. $\sigma^2=0.1$. Dotted lines in (a): Fits of form $\eta = (a + b \ln t)/t$ to optimal η for online learning.

speed. Minimizing $\epsilon_g(t) \approx \epsilon_\infty + \text{const} \cdot \exp(-ct) \approx c_1 + \eta c_2 + c_3 \exp(-c_4 \eta t)$ leads to $\eta_{\text{opt}} = (a + b \ln t)/t$ (with some constants a, b, $c_{1\ldots 4}$). Although derived for small η, this functional form (dotted lines in Fig. 4a) also provides a good description down to fairly small t, where η_{opt} becomes large. The optimal weight decay λ increases[3] with t towards the limiting value σ^2. However, optimizing λ is much less important than choosing the right η: Minimizing $\epsilon_g(t)$ for fixed λ yields almost the same generalization error as optimizing both η and λ (we omit detailed results here[4]). It is encouraging to see from Fig. 4c that after as few as $t = 10$ updates per weight with optimal η, the generalization error is almost indistinguishable from its optimal value for $t \to \infty$ (this also holds if λ is kept fixed). Optimization of the learning rate should therefore be worthwhile in most practical scenarios.

In Fig. 4c, we also compare the performance of online learning to that of offline learning (calculated from the appropriate discrete time version of [3]), again with

---

[3] One might have expected the opposite effect of having larger λ at low t in order to 'contain' potential divergences from the larger optimal learning rates η. However, smaller λ tends to make the asymptotic value ϵ_∞ less sensitive to large values of η as we saw above, and we conclude that this effect dominates.

[4] For fixed $\lambda < \sigma^2$, where $\epsilon_g(t)$ has an over-training minimum (see Fig. 3a), the asymptotic behaviour of η_{opt} changes to $\eta_{\text{opt}} \propto t^{-1}$ (without the $\ln t$ factor), corresponding to a fixed effective learning time ηt required to reach this minimum.

optimized values of η and λ for given t. The performance loss from using online instead of offline learning is seen to be negligible. This may seem surprising given the effective noise on weight updates implied by online learning, in particular for small t. However, comparing the respective optimal learning rates (Fig. 4a), we see that online learning makes up for this deficiency by allowing larger values of η to be used (for large α, for example, $\eta_c(\text{offline}) = 2/\alpha \ll \eta_c(\text{online}) = 2$).

Finally, we compare our finite α results with those for the limiting case $\alpha \to \infty$. Good agreement exists for any learning time t if the asymptotic generalization error $\epsilon_\infty(\alpha < \infty)$ is dominated by the contribution from the nonzero learning rate η (as is the case for $\alpha \to \infty$). In practice, however, one wants η to be small enough to make only a negligible contribution to $\epsilon_\infty(\alpha < \infty)$; in this regime, the $\alpha \to \infty$ results are essentially useless.

4 CONCLUSIONS

The main theoretical contribution of this paper is the extension of the statistical mechanics method of order parameter dynamics to the dynamics of order parameter (generating) functions. The results that we have obtained for a simple linear model system are also of practical relevance. For example, the calculated dependence on η of the asymptotic generalization error ϵ_∞ and the convergence speed shows that, in general, sizable values of η can be used for training sets of limited size ($\alpha \approx 1$), while for larger α it is important to keep learning rates small. We also found a simple functional form for the dependence of the optimal η on a given final learning time t. This could be used, for example, to estimate the optimal η for large t from test runs with only a small number of weight updates. Finally, we found that for optimized η online learning performs essentially as well as offline learning, whether or not the weight decay λ is optimized as well. This is encouraging, since online learning effectively induces noisy weight updates. This allows it to cope better than offline learning with the problem of local (training error) minima in realistic neural networks. Online learning has the further advantage that the critical learning rates are not significantly lowered by input distributions with nonzero mean, whereas for offline learning they are significantly reduced [10]. In the future, we hope to extend our approach to dynamic (t-dependent) optimization of η (although performance improvements over optimal fixed η may be small [6]), and to more complicated network architectures in which the crucial question of local minima can be addressed.

References

[1] See for example: *The dynamics of online learning*. Workshop at *NIPS'95*.
[2] T. Heskes and B. Kappen. *Phys. Rev. A*, 44:2718, 1991.
[3] A. Krogh and J. A. Hertz. *J. Phys. A*, 25:1135, 1992.
[4] D. Saad and S. Solla. *Phys. Rev. E*, 52:4225, 1995; also in *NIPS-8*.
[5] M. Biehl and H. Schwarze. *J. Phys. A*, 28:643–656, 1995.
[6] Z.-Q. Luo. *Neur. Comp.*, 3:226, 1991; T. Heskes and W. Wiegerinck. *IEEE Trans. Neur. Netw.*, 7:919, 1996.
[7] P. Sollich. *J. Phys. A*, 28:6125, 1995.
[8] L. L. Bonilla, F. G. Padilla, G. Parisi and F. Ritort. *Europhys. Lett.*, 34:159, 1996; *Phys. Rev. B*, 54:4170, 1996.
[9] J. A. Hertz, A. Krogh and G. I. Thorbergsson. *J. Phys. A*, 22:2133, 1989.
[10] T. L. H. Watkin, A. Rau and M. Biehl. *Rev. Modern Phys.*, 65:499, 1993.

Support Vector Method for Function Approximation, Regression Estimation, and Signal Processing

Vladimir Vapnik
AT&T Research
101 Crawfords Corner
Holmdel, NJ 07733
vlad@research.att.com

Steven E. Golowich
Bell Laboratories
700 Mountain Ave.
Murray Hill, NJ 07974
golowich@bell-labs.com

Alex Smola*
GMD First
Rudower Shausee 5
12489 Berlin
asm@big.att.com

Abstract

The Support Vector (SV) method was recently proposed for estimating regressions, constructing multidimensional splines, and solving linear operator equations [Vapnik, 1995]. In this presentation we report results of applying the SV method to these problems.

1 Introduction

The Support Vector method is a universal tool for solving multidimensional function estimation problems. Initially it was designed to solve pattern recognition problems, where in order to find a decision rule with good generalization ability one selects some (small) subset of the training data, called the Support Vectors (SVs). Optimal separation of the SVs is equivalent to optimal separation the entire data.

This led to a new method of representing decision functions where the decision functions are a linear expansion on a basis whose elements are nonlinear functions parameterized by the SVs (we need one SV for each element of the basis). This type of function representation is especially useful for high dimensional input space: the number of free parameters in this representation is equal to the number of SVs but does not depend on the dimensionality of the space.

Later the SV method was extended to real-valued functions. This allows us to expand high-dimensional functions using a small basis constructed from SVs. This

---
*smola@prosun.first.gmd.de

novel type of function representation opens new opportunities for solving various problems of function approximation and estimation.

In this paper we demonstrate that using the SV technique one can solve problems that in classical techniques would require estimating a large number of free parameters. In particular we construct one and two dimensional splines with an arbitrary number of grid points. Using linear splines we approximate non-linear functions. We show that by reducing requirements on the accuracy of approximation, one decreases the number of SVs which leads to data compression. We also show that the SV technique is a useful tool for regression estimation. Lastly we demonstrate that using the SV function representation for solving inverse ill-posed problems provides an additional opportunity for regularization.

2 SV method for estimation of real functions

Let $x \in R^n$ and $y \in R^1$. Consider the following set of real functions: a vector x is mapped into some a priori chosen Hilbert space, where we define functions that are linear in their parameters

$$y = f(x, w) = \sum_{i=1}^{\infty} w_i \phi_i(x), \quad w = (w_1, ..., w_N, ...) \in \Omega \qquad (1)$$

In [Vapnik, 1995] the following method for estimating functions in the set (1) based on training data $(x_1, y_1), ..., (x_\ell, y_\ell)$ was suggested: find the function that minimizes the following functional:

$$R(w) = \frac{1}{\ell} \sum_{i=1}^{\ell} |y_i - f(x_i, w)|_\varepsilon + \gamma(w, w), \qquad (2)$$

where

$$|y - f(x, w)|_\varepsilon = \begin{cases} 0 & \text{if } |y - f(x, w)| < \varepsilon, \\ |y - f(x, w)| - \varepsilon & \text{otherwise,} \end{cases} \qquad (3)$$

(w, w) is the inner product of two vectors, and γ is some constant. It was shown that the function minimizing this functional has a form:

$$f(x, \alpha, \alpha^*) = \sum_{i=1}^{\ell} (\alpha_i^* - \alpha_i)(\Phi(x_i), \Phi(x)) + b \qquad (4)$$

where $\alpha_i^*, \alpha_i \geq 0$ with $\alpha_i^* \alpha_i = 0$ and $(\Phi(x_i), \Phi(x))$ is the inner product of two elements of Hilbert space.

To find the coefficients α_i^* and α_i one has to solve the following quadratic optimization problem: maximize the functional

$$W(\alpha^*, \alpha) = -\varepsilon \sum_{i=1}^{\ell} (\alpha_i^* + \alpha_i) + \sum_{i=1}^{\ell} y(\alpha_i^* - \alpha_i) - \frac{1}{2} \sum_{i,j=1}^{\ell} (\alpha_i^* - \alpha_i)(\alpha_j^* - \alpha_j)(\Phi(x_i), \Phi(x_j)), \qquad (5)$$

subject to constraints

$$\sum_{i=1}^{\ell} (\alpha_i^* - \alpha_i) = 0, \quad 0 \leq \alpha_i, \alpha_i^* \leq C, \quad i = 1, ..., \ell. \qquad (6)$$

SV Method for Function Approximation and Regression Estimation

The important feature of the solution (4) of this optimization problem is that only some of the coefficients $(\alpha_i^* - \alpha_i)$ differ from zero. The corresponding vectors x_i are called Support Vectors (SVs). Therefore (4) describes an expansion on SVs.

It was shown in [Vapnik, 1995] that to evaluate the inner products $(\Phi(x_i), \Phi(x))$ both in expansion (4) and in the objective function (5) one can use the general form of the inner product in Hilbert space. According to Hilbert space theory, to guarantee that a symmetric function $K(u,v)$ has an expansion

$$K(u,v) = \sum_{k=1}^{\infty} a_k \phi_k(u) \phi_k(v)$$

with positive coefficients $a_k > 0$, i.e. to guarantee that $K(u,v)$ is an inner product in some feature space Φ, it is necessary and sufficient that the conditions

$$\int K(u,v) g(u) g(v)\, du\, dv > 0 \tag{7}$$

be valid for any non-zero function g on the Hilbert space (Mercer's theorem).

Therefore, in the SV method, one can replace (4) with

$$f(x, \alpha, \alpha^*) = \sum_{i=1}^{\ell} (\alpha_i^* - \alpha_i) K(x, x_i) + b \tag{8}$$

where the inner product $(\Phi(x_i), \Phi(x))$ is defined through a kernel $K(x_i, x)$. To find coefficients α_i^* and α_i one has to maximize the function

$$W(\alpha^*, \alpha) = -\varepsilon \sum_{i=1}^{\ell} (\alpha_i^* + \alpha_i) + \sum_{i=1}^{\ell} y(\alpha_i^* - \alpha_i) - \frac{1}{2} \sum_{i,j=1}^{\ell} (\alpha_i^* - \alpha_i)(\alpha_j^* - \alpha_j) K(x_i, x_j) \tag{9}$$

subject to constraints (6).

3 Constructing kernels for inner products

To define a set of approximating functions one has to define a kernel $K(x_i, x)$ that generates the inner product in some feature space and solve the corresponding quadratic optimization problem.

3.1 Kernels generating splines

We start with the spline functions. According to their definition, splines are piecewise polynomial functions, which we will consider on the set $[0,1]$. Splines of order n have the following representation

$$f_n(x) = \sum_{r=0}^{n} a_r x^r + \sum_{s=1}^{N} w_j (x - t_s)_+^n \tag{10}$$

where $(x-t)_+ = \max\{(x-t), 0\}$, $t_1, ..., t_N \in [0,1]$ are the nodes, and a_r, w_j are real values. One can consider the spline function (10) as a linear function in the $n + N + 1$ dimensional feature space spanned by

$$1, x, ..., x^n, (x-t_1)_+^n, ..., (x-t_N)_+^n.$$

Therefore the inner product that generates splines of order n in one dimension is

$$K(x_i, x_j) = \sum_{r=0}^{n} x_i^r x_j^r + \sum_{s=1}^{N}(x_i - t_s)_+^n (x_j - t_s)_+^n. \quad (11)$$

Two dimensional splines are linear functions in the $(N+n+1)^2$ dimensional space

$$1, x, ..., x^n, y, ..., y^n, ..., (x-t_1)_+^n (y-t_1^*)_+^n, ..., (x-t_N)_+^n (y-t_N^*)_+^n. \quad (12)$$

Let us denote by $u_i = (x_i, y_i)$, $u_j = (x_j, y_j)$ two two-dimensional vectors. Then the generating kernel for two dimensional spline functions of order n is

$$K(u_i, u_j) = K(x_i, x_j) K(y_i, y_j)$$

It is easy to check that the generating kernel for the m-dimensional splines is the product of m one-dimensional generating kernels.

In applications of the SV method the number of nodes does not play an important role. Therefore, we introduce splines of order d with an infinite number of nodes $S_d^{(\infty)}$. To do this in the R^1 case, we map any real value x_i to the element $1, x_i, ..., x_i^n, (x_i - t)_+^n$ of the Hilbert space. The inner product becomes

$$K(x_i, x_j) = \sum_{r=0}^{n} x_i^r x_j^r + \int_0^1 (x_i - t)_+^n (x_j - t)_+^n dt \quad (13)$$

For linear splines $S_1^{(\infty)}$ we therefore have the following generating kernel:

$$K(x_i, x_j) = 1 + x_i x_j + x_i x_j \min(x_i, x_j) - \frac{(x_i + x_j)}{2}(\min(x_i, x_j))^2 + \frac{(\min(x_i, x_j))^3}{3}. \quad (14)$$

In many applications expansions in B_n-splines [Unser & Aldroubi, 1992] are used, where

$$B_n(x) = \sum_{r=0}^{n+1} \frac{(-1)^r}{n!} \binom{n+1}{r} \left(x + \frac{n+1}{2} - r\right)_+^n.$$

One may use B_n-splines to perform a construction similar to the above, yielding the kernel

$$K(x_i, x_j) = \int_{-\infty}^{\infty} B_n(x_i - t) B_n(x_j - t) dt = B_{2n+1}(x_i - x_j).$$

3.2 Kernels generating Fourier expansions

Lastly, Fourier expansion can be considered as a hyperplane in following $2N+1$ dimensional feature space

$$\frac{1}{\sqrt{2}}, \cos x, \sin x, ..., \cos Nx, \sin Nx.$$

The inner product in this space is defined by the Dirichlet formula:

$$K(x_i, x_j) = \frac{1}{2} + \sum_{r=1}^{N}(\cos r x_i \cos r x_j + \sin r x_i \sin r x_j) = \frac{\sin(N+1/2)(x_i - x_j)}{\sin \frac{x_i - x_j}{2}}. \quad (15)$$

4 Function estimation and data compression

In this section we approximate functions on the basis of observations at ℓ points

$$(x_1, y_1), ..., (x_\ell, y_\ell). \tag{16}$$

We demonstrate that to construct an approximation within an accuracy of $\pm \varepsilon$ at the data points, one can use only the subsequence of the data containing the SVs.

We consider approximating the one and two dimensional functions

$$f(x) = \text{sinc}|x| = \frac{\sin|x|}{|x|} \tag{17}$$

on the basis of a sequence of measurements (without noise) on the uniform lattice (100 for the one dimensional case and 2,500 for the two-dimensional case).

For different ε we approximate this function by linear splines from $S_1^{(\infty)}$.

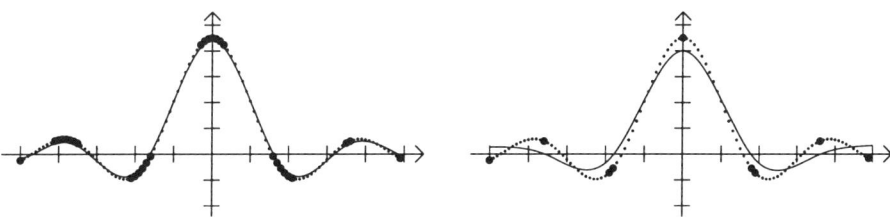

Figure 1: Approximations with different levels of accuracy require different numbers of SV: 31 SV for $\varepsilon = 0.02$ (left) and 9 SV for $\varepsilon = 0.1$. Large dots indicate SVs.

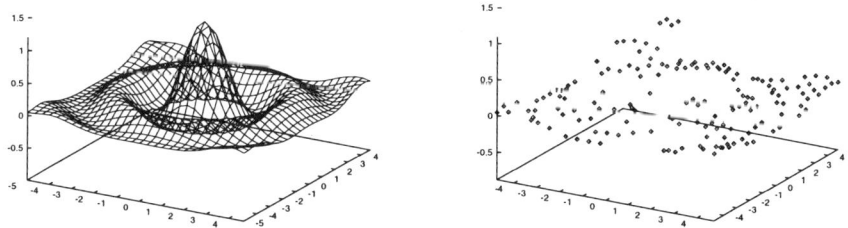

Figure 2: Approximation of $f(x,y) = \text{sinc}\sqrt{x^2 + y^2}$ by two dimensional linear splines with accuracy $\varepsilon = 0.01$ (left) required 157 SV (right)

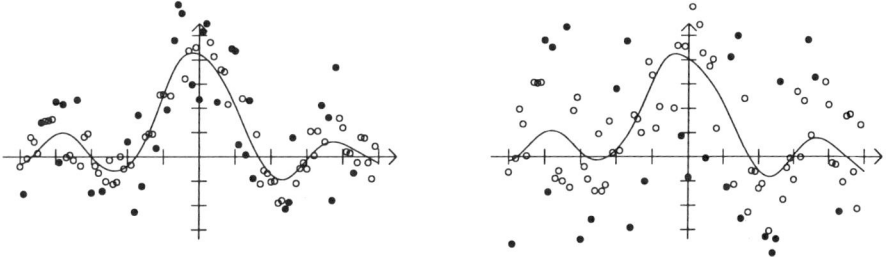

Figure 3: $\text{sinc}x$ function corrupted by different levels of noise ($\sigma = 0.2$ left, 0.5 right) and its regression. Black dots indicate SV, circles non-SV data.

5 Solution of the linear operator equations

In this section we consider the problem of solving linear equations in the set of functions defined by SVs. Consider the problem of solving a linear operator equation

$$Af(t) = F(x), \qquad f(t) \in \Xi, \ F(x) \in \Psi, \tag{18}$$

where we are given measurements of the right hand side

$$(x_1, F_1), ..., (x_\ell, F_\ell). \tag{19}$$

Consider the set of functions $f(t, w) \in \Xi$ linear in some feature space $\{\Phi(t) = (\phi_0(t), ..., \phi_N(t), ...)\}$:

$$f(t, w) = \sum_{r=0}^{\infty} w_r \phi_r(t) = (W, \Phi(t)). \tag{20}$$

The operator A maps this set of functions into

$$F(x, w) = Af(t, w) = \sum_{r=0}^{\infty} w_r A\phi_r(t) = \sum_{r=0}^{\infty} w_r \psi_r(x) = (W, \Psi(x)) \tag{21}$$

where $\psi_r(x) = A\phi_r(t)$, $\Psi(x) = (\psi_1(x), ..., \psi_N(x), ...)$. Let us define the generating kernel in image space

$$K(x_i, x_j) = \sum_{r=0}^{\infty} \psi_r(x_i)\psi_r(x_j) = (\Psi(x_i), \Psi(x_j)) \tag{22}$$

and the corresponding cross-kernel function

$$\mathcal{K}(x_i, t) = \sum_{r=0}^{\infty} \psi_r(x_i)\phi_r(t) = (\Psi(x_i), \Phi(t)). \tag{23}$$

The problem of solving (18) in the set of functions $f(t, w) \in \Xi$ (finding the vector W) is equivalent to the problem of regression estimation (21) using data (19).

To estimate the regression on the basis of the kernel $K(x_i, x_j)$ one can use the methods described in Section 1. The obtained parameters $(\alpha_i^* - \alpha_i, \ i = 1, ...\ell)$ define the approximation to the solution of equation (18) based on data (19):

$$f(t, \alpha) = \sum_{i=1}^{\ell} (\alpha_i^* - \alpha_i) \mathcal{K}(x_i, t).$$

We have applied this method to solution of the Radon equation

$$\int_{-a(m)}^{a(m)} f(m\cos\mu + u\sin\mu, \ m\sin\mu - u\cos\mu) du = p(m, \mu),$$

$$-1 \leq m \leq 1, \quad 0 < \mu < \pi, \quad a(m) = \sqrt{1 - m^2} \tag{24}$$

using noisy observations $(m_1, \mu_1, p_1), ..., (m_\ell, \mu_\ell, p_\ell)$, where $p_i = p(m_i, \mu_i) + \xi_i$ and $\{\xi_i\}$ are independent with $E\xi_i = 0$, $E\xi_i^2 < \infty$.

For two-dimensional linear splines $S_1^{(\infty)}$ we obtained analytical expressions for the kernel (22) and cross-kernel (23). We have used these kernels for solving the corresponding regression problem and reconstructing images based on data that is similar to what one might get from a Positron Emission Tomography scan [Shepp, Vardi & Kaufman, 1985].

A remarkable feature of this solution is that it avoids a pixel representation of the function which would require the estimation of 10,000 to 60,000 parameters. The spline approximation shown here required only 172 SVs.

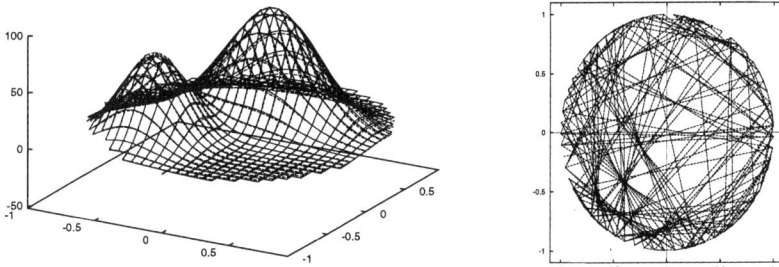

Figure 4: Original image (dashed line) and its reconstruction (solid line) from 2,048 observations (left). 172 SVs (support lines) were used in the reconstruction (right).

6 Conclusion

In this article we present a new method of function estimation that is especially useful for solving multi-dimensional problems. The complexity of the solution of the function estimation problem using the SV representation depends on the complexity of the desired solution (i.e. on the required number of SVs for a reasonable approximation of the desired function) rather than on the dimensionality of the space. Using the SV method one can solve various problems of function estimation both in statistics and in applied mathematics.

Acknowledgments

We would like to thank Chris Burges (Lucent Technologies) and Bernhard Schölkopf (MPIK Tübingen) for help with the code and useful discussions.

This work was supported in part by NSF grant PHY 95-12729 (Steven Golowich) and by ARPA grant N00014-94-C-0186 and the German National Scholarship Foundation (Alex Smola).

References

1. Vladimir Vapnik, "The Nature of Statistical Learning Theory", 1995, Springer Verlag N.Y., 189 p.

2. Michael Unser and Akram Aldroubi, "Polynomial Splines and Wevelets - A Signal Perspectives", In the book: "Wavelets –A tutorial in Theory and Applications", C.K. Chui (ed) pp. 91 – 122, 1992 Academic Press, Inc.

3. L. Shepp, Y. Vardi, and L. Kaufman, "A statistical model for Positron Emission Tomography," *J. Amer. Stat. Assoc.* **80:389** pp. 8-37 1985.

The Learning Dynamics of a Universal Approximator

Ansgar H. L. West[1,2]
A.H.L.West@aston.ac.uk

David Saad[1]
D.Saad@aston.ac.uk

Ian T. Nabney[1]
I.T.Nabney@aston.ac.uk

[1]Neural Computing Research Group, University of Aston
Birmingham B4 7ET, U.K.
http://www.ncrg.aston.ac.uk/
[2]Department of Physics, University of Edinburgh
Edinburgh EH9 3JZ, U.K.

Abstract

The learning properties of a universal approximator, a normalized committee machine with adjustable biases, are studied for on-line back-propagation learning. Within a statistical mechanics framework, numerical studies show that this model has features which do not exist in previously studied two-layer network models without adjustable biases, e.g., attractive suboptimal symmetric phases even for realizable cases and noiseless data.

1 INTRODUCTION

Recently there has been much interest in the theoretical breakthrough in the understanding of the on-line learning dynamics of multi-layer feedforward perceptrons (MLPs) using a statistical mechanics framework. In the seminal paper (Saad & Solla, 1995), a two-layer network with an arbitrary number of hidden units was studied, allowing insight into the learning behaviour of neural network models whose complexity is of the same order as those used in real world applications.

The model studied, a soft committee machine (Biehl & Schwarze, 1995), consists of a single hidden layer with adjustable input-hidden, but fixed hidden-output weights. The average learning dynamics of these networks are studied in the thermodynamic limit of infinite input dimensions in a student-teacher scenario, where a *student* network is presented serially with training examples (ξ^μ, ζ^μ) labelled by a *teacher* network of the same architecture but possibly different number of hidden units. The student updates its parameters *on-line*, i.e., after the presentation of each example, along the gradient of the squared error on that example, an algorithm usually referred to as back-propagation.

Although the above model is already quite similar to real world networks, the approach suffers from several drawbacks. First, the analysis of the mean learning dynamics employs the thermodynamic limit of infinite input dimension — a problem which has been addressed in (Barber et al., 1996), where finite size effects have been studied and it was shown that the thermodynamic limit is relevant in most cases. Second, the hidden-output weights are kept fixed, a constraint which has been removed in (Riegler & Biehl, 1995), where it was shown that the learning dynamics are usually dominated by the input-hidden weights. Third, the biases of the hidden units were fixed to zero, a constraint which is actually more severe than fixing the hidden-output weights. We show in Appendix A that soft committee machines are universal approximators provided one allows for adjustable biases in the hidden layer.

In this paper, we therefore study the model of a normalized soft committee machine with variable biases following the framework set out in (Saad & Solla, 1995). We present numerical studies of a variety of learning scenarios which lead to remarkable effects not present for the model with fixed biases.

2 DERIVATION OF THE DYNAMICAL EQUATIONS

The student network we consider is a normalized soft committee machine of K hidden units with adjustable biases. Each hidden unit i consists of a bias θ_i and a weight vector W_i which is connected to the N-dimensional inputs ξ. All hidden units are connected to a linear output unit with arbitrary but fixed gain γ by couplings of fixed strength. The activation of any unit is normalized by the inverse square root of the number of weight connections into the unit, which allows all weights to be of $\mathcal{O}(1)$ magnitude, independent of the input dimension or the number of hidden units. The implemented mapping is therefore $f_W(\xi) = (\gamma/\sqrt{K}) \sum_{i=1}^{K} g(u_i - \theta_i)$, where $u_i = W_i \cdot \xi/\sqrt{N}$ and $g(\cdot)$ is a sigmoidal transfer function. The teacher network to be learned is of the same architecture except for a possible difference in the number of hidden units M and is defined by the weight vectors B_n and biases ρ_n ($n = 1, \ldots, M$). Training examples are of the form (ξ^μ, ζ^μ), where the input vectors ξ^μ are drawn form the normal distribution and the outputs are $\zeta^\mu = (\gamma/\sqrt{M}) \sum_{n=1}^{M} g(v_n^\mu - \rho_n)$, where $v_n^\mu = B_n \cdot \xi^\mu / \sqrt{N}$.

The weights and biases are updated in response to the presentation of an example (ξ^μ, ζ^μ), along the gradient of the squared error measure $\epsilon = \frac{1}{2}[\zeta^\mu - f_W(\xi^\mu)]^2$

$$W_i^{\mu+1} - W_i^\mu = \eta_W \delta_i^\mu \frac{\xi^\mu}{\sqrt{N}} \quad \text{and} \quad \theta_i^{\mu+1} - \theta_i^\mu = -\frac{\eta_\theta}{N} \delta_i^\mu \quad (1)$$

with $\delta_i^\mu \equiv [\zeta^\mu - f_W(\xi^\mu)]g'(u_i^\mu - \theta_i)$. The two learning rates are η_W for the weights and η_θ for the biases. In order to analyse the mean learning dynamics resulting from the above update equations, we follow the statistical mechanics framework in (Saad & Solla, 1995). Here we will only outline the main ideas and concentrate on the results of the calculation.

As we are interested in the typical behaviour of our training algorithm we average over all possible instances of the examples ξ. We rewrite the update equations (1) in W_i as equations in the order parameters describing the overlaps between pairs of student nodes $Q_{ij} = W_i \cdot W_j / N$, student and teacher nodes $R_{in} = W_i \cdot B_n / N$, and teacher nodes $T_{nm} = B_n \cdot B_m / N$. The generalization error ϵ_g, measuring the typical performance, can be expressed solely in these variables and the biases θ_i and ρ_n. The order parameters Q_{ij}, R_{in} and the biases θ_i are the dynamical variables. These quantities need to be self-averaging with respect to the randomness in the training data in the thermodynamic limit ($N \to \infty$), which enforces two necessary constraints on our calculation. First, the number of hidden units $K \ll N$, whereas one needs $K \sim \mathcal{O}(N)$ for the universal approximation proof to hold. Second, one can show that the updates of the biases have to be of $\mathcal{O}(1/N)$, i.e., the bias learning rate has to be scaled by $1/N$, in order to make the biases self-averaging quantities, a fact that is confirmed by simulations [see Fig. 1]. If we interpret the normalized example number $\alpha = \mu/N$ as a continuous time variable, the update equations for the order parameters and the biases become first order coupled differential equations

$$\frac{dQ_{ij}}{d\alpha} = \eta_w \langle \delta_i u_j + \delta_j u_i \rangle_\xi + \eta_w^2 \langle \delta_i \delta_j \rangle_\xi .$$

$$\frac{dR_{in}}{d\alpha} = \eta_w \langle \delta_i v_n \rangle_\xi, \quad \text{and} \quad \frac{d\theta_i}{d\alpha} = -\eta_\theta \langle \delta_i \rangle_\xi . \quad (2)$$

Choosing $g(x) = \text{erf}(x/\sqrt{2})$ as the sigmoidal transfer, most integrations in Eqs. (2) can be performed analytically, but for single Gaussian integrals remaining for η_w^2-terms and the generalization error. The exact form of the resulting dynamical equations is quite complicated and will be presented elsewhere. Here we only remark, that the gain γ of the linear output unit, which determines the output scale, merely rescales the learning rates with γ^2 and can therefore be set to one without loss of generality. Due to the numerical integrations required, the differential equations can only be solved accurately in moderate times for smaller student networks ($K \leq 5$) but any teacher size M.

3 ANALYSIS OF THE DYNAMICAL EQUATIONS

The dynamical evolution of the overlaps Q_{ij}, R_{in} and the biases θ_i follows from integrating the equations of motion (2) from initial conditions determined by the (random) initialization of the student weights W_i and biases θ_i. For random initialization the resulting norms Q_{ii} of the student vector will be order $\mathcal{O}(1)$, while the overlaps Q_{ij} between different student vectors, and student-teacher vectors R_{in} will be only order $\mathcal{O}(1/\sqrt{N})$. A random initialization of the weights and biases can therefore be simulated by initializing the norms Q_{ii}, the biases θ_i and the normalized overlaps $\hat{Q}_{ij} = Q_{ij}/\sqrt{Q_{ii}Q_{jj}}$ and $\hat{R}_{in} = R_{in}/\sqrt{Q_{ii}T_{nn}}$ from uniform distributions in the $[0,1]$, $[-1,1]$, and $[-10^{-12}, 10^{-12}]$ intervals respectively.

We find that the results of the numerical integration are sensitive to these random initial values, which has not been the case to this extent for fixed biases. Furthermore, the dynamical behaviour can become very complex even for realizable cases ($K = M$) and networks with three or four hidden units. For sake of simplicity, we will therefore restrict our presentation to networks with two hidden units ($K = M = 2$) and uncorrelated isotropic teachers, defined by $T_{nm} = \delta_{nm}$, although larger networks and graded teacher scenarios were investigated extensively as well. We have further limited our scope by investigating a common learning rate ($\eta_0 = \eta_\theta = \eta_w$) for biases and weights. To study the effect of different weight initialization, we have fixed the initial values of the student-student overlaps Q_{ij} and biases θ_i, as these can be manipulated freely in any learning scenario. Only the initial student-teacher overlaps R_{in} are randomized as suggested above.

In Fig. 1 we compare the evolution of the overlaps, the biases and the generalization error for the soft committee machine with and without adjustable bias learning a similar realizable teacher task. The student denoted by $*$ lacks biases, i.e., $\theta_i = 0$, and learns to imitate an isotropic teacher with zero biases ($\rho_n = 0$). The other student features adjustable biases, trained from an isotropic teacher with small biases ($\rho_{1,2} = \mp 0.1$). For both scenarios, the learning rate and the initial conditions were judiciously chosen to be $\eta_0 = 2.0$, $Q_{11} = 0.1$, $Q_{22} = 0.2$, $\hat{R}_{in} = \hat{Q}_{12} = U[-10^{-12}, 10^{-12}]$ with $\theta_1 = 0.0$ and $\theta_2 = 0.5$ for the student with adjustable biases.

In both cases, the student weight vectors (Fig. 1a) are drawn quickly from their initial values into a suboptimal symmetric phase, characterized by the lack of specialization of the student hidden units on a particular teacher hidden unit, as can be depicted from the similar values of R_{in} in Fig. 1b. This symmetry is broken

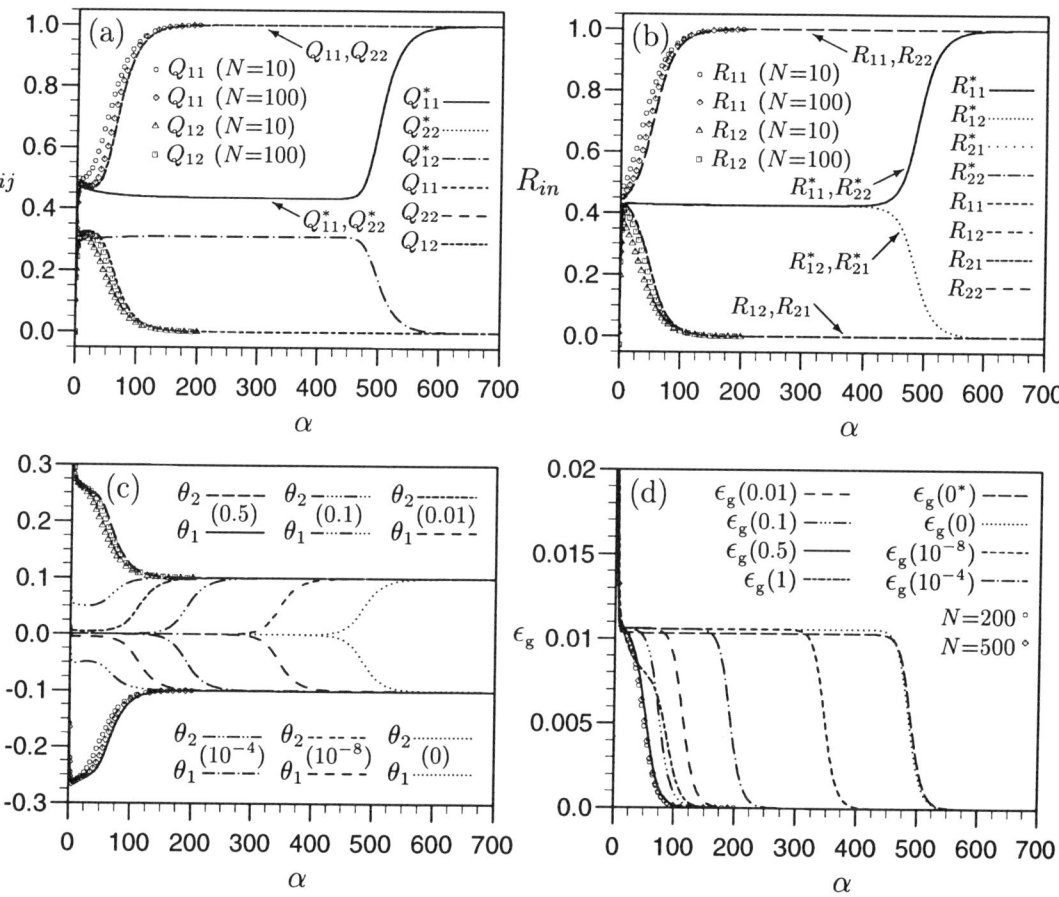

Figure 1: The dynamical evolution of the student-student overlaps Q_{ij} (a), and the student-teacher overlaps R_{in} (b) as a function of the normalized example number α is compared for two student-teacher scenarios: One student (denoted by *) has fixed zero biases, the other has adjustable biases. The influence of the symmetry in the initialization of the biases on the dynamics is shown for the student biases θ_i (c), and the generalization error ϵ_g (d): $\theta_1 = 0$ is kept for all runs, but the initial value of θ_2 varies and is given in brackets in the legends. Finite size simulations for input dimensions $N = 10 \ldots 500$ show that the dynamical variables are self-averaging.

almost immediately in the learning scenario with adjustable biases and the student converges quickly to the optimal solution, characterized by the evolution of the overlap matrices $\mathbf{Q}$, $\mathbf{R}$ and biases θ_i (see Fig. 1c) to their optimal values $\mathbf{T}$ and ρ_n (up to the permutation symmetry due to the arbitrary labeling of the student nodes). Likewise, the generalization error ϵ_g decays to zero in Fig. 1d. The student with fixed biases is trapped for most of its training time in the symmetric phase before it eventually converges.

Extensive simulations for input dimensions $N = 10 \ldots 500$ confirm that the dynamic variables are self-averaging and show that variances decrease with $1/N$. The mean trajectories are in good agreement with the theoretical predictions even for very small input dimensions ($N = 10$) and are virtually indistinguishable for $N = 500$.

The length of the symmetric phase for the isotropic teacher scenario is dominated by the learning rate[1], but also exhibits a logarithmic dependence on the typical

---

[1] The length of the symmetric phase is linearly dependent on η_0 for small learning rates.

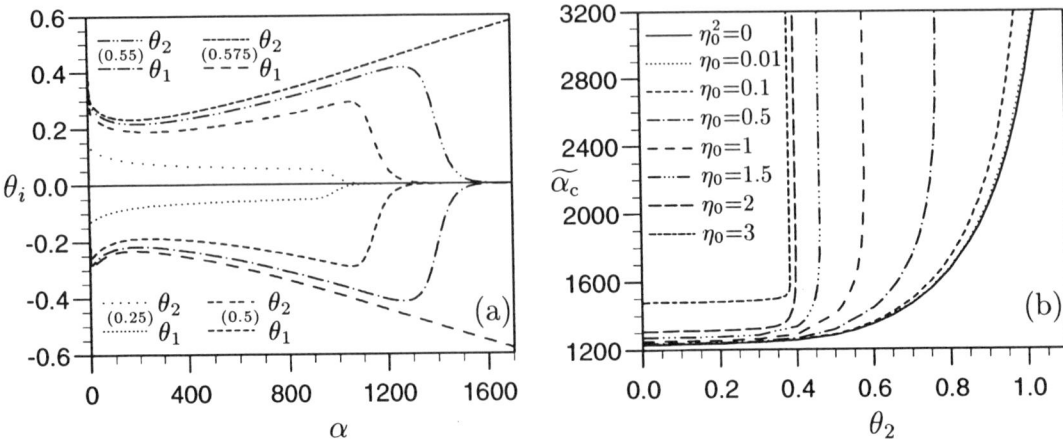

Figure 2: (a) The dynamical evolution of the biases θ_i for a student imitating an isotropic teacher with zero biases. reveals symmetric dynamics for θ_1 and θ_2. The student was randomly initialized identically for the different runs, but for a change in the range of the random initialization of the biases $(U[-b,b])$, with the value of b given in the legend. Above a critical value of b the student remains stuck in a suboptimal phase. (b) The normalized convergence time $\widetilde{\alpha}_c \equiv \eta_0 \alpha_c$ is shown as a function of the initialization of θ_2 for varios learning rates η_0 (see legend, $\eta_0^2 = 0$ symbolizes the dynamics neglecting η_0^2 terms.).

differences in the initial student-teacher overlaps R_{in} (Biehl et al., 1996) which are typically of order $\mathcal{O}(1/\sqrt{N})$ and cannot be influenced in real scenarios without a priori knowledge. The initialization of the biases, however, can be controlled by the user and its influence on the learning dynamics is shown in Figs. 1c and 1d for the biases and the generalization error respectively. For initially identical biases ($\theta_1 = \theta_2 = 0$), the evolution of the order parameters and hence the generalization error is almost indistinguishable from the fixed biases case. A breaking of this symmetry leads to a decrease of the symmetric phase linear in $\log(|\theta_1 - \theta_2|)$ until it has all but disappeared. The dynamics are again slowed down for very large initialization of the biases (see 1d), where the biases have to travel a long way to their optimal values.

This suggests that for a given learning rate the biases have a dominant effect in the learning process and strongly break existent symmetries in weight space. This is arguably due to a steep minimum in the generalization error surface along the direction of the biases. To confirm this, we have studied a range of other learning scenarios including larger networks and non-isotropic teachers, e.g., graded teachers with $T_{nm} = n\delta_{nm}$. Even when the norms of the teacher weight vectors are strongly graded, which also breaks the weight symmetry and reduces the symmetric phase significantly in the case of fixed biases, we have found that the biases usually have the stronger symmetry breaking effect: the trajectories of the biases never cross, provided that they were not initialized too symmetrically.

This would seem to promote initializing the biases of the student hidden units evenly across the input domain, which has been suggested previously on a heuristic basis (Nguyen & Widrow, 1990). However, this can lead to the student being stuck in a suboptimal configuration. In Fig. 2a, we show the dynamics of the student biases θ_i when the teacher biases are symmetric ($\rho_n = 0$). We find that the student progress is inversely related to the magnitude of the bias initialization and finally fails to converge at all. It remains in a suboptimal phase characterized by biases of the same large magnitude but opposite sign and highly correlated weight vectors. In effect, the outputs of the two student nodes cancel out over most of the input domain. In

Fig. 2b, the influence of the learning rate in combination with the bias initialization in determining convergence is illustrated. The convergence time α_c, defined as the example number at which the generalization error has decayed to a small value, here judiciously chosen to be 10^{-8}, is shown as a function of the initial value of θ_2 for various learning rates η_0. For convenience, we have normalized the convergence time with $1/\eta_0$. The initialization of the other order parameters is identical to Fig. 1a. One finds that the convergence time diverges for all learning rates, above a critical initial value of θ_2. For increasing learning rates, this transition becomes sharper and occurs at smaller θ_2, i.e., the dynamics become more sensitive to the bias initialization.

4 SUMMARY AND DISCUSSION

This research has been motivated by recent progress in the theoretical study of on-line learning in realistic two-layer neural network models — the soft-committee machine, trained with back-propagation (Saad & Solla, 1995). The studies so far have excluded biases to the hidden layers, a constraint which has been removed in this paper, which makes the model a universal approximator. The dynamics of the extended model turn out to be very rich and more complex than the original model.

In this paper, we have concentrated on the effect of initialization of student weights and biases. We have further restricted our presentation for simplicity to realizable cases and small networks with two hidden units, although larger networks were studied for comparison. Even in these simple learning scenarios, we find surprising dynamical effects due to the adjustable biases. In the case where the teacher network exhibits distinct biases, unsymmetric initial values of the student biases break the node symmetry in weight space effectively and can speed up the learning process considerably, suggesting that student biases should in practice be initially spread evenly across the input domain if there is no a priori knowledge of the function to be learned. For degenerate teacher biases however such a scheme can be counterproductive as different initial student bias values slow down the learning dynamics and can even lead to the student being stuck in suboptimal fixed points, characterized by student biases being grouped symmetrically around the degenerate teacher biases and strong correlations between the associated weight vectors.

In fact, these attractive suboptimal fixed points exist even for non-degenerate teacher biases, but the range of initial conditions attracted to these suboptimal network configurations decreases in size. Furthermore, this domain is shifted to very large initial student biases as the difference in the values of the teacher biases is increased. We have found these effects also for larger network sizes, where the dynamics and number of attractive suboptimal fixed points with different internal symmetries increases. Although attractive suboptimal fixed points were also found in the original model (Biehl et al., 1996), the basins of attraction of initial values are in general very small and are therefore only of academic interest.

However, our numerical work suggests that a simple rule of thumb to avoid being attracted to suboptimal fixed points is to always initialize the squared norm of a weight vector larger than the magnitude of the corresponding bias. This scheme will still support spreading of the biases across the main input domain in order to encourage node symmetry breaking. This is somewhat similar to previous findings (Nguyen & Widrow, 1990; Kim & Ra, 1991), the former suggesting spreading the biases across the input domain, the latter relating the minimal initial size of each weight with the learning rate. This work provides a more theoretical motivation for these results and also distinguishes between the different rôles of biases and weights.

In this paper we have addressed mainly one important issue for theoreticians and practitioners alike: the initialization of the student network weights and biases. Other important issues, notably the question of optimal and maximal learning rates for different network sizes during convergence, will be reported elsewhere.

A THEOREM

Let S_g denote the class of neural networks defined by sums of the form $\sum_{i=1}^{K} n_i g(u_i - \theta_i)$ where K is arbitrary (representing an arbitrary number of hidden units), $\theta_i \in \mathbb{R}$ and $n_i \in \mathbb{Z}$ (i.e. integer weights). Let $\psi(x) \equiv \partial g(x)/\partial x$ and let $\mathcal{D}_\psi$ denote the class of networks defined by sums of the form $\sum_{i=1}^{K} w_i \psi(u_i - \theta_i)$ where $w_i \in \mathbb{R}$. If g is continuously differentiable and if the class $\mathcal{D}_\psi$ are universal approximators, then S_g is a class of universal approximators; that is, such functions are dense in the space of continuous functions with the L_∞ norm.

As a corollary, the normalized soft committee machine forms a class of universal approximators with both sigmoid and error transfer functions [since radial basis function networks are universal (Park & Sandberg, 1993) and we need consider only the one-dimensional input case as noted in the proof below]. Note that some restriction on g is necessary: if g is the step function, then with arbitrary hidden-output weights, the network is a universal approximator, while with fixed hidden-output weights it is not.

A.1 Proof

By the arguments of (Hornik et al., 1990) which use the properties of trigonometric polynomials, it is sufficient to consider the case of one-dimensional input and output spaces. Let I denote a compact interval in $\mathbb{R}$ and let f be a continuous function defined on I. Because $\mathcal{D}_\psi$ is universal, given any $\epsilon > 0$ we can find weights w_i and biases θ_i such that

$$\left\| f - \sum_{i=1}^{K} w_i \psi(u - \theta_i) \right\|_\infty < \frac{\epsilon}{2} \qquad (i)$$

Because the rationals are dense in the reals, without loss of generality we can assume that the weights $w_i \in \mathbb{Q}$. Since $\psi(x)$ is continuous and I is compact, the convergence of $[g(x+h) - g(x)]/h$ to $\partial g(x)/\partial x$ is uniform and hence for all $n > n\left(\frac{\epsilon}{2K w_i}\right)$ the following inequality holds:

$$\left\| n w_i \left[g\left(u + \frac{1}{n} - \theta_i\right) - g(u - \theta_i) \right] - w_i \psi(u - \theta_i) \right\|_\infty < \frac{\epsilon}{2K} \qquad (ii)$$

Also note that for suitable $n_i > n\left(\frac{\epsilon}{2K w_i}\right)$, $m_i = n_i w_i \in \mathbb{Z}$, as w_i is a rational number. Thus, by the triangle inequality,

$$\left\| \sum_{i=1}^{K} m_i \left[g\left(u + \frac{1}{n_i} - \theta_i\right) - g(u - \theta_i) \right] - \sum_{i=1}^{K} w_i \psi(u - \theta_i) \right\|_\infty < \frac{\epsilon}{2}. \qquad (iii)$$

The result now follows from equations (i) and (iii) and the triangle inequality.

References

Barber, D., Saad, D., & Sollich, P. 1996. *Europhys. Lett.*, **34**, 151–156.

Biehl, M., & Schwarze, H. 1995. *J. Phys. A*, **28**, 643–656.

Biehl, M., Riegler, P., & Wöhler, C. 1996. University of Würzburg Preprint WUE-ITP-96-003.

Hornik, K., Stinchcombe, M., & White, H. 1990. *Neural Networks*, **3**, 551–560.

Kim, Y. K., & Ra, J. B. 1991. Pages 2396–2401 of: *International Joint Conference on Neural Networks 91*.

Nguyen, D., & Widrow, B. 1990. Pages C21–C26 of: *IJCNN International Conference on Neural Networks 90*.

Park, J., & Sandberg, I. W. 1993. *Neural Computation*, **5**, 305–316.

Riegler, P., & Biehl, M. 1995. *J. Phys. A*, **28**, L507–L513.

Saad, D., & Solla, S. A. 1995. *Phys. Rev. E*, **52**, 4225–4243.

Computing with infinite networks

Christopher K. I. Williams
Neural Computing Research Group
Department of Computer Science and Applied Mathematics
Aston University, Birmingham B4 7ET, UK
c.k.i.williams@aston.ac.uk

Abstract

For neural networks with a wide class of weight-priors, it can be shown that in the limit of an infinite number of hidden units the prior over functions tends to a Gaussian process. In this paper analytic forms are derived for the covariance function of the Gaussian processes corresponding to networks with sigmoidal and Gaussian hidden units. This allows predictions to be made efficiently using networks with an infinite number of hidden units, and shows that, somewhat paradoxically, it may be easier to compute with infinite networks than finite ones.

1 Introduction

To someone training a neural network by maximizing the likelihood of a finite amount of data it makes no sense to use a network with an infinite number of hidden units; the network will "overfit" the data and so will be expected to generalize poorly. However, the idea of selecting the network size depending on the amount of training data makes little sense to a Bayesian; a model should be chosen that reflects the understanding of the problem, and then application of Bayes' theorem allows inference to be carried out (at least in theory) after the data is observed.

In the Bayesian treatment of neural networks, a question immediately arises as to how many hidden units are believed to be appropriate for a task. Neal (1996) has argued compellingly that for real-world problems, there is no reason to believe that neural network models should be limited to nets containing only a "small" number of hidden units. He has shown that it is sensible to consider a limit where the number of hidden units in a net tends to infinity, and that good predictions can be obtained from such models using the Bayesian machinery. He has also shown that for fixed hyperparameters, a large class of neural network models will converge to a Gaussian process prior over functions in the limit of an infinite number of hidden units.

Neal's argument is an existence proof—it states that an infinite neural net will converge to a Gaussian process, but does not give the covariance function needed to actually specify the particular Gaussian process. In this paper I show that for certain weight priors and transfer functions in the neural network model, the covariance function which describes the behaviour of the corresponding Gaussian process can be calculated analytically. This allows predictions to be made using neural networks with an infinite number of hidden units in time $O(n^3)$, where n is the number of training examples[1]. The only alternative currently available is to use Markov Chain Monte Carlo (MCMC) methods (e.g. Neal, 1996) for networks with a large (but finite) number of hidden units. However, this is likely to be computationally expensive, and we note possible concerns over the time needed for the Markov chain to reach equilibrium. The availability of an analytic form for the covariance function also facilitates the comparison of the properties of neural networks with an infinite number of hidden units as compared to other Gaussian process priors that may be considered.

The Gaussian process analysis applies for fixed hyperparameters θ. If it were desired to make predictions based on a hyperprior $P(\theta)$ then the necessary θ-space integration could be achieved by MCMC methods. The great advantage of integrating out the weights analytically is that it dramatically reduces the dimensionality of the MCMC integrals, and thus improves their speed of convergence.

1.1 From priors on weights to priors on functions

Bayesian neural networks are usually specified in a hierarchical manner, so that the weights w are regarded as being drawn from a distribution $P(w|\theta)$. For example, the weights might be drawn from a zero-mean Gaussian distribution, where θ specifies the variance of groups of weights. A full description of the prior is given by specifying $P(\theta)$ as well as $P(w|\theta)$. The hyperprior can be integrated out to give $P(w) = \int P(w|\theta)P(\theta)\,d\theta$, but in our case it will be advantageous not to do this as it introduces weight correlations which prevent convergence to a Gaussian process.

In the Bayesian view of neural networks, predictions for the output value y_* corresponding to a new input value x_* are made by integrating over the posterior in weight space. Let $\mathcal{D} = ((x_1,t_1),(x_2,t_2),\ldots,(x_n,t_n))$ denote the n training data pairs, $t = (t_1,\ldots,t_n)^T$ and $f_*(w)$ denote the mapping carried out by the network on input x_* given weights w. $P(w|t,\theta)$ is the weight posterior given the training data[2]. Then the predictive distribution for y_* given the training data and hyperparameters θ is

$$P(y_*|t,\theta) = \int \delta(y_* - f_*(w))P(w|t,\theta)\,dw \quad (1)$$

We will now show how this can also be viewed as making the prediction using priors over functions rather than weights. Let $f(w)$ denote the vector of outputs corresponding to inputs $(x_1,\ldots,x_n)$ given weights w. Then, using Bayes' theorem we have $P(w|t,\theta) = P(t|w)P(w|\theta)/P(t|\theta)$, and $P(t|w) = \int P(t|y)\,\delta(y - f(w))\,dy$. Hence equation 1 can be rewritten as

$$P(y_*|t,\theta) = \frac{1}{P(t|\theta)} \int\int P(t|y)\,\delta(y_* - f_*(w))\delta(y - f(w))\,P(w|\theta)\,dw\,dy \quad (2)$$

However, the prior over $(y_*, y_1, \ldots, y_n)$ is given by $P(y_*, y|\theta) = P(y_*|y,\theta)P(y|\theta) = \int \delta(y_* - f_*(w))\,\delta(y - f(w))P(w|\theta)\,dw$ and thus the predictive distribution can be

---
[1] For large n, various approximations to the exact solution which avoid the inversion of an $n \times n$ matrix are available.

[2] For notational convenience we suppress the x-dependence of the posterior.

written as

$$P(y_*|t,\theta) = \frac{1}{P(t|\theta)}\int P(t|y)P(y_*|y,\theta)P(y|\theta)\,dy = \int P(y_*|y,\theta)P(y|t,\theta)\,dy \quad (3)$$

Hence in a Bayesian view it is the prior over function values $P(y_*,y|\theta)$ which is important; specifying this prior by using weight distributions is one valid way to achieve this goal. In general we can use the weight space or function space view, which ever is more convenient, and for infinite neural networks the function space view is more useful.

2 Gaussian processes

A stochastic process is a collection of random variables $\{Y(x)|x \in X\}$ indexed by a set X. In our case X will be $\mathcal{R}^d$, where d is the number of inputs. The stochastic process is specified by giving the probability distribution for every finite subset of variables $Y(x_1),\ldots,Y(x_k)$ in a consistent manner. A Gaussian process (GP) is a stochastic process which can be fully specified by its mean function $\mu(x) = E[Y(x)]$ and its covariance function $C(x,x') = E[(Y(x) - \mu(x))(Y(x') - \mu(x'))]$; any finite set of Y-variables will have a joint multivariate Gaussian distribution. For a multidimensional input space a Gaussian process may also be called a Gaussian random field.

Below we consider Gaussian processes which have $\mu(x) \equiv 0$, as is the case for the neural network priors discussed in section 3. A non-zero $\mu(x)$ can be incorporated into the framework at the expense of a little extra complexity.

A widely used class of covariance functions is the stationary covariance functions, whereby $C(x,x') = C(x - x')$. These are related to the spectral density (or power spectrum) of the process by the Wiener-Khinchine theorem, and are particularly amenable to Fourier analysis as the eigenfunctions of a stationary covariance kernel are $\exp i\mathbf{k}.\mathbf{x}$. Many commonly used covariance functions are also isotropic, so that $C(\mathbf{h}) = C(h)$ where $\mathbf{h} = x - x'$ and $h = |\mathbf{h}|$. For example $C(h) = \exp(-(h/\sigma)^\nu)$ is a valid covariance function for all d and for $0 < \nu \le 2$. Note that in this case σ sets the correlation length-scale of the random field, although other covariance functions (e.g. those corresponding to power-law spectral densities) may have no preferred length scale.

2.1 Prediction with Gaussian processes

The model for the observed data is that it was generated from the *prior* stochastic process, and that independent Gaussian noise (of variance σ_ν^2) was then added. Given a prior covariance function $C_P(x_i,x_j)$, a noise process $C_N(x_i,x_j) = \sigma_\nu^2 \delta_{ij}$ (i.e. independent noise of variance σ_ν^2 at each data point) and the training data, the prediction for the distribution of y_* corresponding to a test point x_* is obtained simply by applying equation 3. As the prior and noise model are both Gaussian the integral can be done analytically and $P(y_*|t,\theta)$ is Gaussian with mean and variance

$$\hat{y}(x_*) = k_P^T(x_*)(K_P + K_N)^{-1}t \quad (4)$$
$$\sigma_{\hat{y}}^2(x_*) = C_P(x_*,x_*) - k_P^T(x_*)(K_P + K_N)^{-1}k_P(x_*) \quad (5)$$

where $[K_\alpha]_{ij} = C_\alpha(x_i,x_j)$ for $\alpha = P,N$ and $k_P(x_*) = (C_P(x_*,x_1),\ldots,C_P(x_*,x_n))^T$. $\sigma_{\hat{y}}^2(x_*)$ gives the "error bars" of the prediction.

Equations 4 and 5 are the analogue for spatial processes of Wiener-Kolmogorov prediction theory. They have appeared in a wide variety of contexts including geostatistics where the method is known as "kriging" (Journel and Huijbregts, 1978; Cressie 1993), multidimensional spline smoothing (Wahba, 1990), in the derivation of radial basis function neural networks (Poggio and Girosi, 1990) and in the work of Whittle (1963).

3 Covariance functions for Neural Networks

Consider a network which takes an input x, has one hidden layer with H units and then linearly combines the outputs of the hidden units with a bias to obtain $f(x)$. The mapping can be written

$$f(x) = b + \sum_{j=1}^{H} v_j h(x; u_j) \tag{6}$$

where $h(x; u)$ is the hidden unit transfer function (which we shall assume is bounded) which depends on the input-to-hidden weights u. This architecture is important because it has been shown by Hornik (1993) that networks with one hidden layer are universal approximators as the number of hidden units tends to infinity, for a wide class of transfer functions (but excluding polynomials). Let b and the v's have independent zero-mean distributions of variance σ_b^2 and σ_v^2 respectively, and let the weights u_j for each hidden unit be independently and identically distributed. Denoting all weights by w, we obtain (following Neal, 1996)

$$E_w[f(x)] = 0 \tag{7}$$

$$E_w[f(x)f(x')] = \sigma_b^2 + \sum_j \sigma_v^2 E_u[h_j(x; u)h_j(x'; u)] \tag{8}$$

$$= \sigma_b^2 + H\sigma_v^2 E_u[h(x; u)h(x'; u)] \tag{9}$$

where equation 9 follows because all of the hidden units are identically distributed. The final term in equation 9 becomes $\omega^2 E_u[h(x; u)h(x'; u)]$ by letting σ_v^2 scale as ω^2/H.

As the transfer function is bounded, all moments of the distribution will be bounded and hence the Central Limit Theorem can be applied, showing that the stochastic process will become a Gaussian process in the limit as $H \to \infty$.

By evaluating $E_u[h(x)h(x')]$ for all x and x' in the training and testing sets we can obtain the covariance function needed to describe the neural network as a Gaussian process. These expectations are, of course, integrals over the relevant probability distributions of the biases and input weights. In the following sections two specific choices for the transfer functions are considered, (1) a sigmoidal function and (2) a Gaussian. Gaussian weight priors are used in both cases.

It is interesting to note why this analysis cannot be taken a stage further to integrate out any hyperparameters as well. For example, the variance σ_v^2 of the v weights might be drawn from an inverse Gamma distribution. In this case the distribution $P(v) = \int P(v|\sigma_v^2)P(\sigma_v^2)d\sigma_v^2$ is no longer the product of the marginal distributions for each v weight (in fact it will be a multivariate t-distribution). A similar analysis can be applied to the u weights with a hyperprior. The effect is to make the hidden units non-independent, so that the Central Limit Theorem can no longer be applied.

3.1 Sigmoidal transfer function

A sigmoidal transfer function is a very common choice in neural networks research; nets with this architecture are usually called multi-layer perceptrons.

Below we consider the transfer function $h(\boldsymbol{x}; \boldsymbol{u}) = \Phi(u_0 + \sum_{i=1}^d u_j x_i)$, where $\Phi(z) = 2/\sqrt{\pi} \int_0^z e^{-t^2} dt$ is the error function, closely related to the cumulative distribution function for the Gaussian distribution. Appropriately scaled, the graph of this function is very similar to the tanh function which is more commonly used in the neural networks literature.

In calculating $V(\boldsymbol{x}, \boldsymbol{x}') \stackrel{def}{=} E_{\boldsymbol{u}}[h(\boldsymbol{x}; \boldsymbol{u}) h(\boldsymbol{x}'; \boldsymbol{u})]$ we make the usual assumptions (e.g. MacKay, 1992) that $\boldsymbol{u}$ is drawn from a zero-mean Gaussian distribution with covariance matrix Σ, i.e. $\boldsymbol{u} \sim N(0, \Sigma)$. Let $\tilde{\boldsymbol{x}} = (1, x_1, \ldots, x_d)$ be an augmented input vector whose first entry corresponds to the bias. Then $V_{\text{erf}}(\boldsymbol{x}, \boldsymbol{x}')$ can be written as

$$V_{\text{erf}}(\boldsymbol{x}, \boldsymbol{x}') = \frac{1}{(2\pi)^{\frac{d+1}{2}} |\Sigma|^{1/2}} \int \Phi(\boldsymbol{u}^T \tilde{\boldsymbol{x}}) \Phi(\boldsymbol{u}^T \tilde{\boldsymbol{x}}') \exp(-\frac{1}{2} \boldsymbol{u}^T \Sigma^{-1} \boldsymbol{u}) \, d\boldsymbol{u} \quad (10)$$

This integral can be evaluated analytically[3] to give

$$V_{\text{erf}}(\boldsymbol{x}, \boldsymbol{x}') = \frac{2}{\pi} \sin^{-1} \frac{2 \tilde{\boldsymbol{x}}^T \Sigma \tilde{\boldsymbol{x}}'}{\sqrt{(1 + 2 \tilde{\boldsymbol{x}}^T \Sigma \tilde{\boldsymbol{x}})(1 + 2 \tilde{\boldsymbol{x}}'^T \Sigma \tilde{\boldsymbol{x}}')}} \quad (11)$$

We observe that this covariance function is not stationary, which makes sense as the distributions for the weights are centered about zero, and hence translational symmetry is not present.

Consider a diagonal weight prior so that $\Sigma = \text{diag}(\sigma_0^2, \sigma_1^2, \ldots, \sigma_1^2)$, so that the inputs $i = 1, \ldots, d$ have a different weight variance to the bias σ_0^2. Then for $|\boldsymbol{x}|^2, |\boldsymbol{x}'|^2 \gg (1 + 2\sigma_0^2)/2\sigma_1^2$, we find that $V_{\text{erf}}(\boldsymbol{x}, \boldsymbol{x}') \simeq 1 - 2\theta/\pi$, where θ is the angle between $\boldsymbol{x}$ and $\boldsymbol{x}'$. Again this makes sense intuitively; if the model is made up of a large number of sigmoidal functions in random directions (in $\boldsymbol{x}$ space), then we would expect points that lie diametrically opposite (i.e. at $\boldsymbol{x}$ and $-\boldsymbol{x}$) to be anti-correlated, because they will lie in the $+1$ and -1 regions of the sigmoid function for most directions.

3.2 Gaussian transfer function

One other very common transfer function used in neural networks research is the Gaussian, so that $h(\boldsymbol{x}; \boldsymbol{u}) = \exp[-(\boldsymbol{x} - \boldsymbol{u})^T (\boldsymbol{x} - \boldsymbol{u})/2\sigma_g^2]$, where σ_g^2 is the width parameter of the Gaussian. Gaussian basis functions are often used in Radial Basis Function (RBF) networks (e.g. Poggio and Girosi, 1990).

For a Gaussian prior over the distribution of $\boldsymbol{u}$ so that $\boldsymbol{u} \sim N(0, \sigma_u^2 I)$,

$$V_G(\boldsymbol{x}, \boldsymbol{x}') = \frac{1}{(2\pi\sigma_u^2)^{d/2}} \int \exp -\frac{(\boldsymbol{x} - \boldsymbol{u})^T (\boldsymbol{x} - \boldsymbol{u})}{2\sigma_g^2} \exp -\frac{(\boldsymbol{x}' - \boldsymbol{u})^T (\boldsymbol{x}' - \boldsymbol{u})}{2\sigma_g^2} \exp -\frac{\boldsymbol{u}^T \boldsymbol{u}}{2\sigma_u^2} d\boldsymbol{u} \quad (12)$$

By completing the square and integrating out $\boldsymbol{u}$ we obtain

$$V_G(\boldsymbol{x}, \boldsymbol{x}') = \left(\frac{\sigma_e}{\sigma_u}\right)^d \exp\{-\frac{\boldsymbol{x}^T \boldsymbol{x}}{2\sigma_m^2}\} \exp\{-\frac{(\boldsymbol{x} - \boldsymbol{x}')^T (\boldsymbol{x} - \boldsymbol{x}')}{2\sigma_s^2}\} \exp\{-\frac{\boldsymbol{x}'^T \boldsymbol{x}'}{2\sigma_m^2}\} \quad (13)$$

where $1/\sigma_e^2 = 2/\sigma_g^2 + 1/\sigma_u^2$, $\sigma_s^2 = 2\sigma_g^2 + \sigma_g^4/\sigma_u^2$ and $\sigma_m^2 = 2\sigma_u^2 + \sigma_g^2$. This formula can be generalized by allowing covariance matrices Σ_b and Σ_u in place of $\sigma_g^2 I$ and $\sigma_u^2 I$; rescaling each input variable x_i independently is a simple example.

---

[3] Introduce a dummy parameter λ to make the first term in the integrand $\Phi(\lambda \boldsymbol{u}^T \tilde{\boldsymbol{x}})$. Differentiate the integral with respect to λ and then use integration by parts. Finally recognize that $dV_{\text{erf}}/d\lambda$ is of the form $(1 - \theta^2)^{-1/2} d\theta/d\lambda$ and hence obtain the $\sin^{-1}$ form of the result, and evaluate it at $\lambda = 1$.

Again this is a non-stationary covariance function, although it is interesting to note that if $\sigma_u^2 \to \infty$ (while scaling ω^2 appropriately) we find that $V_G(\boldsymbol{x}, \boldsymbol{x}') \propto \exp\{-(\boldsymbol{x}-\boldsymbol{x}')^T(\boldsymbol{x}-\boldsymbol{x}')/4\sigma_g^2\}$ [4]. For a finite value of σ_u^2, $V_G(\boldsymbol{x}, \boldsymbol{x}')$ is a stationary covariance function "modulated" by the Gaussian decay function $\exp(-\boldsymbol{x}^T\boldsymbol{x}/2\sigma_m^2)\exp(-\boldsymbol{x}'^T\boldsymbol{x}'/2\sigma_m^2)$. Clearly if σ_m^2 is much larger than the largest distance in $\boldsymbol{x}$-space then the predictions made with V_G and a Gaussian process with only the stationary part of V_G will be very similar.

It is also possible to view the infinite network with Gaussian transfer functions as an example of a shot-noise process based on an inhomogeneous Poisson process (see Parzen (1962) §4.5 for details). Points are generated from an inhomogeneous Poisson process with the rate function $\propto \exp(-\boldsymbol{x}^T\boldsymbol{x}/2\sigma_u^2)$, and Gaussian kernels of height v are centered on each of the points, where v is chosen iid from a distribution with mean zero and variance σ_v^2.

3.3 Comparing covariance functions

The priors over functions specified by sigmoidal and Gaussian neural networks differ from covariance functions that are usually employed in the literature, e.g. splines (Wahba, 1990). How might we characterize the different covariance functions and compare the kinds of priors that they imply?

The complex exponential $\exp i\boldsymbol{k}.\boldsymbol{x}$ is an eigenfunction of a stationary and isotropic covariance function, and hence the spectral density (or power spectrum) $S(k)$ ($k = |\boldsymbol{k}|$) nicely characterizes the corresponding stochastic process. Roughly speaking the spectral density describes the "power" at a given spatial frequency k; for example, splines have $S(k) \propto k^{-\beta}$. The decay of $S(k)$ as k increases is essential, as it provides a smoothing or damping out of high frequencies. Unfortunately non-stationary processes cannot be analyzed in exactly this fashion because the complex exponentials are not (in general) eigenfunctions of a non-stationary kernel. Instead, we must consider the eigenfunctions defined by $\int C(\boldsymbol{x}, \boldsymbol{x}')\phi(\boldsymbol{x}')d\boldsymbol{x}' = \lambda\phi(\boldsymbol{x})$. However, it may be possible to get some feel for the effect of a non-stationary covariance function by looking at the diagonal elements in its 2d-dimensional Fourier transform, which correspond to the entries in power spectrum for stationary covariance functions.

3.4 Convergence of finite network priors to GPs

From general Central Limit Theorem results one would expect a rate of convergence of $H^{-1/2}$ towards a Gaussian process prior. How many units will be required in practice would seem to depend on the particular values of the weight-variance parameters. For example, for Gaussian transfer functions, σ_m defines the radius over which we expect the process to be significantly different from zero. If this radius is increased (while keeping the variance of the basis functions σ_g^2 fixed) then naturally one would expect to need more hidden units in order to achieve the same level of approximation as before. Similar comments can be made for the sigmoidal case, depending on $(1 + 2\sigma_0^2)/2\sigma_1^2$.

I have conducted some experiments for the sigmoidal transfer function, comparing the predictive performance of a finite neural network with one input unit to the equivalent Gaussian process on data generated from the GP. The finite network simulations were carried out using a slightly modified version of Neal's MCMC Bayesian neural networks code (Neal, 1996) and the inputs were drawn from a

---

[4] Note that this would require $\omega^2 \to \infty$ and hence the Central Limit Theorem would no longer hold, i.e. the process would be non-Gaussian.

$N(0, 1)$ distribution. The hyperparameter settings were $\sigma_I = 10.0$, $\sigma_0 = 2.0$, $\sigma_v = 1.189$ and $\sigma_b = 1.0$. Roughly speaking the results are that 100's of hidden units are required before similar performance is achieved by the two methods, although there is considerable variability depending on the particular sample drawn from the prior; sometimes 10 hidden units appears sufficient for good agreement.

4 Discussion

The work described above shows how to calculate the covariance function for sigmoidal and Gaussian basis functions networks. It is probable similar techniques will allow covariance functions to be derived analytically for networks with other kinds of basis functions as well; these may turn out to be similar in form to covariance functions already used in the Gaussian process literature.

In the derivations above the hyperparameters θ were fixed. However, in a real data analysis problem it would be unlikely that appropriate values of these parameters would be known. Given a prior distribution $P(\theta)$ predictions should be made by integrating over the posterior distribution $P(\theta|t) \propto P(\theta)P(t|\theta)$, where $P(t|\theta)$ is the likelihood of the training data t under the model; $P(t|\theta)$ is easily computed for a Gaussian process. The prediction $\bar{y}(x)$ for test input x is then given by

$$\bar{y}(x) = \int \hat{y}_\theta(x) P(\theta|D) d\theta \qquad (14)$$

where $\hat{y}_\theta(x)$ is the predicted mean (as given by equation 4) for a particular value of θ. This integration is not tractable analytically but Markov Chain Monte Carlo methods such as Hybrid Monte Carlo can be used to approximate it. This strategy was used in Williams and Rasmussen (1996), but for stationary covariance functions, not ones derived from Gaussian processes; it would be interesting to compare results.

Acknowledgements

I thank David Saad and David Barber for help in obtaining the result in equation 11, and Chris Bishop, Peter Dayan, Ian Nabney, Radford Neal, David Saad and Huaiyu Zhu for comments on an earlier draft of the paper. This work was partially supported by EPSRC grant GR/J75425, "Novel Developments in Learning Theory for Neural Networks".

References

Cressie, N. A. C. (1993). *Statistics for Spatial Data*. Wiley.

Hornik, K. (1993). Some new results on neural network approximation. *Neural Networks* **6** (8), 1069–1072.

Journel, A. G. and C. J. Huijbregts (1978). *Mining Geostatistics*. Academic Press.

MacKay, D. J. C. (1992). A Practical Bayesian Framework for Backpropagation Networks. *Neural Computation* **4(3)**, 448–472.

Neal, R. M. (1996). *Bayesian Learning for Neural Networks*. Springer. Lecture Notes in Statistics 118.

Parzen, E. (1962). *Stochastic Processes*. Holden-Day.

Poggio, T. and F. Girosi (1990). Networks for approximation and learning. *Proceedings of IEEE* **78**, 1481–1497.

Wahba, G. (1990). *Spline Models for Observational Data*. Society for Industrial and Applied Mathematics. CBMS-NSF Regional Conference series in applied mathematics.

Whittle, P. (1963). *Prediction and regulation by linear least-square methods*. English Universities Press.

Williams, C. K. I. and C. E. Rasmussen (1996). Gaussian processes for regression. In D. S. Touretzky, M. C. Mozer, and M. E. Hasselmo (Eds.), *Advances in Neural Information Processing Systems 8*, pp. 514–520. MIT Press.

Microscopic Equations in Rough Energy Landscape for Neural Networks

K. Y. Michael Wong
Department of Physics,
The Hong Kong University of Science and Technology,
Clear Water Bay, Kowloon, Hong Kong.
E-mail: phkywong@usthk.ust.hk

Abstract

We consider the microscopic equations for learning problems in neural networks. The aligning fields of an example are obtained from the cavity fields, which are the fields if that example were absent in the learning process. In a rough energy landscape, we assume that the density of the local minima obey an exponential distribution, yielding macroscopic properties agreeing with the first step replica symmetry breaking solution. Iterating the microscopic equations provide a learning algorithm, which results in a higher stability than conventional algorithms.

1 INTRODUCTION

Most neural networks learn iteratively by gradient descent. As a result, closed expressions for the final network state after learning are rarely known. This precludes further analysis of their properties, and insights into the design of learning algorithms. To complicate the situation, metastable states (i.e. local minima) are often present in the energy landscape of the learning space so that, depending on the initial configuration, each one is likely to be the final state.

However, large neural networks are mean field systems since the examples and weights strongly interact with each other during the learning process. This means that when one example or weight is considered, the influence of the rest of the system can be regarded as a background satisfying some averaged properties. The situation is similar to a number of disordered systems such as spin glasses, in which mean field theories are applicable (Mézard, Parisi & Virasoro, 1987). This explains the success of statistical mechanical techniques such as the replica method in deriving the macroscopic properties of neural networks, e.g. the storage capacity (Gardner & Derrida 1988), generalization ability (Watkin, Rau & Biehl 1993). The replica method, though, provides much less information on the microscopic conditions of the individual dynamical variables.

An alternative mean field approach is the cavity method. It is a generalization of the Thouless-Anderson-Palmer approach to spin glasses, which started from microscopic equations of the system elements (Thouless, Anderson & Palmer, 1977). Mézard applied the method to neural network learning (Mézard, 1989). Subsequent extensions were made to the teacher-student perceptron (Bouten, Schietse & Van den Broeck 1995), the AND machine (Griniasty, 1993) and the multiclass perceptron (Gerl & Krey, 1995). They yielded macroscopic properties identical to the replica approach, but the microscopic equations were not discussed, and the existence of local minima was neglected.

Recently, the cavity method was applied to general classes of single and multilayer networks with smooth energy landscapes, i.e. without the local minima (Wong, 1995a). The aligning fields of the examples satisfy a set of microscopic equations. Solving these equations iteratively provides a learning algoirthm, as confirmed by simulations in the maximally stable perceptron and the committee tree. The method is also useful in solving the dynamics of feedforward networks which were unsolvable previously (Wong, 1995b).

Despite its success, the theory is so far applicable only to the regime of smooth energy landscapes. Beyond this regime, a stability condition is violated, and local minima begin to appear (Wong, 1995a). In this paper I present a mean field theory for the regime of rough energy landscapes. The complete analysis will be published elsewhere and here I sketch the derivations, emphasizing the underlying physical picture. As shown below, a similar set of microscopic equations hold in this case, as confirmed by simulations in the committee tree. In fact, we find that the solutions to these equations have a higher stability than other conventional learning algorithms.

2 MICROSCOPIC EQUATIONS FOR SMOOTH ENERGY LANDSCAPES

We proceed by reviewing the cavity method for the case of smooth energy landscapes. For illustration we consider the single layer neural network (for two layer networks see Wong, 1995a). There are $N \gg 1$ input nodes $\{S_j\}$ connecting to a single output node by the synaptic weights $\{J_j\}$. The output state is determined by the sign of the local field at the output node, i.e. $S_{out} = \mathrm{sgn}(\sum_j J_j S_j)$. Learning a set of p examples means to find the weights $\{J_j\}$ such that the network gives the correct input-to-output mapping for the examples. If example μ maps the inputs S_j^μ to the output O^μ, then a successful learning process should find a weight vector J_j such that $\mathrm{sgn}(\sum_j J_j \xi_j^\mu) = 1$, where $\xi_j^\mu = O^\mu S_j^\mu$. Thus the usual approach to learning is to first define an energy function (or error function) $E = \sum_\mu g(\Lambda_\mu)$, where $\Lambda_\mu \equiv \sum_j J_j \xi_j^\mu / \sqrt{N}$ are the aligning fields, i.e. the local fields in the direction of the correct output, normalized by the factor $\sqrt{N}$. For example, the Adatron algorithm uses the energy function $g(\Lambda) = (\kappa - \Lambda)\Theta(\kappa - \Lambda)$ where κ is the stability parameter and Θ is the step function (Anlauf & Biehl, 1989). Next, one should minimize E by gradient descent dynamics. To avoid ambiguity, the weights are normalized to $\sum_j S_j^2 = \sum_j J_j^2 = N$.

The cavity method uses a self-consistency argument to consider what happens when a set of p examples is expanded to $p+1$ examples. The central quantity in this method is the *cavity field*. For an added example labelled 0, the cavity field is the aligning field when it is fed to a network which learns examples 1 to p (but never learns example 0), i.e. $t_0 \equiv \sum_j J_j \xi_j^0 / \sqrt{N}$. Since the original network has no information about example 0, J_j and ξ_j^0 are uncorrelated. Thus the cavity field obeys a Gaussian distribution for random example inputs.

After the network has learned examples 0 to p, the weights adjust from $\{J_j\}$ to $\{J_j^0\}$, and the cavity field t_0 adjusts to the generic aligning field Λ_0. As shown schematically in Fig. 1(a), we assume that the adjustments of the aligning fields of the original examples are small, typically of the order $O(N^{-1/2})$. Perturbative analysis concludes that *the aligning field is a well defined function of the cavity field*, i.e. $\Lambda_0 = \lambda(t_0)$ where $\lambda(t)$ is the inverse function of

$$t = \lambda + \gamma g'(\lambda), \tag{1}$$

and γ is called the *local susceptibility*. The cavity fields satisfy a set of self-consistent equations

$$t_\mu = \sum_{\nu \neq \mu} [\lambda(t_\nu) - t_\nu] Q_{\nu\mu} + \alpha \chi \lambda(t_\mu) \tag{2}$$

where $Q_{\nu\mu} = \sum_j \xi_j^\nu \xi_j^\mu / N$. χ is called *nonlocal susceptibility*, and $\alpha \equiv p/N$. The weights J_j are given by

$$J_j = (1 - \alpha\chi)^{-1} \frac{1}{\sqrt{N}} \sum_\mu [\lambda(t_\mu) - t_\mu] \xi_j^\mu. \tag{3}$$

Noting the Gaussian distribution of the cavity fields, the macroscopic properties of the neural network, such as the storage capacity, can be derived, and the results are identical to those obtained by the replica method (Gardner & Derrida 1988).

However, the real advantage of the cavity method lies in the microscopic information it provides. The above equations can be iterated sequentially, resulting in a general learning algorithm. Simulations confirm that the equations are satisfied in the single layer perceptron, and their generalized version holds in the committee tree at low loading (Wong, 1995a).

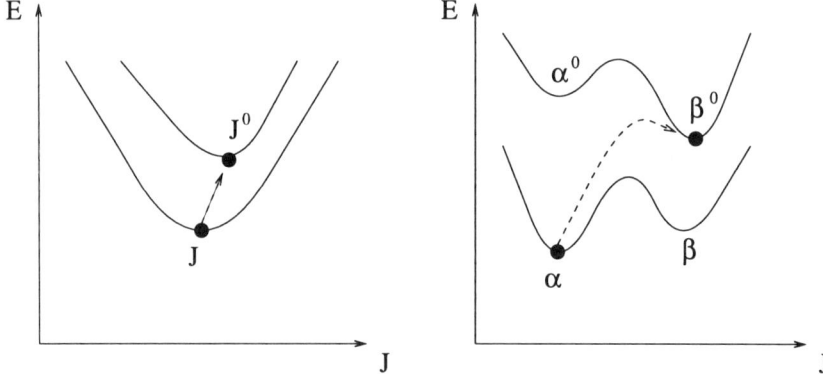

Figure 1: Schematic drawing of the change in the energy landscape in the weight space when example 0 is added, for the regime of (a) smooth energy landscape, (b) rough energy landscape.

3 MICROSCOPIC EQUATIONS FOR ROUGH ENERGY LANDSCAPES

However, the above argument holds under the assumption that the adjustment due to the addition of a new example is controllable. We can derive a stability condition for this assumption, and we find that it is equivalent to the Almeida-Thouless condition in the replica method (Mézard, Parisi & Virasoro, 1987).

An example for such instability occurs in the committee tree, which consists of hidden nodes $a = 1, \ldots, K$ with binary outputs, each fed by K nonoverlapping groups of N/K input nodes. The output of the committee tree is the majority state of the K hidden nodes. The solution in the cavity method minimizes the change from the cavity fields $\{t_a\}$ to the aligning fields $\{\Lambda_a\}$, as measured by $\sum_a (\Lambda_a - t_a)^2$ in the space of correct outputs. Thus for a stability parameter κ, $\Lambda_a = \kappa$ when $t_a < \kappa$ and the value of t_a is above median among the K hidden nodes, otherwise $\Lambda_a = t_a$. Note that a discontinuity exists in the aligning field function. Now suppose $t_a < \kappa$ is the median, but the next highest value t_b happens to be slightly less than t_a. Then the addition of example 0 may induce a change from $t_b < t_a$ to $t_{b0} > t_{a0}$. Hence Λ_{b0} changes from t_b to κ whereas Λ_{a0} changes from κ to t_{a0}. The adjustment of the system is no longer small, and the previous perturbative analysis is not valid. In fact, it has been shown that all networks having a gap in the aligning field function are not stable against the addition of examples (Wong, 1995a).

To consider what happens beyond the stability regime, one has to take into account the rough energy landscape of the learning space. Suppose that the original global minimum for examples 1 to p is α. After adding example 0, a nonvanishing change to the system is induced, and the global minimum shifts to the neighborhood of the local minimum β, as schematically shown in Fig. 1(b). Hence the resultant aligning fields Λ_0^β are no longer well-defined functions of the cavity fields t_0^α. Instead they are well-defined functions of the cavity fields t_0^β. Nevertheless, one may expect that correlations exist between the states α and β.

Let $\sqrt{q_0}$ be the correlation between the network states, i.e. $\langle J_j^\alpha J_j^\beta \rangle = \sqrt{q_0}$. Since both states α and β are determined in the absence of the added example 0, the correlation $\langle t_0^\alpha t_0^\beta \rangle = \sqrt{q_0}$ as well. Knowing that both t_0^α and t_0^β obey Gaussian distributions, the cavity field distribution can be determined if we know the prior distribution of the local minima.

At this point we introduce the central assumption in the cavity method for rough energy landscapes: we assume that the number of local minima at energy E obey an exponential distribution $d\aleph(E) = C \exp(-wE) dE$. Similar assumptions have been used in specifying the density of states in disordered systems (Mézard, Parisi & Virasoro 1987). Thus for single layer networks (and for two layer networks with appropriate generalizations), the cavity field ditribution is given by

$$P(t_0^\beta | t_0^\alpha) = \frac{G(t_0^\beta | t_0^\alpha) \exp[-w \Delta E(\lambda(t_0^\beta))]}{\int dt_0^\beta G(t_0^\beta | t_0^\alpha) \exp[-w \Delta E(\lambda(t_0^\beta))]}, \tag{4}$$

where $G(t_0^\beta | t_0^\alpha)$ is a Gaussian distribution. w is a parameter describing the distribution, and $\lambda(t_0^\beta)$ is the aligning field function. The weights J_j^β are given by

$$J_j^\beta = (1 - \alpha \chi)^{-1} \frac{1}{\sqrt{N}} \sum_\mu [\lambda(t_\mu^\beta) - t_\mu^\beta] \xi_j^\mu. \tag{5}$$

Noting the Gaussian distribution of the cavity fields, self-consistent equations for both q_0 and the local susceptibility γ can be derived.

To determine the distribution of local minima, namely the parameters C and w, we introduce a "free energy" $F(p, N)$ for p examples and N input nodes, given by $d\aleph(E) = \exp[w(F(p, N) - E)]dE$. This "free energy" determines the averaged energy of the local minima and should be an extensive quantity, i.e. it should scale as the system size. Cavity arguments enable us to find an expression $F(p+1, N) - F(p, N)$. Similarly, we may consider a cavity argument for the addition of one input node, expanding the network size from N to $N + 1$. This yields an expression for $F(p, N+1) - F(p, N)$. Since F is an extensive quantity, $F(p, N)$ should scale as N for a given ratio $\alpha = p/N$. This implies

$$\frac{F}{N} = \alpha(F(p+1, N) - F(p, N)) + (F(p, N+1) - F(p, N)). \qquad (6)$$

We have thus obtained an expression for the averaged energy of the local minima. Minimizing the free energy with respect to the parameter w gives a self-consistent equation.

The three equations for q_0, γ and w completely determines the model. The macroscopic properties of the neural network, such as the storage capacity, can be derived, and the results are identical to the first step replica symmetry breaking solution in the replica method.

It remains to check whether the microscopic equations have been modified due to the roughening of the energy landscape. It turns out that while the cavity fields in the *initial* state α do not satisfy the microscopic equations (2), those at the *final* metastable state β do, except that the nonlocal susceptibility χ has to be replaced by its average over the distribution of the local minima. In fact, the nonlocal susceptibility describes the reactive effects due to the background examples, which adjust on the addition of the new example. (Technically, this is called the Onsager reaction.) The adjustments due to hopping between valleys in a rough energy landscape have thus been taken into account.

4 SIMULATION RESULTS

To verify the theory, I simulate a committee tree learning random examples. Learning can be done by the more conventional Least Action algorithm (Nilsson 1965), or by iterating the microscopic equations.

We verify that the Least Action algorithm yields an aligning field function $\lambda(t)$ consistent with the cavity theory. Suppose the weights from input j to hidden node a is given by $J_{aj} = \sum_\mu x_{a\mu} \xi_j^\mu / \sqrt{N}$. Comparing with $J_{aj} = (1 - \alpha\chi)^{-1} \sum_\mu (\Lambda_{a\mu} - t_{a\mu}) \xi_j^\mu / \sqrt{N}$, we estimate the nonlocal susceptibility χ by requiring the distribution of $\tilde{t}_{a\mu} \equiv \Lambda_{a\mu} - (1 - \alpha\chi)x_{a\mu}$ to have a zero first moment. $\tilde{t}_{a\mu}$ is then an estimate of $t_{a\mu}$. Fig. 2 shows the resultant relation between $\Lambda_{a\mu}$ and $\tilde{t}_{a\mu}$. It agrees with the predictions of the cavity theory. Fig. 3 shows the values of the stability parameter κ measured from the Least Action algorithm and the microscopic equations. They have better agreement with the predictions of the rough energy landscape (first step replica symmetry breaking solution) rather than the smooth energy landscape (replica symmetric solution). Note that the microscopic equations yield a higher stability than the Least Action algorithm.

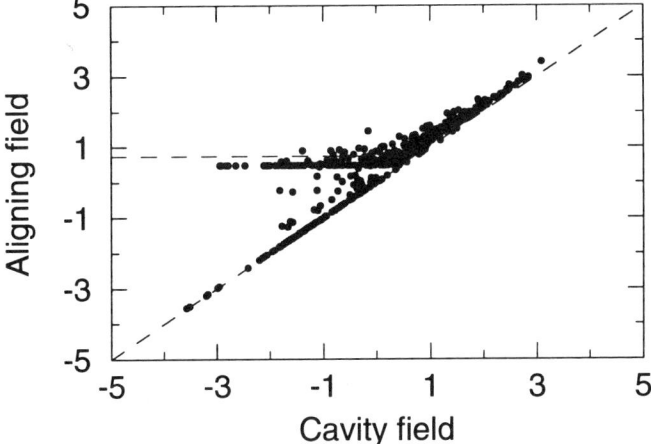

Figure 2: The aligning fields versus the cavity fields for a branch of the committee tree with $K = 3$, $\alpha = 0.8$ and $N = 600$. The dashed line is the prediction of the cavity theory for the regime of rough energy landscape.

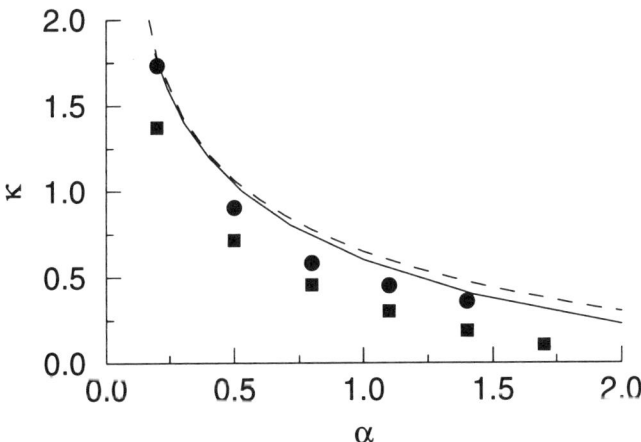

Figure 3: The stability parameter κ versus the storage level α in the committee tree with $K = 3$ for the cavity theory of: (a) smooth energy landscape (dashed line), (b) rough energy landscape (solid line), and the simulation of: (c) iterating the microscopic equations (circles), (d) the Least Action algorithm (squares). Error bars are smaller than the size of the symbols.

5 CONCLUSION

In summary, we have derived the microscopic equations for neural network learning in the regime of rough energy landscapes. They turn out to have the same form as in the case of smooth energy landscape, except that the parameters are averaged over the distribution of local minima. Iterating the equations result in a learning algorithm, which yields a higher stability than more conventional algorithms in the committee tree. However, for high loading, the iterations may not converge.

The success of the present scheme lies its ability to take into account the underlying physical picture of many local minima of comparable energy. It correctly describes the experience that slightly different training sets may lead to vastly different neural networks. The stability parameter predicted by the rough landscape ansatz has a better agreement with simulations than the smooth one. It provides a physical interpretation of the replica symmetry breaking solution in the replica method. It is possible to generalize the theory to the physical picture with hierarchies of clusters of local minima, which corresponds to the infinite step replica symmetry breaking solution, though the mathematics is much more involved.

Acknowledgements

This work is supported by the Hong Kong Telecom Institute of Information Techology, HKUST.

References

Anlauf, J.K., & Biehl, M. (1989) The AdaTron: an adaptive perceptron algorithm. *Europhysics Letters* **10**(7):687-692.

Bouten, M., Schietse, J. & Van den Broeck, C. (1995) Gradient descent learning in perceptrons: A review of its possibilities. *Physical Review E* **52**(2):1958-1967.

Gardner, E. & Derrida, B. (1988) Optimal storage properties of neural network models. *Journal of Physics A: Mathematical and General* **21**(1):271-284.

Gerl, F. & Krey, U. (1995) A Kuhn-Tucker cavity method for generalization with applications to perceptrons with Ising and Potts neurons. *Journal of Physics A: Mathematical and General* **28**(23):6501-6516.

Griniasty, M. (1993) "Cavity-approach" analysis of the neural-network learning problem. *Physical Review E* **47**(6):4496-4513.

Mézard, M. (1989) The space of interactions in neural networks: Gardner's computation with the cavity method. *Journal of Physics A: Mathematical and General* **22**(12):2181-2190.

Mézard, M., Parisi, G. & Virasoro, M. (1987) *Spin Glass Theory and Beyond*. Singapore: World Scientific.

Nilsson, N.J. (1965) *Learning Machines*. New York: McGraw-Hill.

Thouless, D.J., Anderson, P.W. & Palmer, R.G. (1977) Solution of 'solvable model of a spin glass'. *Philosophical Magazine* **35**(3):593-601.

Watkin, T.L.H., Rau, A. & Biehl, M. (1993) The statistical mechanics of learning a rule. *Review of Modern Physics* **65**(2):499-556.

Wong, K.Y.M. (1995a) Microscopic equations and stability conditions in optimal neural networks. *Europhysics Letters* **30**(4):245-250.

Wong, K.Y.M. (1995b) The cavity method: Applications to learning and retrieval in neural networks. In J.-H. Oh, C. Kwon and S. Cho (eds.), *Neural Networks: The Statistical Mechanics Perspective*, pp. 175-190. Singapore: World Scientific.

Time Series Prediction Using Mixtures of Experts

Assaf J. Zeevi
Information Systems Lab
Department of Electrical Engineering
Stanford University
Stanford, CA. 94305
azeevi@isl.stanford.edu

Ron Meir
Department of Electrical Engineering
Technion
Haifa 32000, Israel
rmeir@ee.technion.ac.il

Robert J. Adler
Department of Statistics
University of North Carolina
Chapel Hill, NC. 27599
adler@stat.unc.edu

Abstract

We consider the problem of prediction of stationary time series, using the architecture known as mixtures of experts (MEM). Here we suggest a mixture which blends several autoregressive models. This study focuses on some theoretical foundations of the prediction problem in this context. More precisely, it is demonstrated that this model is a *universal approximator*, with respect to learning the unknown prediction function. This statement is strengthened as upper bounds on the mean squared error are established. Based on these results it is possible to compare the MEM to other families of models (e.g., neural networks and state dependent models). It is shown that a degenerate version of the MEM is in fact *equivalent* to a neural network, and the number of experts in the architecture plays a similar role to the number of hidden units in the latter model.

1 Introduction

In this work we pursue a new family of models for time series, substantially extending, but strongly related to and based on the classic linear autoregressive moving average (ARMA) family. We wish to exploit the linear autoregressive technique in a manner that will enable a substantial increase in modeling power, in a framework which is non-linear and yet mathematically tractable.

The novel model, whose main building blocks are linear AR models, deviates from linearity in the integration process, that is, the way these blocks are combined. This model was first formulated in the context of a regression problem, and an extension to a hierarchical structure was also given [2]. It was termed the mixture of experts model (MEM).

Variants of this model have recently been used in prediction problems both in economics and engineering. Recently, some theoretical aspects of the MEM, in the context of non-linear regression, were studied by Zeevi et al. [8], and an equivalence to a class of neural network models has been noted.

The purpose of this paper is to extend the previous work regarding the MEM in the context of regression, to the problem of prediction of time series. We shall demonstrate that the MEM is a universal approximator, and establish upper bounds on the *approximation error*, as well as the mean squared error, in the setting of *estimation* of the predictor function.

It is shown that the MEM is intimately related to several existing, state of the art, statistical non-linear models encompassing Tong's TAR (threshold autoregressive) model [7], and a certain version of Priestley's [6] state dependent models (SDM). In addition, it is demonstrated that the MEM is equivalent (in a sense that will be made precise) to the class of feedforward, sigmoidal, neural networks.

2 Model Description

The MEM [2] is an architecture composed of n *expert networks*, each being an AR(d) linear model. The experts are combined via a *gating* network, which partitions the input space accordingly. Considering a scalar time series $\{x_t\}$, we associate with each expert a probabilistic model (density function) relating input vectors $\mathbf{x}_{t-d}^{t-1} \equiv [x_{t-1}, x_{t-2}, \ldots, x_{t-d}]$ to an output scalar $x_t \in \mathbb{R}$ and denote these probabilistic models by $p(x_t | \mathbf{x}_{t-d}^{t-1}; \boldsymbol{\theta}_j, \sigma_j)$ $j = 1, 2, \ldots, n$ where $(\boldsymbol{\theta}_j, \sigma_j)$ is the expert parameter vector, taking values in a compact subset of $\mathbb{R}^{d+1}$. In what follows we will use upper case X_t to denote random variables, and lower case x_t to denote values taken by those r.v.'s.

Letting the parameters of each expert network be denoted by $(\boldsymbol{\theta}_j, \sigma_j)$, $j = 1, 2, \ldots, n$, those of the gating network by $\boldsymbol{\theta}_g$ and letting $\Theta = (\{\boldsymbol{\theta}_j, \sigma_j\}_{j=1}^n, \boldsymbol{\theta}_g)$ represent the complete set of parameters specifying the model, we may express the conditional distribution of the model, $p(x_t | \mathbf{x}_{t-d}^{t-1}, \Theta)$, as

$$p(x_t | \mathbf{x}_{t-d}^{t-1}; \Theta) = \sum_{j=1}^{n} g_j(\mathbf{x}_{t-d}^{t-1}; \boldsymbol{\theta}_g) p(x_t | \mathbf{x}_{t-d}^{t-1}; \boldsymbol{\theta}_j, \sigma_j), \qquad (1)$$

together with the constraint that $\sum_{j=1}^{n} g_j(\mathbf{x}_{t-d}^{t-1}; \boldsymbol{\theta}_g) = 1$ and $g_j(\mathbf{x}_{t-d}^{t-1}; \boldsymbol{\theta}_g) \geq$

Time Series Prediction using Mixtures of Experts

$0 \quad \forall \mathbf{x}_{t-d}^{t-1}$. We assume that the parameter vector $\Theta \in \Omega$, a compact subset of $\mathbb{R}^{2n(d+1)}$.

Following the work of Jordan and Jacobs [2] we take the probability density functions to be Gaussian with mean $\boldsymbol{\theta}_j^T \mathbf{x}_{t-d}^{t-1} + \theta_{j,0}$ and variance σ_j (representative of the underlying, *local* AR(d) model). The function $g_j(\mathbf{x}; \boldsymbol{\theta}_g) \equiv \exp\{\boldsymbol{\theta}_{g_j}^T \mathbf{x} + \theta_{g_j,0}\} / (\sum_{i=1}^n \exp\{\boldsymbol{\theta}_{g_i}^T \mathbf{x} + \theta_{g_i,0}\}$, thus implementing a multiple output logistic regression function.

The underlying non-linear mapping (i.e., the conditional expectation, or L_2 prediction function) characterizing the MEM, is described by using (1) to obtain the conditional expectation of X_t,

$$f_n^\theta = \mathrm{E}[X_t | X_{t-d}^{t-1}; \mathcal{M}_n] = \sum_{j=1}^n g_j(X_{t-d}^{t-1}; \boldsymbol{\theta}_g)[\boldsymbol{\theta}_j^T X_{t-d}^{t-1} + \theta_{j,0}], \qquad (2)$$

where $\mathcal{M}_n$ denotes the MEM model. Here the subscript n stands for the number of experts. Thus, we have $\hat{X}_t = f_n^\theta \equiv f_n(X_{t-d}^{t-1}; \Theta)$ where $f_n : \mathbb{R}^d \times \Omega \to \mathbb{R}$, and $\hat{X}_t$ denotes the projection of X_t on the 'relevant past', given the model, thus defining the *model predictor function*.

We will use the notation MEM($n; d$) where n is the number of experts in the model (proportional to the complexity, or number of parameters in the model), and d the lag size. In this work we assume that d is known and given.

3 Main results

3.1 Background

We consider a stationary time series, more precisely a discrete time stochastic process $\{X_t\}$ which is assumed to be strictly stationary. We define the L_2 predictor function

$$f \equiv \mathrm{E}[X_t | X_{-\infty}^{t-1}] = \mathrm{E}[X_t | X_{t-d}^{t-1}] \quad a.s.$$

for some fixed lag size d. Markov chains are perhaps the most widely encountered class of probability models exhibiting this dependence. The NAR(d), that is nonlinear AR(d), model is another example, widely studied in the context of time series (see [4] for details). Assuming additive noise, the NAR(d) model may be expressed as

$$X_t = f(X_{t-1}, X_{t-2}, \ldots, X_{t-d}) + \varepsilon_t . \qquad (3)$$

We note that in this formulation $\{\varepsilon_t\}$ plays the role of the *innovation* process for X_t, and the function $f(\cdot)$ describes the information on X_t contained within its past history.

In what follows, we restrict the discussion to stochastic processes satisfying certain constraints on the memory decay, more precisely we are assuming that $\{X_t\}$ is an exponentially α-mixing process. Loosely stated, this assumption enables the process to have a law of large numbers associated with it, as well as a certain version of the central limit theorem. These results are the basis for analyzing the asymptotic behavior of certain parameter estimators (see, [9] for further details), but other than that this assumption is merely stated here for the sake of completeness. We note in

3.2 Objectives

Knowing the L_2 predictor function, f, allows optimal prediction of future samples, where optimal is meant in the sense that the predicted value is the closest to the true value of the next sample point, in the mean squared error sense. It therefore seems a reasonable strategy, to try and *learn* the optimal predictor function, based on some finite realization of the stochastic process, which we will denote $\mathcal{D}_N = \{X_t\}_{t=0}^{d+N+1}$. Note that for $N \gg d$, the number of sample points is approximately N.

We therefore define our objective as follows. Based on the data $\mathcal{D}_N$, we seek the 'best' approximation to f, the L_2 predictor function, using the MEM(n, d) predictor $f_n^\theta \in \mathcal{M}_n$ as the approximator model.

More precisely, define the least squares (LS) parameter estimator for the MEM(n, d) as

$$\hat{\boldsymbol{\theta}}_{n,N} = \arg\min_{\boldsymbol{\theta} \in \Theta} \sum_{t=d+1}^{N} [X_t - f_n(X_{t-d}^{t-1}, \boldsymbol{\theta})]^2$$

where $f_n(X_{t-d}^{t-1}, \boldsymbol{\theta})$ is f_n^θ evaluated at the point X_{t-d}^{t-1}, and define the LS functional estimator as

$$\hat{f}_{n,N} \equiv f_n^\theta|_{\theta=\hat{\boldsymbol{\theta}}_{n,N}}$$

where $\hat{\boldsymbol{\theta}}_{n,N}$ is the LS parameter estimator.

Now, define the functional estimator risk as

$$\text{MSE}[f, \hat{f}_{n,N}] \equiv \mathbb{E}_\mathcal{D}\left[\int |f - \hat{f}_{n,N}|^2 d\nu\right]$$

where ν is the d fold probability measure of the process $\{X_t\}$. In this work we maintain that the integration is over some compact domain $I^d \subset \mathbb{R}^d$, though recent work [3] has shown that the results can be extended to $\mathbb{R}^d$, at the price of slightly slower convergence rates.

It is reasonable, and quite customary, to expect a 'good' estimator to be one that is asymptotically unbiased. However, growth of the sample size itself need not, and in general does not, mean that the estimator is 'becoming' unbiased. Consequently, as a figure of merit, we may restrict attention to the *approximation capacity* of the model. That is we ask, what is the error in approximating a given class of predictor functions, using the MEM(n, d) (i.e., $\{\mathcal{M}_n\}$) as the approximator class.

To measure this figure, we define the *optimal risk* as

$$\text{MSE}[f, f_n^*] \equiv \int |f - f_n^*|^2 d\nu,$$

where $f_n^* \equiv f_n^\theta|_{\theta=\theta^*}$ and

$$\theta_n^* = \arg\min_{\theta \in \Theta} \int |f - f_n^\theta|^2 d\nu,$$

that is, $\boldsymbol{\theta}_n^*$ is the parameter minimizing the expected L_2 loss function. One may think of f_n^* as the 'best' predictor function in the class of approximators, i.e., the closest approximation to the optimal predictor, given the finite complexity, n, (i.e., finite number of parameters) of the model. Here n is simply the number of experts (AR models) in the architecture.

3.3 Upper Bounds on the Mean Squared Error and Universal Approximation Results

Consider first the case where we are simply interested in approximating the function f, assuming it belongs to some class of functions. The question then arises as to how well one may approximate f by a MEM architecture comprising n experts. The answer to this question is given in the following proposition, the proof of which can be found in [8].

Proposition 3.1 (Optimal risk bounds) *Consider the class of functions $\mathcal{M}_n$ defined in (2) and assume that the optimal predictor f belongs to a Sobolev class containing r continuous derivatives in L_2. Then the following bound holds:*

$$\mathrm{MSE}[f, f_n^*] \leq \frac{c}{n^{2r/d}} \tag{4}$$

where c is a constant independent of n.

PROOF SKETCH: The proof proceeds by first approximating the normalized gating function $g_j()$ by polynomials of finite degree, and then using the fact that polynomials can approximate functions in Sobolev space to within a known degree of approximation.

The following main theorem, establishing upper bounds on the functional estimator risk, constitutes the main result of this paper. The proof is given in [9].

Theorem 3.1 (Upper bounds on the estimator risk)
Suppose the stochastic process obeys the conditions set forth in the previous section. Assume also that the optimal predictor function, f, possesses r smooth derivatives in L_2. Then for N sufficiently large we have

$$\mathrm{MSE}[f, \hat{f}_{n,N}] \leq \frac{c}{n^{2r/d}} + \frac{m_n^*}{2N} + o\left(\frac{1}{N}\right), \tag{5}$$

where r is the number of continuous derivatives in L_2 that f is assumed to possess, d is the lag size, and N is the size of the data set $\mathcal{D}_N$.

PROOF SKETCH: The proof proceeds by a standard stochastic Taylor expansion of the loss around the point $\boldsymbol{\theta}_n^*$. Making common regularity assumptions [1] and using the assumption on the α-mixing nature of the process allows one to establish the usual asymptotic normality results, from which the result follows.

We use the notation m_n^* to denote the *effective number of parameters*. More precisely, $m_n^* = \mathrm{Tr}\{B_n^*(A_n^*)^{-1}\}$ and the matrices A^* and B^* are related to the Fisher information matrix in the case of misspecified estimation (see [1] for further discussion). The upper bound presented in Theorem 3.1 is related to the classic *bias - variance* decomposition in statistics and the obvious tradeoffs are evident by inspection.

3.4 Comments

It follows from Proposition 3.1 that the class of mixtures of experts is a universal approximator, w.r.t. the class of target functions defined for the optimal predictor. Moreover, Proposition 3.1 establishes the rate of convergence of the approximator, and therefore relates the approximation error to the number of experts used in the architecture (n).

Theorem 3.1 enhances this result, as it relates the sample complexity and model complexity, for this class of models. The upper bounds may be used in defining *model selection* criteria, based on upper bound minimization. In this setting, we may use an estimator of the stochastic error bound (i.e., the estimation error), to penalize the complexity of the model, in the spirit of AIC, MDL etc (see [8] for further discussion).

At a first glance it may seem surprising to find that a combination of linear models is a universal function approximator. However, one must keep in mind that the *global* model is nonlinear, due to the gating network. Nevertheless, this result does imply, at least on a theoretical ground, that one may restrict the MEM(n, d) to be locally linear, without loss of generality. Thus, taking a simple local model, enabling efficient and tractable learning algorithms (see [2]), still results in a rich global model.

3.5 Comparison

Recently, Mhaskar [5] proved upper bounds on a feedforward sigmoidal neural network, for target functions in the same class as we consider herein, i.e., the Sobolev class. The bound we have obtained in Proposition 3.1, and its extension in [8], demonstrate that w.r.t. to this particular target class, neural networks and mixtures of experts are equivalent. That is, both models attain optimal precision in the degree of approximation results (see [5] for details of this argument). Keeping in mind the advantages of the MEM with respect to learning and generalization [2], we believe that our results lend further credence to the emerging view as to the superiority of modular architectures over the more standard feedforward neural networks.

Moreover, the detailed proof of Proposition 3.1 (see [8]) actually takes the MEM(n, d) to be made up of local *constants*. That is, the linear experts are degenerated to constant functions. Thus, one may conjecture that mixtures of experts are in fact a more general class than feedforward neural networks, though we have no proof of this as of yet.

Two nonlinear alternatives, generalizing standard statistical linear models, have been pointed out in the introductory section. These are Tong's TAR (threshold autoregressive) model [7], and the more general SDM (state dependent models) introduced by Priestley. The latter models can be reduced to a TAR model by imposing a more restrictive structure (for further details see [6]) . We have shown, based on the results described above (see [9]), that the MEM may be viewed as a generalization of the SDM (and consequently of the TAR model). The relation to the state dependent models is of particular interest, as the mixtures of experts is structured on state dependence as well. Exact statement and proofs of these facts can be found in [9].

We should also note that we have conducted several numerical experiments, comparing the performance of the MEM with other approaches. We tested the model on both synthetic as well as real-world data. Without any fine-tuning of parameters we found the performance of the MEM, with linear expert functions, to compare very favorably with other approaches (such as TAR, ARMA and neural networks). Details of the numerical results may be found in [9]. Moreover, the model also provided a very natural and intuitive segmentation of the process.

4 Discussion

In this work we have pursued a novel non-linear model for prediction in stationary time series. The mixture of experts model (MEM) has been demonstrated to be a rich model, endowed with a sound theoretical basis, and compares favorably with other, state of the art, nonlinear models.

We hope that the results of this study will aid in establishing the MEM as, yet another, powerful tool for the study of time-series applicable to the fields of statistics, economics, and signal processing.

References

[1] Domowitz, I. and White, H. "Misspecified Models with Dependent Observations", *Journal of Econometrics*, vol. 20: 35-58, 1982.

[2] Jordan, M. and Jacobs, R. "Hierarchical Mixtures of Experts and the EM Algorithm", *Neural Computation*, vol. 6, pp. 181-214, 1994.

[3] Maiorov, V. and Meir. V. "Approximation Bounds for Smooth Functions in $C(\mathbb{R}^d)$ by Neural and Mixture Networks", submitted for publication, December 1996.

[4] Meyn, S.P. and Tweedie, R.L. (1993) *Markov Chains and Stochastic Stability*, Springer-Verlag, London.

[5] Mhaskar, H. (1996) "Neural Networks for Optimal Approximation of Smooth and Analytic Functions", *Neural Computation* vol. 8(1), pp. 164-177.

[6] Priestley M.B. *Non-linear and Non-stationary Time Series Analysis*, Academic Press, New York, 1988.

[7] Tong, H. *Threshold Models in Non-linear Time Series Analysis*, Springer Verlag, New York, 1983.

[8] Zeevi, A.J., Meir, R. and Maiorov, V. "Error Bounds for Functional Approximation and Estimation Using Mixtures of Experts", EE Pub. CC-132., Electrical Engineering Department, Technion, 1995.

[9] Zeevi, A.J., Meir, R. and Adler, R.J. "Non-linear Models for Time Series Using Mixtures of Experts", EE Pub. CC-150, Electrical Engineering Department, Technion, 1996.

Part IV
Algorithms and Architecture

Genetic Algorithms and Explicit Search Statistics

Shumeet Baluja
baluja@cs.cmu.edu
Justsystem Pittsburgh Research Center &
School of Computer Science, Carnegie Mellon University

Abstract

The genetic algorithm (GA) is a heuristic search procedure based on mechanisms abstracted from population genetics. In a previous paper [Baluja & Caruana, 1995], we showed that much simpler algorithms, such as hillclimbing and Population-Based Incremental Learning (PBIL), perform comparably to GAs on an optimization problem custom designed to benefit from the GA's operators. This paper extends these results in two directions. First, in a large-scale empirical comparison of problems that have been reported in GA literature, we show that on many problems, simpler algorithms can perform significantly better than GAs. Second, we describe when crossover is useful, and show how it can be incorporated into PBIL.

1 IMPLICIT VS. EXPLICIT SEARCH STATISTICS

Although there has recently been controversy in the genetic algorithm (GA) community as to whether GAs should be used for static function optimization, a large amount of research has been, and continues to be, conducted in this direction [De Jong, 1992]. Since much of GA research focuses on optimization (most often in static environments), this study examines the performance of GAs in these domains.

In the standard GA, candidate solutions are encoded as fixed length binary vectors. The initial group of potential solutions is chosen randomly. At each generation, the fitness of each solution is calculated; this is a measure of how well the solution optimizes the objective function. The subsequent generation is created through a process of selection, recombination, and mutation. Recombination operators merge the information contained within pairs of selected "parents" by placing random subscts of the information from both parents into their respective positions in a member of the subsequent generation. The fitness proportional selection works as selective pressure; higher fitness solution strings have a higher probability of being selected for recombination. Mutations are used to help preserve diversity in the population by introducing random changes into the solution strings. The GA uses the population to *implicitly* maintain statistics about the search space. The selection, crossover, and mutation operators can be viewed as mechanisms of extracting the implicit statistics from the population to choose the next set of points to sample. Details of GAs can be found in [Goldberg, 1989] [Holland, 1975].

Population-based incremental learning (PBIL) is a combination of genetic algorithms and competitive learning [Baluja, 1994]. The PBIL algorithm attempts to *explicitly* maintain statistics about the search space to decide where to sample next. The object of the algorithm is to create a real valued probability vector which, when sampled, reveals high quality solution vectors with high probability. For example, if a good solution can be encoded as a string of alternating 0's and 1's, a suitable final probability vector would be 0.01, 0.99, 0.01, 0.99, etc. The PBIL algorithm and parameters are shown in Figure 1.

Initially, the values of the probability vector are initialized to 0.5. Sampling from this vector yields random solution vectors because the probability of generating a 1 or 0 is equal. As search progresses, the values in the probability vector gradually shift to represent high

```
****** Initialize Probability Vector *****
for i :=1 to LENGTH do P[i] = 0.5;

while (NOT termination condition)
        ***** Generate Samples *****
        for i :=1 to SAMPLES do
                sample_vectors[i] := generate_sample_vector_according_to_probabilities (P);
                evaluations[i] := evaluate(sample_vectors[i]);

        best_vector := find_vector_with_best_evaluation (sample_vectors, evaluations);
        worst_vector := find_vector_with_worst_evaluation (sample_vectors, evaluations);

        ***** Update Probability Vector Towards Best Solution *****
        for i :=1 to LENGTH do
                P[i] := P[i] * (1.0 - LR) + best_vector[i] * (LR);

        ***** Update Probability Vector Away from Worst Solution *****
        for i :=1 to LENGTH do
                if (best_vector[i] ≠ worst_vector[i]) then
                        P[i] := P[i] * (1.0 - NEGATIVE_LR) + best_vector[i] * (NEGATIVE_LR);
```

PBIL: USER DEFINED CONSTANTS (Values Used in this Study):
SAMPLES: the number of vectors generated before update of the probability vector (100).
LR: the learning rate, how fast to exploit the search performed (0.1).
NEGATIVE_LR: negative learning rate, how much to learn from negative examples (PBIL1=0.0, PBIL2= 0.075).
LENGTH: the number of bits in a generated vector (problem specific).

Figure 1: PBIL1/PBIL2 algorithm for a binary alphabet. PBIL2 includes shaded region. Mutations not shown.

evaluation solution vectors through the following process. A number of solution vectors are generated based upon the probabilities specified in the probability vector. The probability vector is pushed towards the generated solution vector with the highest evaluation. After the probability vector is updated, a new set of solution vectors is produced by sampling from the updated probability vector, and the cycle is continued. As the search progresses, entries in the probability vector move away from their initial settings of 0.5 towards either 0.0 or 1.0.

One key feature of the *early* generations of genetic optimization is the parallelism in the search; many diverse points are represented in the population of points during the early generations. When the population is diverse, crossover can be an effective means of search, since it provides a method to explore novel solutions by combining different members of the population. Because PBIL uses a single probability vector, it may seem to have less expressive power than a GA using a full population, since a GA can *represent* a large number of points simultaneously. A traditional single population GA, however, would not be able to *maintain* a large number of points. Because of sampling errors, the population will converge around a single point. This phenomenon is summarized below:

> "... the theorem [Fundamental Theorem of Genetic Algorithms [Goldberg, 1989]], assumes an infinitely large population size. In a finite size population, even when there is no selective advantage for either of two competing alternatives... the population will converge to one alternative or the other in finite time (De Jong, 1975; [Goldberg & Segrest, 1987]). This problem of finite populations is so important that geneticists have given it a special name, genetic drift. Stochastic errors tend to accumulate, ultimately causing the population to converge to one alternative or another" [Goldberg & Richardson, 1987].

Diversity in the population is crucial for GAs. By maintaining a population of solutions, the GA is able—in theory at least—to maintain samples in many different regions. Crossover is used to merge these different solutions. A necessary (although not sufficient) condition for crossover to work well is diversity in the population. When diversity is lost, crossover begins to behave like a mutation operator that is sensitive to the convergence of the value of each bit [Eshelman, 1991]. If all individuals in the population converge at some bit position, crossover leaves those bits unaltered. At bit positions where individuals have not converged, crossover will effectively mutate values in those positions. Therefore, crossover creates new individuals that differ from the individuals it combines only at the bit positions where the mated individuals disagree. This is analogous to PBIL which creates new trials that differ mainly in positions where prior good performers have disagreed.

As an example of how the PBIL algorithm works, we can examine the values in the probability vector through multiple generations. Consider the following maximization problem: $1.0/|(366503875925.0 - X)|$, $0 \leq X < 2^{40}$. Note that 366503875925 is represented in binary as a string of 20 pairs of alternating '01'. The evolution of the probability vector is shown in Figure 2. Note that the most significant bits are pinned to either 0 or 1 very quickly, while the least significant bits are pinned last. This is because during the early portions of the search, the most significant bits yield more information about high evaluation regions of the search space than the least significant bits.

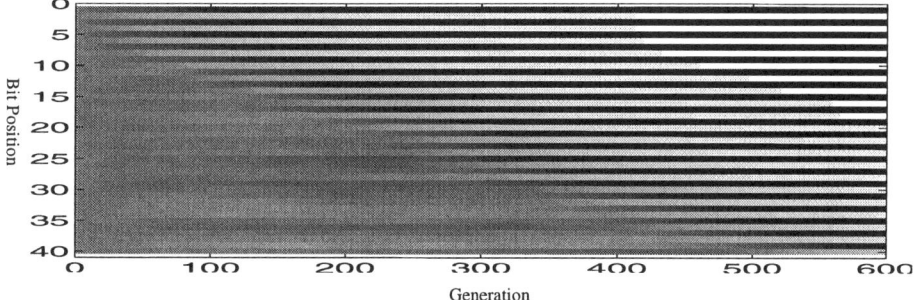

Figure 2: Evolution of the probability vector over successive generations. White represents a high probability of generating a 1, black represents a high probability of generating a 0. Intermediate grey represent probabilities close to 0.5 - equal chances of generating a 0 or 1. Bit 0 is the most significant, bit 40 the least.

2 AN EMPIRICAL COMPARISON

This section provides a summary of the results obtained from a large scale empirical comparison of seven iterative and evolution-based optimization heuristics. Thirty-four static optimization problems, spanning six sets of problem classes which are commonly explored in the genetic algorithm literature, are examined. The search spaces in these problems range from 2^{128} to 2^{2040}. The results indicate that, on many problems, using standard GAs for optimizing static functions does not yield a benefit, in terms of the final answer obtained, over simple hillclimbing or PBIL. Recently, there have been other studies which have examined the performance of GAs in comparison to hillclimbing on a few problems; they have shown similar results [Davis, 1991][Juels & Wattenberg, 1996].

Three variants of Multiple-Restart Stochastic Hillclimbing (MRSH) are explored in this paper. The first version, MRSH-1, maintains a list of the position of the bit flips which were attempted without improvement. These bit flips are not attempted again until a better solution is found. When a better solution is found, the list is emptied. If the list becomes as large as the solution encoding, MRSH-1 is restarted at a random solution with an empty list. MRSH-2 and MRSH-3 allow moves to regions of higher and equal evaluation. In MRSH-2, the number of evaluations before restart depends upon the length of the encoded solution. MRSH-2 allows 10*(length of solution) evaluations without improvement before search is restarted. When a solution with a higher evaluation is found, the count is reset. In MRSH-3, after the total number of iterations is specified, restart is forced 5 times during search, at equally spaced intervals.

Two variants of the standard GA are tested in this study. The first, termed SGA, has the following parameters: Two-Point crossover, with a crossover rate of 100% (% of times crossover occurs, otherwise the individuals are copied without crossover), mutation probability of 0.001 per bit, population size of 100, and elitist selection (the best solution in generation N replaces the worst solution in generation N+1). The second GA used, termed GA-Scale, uses the same parameters except: uniform crossover with a crossover rate of 80% and the fitness of the worst member in a generation is subtracted from the fitnesses of each member of the generation before the probabilities of selection are determined.

Two variants of PBIL are tested. Both move the probability vector towards the best example in each generated population. PBIL2 also moves the probability vector away from the worst example in each generation. Both variants are shown in Figure 1. A small mutation, analogous to the mutation used in genetic algorithms, is also used in both PBILs. The mutation is directly applied to the probability vector.

The results obtained in this study should *not* be considered to be state-of-the-art. The problem encodings were chosen to be easily reproducible and to allow easy comparison with other studies. Alternate encodings may yield superior results. In addition, no problem-specific information was used for any of the algorithms. Problem-specific information, when available, could help all of the algorithms examined.

All of the variables in the problems were encoded in binary, either with standard Gray-code or base-2 representation. The variables were represented in non-overlapping, contiguous regions within the solution encoding. The results reported are the best evaluations found through the search of each algorithm, averaged over at least 20 independent runs per algorithm per problem; the results for GA-SCALE and PBIL2 algorithms are the average of at least 50 runs. All algorithms were given 200,000 evaluations per run. In each run, the GA and PBIL algorithms were given 2000 generations, with 100 function evaluations per generation. In each run, the MRSH algorithms were restarted in random locations as many times as needed until 200,000 evaluations were performed. The best answer found in the 200,000 evaluations was returned as the answer found in the run.

Brief notes about the encodings are given below. Since the numerical results are not useful without the exact problems, *relative* results are provided in Table I. For most of the problems, exact results and encodings are in [Baluja, 1995]. To measure the significance of the difference between the results obtained by PBIL2 and GA-SCALE, the Mann-Whitney test is used. This is a non-parametric equivalent to the standard two-sample pooled *t*-tests.

- **TSP:** 128, 200 & 255 city problems were tried. The "sort" encoding [Syswerda, 1989] was used. The last problem was tried with the encoding in binary and Gray-Code.

- **Jobshop:** Two standard JS problems were tried with two encodings. The first encoding is described in [Fang *et. al*, 1993]. The second encoding is described in [Baluja, 1995]. An additional, randomly generated, problem was also tried with the second encoding.

- **Knapsack:** Problem 1&2: a unique element is represented by each bit. Problem 3&4: there are 8 and 32 copies of each element respectively. The encoding specified the number of copies of each element to include. Each element is assigned a "value" and "weight". Object: maximize value while staying under pre-specified weight.

- **Bin-Packing/Equal Piles:** The solution is encoded in a bit vector of length $M * \log_2 N$ (N bins, M elem.). Each element is assigned a substring of length $\log_2 N$, which specifies a bin. Object: pack the given bins as tightly as possible. Because of the large variation in results which is found by varying the number of bins and elements, the results from 8 problems are reported.

- **Neural-Network Weight Optimization:** Problem 1&2: identify the parity of 7 inputs. Problem 3&4: determine whether a point falls within the middle of 3 concentric squares. For problems 3&4, 5 extra inputs, which contained noise, were used. The networks had 8 inputs (including bias), 5 hidden units, and 1 output. The network was fully connected between sequential layers.

- **Numerical Function Optimization (F1-F3):** Problems 1&2: the variables in the first portions of the solution string have a large influence on the quality of the rest of the solution. In the third problem, each variable can be set independently. See [Baluja, 1995] for details.

- **Graph Coloring:** Select 1 of 4 colors for nodes of a partially connected graph such that connected nodes are not the same color. The graphs used were not necessarily planar.

Table I: Summary of Empirical Results - Relative Ranks (1=best, 7=worst).

	Encoding Length (bits)	MRSH 1	MRSH 2	MRSH 3	PBIL 1	PBIL 2	SGA	GA Scale	MRSH BEST	PBIL BEST	GA BEST	Confidence (GA-Scale ≠ PBIL2)
TSP 128 city (binary)	896	6	3	4	2	1	7	5		•		>99%
TSP 200 city (binary)	1600	5	4	3	2	1	7	6		•		>99%
TSP 255 city (binary)	2040	5	1	2	4	3	7	6	•			>99%
TSP 255 city (Gray-Code)	2040	5	1	2	4	3	7	6	•			>99%
Jobshop 10x10 (Fang)	500	7	5	6	2	1	4	3		•		>99%
Jobshop 20x5 (Fang)	500	7	6	5	2	1	4	3		•		>99%
Jobshop 10x10 (Baluja)	700	7	5	6	3	1	4	2		•		93%
Jobshop 20x5 (Baluja)	700	7	5	4	2	1	6	3		•		>99%
Jobshop 20x5 - random. (Baluja)	700	7	5	4	2	1	6	3		•		>99%
Knapsack (512 elem., 1 copy)	512	5	7	6	2	1	4	3		•		>99%
Knapsack (2000 elem., 1 copy)	2000	4	5	6	1	3	7	2		•		>99%
Knapsack (100 elem., 8 copies)	300	4	5	6	3	2	7	1			•	Not Avail.
Knapsack (120 elem., 32 copies)	600	4	5	6	2	1	7	3		•		>99%
Bin (2 bins, 1600 elements)	1600	1	5	6	3	4	7	2	•			97%
Bin (2 bins, 128 elements)	128	1	3	7	4	2	5	6	•			>99%
Bin (4 bins, 512 elements)	1024	4	3	5	6	7	2	1			•	>99%
Bin (8 bins, 128 elements)	384	6	5	7	2	1	4	3		•		>99%
Bin (16 bins, 128 elements)	512	7	5	6	3	1	2	4		•		>99%
Bin (32 bins, 128 elements)	640	5	6	7	3	1	4	2		•		96%
Bin (32 bins, 256 elements)	1280	2	4	5	6	7	3	1			•	>99%
Bin (64 bins, 128 elements)	768	4	6	7	3	1	5	2		•		>99%
Neural Net PARITY 7 (binary)	368	5	5	7	2	1	4	3		•		>99%
Neural Net PARITY 7 (gray)	368	5	6	7	2	1	3	4		•		>99%
Neural Net SQUARE (binary)	368	5	6	7	2	1	3	4		•		>99%
Neural Net SQUARE (gray)	368	4	2	7	1	3	5	6		•		>99%
F1 (Encoded in Binary)	900	5	6	7	3	1	2	4		•		>99%
F1 (Encoded in Gray Code)	900	5	6	7	2	1	3	4		•		>99%
F2 (Encoded in Binary)	900	5	6	7	2	1	4	3		•		>99%
F2 (Encoded in Gray Code)	900	5	4	6	2	1	7	3		•		>99%
F3 (Encoded in Binary)	900	6	5	7	2	1	4	3		•		>99%
F3 (Encoded in Gray Code)	900	1	1	1	5	4	7	6	•			>99%
G.Color - 200 node, 1000 connx.	400	6	2	1	4	3	7	5	•			>99%
G.Color - 200 node, 2000 connx.	400	6	1	2	5	3	7	4	•			>99%
G.Color - 400 node, 8000 connx.	800	5	1	2	4	3	7	6	•			>99%
TOTAL (34 Problems)									8	23	3	

3 EXPLICITLY PRESERVING DIVERSITY

Although the results in the previous section showed that PBIL often outperformed GAs and hillclimbing, PBIL may not surpass GAs at all population sizes. As the population size increases, the observed behavior of a GA more closely approximates the ideal behavior predicted by theory [Holland, 1975]. The population may contain sufficient samples from distinct regions for crossover to effectively combine "building blocks" from multiple solutions. However, the desire to minimize the total number of function evaluations often prohibits the use of large enough populations to make crossover behave ideally.

One method of avoiding the cost of using a very large population is to use a parallel GA (pGA). Many studies have found pGAs to be very effective for preserving diversity for function optimization [Cohoon et al., 1988][Whitley et al., 1990]. In the pGA, a collection of independent GAs, each maintaining separate populations, communicate with each other via infrequent inter-population (as opposed to intra-population) matings. pGAs suffer less from premature convergence than single population GAs. Although the individual populations typically converge, different populations converge to different solutions, thus preserving diversity across the populations. Inter-population mating permits crossover to combine solutions found in different regions of the search space.

We would expect that employing multiple PBIL evolutions, parallel PBIL (pPBIL), has the potential to yield performance improvements similar to those achieved in pGAs. Multiple PBIL evolutions are simulated by using multiple probability vectors to generate solutions. To keep the evolutions independent, each probability vector is only updated with solutions which are generated by sampling it.

The benefit of parallel populations (beyond just multiple runs) is in using crossover to combine dissimilar solutions. There are many ways of introducing crossover into PBIL. The method which is used here is to sample two probability vectors for the creation of each solution vector, see Figure 3. The figure shows the algorithm with uniform crossover; nonetheless, many other crossover operators can be used.

The randomized nature of crossover often yields unproductive results. If crossover is to be used, it is important to simulate the crossover operation many times. Therefore, crossover is used to create each member of the population (this is in contrast to crossing over the probability vectors once, and generating the entire population from the newly created probability vector). More details on integrating crossover and PBIL, and its use in combinatorial problems in robotic surgery can be found in [Baluja & Simon, 1996].

Results with using pPBIL in comparison to PBIL, GA, and pGA are shown in Table II. For many of the problems explored here, parallel versions of GAs and PBIL work better than the sequential versions, and the parallel PBIL models work better than the parallel GA models. In each of these experiments, the parameters were hand-tuned for each algorithms. *In every case, the GA was given at least twice as many function evaluations as PBIL.* The crossover operator was chosen by trying several operators on the GA, and selecting the best one. The same crossover operator was then used for PBIL. For the pGA and pPBIL experiments, 10 subpopulations were always used.

```
***** Generate Samples With Two Probability Vectors *****
for i :=1 to SAMPLES do
    vector1 := generate_sample_vector_with_probabilities (P1);
    vector2 := generate_sample_vector_with_probabilities (P2);
    for j := 1 to LENGTH_do
        if (random (2) = 0) sample_vector[i][j] := vector1[j]
        else  sample_vector[i][j] := vector2[j]
    evaluations[i] := Evaluate_Solution (sample[i]);
best_vector := best_evaluation (sample_vectors, evaluations);

***** Update Both Probability Vectors Towards Best Solution *****
for i :=1 to LENGTH do
    P1[i] := P1[i] * (1.0 - LR) + best_vector[i] * (LR);
    P2[i] := P2[i] * (1.0 - LR) + best_vector[i] * (LR);
```

Figure 3: Generating samples based on two probability vectors. Shown with uniform crossover [Syswerda, 1989] (50% chance of using probability vector 1 or vector 2 for each bit position). Every 100 generations, each population makes a local copy of another population's probability vector (to replace **vector2**). In these experiments, there are a total of 10 subpopulations.

Table II: Sequential & Parallel, GA & PBIL, Avg. 25 runs

Problem (Minimize or Maximize Solution)	GA	pGA	PBIL	pPBIL
TSP - 128 city (minimize tour length)	3256	2832	1718	1344
TSP - 200 city (minimize tour length)	14501	11633	6993	5012
Numerical Optim. Highly Correlated Parameters - Base-2 Code (max)	0.15	0.30	0.19	0.30
Numerical Optim. Highly Correlated Parameters - Gray Code (max)	0.18	0.31	0.18	1.6
Numerical Optim. Independent Parameters - Base-2 Code (max)	0.68	2.91	0.71	4.45
Numerical Optim. Independent Parameters - Gray Code (max)	8.33	8.33	8.33	8.33
Checkerboard (Problem with many maxima, see [Baluja, 1994]) (max)	1119	1150	1206	1256

4 SUMMARY & CONCLUSIONS

PBIL was examined on a very large set of problems drawn from the GA literature. The effectiveness of PBIL for finding good solutions for static optimization functions was compared with a variety of GA and hillclimbing techniques. Second, Parallel-PBIL was introduced. pPBIL is designed to explicitly preserve diversity by using multiple parallel evolutions. Methods for reintroducing crossover into pPBIL were given.

With regard to the empirical results, it should be noted that it is incorrect to say that one procedure will always perform better than another. The results *do not* indicate that PBIL will always outperform a GA. For example, we have presented problems on which GAs work better. Further, on problems such as binpacking, the relative results can change drastically depending upon the number of bins and elements. The conclusion which should be reached from these results is that algorithms, like PBIL and MRSH, which are much simpler than GAs, can outperform standard GAs on many problems of interest.

The PBIL algorithm presented here is very simple and should serve as a prototype for future study. Three directions for future study are presented here. First, the most obvious extension to PBIL is to track more detailed statistics, such as pair-wise covariances of bit positions in high-evaluation vectors. Preliminary work in this area has been conducted, and the results are very promising. Second, another extension is to quickly determine which probability vectors, in the pPBIL model, are unlikely to yield promising answers; methods such as Hoeffding Races may be adapted here [Maron & Moore, 1994]. Third, the manner in which the updates to the probability vector occur is similar to the weight update rules used in Learning Vector Quantization (LVQ). Many of the heuristics used in LVQ can be incorporated into the PBIL algorithm.

Perhaps the most important contribution of the PBIL algorithm is a novel way of examining GAs. In many previous studies of the GA, the GA was examined at a micro-level, analyzing the preservation of building blocks and frequency of sampling hyperplanes. In this study, the statistics at the population level were examined. In the standard GA, the population serves to *implicitly* maintain statistics about the search space. The selection and crossover mechanisms are ways of extracting these statistics from the population. PBIL's population does not maintain the information that is carried from one generation to the next. The statistics of the search are *explicitly* kept in the probability vector.

References

Baluja, S. (1995) "An Empirical Comparison of Seven Iterative and Evolutionary Function Optimization Heuristics," CMU-CS-95-193. Available via. http://www.cs.cmu.edu/~baluja.

Baluja, S. (1994) "Population-Based Incremental Learning". Carnegie Mellon University. Technical Report. CMU-CS-94-163.

Baluja, S. & Caruana, R. (1995) "Removing the Genetics from the Standard Genetic Algorithm", *Inter.Conf. Mach. Learning-12*.

Baluja, S. & Simon, D. (1996) "Evolution-Based Methods for Selecting Point Data for Object Localization: Applications to Computer Assisted Surgery". CMU-CS-96-183.

Cohoon, J., Hedge, S., Martin, W., Richards, D., (1988) "Distributed Genetic Algorithms for the Floor Plan Design Problem," School of Engineering and Applied Science, Computer Science Dept., University of Virginia, TR-88-12.

Davis, L.J. (1991) "Bit-Climbing, Representational Bias and Test Suite Design". *International Conf. on Genetic Algorithms 4*.

De Jong, K. (1975) *An Analysis of the Behavior of a Class of Genetic Adaptive Systems*. Ph.D. Dissertation.

De Jong, K. (1993) "Genetic Algorithms are NOT Function Optimizers". In Whitley (ed.) *Foundations of GAs-2*. 5-17.

Eshelman, L.J. (1991) "The CHC Adaptive Search Algorithm," in Rawlings (ed.) *Foundations of GAs-1*. 265-283.

Fang, H.L, Ross, P., Corne, D. (1993) "A Promising Genetic Algorithm Approach to Job-Shop Scheduling, Rescheduling, and Open- Shop Scheduling Problems". In Forrest, S. *International Conference on Genetic Algorithms 5*.

Goldberg, D.E. (1989) *Genetic Algorithms in Search, Optimization, and Machine Learning*. Addison-Wesley.

Goldberg & Richardson (1987) "Genetic Algorithms with Sharing for Multimodal Function Optimization" - *Proceedings of the Second International Conference on Genetic Algorithms*.

Holland, J. H. (1975) *Adaptation in Natural and Artificial Systems*. Ann Arbor: The University of Michigan Press.

Juels, A. & Wattenberg, M. (1994) "Stochastic Hillclimbing as a Baseline Method for Evaluating Genetic Algorithms" *NIPS 8*.

Maron, O. & Moore, A.(1994) "Hoeffding Races:Accelerating Model Selection for Classification and Function Approx." *NIPS 6*

Mitchell, M., Holland, J. & Forrest, S. (1994) "When will a Genetic Algorithm Outperform Hill Climbing" *NIPS 6*.

Syswerda, G. (1989) "Uniform Crossover in Genetic Algorithms," *International Conference on Genetic Algorithms 3*. 2-9.

Whitley, D., & Starkweather, T. "Genitor II: A Distributed Genetic Algorithm". *JETAI* 2: 189-214.

Consistent Classification, Firm and Soft

Yoram Baram*
Department of Computer Science
Technion, Israel Institute of Technology
Haifa 32000, Israel
baram@cs.technion.ac.il

Abstract

A classifier is called *consistent* with respect to a given set of class–labeled points if it correctly classifies the set. We consider classifiers defined by unions of local separators and propose algorithms for consistent classifier reduction. The expected complexities of the proposed algorithms are derived along with the expected classifier sizes. In particular, the proposed approach yields a consistent reduction of the nearest neighbor classifier, which performs "firm" classification, assigning each new object to a class, regardless of the data structure. The proposed reduction method suggests a notion of "soft" classification, allowing for indecision with respect to objects which are insufficiently or ambiguously supported by the data. The performances of the proposed classifiers in predicting stock behavior are compared to that achieved by the nearest neighbor method.

1 Introduction

Certain classification problems, such as recognizing the digits of a hand written zip–code, require the assignment of each object to a class. Others, involving relatively small amounts of data and high risk, call for indecision until more data become available. Examples in such areas as medical diagnosis, stock trading and radar detection are well known. The training data for the classifier in both cases will correspond to firmly labeled members of the competing classes. (A patient may be

---

*Presently a Senior Research Associate of the National Research Council at M. S. 210-9, NASA Ames Research Center, Moffett Field, CA 94035, on sabbatical leave from the Technion.

either ill or healthy. A stock price may increase, decrease or stay the same). Yet, the classification of new objects need not be firm. (A given patient may be kept in hospital for further observation. A given stock need not be bought or sold every day). We call classification of the first kind "firm" and classification of the second kind "soft". The latter is not the same as training the classifier with a "don't care" option, which would be just another firm labeling option, as "yes" and "no", and would require firm classification. A classifier that correctly classifies the training data is called "consistent". Consistent classifier reductions have been considered in the contexts of the nearest neighbor criterion (Hart, 1968) and decision trees (Holte, 1993, Webb, 1996).

In this paper we present a geometric approach to consistent firm and soft classification. The classifiers are based on unions of local separators, which cover all the labeled points of a given class, and separate them from the others. We propose a consistent reduction of the nearest neighbor classifier and derive its expected design complexity and the expected classifier size. The nearest neighbor classifier and its consistent derivatives perform "firm" classification. Soft classification is performed by unions of maximal–volume spherical local separators. A domain of indecision is created near the boundary between the two sets of class–labeled points, and in regions where there is no data. We propose an economically motivated *benefit* function for a classifier as the difference between the probabilities of success and failure. Employing the respective benefit functions, the advantage of soft classification over firm classification is shown to depend on the rate of indecision. The performances of the proposed algorithms in predicting stock behavior are compared to those of the nearest neighbor method.

2 Consistent Firm Classification

Consider a finite set of points $X = \{x^{(i)}, i = 1, \ldots, N\}$ in some subset of R^n, the real space of dimension n. Suppose that each point of X is assigned to one of two classes, and let the corresponding subsets of X, having N_1 and N_2 points, respectively, be denoted X_1 and X_2. We shall say that the two sets are labeled L_1 and L_2, respectively. It is desired to divide R^n into labeled regions, so that new, unlabeled points can be assigned to one of the two classes.

We define a *local separator* of a point x of X_1 with respect to X_2 as a convex set, $s(x|2)$, which contains x and no point of X_2. A *separator family* is defined as a rule that produces local separators for class–labeled points.

We call the set of those points of R^n that are closer to a point $x \in X_1$ than to any point of X_2 the *minimum–distance* local separator of x with respect to X_2.

We define the *local clustering degree*, c, of the data as the expected fraction of data points that are covered by a local minimum–distance separator.

The *nearest neighbor* criterion extends the class assignment of a point $x \in X_1$ to its minimum–distance local separator. It is clearly a consistent and firm classifier whose memory size is $O(N)$.

Hart's **Condensed Nearest Neighbor (CNN)** classifier (Hart, 1968) is a *consistent subset* of the data points that correctly classifies the entire data by the nearest neighbor method. It is not difficult to show that the complexity of the algorithm proposed by Hart for finding such a subset is $O(N^3)$. The expected memory requirement (or classifier size) has remained an open question.

We propose the following **Reduced Nearest Neighbor (RNN)** classifier: include a labeled point in the consistent subset only if it is not covered by the minimum–distance local separator of any of the points of the same class already in the subset.

It can be shown (Baram, 1996) that the complexity of the RNN algorithm is $O(N^2)$. and that the expected classifier size is $O(\log_{1/(1-c)} N)$. It can also be shown that the latter bounds the expected size of the CNN classifier as well.

It has been suggested that the utility of the Occam's razor in classification would be (Webb, 1996):

"Given a choice between two plausible classifiers that perform identically on the data set, the simpler classifier is expected to classify correctly more objects outside the training set".

The above statement is disproved by the CNN and the RNN classifiers, which are strict consistent reductions of the nearest neighbor classifier, likely to produce more errors.

3 Soft Classification: Indecision Pays, Sometimes

When a new, unlabeled, point is closely surrounded by many points of the same class, its assignment to the same class can be said to be unambiguously supported by the data. When a new point is surrounded by points of different classes, or when it is relatively far from any of the labeled points, its assignment to either class can be said to be unsupported or ambiguously supported by the data. In the latter cases, it may be more desirable to have a certain indecision domain, where new points will not be assigned to a class. This will translate into the creation of indecision domains near the boundary between the two sets of labeled points and where there is no data.

We define a *separator* $S(1|2)$ of X_1 with respect to X_2 as a set that includes X_1 and excludes X_2.

Given a separator family, the union of local separators $s(x^{(i)}|2)$ of the points $x^{(i)}$, $i = 1\ldots, N_1$, of X_1 with respect to X_2,

$$S(1|2) = \cup_{x^{(i)} \in X_1} s(x^{(i)}|2) \qquad (1)$$

is a separator of X_1 with respect to X_2. It consists of N_1 local separators.

Let $X_{1,c}$ be a subset of X_1. The set

$$S_c(1|2) = \cup_{x^{(i)} \in X_{1,c}} s(x^{(i)}|2) \qquad (2)$$

will be called a *consistent* separator of X_1 with respect to X_2 if it contains all the points of X_1. The set $X_{1,c}$ will then be called a *consistent subset* with respect to the given separator family.

Let us extend the class assignment of each of the labeled points to a local separator of a given family and maximize the volume of each of the local separators without including in it any point of the competing class. Let $S_c(1|2)$ and $S_c(2|1)$ be consistent separators of the two sets, consisting of maximal–volume (or, simply, *maximal*) local separators of labeled points of the corresponding classes. The intersection of $S_c(1|2)$ and $S_c(2|1)$ defines a conflict and will be called a *domain of ambiguity of the first kind*. A region uncovered by either separator will be called a *domain of ambiguity of the second kind*. The union of the domains of ambiguity will be designated the *domain of indecision*. The remainders of the two separators, excluding their intersection, define the conflict–free domains assigned to the two classes.

The resulting "soft" classifier rules out hard conflicts, where labeled points of one class are included in the separator of the other. Yet, it allows for indecision in areas which are either claimed by both separators or claimed by neither.

Let the true class be denoted y (with possible values, e.g., y=1 or y=2) and let the classification outcome be denoted $\hat{y}$. Let the probabilities of decision and indecision by the soft classifier be denoted P_d and P_{id}, respectively (of course, $P_{id} = 1 - P_d$), and let the probabilities of correct and incorrect decisions by the firm and the soft classifiers be denoted $P_{\text{firm}}\{\hat{y}=y\}$, $P_{\text{firm}}\{\hat{y} \neq y\}$, $P_{\text{soft}}\{\hat{y}=y\}$ and $P_{\text{soft}}\{\hat{y} \neq y\}$, respectively. Finally, let the joint probabilities of a decision being made by the soft classifier and the correctness or incorrectness of the decision be denoted, respectively, $P_{\text{soft}}\{d, \hat{y}=y\}$ and $P_{\text{soft}}\{d, \hat{y} \neq y\}$ and let the corresponding conditional probabilities be denoted $P_{\text{soft}}\{\hat{y}=y \mid d\}$ and $P_{\text{soft}}\{\hat{y} \neq y \mid d\}$, respectively.

We define the *benefit* of using the firm classifier as the difference between the probability that a point is classified correctly by the classifier and the probability that it is misclassified:

$$B_{\text{firm}} = P_{\text{firm}}\{\hat{y}=y\} - P_{\text{firm}}\{\hat{y} \neq y\} = 2P_{\text{firm}}\{\hat{y}=y\} - 1. \quad (3)$$

This definition is motivated by economic consideration: the profit produced by an investment will be, on average, proportional to the benefit function. This will become more evident in a later section, were we consider the problem of stock trading.

For a soft classifier, we similarly define the benefit as the difference between the probability of a correct classification and that of an incorrect one (which, in an economic context, assumes that indecision has no cost, other than the possible loss of profit). Now, however, these probabilities are for the joint events that a classification is made, and that the outcome is correct or incorrect, respectively:

$$\begin{aligned} B_{\text{soft}} &= P_{\text{soft}}\{d, \hat{y}=y\} - P_{\text{soft}}\{d, \hat{y} \neq y\} \\ &= [2P_{\text{soft}}\{\hat{y}=y \mid d\} - 1]P_d \end{aligned} \quad (4)$$

Soft classification will be more beneficial than firm classification if $B_{\text{soft}} > B_{\text{firm}}$, which may be written as

$$P_{id} < 1 - \frac{P_{\text{firm}}\{\hat{y}=y\} - 0.5}{P_{\text{soft}}\{\hat{y}=y \mid d\} - 0.5} \quad (5)$$

For the latter to be a useful condition, it is necessary that $P_{\text{firm}}\{\hat{y}=y\} > 0.5$, $P_{\text{soft}}\{\hat{y}=y \mid d\} > 0.5$ and $P_{\text{soft}}\{\hat{y}=y \mid d\} > P_{\text{firm}}\{\hat{y}=y\}$. The latter will be normally satisfied, since points of the same class can be expected to be denser under the corresponding separator than in the indecision domain. In other words, the error ratio produced by the soft classifier on the decided cases can be expected to be smaller than the error ratio produced by the firm classifier, which decides on all the cases. The satisfaction of condition (5) would depend on the geometry of the data. It will be satisfied for certain cases, and will not be satisfied for others. This will be numerically demonstrated for the stock trading problem.

The maximal local spherical separator of x is defined by the open sphere centered at x, whose radius $r(x|2)$ is the distance between x and the point of X_2 nearest to x. Denoting by $s(x, r)$ the sphere of radius r in R^n centered at x, the maximal local separator is then $s_M(x|2) = s(x, r(x|2))$.

A separator construction algorithm employing maximal local spherical separators is described below. Its complexity is clearly $O(N^2)$.

Let $\tilde{X}_1 = X_1$. For each of the points $x^{(i)}$ of $\tilde{X}_1$, find the minimal distance to the points of X_2. Call it $r(x^{(i)}|2)$. Select the point $x^{(i)}$ for which $r(x^{(i)}|2) \geq r(x^{(j)}|2)$, $j \neq i$, for the consistent subset. Eliminate from $\tilde{X}_1$ all the points that are covered by $s_M(x^{(i)}|2)$. Denote the remaining set $\tilde{X}_1$. Repeat the procedure while $\tilde{X}_1$ is non–empty. The union of the maximal local spherical separators is a separator for X_1 with respect to X_2.

4 Example: Firm and soft prediction of stock behaviour

Given a sequence of k daily trading ("close") values of a stock, it is desired to predict whether the next day will show an increase or a decrease with respect to the last day in the sequence. Records for ten different stocks, each containing, on average, 1260 daily values were used. About 60 percent of the data were used for training and the rest for testing. The CNN algorithm reduced the data by 40% while the RNN algorithm reduced the data by 35%. Results are show in Fig. 1. It can be seen that, on average, the nearest neighbor method has produced the best results. The performances of the CNN and the RNN classifiers (the latter producing only slightly better results) are somewhat lower. It has been argued that performance within a couple of percentage points by a reduced classifier supports the utility of Occam's razor (Holte, 1993). However, a couple of percentage points can be quite meaningful in stock trading.

In order to evaluate the utility of soft classification in stock trading, let the prediction success rate of a firm classifier, be denoted f and that of a soft classifier for the decided cases s. For a given trade, let the gain or loss per unit invested be denoted q, and the rate of indecision of the soft classifier ir. Suppose that, employing the firm classifier, a stock is traded once every day (say, at the "close" value), and that, employing the soft classifier, it is traded on a given day only if a trade is decided by the classifier (that is, the input does not fall in the indecision domain). The expected profit for M days per unit invested is $2(f - 0.5)qM$ for the firm classifier and $2(s - 0.5)q(1 - ir)M$ for the soft classifier (these values disregard possible commission and slippage costs). The soft classifier will be preferred over the firm one if the latter quantity is greater than the former, that is, if

$$ir < 1 - \frac{f - 0.5}{s - 0.5} \tag{6}$$

which is the sample representation of condition (5) for the stock trading problem.

	NN	CNN	RNN	soft classifier		benefit
				indecision	success	
xaip	61.4%	58.4%	57.0%	48.4%	70.1%	-
xaldnf	51.7%	52.3%	50.1%	74.6%	51.3%	-
xddddf	52.0%	49.6%	51.8%	44.3%	53.3%	-
xdssi	48.3%	47.7%	48.6%	43.6%	52.6%	+
xecilf	53.0%	50.9%	52.6%	47.6%	48.8%	-
xedusf	80.7%	74.7%	76.3%	30.6%	89.9%	-
xelbtf	53.7%	55.6%	52.5%	42.2%	50.1%	-
xetz	66.0%	61.0%	61.0%	43.8%	68.6%	-
xelrnf	51.5%	49.0%	49.2%	39.2%	56.0%	+
xelt	85.6%	82.7%	84.2%	32.9%	93.0%	-
Average	60.4%	58.2%	58.3%	44.7%	63.4%	

Figure 1: Success rates in the prediction of rize and fall in stock values.

Results for the soft classifier, applied to the stock data, are presented in Fig. 1. The indecision rates and the success rates in the decided cases are then specified along with a benefit sign. A positive benefit represents a satisfaction of condition (6), with ir, f and s replaced by the corresponding sample values given in the table. This indicates a higher profit in applying the soft classifier over the application of the nearest neighbor classifier. A negative benefit indicates that a higher profit is produced by the nearest neighbor classifier. It can be seen that for two of the stocks (xdssi and xelrnf) soft classification has produced better results than firm classification, and for the remaining eight stocks firm classification by the nearest neighbor method has produced better results.

5 Conclusion

Solutions to the consistent classification problem have been specified in terms of local separators of data points of one class with respect to the other. The expected complexities of the proposed algorithms have been specified, along with the expected sizes of the resulting classifiers. Reduced consistent versions of the nearest neighbor classifier have been specified and their expected complexities have been derived. A notion of "soft" classification has been introduced an algorithm for its implementation have been presented and analyzed. A criterion for the utility of such classification has been presented and its application in stock trading has been demonstrated.

Acknowledgment

The author thanks Dr. Amir Atiya of Cairo University for providing the stock data used in the examples and for valuable discussions of the corresponding results.

References

Baram Y. (1996) Consistent Classification, Firm and Soft, CIS Report No. 9627, Center for Intelligent Systems, Technion, Israel Institute of Technology, Haifa 32000, Israel.

Baum, E. B. (1988) On the Capabilities of Multilayer Perceptrons, J. Complexity, Vol. 4, pp. 193 – 215.

Hart, P. E. (1968) The Condensed Nearest Neighbor Rule, IEEE Trans. on Information Theory, Vol. IT–14, No. 3, pp. 515 – 516.

Holte, R. C. (1993) Very Simple Classification Rules Perform Well on Most Commonly Used databases, Machine Learning, Vol. 11, No. 1 pp. 63 – 90.

Rosenblatt, F. (1958) The Perceptron: A Probabilistic Model for Information Storage and Organization in the Brain, Psychological Review, Vol. 65, pp. 386 – 408.

Webb, G. I. (1996) Further Experimental Evidence against the Utility of Occam's Razor, J. of Artificial Intelligence Research 4, pp. 397 – 147.

Bayesian Model Comparison by Monte Carlo Chaining

David Barber
D.Barber@aston.ac.uk

Christopher M. Bishop
C.M.Bishop@aston.ac.uk

Neural Computing Research Group
Aston University, Birmingham, B4 7ET, U.K.
http://www.ncrg.aston.ac.uk/

Abstract

The techniques of Bayesian inference have been applied with great success to many problems in neural computing including evaluation of regression functions, determination of error bars on predictions, and the treatment of hyper-parameters. However, the problem of model comparison is a much more challenging one for which current techniques have significant limitations. In this paper we show how an extended form of Markov chain Monte Carlo, called *chaining*, is able to provide effective estimates of the relative probabilities of different models. We present results from the robot arm problem and compare them with the corresponding results obtained using the standard Gaussian approximation framework.

1 Bayesian Model Comparison

In a Bayesian treatment of statistical inference, our state of knowledge of the values of the parameters $\mathbf{w}$ in a model $\mathcal{M}$ is described in terms of a probability distribution function. Initially this is chosen to be some prior distribution $p(\mathbf{w}|\mathcal{M})$, which can be combined with a likelihood function $p(D|\mathbf{w}, \mathcal{M})$ using Bayes' theorem to give a posterior distribution $p(\mathbf{w}|D, \mathcal{M})$ in the form

$$p(\mathbf{w}|D, \mathcal{M}) = \frac{p(D|\mathbf{w}, \mathcal{M}) p(\mathbf{w}|\mathcal{M})}{p(D|\mathcal{M})} \tag{1}$$

where D is the data set. Predictions of the model are obtained by performing integrations weighted by the posterior distribution.

The comparison of different models $\mathcal{M}_i$ is based on their relative probabilities, which can be expressed, again using Bayes' theorem, in terms of prior probabilities $p(\mathcal{M}_i)$ to give

$$\frac{p(\mathcal{M}_i|D)}{p(\mathcal{M}_j|D)} = \frac{p(D|\mathcal{M}_i)p(\mathcal{M}_i)}{p(D|\mathcal{M}_j)p(\mathcal{M}_j)} \qquad (2)$$

and so requires that we be able to evaluate the *model evidence* $p(D|\mathcal{M}_i)$, which corresponds to the denominator in (1). The relative probabilities of different models can be used to select the single most probable model, or to form a committee of models, weighed by their probabilities.

It is convenient to write the numerator of (1) in the form $\exp\{-E(\mathbf{w})\}$, where $E(\mathbf{w})$ is an error function. Normalization of the posterior distribution then requires that

$$p(D|\mathcal{M}) = \int \exp\{-E(\mathbf{w})\}\,d\mathbf{w}. \qquad (3)$$

Generally, it is straightforward to evaluate $E(\mathbf{w})$ for a given value of $\mathbf{w}$, although it is extremely difficult to evaluate the corresponding model evidence using (3) since the posterior distribution is typically very small except in narrow regions of the high-dimensional parameter space, which are unknown a-priori. Standard numerical integration techniques are therefore inapplicable.

One approach is based on a local Gaussian approximation around a mode of the posterior (MacKay, 1992). Unfortunately, this approximation is expected to be accurate only when the number of data points is large in relation to the number of parameters in the model. In fact it is for relatively complex models, or problems for which data is scarce, that Bayesian methods have the most to offer. Indeed, Neal (1996) has argued that, from a Bayesian perspective, there is no reason to limit the number of parameters in a model, other than for computational reasons. We therefore consider an approach to the evaluation of model evidence which overcomes the limitations of the Gaussian framework. For additional techniques and references to Bayesian model comparison, see Gilks *et al.* (1995) and Kass and Raftery (1995).

2 Chaining

Suppose we have a simple model $\mathcal{M}_0$ for which we can evaluate the evidence analytically, and for which we can easily generate a sample $\mathbf{w}^l$ (where $l = 1, \ldots, L$) from the corresponding distribution $p(\mathbf{w}|D, \mathcal{M}_0)$. Then the evidence for some other model $\mathcal{M}$ can be expressed in the form

$$\begin{aligned}\frac{p(D|\mathcal{M})}{p(D|\mathcal{M}_0)} &= \int \exp\{-E(\mathbf{w}) + E_0(\mathbf{w})\}p(\mathbf{w}|D, \mathcal{M}_0)\,d\mathbf{w} \\ &\simeq \frac{1}{L}\sum_{l=1}^{L}\exp\{-E(\mathbf{w}^l) + E_0(\mathbf{w}^l)\}.\end{aligned} \qquad (4)$$

Unfortunately, the Monte Carlo approximation in (4) will be poor if the two error functions are significantly different, since the exponent is dominated by regions where E is relatively small, for which there will be few samples unless E_0 is also small in those regions. A simple Monte Carlo approach will therefore yield poor results. This problem is equivalent to the evaluation of free energies in statistical physics, which is known to be a challenging problem, and where a number of approaches have been developed Neal (1993).

Here we discuss one such approach to this problem based on a chain of K successive models $\mathcal{M}_i$ which interpolate between $\mathcal{M}_0$ and $\mathcal{M}$, so that the required evidence can be written as

$$p(D|\mathcal{M}) = p(D|\mathcal{M}_0)\frac{p(D|\mathcal{M}_1)}{p(D|\mathcal{M}_0)}\frac{p(D|\mathcal{M}_2)}{p(D|\mathcal{M}_1)}\cdots\frac{p(D|\mathcal{M})}{p(D|\mathcal{M}_K)}. \tag{5}$$

Each of the ratios in (5) can be evaluated using (4). The goal is to devise a chain of models such that each successive pair of models has probability distributions which are reasonably close, so that each of the ratios in (5) can be evaluated accurately, while keeping the total number of links in the chain fairly small to limit the computational costs.

We have chosen the technique of hybrid Monte Carlo (Duane et al., 1987; Neal, 1993) to sample from the various distributions, since this has been shown to be effective for sampling from the complex distributions arising with neural network models (Neal, 1996). This involves introducing Hamiltonian equations of motion in which the parameters $\mathbf{w}$ are augmented by a set of fictitious 'momentum' variables, which are then integrated using the leapfrog method. At the end of each trajectory the new parameter vector is accepted with a probability governed by the Metropolis criterion, and the momenta are replaced using Gibbs sampling. As a check on our software implementation of chaining, we have evaluated the evidence for a mixture of two non-isotropic Gaussian distributions, and obtained a result which was within 10% of the analytical solution.

3 Application to Neural Networks

We now consider the application of the chaining method to regression problems involving neural network models. The network corresponds to a function $y(\mathbf{x},\mathbf{w})$, and the data set consists of N pairs of input vectors $\mathbf{x}_n$ and corresponding targets t_n where $n = 1,\ldots,N$. Assuming Gaussian noise on the target data, the likelihood function takes the form

$$p(D|\mathbf{w},\mathcal{M}) = \left(\frac{\beta}{2\pi}\right)^{N/2}\exp\left\{-\frac{\beta}{2}\sum_{n=1}^{N}\|y(\mathbf{x}_n;\mathbf{w}) - t_n\|^2\right\} \tag{6}$$

where β is a hyper-parameter representing the inverse of the noise variance. We consider networks with a single hidden layer of 'tanh' units, and linear output units. Following Neal (1996) we use a diagonal Gaussian prior in which the weights are divided into groups $\mathbf{w}_k$, where $k = 1,\ldots,4$ corresponding to input-to-hidden weights, hidden-unit biases, hidden-to-output weights, and output biases. Each group is governed by a separate 'precision' hyper-parameter α_k, so that the prior takes the form

$$p(\mathbf{w}|\{\alpha_k\}) = \frac{1}{Z_W}\exp\left\{-\frac{1}{2}\sum_k \alpha_k \mathbf{w}_k^T \mathbf{w}_k\right\} \tag{7}$$

where Z_W is the normalization coefficient. The hyper-parameters $\{\alpha_k\}$ and β are themselves each governed by hyper-priors given by Gamma distributions of the form

$$p(\alpha) \propto \alpha^s \exp(-\alpha s/2\omega) \tag{8}$$

in which the mean ω and variance $2\omega^2/s$ are chosen to give very broad hyper-priors in reflection of our limited prior knowledge of the values of the hyper-parameters. We use the hybrid Monte Carlo algorithm to sample from the joint distribution of parameters and hyper-parameters. For the evaluation of evidence ratios, however, we consider only the parameter samples, and perform the integrals over hyper-parameters analytically, using the fact that the gamma distribution is conjugate to the Gaussian.

In order to apply chaining to this problem, we choose the prior as our reference distribution, and then define a set of intermediate distributions based on a parameter λ which governs the effective contribution from the data term, so that

$$E(\lambda, \mathbf{w}) = \lambda \phi(\mathbf{w}) + E_0(\mathbf{w}) \qquad (9)$$

where $\phi(\mathbf{w})$ arises from the likelihood term (6) while $E_0(\mathbf{w})$ corresponds to the prior (7). We select a set of 18 values of λ which interpolate between the reference distribution ($\lambda = 0$) and the desired model distribution ($\lambda = 1$). The evidence for the prior alone is easily evaluated analytically.

4 Gaussian Approximation

As a comparison against the method of chaining, we consider the framework of MacKay (1992) based on a local Gaussian approximation to the posterior distribution. This approach makes use of the *evidence approximation* in which the integration over hyper-parameters is approximated by setting them to specific values which are themselves determined by maximizing their evidence functions.

This leads to a hierarchical treatment as follows. At the lowest level, the maximum $\widehat{\mathbf{w}}$ of the posterior distribution over weights is found for fixed values of the hyper-parameters by minimizing the error function. Periodically the hyper-parameters are re-estimated by evidence maximization, where the evidence is obtained analytically using the Gaussian approximation. This gives the following re-estimation formulae

$$\frac{1}{\beta} := \frac{1}{N-\gamma} \sum_{n=1}^{N} \|y(\mathbf{x}_n; \widehat{\mathbf{w}}) - t_n\|^2 \qquad \alpha_k := \frac{\gamma_k}{\widehat{\mathbf{w}}_k^T \widehat{\mathbf{w}}_k} \qquad (10)$$

where $\gamma_k = W_k - \alpha_k \text{Tr}_k(\mathbf{A}^{-1})$, W_k is the total number of parameters in group k, $\mathbf{A} = \nabla\nabla E(\widehat{\mathbf{w}})$, $\gamma = \sum_k \gamma_k$, and $\text{Tr}_k(\cdot)$ denotes the trace over the kth group of parameters. The weights are updated in an inner loop by minimizing the error function using a conjugate gradient optimizer, while the hyper-parameters are periodically re-estimated using (10)[1].

Once training is complete, the model evidence is evaluated by making a Gaussian approximation around the converged values of the hyper-parameters, and integrating over this distribution analytically. This gives the model log evidence as

$$\ln p(D|\mathcal{M}) = -E(\widehat{\mathbf{w}}) - \frac{1}{2}\ln|\mathbf{A}| + \frac{1}{2}\sum_k W_k \ln \alpha_k +$$
$$\frac{N}{2}\ln \beta + \ln h! + 2\ln h + \frac{1}{2}\sum_k \ln(2/\gamma_k) + \frac{1}{2}\ln(2/(N-\gamma)). \qquad (11)$$

---

[1] Note that we are assuming that the hyper-priors (8) are sufficiently broad that they have no effect on the location of the evidence maximum and can therefore be neglected.

Here h is the number of hidden units, and the terms $\ln h! + 2\ln h$ take account of the many equivalent modes of the posterior distribution arising from sign-flip and hidden unit interchange symmetries in the network model. A derivation of these results can be found in Bishop (1995; pages 434–436).

The result (11) corresponds to a single mode of the distribution. If we initialize the weight optimization algorithm with different random values we can find distinct solutions. In order to compute an overall evidence for the particular network model with a given number of hidden units, we make the assumption that we have found all of the distinct modes of the posterior distribution precisely once each, and then sum the evidences to arrive at the total model evidence. This neglects the possibility that some of the solutions found are related by symmetry transformations (and therefore already taken into account) or that we have missed important modes. While some attempt could be made to detect degenerate solutions, it will be difficult to do much better than the above within the framework of the Gaussian approximation.

5 Results: Robot Arm Problem

As an illustration of the evaluation of model evidence for a larger-scale problem we consider the modelling of the forward kinematics for a two-link robot arm in a two-dimensional space, as introduced by MacKay (1992). This problem was chosen as MacKay reports good results in using the Gaussian approximation framework to evaluate the evidences, and provides a good opportunity for comparison with the chaining approach. The task is to learn the mapping $(x_1, x_2) \to (y_1, y_2)$ given by

$$y_1 = 2.0\cos(x_1) + 1.3\cos(x_1 + x_2) \qquad y_2 = 2.0\sin(x_1) + 1.3\sin(x_1 + x_2) \quad (12)$$

where the data set consists of 200 input-output pairs with outputs corrupted by zero mean Gaussian noise with standard deviation $\sigma = 0.05$. We have used the original training data of MacKay, but generated our own test set of 1000 points using the same prescription. The evidence is evaluated using both chaining and the Gaussian approximation, for networks with various numbers of hidden units.

In the chaining method, the particular form of the gamma priors for the precision variables are as follows: for the input-to-hidden weights and hidden-unit biases, $\omega = 1$, $s = 0.2$; for the hidden-to-output weights, $\omega = h$, $s = 0.2$; for the output biases, $\omega = 0.2$, $s = 1$. The noise level hyper-parameters were $\omega = 400$, $s = 0.2$. These settings follow closely those used by Neal (1996) for the same problem. The hidden-to-output precision scaling was chosen by Neal such that the limit of an infinite number of hidden units is well defined and corresponds to a Gaussian process prior. For each evidence ratio in the chain, the first 100 samples from the hybrid Monte Carlo run, obtained with a trajectory length of 50 leapfrog iterations, are omitted to give the algorithm a chance to reach the equilibrium distribution. The next 600 samples are obtained using a trajectory length of 300 and are used to evaluate the evidence ratio.

In Figure 1 (a) we show the error values of the sampling stage for 24 hidden units, where we see that the errors are largely uncorrelated, as required for effective Monte Carlo sampling. In Figure 1 (b), we plot the values of $\ln\{p(D|\mathcal{M}_i)/p(D|\mathcal{M}_{i-1})\}$ against λ_i $i = 1..18$. Note that there is a large change in the evidence ratios at the beginning of the chain, where we sample close to the reference distribution. For this

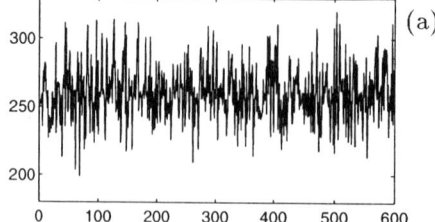 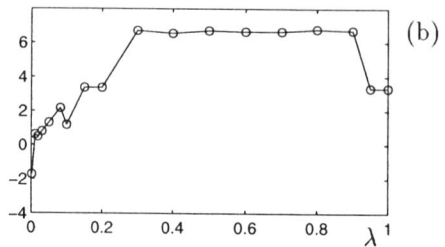

Figure 1: (a) error $E(\lambda = 0.6, \mathbf{w})$ for $h = 24$, plotted for 600 successive Monte Carlo samples. (b) Values of the ratio $\ln\{p(D|\mathcal{M}_i)/p(D|\mathcal{M}_{i-1})\}$ for $i = 1, \ldots, 18$ for $h = 24$.

reason, we choose the λ_i to be dense close to $\lambda = 0$. We are currently researching more principled approaches to the partitioning selection. Figure 2 (a) shows the log model evidence against the number of hidden units. Note that the chaining approach is computationally expensive: for $h=24$, a complete chain takes 48 hours in a Matlab implementation running on a Silicon Graphics Challenge L.

We see that there is no decline in the evidence as the number of hidden units grows. Correspondingly, in Figure 2 (b), we see that the test error performance does not degrade as the number of hidden units increases. This indicates that there is no over-fitting with increasing model complexity, in accordance with Bayesian expectations.

The corresponding results from the Gaussian approximation approach are shown in Figure 3. We see that there is a characteristic 'Occam hill' whereby the evidence shows a peak at around $h = 12$, with a strong decrease for smaller values of h and a slower decrease for larger values. The corresponding test set errors similarly show a minimum at around $h = 12$, indicating that the Gaussian approximation is becoming increasingly inaccurate for more complex models.

6 Discussion

We have seen that the use of chaining allows the effective evaluation of model evidences for neural networks using Monte Carlo techniques. In particular, we find that there is no peak in the model evidence, or the corresponding test set error, as the number of hidden units is increased, and so there is no indication of over-fitting. This is in accord with the expectation that model complexity should not be limited by the size of the data set, and is in marked contrast to the conventional

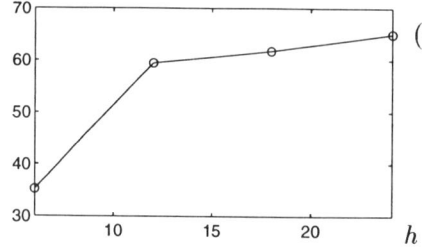 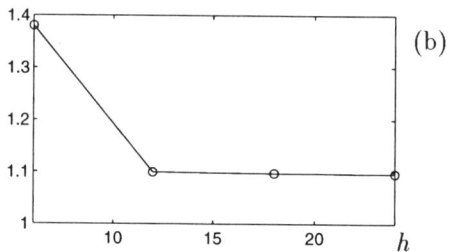

Figure 2: (a) Plot of $\ln p(D|\mathcal{M})$ for different numbers of hidden units. (b) Test error against the number of hidden units. Here the theoretical minimum value is 1.0. For $h = 64$ the test error is 1.11

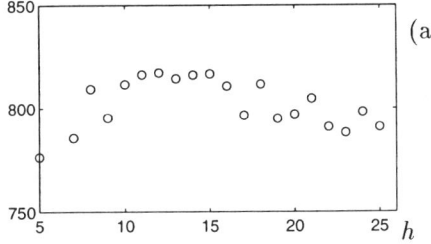 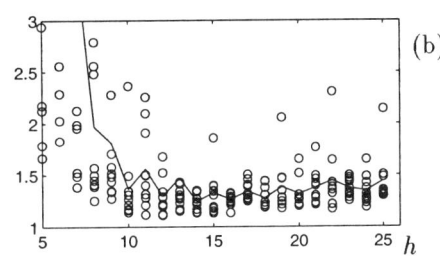

Figure 3: (a) Plot of the model evidence for the robot arm problem versus the number of hidden units, using the Gaussian approximation framework. This clearly shows the characteristic 'Occam hill' shape. Note that the evidence is computed up to an additive constant, and so the origin of the vertical axis has no significance. (b) Corresponding plot of the test set error versus the number of hidden units. Individual points correspond to particular modes of the posterior weight distribution, while the line shows the mean test set error for each value of h.

maximum likelihood viewpoint. It is also consistent with the result that, in the limit of an infinite number of hidden units, the prior over network weights leads to a well-defined Gaussian prior over functions (Williams, 1997).

An important advantage of being able to make accurate evaluations of the model evidence is the ability to compare quite distinct kinds of model, for example radial basis function networks and multi-layer perceptrons. This can be done either by chaining both models back to a common reference model, or by evaluating normalized model evidences explicitly.

Acknowledgements

We would like to thank Chris Williams and Alastair Bruce for a number of useful discussions. This work was supported by EPSRC grant GR/J75425: *Novel Developments in Learning Theory for Neural Networks*.

References

Bishop, C. M. (1995). *Neural Networks for Pattern Recognition*. Oxford University Press.

Duane, S., A. D. Kennedy, B. J. Pendleton, and D. Roweth (1987). Hybrid Monte Carlo. *Physics Letters B* **195** (2), 216–222.

Gilks, W. R., S. Richardson, and D. J. Spiegelhalter (1995). *Markov Chain Monte Carlo in Practice*. Chapman and Hall.

Kass, R. E. and A. E. Raftery (1995). Bayes factors. *J. Am. Statist. Ass.* **90**, 773–795.

MacKay, D. J. C. (1992). A practical Bayesian framework for back-propagation networks. *Neural Computation* **4** (3), 448–472.

Neal, R. M. (1993). Probabilistic inference using Markov chain Monte Carlo methods. Technical Report CRG-TR-93-1, Department of Computer Science, University of Toronto, Cananda.

Neal, R. M. (1996). *Bayesian Learning for Neural Networks*. Springer. Lecture Notes in Statistics 118.

Williams, C. K. I. (1997). Computing with infinite networks. This volume.

Gaussian Processes for Bayesian Classification via Hybrid Monte Carlo

David Barber and Christopher K. I. Williams
Neural Computing Research Group
Department of Computer Science and Applied Mathematics
Aston University, Birmingham B4 7ET, UK
d.barber@aston.ac.uk   c.k.i.williams@aston.ac.uk

Abstract

The full Bayesian method for applying neural networks to a prediction problem is to set up the prior/hyperprior structure for the net and then perform the necessary integrals. However, these integrals are not tractable analytically, and Markov Chain Monte Carlo (MCMC) methods are slow, especially if the parameter space is high-dimensional. Using Gaussian processes we can approximate the weight space integral analytically, so that only a small number of hyperparameters need be integrated over by MCMC methods. We have applied this idea to classification problems, obtaining excellent results on the real-world problems investigated so far.

1 INTRODUCTION

To make predictions based on a set of training data, fundamentally we need to combine our prior beliefs about possible predictive functions with the data at hand. In the Bayesian approach to neural networks a prior on the weights in the net induces a prior distribution over functions. This leads naturally to the idea of specifying our beliefs about functions more directly. Gaussian Processes (GPs) achieve just that, being examples of stochastic process priors over functions that allow the efficient computation of predictions. It is also possible to show that a large class of neural network models converge to GPs in the limit of an infinite number of hidden units (Neal, 1996). In previous work (Williams and Rasmussen, 1996) we have applied GP priors over functions to the problem of predicting a real-valued output, and found that the method has comparable performance to other state-of-the-art methods. This paper extends the use of GP priors to classification problems.

The GPs we use have a number of adjustable hyperparameters that specify quantities like the length scale over which smoothing should take place. Rather than optimizing these parameters (e.g. by maximum likelihood or cross-validation methods) we place priors over them and use a Markov Chain Monte Carlo (MCMC) method to obtain a sample from the posterior which is then used for making predictions. An important advantage of using GPs rather than neural networks arises from the fact that the GPs are characterized by a few (say ten or twenty) hyperparameters, while the networks have a similar number of hyperparameters but many (e.g. hundreds) of weights as well, so that MCMC integrations for the networks are much more difficult.

We first briefly review the regression framework as our strategy will be to transform the classification problem into a corresponding regression problem by dealing with the input values to the logistic transfer function. In section 2.1 we show how to use Gaussian processes for classification when the hyperparameters are fixed, and then describe the integration over hyperparameters in section 2.3. Results of our method as applied to some well known classification problems are given in section 3, followed by a brief discussion and directions for future research.

1.1 Gaussian Processes for regression

We outline the GP method as applied to the prediction of a real valued output $y_* = y(\boldsymbol{x}_*)$ for a new input value $\boldsymbol{x}_*$, given a set of training data $\mathcal{D} = \{(\boldsymbol{x}_i, t_i),\ i = 1\ldots n\}$

Given a set of inputs $\boldsymbol{x}_*, \boldsymbol{x}_1, \ldots \boldsymbol{x}_n$, a GP allows us to specify how correlated we expect their corresponding outputs $\boldsymbol{y} = (y(\boldsymbol{x}_1), y(\boldsymbol{x}_2), \ldots, y(\boldsymbol{x}_n))$ to be. We denote this prior over functions as $P(\boldsymbol{y})$, and similarly, $P(y_*, \boldsymbol{y})$ for the joint distribution including y_*. If we also specify $P(\boldsymbol{t}|\boldsymbol{y})$, the probability of observing the particular values $\boldsymbol{t} = (t_1, \ldots t_n)^T$ given actual values $\boldsymbol{y}$ (i.e. a noise model) then

$$P(y_*|\boldsymbol{t}) = \int P(y_*, \boldsymbol{y}|\boldsymbol{t})d\boldsymbol{y} = \frac{1}{P(\boldsymbol{t})} \int P(y_*, \boldsymbol{y})P(\boldsymbol{t}|\boldsymbol{y})d\boldsymbol{y} \qquad (1)$$

Hence the predictive distribution for y_* is found from the marginalization of the product of the prior and the noise model. If $P(\boldsymbol{t}|\boldsymbol{y})$ and $P(y_*, \boldsymbol{y})$ are Gaussian then $P(y_*|\boldsymbol{t})$ is a Gaussian whose mean and variance can be calculated using matrix computations involving matrices of size $n \times n$. Specifying $P(y_*, \boldsymbol{y})$ to be a multidimensional Gaussian (for all values of n and placements of the points $\boldsymbol{x}_*, \boldsymbol{x}_1, \ldots \boldsymbol{x}_n$) means that the prior over functions is a GP. More formally, a stochastic process is a collection of random variables $\{Y(\boldsymbol{x})|\boldsymbol{x} \in X\}$ indexed by a set X. In our case X will be the input space with dimension d, the number of inputs. A GP is a stochastic process which can be fully specified by its mean function $\mu(\boldsymbol{x}) = E[Y(\boldsymbol{x})]$ and its covariance function $C(\boldsymbol{x}, \boldsymbol{x}') = E[(Y(\boldsymbol{x}) - \mu(\boldsymbol{x}))(Y(\boldsymbol{x}') - \mu(\boldsymbol{x}'))]$; any finite set of Y-variables will have a joint multivariate Gaussian distribution. Below we consider GPs which have $\mu(\boldsymbol{x}) \equiv 0$.

2 GAUSSIAN PROCESSES FOR CLASSIFICATION

For simplicity of exposition, we will present our method as applied to two class problems as the extension to multiple classes is straightforward.

By using the logistic transfer function σ to produce an output which can be interpreted as $\pi(\boldsymbol{x})$, the probability of the input $\boldsymbol{x}$ belonging to class 1, the job of specifying a prior over functions π can be transformed into that of specifying a prior over the input to the transfer function. We call the input to the transfer function the *activation*, and denote it by y, with $\pi(\boldsymbol{x}) = \sigma(y(\boldsymbol{x}))$. For input $\boldsymbol{x}_i$, we will denote the corresponding probability and activation by π_i and y_i respectively.

To make predictions when using fixed hyperparameters we would like to compute $\hat{\pi}_* = \int \pi_* P(\pi_*|t) \, d\pi_*$, which requires us to find $P(\pi_*|t) = P(\pi(x_*)|t)$ for a new input x_*. This can be done by finding the distribution $P(y_*|t)$ (y_* is the activation of π_*) and then using the appropriate Jacobian to transform the distribution. Formally the equations for obtaining $P(y_*|t)$ are identical to equation 1. However, even if we use a GP prior so that $P(y_*, y)$ is Gaussian, the usual expression for $P(t|y) = \prod_i \pi_i^{t_i}(1-\pi_i)^{1-t_i}$ for classification data (where the t's take on values of 0 or 1), means that the marginalization to obtain $P(y_*|t)$ is no longer analytically tractable.

We will employ Laplace's approximation, i.e. we shall approximate the integrand $P(y_*, y|t, \theta)$ by a Gaussian distribution centred at a maximum of this function with respect to y_*, y with an inverse covariance matrix given by $-\nabla\nabla \log P(y_*, y|t, \theta)$. The necessary integrations (marginalization) can then be carried out analytically (see, e.g. Green and Silverman (1994) §5.3) and we provide a derivation in the following section.

2.1 Maximizing $P(y_*, y|t)$

Let y_+ denote (y_*, y), the complete set of activations. By Bayes' theorem $\log P(y_+|t) = \log P(t|y) + \log P(y_+) - \log P(t)$, and let $\Psi_+ = \log P(t|y) + \log P(y_+)$. As $P(t)$ does not depend on y_+ (it is just a normalizing factor), the maximum of $P(y_+|t)$ is found by maximizing Ψ_+ with respect to y_+. We define Ψ similarly in relation to $P(y|t)$. Using $\log P(t_i|y_i) = t_i y_i - \log(1 + e^{y_i})$, we obtain

$$\Psi_+ = t^T y - \sum_{i=1}^{n} \log(1 + e^{y_i}) - \frac{1}{2} y_+^T K_+^{-1} y_+ - \frac{1}{2} \log|K_+| - \frac{n+1}{2} \log 2\pi \quad (2)$$

$$\Psi = t^T y - \sum_{i=1}^{n} \log(1 + e^{y_i}) - \frac{1}{2} y^T K^{-1} y - \frac{1}{2} \log|K| - \frac{n}{2} \log 2\pi \quad (3)$$

where K_+ is the covariance matrix of the GP evaluated at $x_1, \ldots x_n, x_*$. K_+ can be partitioned in terms of an $n \times n$ matrix K, a $n \times 1$ vector k and a scalar k_*, viz.

$$K_+ = \begin{pmatrix} K & k \\ k^T & k_* \end{pmatrix} \quad (4)$$

As y_* only enters into equation 2 in the quadratic prior term and has no data point associated with it, maximizing Ψ_+ with respect to y_+ can be achieved by first maximizing Ψ with respect to y and then doing the further quadratic optimization to determine the posterior mean $\hat{y}_*$. To find a maximum of Ψ we use the Newton-Raphson (or Fisher scoring) iteration $y^{new} = y - (\nabla\nabla\Psi)^{-1}\nabla\Psi$. Differentiating equation 3 with respect to y we find

$$\nabla\Psi = (t - \pi) - K^{-1} y \quad (5)$$
$$\nabla\nabla\Psi = -K^{-1} - W \quad (6)$$

where $W = diag(\pi_1(1-\pi_1), .., \pi_n(1-\pi_n))$, which gives the iterative equation[1],

$$y^{new} = (K^{-1} + W)^{-1} W(y + W^{-1}(t - \pi)) \quad (7)$$

---
[1] The complexity of calculating each iteration using standard matrix methods is $O(n^3)$. In our implementation, however, we use conjugate gradient methods to avoid explicitly inverting matrices. In addition, by using the previous iterate y as an initial guess for the conjugate gradient solution to equation 7, the iterates are computed an order of magnitude faster than using standard algorithms.

Given a converged solution $\tilde{y}$ for y, $\hat{y}_*$ can easily be found using $y_* = k^T K^{-1} \tilde{y} = k^T(t - \tilde{\pi})$. $var(y_*)$ is given by $(K_+^{-1} + W_+)^{-1}_{(n+1)(n+1)}$, where W_+ is the W matrix with a zero appended in the $(n+1)$th diagonal position.

Given the (Gaussian) distribution of y_* we then wish to find the mean of the distribution of $P(\pi_*|t)$ which is found from $\hat{\pi}_* = \int \sigma(y_*) P(y_*|t)$. We calculate this by approximating the sigmoid by a set of five cumulative normal densities (erf) that interpolate the sigmoid at chosen points. This leads to a very fast and accurate analytic approximation for the mean class prediction.

The justification of Laplace's approximation in our case is somewhat different from the argument usually put forward, e.g. for asymptotic normality of the maximum likelihood estimator for a model with a finite number of parameters. This is because the dimension of the problem grows with the number of data points. However, if we consider the "infill asymptotics", where the number of data points in a *bounded* region increases, then a local average of the training data at any point x will provide a tightly localized estimate for $\pi(x)$ and hence $y(x)$, so we would expect the distribution $P(y)$ to become more Gaussian with increasing data.

2.2 Parameterizing the covariance function

There are many reasonable choices for the covariance function. Formally, we are required to specify functions which will generate a non-negative definite covariance matrix for any set of points $(x_1, \ldots, x_k)$. From a modelling point of view we wish to specify covariances so that points with nearby inputs will give rise to similar predictions. We find that the following covariance function works well:

$$C(x, x') = v_0 \exp\left\{-\frac{1}{2} \sum_{l=1}^{d} w_l (x_l - x'_l)^2\right\} \tag{8}$$

where x_l is the lth component of x and $\theta = \log(v_0, w_1, \ldots, w_d)$ plays the role of hyperparameters[2].

We define the hyperparameters to be the log of the variables in equation 8 since these are positive scale-parameters. This covariance function has been studied by Sacks *et al* (1989) and can be obtained from a network of Gaussian radial basis functions in the limit of an infinite number of hidden units (Williams, 1996).

The w_l parameters in equation 8 allow a different length scale on each input dimension. For irrelevant inputs, the corresponding w_l will become small, and the model will ignore that input. This is closely related to the Automatic Relevance Determination (ARD) idea of MacKay and Neal (Neal, 1996). The v_0 variable gives the overall scale of the prior; in the classification case, this specifies if the π values will typically be pushed to 0 or 1, or will hover around 0.5.

2.3 Integration over the hyperparameters

Given that the GP contains adjustable hyperparameters, how should they be adapted given the data? Maximum likelihood or (generalized) cross-validation methods are often used, but we will prefer a Bayesian solution. A prior distribution over the hyperparameters $P(\theta)$ is modified using the training data to obtain the posterior distribution $P(\theta|t) \propto P(t|\theta)P(\theta)$. To make predictions we integrate

---

[2] We call θ the hyperparameters rather than parameters as they correspond closely to hyperparameters in neural networks.

the predicted probabilities over the posterior; for example, the mean value $\bar{\pi}(x_*)$ for test input x_* is given by

$$\bar{\pi}(x_*) = \int \hat{\pi}(x_*|\theta) P(\theta|t) d\theta, \qquad (9)$$

where $\hat{\pi}(x_*|\theta)$ is the mean prediction for a fixed value of the hyperparameters, as given in section 2.

For the regression problem $P(t|\theta)$ can be calculated exactly using $P(t|\theta) = \int P(t|y) P(y|\theta) dy$, but this integral is not analytically tractable for the classification problem. Again we use Laplace's approximation and obtain[3]

$$\log P(t|\theta) \simeq \Psi(\tilde{y}) + \frac{1}{2} |K^{-1} + W| + \frac{n}{2} \log 2\pi \qquad (10)$$

where $\tilde{y}$ is the converged iterate of equation 7. We denote the right-hand side of equation 10 by $\log P_a(t|\theta)$ (where a stands for approximate).

The integration over θ-space also cannot be done analytically, and we employ a Markov Chain Monte Carlo method. We have used the Hybrid Monte Carlo (HMC) method of Duane et al (1987), with broad Gaussian hyperpriors on the parameters.

HMC works by creating a fictitious dynamical system in which the hyperparameters are regarded as position variables, and augmenting these with momentum variables p. The purpose of the dynamical system is to give the hyperparameters "inertia" so that random-walk behaviour in θ-space can be avoided. The total energy, $\mathcal{H}$, of the system is the sum of the kinetic energy, $\mathcal{K} = p^T p/2$ and the potential energy, $\mathcal{E}$. The potential energy is defined such that $p(\theta|D) \propto \exp(-\mathcal{E})$, i.e. $\mathcal{E} = -\log P(t|\theta) - \log P(\theta)$. In practice $\log P_a(t|\theta)$ is used instead of $\log P(t|\theta)$. We sample from the joint distribution for θ and p given by $P(\theta, p) \propto \exp(-\mathcal{E} - \mathcal{K})$; the marginal of this distribution for θ is the required posterior. A sample of hyperparameters from the posterior can therefore be obtained by simply ignoring the momenta.

Sampling from the joint distribution is achieved by two steps: (i) finding new points in phase space with near-identical energies $\mathcal{H}$ by simulating the dynamical system using a discretised approximation to Hamiltonian dynamics, and (ii) changing the energy $\mathcal{H}$ by Gibbs sampling the momentum variables.

Hamilton's first order differential equations for $\mathcal{H}$ are approximated using the leapfrog method which requires the derivatives of $\mathcal{E}$ with respect to θ. Given a Gaussian prior on θ, $\log P(\theta)$ is straightforward to differentiate. The derivative of $\log P_a(\theta)$ is also straightforward, although implicit dependencies of $\tilde{y}$ (and hence $\tilde{\pi}$) on θ must be taken into account by using equation 5 at the maximum point to obtain $\partial \tilde{y}/\partial \theta = (I + KW)^{-1} (\partial K/\partial \theta)(t - \pi)$. The computation of the energy can be quite expensive as for each new θ, we need to perform the maximization required for Laplace's approximation, equation 10. The Newton-Raphson iteration was initialized each time with $\pi = 0.5$, and continued until the mean relative difference of the elements of W between consecutive iterations was less than 10^{-4}.

The same step size ε is used for all hyperparameters, and should be as large as possible while keeping the rejection rate low. We have used a trajectory made up of $L = 20$ leapfrog steps, which gave a low correlation between successive states[4]. This proposed state is then accepted or rejected using the Metropolis rule depending on

---

[3] This requires $O(n^3)$ computation.

[4] In our experiments, where θ is only 7 or 8 dimensional, we found the trajectory length needed is much shorter than that for neural network HMC implementations.

the final energy $\mathcal{H}^*$ (which is not necessarily equal to the initial energy $\mathcal{H}$ because of the discretization of Hamilton's equations).

The priors over hyperparameters were set to be Gaussian with a mean of -3 and a standard deviation of 3. In all our simulations a step size $\varepsilon = 0.1$ produced a very low rejection rate ($< 5\%$). The hyperparameters corresponding to the w_l's were initialized to -2 and that for v_0 to 0. The sampling procedure was run for 200 iterations, and the first third of the run was discarded; this "burn-in" is intended to give the hyperparameters time to come close to their equilibrium distribution.

3 RESULTS

We have tested our method on two well known two-class classification problems, the Leptograpsus crabs and Pima Indian diabetes datasets and the multiclass Forensic Glass dataset[5]. We first rescale the inputs so that they have mean zero and unit variance on the training set. Our Matlab implementations for the HMC simulations for both tasks each take several hours on a SGI Challenge machine (R10000), although good results can be obtained in less time. We also tried a standard Metropolis MCMC algorithm for the Crabs problem, and found similar results, although the sampling by this method is slower than that for HMC. Comparisons with other methods are taken from Ripley (1994) and Ripley (1996).

Our results for the two-class problems are presented in Table 1: In the Leptograpsus crabs problem we attempt to classify the sex of crabs on the basis of five anatomical attributes. There are 100 examples available for crabs of each sex, making a total of 200 labelled examples. These are split into a training set of 40 crabs of each sex, making 80 training examples, with the other 120 examples used as the test set. The performance of the GP is equal to the best of the other methods reported in Ripley (1994), namely a 2 hidden unit neural network with direct input to output connections and a logistic output unit which was trained with maximum likelihood (Network(1) in Table 1).

For the Pima Indians diabetes problem we have used the data as made available by Prof. Ripley, with his training/test split of 200 and 332 examples respectively (Ripley, 1996). The baseline error obtained by simply classifying each record as coming from a diabetic gives rise to an error of 33%. Again, the GP method is comparable with the best alternative performance, with an error of around 20%.

Table 1	Pima	Crabs
Neural Network(1)	-	3
Neural Network(2)	-	3
Neural Network(3)	75+	-
Linear Discriminant	67	8
Logistic regression	66	4
MARS (degree = 1)	75	4
PP (4 ridge functions)	75	6
2 Gaussian Mixture	64	-
Gaussian Process (HMC)	68	3
Gaussian Process (MAP)	69	3

Table 2	Forensic Glass
Neural Network (4HU)	23.8%
Linear Discriminant	36%
MARS (degree = 1)	32.2%
PP (5 ridge functions)	35%
Gaussian Mixture	30.8%
Decision Tree	32.2%
Gaussian Process (MAP)	23.3%

Table 1: Number of test errors for the Pima Indian diabetes and Leptograpsus crabs tasks. Network(2) used two hidden units and the predictive approach (Ripley, 1994), which uses Laplace's approximation to weight each network local minimum. Network(3) had one hidden unit and was trained with maximum likelihood; the results were worse for nets with two or more hidden units (Ripley, 1996). Table 2: Percentage classification error on the Forensic Glass task.

---

[5] All available from http://markov.stats.ox.ac.uk/pub/PRNN.

Our method is readily extendable to multiple class problems by using the softmax function. The details of this work which will be presented elsewhere, and we simply report here our initial findings on the Forensic Glass problem (Table 2). This is a 6 class problem, consisting of 214 examples containing 9 attributes. The performance is estimated using 10 fold cross validation. Computing the MAP estimate took $\approx$ 24 hours and gave a classification error of 23.3%, comparable with the best of the other presented methods.

4 DISCUSSION

We have extended the work of Williams and Rasmussen (1996) to classification problems, and have demonstrated that it performs well on the datasets we have tried so far. One of the main advantages of this approach is that the number of parameters used in specifying the covariance function is typically much smaller than the number of weights and hyperparameters that are used in a neural network, and this greatly facilitates the implementation of Monte Carlo methods. Furthermore, because the Gaussian Process is a prior on function space (albeit in the activation function space), we are able to interpret our prior more readily than for a model in which the priors are on the parametrization of the function space, as in neural network models. Some of the elegance that is present using Gaussian Processes for regression is lost due to the inability to perform the required marginalisation exactly. Nevertheless, our simulation results suggest that Laplace's approximation is accurate enough to yield good results in practice. As methods based on GPs require the inversion of $n \times n$ matrices, where n is the number of training examples, we are looking into methods such as query selection for large dataset problems. Other future research directions include the investigation of different covariance functions and improvements on the approximations employed.

We hope to make our MATLAB code available from http://www.ncrg.aston.ac.uk/

Acknowledgements

We thank Prof. B. Ripley for making available the Leptograpsus crabs and Pima Indian diabetes datasets. This work was partially supported by EPSRC grant GR/J75425, "Novel Developments in Learning Theory for Neural Networks".

References

Duane, S., A. D. Kennedy, B. J. Pendleton, and D. Roweth (1987). Hybrid Monte Carlo. *Physics Letters B* **195**, 216–222.

Green, P. J.and Silverman, B. W. (1994). *Nonparametric regression and generalized linear models*. Chapman and Hall.

Neal, R. M. (1996). *Bayesian Learning for Neural Networks*. Springer. Lecture Notes in Statistics 118.

Ripley, B. (1996). *Pattern Recognition and Neural Networks*. Cambridge.

Ripley, B. D. (1994). Flexible Non-linear Approaches to Classification. In V. Cherkassy, J. H. Friedman, and H. Wechsler (Eds.), *From Statistics to Neural Networks*, pp. 105–126. Springer.

Sacks, J., W. J. Welch, T. J. Mitchell, and H. P. Wynn (1989). Design and analysis of computer experiments. *Statistical Science* **4**(4), 409–435.

Williams, C. K. I. Computing with infinite networks. This volume.

Williams, C. K. I. and C. E. Rasmussen (1996). Gaussian processes for regression. In D. S. Touretzky, M. C. Mozer, and M. E. Hasselmo (Eds.), *Advances in Neural Information Processing Systems 8*, pp. 514–520. MIT Press.

Regression with Input-Dependent Noise: A Bayesian Treatment

Christopher M. Bishop
C.M.Bishop@aston.ac.uk

Cazhaow S. Qazaz
qazazcs@aston.ac.uk

Neural Computing Research Group
Aston University, Birmingham, B4 7ET, U.K.
http://www.ncrg.aston.ac.uk/

Abstract

In most treatments of the regression problem it is assumed that the distribution of target data can be described by a deterministic function of the inputs, together with additive Gaussian noise having constant variance. The use of maximum likelihood to train such models then corresponds to the minimization of a sum-of-squares error function. In many applications a more realistic model would allow the noise variance itself to depend on the input variables. However, the use of maximum likelihood to train such models would give highly biased results. In this paper we show how a Bayesian treatment can allow for an input-dependent variance while overcoming the bias of maximum likelihood.

1 Introduction

In regression problems it is important not only to predict the output variables but also to have some estimate of the error bars associated with those predictions. An important contribution to the error bars arises from the intrinsic noise on the data. In most conventional treatments of regression, it is assumed that the noise can be modelled by a Gaussian distribution with a constant variance. However, in many applications it will be more realistic to allow the noise variance itself to depend on the input variables. A general framework for modelling the conditional probability density function of the target data, given the input vector, has been introduced in the form of *mixture density networks* by Bishop (1994, 1995). This uses a feed-forward network to set the parameters of a mixture kernel distribution, following Jacobs *et al.* (1991). The special case of a single isotropic Gaussian kernel function was discussed by Nix and Weigend (1995), and its generalization to allow for an arbitrary covariance matrix was given by Williams (1996).

These approaches, however, are all based on the use of maximum likelihood, which can lead to the noise variance being systematically under-estimated. Here we adopt an approximate hierarchical Bayesian treatment (MacKay, 1991) to find the most probable interpolant and most probable input-dependent noise variance. We compare our results with maximum likelihood and show how this Bayesian approach leads to a significantly reduced bias.

In order to gain some insight into the limitations of the maximum likelihood approach, and to see how these limitations can be overcome in a Bayesian treatment, it is useful to consider first a much simpler problem involving a single random variable (Bishop, 1995). Suppose that a variable z is known to have a Gaussian distribution, but with unknown mean μ and unknown variance σ^2. Given a sample $D \equiv \{z_n\}$ drawn from that distribution, where $n = 1, \ldots, N$, our goal is to infer values for the mean and variance. The likelihood function is given by

$$p(D|\mu, \sigma^2) = \frac{1}{(2\pi\sigma^2)^{N/2}} \exp\left\{-\frac{1}{2\sigma^2} \sum_{n=1}^{N}(z_n - \mu)^2\right\}. \tag{1}$$

A non-Bayesian approach to finding the mean and variance is to maximize the likelihood jointly over μ and σ^2, corresponding to the intuitive idea of finding the parameter values which are most likely to have given rise to the observed data set. This yields the standard result

$$\widehat{\mu} = \frac{1}{N} \sum_{n=1}^{N} z_n, \qquad \widehat{\sigma}^2 = \frac{1}{N} \sum_{n=1}^{N} (z_n - \widehat{\mu})^2. \tag{2}$$

It is well known that the estimate $\widehat{\sigma}^2$ for the variance given in (2) is *biased* since the expectation of this estimate is not equal to the true value

$$\mathcal{E}[\widehat{\sigma}^2] = \frac{N-1}{N}\sigma_0^2 \tag{3}$$

where σ_0^2 is the true variance of the distribution which generated the data, and $\mathcal{E}[\cdot]$ denotes an average over data sets of size N. For large N this effect is small. However, in the case of regression problems there are generally much larger number of degrees of freedom in relation to the number of available data points, in which case the effect of this bias can be very substantial.

The problem of bias can be regarded as a symptom of the maximum likelihood approach. Because the mean $\widehat{\mu}$ has been estimated from the data, it has fitted some of the noise on the data and this leads to an under-estimate of the variance. If the true mean is used in the expression for $\widehat{\sigma}^2$ in (2) instead of the maximum likelihood expression, then the estimate is unbiased.

By adopting a Bayesian viewpoint this bias can be removed. The marginal likelihood of σ^2 should be computed by *integrating* over the mean μ. Assuming a 'flat' prior $p(\mu)$ we obtain

$$p(D|\sigma^2) = \int p(D|\sigma^2, \mu)p(\mu) \, d\mu \tag{4}$$

Regression with Input-Dependent Noise: A Bayesian Treatment

$$\propto \frac{1}{\sigma^{N-1}} \exp\left\{-\frac{1}{2\sigma^2}\sum_{n=1}^{N}(z_n - \widehat{\mu})^2\right\}. \tag{5}$$

Maximizing (5) with respect to σ^2 then gives

$$\widetilde{\sigma}^2 = \frac{1}{N-1}\sum_{n=1}^{N}(z_n - \widehat{\mu})^2 \tag{6}$$

which is unbiased.

This result is illustrated in Figure 1 which shows contours of $p(D|\mu,\sigma^2)$ together with the marginal likelihood $p(D|\sigma^2)$ and the conditional likelihood $p(D|\widehat{\mu},\sigma^2)$ evaluated at $\mu = \widehat{\mu}$.

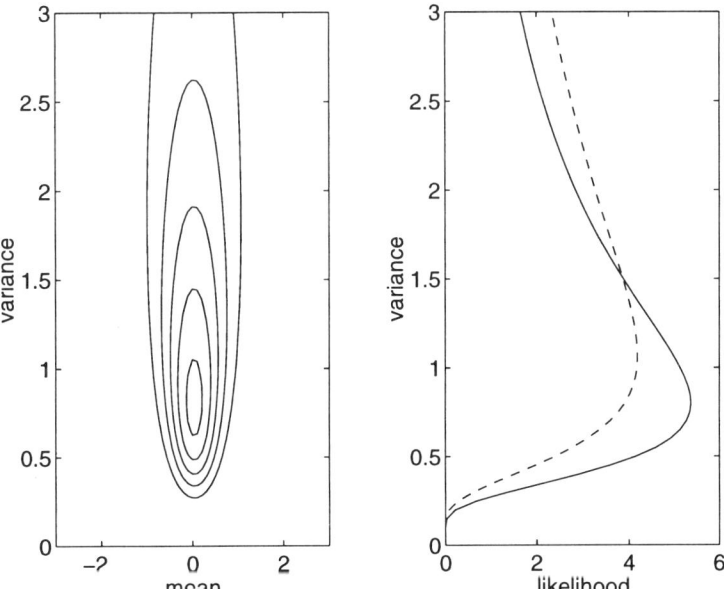

Figure 1: The left hand plot shows contours of the likelihood function $p(D|\mu,\sigma^2)$ given by (1) for 4 data points drawn from a Gaussian distribution having zero mean and unit variance. The right hand plot shows the marginal likelihood function $p(D|\sigma^2)$ (dashed curve) and the conditional likelihood function $p(D|\widehat{\mu},\sigma^2)$ (solid curve). It can be seen that the skewed contours result in a value of $\widehat{\sigma}^2$, which maximizes $p(D|\widehat{\mu},\sigma^2)$, which is smaller than $\widetilde{\sigma}^2$ which maximizes $p(D|\sigma^2)$.

2 Bayesian Regression

Consider a regression problem involving the prediction of a noisy variable t given the value of a vector $\mathbf{x}$ of input variables[1]. Our goal is to predict both a regression function and an input-dependent noise variance. We shall therefore consider two networks. The first network takes the input vector $\mathbf{x}$ and generates an output

---

[1]For simplicity we consider a single output variable. The extension of this work to multiple outputs is straightforward.

$y(\mathbf{x}; \mathbf{w})$ which represents the regression function, and is governed by a vector of weight parameters $\mathbf{w}$. The second network also takes the input vector $\mathbf{x}$, and generates an output function $\beta(\mathbf{x}; \mathbf{u})$ representing the inverse variance of the noise distribution, and is governed by a vector of weight parameters $\mathbf{u}$. The conditional distribution of target data, given the input vector, is then modelled by a normal distribution $p(t|\mathbf{x}, \mathbf{w}, \mathbf{u}) = \mathcal{N}(t|y, \beta^{-1})$. From this we obtain the likelihood function

$$p(D|\mathbf{w}, \mathbf{u}) = \frac{1}{Z_D} \exp\left\{-\sum_{n=1}^{N} \beta_n E_n\right\} \quad (7)$$

where $\beta_n = \beta(\mathbf{x}_n; \mathbf{u})$,

$$Z_D = \prod_{n=1}^{N} \left(\frac{2\pi}{\beta_n}\right)^{1/2}, \qquad E_n = \frac{1}{2}(y(\mathbf{x}_n; \mathbf{w}) - t_n)^2 \quad (8)$$

and $D \equiv \{\mathbf{x}_n, t_n\}$ is the data set.

Some simplification of the subsequent analysis is obtained by taking the regression function, and $\ln \beta$, to be given by linear combinations of fixed basis functions, as in MacKay (1995), so that

$$y(\mathbf{x}; \mathbf{w}) = \mathbf{w}^T \boldsymbol{\phi}(\mathbf{x}), \qquad \beta(\mathbf{x}; \mathbf{u}) = \exp\left(\mathbf{u}^T \boldsymbol{\psi}(\mathbf{x})\right) \quad (9)$$

where choose one basis function in each network to be a constant $\phi_0 = \psi_0 = 1$ so that the corresponding weights w_0 and u_0 represent bias parameters.

The maximum likelihood procedure chooses values $\hat{\mathbf{w}}$ and $\hat{\mathbf{u}}$ by finding a joint maximum over $\mathbf{w}$ and $\mathbf{u}$. As we have already indicated, this will give a biased result since the regression function inevitably fits part of the noise on the data, leading to an over-estimate of $\beta(\mathbf{x})$. In extreme cases, where the regression curve passes exactly through a data point, the corresponding estimate of β can go to infinity, corresponding to an estimated noise variance of zero.

The solution to this problem has already been indicated in Section 1 and was first suggested in this context by MacKay (1991, Chapter 6). In order to obtain an unbiased estimate of $\beta(\mathbf{x})$ we must find the marginal distribution of β, or equivalently of $\mathbf{u}$, in which we have integrated out the dependence on $\mathbf{w}$. This leads to a hierarchical Bayesian analysis.

We begin by defining priors over the parameters $\mathbf{w}$ and $\mathbf{u}$. Here we consider isotropic Gaussian priors of the form

$$p(\mathbf{w}|\alpha_w) = \left(\frac{\alpha_w}{2\pi}\right)^{1/2} \exp\left\{-\frac{\alpha_w}{2}\|\mathbf{w}\|^2\right\} \quad (10)$$

$$p(\mathbf{u}|\alpha_u) = \left(\frac{\alpha_u}{2\pi}\right)^{1/2} \exp\left\{-\frac{\alpha_u}{2}\|\mathbf{u}\|^2\right\} \quad (11)$$

where α_w and α_u are *hyper-parameters*. At the first stage of the hierarchy, we assume that $\mathbf{u}$ is fixed to its most probable value $\mathbf{u}_{MP}$, which will be determined shortly. The most probable value of $\mathbf{w}$, denoted by $\mathbf{w}_{MP}$, is then found by maximizing the posterior distribution[2]

$$p(\mathbf{w}|D, \mathbf{u}_{\text{MP}}, \alpha_w) = \frac{p(D|\mathbf{w}, \mathbf{u}_{\text{MP}})p(\mathbf{w}|\alpha_w)}{p(D|\mathbf{u}_{\text{MP}}, \alpha_w)} \qquad (12)$$

where the denominator in (12) is given by

$$p(D|\mathbf{u}_{\text{MP}}, \alpha_w) = \int p(D|\mathbf{w}, \mathbf{u}_{\text{MP}})p(\mathbf{w}|\alpha_w)\, d\mathbf{w}. \qquad (13)$$

Taking the negative log of (12), and dropping constant terms, we see that $\mathbf{w}_{\text{MP}}$ is obtained by minimizing

$$S(\mathbf{w}) = \sum_{n=1}^{N} \beta_n E_n + \frac{\alpha_w}{2} \|\mathbf{w}\|^2 \qquad (14)$$

where we have used (7) and (10). For the particular choice of model (9) this minimization represents a linear problem which is easily solved (for a given $\mathbf{u}$) by standard matrix techniques.

At the next level of the hierarchy, we find $\mathbf{u}_{\text{MP}}$ by maximizing the marginal posterior distribution

$$p(\mathbf{u}|D, \alpha_u, \alpha_w) = \frac{p(D|\mathbf{u}, \alpha_w)p(\mathbf{u}|\alpha_u)}{p(D|\alpha_w, \alpha_u)}. \qquad (15)$$

The term $p(D|\mathbf{u}, \alpha_w)$ is just the denominator from (12) and is found by integrating over $\mathbf{w}$ as in (13). For the model (9) and prior (10) this integral is Gaussian and can be performed analytically without approximation. Again taking logarithms and discarding constants, we have to minimize

$$M(\mathbf{u}) = \sum_{n=1}^{N} \beta_n E_n + \frac{\alpha_u}{2} \|\mathbf{u}\|^2 - \frac{1}{2} \sum_{n=1}^{N} \ln \beta_n + \frac{1}{2} \ln |\mathbf{A}| \qquad (16)$$

where $|\mathbf{A}|$ denotes the determinant of the Hessian matrix $\mathbf{A}$ given by

$$\mathbf{A} = \sum_{n=1}^{N} \beta_n \boldsymbol{\phi}(\mathbf{x}_n)\boldsymbol{\phi}(\mathbf{x}_n)^{\text{T}} + \alpha_w \mathbf{I} \qquad (17)$$

and $\mathbf{I}$ is the unit matrix. The function $M(\mathbf{u})$ in (16) can be minimized using standard non-linear optimization algorithms. We use scaled conjugate gradients, in which the necessary derivatives of $\ln |\mathbf{A}|$ are easily found in terms of the eigenvalues of $\mathbf{A}$.

In summary, the algorithm requires an outer loop in which the most probable value $\mathbf{u}_{\text{MP}}$ is found by non-linear minimization of (16), using the scaled conjugate gradient algorithm. Each time the optimization code requires a value for $M(\mathbf{u})$ or its gradient, for a new value of $\mathbf{u}$, the optimum value for $\mathbf{w}_{\text{MP}}$ must be found by minimizing (14). In effect, $\mathbf{w}$ is evolving on a fast time-scale, and $\mathbf{u}$ on a slow time-scale. The corresponding maximum (penalized) likelihood approach consists of a joint non-linear optimization over $\mathbf{u}$ and $\mathbf{w}$ of the posterior distribution $p(\mathbf{w}, \mathbf{u}|D)$ obtained from (7), (10) and (11). Finally, the hyperparameters are given fixed values $\alpha_w = \alpha_u = 0.1$ as this allows the maximum likelihood and Bayesian approaches to be treated on an equal footing.

---

[2] Note that the result will be dependent on the choice of parametrization since the maximum of a distribution is not invariant under a change of variable.

3 Results and Discussion

As an illustration of this algorithm, we consider a toy problem involving one input and one output, with a noise variance which has an x^2 dependence on the input variable. Since the estimated quantities are noisy, due to the finite data set, we consider an averaging procedure as follows. We generate 100 independent data sets each consisting of 10 data points. The model is trained on each of the data sets in turn and then tested on the remaining 99 data sets. Both the $y(\mathbf{x}; \mathbf{w})$ and $\beta(\mathbf{x}; \mathbf{u})$ networks have 4 Gaussian basis functions (plus a bias) with width parameters chosen to equal the spacing of the centres.

Results are shown in Figure 2. It is clear that the maximum likelihood results are biased and that the noise variance is systematically underestimated. By contrast,

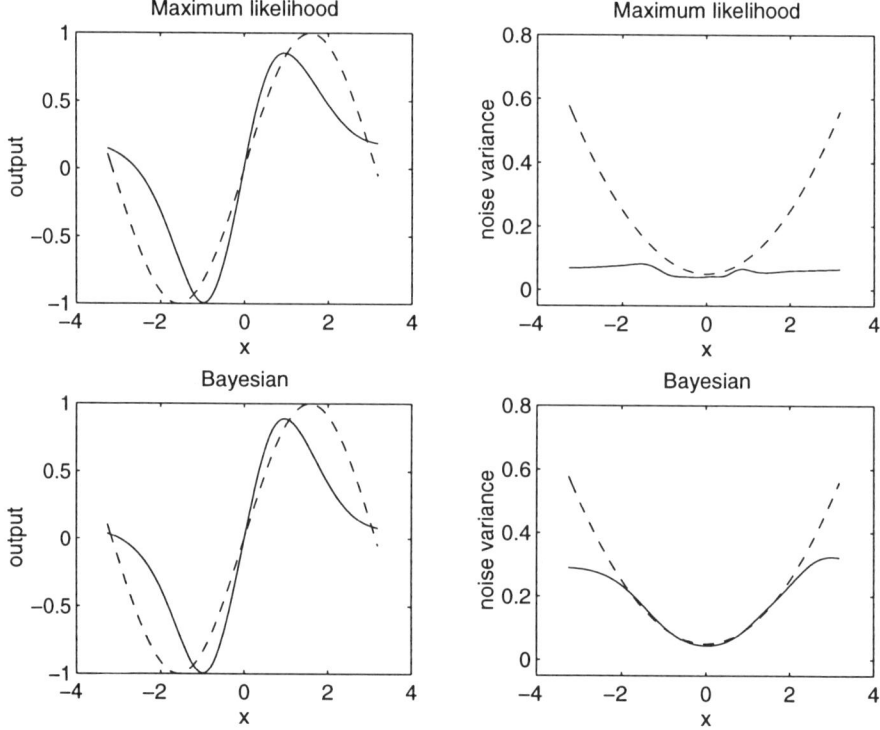

Figure 2: The left hand plots show the sinusoidal function (dashed curve) from which the data were generated, together with the regression function averaged over 100 training sets. The right hand plots show the true noise variance (dashed curve) together with the estimated noise variance, again averaged over 100 data sets.

the Bayesian results show an improved estimate of the noise variance. This is borne out by evaluating the log likelihood for the test data under the corresponding predictive distributions. The Bayesian approach gives a log likelihood per data point, averaged over the 100 runs, of -1.38. Due to the over-fitting problem, maximum likelihood occasionally gives extremely large negative values for the log likelihood (when β has been estimated to be very large, corresponding to a regression curve which passes close to an individual data point). Even omitting these extreme values, the maximum likelihood still gives an average log likelihood per data point of

-17.1 which is substantially smaller than the Bayesian result.

We are currently exploring the use of Markov chain Monte Carlo methods (Neal, 1993) to perform the integrations required by the Bayesian analysis numerically, without the need to introduce the Gaussian approximation or the evidence framework. Recently, MacKay (1995) has proposed an alternative technique based on Gibbs sampling. It will be interesting to compare these various approaches.

Acknowledgements: This work was supported by EPSRC grant GR/K51792, *Validation and Verification of Neural Network Systems.*

References

Bishop, C. M. (1994). Mixture density networks. Technical Report NCRG/94/001, Neural Computing Research Group, Aston University, Birmingham, UK.

Bishop, C. M. (1995). *Neural Networks for Pattern Recognition.* Oxford University Press.

Jacobs, R. A., M. I. Jordan, S. J. Nowlan, and G. E. Hinton (1991). Adaptive mixtures of local experts. *Neural Computation* **3** (1), 79–87.

MacKay, D. J. C. (1991). *Bayesian Methods for Adaptive Models.* Ph.D. thesis, California Institute of Technology.

MacKay, D. J. C. (1995). Probabilistic networks: new models and new methods. In F. Fogelman-Soulié and P. Gallinari (Eds.), *Proceedings ICANN'95 International Conference on Artificial Neural Networks*, pp. 331–337. Paris: EC2 & Cie.

Neal, R. M. (1993). Probabilistic inference using Markov chain Monte Carlo methods. Technical Report CRG-TR-93-1, Department of Computer Science, University of Toronto, Cananda.

Nix, A. D. and A. S. Weigend (1995). Learning local error bars for nonlinear regression. In G. Tesauro, D. S. Touretzky, and T. K. Leen (Eds.), *Advances in Neural Information Processing Systems*, Volume 7, pp. 489–496. Cambridge, MA: MIT Press.

Williams, P. M. (1996). Using neural networks to model conditional multivariate densities. *Neural Computation* **8** (4), 843–854.

GTM: A Principled Alternative to the Self-Organizing Map

Christopher M. Bishop
C.M.Bishop@aston.ac.uk

Markus Svensén
svensjfm@aston.ac.uk

Christopher K. I. Williams
C.K.I.Williams@aston.ac.uk

Neural Computing Research Group
Aston University, Birmingham, B4 7ET, UK
http://www.ncrg.aston.ac.uk/

Abstract

The Self-Organizing Map (SOM) algorithm has been extensively studied and has been applied with considerable success to a wide variety of problems. However, the algorithm is derived from heuristic ideas and this leads to a number of significant limitations. In this paper, we consider the problem of modelling the probability density of data in a space of several dimensions in terms of a smaller number of latent, or hidden, variables. We introduce a novel form of latent variable model, which we call the GTM algorithm (for *Generative Topographic Mapping*), which allows general non-linear transformations from latent space to data space, and which is trained using the EM (expectation-maximization) algorithm. Our approach overcomes the limitations of the SOM, while introducing no significant disadvantages. We demonstrate the performance of the GTM algorithm on simulated data from flow diagnostics for a multi-phase oil pipeline.

1 Introduction

The Self-Organizing Map (SOM) algorithm of Kohonen (1982) represents a form of unsupervised learning in which a set of unlabelled data vectors t_n ($n = 1, \ldots, N$) in a D-dimensional data space is summarized in terms of a set of reference vectors having a spatial organization corresponding (generally) to a two-dimensional sheet[1].

---

[1] Biological metaphor is sometimes invoked when motivating the SOM procedure. It should be stressed that our goal here is not neuro-biological modelling, but rather the development of effective algorithms for data analysis.

While this algorithm has achieved many successes in practical applications, it also suffers from some major deficiencies, many of which are highlighted in Kohonen (1995) and reviewed in this paper.

From the perspective of statistical pattern recognition, a fundamental goal in unsupervised learning is to develop a representation of the distribution $p(\mathbf{t})$ from which the data were generated. In this paper we consider the problem of modelling $p(\mathbf{t})$ in terms of a number (usually two) of *latent* or *hidden* variables. By considering a particular class of such models we arrive at a formulation in terms of a constrained Gaussian mixture which can be trained using the EM (expectation-maximization) algorithm. The topographic nature of the representation is an intrinsic feature of the model and is not dependent on the details of the learning process. Our model defines a *generative* distribution $p(\mathbf{t})$ and will be referred to as the GTM (*Generative Topographic Mapping*) algorithm (Bishop et al., 1996a).

2 Latent Variables

The goal of a latent variable model is to find a representation for the distribution $p(\mathbf{t})$ of data in a D-dimensional space $\mathbf{t} = (t_1, \ldots, t_D)$ in terms of a number L of latent variables $\mathbf{x} = (x_1, \ldots, x_L)$. This is achieved by first considering a non-linear function $\mathbf{y}(\mathbf{x}; \mathbf{W})$, governed by a set of parameters $\mathbf{W}$, which maps points $\mathbf{x}$ in the latent space into corresponding points $\mathbf{y}(\mathbf{x}; \mathbf{W})$ in the data space. Typically we are interested in the situation in which the dimensionality L of the latent space is less than the dimensionality D of the data space, since our premise is that the data itself has an intrinsic dimensionality which is less than D. The transformation $\mathbf{y}(\mathbf{x}; \mathbf{W})$ then maps the latent space into an L-dimensional non-Euclidean manifold embedded within the data space.

If we define a probability distribution $p(\mathbf{x})$ on the latent space, this will induce a corresponding distribution $p(\mathbf{y}|\mathbf{W})$ in the data space. We shall refer to $p(\mathbf{x})$ as the prior distribution of $\mathbf{x}$ for reasons which will become clear shortly. Since $L < D$, the distribution in $\mathbf{t}$-space would be confined to a manifold of dimension L and hence would be singular. Since in reality the data will only approximately live on a lower-dimensional manifold, it is appropriate to include a noise model for the $\mathbf{t}$ vector. We therefore define the distribution of $\mathbf{t}$, for given $\mathbf{x}$ and $\mathbf{W}$, to be a spherical Gaussian centred on $\mathbf{y}(\mathbf{x}; \mathbf{W})$ having variance β^{-1} so that $p(\mathbf{t}|\mathbf{x}, \mathbf{W}, \beta) \sim \mathcal{N}(\mathbf{t}|\mathbf{y}(\mathbf{x}; \mathbf{W}), \beta^{-1}\mathbf{I})$. The distribution in $\mathbf{t}$-space, for a given value of $\mathbf{W}$, is then obtained by integration over the $\mathbf{x}$-distribution

$$p(\mathbf{t}|\mathbf{W}, \beta) = \int p(\mathbf{t}|\mathbf{x}, \mathbf{W}, \beta) p(\mathbf{x}) \, d\mathbf{x}. \tag{1}$$

For a given a data set $\mathcal{D} = (\mathbf{t}_1, \ldots, \mathbf{t}_N)$ of N data points, we can determine the parameter matrix $\mathbf{W}$, and the inverse variance β, using maximum likelihood, where the log likelihood function is given by

$$L(\mathbf{W}, \beta) = \sum_{n=1}^{N} \ln p(\mathbf{t}_n | \mathbf{W}, \beta). \tag{2}$$

In principle we can now seek the maximum likelihood solution for the weight matrix, once we have specified the prior distribution $p(\mathbf{x})$ and the functional form of the

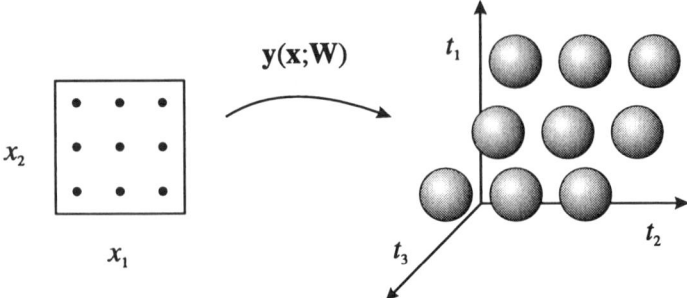

Figure 1: We consider a prior distribution $p(\mathbf{x})$ consisting of a superposition of delta functions, located at the nodes of a regular grid in latent space. Each node $\mathbf{x}_l$ is mapped to a point $\mathbf{y}(\mathbf{x}_l; \mathbf{W})$ in data space, which forms the centre of the corresponding Gaussian distribution.

mapping $\mathbf{y}(\mathbf{x}; \mathbf{W})$, by maximizing $L(\mathbf{W}, \beta)$. The latent variable model can be related to the Kohonen SOM algorithm by choosing $p(\mathbf{x})$ to be a sum of delta functions centred on the nodes of a regular grid in latent space $p(\mathbf{x}) = 1/K \sum_{l=1}^{K} \delta(\mathbf{x} - \mathbf{x}_l)$. This form of $p(\mathbf{x})$ allows the integral in (1) to be performed analytically. Each point $\mathbf{x}_l$ is then mapped to a corresponding point $\mathbf{y}(\mathbf{x}_l; \mathbf{W})$ in data space, which forms the centre of a Gaussian density function, as illustrated in Figure 1. Thus the distribution function in data space takes the form of a Gaussian mixture model $p(\mathbf{t}|\mathbf{W}, \beta) = 1/K \sum_{l=1}^{K} p(\mathbf{t}|\mathbf{x}_l, \mathbf{W}, \beta)$ and the log likelihood function (2) becomes

$$L(\mathbf{W}, \beta) = \sum_{n=1}^{N} \ln \left\{ \frac{1}{K} \sum_{l=1}^{K} p(\mathbf{t}_n|\mathbf{x}_l, \mathbf{W}, \beta) \right\}. \qquad (3)$$

This distribution is a *constrained* Gaussian mixture since the centres of the Gaussians cannot move independently but are related through the function $\mathbf{y}(\mathbf{x}; \mathbf{W})$. Note that, provided the mapping function $\mathbf{y}(\mathbf{x}; \mathbf{W})$ is smooth and continuous, the projected points $\mathbf{y}(\mathbf{x}_l; \mathbf{W})$ will necessarily have a topographic ordering.

2.1 The EM Algorithm

If we choose a particular parametrized form for $\mathbf{y}(\mathbf{x}; \mathbf{W})$ which is a differentiable function of $\mathbf{W}$ we can use standard techniques for non-linear optimization, such as conjugate gradients or quasi-Newton methods, to find a weight matrix $\mathbf{W}^*$, and inverse variance β^*, which maximize $L(\mathbf{W}, \beta)$. However, our model consists of a mixture distribution which suggests that we might seek an EM algorithm (Dempster et al., 1977). By making a careful choice of model $\mathbf{y}(\mathbf{x}; \mathbf{W})$ we will see that the M-step can be solved exactly. In particular we shall choose $\mathbf{y}(\mathbf{x}; \mathbf{W})$ to be given by a generalized linear network model of the form

$$\mathbf{y}(\mathbf{x}; \mathbf{W}) = \mathbf{W}\boldsymbol{\phi}(\mathbf{x}) \qquad (4)$$

where the elements of $\boldsymbol{\phi}(\mathbf{x})$ consist of M fixed basis functions $\phi_j(\mathbf{x})$, and $\mathbf{W}$ is a $D \times M$ matrix with elements w_{kj}. Generalized linear networks possess the same universal approximation capabilities as multi-layer adaptive networks, provided the basis functions $\phi_j(\mathbf{x})$ are chosen appropriately.

By setting the derivatives of (3) with respect to w_{kj} to zero, we obtain

$$\mathbf{\Phi}^T \mathbf{G} \mathbf{\Phi} \mathbf{W}^T = \mathbf{\Phi}^T \mathbf{R} \mathbf{T} \qquad (5)$$

where $\mathbf{\Phi}$ is a $K \times M$ matrix with elements $\Phi_{lj} = \phi_j(\mathbf{x}_l)$, $\mathbf{T}$ is a $N \times D$ matrix with elements t_{kn}, and $\mathbf{R}$ is a $K \times N$ matrix with elements R_{ln} given by

$$R_{ln}(\mathbf{W}, \beta) = \frac{p(\mathbf{t}_n | \mathbf{x}_l, \mathbf{W}, \beta)}{\sum_{l'=1}^{K} p(\mathbf{t}_n | \mathbf{x}_{l'}, \mathbf{W}, \beta)} \qquad (6)$$

which represents the posterior probability, or *responsibility*, of the mixture components l for the data point n. Finally, $\mathbf{G}$ is a $K \times K$ diagonal matrix, with elements $G_{ll} = \sum_{n=1}^{N} R_{ln}(\mathbf{W}, \beta)$. Equation (5) can be solved for $\mathbf{W}$ using standard matrix inversion techniques. Similarly, optimizing with respect to β we obtain

$$\frac{1}{\beta} = \frac{1}{ND} \sum_{l=1}^{K} \sum_{n=1}^{N} R_{ln}(\mathbf{W}, \beta) \| \mathbf{y}(\mathbf{x}_l; \mathbf{W}) - \mathbf{t}_n \|^2 . \qquad (7)$$

Here (6) corresponds to the E-step, while (5) and (7) correspond to the M-step. Typically the EM algorithm gives satisfactory convergence after a few tens of cycles. An on-line version of this algorithm can be obtained by using the Robbins-Monro procedure to find a zero of the objective function gradient, or by using an on-line version of the EM algorithm.

3 Relation to the Self-Organizing Map

The list below describes some of the problems with the SOM procedure and how the GTM algorithm solves them.

1. The SOM algorithm is not derived by optimizing an objective function, unlike GTM. Indeed it has been proven (Erwin et al., 1992) that such an objective function cannot exist for the SOM algorithm.

2. In GTM the neighbourhood-preserving nature of the mapping is an automatic consequence of the choice of a smooth, continuous function $\mathbf{y}(\mathbf{x}; \mathbf{W})$. Neighbourhood-preservation is not guaranteed by the SOM procedure.

3. There is no assurance that the code-book vectors will converge using SOM. Convergence of the batch GTM algorithm is guaranteed by the EM algorithm, and the Robbins-Monro theorem provides a convergence proof for the on-line version.

4. GTM defines an explicit probability density function in data space. In contrast, SOM does not define a density model. Attempts have been made to interpret the density of codebook vectors as a model of the data distribution but with limited success. The advantages of having a density model include the ability to deal with missing data in a principled way, and the straightforward possibility of using a mixture of such models, again trained using EM.

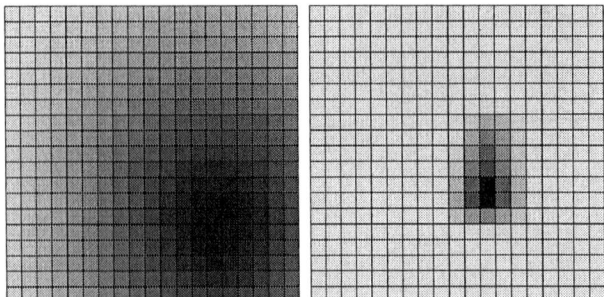

Figure 2: Examples of the posterior probabilities (responsibilities) of the latent space points at an early stage (left) and late stage (right) during the convergence of the GTM algorithm, evaluated for a single data point from the training set in the oil-flow problem discussed in Section 4. Note how the probabilities form a localized 'bubble' whose size shrinks *automatically* during training, in contrast to the hand-crafted shrinkage of the neighbourhood function in the SOM.

5. For SOM the choice of how the neighbourhood function should shrink over time during training is arbitrary, and so this must be optimized empirically. There is no neighbourhood function to select for GTM.

6. It is difficult to know by what criteria to compare different runs of the SOM procedure. For GTM one simply compares the likelihood of the data under the model, and standard statistical tests can be used for model comparison.

Notwithstanding these key differences, there are very close similarities between the SOM and GTM techniques. Figure 2 shows the posterior probabilities (responsibilities) corresponding to the oil flow problem considered in Section 4. At an early stage of training the responsibility for representing a particular data point is spread over a relatively large region of the map. As the EM algorithm proceeds so this responsibility 'bubble' shrinks automatically. The responsibilities (computed in the E-step) govern the updating of $\mathbf{W}$ and β in the M-step and, together with the smoothing effect of the basis functions $\phi_j(\mathbf{x})$, play an analogous role to the neighbourhood function in the SOM procedure. While the SOM neighbourhood function is arbitrary, however, the shrinking responsibility bubble in GTM arises directly from the EM algorithm.

4 Experimental Results

We present results from the application of this algorithm to a problem involving 12-dimensional data arising from diagnostic measurements of oil flows along multiphase pipelines (Bishop and James, 1993). The three phases in the pipe (oil, water and gas) can belong to one of three different geometrical configurations, corresponding to stratified, homogeneous, and annular flows, and the data set consists of 1000 points drawn with equal probability from the 3 classes. We take the latent variable space to be two-dimensional, since our goal in this application is data visualization. Each data point $\mathbf{t}_n$ induces a posterior distribution $p(\mathbf{x}|\mathbf{t}_n, \mathbf{W}, \beta)$ in x-space. However, it is often convenient to project each data point down to a unique point in x-space, which can be done by finding the mean of the posterior distribution.

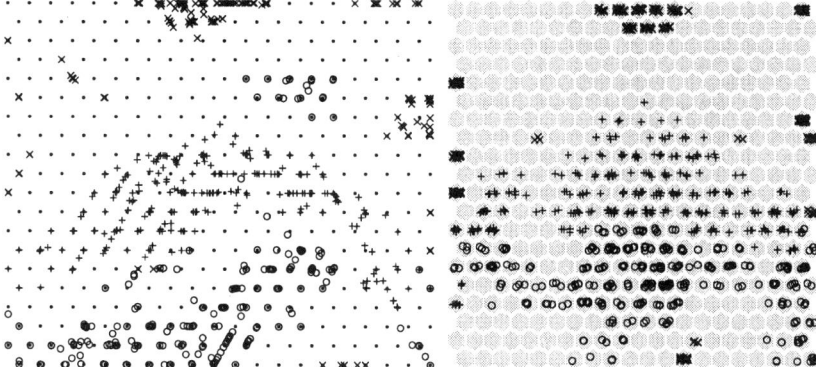

Figure 3: The left plot shows the posterior-mean projection of the oil flow data in the latent space of the non-linear model. The plot on the right shows the same data set visualized using the batch SOM procedure, in which each data point is assigned to the point on the feature map corresponding to the codebook vector to which it is nearest. In both plots, crosses, circles and plus-signs represent the three different oil-flow configurations.

Figure 3 shows the oil data visualized with GTM and SOM. The CPU times taken for the GTM, SOM with a Gaussian neighbourhood, and SOM with a 'top-hat' neighbourhood were 644, 1116 and 355 seconds respectively. In each case the algorithms were run for 25 complete passes through the data set.

5 Discussion

In the fifteen years since the SOM procedure was first proposed, it has been used with great success in a wide variety of applications. It is, however, based on heuristic concepts, rather than statistical principles, and this leads to a number of serious deficiencies in the algorithm. There have been several attempts to provide algorithms which are similar in spirit to the SOM but which overcome its limitations, and it is useful to compare these to the GTM algorithm.

The formulation of the elastic net algorithm described by Durbin et al. (1989) also constitutes a Gaussian mixture model in which the Gaussian centres acquire a spatial ordering during training. The principal difference compared with GTM is that in the elastic net the centres are independent parameters but are encouraged to be spatially close by the use of a quadratic regularization term, whereas in GTM there is no regularizer on the centres and instead the centres are constrained to lie on a manifold given by the non-linear projection of the latent-variable space. The existence of a well-defined manifold means that the local magnification factors can be evaluated explicitly as continuous functions of the latent variables (Bishop et al., 1996b). By contrast, in algorithms such as SOM and the elastic net, the embedded manifold is defined only indirectly as a discrete approximation by the locations of the code-book vectors or Gaussian centres.

One version of the principal curves algorithm (Tibshirani, 1992) introduces a generative distribution based on a mixture of Gaussians, with a well-defined likelihood function, which is trained by the EM algorithm. However, the number of Gaussian components is equal to the number of data points, and the algorithm has been formulated for one-dimensional manifolds, making this algorithm further removed from the SOM.

MacKay (1995) considers convolutional models of the form (1) using multi-layer network models in which a discrete sample from the latent space is interpreted as a Monte Carlo approximation to the integration over a continuous distribution. Although an EM approach could be applied to such a model, the M-step of the corresponding EM algorithm would itself require a non-linear optimization.

In conclusion, we have provided an alternative algorithm to the SOM which overcomes its principal deficiencies while retaining its general characteristics. We know of no significant disadvantage in using the GTM algorithm in place of the SOM. While we believe the SOM procedure is superseded by the GTM algorithm, is should be noted that the SOM has provided much of the inspiration for developing GTM.

A web site for GTM is provided at:

http://www.ncrg.aston.ac.uk/GTM/

which includes postscript files of relevant papers, software implementations in Matlab and C, and example data sets used in the development of the GTM algorithm.

Acknowledgements

This work was supported by EPSRC grant GR/K51808: *Neural Networks for Visualisation of High-Dimensional Data*. Markus Svensén would like to thank the staff of the SANS group in Stockholm for their hospitality during part of this project.

References

Bishop, C. M. and G. D. James (1993). Analysis of multiphase flows using dual-energy gamma densitometry and neural networks. *Nuclear Instruments and Methods in Physics Research* **A327**, 580–593.

Bishop, C. M., M. Svensén, and C. K. I. Williams (1996a). Gtm: The generative topographic mapping. Technical Report NCRG/96/015, Neural Computing Research Group, Aston University, Birmingham, UK. Submitted to Neural Computation.

Bishop, C. M., M. Svensén, and C. K. I. Williams (1996b). Magnification factors for the GTM algorithm. In preparation.

Dempster, A. P., N. M. Laird, and D. B. Rubin (1977). Maximum likelihood from incomplete data via the EM algorithm. *Journal of the Royal Statistical Society, B* **39** (1), 1–38.

Durbin, R., R. Szeliski, and A. Yuille (1989). An analysis of the elastic net approach to the travelling salesman problem. *Neural Computation* **1** (3), 348–358.

Erwin, E., K. Obermayer, and K. Schulten (1992). Self-organizing maps: ordering, convergence properties and energy functions. *Biological Cybernetics* **67**, 47–55.

Kohonen, T. (1982). Self-organized formation of topologically correct feature maps. *Biological Cybernetics* **43**, 59–69.

Kohonen, T. (1995). *Self-Organizing Maps*. Berlin: Springer-Verlag.

MacKay, D. J. C. (1995). Bayesian neural networks and density networks. *Nuclear Instruments and Methods in Physics Research, A* **354** (1), 73–80.

Tibshirani, R. (1992). Principal curves revisited. *Statistics and Computing* **2**, 183–190.

The CONDENSATION algorithm — conditional density propagation and applications to visual tracking

A. Blake and M. Isard*
Department of Engineering Science,
University of Oxford,
Oxford OX1 3PJ, UK.

Abstract

The power of sampling methods in Bayesian reconstruction of noisy signals is well known. The extension of sampling to temporal problems is discussed. Efficacy of sampling over time is demonstrated with visual tracking.

1 INTRODUCTION

The problem of tracking curves in dense visual clutter is a challenging one. Trackers based on Kalman filters are of limited power; because they are based on Gaussian densities which are unimodal they cannot represent simultaneous alternative hypotheses. Extensions to the Kalman filter to handle multiple data associations (Bar-Shalom and Fortmann, 1988) work satisfactorily in the simple case of point targets but do not extend naturally to continuous curves.

Tracking is the propagation of shape and motion estimates over time, driven by a temporal stream of observations. The noisy observations that arise in realistic problems demand a robust approach involving propagation of probability distributions over time. Modest levels of noise may be treated satisfactorily using Gaussian densities, and this is achieved effectively by Kalman filtering (Gelb, 1974). More pervasive noise distributions, as commonly arise in visual background clutter, demand a more powerful, non-Gaussian approach.

One very effective approach is to use random sampling. The CONDENSATION algorithm, described here, combines random sampling with learned dynamical models to propagate an entire probability distribution for object position and shape, over time. The result is accurate tracking of agile motion in clutter, decidedly more

---
*Web: http://www.robots.ox.ac.uk/~ab/

robust than what has previously been attainable by Kalman filtering. Despite the use of random sampling, the algorithm is efficient, running in near real-time when applied to visual tracking.

2 SAMPLING METHODS

A standard problem in statistical pattern recognition is to find an object parameterised as $\mathbf{x}$ with prior $p(\mathbf{x})$, using data $\mathbf{z}$ from a single image. The posterior density $p(\mathbf{x}|\mathbf{z})$ represents all the knowledge about $\mathbf{x}$ that is deducible from the data. It can be evaluated in principle by applying Bayes' rule (Papoulis, 1990) to obtain

$$p(\mathbf{x}|\mathbf{z}) = kp(\mathbf{z}|\mathbf{x})p(\mathbf{x}) \qquad (1)$$

where k is a normalisation constant that is independent of $\mathbf{x}$. However $p(\mathbf{z}|\mathbf{x})$ may become sufficiently complex that $p(\mathbf{x}|\mathbf{z})$ cannot be evaluated simply in closed form. Such complexity arises typically in visual clutter, when the superfluity of observable features tends to suggest multiple, competing hypotheses for $\mathbf{x}$. A one-dimensional illustration of the problem is illustrated in figure 1 in which multiple features give

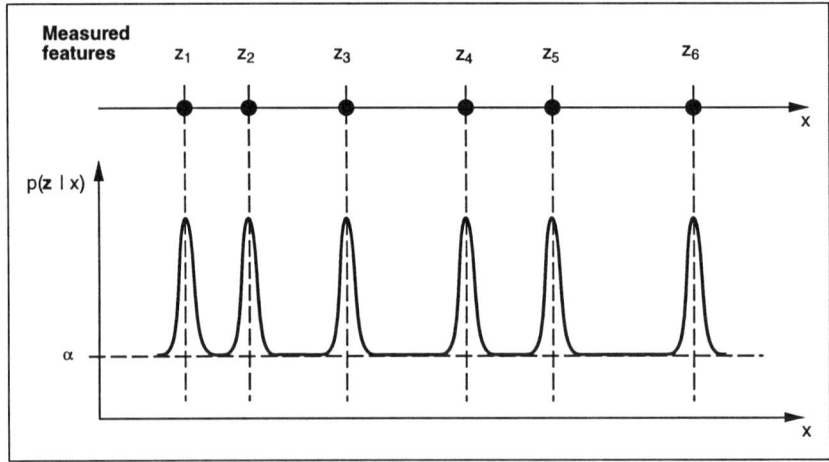

Figure 1: **One-dimensional observation model.** *A probabilistic observation model allowing for clutter and the possibility of missing the target altogether is specified here as a conditional density $p(\mathbf{z}|x)$.*

rise to a multimodal observation density function $p(\mathbf{z}|\mathbf{x})$.

When direct evaluation of $p(\mathbf{x}|\mathbf{z})$ is infeasible, iterative sampling techniques can be used (Geman and Geman, 1984; Ripley and Sutherland, 1990; Grenander et al., 1991; Storvik, 1994). The *factored sampling* algorithm (Grenander et al., 1991). generates a random variate $\mathbf{x}$ from a distribution $\tilde{p}(\mathbf{x})$ that approximates the posterior $p(\mathbf{x}|\mathbf{z})$. First a sample-set $\{\mathbf{s}^{(1)}, \ldots, \mathbf{s}^{(N)}\}$ is generated from the prior density $p(\mathbf{x})$ and then a sample $\mathbf{x} = \mathbf{x}_i$, $i \in \{1, \ldots, N\}$ is chosen with probability

$$\pi_i = \frac{p(\mathbf{z}|\mathbf{x} = \mathbf{s}^{(i)})}{\sum_{j=1}^{N} p(\mathbf{z}|\mathbf{x} = \mathbf{s}^{(j)})}.$$

Sampling methods have proved remarkably effective for recovering static objects from cluttered images. For such problems $\mathbf{x}$ is multi-dimensional, a set of parameters for curve position and shape. In that case the sample-set $\{\mathbf{s}^{(1)}, \ldots, \mathbf{s}^{(N)}\}$ represents a distribution of **x**-values which can be seen as a distribution of curves in the image plane, as in figure 2.

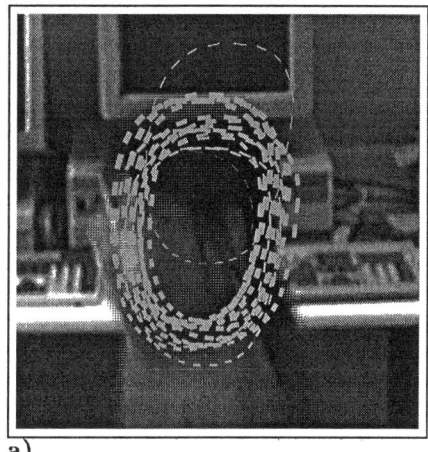
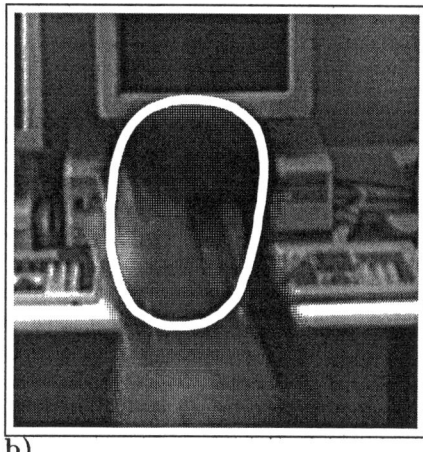

Figure 2: **Sample-set representation of shape distributions** *for a curve with parameters* **x**, *modelling the outline (a) of the head of a dancing girl. Each sample* $s^{(n)}$ *is shown as a curve (of varying position and shape) with a thickness proportional to the weight* $\pi^{(n)}$. *The weighted mean of the sample set (b) serves as an estimator of mean shape*

3 THE CONDENSATION ALGORITHM

The CONDENSATION algorithm is based on factored sampling but extended to apply iteratively to successive images in a sequence. Similar sampling strategies have appeared elsewhere (Gordon et al., 1993; Kitigawa, 1996), presented as developments of Monte-Carlo methods. The methods outlined here are described in detail elsewhere. Fuller descriptions and derivation of the CONDENSATION algorithm are in (Isard and Blake, 1996; Blake and Isard, 1997) and details of the learning of dynamical models, which is crucial to the effective operation of the algorithm are in (Blake et al., 1995).

Given that the estimation process at each time-step is a self-contained iteration of factored sampling, the output of an iteration will be a weighted, time-stamped sample-set, denoted $s_t^{(n)}$, $n = 1, \ldots, N$ with weights $\pi_t^{(n)}$, representing approximately the conditional state-density $p(\mathbf{x}_t|\mathcal{Z}_t)$ at time t, where $\mathcal{Z}_t = (\mathbf{z}_1, \ldots, \mathbf{z}_t)$. How is this sample-set obtained? Clearly the process must begin with a prior density and the effective prior for time-step t should be $p(\mathbf{x}_t|\mathcal{Z}_{t-1})$. This prior is of course multi-modal in general and no functional representation of it is available. It is derived from the sample set representation $(s_{t-1}^{(n)}, \pi_{t-1}^{(n)})$, $n = 1, \ldots, N$ of $p(\mathbf{x}_{t-1}|\mathcal{Z}_{t-1})$, the output from the previous time-step, to which prediction must then be applied.

The iterative process applied to the sample-sets is depicted in figure 3. At the top of the diagram, the output from time-step $t - 1$ is the weighted sample-set $\{(s_{t-1}^{(n)}, \pi_{t-1}^{(n)}), n = 1, \ldots, N\}$. The aim is to maintain, at successive time-steps, sample sets of fixed size N, so that the algorithm can be guaranteed to run within a given computational resource. The first operation therefore is to sample (with

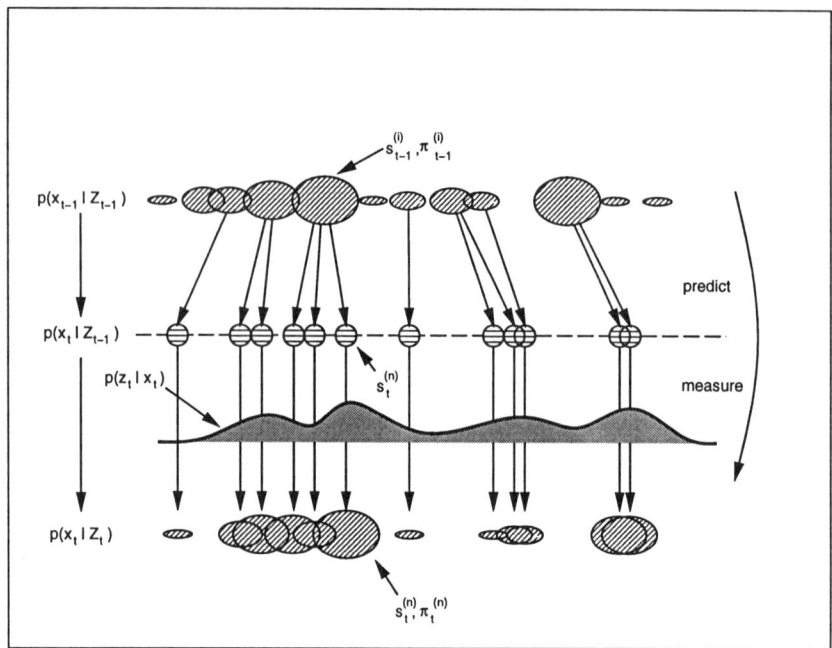

Figure 3: **One time-step in the CONDENSATION algorithm.** *Blob centres represent sample values and sizes depict sample weights.*

replacement) N times from the set $\{s_{t-1}^{(n)}\}$, choosing a given element with probability $\pi_{t-1}^{(n)}$. Some elements, especially those with high weights, may be chosen several times, leading to identical copies of elements in the new set. Others with relatively low weights may not be chosen at all.

Each element chosen from the new set is now subjected to a predictive step. (The dynamical model we generally use for prediction is a linear stochastic differential equation (s.d.e.) learned from training sets of sample object motion (Blake et al., 1995).) The predictive step includes a random component, so identical elements may now split as each undergoes its own independent random motion step. At this stage, the sample set $\{s_t^{(n)}\}$ for the new time-step has been generated but, as yet, without its weights; it is approximately a fair random sample from the effective prior density $p(\mathbf{x}_t|\mathcal{Z}_{t-1})$ for time-step t. Finally, the observation step from factored sampling is applied, generating weights from the observation density $p(\mathbf{z}_t|\mathbf{x}_t)$ to obtain the sample-set representation $\{(s_t^{(n)}, \pi_t^{(n)})\}$ of state-density for time t.

The algorithm is specified in detail in figure 4. The process for a single time-step consists of N iterations to generate the N elements of the new sample set. Each iteration has three steps, detailed in the figure, and we comment below on each.

1. **Select** nth new sample $s_t'^{(n)}$ to be some $s_{t-1}^{(j)}$ from the old sample set, sampled with replacement with probability $\pi_{t-1}^{(j)}$. This is achieved efficiently by using *cumulative* weights $c_{t-1}^{(j)}$ (constructed in step 3).

2. **Predict** by sampling randomly from the conditional density for the dynamical model to generate a sample for the new sample-set.

3. **Measure** in order to generate weights $\pi_t^{(n)}$ for the new sample. Each weight

is evaluated from the observation density function which, being multimodal in general, "infuses" multimodality into the state density.

Iterate

From the "old" sample-set $\{s_{t-1}^{(n)}, \pi_{t-1}^{(n)}, c_{t-1}^{(n)}, n = 1, \ldots, N\}$ at time-step $t - 1$, construct a "new" sample-set $\{s_t^{(n)}, \pi_t^{(n)}, c_t^{(n)}\}, n = 1, \ldots, N$ for time t.

Construct the nth of N new samples as follows:

1. **Select** a sample $s_t'^{(n)}$ as follows:
   (a) generate a random number $r \in [0, 1]$, uniformly distributed.
   (b) find, by binary subdivision, the smallest j for which $c_{t-1}^{(j)} \geq r$
   (c) set $s_t'^{(n)} = s_{t-1}^{(j)}$

2. **Predict** by sampling from
$$p(\mathbf{x}_t | \mathbf{x}_{t-1} = s'^{(n)}_{t-1})$$
to choose each $s_t^{(n)}$.

3. **Measure** and weight the new position in terms of the measured features $\mathbf{z}_t$:
$$\pi_t^{(n)} = p(\mathbf{z}_t | \mathbf{x}_t = s_t^{(n)})$$
then normalise so that $\sum_n \pi_t^{(n)} = 1$ and store together with cumulative probability as $(s_t^{(n)}, \pi_t^{(n)}, c_t^{(n)})$ where
$$c_t^{(0)} = 0,$$
$$c_t^{(n)} = c_t^{(n-1)} + \pi_t^{(n)} \quad (n = 1 \ldots N).$$

Figure 4: The CONDENSATION algorithm.

At any time-step, it is possible to "report" on the current state, for example by evaluating some moment of the state density as

$$\mathcal{E}[f(\mathbf{x}_t)] = \sum_{n=1}^{N} \pi_t^{(n)} f\left(s_t^{(n)}\right). \qquad (2)$$

4 RESULTS

A good deal of experimentation has been performed in applying the CONDENSATION algorithm to the tracking of visual motion, including moving hands and dancing figures. Perhaps one of the most stringent tests was the tracking of a leaf on a bush, in which the foreground leaf is effectively camouflaged against the background.

A 12 second (600 field) sequence shows a bush blowing in the wind, the task being to track one particular leaf. A template was drawn by hand around a still of one chosen leaf and allowed to undergo affine deformations during tracking. Given that a clutter-free training sequence is not available, the motion model was learned by means of a bootstrap procedure (Blake et al., 1995). A tracker with default dynamics proved capable of tracking the first 150 fields of a training sequence before losing the leaf, and those tracked positions allowed a first approximation to the model to be learned. Installing that in a CONDENSATION tracker, the entire sequence could be tracked, though with occasional misalignments. Finally a third learned model was sufficient to track accurately the entire 12-second training sequence. Despite occasional violent gusts of wind and temporary obscuration by another leaf, the CONDENSATION algorithm successfully followed the object. In fact, tracking is accurate enough using $N = 1200$ samples to separate the foreground leaf from the background reliably, an effect which can otherwise only be achieved using "bluescreening". Having obtained the model iteratively as above, independent test sequences could be tracked without further training. With $N = 1200$ samples per time-step the tracker runs at 6.5 Hz on a SGI Indy SC4400 200MHz workstation. Reducing this to $N = 200$ increases processing speed to video frame-rate (25 Hz), at the cost of occasional misalignments in the mean configuration of the contour.

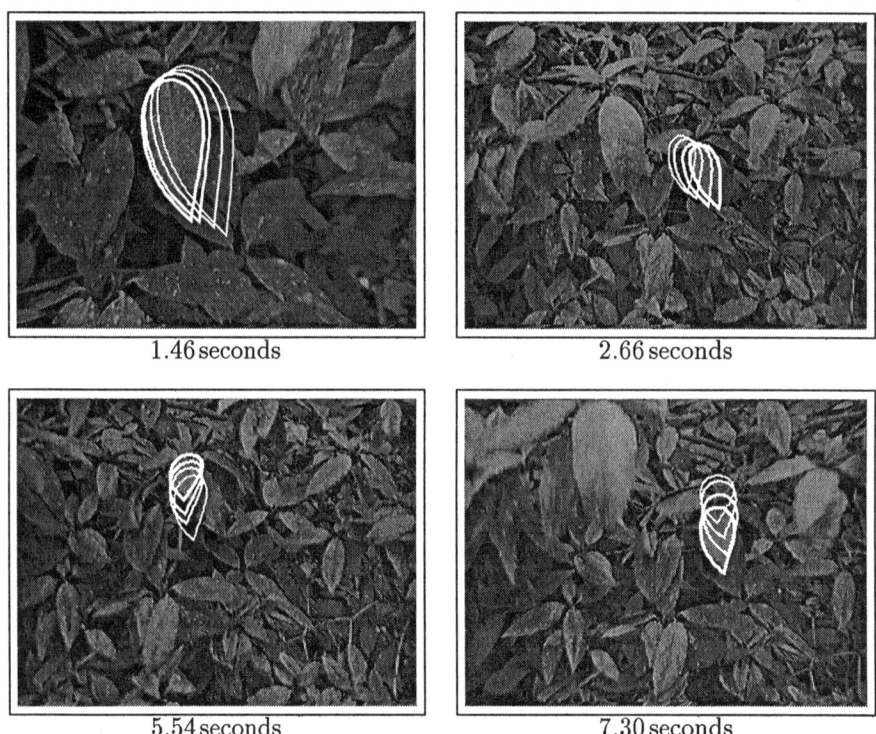

Figure 5: **Tracking with camouflage.** *Stills depict mean contour configurations, with preceding tracked leaf positions plotted at 40 ms intervals to indicate motion.*

5 CONCLUSIONS

Tracking in clutter is hard because of the essential multi-modality of the conditional observation density $p(z|x)$. In the case of curves multiple-hypothesis tracking is inapplicable and a new approach is needed. The CONDENSATION algorithm is a fusion of the statistical factored sampling algorithm for static, non-Gaussian problems with a stochastic model for object motion. The result is an algorithm for tracking rigid and non-rigid motion which has been demonstrated to be far more effective in clutter than comparable Kalman filters (Blake et al., 1993).

The new approach raises a number of questions. One is how densities represented as sample sets can be interrogated in a more general way than simply computing their moments as in (2). For example it is often desirable to locate local modes in the state density, representing leading hypotheses. We are seeking therefore to construct a satisfactory theory of "operators" to interrogate densities in a more general fashion.

Secondly, it is striking that the density propagation equation in the CONDENSATION algorithm is a continuous form of the propagation rule of the "forward algorithm" for Hidden Markov Models (HMMs) (Rabiner and Bing-Hwang, 1993). This suggests the use of mixed discrete/continuous states, propagating over time. Mixed states would allow switching between multiple models, for instance walk-trot-canter-gallop, each model represented by a stochastic differential equation, with transitions governed by a discrete conditional probability matrix.

Acknowledgements

The authors would like to acknowledge the support of the EPSRC. They are also grateful for discussions with Roger Brockett and David Reynard.

References

Bar-Shalom, Y. and Fortmann, T. (1988). *Tracking and Data Association*. Academic Press.

Blake, A., Curwen, R., and Zisserman, A. (1993). A framework for spatio-temporal control in the tracking of visual contours. *Int. Journal of Computer Vision*, 11(2):127–145.

Blake, A. and Isard, M. (1994). 3D position, attitude and shape input using video tracking of hands and lips. In *Proc. Siggraph* 185–192. ACM.

Blake, A. and Isard, M. (1997). Condensation — conditional density propagation for visual tracking. *Int. Journal of Computer Vision*, in press.

Blake, A., Isard, M., and Reynard, D. (1995). Learning to track the visual motion of contours. *Artificial Intelligence*, 78:101–134.

Gelb, A., editor (1974). *Applied Optimal Estimation*. MIT Press, Cambridge, MA.

Geman, S. and Geman, D. (1984). Stochastic Relaxation, Gibbs Distributions, and the Bayesian Restoration of Images. *IEEE Trans. Pattern Analysis and Machine Intelligence*, 6(6):721–741.

Gordon, N., Salmond, D., and Smith, A. (1993). Novel approach to nonlinear/non-gaussian bayesian state estimation. *IEE Proc. F*, 140(2):107–113.

Grenander, U., Chow, Y., and Keenan, D. M. (1991). *HANDS. A Pattern Theoretical Study of Biological Shapes*. Springer-Verlag. New York.

Isard, M. and Blake, A. (1996). Visual tracking by stochastic propagation of conditional density. In *Proc. 4th European Conf. on Computer Vision* 343–356, Cambridge, England.

Kitigawa, G. (1996). Monte-carlo filter and smoother for non-Gaussian nonlinear state space models. *J. Computational and Graphical Statistics*, 5(1):1–25.

Papoulis, A. (1990). *Probability and Statistics*. Prentice-Hall.

Rabiner, L. and Bing-Hwang, J. (1993). *Fundamentals of speech recognition*. Prentice-Hall.

Ripley, B. and Sutherland, A. (1990). Finding spiral structures in images of galaxies. *Phil. Trans. R. Soc. Lond. A.*, 332(1627):477–485.

Storvik, G. (1994). A Bayesian approach to dynamic contours through stochastic sampling and simulated annealing. *IEEE Trans. Pattern Analysis and Machine Intelligence*, 16(10):976–986.

Clustering via Concave Minimization

P. S. Bradley and O. L. Mangasarian
Computer Sciences Department
University of Wisconsin
1210 West Dayton Street
Madison, WI 53706
email: *paulb@cs.wisc.edu, olvi@cs.wisc.edu*

W. N. Street
Computer Science Department
Oklahoma State University
205 Mathematical Sciences
Stillwater, OK 74078
email:*nstreet@cs.okstate.edu*

Abstract

The problem of assigning m points in the n-dimensional real space R^n to k clusters is formulated as that of determining k centers in R^n such that the sum of distances of each point to the nearest center is minimized. If a polyhedral distance is used, the problem can be formulated as that of minimizing a piecewise-linear concave function on a polyhedral set which is shown to be equivalent to a bilinear program: minimizing a bilinear function on a polyhedral set. A fast finite k-Median Algorithm consisting of solving few linear programs in closed form leads to a stationary point of the bilinear program. Computational testing on a number of real-world databases was carried out. On the Wisconsin Diagnostic Breast Cancer (WDBC) database, k-Median training set correctness was comparable to that of the k-Mean Algorithm, however its testing set correctness was better. Additionally, on the Wisconsin Prognostic Breast Cancer (WPBC) database, distinct and clinically important survival curves were extracted by the k-Median Algorithm, whereas the k-Mean Algorithm failed to obtain such distinct survival curves for the same database.

1 Introduction

The unsupervised assignment of elements of a given set to groups or clusters of like points, is the objective of cluster analysis. There are many approaches to this problem, including statistical [9], machine learning [7], integer and mathematical programming [18, 1]. In this paper we concentrate on a simple concave minimization formulation of the problem that leads to a finite and fast algorithm. Our point of departure is the following explicit description of the problem: given m points in the n-dimensional real space R^n, and a fixed number k of clusters, determine k centers in R^n such that the sum of "distances" of each point to the nearest center is minimized. If the 1-norm is used, the problem can be formulated as the minimization of a piecewise-linear concave function on a polyhedral set. This is a hard problem to solve because a local minimum is not necessarily a global minimum. However, by converting this problem to a bilinear program, a fast successive-linearization k-Median Algorithm terminates after a few linear programs (each explicitly solvable in closed form) at a point satisfying the minimum principle necessary optimality condition for the problem. Although there is no guarantee that such a point is a global solution to our original problem, numerical tests on five real-world databases indicate that the k-Median Algorithm is comparable to or better than the k-Mean Algorithm [18, 9, 8]. This may be due to the fact that outliers have less influence on the k-Median Algorithm which utilizes the 1-norm distance. In contrast the k-Mean Algorithm uses squares of 2-norm distances to generate cluster centers which may be inaccurate if outliers are present. We also note that clustering algorithms based on statistical assumptions that minimize some function of scatter matrices do not appear to have convergence proofs [8, pp. 508-515], however convergence to a partial optimal solution is given in [18] for k-Mean type algorithms.

We outline now the contents of the paper. In Section 2, we formulate the clustering problem for a fixed number of clusters, as that of minimizing the sum of the 1-norm distances of each point to the nearest cluster center. This piecewise-linear concave function minimization on a polyhedral set turns out to be equivalent to a bilinear program [3]. We use an effective linearization of the bilinear program proposed in [3, Algorithm 2.1] to solve our problem by solving a few linear programs. Because of the simple structure, these linear programs can be explicitly solved in closed form, thus leading to the finite k-Median Algorithm 2.3 below. In Section 3 we give computational results on five real-world databases. Section 4 concludes the paper.

A word about our notation now. All vectors are column vectors unless otherwise specified. For a vector $x \in R^n$, x_i, $i = 1, \ldots, n$, will denote its components. The norm $\|\cdot\|_p$ will denote the p norm, $1 \leq p \leq \infty$, while $A \in R^{m \times n}$ will signify a real $m \times n$ matrix. For such a matrix, A^T will denote the transpose, and A_i will denote row i. A vector of ones in a real space of arbitrary dimension will be denoted by e.

2 Clustering as Bilinear Programming

Given a set $\mathcal{A}$ of m points in R^n represented by the matrix $A \in R^{m \times n}$ and a number k of desired clusters, we formulate the clustering problem as follows. Find cluster centers C_ℓ, $\ell = 1, \ldots, k$, in R^n such that the sum of the minima over $\ell \in \{1, \ldots, k\}$ of the 1-norm distance between each point A_i, $i = 1, \ldots, m$, and the cluster centers C_ℓ, $\ell = 1, \ldots, k$, is minimized. More specifically we need to solve the following mathematical program:

$$\begin{aligned}
& \underset{C,D}{\text{minimize}} && \sum_{i=1}^{m} \min_{\ell=1,\ldots,k} \{e^T D_{i\ell}\} \\
& \text{subject to} && -D_{i\ell} \leq A_i^T - C_\ell \leq D_{i\ell},\ i = 1, \ldots, m,\ \ell = 1, \ldots k
\end{aligned} \quad (1)$$

Here $D_{i\ell} \in R^n$, is a dummy variable that bounds the components of the difference

$A_i^T - C_\ell$ between point A_i^T and center C_ℓ, and e is a vector of ones in R^n. Hence $e^T D_{i\ell}$ bounds the 1-norm distance between A_i and C_ℓ. We note immediately that since the objective function of (1) is the sum of minima of k linear (and hence concave) functions, it is a piecewise-linear concave function [13, Corollary 4.1.14]. If the 2-norm or p-norm, $p \neq 1, \infty$, is used, the objective function will be neither concave nor convex. Nevertheless, minimizing a piecewise-linear concave function on a polyhedral set is NP-hard, because the general linear complementarity problem, which is NP-complete [4], can be reduced to such a problem [11, Lemma 1]. Given this fact we try to look for effective methods for processing this problem. We propose reformulation of problem (1) as a bilinear program. Such reformulations have been very effective in computationally solving NP-complete linear complementarity problems [14] as well as other difficult machine learning [12] and optimization problems with equilibrium constraints [12]. In order to carry out this reformulation we need the following simple lemma.

Lemma 2.1 Let $a \in R^k$. Then

$$\min_{1 \leq \ell \leq k} \{a_\ell\} = \min_{t \in R^k} \left\{ \sum_{\ell=1}^{k} a_\ell t_\ell \,\middle|\, \sum_{\ell=1}^{k} t_\ell = 1,\, t_\ell \geq 0,\, \ell = 1,\ldots,k \right\} \qquad (2)$$

Proof This essentially obvious result follows immediately upon writing the dual of the linear program appearing on the right-hand side of (2) which is

$$\max_{h \in R} \{h \mid h \leq a_\ell,\, \ell = 1, \ldots k\} \qquad (3)$$

Obviously, the maximum of this dual problem is $h = \min_{1 \leq \ell \leq k}\{a_\ell\}$. By linear programming duality theory, this maximum equals the minimum of the primal linear program in the right hand side of (2). This establishes the equality of (2). □

By defining $a_\ell^i = e^T D_{i\ell}$, $i = 1,\ldots, m$, $\ell = 1, \ldots, k$, Lemma 2.1 can be used to reformulate the clustering problem (1) as a bilinear program as follows.

Proposition 2.2 Clustering as a Bilinear Program *The clustering problem (1) is equivalent to the following bilinear program:*

$$\begin{array}{ll}
\underset{C_\ell \in R^n,\, D_{i\ell} \in R^n,\, T_{i\ell} \in R}{\text{minimize}} & \sum_{i=1}^{m} \sum_{\ell=1}^{k} e^T D_{i\ell} T_{i\ell} \\
\text{subject to} & -D_{i\ell} \leq A_i^T - C_\ell \leq D_{i\ell},\, i = 1\ldots, m,\, \ell = 1, \ldots, k \\
& \sum_{\ell=1}^{k} T_{i\ell} = 1 \quad T_{i\ell} \geq 0,\, i = 1,\ldots, m,\, \ell = 1,\ldots, k
\end{array} \qquad (4)$$

Note that the constraints of (4) are uncoupled in the variables (C, D) and the variable T. Hence the Uncoupled Bilinear Program Algorithm UBPA [3, Algorithm 2.1] is applicable. Simply stated, this algorithm alternates between solving a linear program in the variable T and a linear program in the variables (C, D). The algorithm terminates in a finite number of iterations at a stationary point satisfying the minimum principle necessary optimality condition for problem (4) [3, Theorem 2.1]. We note however, because of the simple structure the bilinear program (4), the two linear programs can be solved explicitly in closed form. This leads to the following algorithmic implementation.

Algorithm 2.3 k-Median Algorithm *Given $C_1^j, \ldots, C_k^j$ at iteration j, compute $C_1^{j+1}, \ldots, C_k^{j+1}$ by the following two steps:*

(a) **Cluster Assignment:** *For each A_i^T, $i = 1, \ldots m$, determine $\ell(i)$ such that $C_{\ell(i)}^j$ is closest to A_i^T in the 1-norm.*

(b) **Cluster Center Update:** *For $\ell = 1, \ldots, k$ choose C_ℓ^{j+1} as a median of all A_i^T assigned to C_ℓ^j.*

Stop when $C_\ell^{j+1} = C_\ell^j$, $\ell = 1, \ldots, k$.

Although the k-Median Algorithm is similar to the k-Mean Algorithm wherein the 2-norm distance is used [18, 8, 9], it differs from it computationally, and theoretically. In fact, the underlying problem (1) of the k-Median Algorithm is a concave minimization on a polyhedral set while the corresponding problem for the p-norm, $p \neq 1$, is:

$$\underset{C,D}{\text{minimize}} \quad \sum_{i=1}^{m} \min_{\ell=1,\ldots,k} \|D_{i\ell}\|_p \tag{5}$$
$$\text{subject to} \quad -D_{i\ell} \leq A_i^T - C_\ell \leq D_{i\ell}, i = 1 \ldots, m, \ \ell = 1, \ldots, k.$$

This is not a concave minimization on a polyhedral set, because the minimum of a set of convex functions is not in general concave. The concave minimization problem of [18] is not in the original space of the problem variables, that is, the cluster center variables, (C, D), but merely in the space of variables T that assign points to clusters. We also note that the k-Mean Algorithm finds a stationary point not of problem (5) with $p = 2$, but of the same problem except that $\|D_{i\ell}\|_2$ is replaced by $\|D_{i\ell}\|_2^2$. Without this squared distance term, the subproblem of the k-Mean Algorithm becomes the considerably harder Weber problem [17, 5] which locates a center in R^n closest in sum of Euclidean distances (not their squares!) to a finite set of given points. The Weber problem has no closed form solution. However, using the mean as a cluster center of points assigned to the cluster, minimizes the sum of the *squares* of the distances from the cluster center to the points. It is precisely the mean that is used in the k-Mean Algorithm subproblem.

Because there is no guaranteed way to ensure global optimality of the solution obtained by either the k-Median or k-Mean Algorithms, different starting points can be used to initiate the algorithm. Random starting cluster centers or some other heuristic can be used such as placing k initial centers along the coordinate axes at densest, second densest, ..., k densest intervals on the axes.

3 Computational Results

An important computational issue is how to measure the correctness of the results obtained by the proposed algorithm. We decided on the following three ways.

Remark 3.1 Training Set Correctness *The k-Median algorithm ($k = 2$) is applied to a database with two known classes to obtain centers. Training correctness is measured by the ratio of the sum of the number examples of the majority class in each cluster to the total number of points in the database. The k-Median training set correctness is compared to that of the k-Mean Algorithm as well as the training correctness of a supervised learning method, a perceptron trained by robust linear programming [2]. Table 1 shows results averaged over ten random starts for the* publicly available Wisconsin Diagnostic Breast Cancer (WDBC) database as well as three others [15, 16]. We note that for two of the databases k-Median outperformed k-Mean, and for the other two k-Mean was better.

Algorithm ↓ Database →	WDBC	Cleveland	Votes	Star/Galaxy-Bright
Unsupervised k-Median	93.2%	80.6%	84.6%	87.6%
Unsupervised k-Mean	91.1%	83.1%	85.5%	85.6%
Supervised Robust LP	100%	86.5%	95.6%	99.7%

Table 1 Training set correctness using the unsupervised k-Median and k-Mean Algorithms and the supervised Robust LP on four databases

Remark 3.2 Testing Set Correctness

The idea behind this approach is that supervised learning may be costly due to problem size, difficulty in obtaining true classification, etc., hence the importance of good performance of an unsupervised learning algorithm on a testing subset of a database. The WDBC database [15] is split into training and testing subsets of different proportions. The k-Median and k-Mean Algorithms ($k = 2$) are applied to the training subset. The centers are given class labels determined by the majority class of training subset points assigned to the cluster. Class labels are assigned to the testing subset by the label of the closest center. Testing correctness is determined by the number of points in testing subset correctly classified by this assignment. This is compared to the correctness of a supervised learning method, a perceptron trained via robust linear programming [2], using the leave-one-out strategy applied to the testing subset only. This comparison is then carried out for various sizes of the testing subset. Figure 1 shows the results averaged over 50 runs for each of 7 testing subset sizes. As expected, the performance of the supervised learning algorithm (Robust LP) improved as the size of the testing subset increases. The k-Median Algorithm test set correctness remained fairly constant in the range of 92.3% to 93.5%, while the k-Mean Algorithm test set correctness was lower and more varied in the range 88.0% to 91.3%.

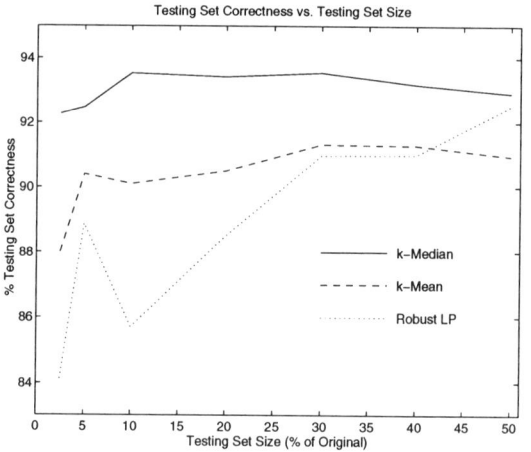

Figure 1: Correctness on variable-size test set of unsupervised k-Median & k-Mean Algorithms versus correctness of the supervised Robust LP on WDBC

Remark 3.3 Separability of Survival Curves
In mining medical databases, survival curves [10] are important prognostic tools. We applied the k-Median and k-Mean ($k = 3$) Algorithms, as knowledge discovery in database (KDD) tools [6], to the Wisconsin Prognostic Breast Cancer Database (WPBC) [15] using only two features: tumor size and lymph node status. Survival curves were constructed for

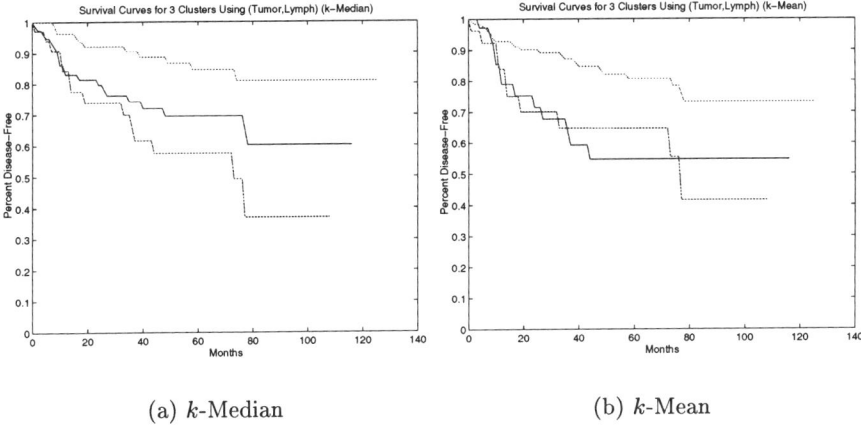

(a) k-Median (b) k-Mean

Figure 2: Survival curves for the 3 clusters obtained by k-Median and k-Mean Algorithms

each cluster, representing expected percent of surviving patients as a function of time, for patients in that cluster. Figure 2(a) depicts the survival curves from clusters obtained from the k-Median Algorithm, Figure 2(b) depicts curves for the k-Mean Algorithm. The key observation to make here is that curves in Figure 2(a) are well separated, and hence the clusters can be used as prognostic indicators. In contrast, the curves in Figure 2(b) are poorly separated, and hence are not useful for prognosis.

4 Conclusion

We have proposed a new approach for assigning points to clusters based on a simple concave minimization model. Although a global solution to the problem cannot be guaranteed, a finite and simple k-Median Algorithm quickly locates a very useful stationary point. Utility of the proposed algorithm lies in its ability to handle large databases and hence would be a useful tool for data mining. Comparing it with the k-Mean Algorithm, we have exhibited instances where the k-Median Algorithm is superior, and hence preferable. Further research is needed to pinpoint types of problems for which the k-Median Algorithm is best.

5 Acknowledgements

Our colleague Jude Shavlik suggested the testing set strategy used in Remark 3.2. This research is supported by National Science Foundation Grants CCR-9322479 and National Institutes of Health INRSA Fellowship 1 F32 CA 68690-01.

References

[1] K. Al-Sultan. A Tabu search approach to the clustering problem. *Pattern Recognition*, 28(9):1443–1451, 1995.

[2] K. P. Bennett and O. L. Mangasarian. Robust linear programming discrimination of two linearly inseparable sets. *Optimization Methods and Software*, 1:23–34, 1992.

[3] K. P. Bennett and O. L. Mangasarian. Bilinear separation of two sets in n-space. *Computational Optimization & Applications*, 2:207–227, 1993.

[4] S.-J. Chung. NP-completeness of the linear complementarity problem. *Journal of Optimization Theory and Applications*, 60:393–399, 1989.

[5] F. Cordellier and J. Ch. Fiorot. On the Fermat-Weber problem with convex cost functionals. *Mathematical Programming*, 14:295–311, 1978.

[6] U. Fayyad, G. Piatetsky-Shapiro, and P. Smyth. The KDD process for extracting useful knowledge from volumes of data. *Communications of the ACM*, 39:27–34, 1996.

[7] D. Fisher. Knowledge acquisition via incremental conceptual clustering. *Machine Learning*, 2:139–172, 1987.

[8] K. Fukunaga. *Statistical Pattern Recognition*. Academic Press, NY, 1990.

[9] A. K. Jain and R. C. Dubes. *Algorithms for Clustering Data*. Prentice-Hall, Inc, Englewood Cliffs, NJ, 1988.

[10] E. L. Kaplan and P. Meier. Nonparametric estimation from incomplete observations. *J. Am. Stat. Assoc.*, 53:457–481, 1958.

[11] O. L. Mangasarian. Characterization of linear complementarity problems as linear programs. *Mathematical Programming Study*, 7:74–87, 1978.

[12] O. L. Mangasarian. Misclassification minimization. *Journal of Global Optimization*, 5:309–323, 1994.

[13] O. L. Mangasarian. *Nonlinear Programming*. SIAM, Philadelphia, PA, 1994.

[14] O. L. Mangasarian. The linear complementarity problem as a separable bilinear program. *Journal of Global Optimization*, 6:153–161, 1995.

[15] P. M. Murphy and D. W. Aha. UCI repository of machine learning databases. Department of Information and Computer Science, University of California, Irvine, www.ics.uci.edu/AI/ML/MLDBRepository.html, 1992.

[16] S. Odewahn, E. Stockwell, R. Pennington, R. Hummphreys, and W. Zumach. Automated star/galaxy discrimination with neural networks. *Astronomical Journal*, 103(1):318–331, 1992.

[17] M. L. Overton. A quadratically convergent method for minimizing a sum of euclidean norms. *Mathematical Programming*, 27:34–63, 1983.

[18] S. Z. Selim and M. A. Ismail. K-Means-Type algorithms: a generalized convergence theorem and characterization of local optimality. *IEEE Transactions on Pattern Analysis and Machine Intelligence*, PAMI-6:81–87, 1984.

Improving the Accuracy and Speed of Support Vector Machines

Chris J.C. Burges
Bell Laboratories
Lucent Technologies, Room 3G429
101 Crawford's Corner Road
Holmdel, NJ 07733-3030
burges@bell-labs.com

Bernhard Schölkopf*
Max–Planck–Institut für
biologische Kybernetik,
Spemannstr. 38
72076 Tübingen, Germany
bs@mpik-tueb.mpg.de

Abstract

Support Vector Learning Machines (SVM) are finding application in pattern recognition, regression estimation, and operator inversion for ill-posed problems. Against this very general backdrop, any methods for improving the generalization performance, or for improving the speed in test phase, of SVMs are of increasing interest. In this paper we combine two such techniques on a pattern recognition problem. The method for improving generalization performance (the "virtual support vector" method) does so by incorporating known invariances of the problem. This method achieves a drop in the error rate on 10,000 NIST test digit images of 1.4% to 1.0%. The method for improving the speed (the "reduced set" method) does so by approximating the support vector decision surface. We apply this method to achieve a factor of fifty speedup in test phase over the virtual support vector machine. The combined approach yields a machine which is both 22 times faster than the original machine, and which has better generalization performance, achieving 1.1% error. The virtual support vector method is applicable to any SVM problem with known invariances. The reduced set method is applicable to any support vector machine.

1 INTRODUCTION

Support Vector Machines are known to give good results on pattern recognition problems despite the fact that they do not incorporate problem domain knowledge.

---

*Part of this work was done while B.S. was with AT&T Research, Holmdel, NJ.

However, they exhibit classification speeds which are substantially slower than those of neural networks (LeCun et al., 1995).

The present study is motivated by the above two observations. First, we shall improve accuracy by incorporating knowledge about invariances of the problem at hand. Second, we shall increase classification speed by reducing the complexity of the decision function representation. This paper thus brings together two threads explored by us during the last year (Schölkopf, Burges & Vapnik, 1996; Burges, 1996).

The method for incorporating invariances is applicable to any problem for which the data is expected to have known symmetries. The method for improving the speed is applicable to any support vector machine. Thus we expect these methods to be widely applicable to problems beyond pattern recognition (for example, to the regression estimation problem (Vapnik, Golowich & Smola, 1996)).

After a brief overview of Support Vector Machines in Section 2, we describe how problem domain knowledge was used to improve generalization performance in Section 3. Section 4 contains an overview of a general method for improving the classification speed of Support Vector Machines. Results are collected in Section 5. We conclude with a discussion.

2 SUPPORT VECTOR LEARNING MACHINES

This Section summarizes those properties of Support Vector Machines (SVM) which are relevant to the discussion below. For details on the basic SVM approach, the reader is referred to (Boser, Guyon & Vapnik, 1992; Cortes & Vapnik, 1995; Vapnik, 1995). We end by noting a physical analogy.

Let the training data be elements $\mathbf{x}_i \in \mathcal{L}, \mathcal{L} = \mathbf{R}^d, i = 1, \ldots, \ell$, with corresponding class labels $y_i \in \{\pm 1\}$. An SVM performs a mapping $\Phi : \mathcal{L} \to \mathcal{H}, \mathbf{x} \mapsto \bar{\mathbf{x}}$ into a high (possibly infinite) dimensional Hilbert space $\mathcal{H}$. In the following, vectors in $\mathcal{H}$ will be denoted with a bar. In $\mathcal{H}$, the SVM decision rule is simply a separating hyperplane: the algorithm constructs a decision surface with normal $\bar{\Psi} \in \mathcal{H}$ which separates the $\mathbf{x}_i$ into two classes:

$$\bar{\Psi} \cdot \bar{\mathbf{x}}_i + b \geq k_0 - \xi_i, \quad y_i = +1 \quad (1)$$
$$\bar{\Psi} \cdot \bar{\mathbf{x}}_i + b \leq k_1 + \xi_i, \quad y_i = -1 \quad (2)$$

where the ξ_i are positive slack variables, introduced to handle the non-separable case (Cortes & Vapnik, 1995), and where k_0 and k_1 are typically defined to be $+1$ and -1, respectively. $\bar{\Psi}$ is computed by minimizing the objective function

$$\frac{\bar{\Psi} \cdot \bar{\Psi}}{2} + C(\sum_{i=1}^{\ell} \xi_i)^p \quad (3)$$

subject to (1), (2), where C is a constant, and we choose $p = 2$. In the separable case, the SVM algorithm constructs that separating hyperplane for which the margin between the positive and negative examples in $\mathcal{H}$ is maximized. A test vector $\mathbf{x} \in \mathcal{L}$ is then assigned a class label $\{+1, -1\}$ depending on whether $\bar{\Psi} \cdot \Phi(\mathbf{x}) + b$ is greater or less than $(k_0 + k_1)/2$. Support vectors $\mathbf{s}_j \in \mathcal{L}$ are defined as training samples for which one of Equations (1) or (2) is an equality. (We name the support vectors s to distinguish them from the rest of the training data). The solution $\bar{\Psi}$ may be expressed

$$\bar{\Psi} = \sum_{j=1}^{N_S} \alpha_j y_j \Phi(\mathbf{s}_j) \quad (4)$$

where $\alpha_j \geq 0$ are the positive weights, determined during training, $y_j \in \{\pm 1\}$ the class labels of the s_j, and N_S the number of support vectors. Thus in order to classify a test point $\mathbf{x}$ one must compute

$$\bar{\Psi} \cdot \bar{\mathbf{x}} = \sum_{j=1}^{N_S} \alpha_j y_j \bar{s}_j \cdot \bar{\mathbf{x}} = \sum_{j=1}^{N_S} \alpha_j y_j \Phi(s_j) \cdot \Phi(\mathbf{x}) = \sum_{j=1}^{N_S} \alpha_j y_j K(s_j, \mathbf{x}). \quad (5)$$

One of the key properties of support vector machines is the use of the kernel K to compute dot products in $\mathcal{H}$ without having to explicitly compute the mapping Φ.

It is interesting to note that the solution has a simple physical interpretation in the high dimensional space $\mathcal{H}$. If we assume that each support vector $\bar{s}_j$ exerts a perpendicular force of size α_j and sign y_j on a solid plane sheet lying along the hyperplane $\bar{\Psi} \cdot \bar{\mathbf{x}} + b = (k_0 + k_1)/2$, then the solution satisfies the requirements of mechanical stability. At the solution, the α_j can be shown to satisfy $\sum_{j=1}^{N_S} \alpha_j y_j = 0$, which translates into the forces on the sheet summing to zero; and Equation (4) implies that the torques also sum to zero.

3 IMPROVING ACCURACY

This section follows the reasoning of (Schölkopf, Burges, & Vapnik, 1996). Problem domain knowledge can be incorporated in two different ways: the knowledge can be directly built into the algorithm, or it can be used to generate artificial training examples ("virtual examples"). The latter significantly slows down training times, due to both correlations in the artificial data and to the increased training set size (Simard et al., 1992); however it has the advantage of being readily implemented for any learning machine and for any invariances. For instance, if instead of Lie groups of symmetry transformations one is dealing with discrete symmetries, such as the bilateral symmetries of Vetter, Poggio, & Bülthoff (1994), then derivative-based methods (c.g. Simard et al., 1992) are not applicable.

For support vector machines, an intermediate method which combines the advantages of both approaches is possible. The support vectors characterize the solution to the problem in the following sense: If all the other training data were removed, and the system retrained, then the solution would be unchanged. Furthermore, those support vectors $\bar{s}_i$ which are not errors are close to the decision boundary in $\mathcal{H}$, in the sense that they either lie exactly on the margin ($\xi_i = 0$) or close to it ($\xi_i < 1$). Finally, different types of SVM, built using different kernels, tend to produce the same set of support vectors (Schölkopf, Burges, & Vapnik, 1995). This suggests the following algorithm: first, train an SVM to generate a set of support vectors $\{s_1, \ldots, s_{N_s}\}$; then, generate the artificial examples (*virtual support vectors*) by applying the desired invariance transformations to $\{s_1, \ldots, s_{N_s}\}$; finally, train another SVM on the new set. To build a ten-class classifier, this procedure is carried out separately for ten binary classifiers.

Apart from the increase in overall training time (by a factor of two, in our experiments), this technique has the disadvantage that many of the virtual support vectors become support vectors for the second machine, increasing the number of summands in Equation (5) and hence decreasing classification speed. However, the latter problem can be solved with the reduced set method, which we describe next.

4 IMPROVING CLASSIFICATION SPEED

The discussion in this Section follows that of (Burges, 1996). Consider a set of vectors $\mathbf{z}_k \in \mathcal{L}, k = 1, \ldots, N_Z$ and corresponding weights $\gamma_k \in \mathbf{R}$ for which

$$\bar{\Psi}' \equiv \sum_{k=1}^{N_Z} \gamma_k \Phi(\mathbf{z}_k) \qquad (6)$$

minimizes (for fixed N_Z) the Euclidean distance to the original solution:

$$\rho = \|\bar{\Psi} - \bar{\Psi}'\|. \qquad (7)$$

Note that ρ, expressed here in terms of vectors in $\mathcal{H}$, can be expressed entirely in terms of functions (using the kernel K) of vectors in the input space $\mathcal{L}$. The $\{(\gamma_k, \mathbf{z}_k) \mid k = 1, \ldots, N_Z\}$ is called the *reduced set*. To classify a test point $\mathbf{x}$, the expansion in Equation (5) is replaced by the approximation

$$\bar{\Psi}' \cdot \bar{\mathbf{x}} = \sum_{k=1}^{N_Z} \gamma_k \bar{\mathbf{z}}_k \cdot \bar{\mathbf{x}} = \sum_{k=1}^{N_Z} \gamma_k K(\mathbf{z}_k, \mathbf{x}). \qquad (8)$$

The goal is then to choose the smallest $N_Z \ll N_S$, and corresponding reduced set, such that any resulting loss in generalization performance remains acceptable. Clearly, by allowing $N_Z = N_S$, ρ can be made zero. Interestingly, there are non-trivial cases where $N_Z < N_S$ and $\rho = 0$, in which case the reduced set leads to an increase in classification speed with no loss in generalization performance. Note that reduced set vectors are not support vectors, in that they do not necessarily lie on the separating margin and, unlike support vectors, are not training samples.

While the reduced set can be found exactly in some cases, in general an unconstrained conjugate gradient method is used to find the $\mathbf{z}_k$ (while the corresponding optimal γ_k can be found exactly, for all k). The method for finding the reduced set is computationally very expensive (the final phase constitutes a conjugate gradient descent in a space of $(d+1) \cdot N_Z$ variables, which in our case is typically of order 50,000).

5 EXPERIMENTAL RESULTS

In this Section, by "accuracy" we mean generalization performance, and by "speed" we mean classification speed. In our experiments, we used the MNIST database of 60000+10000 handwritten digits, which was used in the comparison investigation of LeCun et al (1995). In that study, the error rate record of 0.7% is held by a boosted convolutional neural network ("LeNet4").

We start by summarizing the results of the virtual support vector method. We trained ten binary classifiers using $C = 10$ in Equation (3). We used a polynomial kernel $K(\mathbf{x}, \mathbf{y}) = (\mathbf{x} \cdot \mathbf{y})^5$. Combining classifiers then gave 1.4% error on the 10,000 test set; this system is referred to as ORIG below. We then generated new training data by translating the resulting support vectors by one pixel in each of four directions, and trained a new machine (using the same parameters). This machine, which is referred to as VSV below, achieved 1.0% error on the test set. The results for each digit are given in Table 1.

Note that the improvement in accuracy comes at a cost in speed of approximately a factor of 2. Furthermore, the speed of ORIG was comparatively slow to start with (LeCun et al., 1995), requiring approximately 14 million multiply adds for one

Table 1: Generalization Performance Improvement by Incorporating Invariances. N_E and N_{SV} are the number of errors and number of support vectors respectively; "ORIG" refers to the original support vector machine, "VSV" to the machine trained on virtual support vectors.

Digit	N_E ORIG	N_E VSV	N_{SV} ORIG	N_{SV} VSV
0	17	15	1206	2938
1	15	13	757	1887
2	34	23	2183	5015
3	32	21	2506	4764
4	30	30	1784	3983
5	29	23	2255	5235
6	30	18	1347	3328
7	43	39	1712	3968
8	47	35	3053	6978
9	56	40	2720	6348

Table 2: Dependence of Performance of Reduced Set System on Threshold. The numbers in parentheses give the corresponding number of errors on the test set. Note that Thrsh Test gives a lower bound for these numbers.

Digit	Thrsh VSV	Thrsh Bayes	Thrsh Test
0	1.39606 (19)	1.48648 (18)	1.54696 (17)
1	3.98722 (24)	4.43154 (12)	4.32039 (10)
2	1.27175 (31)	1.33081 (30)	1.26466 (29)
3	1.26518 (29)	1.42589 (27)	1.33822 (26)
4	2.18764 (37)	2.3727 (35)	2.30899 (33)
5	2.05222 (33)	2.21349 (27)	2.27403 (24)
6	0.95086 (25)	1.06629 (24)	0.790952 (20)
7	3.0969 (59)	3.34772 (57)	3.27419 (54)
8	-1.06981 (39)	-1.19615 (40)	-1.26365 (37)
9	1.10586 (40)	1.10074 (40)	1.13754 (39)

classification (this can be reduced by caching results of repeated support vectors (Burges, 1996)). In order to become competitive with systems with comparable accuracy, we will need approximately a factor of fifty improvement in speed. We therefore approximated VSV with a reduced set system RS with a factor of fifty fewer vectors than the number of support vectors in VSV.

Since the reduced set method computes an *approximation* to the decision surface in the high dimensional space, it is likely that the accuracy of RS could be improved by choosing a different threshold b in Equations (1) and (2). We computed that threshold which gave the empirical Bayes error for the RS system, measured on the training set. This can be done easily by finding the maximum of the difference between the two un-normalized cumulative distributions of the values of the dot products $\bar{\Psi} \cdot \bar{\mathbf{x}}_i$, where the $\mathbf{x}_i$ are the *original* training data. Note that the effects of bias are reduced by the fact that VSV (and hence RS) was trained only on shifted data, and not on any of the original data. Thus, in the absence of a validation set, the original training data provides a reasonable means of estimating the Bayes threshold. This is a serendipitous bonus of the VSV approach. Table 2 compares results obtained using the threshold generated by the training procedure for the VSV system; the estimated Bayes threshold for the RS system; and, for comparison

Table 3: Speed Improvement Using the Reduced Set method. The second through fourth columns give numbers of errors on the test set for the original system, the virtual support vector system, and the reduced set system. The last three columns give, for each system, the number of vectors whose dot product must be computed in test phase.

Digit	ORIG Err	VSV Err	RS Err	ORIG # SV	VSV # SV	# RSV
0	17	15	18	1206	2938	59
1	15	13	12	757	1887	38
2	34	23	30	2183	5015	100
3	32	21	27	2506	4764	95
4	30	30	35	1784	3983	80
5	29	23	27	2255	5235	105
6	30	18	24	1347	3328	67
7	43	39	57	1712	3968	79
8	47	35	40	3053	6978	140
9	56	40	40	2720	6348	127

purposes only (to see the maximum possible effect of varying the threshold), the Bayes error computed on the *test* set.

Table 3 compares results on the test set for the three systems, where the Bayes threshold (computed with the training set) was used for RS. The results for all ten digits combined are 1.4% error for ORIG, 1.0% for VSV (with roughly twice as many multiply adds) and 1.1% for RS (with a factor of 22 fewer multiply adds than ORIG).

The reduced set conjugate gradient algorithm does not reduce the objective function ρ^2 (Equation (7)) to zero. For example, for the first 5 digits, ρ^2 is only reduced on average by a factor of 2.4 (the algorithm is stopped when progress becomes too slow). It is striking that nevertheless, good results are achieved.

6 DISCUSSION

The only systems in LeCun et al (1995) with better than 1.1% error are LeNet5 (0.9% error, with approximately 350K multiply-adds) and boosted LeNet4 (0.7% error, approximately 450K multiply-adds). Clearly SVMs are not in this league yet (the RS system described here requires approximately 650K multiply-adds).

However, SVMs present clear opportunities for further improvement. (In fact, we have since trained a VSV system with 0.8% error, by choosing a different kernel). More invariances (for example, for the pattern recognition case, small rotations, or varying ink thickness) could be added to the virtual support vector approach. Further, one might use only those virtual support vectors which provide new information about the decision boundary, or use a measure of such information to keep only the most important vectors. Known invariances could also be built directly into the SVM objective function.

Viewed as an approach to function approximation, the reduced set method is currently restricted in that it assumes a decision function with the same functional form as the original SVM. In the case of quadratic kernels, the reduced set can be computed both analytically and efficiently (Burges, 1996). However, the conjugate gradient descent computation for the general kernel is very inefficient. Perhaps relaxing the above restriction could lead to analytical methods which would apply to more complex kernels also.

Acknowledgements

We wish to thank V. Vapnik, A. Smola and H. Drucker for discussions. C. Burges was supported by ARPA contract N00014-94-C-0186. B. Schölkopf was supported by the Studienstiftung des deutschen Volkes.

References

[1] Boser, B. E., Guyon, I. M., Vapnik, V., *A Training Algorithm for Optimal Margin Classifiers*, Fifth Annual Workshop on Computational Learning Theory, Pittsburgh ACM (1992) 144–152.

[2] Bottou, L., Cortes, C., Denker, J. S., Drucker, H., Guyon, I., Jackel, L. D., Le Cun, Y., Müller, U. A., Säckinger, E., Simard, P., Vapnik, V., *Comparison of Classifier Methods: a Case Study in Handwritten Digit Recognition*, Proceedings of the 12th International Conference on Pattern Recognition and Neural Networks, Jerusalem (1994)

[3] Burges, C. J. C., *Simplified Support Vector Decision Rules*, 13th International Conference on Machine Learning (1996), pp. 71 – 77.

[4] Cortes, C., Vapnik, V., *Support Vector Networks*, Machine Learning **20** (1995) pp. 273 – 297

[5] LeCun, Y., Jackel, L., Bottou, L., Brunot, A., Cortes, C., Denker, J., Drucker, H., Guyon, I., Müller, U., Säckinger, E., Simard, P., and Vapnik, V., *Comparison of Learning Algorithms for Handwritten Digit Recognition*, International Conference on Artificial Neural Networks, Ed. F. Fogelman, P. Gallinari, pp. 53-60, 1995.

[6] Schölkopf, B., Burges, C.J.C., Vapnik, V., *Extracting Support Data for a Given Task*, in Fayyad, U. M., Uthurusamy, R. (eds.), Proceedings, First International Conference on Knowledge Discovery & Data Mining, AAAI Press, Menlo Park, CA (1995)

[7] Schölkopf, B., Burges, C.J.C., Vapnik, V., *Incorporating Invariances in Support Vector Learning Machines*, in Proceedings ICANN'96 International Conference on Artificial Neural Networks. Springer Verlag, Berlin, (1996)

[8] Simard, P., Victorri, B., Le Cun, Y., Denker, J., *Tangent Prop — a Formalism for Specifying Selected Invariances in an Adaptive Network*, in Moody, J. E., Hanson, S. J., Lippmann, R. P., *Advances in Neural Information Processing Systems 4*, Morgan Kaufmann, San Mateo, CA (1992)

[9] Vapnik, V., *Estimation of Dependences Based on Empirical Data*, [in Russian] Nauka, Moscow (1979); English translation: Springer Verlag, New York (1982)

[10] Vapnik, V., *The Nature of Statistical Learning Theory*, Springer Verlag, New York (1995)

[11] Vapnik, V., Golowich, S., and Smola, A., *Support Vector Method for Function Approximation, Regression Estimation, and Signal Processing*, Submitted to Advances in Neural Information Processing Systems, 1996

[12] Vetter, T., Poggio, T., and Bülthoff, H., *The Importance of Symmetry and Virtual Views in Three-Dimensional Object Recognition*, Current Biology **4** (1994) 18–23

Estimating Equivalent Kernels For Neural Networks: A Data Perturbation Approach

A. Neil Burgess

Department of Decision Science
London Business School
London, NW1 4SA, UK

(N.Burgess@lbs.lon.ac.uk)

ABSTRACT

We describe the notion of "equivalent kernels" and suggest that this provides a framework for comparing different classes of regression models, including neural networks and both parametric and non-parametric statistical techniques. Unfortunately, standard techniques break down when faced with models, such as neural networks, in which there is more than one "layer" of adjustable parameters. We propose an algorithm which overcomes this limitation, estimating the equivalent kernels for neural network models using a data perturbation approach. Experimental results indicate that the networks do not use the maximum possible number of degrees of freedom, that these can be controlled using regularisation techniques and that the equivalent kernels learnt by the network vary both in "size" and in "shape" in different regions of the input space.

1 INTRODUCTION

The dominant approaches within the statistical community, such as multiple linear regression but even extending to advanced techniques such as generalised additive models (Hastie and Tibshirani, 1990), projection pursuit regression (Friedman and Stuetzle, 1981), and classification and regression trees (Breiman et al., 1984), tend to err, when they do, on the high-bias side due to restrictive assumptions regarding either the functional form of the response to individual variables and/or the limited nature of the interaction effects which can be accommodated. Other classes of models, such as multi-variate adaptive regression spline models of high-order (Friedman, 1991), interaction splines (Wahba, 1990) and especially non-parametric regression techniques (Hardle, 1990) are capable of relaxing some or all of these restrictive assumptions, but run the converse risk of suffering high-variance, or "over fitting".

A large literature of experimental results suggests that, under the right conditions, the flexibility of neural networks allows them to out-perform other techniques. Where the current understanding is limited, however, is in analysing trained neural networks to understand how the degrees of freedom have been allocated, in a way which allows meaningful comparisons with other classes of models. We propose that the notion of "equivalent kernels" [eg. (Hastie and Tibshirani, 1990)] can provide a unifying framework for neural networks and other classes of regression model, as well as providing important information about the neural network itself. We describe an algorithm for estimating equivalent kernels for neural networks which overcomes the limitations of existing analytical methods.

In the following section we describe the concept of equivalent kernels. In Section 3 we describe an algorithm which estimates how the response function learned by the neural network would change if the training data were modified slightly, from which we derive the equivalent kernels for the network. Section 4 provides simulation results for two controlled experiments. Section 5 contains a brief discussion of some of the implications of this work, and highlights a number of interesting directions for further research. A summary of the main points of the paper is presented in Section 6.

2 EQUIVALENT KERNELS

Non-parametric regression techniques, such as kernel smoothing, local regression and nearest neighbour regression, can all be expressed in the form:

$$y(z) = \int_{x=-\infty}^{\infty} \varphi(z,x) . f(x) . t(x) \, dx \tag{1}$$

where $y(z)$ is the response at the query point z, $\varphi(z, x)$ is the weighting, or *kernel*, which is "centred" at z, $f(x)$ is the input density and $t(x)$ is the target function.

In finite samples, this is approximated by:

$$y(x_i) = \sum_{j=1}^{n} \varphi(x_i, x_j) . t_j \tag{2}$$

and the response at point x_i is a weighted average of the sampled target values across the entire dataset. Furthermore, the response can be viewed as a *least squares estimate* for $y(x_i)$ because we can write it as a solution to the minimization problem:

$$\min_{y(x_i)} \left(\sum_{j=1}^{n} \varphi(x_i, x_j) . t_j - y(x_i) \right)^2 \tag{3}$$

We can combine the kernel functions to define the smoother matrix S, given by:

$$S = \begin{bmatrix} \varphi(x_1, x_1) & \varphi(x_1, x_2) & \cdots & \varphi(x_1, x_n) \\ \varphi(x_2, x_1) & \varphi(x_2, x_2) & & \vdots \\ \vdots & & \ddots & \vdots \\ \varphi(x_n, x_1) & \cdots & \cdots & \varphi(x_n, x_n) \end{bmatrix} \tag{4}$$

From which we obtain:

$$\mathbf{y} = \mathbf{S}.\mathbf{t} \tag{5}$$

Where $\mathbf{y} = (y(x_1), y(x_2), \ldots, y(x_n))^T$, and $\mathbf{t} = (t_1, t_2, \ldots, t_n)^T$ is the vector of target values.

From the smoother matrix S, we can derive many kinds of important information. The model is represented in terms of the influence of each observation on the response at each sample point, allowing us to quantify the effect of outliers for instance. It is also possible to calculate the model bias and variance at each sample point [see (Hardle, 1990) for details]. One important measure which we will return to below is the number of degrees of freedom which are absorbed by the model; a number of definitions can be motivated, but in the case of least squares estimators they turn out to be equivalent [see pp 52-55 of (Hastie and Tibshirani, 1990)], perhaps the most intuitive is:

$$\text{dof}_s = \text{trace}(S) \qquad (6)$$

thus a model which is a look up table, i.e. $y(x_i) = t_i$, absorbs all 'n' degrees of freedom, whereas the sample mean, $y(x_i) = 1/n \, \Sigma \, t_i$, absorbs only one degree of freedom. The degrees of freedom can be taken as a natural measure of model complexity, which formulated with respect to the data itself, rather than to the number of parameters.

The discussion above relates only to models which can be expressed in the form given by equation (2), i.e. where the "kernel functions" can be computed. Fortunately, many types of parametric models can be "inverted" in this manner, providing what are known as "equivalent kernels". Consider a model of the form:

$$y(x) = \Sigma_j \, \phi_j(x).w_j \qquad (7)$$

i.e. a weighted function of some arbitrary transformations of the input variables. In the case of fitting using a least squares approach, then the optimal weights $\mathbf{w} = (w_1, w_2, \ldots, w_n)^T$ are given by:

$$\mathbf{w} = \Phi^+ \mathbf{t} \qquad (8)$$

where Φ^+ is the pseudo-inverse of the transformed data matrix Φ. The network output can then be expressed as:

$$y(x_i) = \Sigma_j \, \phi_j(x_i).(\Sigma_{k=1..n} \, [\Phi^+]_{j,k}.t_k) \qquad (9)$$

$$= \Sigma_k [\Sigma_j \, \phi_j(x_i)[\Phi^+]_{j,k}].t_k$$

$$= \Sigma_k \, \varphi(x_i, x_k).t_k$$

and the $\varphi(x_i, x_k)$ are then the "equivalent kernels" of the original model which is now in the same form as equation (2). Examples of equivalent kernels for different classes of parametric and non-parametric models are given by (Hastie and Tibshirani, 1990) whilst a treatment for Radial Basis Function (RBF) networks is presented in (Lowe, 1995).

3 EQUIVALENT KERNELS FOR NEURAL NETWORKS

The analytic approach described above relies on the ability to calculate the optimal weights using the pseudo-inverse of the data matrix. This is only possible if the transformations, $\phi(x)$, are fixed functions, as is typically the case in parametric models or single-layer neural networks. However, for a neural network with more than one layer of adjustable weights, the basis functions are parametrised rather than fixed and are thus themselves a function of the training data. Consequently the equivalent kernels are also dependent on the data, and the problem of finding the equivalent kernels becomes non-linear.

We adopt a solution to this problem which is based on the following observation. In the case where the equivalent kernels are independent of the observed values t_i, we notice from equation (2):

$$\frac{\partial y_i}{\partial t_j} = \varphi(x_i, x_j) \tag{10}$$

i.e. the basis function $\varphi(x_i, x_j)$ is equal to the sensitivity of the response $y(x_i)$ to a small change in the observed value t_j. This suggests that we approximate the equivalent kernels by turning the above expression around:

$$\varphi(x_i, x_j) = \bigl(\psi(x_i) - y(x_i)\bigr)/\varepsilon \tag{11}$$

where ε is a small perturbation of the training data and $\varphi(x_i)$ is the response of the re-optimised network:

$$\psi(x_i) = \varphi^*(x_i, x_j) \cdot (t_j + \varepsilon) + \sum_{k \neq j} \varphi^*(x_i, x_k) \cdot t_k \tag{12}$$

The notation φ^* indicates that the new kernel functions derive from the network fitted to perturbed data. Note that this takes into account **all** of the adjustable parameters in the network. Whereas treating the basis functions as fixed would give simply the number of additive terms in the final layer of the network.

Calculating the equivalent kernels in this fashion is a computationally intensive procedure, with the network needing to be retrained after perturbing each point in turn. Note that regularisation techniques such as weight decay should be incorporated within this procedure as with initial training and are thus correctly accounted for by the algorithm. The retraining step is facilitated by using the optimised weights from the unperturbed data, causing the network to re-train from weights which are initially almost optimal (especially if the perturbation is small).

4   SIMULATION RESULTS

In order to investigate the practical viability of estimating equivalent kernels using the perturbation approach, we performed a controlled experiment on simulated data. The target function used was the first two periods of a sine-wave, sampled at 41 points evenly spaced between 0 and 4π. This function was estimated using a neural network with a single layer of four sigmoid units, a shortcut connection from input to output, and a linear output unit, trained using standard backpropogation.

From the trained network we then estimated the equivalent kernels using the perturbation method described in the previous section. The resulting kernels for points 0, π, and 2π are shown in figure 2, below.

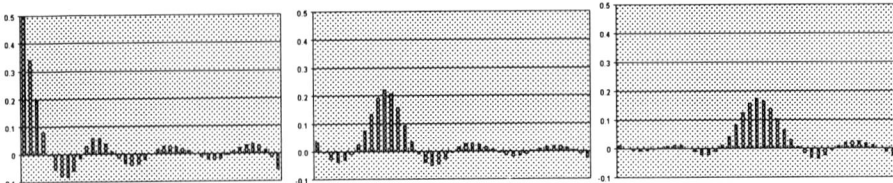

Figure 2: Equivalent Kernels for sine-wave problem

As discussed in the previous section, we can combine the estimated kernels to construct a linear smoother. The correlation coefficient between the function reconstructed from the approximated smoother matrix and the original neural network is found to be 0.995.

From equation (6) we find that the network contains approx. 8.2 degrees of freedom; this compares to the 10 *potential* degrees of freedom, and also to the 6 degrees of freedom which we would expect for an equivalent model with fixed transfer functions. Clearly, to some degreee, perturbations in the training data are accommodated by adjustments to the sigmoid functions.

Using this approach we can also investigate the effects of weight decay on (a) the ability of the network to reproduce the target function, (b) the number of degrees of freedom absorbed by the network, and (c) the kernel functions themselves. We use a standard quadratic weight decay, leading to a cost function of the form:

$$C = (y - f(x))^2 + \gamma.\Sigma w^2 \qquad (13)$$

The effect of gradually increasing the weight decay factor, γ, on both network performance and capacity is shown in figure 3(b), below:

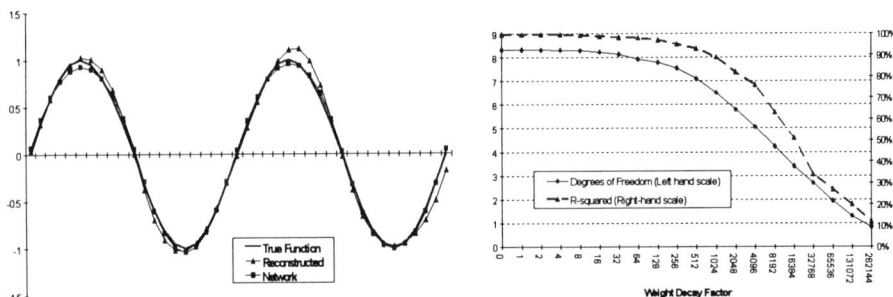

Figure 3: (a) Comparison of network and reconstructed functions with target, and (b) effect of weight decay

Looking at figure 3(b) we note that the two curves follow each other very closely. As the weight decay factor is increased, the effective capacity of the network is reduced and the performance drops off accordingly.

In one dimension, the main flexibility for the equivalent kernels is one of scale: narrow, concentrated kernels which rely heavily on nearby observations versus broad, diffuse kernels in which the response is conditioned on a larger number of observations. In higher dimensions, however, the real power of neural networks as function estimators lies in the fact that the sensitivity of the estimated network function is itself a flexible function of the input vector. Viewed from the perspective of equivalent kernels, this property might be expected to manifest itself in a change in the *shape* of the kernels in different regions of the input space. In order to investigate this effect we applied the perturbation approach in estimating equivalent kernels for a network trained to reproduce a two-dimensional function; the function chosen was a "ring" defined by:

$$z = 1/ (1 + 30.(x^2 + y^2 - 0.5)^2) \tag{14}$$

For ease of visualisation the input points were chosen on a regular 15 by 15 grid running between plus and minus one. This function was approximated using a 2(+1)-8-1 network with sigmoidal hidden units and a linear output unit. Selected kernel functions, estimated from this network, are shown in figure 4, below:

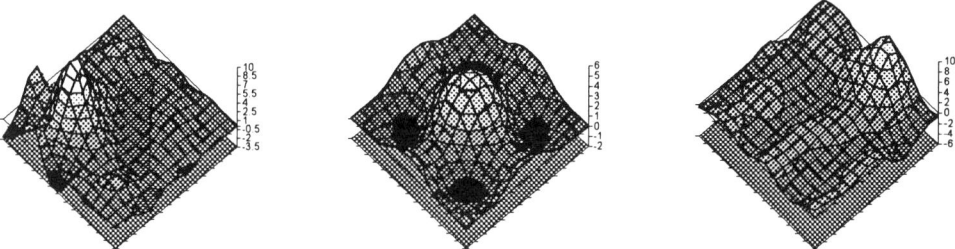

Figure 4: Equivalent Kernels: approximated using the perturbation method

This result clearly shows the changing shape of the kernel functions in different parts of the input space. The function reconstructed from the estimated smoother matrix has a correlation coefficient of 0.987 with the original network function.

5. Discussion

The ability to transform neural network regression models into an equivalent kernel representation raises the possibility of harnessing the whole battery of statistical methods which have been developed for non-parametric techniques: model selection procedures, prediction interval estimation, calculation of degrees of freedom, and statistical significance testing amongst others. The algorithm described in this paper raises the possibility of applying these techniques to more-powerful networks with two or more layers of adaptable weights, be they based on sigmoids, radial functions, splines or whatever, albeit at the price of significant computational effort.

Another opportunity is in the area of model combination where the added value from combining models in an *ensemble* is related to the degree of correlation between the different models (Krogh and Vedelsby, 1995). Typically the pointwise correlation between two models will be related to the similarity between their equivalent kernels and so the equivalent kernel approach opens new possibilities for conditionally modifying the ensemble weights without a need for an additional level of learning.

The influence-based method for estimating the number of degrees of freedom absorbed by a neural network model, focuses attention on uncertainty in the data itself, rather than taking the indirect route based on uncertainty in the model parameters; in future work we propose to investigate the similarities and differences between our approach and those based on the "effective number of parameters" (Moody, 1992) and Bayesian methods (MacKay, 1992).

6. Summary

We suggest that equivalent kernels provide an important tool for understanding *what* neural networks do and *how* they go about doing it; in particular a large battery of existing statistical tools use information derived from the smoother matrix.

The perturbation method which we have presented overcomes the limitations of standard approaches, which are only appropriate for models with a single layer of adjustable weights, albeit at considerable computational expense. It has the added bonus of automatically taking into account the effect of regularisation techniques such as weight decay.

The experimental results illustrate the application of the technique to two simple problems. As expected the number of degrees of freedom in the models is found to be related to the amount of weight decay used during training. The equivalent kernels are found to vary significantly in different regions of input space and the functions reconstructed from the estimated smoother matrices closely match the orignal networks.

7. References

Breiman, L., Friedman, J. H., Olshen, R. A., and Stone C. J., 1984, *Classification and Regression Trees*, Wadsworth and Brooks/Cole, Monterey.

Friedman, J.H. and Stuetzle, W., 1981. Projection pursuit regression. *Journal of the American Statistical Association*. Vol. 76, pp. 817-823.

Friedman, J.H., 1991. Multivariate Adaptive Regression Splines (with discussion). *Annals of Statistics*. Vol 19, num. 1, pp. 1-141.

Hardle, W., 1990. *Applied nonparametric regression*. Cambridge University Press.

Hastie, T.J. and Tibshirani, R.J., 1990. *Generalised Additive Models*. Chapman and Hall, London.

Krogh, A, and Vedelsby, J., Neural network ensembles, cross-validation and active learning, *NIPS 7*, pp231-238.

Lowe, D., 1995, On the use of nonlocal and non positive definite basis functions in radial basis function networks, *Proceedings of the Fourth IEE Conference on Artificial Neural Networks*, pp. 206-211.

MacKay, D. J. C., 1992, A practical Bayesian framework for backprop networks, *Neural Computation*, 4, 448-472.

Moody, J. E., 1992, The effective number of parameters: an analysis of generalisation and regularization in nonlinear learning systems, *NIPS 4*, 847-54, Morgan Kaufmann, San Mateo

Wahba, G., 1990, *Spline Models for Observational Data*. Society for Industrial and Applied Mathematics, Philadelphia.

Promoting Poor Features to Supervisors: Some Inputs Work Better as Outputs

Rich Caruana
JPRC and
Carnegie Mellon University
Pittsburgh, PA 15213
caruana@cs.cmu.edu

Virginia R. de Sa
Sloan Center for Theoretical Neurobiology and
W. M. Keck Center for Integrative Neuroscience
University of California, San Francisco CA 94143
desa@phy.ucsf.edu

Abstract

In supervised learning there is usually a clear distinction between inputs and outputs — inputs are what you will measure, outputs are what you will predict from those measurements. This paper shows that the distinction between inputs and outputs is not this simple. Some features are more useful as extra *outputs* than as *inputs*. By using a feature as an output we get more than just the case values but can learn a mapping from the other inputs to that feature. For many features this mapping may be more useful than the feature value itself. We present two regression problems and one classification problem where performance improves if features that could have been used as inputs are used as extra outputs instead. This result is surprising since a feature used as an output is not used during testing.

1 Introduction

The goal in supervised learning is to learn functions that map inputs to outputs with high predictive accuracy. The standard practice in neural nets is to use all features that will be available for the test cases as inputs, and use as outputs only the features to be predicted.

Extra features available for training cases that *won't* be available during testing can be used as extra *outputs* that often benefit the original output[2][5]. Other ways of adding information to supervised learning through outputs include hints[1], tangent-prop[7], and EBNN[8]. In unsupervised learning it has been shown that inputs arising from different modalities can provide supervisory signals (outputs for the other modality) to each other and thus aid learning [3][6].

If outputs are so useful, and since any input could be used as an output, would some inputs be more useful as outputs? Yes. In this paper we show that in supervised backpropagation learning, some features are more useful as outputs than as inputs. This is surprising since using a feature as an output only extracts information from it during training; during testing it is not used.

This paper uses the following terms: The Main Task is the output to be learned. The goal is to improve performance on the Main Task. Regular Inputs are the features provided as inputs in all experiments. Extra Inputs (Extra Outputs) are the extra features when used as inputs (outputs). STD is standard backpropagation using the Regular Inputs as inputs and the Main Task as outputs. STD+IN uses the Extra Features as Extra Inputs to learn the Main Task. STD+OUT uses the Extra Features, but as Extra Outputs learned in parallel with the Main Task, using just the Regular Inputs as inputs.

2 Poorly Correlated Features

This section presents a simple synthetic problem where it is easy to see why using a feature as an extra output is better than using that same feature as an extra input.

Consider the following function:

$$F1(A,B) = \text{SIGMOID}(A+B), \qquad \text{SIGMOID}(x) = 1/(1+e^{(-x)})$$

The STD net in Figure 1a has 20 inputs, 16 hidden units, and one output. We use backpropagation on this net to learn F1(). A and B are uniformly sampled from the interval [-5,5]. The network's input is binary codes for A and B. The range [-5,5] is discretized into 2^{10} bins and the binary code of the resulting bin number is used as the input coding. The first 10 input units receive the code for A and the second 10 that for B. The target output is the unary real (unencoded) value F1(A,B).

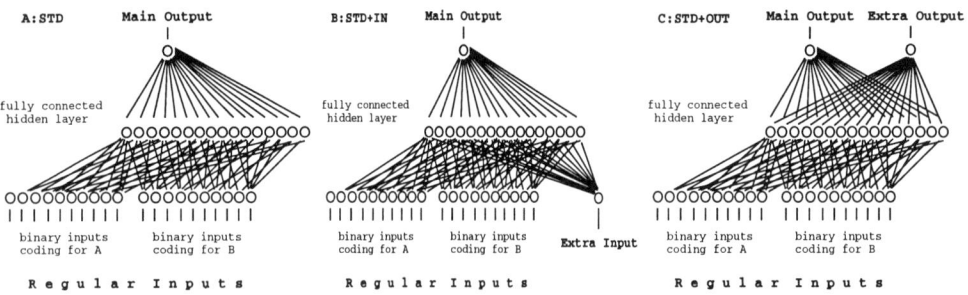

Figure 1: Three Neural Net Architectures for Learning F1

Backpropagation is done with per-epoch updating and early stopping. Each trial uses new random training, halt, and test sets. Training sets contain 50 patterns. This is enough data to get good performance, but not so much that there is not room for improvement. We use large halt and test sets — 1000 cases each — to minimize the effect of sampling error in the measured performances. Larger halt and test sets yield similar results. We use this methodology for all the experiments in this paper.

Table 1 shows the mean performance of 50 trials of STD Net 1a with backpropagation and early stopping.

Now consider a similar function:

$$F2(A,B) = \text{SIGMOID}(A-B).$$

Suppose, in addition to the 10-bit codings for A and B, you are given the unencoded unary value F2(A,B) as an extra input feature. Will this extra input help you learn F1(A,B) better? Probably not. A+B and A-B do not correlate for random A and B. The correlation coefficient for our training sets is typically less than ±0.01. Because

Table 1: Mean Test Set Root-Mean-Squared-Error on F1

Network	Trials	Mean RMSE	Significance
STD	50	0.0648	-
STD+IN	50	0.0647	ns
STD+OUT	50	0.0631	0.013*

of this, knowing the value of F2(A,B) does not tell you much about the target value F1(A,B) (and vice-versa).

F1(A,B)'s poor correlation with F2(A,B) hurts backprop's ability to learn to use F2(A,B) to predict F1(A,B). The STD+IN net in Figure 1b has 21 inputs — 20 for the binary codes for A and B, and an extra input for F2(A,B). The 2nd line in Table 1 shows the performance of STD+IN for the same training, halting, and test sets used by STD; the only difference is that there is an extra input feature in the data sets for STD+IN. Note that the performance of STD+IN is not significantly different from that of STD — the extra information contained in the feature F2(A,B) does not help backpropagation learn F1(A,B) *when used as an extra input.*

If F2(A,B) does not help backpropagation learn F1(A,B) when used as an input, should we ignore it altogether? No. F1(A,B) and F2(A,B) are strongly related. They both benefit from decoding the binary input encoding to compute the subfeatures A and B. If, instead of using F2(A,B) as an extra input, it is used as an extra output trained with backpropagation, it will bias the shared hidden layer to learn A and B better, and this will help the net better learn to predict F1(A,B).

Figure 1c shows a net with 20 inputs for A and B, and 2 outputs, one for F1(A,B) and one for F2(A,B). Error is back-propagated from both outputs, but the performance of this net is evaluated only on the output F1(A,B) and early stopping is done using only the performance of this output. The 3rd line in Table 1 shows the mean performance of 50 trials of this multitask net on F1(A,B). Using F2(A,B) as an extra output significantly improves performance on F1(A,B). Using the extra feature as an extra output is better than using it as an extra input. *By using F2(A,B) as an output we make use of more than just the individual output values F2(A,B) but learn to extract information about the function mapping the inputs to F2(A,B). This is a key difference between using features as inputs and outputs.*

The increased performance of STD+OUT over STD and STD+IN is not due to STD+OUT reducing the capacity available for the main task F1(). All three nets — STD, STD+IN, STD+OUT — perform better with *more* hidden units. (Because larger capacity favors STD+OUT over STD and STD+IN, we report results for the moderate sized 16 hidden unit nets to be fair to STD and STD+IN.)

3 Noisy Features

This section presents two problems where extra features are more useful as inputs if they have low noise, but which become more useful as outputs as their noise increases. Because the extra features are ideal features for these problems, this demonstrates that what we observed in the previous section does not depend on the extra features being contrived so that their correlation with the main task is low – features with high correlation can still be more useful as outputs.

Once again, consider the main task from the previous section:

F1(A,B) = SIGMOID(A+B)

Now consider these extra features:

EF(A) = A + NOISE_SCALE * Noise1

EF(B) = B + NOISE_SCALE * Noise2

Noise1 and Noise2 are uniformly sampled on [-1,1]. If NOISE_SCALE is not too large, EF(A) and EF(B) are excellent input features for learning F1(A,B) because the net can avoid learning to decode the binary input representations. However, as NOISE_SCALE increases, EF(A) and EF(B) become less useful and it is better for the net to learn F1(A,B) from the binary inputs for A and B.

As before, we try using the extra features as either extra inputs or as extra outputs. Again, the training sets have 50 patterns, and the halt and test sets have 1000 patterns. Unlike before, however, we ran preliminary tests to find the best net size. The results showed 256 hidden units to be about optimal for the STD nets with early stopping on this problem.

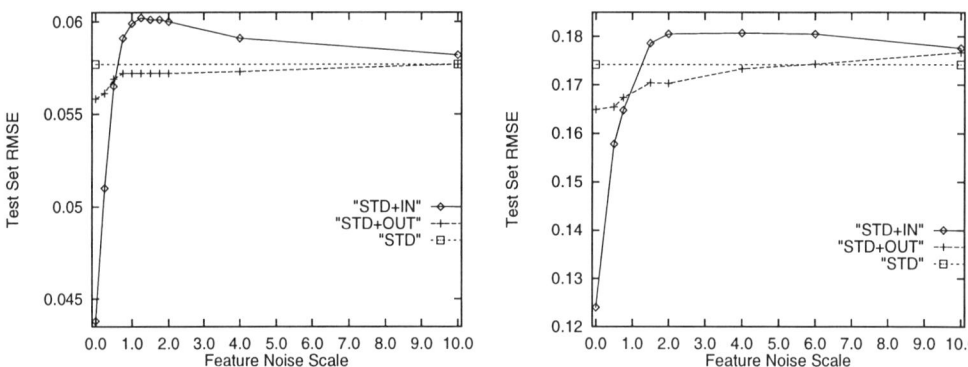

Figure 2: STD, STD+IN, and STD+OUT on F1 (left) and F3 (right)

Figure 2a plots the average performance of 50 trials of STD+IN and STD+OUT as NOISE_SCALE varies from 0.0 to 10.0. The performance of STD, which does not use EF(A) and EF(B), is shown as a horizontal line; it is independent of NOISE_SCALE. Let's first examine the results of STD+IN which uses EF(A) and EF(B) as extra inputs. As expected, when the noise is small, using EF(A) and EF(B) as extra inputs improves performance considerably. As the noise increases, however, this improvement decreases. Eventually there is so much noise in EF(A) and EF(B) that they no longer help the net if used as inputs. And, if the noise increases further, using EF(A) and EF(B) as extra inputs actually hurts. Finally, as the noise gets very large, performance asymptotes back towards the baseline.

Using EF(A) and EF(B) as extra outputs yields quite different results. When the noise is low, they do not help as much as they did as extra inputs. As the noise increases, however, at some point they help more as extra outputs than as extra inputs, and never hurt performance the way the noisy extra inputs did.

Why does noise cause STD+IN to perform worse than STD? With a finite training sample, correlations between noisy inputs and the main task cause the network to use the noisy inputs. To the extent that the main task is a function of the noisy inputs, it must pass the noise to the output, causing the output to be noisy. Also, as the net comes to depend on the noisy inputs, it depends less on the noise-free binary inputs. The noisy inputs *explain away* some of the training signal, so less is available to encourage learning to decode the binary inputs.

Why does noise not hurt STD+OUT as much as it hurts STD+IN? As outputs, the net is learning the mapping from the regular inputs to EF(A) and EF(B). Early in training, the net learns to interpolate through the noise and thus learns smooth functions for EF(A) and EF(B) that have reasonable fidelity to the true mapping. This makes learning less sensitive to the noise added to these features.

3.1 Another Problem

F1(A,B) is only mildly nonlinear because A and B do not go far into the tails of the SIGMOID. Do the results depend on this smoothness? To check, we modified F1(A,B) to make it more nonlinear. Consider this function:

F3(A,B) = SIGMOID(EXPAND(SIGMOID(A)–SIGMOID(B)))

where EXPAND scales the inputs from (SIGMOID(A)–SIGMOID(B)) to the range [-12.5,12.5], and A and B are drawn from [-12.5,12.5]. F3(A,B) is significantly more nonlinear than F1(A,B) because the expanded scales of A and B, and expanding the difference to [-12.5,12.5] before passing it through another sigmoid, cause much of the data to fall in the tails of either the inner or outer sigmoids.

Consider these extra features:

EF(A) = SIGMOID(A) + NOISE_SCALE * Noise1

EF(B) = SIGMOID(B) + NOISE_SCALE * Noise2

where Noises are sampled as before. Figure 2B shows the results of using extra features EF(A) and EF(B) as extra inputs or as extra outputs. The trend is similar to that in Figure 2A but the benefit of STD+OUT is even larger at low noise. The data for 2a and 2b are generated using different seeds, 2a used steepest descent and Mitre's Aspirin simulator, 2b used conjugate gradient and Toronto's Xerion simulator, and F1 and F3 do not behave as similarly as their definitions might suggest. The similarity between the two graphs is due to the ubiquity of the phenomena, not to some small detail of the test functions or how the experiments were run.

4 A Classification Problem

This section presents a problem that combines feature correlation (Section 1) and feature noise (Section 2) into one problem. Consider the 1-D classification problem, shown in Figure 3, of separating two Gaussian distributions with means 0 and 1, and standard deviations of 1. This problem is simple to learn if the 1-D input is coded as a single, continuous input but can be made harder by embedding it non-linearly in a higher dimensional space. Consider encoding input values defined on [0.0,15.0] using an *interpolated* 4-D Gray code($\overline{GC}$); integer values are mapped to a 4-D binary Gray code and intervening non-integers are mapped linearly to intervening 4-D vectors between the binary Gray codes for the bounding integers. As the Gray code flips only one bit between neighboring integers this involves simply interpolating along the 1 dimension in the 4-D unit cube that changes. Thus 3.4 is encoded as $.4(\overline{GC}(4) - \overline{GC}(3)) + \overline{GC}(3)$.

The extra feature is a 1-D value correlated (with correlation ρ) with the original unencoded regular input, X. The extra feature is drawn from a Gaussian distribution with mean $\rho \times (X - .5) + .5$ and standard deviation $\sqrt{(1 - \rho^2)}$. Examples of the distributions of the unencoded original dimension and the extra feature for various correlations are shown in Figure 3. This problem has been carefully constructed so that the optimal classification boundary does not change as ρ varies.

Consider the extreme cases. At $\rho = 1$, the extra feature is exactly an unencoded

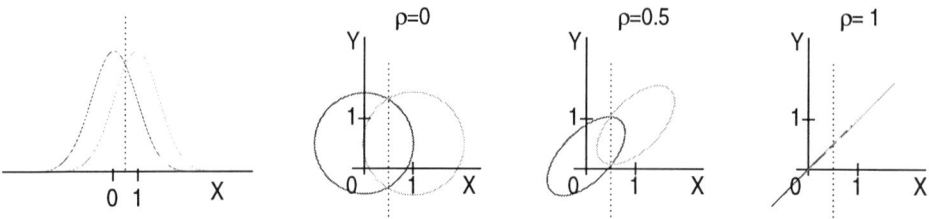

Figure 3: Two Overlapped Gaussian Classes (left), and An Extra Feature (y-axis) Correlated Different Amounts ($\rho = 0$: no correlation, $\rho = 1$: perfect correlation) With the unencoded version of the Regular Input (x-axis)

version of the regular input. A STD+IN net using this feature as an extra input could ignore the encoded inputs and solve the problem using this feature alone. An STD+OUT net using this extra feature as an extra output would have its hidden layer biased towards representations that decode the Gray code, which is useful to the main classification task. At the other extreme ($\rho = 0$), we expect nets using the extra feature to learn no better than one using just the regular inputs because there is no useful information provided by the uncorrelated extra feature. The interesting case is between the two extremes. We can imagine a situation where as an output, the extra feature is still able to help STD+OUT by guiding it to decode the Gray code but does not help STD+IN because of the high level of noise.

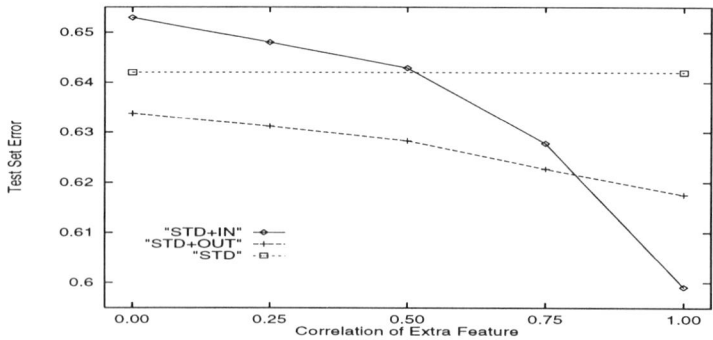

Figure 4: STD, STD+IN, and STD+OUT vs. ρ on the Classification Problem

The class output unit uses a sigmoid transfer function and cross-entropy error measure. The output unit for the correlated extra feature uses a linear transfer function and squared error measure. Figure 4 shows the average performance of 50 trials of STD, STD+IN, and STD+OUT as a function of ρ using networks with 20 hidden units, 70 training patterns, and halt and test sets of 1000 patterns each. As in the previous section, STD+IN is much more sensitive to changes in the extra feature than STD+OUT, so that by $\rho = 0.75$ the curves cross and for ρ less than 0.75, the dimension is actually more useful as an output dimension than an extra input.

5 Discussion

Are the benefits of using some features as extra outputs instead of as inputs large enough to be interesting? Yes. Using only 1 or 2 features as extra outputs instead of as inputs reduced error 2.5% on the problem in Section 1, more than 5% in regions of the graphs in Section 2, and more than 2.5% in regions of the graph in Section

3. In domains where many features might be moved, the net effect may be larger.

Are some features more useful as outputs than as inputs only on contrived problems? No. In this paper we used the simplest problems we could devise where a few features worked better as outputs than as inputs. But our findings explain a result we noted previously, but did not understand, when applying multitask learning to pneumonia risk prediction[4]. There, we had the choice of using lab tests that would be unavailable on future patients as extra outputs, or using poor — i.e., noisy — predictions of them as extra inputs. Using the lab tests as extra outputs worked better. If one compares the zero noise points for STD+OUT (there's no noise in a feature when used as an output because we use the values in the training set, not predicted values) with the high noise points for STD+IN in the graphs in Section 2, it is easy to see why STD+OUT could perform much better.

This paper shows that the benefit of using a feature as an extra output is different from the benefit of using that feature as an input. As an input, the net has access to the values on the training and test cases to use for prediction. As an output, however, the net is instead biased to learn a mapping from the other inputs in the training set to that output. From the graphs it is clear that some features help when used either as an input, or as an output. Given that the benefit of using a feature as an extra output is different from that of using it as an input, can we get both benefits? Our early results with techniques that reap both benefits by allowing some features to be used simultaneously as both inputs and outputs while preventing learning direct feedthrough identity mappings are promising.

Acknowledgements

R. Caruana was supported in part by ARPA grant F33615-93-1-1330, NSF grant BES-9315428, and Agency for Health Care Policy and Research grant HS06468. V. de Sa was supported by postdoctoral fellowships from NSERC (Canada) and the Sloan Foundation. We thank Mitre Group for the Aspirin/Migraines Simulator and The University of Toronto for the Xerion Simulator.

References

[1] Y.S. Abu-Mostafa, "Learning From Hints in Neural Networks," *Journal of Complexity* 6:2, pp. 192–198, 1989.

[2] S. Baluja, and D.A. Pomerleau, "Using the Representation in a Neural Network's Hidden Layer for Task-Specific Focus of Attention". In C. Mellish (ed.) The International Joint Conference on Artificial Intelligence 1995 (IJCAI-95): Montreal, Canada. IJCAII & Morgan Kaufmann. San Mateo, CA. pp 133-139, 1995.

[3] S. Becker and G. E. Hinton, "A self-organizing neural network that discovers surfaces in random-dot stereograms," *Nature* **355** pp. 161-163, 1992.

[4] R. Caruana, S. Baluja, and T. Mitchell, "Using the Future to Sort Out the Present: Rankprop and Multitask Learning for Pneumnia Risk Prediction," *Advances in Neural Information Processing Systems 8*, 1996.

[5] R. Caruana, "Learning Many Related Tasks at the Same Time With Backpropagation," *Advances in Neural Information Processing Systems 7*, 1995.

[6] V. R. de Sa, "Learning classification with unlabeled data," *Advances in Neural Information Processing Systems 6*, pp. 112-119, Morgan Kaufmann, 1994.

[7] P. Simard, B. Victorri, Y. L. Cun, and J. Denker, "Tangent prop — a formalism for specifying selected invariances in an adaptive network," *Advances in Neural Information Processing Systems 4*, pp. 895-903, Morgan Kaufmann, 1992.

[8] S. Thrun and T. Mitchell, "Learning One More Thing," CMU TR: CS-94-184, 1994.

Self-Organizing and Adaptive Algorithms for Generalized Eigen-Decomposition

Chanchal Chatterjee
Newport Corporation
1791 Deere Avenue, Irvine, CA 92606

Vwani P. Roychowdhury
Electrical Engineering Department
UCLA, Los Angeles, CA 90095

ABSTRACT

The paper is developed in two parts where we discuss a new approach to self-organization in a single-layer linear feed-forward network. First, two novel algorithms for self-organization are derived from a two-layer linear hetero-associative network performing a one-of-m classification, and trained with the constrained least-mean-squared classification error criterion. Second, two adaptive algorithms are derived from these self-organizing procedures to compute the principal generalized eigenvectors of two correlation matrices from two sequences of random vectors. These novel adaptive algorithms can be implemented in a single-layer linear feed-forward network. We give a rigorous convergence analysis of the adaptive algorithms by using *stochastic approximation theory*. As an example, we consider a problem of online signal detection in digital mobile communications.

1. INTRODUCTION

We study the problems of hetero-associative training, linear discriminant analysis, generalized eigen-decomposition and their theoretical connections. The paper is divided into two parts. In the first part, we study the relations between hetero-associative training with a linear feed-forward network, and feature extraction by the linear discriminant analysis (LDA) criterion. Here we derive two novel algorithms that unify the two problems. In the second part, we generalize the self-organizing algorithm for LDA to obtain adaptive algorithms for generalized eigen-decomposition, for which we provide a rigorous proof of convergence by using *stochastic approximation theory*.

1.1 HETERO-ASSOCIATION AND LINEAR DISCRIMINANT ANALYSIS

In this discussion, we consider a special case of hetero-association that deals with the classification problems. Here the inputs belong to a finite m-set of pattern classes, and the outputs indicate the classes to which the inputs belong. Usually, the ith standard basis vector e_i is chosen to indicate that a particular input vector x belongs to class i.

The LDA problem, on the other hand, aims at projecting a multi-class data in a lower dimensional subspace such that it is grouped into well-separated clusters for the m classes. The method is based upon a set of scatter matrices commonly known as the mixture scatter S_m and between class scatter S_b (Fukunaga, 1990). These matrices are used to formulate criteria such as $\text{tr}(S_m^{-1}S_b)$ and $\det(S_b)/\det(S_m)$ which yield a linear transform Φ that satisfy the generalized eigenvector problem $S_b\Phi=S_m\Phi\Lambda$, where Λ is the generalized eigenvalue matrix. If S_m is positive definite, we obtain a Φ such that $\Phi^T S_m \Phi = I$ and $\Phi^T S_b \Phi = \Lambda$. Furthermore, the significance of each eigenvector (for class separability) is determined by the corresponding generalized eigenvalue.

A relation between hetero-association and LDA was demonstrated by Gallinari et al. (1991). Their work made explicit that for a linear multi-layer perceptron performing a one-from-m classification that minimized the total mean square error (MSE) at the network output, also maximized a criterion $\det(S_b)/\det(S_m)$ for LDA at the final hidden layer. This study was generalized by Webb and Lowe (1990) by using a nonlinear transform from the input data to the final hidden units, and a linear transform in the final layer. This has been further generalized by Chatterjee and Roychowdhury (1996) by including the Bayes cost for misclassification into the criteria $\text{tr}(S_m^{-1}S_b)$.

Although the above studies offer useful insights into the relations between hetero-association and LDA, they do not suggest an *algorithm* to extract the optimal LDA transform Φ. Since the criteria for class separability are insensitive to multiplication by nonsingular matrices, the above studies suggest that any training procedure that minimizes the MSE at the network output will yield a nonsingular transformation of Φ; i.e., we obtain $Q\Phi$ where Q is a nonsingular matrix. Since $Q\Phi$ does not satisfy the generalized eigenvector problem $S_b\Phi=S_m\Phi\Lambda$ for any arbitrary nonsingular matrix Q, we need to determine an algorithm that will yield $Q=I$.

In order to obtain the optimum linear transform Φ, we constrain the training of a two-layer linear feed-forward network, such that at convergence, the weights for the first layer simultaneously diagonalizes S_m and S_b. Thus, the hetero-associative network is trained by minimizing a *constrained MSE* at the network output. This training procedure yields two novel algorithms for LDA.

1.2 LDA AND GENERALIZED EIGEN-DECOMPOSITION

Since the LDA problem is a generalized eigen-decomposition problem for the symmetric-definite case, the self-organizing algorithms derived from the hetero-associative networks lead us to construct *adaptive algorithms* for generalized eigen-decomposition. Such adaptive algorithms are required in several applications of image and signal processing. As an example, we consider the problem of online interference cancellation in digital mobile communications.

Similar to the LDA problem $S_b\Phi=S_m\Phi\Lambda$, the generalized eigen-decomposition problem $A\Phi=B\Phi\Lambda$ involves the matrix pencil (A,B), where A and B are assumed to be real, symmetric and positive definite. Although a solution to the problem can be obtained by a conventional method, there are several applications in image and signal processing where an online solution of generalized eigen-decomposition is desired. In these real-time situations, the matrices A and B are themselves unknown. Instead, there are available two sequences of random vectors $\{\mathbf{x}_k\}$ and $\{\mathbf{y}_k\}$ with $\lim_{k\to\infty} E[\mathbf{x}_k\mathbf{x}_k^T] = A$ and $\lim_{k\to\infty} E[\mathbf{y}_k\mathbf{y}_k^T] = B$, where $\mathbf{x}_k$ and $\mathbf{y}_k$ represent the online observations of the application. For every sample $(\mathbf{x}_k, \mathbf{y}_k)$, we need to obtain the current estimates Φ_k and Λ_k of Φ and Λ respectively, such that Φ_k and Λ_k converge strongly to their true values.

The conventional approach for evaluating Φ and Λ requires the computation of (A,B) after collecting all of the samples, and then the application of a numerical procedure; i.e., the approach works in a *batch* fashion. There are two problems with this approach. Firstly, the dimension of the samples may be large so that even if all of the samples are available, performing the generalized eigen-decomposition may take prohibitively large amount of computational time. Secondly, the conventional schemes can not adapt to slow or small changes in the data. So the approach is not suitable for real-time applications where the samples come in an *online* fashion.

Although the adaptive generalized eigen-decomposition algorithms are natural generalizations of the self-organizing algorithms for LDA, their derivations do not constitute a proof of convergence. We, therefore, give a rigorous proof of convergence by *stochastic approximation theory*, that shows that the estimates obtained from our adaptive algorithms converge with probability one to the generalized eigenvectors.

In summary, the study offers the following contributions: (1) we present two novel algorithms that unify the problems of hetero-associative training and LDA feature extraction; and (2) we discuss two single-stage adaptive algorithms for generalized eigen-decomposition from two sequences of random vectors.

In our experiments, we consider an example of online interference cancellation in digital mobile communications. In this problem, the signal from a desired user at a far distance from the receiver is corrupted by another user very near to the base. The optimum linear transform $\mathbf{w}$ for weighting the signal is the first principal generalized eigenvector of the signal correlation matrix with respect to the interference correlation matrix. Experiments with our algorithm suggest a rapid convergence within four bits of transmitted signal, and provides a significant advantage over many current methods.

2. HETERO-ASSOCIATIVE TRAINING AND LDA

We consider a two-layer linear network performing a one-from-m classification. Let $\mathbf{x} \in \Re^n$ be an input to the network to be classified into one out of m classes $\omega_1,...,\omega_m$. If $\mathbf{x} \in \omega_i$ then the desired output $\mathbf{d} = \mathbf{e}_i$ (i^{th} std. basis vector). Without loss of generality, we assume the inputs to be a zero-mean stationary process with a nonsingular covariance matrix.

2.1 EXTRACTING THE PRINCIPAL LDA COMPONENTS

In the two-layer linear hetero-associative network, let there be p neurons in the hidden layer, and m output units. The aim is to develop an algorithm so that individual weight vectors for the first layer converge to the first $p \leq m$ generalized eigenvectors corresponding to the p significant generalized eigenvalues arranged in decreasing order. Let $\mathbf{w}_i \in \Re^n$ ($i=1,...,n$) be the weight vectors for the input layer, and $\mathbf{v}_i \in \Re^m$ ($i=1,...,m$) be the weight vectors for the output layer.

The neurons are trained sequentially; i.e., the training of the jth neuron is started only after the weight vector of the $(j-1)^{th}$ neuron has converged. Assume that all the $j-1$ previous neurons have already been trained and their weights have converged to the optimal weight vectors $\mathbf{w}_i$ for $i \in [1, j-1]$. To extract the jth generalized eigenvector in the output of the jth neuron, the updating model for this neuron should be constructed by subtracting the results from all previously computed $j-1$ generalized eigenvectors from the desired output $\mathbf{d}_j$ as below

$$\tilde{\mathbf{d}}_j = \mathbf{d}_j - \sum_{i=1}^{j-1} \mathbf{v}_i \mathbf{w}_i^T \mathbf{x}. \quad (1)$$

This process is equivalent to the *deflation* of the desired output.

The scatter matrices S_m and S_b can be obtained from $\mathbf{x}$ and $\mathbf{d}$ as $S_m = E[\mathbf{xx}^T]$ and $S_b = MM^T$, where $M = E[\mathbf{xd}^T]$. We need to extract the jth LDA transform $\mathbf{w}_j$ that satisfies the generalized eigenvector equation $S_b \mathbf{w}_j = \lambda_j S_m \mathbf{w}_j$ such that λ_j is the jth largest generalized eigenvalue. The constrained MSE criterion at the network output is

$$J(\mathbf{w}_j, \mathbf{v}_j) = E\left[\left\| \mathbf{d}_j - \sum_{i=1}^{j-1} \mathbf{v}_i \mathbf{w}_i^T \mathbf{x} - \mathbf{v}_j \mathbf{w}_j^T \mathbf{x} \right\|^2 \right] + \mu(\mathbf{w}_j^T S_m \mathbf{w}_j - 1). \quad (2)$$

Using (2), we obtain the update equation for $\mathbf{w}_j$ as

$$\mathbf{w}_{k+1}^{(j)} = \mathbf{w}_k^{(j)} + \eta \left(M\mathbf{v}_k^{(j)} - S_m \mathbf{w}_k^{(j)} \left(\mathbf{w}_k^{(j)T} M\mathbf{v}_k^{(j)} \right) - S_m \sum_{i=1}^{j-1} \mathbf{w}_k^{(j)} \mathbf{v}_k^{(i)T} \mathbf{v}_k^{(j)} \right). \quad (3)$$

Differentiating (2) with respect to $\mathbf{v}_j$, and equating it to zero, we obtain the optimum value of $\mathbf{v}_j$ as $M^T \mathbf{w}_j$. Substituting this $\mathbf{v}_j$ in (3) we obtain

$$\mathbf{w}_{k+1}^{(j)} = \mathbf{w}_k^{(j)} + \eta \left(S_b \mathbf{w}_k^{(j)} - S_m \mathbf{w}_k^{(j)} \left(\mathbf{w}_k^{(j)T} S_b \mathbf{w}_k^{(j)} \right) - S_m \sum_{i=1}^{j-1} \mathbf{w}_k^{(i)} \mathbf{w}_k^{(i)T} S_b \mathbf{w}_k^{(j)} \right). \quad (4)$$

Let W_k be the matrix whose i^{th} column is $\mathbf{w}_k^{(i)}$. Then (4) can be written in matrix form as

$$W_{k+1} = W_k + \eta \left(S_b W_k - S_m W_k \text{UT}\left[W_k^T S_b W_k \right] \right), \quad (5)$$

where UT[·] sets all elements below the diagonal of its matrix argument to zero, thereby making it upper triangular.

2.2 ANOTHER SELF-ORGANIZING ALGORITHM FOR LDA

In the previous analysis for a two-layer linear hetero-associative network, we observed that the optimum value for $V = W^T M$, where the ith column of W and row of V are formed by $\mathbf{w}_i$ and $\mathbf{v}_i$ respectively. It is, therefore, worthwhile to explore the gradient descent procedure on the error function below instead of (2)

$$J(W) = E\left[\left\| \mathbf{d} - M^T W W^T \mathbf{x} \right\|^2 \right]. \quad (6)$$

By differentiating this error function with respect to W, and including the deflation process, we obtain the following update procedure for W instead of (5)

$$W_{k+1} = W_k + \eta \left(2 S_b W_k - S_m W_k \text{UT}\left[W_k^T S_b W_k \right] - S_b W_k \text{UT}\left[W_k^T S_m W_k \right] \right). \quad (7)$$

3. LDA AND GENERALIZED EIGEN-DECOMPOSITION

Since LDA consists of solving the generalized eigenvector problem $S_b \Phi = S_m \Phi \Lambda$, we can naturally generalize algorithms (5) and (7) to obtain adaptive algorithms for the generalized eigen-decomposition problem $A\Phi = B\Phi\Lambda$, where A and B are assumed to be symmetric and positive definite. Here, we do not have the matrices A and B. Instead, there are available two sequences of random vectors $\{x_k\}$ and $\{y_k\}$ with $\lim_{k\to\infty} E[x_k x_k^T] = A$ and $\lim_{k\to\infty} E[y_k y_k^T] = B$, where x_k and y_k represent the online observations.

From (5), we obtain the following adaptive algorithm for generalized eigen-decomposition

$$W_{k+1} = W_k + \eta_k \left(A_k W_k - B_k W_k \mathrm{UT}\left[W_k^T A_k W_k \right] \right). \tag{8}$$

Here $\{\eta_k\}$ is a sequence of scalar gains, whose properties are described in Section 4. The sequences $\{A_k\}$ and $\{B_k\}$ are instantaneous values of the matrices A and B respectively. Although the A_k and B_k values can be obtained from x_k and y_k as $x_k x_k^T$ and $y_k y_k^T$ respectively, our algorithm requires that at least one of the $\{A_k\}$ or $\{B_k\}$ sequences have a dominated convergence property. Thus, the $\{A_k\}$ and $\{B_k\}$ sequences may be obtained from $x_k x_k^T$ and $y_k y_k^T$ from the following algorithms

$$A_k = A_{k-1} + \gamma_k \left(x_k x_k^T - A_{k-1} \right) \text{ and } B_k = B_{k-1} + \gamma_k \left(y_k y_k^T - B_{k-1} \right), \tag{9}$$

where A_0 and B_0 are symmetric, and $\{\gamma_k\}$ is a scalar gain sequence.
As done before, we can generalize (7) to obtain the following adaptive algorithm for generalized eigen-decomposition from a sequence of samples $\{A_k\}$ and $\{B_k\}$

$$W_{k+1} = W_k + \eta_k \left(2 A_k W_k - B_k W_k \mathrm{UT}\left[W_k^T A_k W_k \right] - A_k W_k \mathrm{UT}\left[W_k^T B_k W_k \right] \right). \tag{10}$$

Although algorithms (8) and (10) were derived from the network MSE by the gradient descent approach, this derivation does not guarantee their convergence. In order to prove their convergence, we use *stochastic approximation theory*. We give the convergence results only for algorithm (10).

4. STOCHASTIC APPROX. CONVG. PROOF FOR ALG. (10)

In order to prove the convergence of (10), we use stochastic approximation theory due to Ljung (1977). In stochastic approximation theory, we study the asymptotic properties of (10) in terms of the ordinary differential equation (ODE)

$$\frac{d}{dt} W(t) = \lim_{k\to\infty} E\left[2 A_k W - B_k W \mathrm{UT}\left[W^T A_k W \right] - A_k W \mathrm{UT}\left[W^T B_k W \right] \right],$$

where $W(t)$ is the continuous time counterpart of W_k with t denoting continuous time. The method of proof requires the following steps: (1) establishing a set of conditions to be imposed on A, B, A_k, B_k, and η_k, (2) finding the stable stationary points of the ODE; and (3) demonstrating that W_k visits a compact subset of the domain of attraction of a stable stationary point infinitely often.

We use Theorem 1 of Ljung (1977) for the convergence proof. The following is a general set of assumptions for the convergence proof of (10):

Assumption (A1). Each x_k and y_k is bounded with probability one, and $\lim_{k\to\infty} E[x_k x_k^T] = A$ and $\lim_{k\to\infty} E[y_k y_k^T] = B$, where A and B are positive definite.

Assumption (A2). $\{\eta_k \in \Re^+\}$ satisfies $\eta_k \downarrow 0$, $\sum_{k=0}^{\infty} \eta_k = \infty$, $\sum_{k=0}^{\infty} \eta_k^r < \infty$ for some $r > 1$ and $\lim_{k\to\infty} \sup(\eta_k^{-1} - \eta_{k-1}^{-1}) < \infty$.

Assumption (A3). The p largest generalized eigenvalues of A with respect to B are each of unit multiplicity.

Lemma 1. *Let A1 and A2 hold. Let W^* be a locally asymptotically stable (in the sense of Liapunov) solution to the ordinary differential equation (ODE):*

$$\frac{d}{dt}W(t) = 2AW(t) - BW(t)\text{UT}\left[W(t)^T AW(t)\right] - AW(t)\text{UT}\left[W(t)^T BW(t)\right], \quad (11)$$

with domain of attraction $D(W^*)$. Then if there is a compact subset S of $D(W^*)$ such that $W_k \in S$ infinitely often, then we have $W_k \to W^*$ with probability one as $k \to \infty$. ∎

We denote $\lambda_1 > \lambda_2 > ... > \lambda_p \geq ... \geq \lambda_n > 0$ as the generalized eigenvalues of A with respect to B, and ϕ_i as the generalized eigenvector corresponding to λ_i such that $\phi_1,...,\phi_n$ are orthonormal with respect to B. Let $\Phi=[\phi_1...\phi_n]$ and $\Lambda=\text{diag}(\lambda_1,...,\lambda_n)$ denote the matrix of generalized eigenvectors and eigenvalues of A with respect to B. Note that if ϕ_i is a generalized eigenvector, then $d_i\phi_i$ ($|d_i|=1$) is also a generalized eigenvector.

In the next two lemmas, we first prove that all the possible equilibrium points of the ODE (11) are up to an arbitrary permutation of the p generalized eigenvectors of A with respect to B corresponding to the p largest generalized eigenvalues. We next prove that all these equilibrium points of the ODE (11) are unstable equilibrium points, except for $[d_1\phi_1 ... d_n\phi_n]$, where $|d_i|=1$ for $i=1,...,p$.

Lemma 2. *For the ordinary differential equation (11), let A1 and A3 hold. Then $W=\Phi DP$ are equilibrium points of (11), where $D=[D_1|0]^T$ is a nXp matrix with D_1 being a pXp diagonal matrix with diagonal elements d_i such that $|d_i|=1$ or $d_i=0$, and P is a nXn arbitrary permutation matrix.* ∎

Lemma 3. *Let A1 and A3 hold. Then $W=\Phi D$ (where $D=[D_1|0]^T$, $D_1=\text{diag}(d_1,...,d_p)$, $|d_i|=1$) are stable equilibrium points of the ODE (11). In addition, $W=\Phi DP$ ($d_i=0$ for $i \leq p$ or $P \neq I$) are unstable equilibrium points of the ODE (11).* ∎

Lemma 4. *For the ordinary differential equation (11), let A1 and A3 hold. Then the points $W=\Phi D$ (where $D=[D_1|0]^T$, $D_1=\text{diag}(d_1,...,d_p)$, $|d_i|=1$ for $i=1,...,p$) are asymptotically stable.* ∎

Lemma 5. *Let A1-A3 hold. Then there exists a uniform upper bound for η_k such that W_k is uniformly bounded w.p.1.* ∎

The convergence of alg. (10) can now be established by referring to Theorem 1 of Ljung.

Theorem 1. *Let A1-A3 hold. Assume that with probability one the process $\{W_k\}$ visits infinitely often a compact subset of the domain of attraction of one of the asymptotically stable points ΦD. Then with probability one*

$$\lim_{k \to \infty} W_k = \Phi D.$$

Proof. By Lemma 2, ΦD ($|d_i|=1$) are asymptotically stable points of the ODE (11). Since we assume that $\{W_k\}$ visits a compact subset of the domain of attraction of ΦD infinitely often, Lemma 1 then implies the theorem. ∎

5. EXPERIMENTAL RESULTS

We describe the performance of algorithms (8) and (10) with an example of online interference cancellation in a high-dimensional signal, in a digital mobile communication problem. The problem occurs when the desired user transmits a signal from a far distance to the receiver, while another user simultaneously transmits very near to the base. For common receivers, the quality of the received signal from the desired user is dominated by interference from the user close to the base. Due to the high rate and large dimension of the data, the system demands an accurate detection method for just a few data samples.

If we use conventional (numerical analysis) methods, signal detection will require a significant part of the time slot allotted to a receiver, accordingly reducing the effective communication rate. Adaptive generalized eigen-decomposition algorithms, on the other hand, allow the tracking of slow changes, and directly performs signal detection.

The details of the data model can be found in Zoltowski et al. (1996). In this application, the duration for each transmitted code is 127 μs, within which we have 10μs of signal and 117μs of interference. We take 10 frequency samples equi-spaced between –0.4MHz to +0.4MHz. Using 6 antennas, the signal and interference correlation matrices are of dimension 60X60 in the complex domain.

We use both algorithms (8) and (10) for the cancellation of the interference. Figure 1 shows the convergence of the principal generalized eigenvector and eigenvalue. The closed form solution is obtained after collecting all of the signal and interference samples. In order to measure the accuracy of the algorithms, we compute the direction cosine of the estimated principal generalized eigenvector and the generalized eigenvector computed by the conventional method. The optimum value is one. We also show the estimated principal generalized eigenvalue in Figure 1b. The results show that both algorithms converge after the 4th bit of signal.

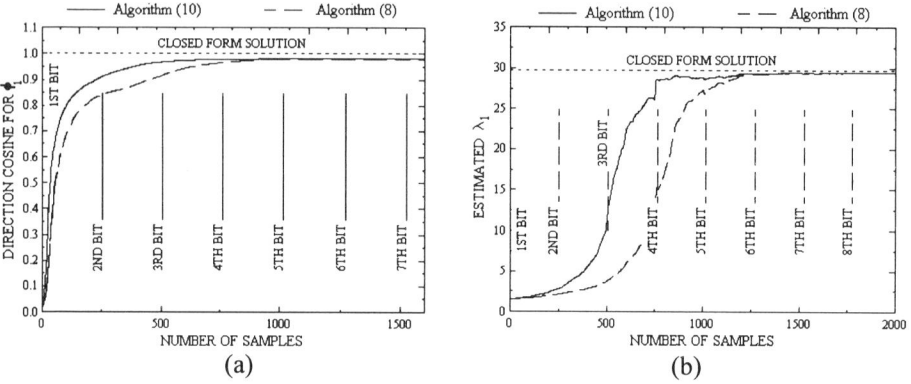

Figure 1. (a) Direction Cosine of Estimated First Principal Generalized Eigenvector, and (b) Estimated First Principal Generalized Eigenvalue.

References

C.Chatterjee and V.Roychowdhury (1996), "Statistical Risk Analysis for Classification and Feature Extraction by Multilayer Perceptrons", *Proceedings IEEE Int'l Conference on Neural Networks*, Washington D.C.

K.Fukunaga (1990), *Introduction to Statistical Pattern Recognition*, 2nd Edition, New York: Academic Press.

P.Gallinari, S.Thiria, F.Badran, F.Fogelman-Soulie (1991), "On the Relations Between Discriminant Analysis and Multilayer Perceptrons", *Neural Networks*, Vol. 4, pp. 349-360.

L.Ljung (1977), "Analysis of Recursive Stochastic Algorithms", *IEEE Transactions on Automatic Control*, Vol. AC-22, No. 4, pp. 551-575.

A.R.Webb and D.Lowe (1990), "The Optimised Internal Representation of Multilayer Classifier Networks Performs Nonlinear Discriminant Analysis", *Neural Networks*, Vol. 3, pp. 367-375.

M.D.Zoltowski, C.Chatterjee, V.Roychowdhury and J.Ramos (1996), "Blind Adaptive 2D RAKE Receiver for CDMA Based on Space-Time MVDR Processing", submitted to *IEEE Transactions on Signal Processing*.

Representation and Induction of Finite State Machines using Time-Delay Neural Networks

Daniel S. Clouse
Computer Science & Engineering Dept.
University of California, San Diego
La Jolla, CA 92093-0114
dclouse@ucsd.edu

C. Lee Giles
NEC Research Institute
4 Independence Way
Princeton, NJ 08540
giles@research.nj.nec.com

Bill G. Horne
NEC Research Institute
4 Independence Way
Princeton, NJ 08540
horne@research.nj.nec.com

Garrison W. Cottrell
Computer Science & Engineering Dept.
University of California, San Diego
La Jolla, CA 92093-0114
gcottrell@ucsd.edu

Abstract

This work investigates the representational and inductive capabilities of *time-delay neural networks* (TDNNs) in general, and of two subclasses of TDNN, those with delays only on the inputs (IDNN), and those which include delays on hidden units (HDNN). Both architectures are capable of representing the same class of languages, the *definite memory machine* (DMM) languages, but the delays on the hidden units in the HDNN helps it outperform the IDNN on problems composed of repeated features over short time windows.

1 Introduction

In this paper we consider the representational and inductive capabilities of *time-delay neural networks* (TDNN) [Waibel et al., 1989] [Lang et al., 1990], also known as NNFIR [Wan, 1993]. A TDNN is a feed-forward network in which the set of inputs to any node i may include the output from previous layers not only in the current time step t, but from d earlier time steps as well. The activation function for node i at time t in such a network is given by equation 1:

$$y_i^t = h(\sum_{j=1}^{i-1} \sum_{k=0}^{d} y_j^{t-k} w_{ijk}) \quad (1)$$

where y_i^t is the activation of node i at time t, w_{ijk} is the connection strength from node j to node i at delay k, and h is the squashing function.

TDNNs have been used in speech recognition [Waibel et al., 1989], and time series prediction [Wan, 1993]. In this paper we concentrate on the language induction problem. A training set of variable-length strings taken from a discrete alphabet $\{0,1\}$ is generated. Each string is labeled as to whether it is in some language L or not. The network must learn to discriminate strings which are in the language from those which are not, not only for the training set strings, but for strings the network has never seen before. The language induction problem provides a simple, familiar domain in which to gain insight into the capabilities of different network architectures.

Specifically, in this paper, we will look at the representational and inductive capabilities of the general class of TDNNs versus a subclass of TDNNs, the *input-delay neural networks* (IDNNs). An IDNN is a TDNN in which delays are limited to the network inputs. In section 2, we will show that the classes of functions representable by general TDNNs and IDNNs are equivalent. In section 3, we will show that the class of languages representable by the TDNNs, are the *definite memory machine* (DMM) languages. In section 4, we will demonstrate the inductive capability of the TDNNs in a simulation in which a large DMM is learned using a small percentage of the possible, short training examples. In section 5, a second set of simulations will show the difference between *representational* and *inductive bias*, and will demonstrate the utility of internal delays in a TDNN network.

2 TDNNs and IDNNs Are Functionally Equivalent

Since every IDNN is also a TDNN, the set of functions computable by any TDNN includes all those computable by the IDNNs. [Wan, 1993] also shows that the IDNNs can compute any function computable by the TDNNs making these two classes of network architectures functionally equivalent. For completeness, here we include a description of how to construct from a TDNN, an equivalent IDNN.

Figure 1a shows a TDNN with a single input u at the current time (u_t), and at four earlier time steps $(u_{t-1} \ldots u_{t-4})$. The inputs to node R consist of the outputs of nodes P and Q at the current time step along with one or two previous time steps. At time t, node P computes $f_P(u_t, \ldots u_{t-4})$, a function of the current input and four delays. At time $t-1$, node P computes $f_P(u_{t-1}, \ldots u_{t-5})$. This serves as one of the delayed inputs to node R. This value could also be computed by sliding node P over one step in the input tap-delay line along with its incoming weights as shown in figure 1b. Using this construction, all the internal delays can be removed, and replaced by copies of the original nodes P and Q, along with their incoming weights. This method can be applied recursively to remove any internal delay in any TDNN network. Thus, for any function computable by a TDNN, we can construct an IDNN which computes the same function.

3 TDNNs Can Represent the DMM Languages

In this section, we show that the set of languages which are representable by some TDNN are exactly those languages representable by the *definite memory machines*

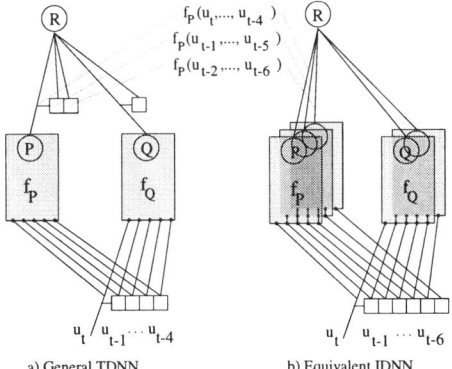

Figure 1: Constructing an IDNN equivalent to a given TDNN

(DMMs). According to Kohavi (1978) a DMM of order d is a *finite state machine* (FSM) whose present state can always be determined uniquely from the knowledge of the most recent d inputs. We equivalently define a DMM of order d as an FSM whose accepting/rejecting behavior is a function of only the most recent d inputs.

To fit TDNNs and IDNNs into the language induction framework, we consider only networks with a single 0/1 input. Since any boolean function can be represented by a feed-forward network with enough hidden units [Horne and Hush, 1994], an IDNN exists which can perform the mapping from d most recent inputs to any accepting/rejecting behavior. Therefore, any DMM language can be represented by some IDNN. Since every IDNN computes a function of its most recent d inputs, by the definition of DMM, there is no boolean output IDNN which represents a non-DMM language. Therefore, the IDNNs represent exactly the DMM languages. Since the TDNN and IDNN classes are functionally equivalent, TDNNs implement exactly the DMM languages as well.

The shift register behavior of the input tap-delay line in an IDNN completely determines the state transition behavior of any machine represented by the network. This state transition behavior is fixed by the architecture. For example, figure 2a shows the state transition diagram for any machine representable by an IDNN with two input delays. The mapping from the current state to "accept" or "reject" is all that can be changed with training. Clouse et al. (1994) describes the conditions under which such a mapping results in a minimal FSM. All mappings used in the subsequent simulations are minimal FSM mappings.

4 Simulation 1: Large DMM

To demonstrate the close relationship between TDNNs and DMMs, here we present the results of a simulation in which we trained an IDNN to reproduce the behavior of a DMM of order 11. The mapping function for the DMM is given in equation 2. Figure 2b shows the minimal 2048 state transition diagram required to represent the DMM. The symbol $\leftrightarrow$ in equation 2 represents the *if-and-only-if* function. The overbar notation, $\bar{u}_k$, represents the negation of u_k, the input at time k. Y_k is the network output at time k. $Y_k > 0.5$ is interpreted as "accept the string seen so far." $Y_k \leq 0.5$ means "reject."

$$y_k = u_{k-10} \leftrightarrow (\bar{u}_k \bar{u}_{k-1} \bar{u}_{k-2} + \bar{u}_{k-2} u_{k-3} + u_{k-1} u_{k-2}) \tag{2}$$

To create training and test sets, we randomly split in two the set of all 4094

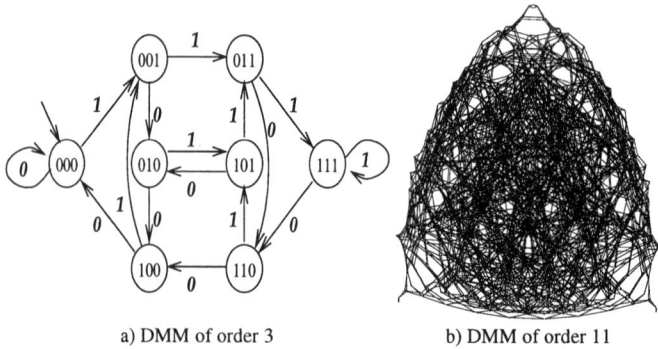

a) DMM of order 3   b) DMM of order 11

Figure 2: Transition diagrams for two DMMs.

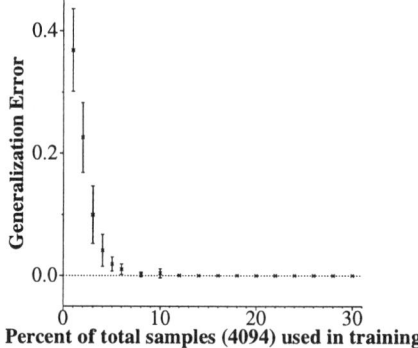

Figure 3: Generalization error on 2048 state DMM.

strings of length 11 or less. We will report results using various percentages of possible strings for the training set. The IDNN had 10 input tap-delays, and seven hidden units. All tap-delays were cleared to 0 before introduction of a new input string. Weights were trained using online back propagation with learning rate 0.25, and momentum 0.25. To speed up the algorithm, weights were updated only if the absolute error on an example was greater than 0.2. Training was stopped when weight updates were required for no examples in the training set. This generally required 200 epochs or fewer, though there were trials which required almost 4000 epochs.

Each point in figure 3 represents the mean classification error on the test set across 20 trials. Error bars indicate one standard deviation on each side of the mean. Each trial consists of a different randomly-chosen training set. The graph plots error at various training set sizes. Note that with training sets as small as 12 percent of possible strings the network generalizes perfectly to the remaining 88 percent. This kind of performance is possible because of the close match between the representational bias of the IDNN and this specific problem.

5   Simulation 2: Inductive biases of IDNNs and HDNNs

In section 2, we showed that the IDNNs and general TDNNs can *represent* the same class of functions. It does not follow that these two architectures are equally capable of *learning* the same functions. In this section, we show that the inductive biases are indeed different. We will present our intuitions about the kinds of problems each architecture is well suited to learning, then back up our intuitions with supporting simulations.

In the following simulations, we compare two specific networks. The network representing the general TDNNs includes delays on hidden layer outputs. We'll refer to this as the *hidden delay neural network* or HDNN. All delays in the second network are confined to the network inputs, and so we call this the IDNN.

We have been careful to design the two networks to be comparable in size. Each of the networks contains two hidden layers. The first hidden layer of the IDNN has four units, and the second five. The IDNN has eight input delays. Each of the two hidden layers of the HDNN has three units. The HDNN has three input delays, and five delays on the output of each node of the first hidden layer. Note that in each network the longest path from input to output requires eight delays. The number of weights, including bias weights, are also similar – 76 for the HDNN, and 79 for the IDNN.

In order for the size of the two networks to be similar, the HDNN must have fewer delays on the network inputs. If we think of each unit in the first hidden layer as a feature detector, the feature detectors in the HDNN will span a smaller time window than the IDNN. On the other hand, the HDNN has a second set of delays which saves the output of the feature detectors over several time steps. If some narrow feature repeats over time, this second set of delays should help the HDNN to pick up this regularity. The IDNN, lacking the internal delays, should find it more difficult to detect this kind of repeated regularity.

To test these ideas, we generated four DMM problems. We call equation 3 the *narrow-repeated* problem because it contains a number of identical terms shifted in time, and because each of these terms is narrow enough to fit in the time window of the HDNN first layer feature detectors.

$$y_k = u_{k-8} \leftrightarrow (u_k u_{k-2} \overline{u}_{k-3} + u_{k-1} u_{k-3} \overline{u}_{k-4} + u_{k-3} u_{k-5} \overline{u}_{k-6} + u_{k-4} u_{k-6} \overline{u}_{k-7}) \tag{3}$$

The *wide-repeated* problem, represented by equation 4, is identical to the narrow-repeated problem except that each term has been stretched so that it will no longer fit in the HDNN feature detector time window.

$$y_k = u_{k-8} \leftrightarrow (u_k u_{k-2} \overline{u}_{k-4} + u_{k-1} u_{k-3} \overline{u}_{k-5} + u_{k-2} u_{k-4} \overline{u}_{k-6} + u_{k-3} u_{k-5} \overline{u}_{k-7}) \tag{4}$$

The *narrow-unrepeated* problem, represented by equation 5, is composed of narrow terms, but none of these terms is simply a shifted reproduction of another.

$$y_k = u_{k-8} \leftrightarrow (u_k u_{k-2} \overline{u}_{k-3} + \overline{u}_{k-1} u_{k-3} u_{k-4} + u_{k-3} \overline{u}_{k-5} u_{k-6} + \overline{u}_{k-4} \overline{u}_{k-6} \overline{u}_{k-7}) \tag{5}$$

Lastly, the *wide-unrepeated* problem of equation 6 contains wide terms which do not repeat.

$$y_k = u_{k-8} \leftrightarrow (u_k u_{k-3} \overline{u}_{k-4} + \overline{u}_{k-1} u_{k-4} u_{k-5} + u_{k-2} \overline{u}_{k-5} u_{k-6} + \overline{u}_{k-3} \overline{u}_{k-6} \overline{u}_{k-7}) \tag{6}$$

Each problem in this section requires a minimum of 512 states to represent.

Similar to the simulation of section 3, we trained both networks on subsets of all possible strings of length 9 or less. Since these problems were more difficult than that of section 3, often the networks were unable to find a solution which performed perfectly on the training set. In this case, training was stopped after 8000 epochs. The results reported later include these trials as well as trials in which training ended because of perfect performance on the training set. Training for the HDNN

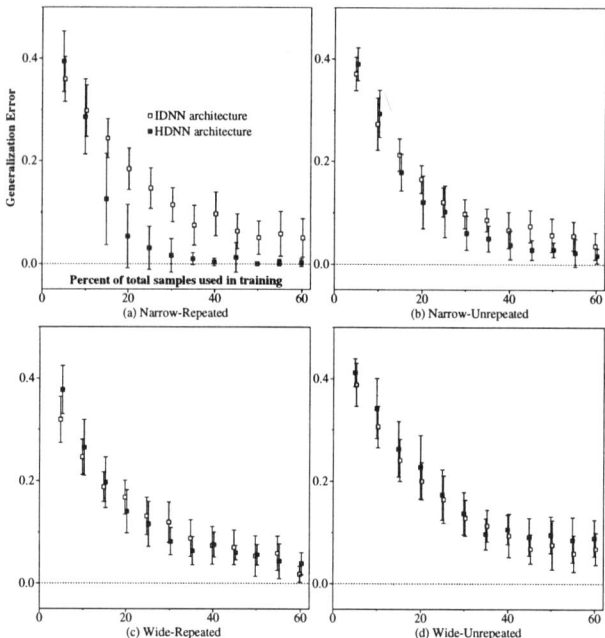

Figure 4: Generalization of a HDNN and an IDNN on four DMM problems

was identical to that of the IDNN except that error was propagated back across the internal delays as in Wan (1993).

Figure 4 plots generalization error versus percentage of possible strings used in training for the two networks for each of the four DMM problems. If our intuitions were correct we would expect to see evidence here that the effect of wider terms, and lack of repetition would have a stronger adverse effect on the HDNN network than on the IDNN. This is exactly what we see. The position of the curve for the IDNN network is stable compared to that of the HDNN when changes are made to the width and repetition factors.

Statistical analysis supports this conclusion. We ran an ANOVA test [Rice, 1988] with four factors (which network, term width, term repetition, and training set size) on the data summarized by the graphs of figure 4. The test detected a significant interaction between the network and width factors ($MS_{net \times wid} = 0.3430$, $F(1, 1824) = 234.4$), and between the network and repetition factors ($MS_{net \times rep} = 0.1181$, $F(1, 1824) = 80.694$). These two interactions are significant at $p < 0.001$, agreeing with our conclusion that width and repetition each has a stronger effect on the performance of the HDNN network.

Further planned tests reveal that the effects of width and repetition are strong enough to change which network generalizes better. We ran a one-way ANOVA test on each problem individually to see which network performs better across the entire curve. The tests reveal that the HDNN performs with significantly less error than the IDNN in the narrow-repeated problem ($MS_{error} = 0.0015$, $MS_{net} = 0.5400$, $F(1, 1824) = 369.0$), and in the narrow-unrepeated problem ($MS_{net} = 0.0683$, $F(1, 1824) = 46.7$). Performance of the IDNN is significantly better in the wide-unrepeated problem ($MS_{net} = 0.0378$, $F(1, 1824) = 25.83$). All of these comparisons are significant at $p < 0.001$. The test on the wide-repeated problem finds no significant difference in performance of the two networks ($MS_{net} = 0.0004$,

$F(1, 1824) = 0.273, p > 0.05)$.

In addition to confirming our intuitions about the kinds of problems that internal delays should be helpful in solving, this set of simulations demonstrates the difference between representational and inductive bias. For all DMM problems except for the wide-unrepeated one, we were able to find, for each network, at least one set of weights which solve the problem perfectly. Despite the fact that the two networks are both capable of representing the problems, the differing way in which they respond to the width and repetition factors demonstrates a difference in their learning biases.

6 Conclusions

This paper presents a number of interesting ideas concerning TDNNs using both theoretical and empirical techniques. On the theoretical side, we have precisely defined the subclass of FSMs which can be represented by TDNNs, the DMM languages. It is interesting to note that this network architecture which has no recurrent connections is capable of representing languages whose transition diagrams require loops.

Other ideas were demonstrated using empirical techniques. First, we have shown that the number of states required to represent an FSM may be a poor predictor of how difficult the language is to learn. We were able to learn a 2048-state FSM using a small percentage of the possible training examples. This is possible because of the close match between the representational bias of the network, and the language learned.

Second, we presented a set of simulations which demonstrated the utility of internal delays in a TDNN. These delays were shown to improve generalization on problems composed of features over short time intervals which reappear repeatedly.

Third, that same set of simulations highlights the difference between representational bias, and inductive bias. Though these two terms are sometimes used interchangeably in the theoretical literature, this work shows that the two concepts are, in fact, separable.

References

[Clouse et al., 1994] Clouse, D. S., Giles, C. L., Horne, B. G., and Cottrell, G. W. (1994). Learning large debruijn automata with feed-forward neural networks. Technical Report CS94-398, University of California, San Diego, Computer Science and Engineering Dept.

[Horne and Hush, 1994] Horne, B. G. and Hush, D. R. (1994). On the node complexity of neural networks. *Neural Networks*, 7(9):1413–1426.

[Kohavi, 1978] Kohavi, Z. (1978). *Switching and Finite Automata Theory*. McGraw-Hill, Inc., New York, NY, second edition.

[Lang et al., 1990] Lang, K., Waibel, A., and Hinton, G. (1990). A time-delay neural network architecture for isolated word recognition. *Neural Networks*, 3(1):23–44.

[Rice, 1988] Rice, J. A. (1988). *Mathematical Statistics and Data Analysis*. Brooks/Cole Publishing Company, Monterey, California.

[Waibel et al., 1989] Waibel, A., Hanazawa, T., Hinton, G., Shikano, K., and Lang, K. (1989). Phoneme recognition using time–delay neural networks. *IEEE Transactions on Acoustics, Speech and Signal Processing*, 37(3):328–339.

[Wan, 1993] Wan, E. A. (1993). Time series prediction by using a connectionist network with internal delay lines. In Weigend, A. S. and Gershenfeld, N. A., editors, *Time Series Prediction: Forecasting the Future and Understanding the Past*. Addison Wesley.

488 Solutions to the XOR Problem

Frans M. Coetzee *
coetzee@ece.cmu.edu
Department of Electrical Engineering
Carnegie Mellon University
Pittsburgh, PA 15213

Virginia L. Stonick
ginny@ece.cmu.edu
Department of Electrical Engineering
Carnegie Mellon University
Pittsburgh, PA 15213

Abstract

A globally convergent homotopy method is defined that is capable of sequentially producing large numbers of stationary points of the multi-layer perceptron mean-squared error surface. Using this algorithm large subsets of the stationary points of two test problems are found. It is shown empirically that the MLP neural network appears to have an extreme ratio of saddle points compared to local minima, and that even small neural network problems have extremely large numbers of solutions.

1 Introduction

The number and type of stationary points of the error surface provide insight into the difficulties of finding the optimal parameters of the network, since the stationary points determine the degree of the system[1]. Unfortunately, even for the small canonical test problems commonly used in neural network studies, it is still unknown how many stationary points there are, where they are, and how these are divided into minima, maxima and saddle points.

Since solving the neural equations explicitly is currently intractable, it is of interest to be able to numerically characterize the error surfaces of standard test problems. To perform such a characterization is non-trivial, requiring methods that reliably converge and are capable of finding large subsets of distinct solutions. It can be shown[2] that methods which produce only one solution set on a given trial become inefficient (at a factorial rate) at finding large sets of multiple distinct solutions, since the same solutions are found repeatedly. This paper presents the first provably globally convergent homotopy methods capable of finding large subsets of the

---

*Currently with Siemens Corporate Research, Princeton NJ 08540

stationary points of the neural network error surface. These methods are used to empirically quantify not only the number but also the type of solutions for some simple neural networks.

1.1 Sequential Neural Homotopy Approach Summary

We briefly acquaint the reader with the principles of homotopy methods, since these approaches differ significantly from standard descent procedures.

Homotopy methods solve systems of nonlinear equations by mapping the known solutions from an initial system to the desired solution of the unsolved system of equations. The basic method is as follows: Given a *final* set of equations $f(x) = 0, x \in D \subseteq \Re^n$ whose solution is sought, a *homotopy* function $h : D \times T \to \Re^n$ is defined in terms of a parameter $\tau \in T \subset \Re$, such that

$$h(x, \tau) = \begin{cases} g(x) & \text{when } \tau = 0 \\ f(x) & \text{when } \tau = 1 \end{cases}$$

where the *initial system* of equations $g(x) = 0$ has a known solution. For optimization problems $f(x) = \nabla_x \epsilon^2(x)$ where $\epsilon^2(x)$ is the error measure. Conceptually, $h(x, \tau) = 0$ is solved numerically for x for increasing values of τ, starting at $\tau = 0$ at the known solution, and incrementally varying τ and correcting the solution x until $\tau = 1$, thereby tracing a path from the initial to the final solutions.

The power and the problems of homotopy methods lie in constructing a suitable function h. Unfortunately, for a given f most choices of h will fail, and, with the exception of polynomial systems, no guaranteed procedures for selecting h exist. Paths generally do not connect the initial and final solutions, either due to non-existence of solutions, or due to paths diverging to infinity. However, if a theoretical proof of existence of a suitable trajectory can be constructed, well-established numerical procedures exist that reliably track the trajectory.

The following theorem, proved in [2], establishes that a suitable homotopy exists for the standard feed-forward backpropagation neural networks:

Theorem 1.1 *Let ϵ^2 be the unregularized mean square error (MSE) problem for the multi-layer perceptron network, with weights $\beta \in \Re^n$. Let $\beta_0 \in U \subset \Re^n$ and $a \in V \subset \Re^n$, where U and V are open bounded sets. Then except for a set of measure zero $(\beta, a) \in U \times V$, the solutions (β, τ) of the set of equations*

$$h(\beta, \tau) = (1 - \tau)(\beta - \beta_0) + \tau D_\beta \left(\epsilon^2 + \mu \psi(||\beta - a||^2) \right) = 0 \qquad (1)$$

where $\mu > 0$ and $\psi : \Re \to \Re$ satisfies $2\psi''(\alpha^2)\alpha^2 + \psi'(\alpha^2) > 0$ as $\alpha \to \infty$, form non-crossing one dimensional trajectories for all $\tau \in \Re$, which are bounded $\forall \tau \in [0, 1]$. Furthermore, the path through $(\beta_0, 0)$ connects to at least one solution $(\beta^*, 1)$ of the regularized MSE error problem

$$\min_\beta \left(\epsilon^2 + \mu \psi(||\beta - a||^2) \right) \qquad (2)$$

On $\tau \in [0, 1]$ the approach corresponds to a pseudo-quadratic error surface being deformed continuously into the final neural network error surface[1]. Multiple solu-

---

[1] The common engineering heuristic whereby some arbitrary error surface is relaxed into another error surface generally does *not* yield well defined trajectories.

tions can be obtained by choosing different initial values β_0. Every desired solution β^* is accessible via an appropriate choice of a, since $\beta_0 = \beta^*$ suffices.

Figure 1 qualitatively illustrates typical paths obtained for this homotopy[2]. The paths typically contain only a few solutions, are disconnected and diverge to infinity. A novel two-stage homotopy[2, 3] is used to overcome these problems by constructing and solving *two* homotopy equations. The first homotopy system is as described above. A synthetic second homotopy solves an auxiliary set of equations on a non-Euclidean compact manifold $(S^n(0;R) \times \Lambda$, where Λ is a compact subset of $R)$ and is used to move between the disconnected trajectories of the first homotopy. The method makes use of the topological properties of the compact manifold to ensure that the secondary homotopy paths do not diverge.

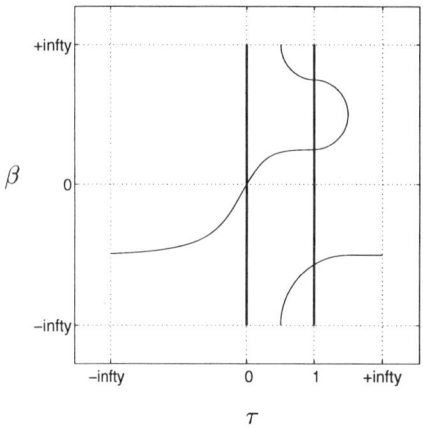
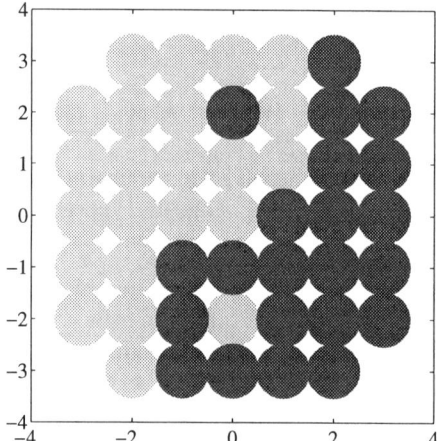

Figure 1: (a) Typical homotopy trajectories, illustrating divergence of paths and multiple solutions occurring on one path. (b) Plot of two-dimensional vectors used as training data for the second test problem (Yin-Yang problem).

2 Test Problems

The test problems described in this paper are small to allow for (i) a large number of repeated runs, and (ii) to make it possible to numerically distinguish between solutions. Classification problems were used since these present the only interesting small problems, even though the MSE criterion is not necessarily best for classification. Unlike most classification tasks, all algorithms were forced to approximate the stationary point accurately by requiring the l_1 norm of the gradient to be less than 10^{-10}, and ensuring that solutions differed in l_1 by more than 0.01.

The historical XOR problem is considered first. The data points $(-1,-1)$, $(1,1)$, $(-1,1)$ and $(1,-1)$ were trained to the target values $-0.8, -0.8, 0.8$ and 0.8. A network with three inputs (one constant), two hidden layer nodes and one output node were used, with hyperbolic tangent transfer functions on the hidden and final

---

[2] Note that the homotopy equation and its trajectories exist outside the interval $\tau = [0, 1]$.

nodes. The regularization used $\mu = 0.05$, $\psi(x) = x$ and $a = 0$ (no bifurcations were found for this value during simulations). This problem was chosen since it is small enough to serve as a benchmark for comparing the convergence and performance of the different algorithms. The second problem, referred to as the Yin-Yang problem, is shown in Figure 1. The problem has 23 and 22 data points in classes one and two respectively, and target values ±0.7. Empirical evidence indicates that the smallest single hidden layer network capable of solving the problem has five hidden nodes. We used a net with three inputs, five hidden nodes and one output. This problem is interesting since relatively high classification accuracy is obtained using only a single neuron, but a 100% classification performance requires at least five hidden nodes and one of only a few global weight solutions.

The stationary points form equivalence classes under renumbering of the weights or appropriate interchange of weight signs. For the XOR problem each solution class contains up to $2^2 \, 2! = 8$ distinct solutions; for the Yin-Yang network, there are $2^5 \, 5! = 3840$ symmetries. *The equivalence classes are reported in the following sections.*

3 Test Results

A Ribak-Poliere conjugate gradient (CG) method was used as a control since this method can find only minima, as contrasted to the other algorithms, all of which are attracted by all stationary points. In the second algorithm, the homotopy equation (1) was solved by following the main path until divergence. A damped Newton (DN) method and the two-stage homotopy method completed the set of four algorithms considered. The different algorithms were initialized with the same n random weights $\beta_0 \in S^{n-1}(0; \sqrt{2n})$.

3.1 Control - The XOR problem

The total number and classification of the solutions obtained for 250 iterations on each algorithm are shown in Table 1.

Table 1: Number of equivalence class solutions obtained. XOR Problem

Algorithm	# Solutions	#Minima	# Maxima	#Saddle Points
CG	17	17	0	0
DN	44	6	0	38
One Stage	28	16	0	12
Two Stage	61	17	0	44
Total Distinct	61	17	0	44

The probability of finding a given solution on a trial is shown in Figure 2. The two-stage homotopy method finds almost every solution from every initial point. In contrast to the homotopy approaches, the Newton method exhibits poor convergence, even when heavily damped. The sets of saddle points found by the DN algorithm and the homotopy algorithms are to a large extent disjoint, even though the same initial weights were used. For the Newton method solutions close to the initial point are typically obtained, while the initial point for the homotopy algo-

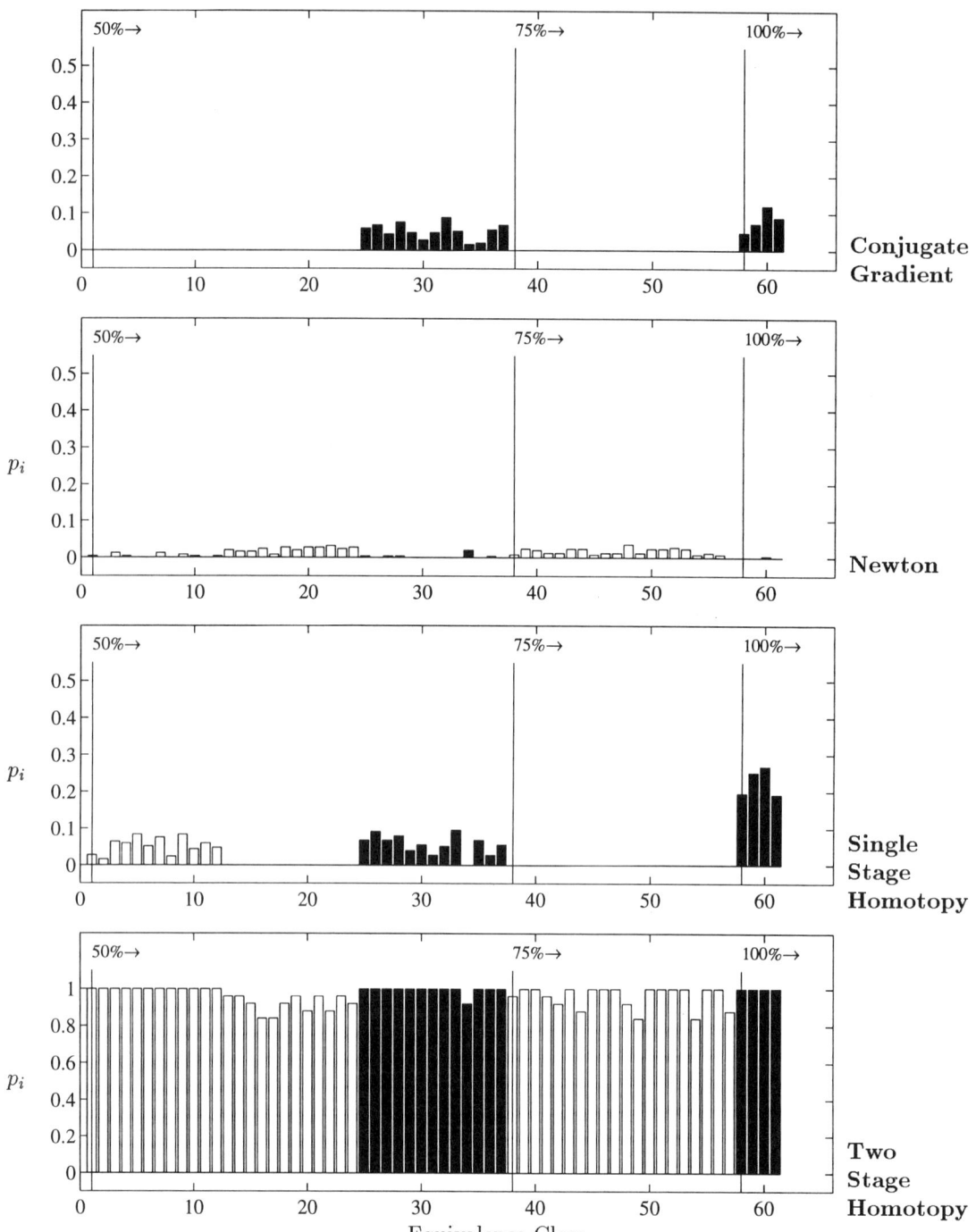

Figure 2: Probability of finding equivalence class i on a trial. Solutions have been sorted based on percentage of the training set correctly classified. Dark bars indicate local minima, light bars saddle points. XOR problem

Table 2: Number of solutions correctly classifying $x\%$ of target data.

Classification	25 %	50 %	75 %	100 %
Minimum	17	17	4	4
Saddle	44	44	20	0
Total Distinct	61	61	24	4

rithm might differ significantly from the final solution. This difference illustrates that homotopy arrives at solutions in a fundamentally different way than descent approaches.

Based on these results we conclude that the two-stage homotopy meets its objective of significantly increasing the number of solutions produced on a single trial. The homotopy algorithms converge more reliably than Newton methods, in theory and in practise. These properties make homotopy attractive for characterizing error surfaces. Finally, due to the large number of trials and significant overlap between the solution sets for very different algorithms, we believe that Tables 1-2 represent accurate estimates for the number and types of solutions to the regularized XOR problem.

3.2 Results on the Yin-Yang problem

The first three algorithms for the Yin-Yang problem were evaluated for 100 trials. The conjugate gradient method showed excellent stability, while the Newton method exhibited serious convergence problems, even with heavy damping. The two-stage algorithm was still producing solutions when the runs were terminated after multiple weeks of computer time, allowing evaluation of only ten different initial points.

Table 3: Number of equivalence class solutions obtained. Yin-Yang Problem

Algorithm	# Solutions	#Minima	# Maxima	#Saddle Points
Conjugate Gradient	14	14	0	0
Damped Newton	10	0	0	10
One Stage Homotopy	78	15	0	63
Two Stage Homotopy	1633	12	0	1621
Total Distinct	1722	28	0	1694

Table 4: Number of solutions correctly classifying $x\%$ of target data.

Classification	75	80	90	95	96	97	98	99	100 %
Minimum	28	28	28	26	26	5	5	2	2
Saddle	1694	1694	1682	400	400	13	13	3	3
Total Distinct	1722	1722	1710	426	426	18	18	5	5

The results in Tables 3-4 for the number of minima are believed to be accurate, due to verification provided by the conjugate gradient method. The number of saddle points should be seen as a *lower bound*. The regularization ensured that the saddle points were well conditioned, *i.e.* the Hessian was not rank deficient, and these solutions are therefore distinct point solutions.

4 Conclusions

The homotopy methods introduced in this paper overcome the difficulties of poor convergence and the problem of repeatedly finding the same solutions. The use of these methods therefore produces significant new empirical insight into some extraordinary unsuspected properties of the neural network error surface.

The error surface appears to consist of relatively few minima, separated by an extraordinarily large number of saddle points. While one recent paper by Goffe *et al* [4] had given some numerical estimates based on which it was concluded that a large number of minima in neural nets exist (they did not find a significant number of these), this extreme *ratio* of saddle points to minima appears to be unexpected. No maxima were discovered in the above runs; in fact none appear to exist within the sphere where solutions were sought (this seems likely given the regularization). The numerical results reveal astounding complexity in the neural network problem. If the equivalence classes are complete, then 488 solutions for the XOR problem are implied, of which 136 are minima. For the Yin-Yang problem, 6,600,000+ solutions and 107,250+ minima were characterized. For the simple architectures considered, these numbers appear extremely high. We are unaware of any other system of equations having these remarkable properties.

Finally, it should be noted that the large number of saddle points and the small ratio of minima to saddle points in neural problems can create tremendous computational difficulties for approaches which produce stationary points, rather than simple minima. The efficiency of any such algorithm at producing solutions will be negated by the fact that, from an optimization perspective, most of these solutions will be useless.

Acknowledgements. The partial support of the National Science Foundation by grant MIP-9157221 is gratefully acknowledged.

References

[1] E. H. Rothe, *Introduction to Various Aspects of Degree Theory in Banach Spaces*. Mathematical Surveys and Monographs (23), Providence, Rhode Island: American Mathematical Society, 1986. ISBN 0-82218-1522-9.

[2] F. M. Coetzee, *Homotopy Approaches for the Analysis and Solution of Neural Network and Other Nonlinear Systems of Equations*. PhD thesis, Carnegie Mellon University, Pittsburgh, PA, May 1995.

[3] F. M. Coetzee and V. L. Stonick, "Sequential homotopy-based computation of multiple solutions to nonlinear equations," in *Proc. IEEE ICASSP*, (Detroit), IEEE, May 1995.

[4] W. L. Goffe, G. D. Ferrier, and J. Rogers, "Global optimization of statistical functions with simulated annealing," *Jour. Econometrics*, vol. 60, no. 1-2, pp. 65–99, 1994.

Minimizing Statistical Bias with Queries

David A. Cohn
Adaptive Systems Group
Harlequin, Inc.
One Cambridge Center
Cambridge, MA 02142
cohn@harlequin.com

Abstract

I describe a querying criterion that attempts to minimize the error of a learner by minimizing its estimated squared bias. I describe experiments with locally-weighted regression on two simple problems, and observe that this "bias-only" approach outperforms the more common "variance-only" exploration approach, even in the presence of noise.

1 INTRODUCTION

In recent years, there has been an explosion of interest in "active" machine learning systems. These are learning systems that make queries, or perform experiments to gather data that are expected to maximize performance. When compared with "passive" learning systems, which accept given, or randomly drawn data, active learners have demonstrated significant decreases in the amount of data required to achieve equivalent performance. In industrial applications, where each experiment may take days to perform and cost thousands of dollars, a method for optimally selecting these points would offer enormous savings in time and money.

An active learning system will typically attempt to select data that will minimize its predictive error. This error can be decomposed into bias and variance terms. Most research in selecting optimal actions or queries has assumed that the learner is approximately unbiased, and that to minimize learner error, variance is the only thing to minimize (e.g. Fedorov [1972], MacKay [1992], Cohn [1996], Cohn et al., [1996], Paass [1995]). In practice, however, there are very few problems for which we have unbiased learners. Frequently, bias constitutes a large portion of a learner's error; if the learner is deterministic and the data are noise-free, then bias is the *only* source of error. Note that the bias term here is a *statistical* bias, distinct from the *inductive* bias discussed in some machine learning research [Dietterich and Kong, 1995].

In this paper I describe an algorithm which selects actions/queries designed to minimize the bias of a locally weighted regression-based learner. Empirically, "variance-minimizing" strategies which ignore bias seem to perform well, even in cases where, strictly speaking, there is no variance to minimize. In the tasks considered in this paper, the bias-minimizing strategy consistently outperforms variance minimization, even in the presence of noise.

1.1 BIAS AND VARIANCE

Let us begin by defining $P(x,y)$ to be the unknown joint distribution over x and y, and $P(x)$ to be the known marginal distribution of x (commonly called the *input distribution*). We denote the learner's output on input x, given training set $\mathcal{D}$ as $\hat{y}(x;\mathcal{D})$. We can then write the expected error of the learner as

$$\int_x E\left[(\hat{y}(x;\mathcal{D}) - y(x))^2 \,|\, x\right] P(x)dx, \qquad (1)$$

where $E[\cdot]$ denotes the expectation over P and over training sets $\mathcal{D}$. The expectation inside the integral may be decomposed as follows (Geman et al., 1992):

$$\begin{aligned} E\left[(\hat{y}(x;\mathcal{D}) - y(x))^2 \,|\, x\right] &= E\left[(y(x) - E[y|x])^2\right] \\ &\quad + (E_\mathcal{D}[y(x;\mathcal{D})] - E[y|x])^2 \\ &\quad + E_\mathcal{D}\left[(\hat{y}(x;\mathcal{D}) - E_\mathcal{D}[\hat{y}(x;\mathcal{D})])^2\right] \end{aligned} \qquad (2)$$

where $E_\mathcal{D}[\cdot]$ denotes the expectation over training sets. The first term in Equation 2 is the variance of y given x – it is the *noise* in the distribution, and does not depend on our learner or how the training data are chosen. The second term is the learner's *squared bias*, and the third is its *variance*; these last two terms comprise the expected squared error of the learner with respect to the regression function $E[y|x]$.

Most research in active learning assumes that the second term of Equation 2 is approximately zero, that is, that the learner is *unbiased*. If this is the case, then one may concentrate on selecting data so as to minimize the variance of the learner. Although this "all-variance" approach is optimal when the learner is unbiased, truly unbiased learners are rare. Even when the learner's representation class is able to match the target function exactly, bias is generally introduced by the learning algorithm and learning parameters. From the Bayesian perspective, a learner is only unbiased if its priors are *exactly* correct.

The optimal choice of query would, of course, minimize *both* bias and variance, but I leave that for future work. For the purposes of this paper, I will only be concerned with selecting queries that are expected to minimize learner bias. This approach is justified in cases where noise is believed to be only a small component of the learner's error. If the learner is deterministic and there is no noise, then strictly speaking, there *is* no error due to variance — all the error must be due to learner bias. In cases with non-determinism or noise, all-bias minimization, like all-variance minimization, becomes an approximation of the optimal approach.

The learning model discussed in this paper is a form of locally weighted regression (LWR) [Cleveland et al., 1988], which has been used in difficult machine learning tasks, notably the "robot juggler" of Schaal and Atkeson [1994]. Previous work [Cohn et al., 1996] discussed all-variance query selection for LWR; in the remainder of this paper, I describe a method for performing all-bias query selection. Section 2 describes the criterion that must be optimized for all-bias query selection. Section 3 describes the locally weighted regression learner used in this paper and describes how the all-bias criterion may be computed for it. Section 4 describes the results of experiments using this criterion on several simple domains. Directions for future work are discussed in Section 5.

2   ALL-BIAS QUERY SELECTION

Let us assume for the moment that we have a source of noise-free examples (x_i, y_i) and a deterministic learner which, given input x, outputs estimate $\hat{y}(x)$.[1] Let us also assume that we have an accurate estimate of the bias of $\hat{y}$ which can be used to estimate the true function $y(x) = \hat{y}(x) - bias(x)$. We will break these rather strong assumptions of noise-free examples and accurate bias estimates in Section 4, but they are useful for deriving the theoretical approach described below.

Given an accurate bias estimate, we must force the biased estimator into the best approximation of $y(x)$ with the fewest number of examples. This, in effect, transforms the query selection problem into an example filter problem similar to that studied by Plutowski and White [1993] for neural networks. Below, I derive this criterion for estimating the change in error at x given a new queried example at $\tilde{x}$.

Since we have (temporarily) assumed a deterministic learner and noise-free data, the expected error in Equation 2 simplifies to:

$$E\left[(\hat{y}(x;\mathcal{D}) - y(x))^2 | x, \mathcal{D}\right] = (\hat{y}(x;\mathcal{D}) - y(x))^2 \qquad (3)$$

We want to select a new $\tilde{x}$ such that when we add $(\tilde{x}, \tilde{y})$, the resulting squared bias is minimized:

$$(\hat{y}' - y)^2 \equiv (\hat{y}(x; \mathcal{D} \cup (\tilde{x}, \tilde{y})) - y(x))^2 . \qquad (4)$$

I will, for the remainder of the paper, use the "'" to indicate estimates based on the initial training set plus the additional example $(\tilde{x}, \tilde{y})$. To minimize Expression 4, we need to compute how a query at $\tilde{x}$ will change the learner's bias at x. If we assume that we know the input distribution,[2] then we can integrate this change over the entire domain (using Monte Carlo procedures) to estimate the resulting average change, and select a $\tilde{x}$ such that the expected squared bias is minimized. Defining $bias \equiv \hat{y} - y$ and $\Delta \hat{y} = \hat{y}' - \hat{y}$, we can write the new squared bias as:

$$\begin{aligned} bias'^2 &= (\hat{y}' - y)^2 = (\hat{y} + \Delta\hat{y} - y)^2 \\ &= \Delta\hat{y}^2 + 2\Delta\hat{y} \cdot bias + bias^2 \end{aligned} \qquad (5)$$

Note that since $bias$ as defined here is independent of $\tilde{x}$, minimizing the bias is equivalent to minimizing $\Delta\hat{y}^2 + 2\Delta\hat{y} \cdot bias$.

The estimate of $bias'$ tells us how much our bias will change for a given $\tilde{x}$. We may optimize this value over $\tilde{x}$ in one of a number of ways. In low dimensional spaces, it is often sufficient to consider a set of "candidate" $\tilde{x}$ and select the one promising the smallest resulting error. In higher dimensional spaces, it is often more efficient to search for an optimal $\tilde{x}$ with a response surface technique [Box and Draper, 1987], or hillclimb on $\partial bias'^2 / \partial \tilde{x}$.

Estimates of $bias$ and $\Delta\hat{y}$ depend on the specific learning model being used. In Section 3, I describe a locally weighted regression model, and show how differentiable estimates of $bias$ and $\Delta\hat{y}$ may be computed for it.

---

[1] For clarity, I will drop the argument x except where required for disambiguation. I will also denote only the univariate case; the results apply in higher dimensions as well.

[2] This assumption is contrary to the assumption normally made in some forms of learning, e.g. PAC-learning, but it is appropriate in many domains.

2.1 AN ASIDE: WHY NOT JUST USE $\hat{y} - \widehat{bias}$?

If we have an accurate bias estimate, it is reasonable to ask why we do not simply use the corrected $\hat{y} - \widehat{bias}$ as our predictor. The answer has two parts, the first of which is that for most learners, there are no perfect bias estimators — they introduce their own bias and variance, which must be addressed in data selection.

Second, we *can* define a composite learner $\hat{y}_c \equiv \hat{y} - \widehat{bias}$. Given a random training sample then, we would expect $\hat{y}_c$ to outperform $\hat{y}$. However, there is no obvious way to select data for this composite learner other than selecting to maximize the performance of its two components. In our case, the second component (the bias estimate) is non-analytic, which leaves us selecting data so as to maximize the performance of the first component (the uncorrected estimator). We are now back to our original problem: we can select data so as to minimize either the bias or variance of the uncorrected LWR-based learner. Since the purpose of the correction is to give an unbiased estimator, intuition suggests that variance minimization would be the more sensible route in this case. Empirically, this approach does not appear to yield any benefit over uncorrected variance minimization (see Figure 1).

3 LOCALLY WEIGHTED REGRESSION

The type of learner I consider here is a form of locally weighted regression (LWR) that is a slight variation on the LOESS model of Cleveland et al. [1988] (see Cohn et al., [1996] for details). The LOESS model performs a linear regression on points in the data set, weighted by a kernel centered at x. The kernel shape is a design parameter: the original LOESS model uses a "tricubic" kernel; in my experiments I use the more common Gaussian

$$h_i(x) \equiv h(x - x_i) = \exp(-k(x - x_i)^2),$$

where k is a smoothing parameter. For brevity, I will drop the argument x for $h_i(x)$, and define $n = \sum_i h_i$. We can then write the weighted means and covariances as:

$$\mu_x = \sum_i h_i \frac{x_i}{n}, \quad \sigma_x^2 = \sum_i h_i \frac{(x_i - x)^2}{n}, \quad \sigma_{y|x}^2 = \sigma_y^2 - \frac{\sigma_{xy}^2}{\sigma_x^2},$$

$$\mu_y = \sum_i h_i \frac{y_i}{n}, \quad \sigma_y^2 = \sum_i h_i \frac{(y_i - \mu_y)^2}{n}, \quad \sigma_{xy} = \sum_i h_i \frac{(x_i - x)(y_i - \mu_y)}{n}.$$

We use these means and covariances to produce an estimate $\hat{y}$ at the x around which the kernel is centered, with a confidence term in the form of a variance estimate:

$$\hat{y} = \mu_y + \frac{\sigma_{xy}}{\sigma_x^2}(x - \mu_x) \quad \sigma_{\hat{y}}^2 = \sigma_{y|x}^2 \frac{\sum_i h_i^2}{n^2}\left[1 + \frac{(x - \mu_x)(x_i - \mu_x)}{\sigma_x^2}\right]^2.$$

In all the experiments discussed in this paper, the smoothing parameter k was set so as to minimize $\sigma_{\hat{y}}^2$.

The low cost of incorporating new training examples makes this form of locally weighted regression appealing for learning systems which must operate in real time, or with time-varying target functions (e.g. [Schaal and Atkeson 1994]).

3.1 COMPUTING $\Delta \hat{y}$ FOR LWR

If we know what new point $(\tilde{x}, \tilde{y})$ we're going to add, computing $\Delta \hat{y}$ for LWR is straightforward. Defining $\tilde{h}$ as the weight given to $\tilde{x}$, and $\tilde{n}$ as $n + \tilde{h}$ we can write

$$\Delta \hat{y} = \hat{y}' - \hat{y} = \mu'_y + \frac{\sigma'_{xy}}{\sigma'^2_x}(x - \mu'_x) - \mu_y - \frac{\sigma_{xy}}{\sigma^2_x}(x - \mu_x)$$

$$= \tilde{h}\frac{(\tilde{y} - \mu_y)}{\tilde{n}} - \frac{\sigma_{xy}}{\sigma^2_x}(x - \mu_x) + \left(x - \frac{n\mu_x}{\tilde{n}} - \frac{\tilde{h}\tilde{x}}{\tilde{n}}\right) \cdot \frac{\tilde{n}\sigma_{xy} + \tilde{h} \cdot (\tilde{x} - \mu_x)(\tilde{y} - \mu_y)}{\tilde{n}\sigma^2_x + \tilde{h} \cdot (\tilde{x} - \mu_x)^2}$$

Note that computing $\Delta \hat{y}$ requires us to know both the $\tilde{x}$ and $\tilde{y}$ of the new point. In practice, we only know $\tilde{x}$. If we assume, however, that we can estimate the learner's bias at any x, then we can also estimate the unknown value $\tilde{y} \approx \hat{y}(\tilde{x}) - bias(\tilde{x})$. Below, I consider how to compute the bias estimate.

3.2 ESTIMATING BIAS FOR LWR

The most common technique for estimating bias is cross-validation. Standard cross-validation however, only gives estimates of the bias at our specific training points, which are usually combined to form an average bias estimate. This is sufficient if one assumes that the training distribution is representative of the test distribution (which it isn't in query learning) and if one is content to just estimate the bias where one already has training data (which we can't be).

In the query selection problem, we must be able to estimate the bias at all possible x. Box and Draper [1987] suggest fitting a higher order model and measuring the difference. For the experiments described in this paper, this method yielded poor results; two other bias-estimation techniques, however, performed very well.

One method of estimating bias is by bootstrapping the residuals of the training points. One produces a "bootstrap sample" of the learner's residuals on the training data, and adds them to the original predictions to create a synthetic training set. By averaging predictions over a number of bootstrapped training sets and comparing the average prediction with that of the original predictor, one arrives at a first-order bootstrap estimate of the predictor's bias [Connor 1993; Efron and Tibshirani, 1993]. It is known that this estimate is itself biased towards zero; a standard heuristic is to divide the estimate by 0.632 [Efron, 1983].

Another method of estimating bias of a learner is by fitting its own cross-validated residuals. We first compute the cross-validated residuals on the training examples. These produce estimates of the learner's bias at each of the training points. We can then use these residuals as training examples for another learner (again LWR) to produce estimates of what the cross-validated error would be in places where we don't have training data.

4 EMPIRICAL RESULTS

In the previous two sections, I have explained how having an estimate of $\Delta \hat{y}$ and $bias$ for a learner allows one to compute the learner's change in bias given a new query, and have shown how these estimates may be computed for a learner that uses locally weighted regression. Here, I apply these results to two simple problems and demonstrate that they may actually be used to select queries that minimize the statistical bias (and the error) of the learner. The problems involve learning the kinematics of a planar two-jointed robot arm: given the shoulder and elbow joint angles, the learner must predict the tip position.

4.1 BIAS ESTIMATES

I tested the accuracy of the two bias estimators by observing their correlations on 64 reference inputs, given 100 random training examples from the planar arm problem. The bias estimates had a correlation with actual biases of 0.852 for the bootstrap method, and 0.871 for the cross-validation method.

4.2 BIAS MINIMIZATION

I ran two sets of experiments using the bias-minimizing criterion in conjunction with the bias estimation technique of the previous section on the planar arm problem. The bias minimization criterion was used as follows: At each time step, the learner was given a set of 64 randomly chosen candidate queries and 64 uniformly chosen reference points. It evaluated $E'(x)$ for each reference point given each candidate point and selected for its next query the candidate point with the smallest average $E'(x)$ over the reference points. I compared the bias-minimizing strategy (using the cross-validation and bootstrap estimation techniques) against random sampling and the variance-minimizing strategy discussed in Cohn et al. [1996]. On a Sparc 10, with m training examples, the average evaluation times per candidate per reference point were $58 + 0.16m$ μseconds for the variance criterion, $65 + 0.53m$ μseconds for the cross-validation-based bias criterion, and $83 + 3.7m$ μseconds for the bootstrap-based bias criterion (with 20x resampling).

To test whether the bias-only assumption was robust against the presence of noise, 1% Gaussian noise was added to the input values of the training data in all experiments. This simulates noisy position effectors on the arm, and results in non-Gaussian noise in the output coordinate system.

In the first series of experiments, the candidate shoulder and elbow joint angles were drawn uniformly over $(U[0, 2\pi], U[0, \pi])$. In unconstrained domains like this, random sampling is a fairly good default strategy. The bias minimization strategies still significantly outperform both random sampling and the variance minimizing strategy in these experiments (see Figure 1).

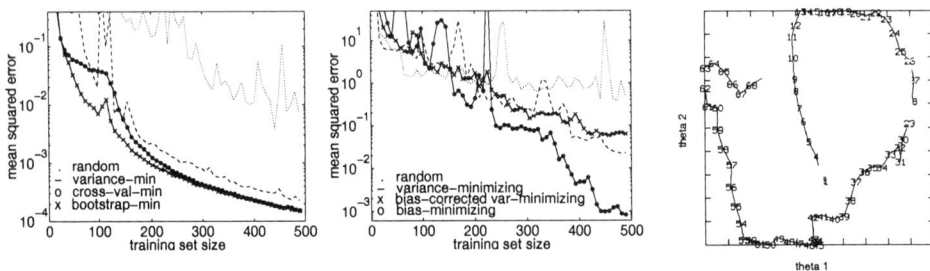

Figure 1: (left) MSE as a function of number of noisy training examples for the unconstrained arm problem. Errors are averaged over 10 runs for the bootstrap method and 15 runs for all others. One run with the cross-validation-based method was excluded when k failed to converge to a reasonable value. (center) MSE as a function of number of noisy training examples for the constrained arm problem. The bias correction strategy discussed in Section 2.1 does no better than the uncorrected variance-minimizing strategy, and much worse than the bias-minimization strategy. (right) Sample exploration trajectory in joint-space for the constrained arm problem, explored according to the bias minimizing criterion.

In the second series of experiments, candidates were drawn uniformly from a region local to the previously selected query: $(\hat{\theta}_1 \pm 0.2\pi, \hat{\theta}_2 \pm 0.1\pi)$. This corresponds to restricting the arm to local motions. In a constrained problem such as this, random sampling is a poor strategy; both the bias and variance-reducing strategies outperform it at least an order of magnitude. Further, the bias-minimization strategy outperforms variance minimization by a large margin (Figure 1). Figure 1 also shows an exploration trajectory produced by pursuing the bias-minimizing criterion. It is noteworthy that, although the implementation in this case was a greedy (one-step) minimization, the trajectory results in globally good exploration.

5 DISCUSSION

I have argued in this paper that, in many situations, selecting queries to minimize learner bias is an appropriate and effective strategy for active learning. I have given empirical evidence that, with a LWR-based learner and the examples considered here, the strategy is effective even in the presence of noise.

Beyond minimizing either bias or variance, an important next step is to explicitly minimize them together. The bootstrap-based estimate should facilitate this, as it produces a complementary variance estimate with little additional computation. By optimizing over both criteria simultaneously, we expect to derive a criterion that that, in terms of statistics, is truly optimal for selecting queries.

REFERENCES

Box, G., & Draper, N. (1987). *Empirical model-building and response surfaces*, Wiley, New York.
Cleveland, W., Devlin, S., & Grosse, E. (1988). Regression by local fitting. *Journal of Econometrics*, **37**, 87–114.
Cohn, D. (1996) Neural network exploration using optimal experiment design. *Neural Networks*, **9(6)**:1071–1083.
Cohn, D., Ghahramani, Z., & Jordan, M. (1996). Active learning with statistical models. *Journal of Artificial Inteligence Research* **4**:129–145.
Connor, J. (1993). Bootstrap Methods in Neural Network Time Series Prediction. In J. Alspector et al., eds., *Proc. of the Int. Workshop on Applications of Neural Networks to Telecommunications*, Lawrence Erlbaum, Hillsdale, N.J.
Dietterich, T., & Kong, E. (1995). Error-correcting output coding corrects bias and variance. In S. Prieditis and S. Russell, eds., *Proceedings of the 12th International Conference on Machine Learning*.
Efron, B. (1983) Estimating the error rate of a prediction rule: some improvements on cross-validation. *J. Amer. Statist. Assoc.* **78**:316–331.
Efron, B. & Tibshirani, R. (1993). *An introduction to the bootstrap.* Chapman & Hall, New York.
Fedorov, V. (1972). *Theory of Optimal Experiments.* Academic Press, New York.
Geman, S., Bienenstock, E., & Doursat, R. (1992). Neural networks and the bias/variance dilemma. *Neural Computation*, **4**, 1–58.
MacKay, D. (1992). Information-based objective functions for active data selection, *Neural Computation*, **4**, 590–604.
Paass, G., and Kindermann, J. (1994). Bayesian Query Construction for Neural Network Models. In G. Tesauro et al., eds., *Advances in Neural Information Processing Systems 7*, MIT Press.
Plutowski, M., & White, H. (1993). Selecting concise training sets from clean data. *IEEE Transactions on Neural Networks*, **4**, 305–318.
Schaal, S. & Atkeson, C. (1994). Robot Juggling: An Implementation of Memory-based Learning. *Control Systems* **14**, 57–71.

MIMIC: Finding Optima by Estimating Probability Densities

Jeremy S. De Bonet, Charles L. Isbell, Jr., Paul Viola
Artificial Intelligence Laboratory
Massachusetts Institute of Technology
Cambridge, MA 02139

Abstract

In many optimization problems, the structure of solutions reflects complex relationships between the different input parameters. For example, experience may tell us that certain parameters are closely related and should not be explored independently. Similarly, experience may establish that a subset of parameters must take on particular values. Any search of the cost landscape should take advantage of these relationships. We present MIMIC, a framework in which we analyze the global structure of the optimization landscape. A novel and efficient algorithm for the estimation of this structure is derived. We use knowledge of this structure to guide a randomized search through the solution space and, in turn, to refine our estimate of the structure. Our technique obtains significant speed gains over other randomized optimization procedures.

1 Introduction

Given some cost function $C(x)$ with local minima, we may search for the optimal x in many ways. Variations of gradient descent are perhaps the most popular. When most of the minima are far from optimal, the search must either include a brute-force component or incorporate randomization. Classical examples include Simulated Annealing (SA) and Genetic Algorithms (GAs) (Kirkpatrick, Gelatt and Vecchi, 1983; Holland, 1975). In all cases, in the process of optimizing $C(x)$ many thousands or perhaps millions of samples of $C(x)$ are evaluated. Most optimization algorithms take these millions of pieces of information, and compress them into a single point x—the current estimate of the solution (one notable exception are GAs to which we will return shortly). Imagine splitting the search process into two parts, both taking $t/2$ time steps. Both parts are structurally identical: taking a description of $C()$, they start their search from some initial point. The sole benefit enjoyed by the second part of the search over the first is that the initial point is perhaps closer to the optimum. Intuitively, there must be some additional information that could be learned from the first half of the search, if only to warn the second half about avoidable mistakes and pitfalls.

We present an optimization algorithm called Mutual-Information-Maximizing Input Clustering (MIMIC). It attempts to communicate information about the cost function obtained from one iteration of the search to later iterations of the search directly. It does this in an efficient and principled way. There are two main components of MIMIC: first, a randomized optimization algorithm that samples from those regions of the input space most likely to contain the minimum for $C()$; second, an effective density estimator that can be used to capture a wide variety of structure on the input space, yet is computable from simple second order statistics on the data. MIMIC's results on simple cost functions indicate an order of magnitude improvement in performance over related approaches. Further experiments on a k-color map coloring problem yield similar improvements.

2 Related Work

Many well known optimization procedures neither represent nor utilize the structure of the optimization landscape. In contrast, Genetic Algorithms (GA) attempt to capture this structure by an ad hoc embedding of the parameters onto a line (the chromosome). The intent of the crossover operation in standard genetic algorithms is to preserve and propagate a group of parameters that *might* be partially responsible for generating a favorable evaluation. Even when such groups exist, many of the offspring generated do not preserve the structure of these groups because the choice of crossover point is random.

In problems where the benefit of a parameter is completely independent of the value of all other parameters, the population simply encodes information about the probability distribution over each parameter. In this case, the crossover operation is equivalent to sampling from this distribution; the more crossovers the better the sample. Even in problems where fitness is obtained through the combined effects of clusters of inputs, the GA crossover operation is beneficial only when its randomly chosen clusters happen to closely match the underlying structure of the problem. Because of the rarity of such a fortuitous occurrence, the benefit of the crossover operation is greatly diminished. As as result, GAs have a checkered history in function optimization (Baum, Boneh and Garrett, 1995; Lang, 1995). One of our goals is to incorporate insights from GAs in a principled optimization framework.

There have been other attempts to capture the advantages of GAs. Population Based Incremental Learning (PBIL) attempts to incorporate the notion of a candidate population by replacing it with a single probability vector (Baluja and Caruana, 1995). Each element of the vector is the probability that a particular bit in a solution is on. During the learning process, the probability vector can be thought of as a simple model of the optimization landscape. Bits whose values are firmly established have probabilities that are close to 1 or 0. Those that are still unknown have probabilities close to 0.5.

When it is the *structure* of the components of a candidate rather than the particular values of the components that determines how it fares, it can be difficult to move PBIL's representation towards a viable solution. Nevertheless, even in these sorts of problems PBIL often out-performs genetic algorithms because those algorithms are hindered by the fact that random crossovers are infrequently beneficial.

A very distinct, but related technique was proposed by Sabes and Jordan for a reinforcement learning task (Sabes and Jordan, 1995). In their framework, the learner must generate actions so that a reinforcement function can be completely explored. Simultaneously, the learner must exploit what it has learned so as to optimize the long-term reward. Sabes and Jordan chose to construct a Boltzmann distribution from the reinforcement function: $p(x) = \frac{\exp(\frac{R(x)}{T})}{Z_T}$ where $R(x)$ is the reinforcement function for action X, T is the temperature, and Z_T is a normalization factor. They use this distribution to generate actions. At high temperatures this distribution approaches the uniform distribution, and results in random exploration of $R()$. At low temperatures only those actions which garner large reinforcement are generated. By reducing T, the learner progresses from an initially randomized search to a more directed search about the true optimal action. Interestingly, their estimate for $p(x)$ is to some extent a model of the optimization landscape which is constructed during the learning process. To our knowledge, Sabes and Jordan have neither attempted optimization over high dimensional spaces, nor attempted to fit $p(x)$ with a complex model.

3 MIMIC

Knowing nothing else about $C(x)$ it might not be unreasonable to search for its minimum by generating points from a uniform distribution over the inputs $p(x)$. Such a search allows none of the information generated by previous samples to effect the generation of subsequent samples. Not surprisingly, much less work might be necessary if samples were generated from a distribution, $p^\theta(x)$, that is uniformly distributed over those x's where $C(x) \leq \theta$ and has a probability of 0 elsewhere. For example, if we had access to $p^{\theta_M}(x)$ for $\theta_M = \min_x C(x)$ a single sample would be sufficient to find an optimum.

This insight suggests a process of successive approximation: given a collection of points for which $C(x) \leq \theta_0$ a density estimator for $p^{\theta_0}(x)$ is constructed. From this density estimator additional samples are generated, a new threshold established, $\theta_1 = \theta_0 - \epsilon$, and a new density estimator created. The process is repeated until the values of $C(x)$ cease to improve.

The MIMIC algorithm begins by generating a random population of candidates choosen uniformly from the input space. From this population the median fitness is extracted and is denoted θ_0. The algorithm then proceeds:

1. Update the parameters of the density estimator of $p^{\theta_i}(x)$ from a sample.
2. Generate more samples from the distribution $p^{\theta_i}(x)$.
3. Set θ_{i+1} equal to the Nth percentile of the data. Retain only the points less than θ_{i+1}.

The validity of this approach is dependent on two critical assumptions: $p^\theta(x)$ can be successfully approximated with a finite amount of data; and $D(p^{\theta-\epsilon}(x)||p^\theta(x))$ is small enough so that samples from $p^\theta(x)$ are also likely to be samples from $p^{\theta-\epsilon}(x)$ (where $D(p||q)$ is the Kullback-Liebler divergence between p and q). Bounds on these conditions can be used to prove convergence in a finite number of successive approximation steps.

The performance of this approach is dependent on the nature of the density approximator used. We have chosen to estimate the conditional distributions for every pair of parameters in the representation, a total of $O(n^2)$ numbers. In the next section we will show how we use these conditionals distributions to construct a joint distribution which is closest in the KL sense to the true joint distribution. Such an approximator is capable of representing clusters of highly related parameters. While this might seem similar to the intuitive behavior of crossover, this representation is strictly more powerful. More importantly, our clusters are *learned* from the data, and are not pre-defined by the programmer.

4 Generating Events from Conditional Probabilities

The joint probability distribution over a set of random variables, $X = \{X_i\}$, is:

$$p(X) = p(X_1|X_2\ldots X_n)p(X_2|X_3\ldots X_n)\ldots p(X_{n-1}|X_n)p(X_n). \quad (1)$$

Given only pairwise conditional probabilities, $p(X_i|X_j)$ and unconditional probabilities, $p(X_i)$, we are faced with the task of generating samples that match as closely as possible the true joint distribution, $p(X)$. It is not possible to capture all possible joint distributions of n variables using only the unconditional and pairwise conditional probabilities; however, we would like to describe the true joint distribution as closely as possible. Below, we derive an algorithm for choosing such a description.

Given a permutation of the numbers between 1 and n, $\pi = i_1 i_2 \ldots i_n$, we define a class of probability distributions, $\hat{p}_\pi(X)$:

$$\hat{p}_\pi(X) = p(X_{i_1}|X_{i_2})p(X_{i_2}|X_{i_3})\ldots p(X_{i_{n-1}}|X_{i_n})p(X_{i_n}). \quad (2)$$

The distribution $\hat{p}_\pi(X)$ uses π as an ordering for the pairwise conditional probabilities. Our goal is to choose the permutation π that maximizes the agreement between $\hat{p}_\pi(X)$ and the true distribution $p(X)$. The agreement between two distributions can be measured by the Kullback-Liebler divergence:

$$\begin{aligned}D(p||\hat{p}_\pi) &= \int_X p[\log p - \log \hat{p}_\pi]dX \\ &= E_p[\log p] - E_p[\log \hat{p}_\pi] \\ &= -h(p) - E_p[\log p(X_{i_1}|X_{i_2})p(X_{i_2}|X_{i_3})\ldots p(X_{i_{n-1}}|X_{i_n})p(X_{i_n})] \\ &= -h(p) + h(X_{i_1}|X_{i_2}) + h(X_{i_2}|X_{i_3}) + \ldots + h(X_{i_{n-1}}|X_{i_n}) + h(X_{i_n}).\end{aligned}$$

This divergence is always non-negative, with equality only in the case where $\hat{p}(\pi)$ and $p(X)$ are identical distributions. The optimal π is defined as the one that minimizes this divergence. For a distribution that can be completely described by pairwise conditional probabilities, the optimal π will generate a distribution that will be identical to the true distribution. Insofar as the true distribution cannot be captured this way, the optimal $\hat{p}_\pi(X)$ will diverge from that distribution.

The first term in the divergence does not depend on π. Therefore, the cost function, $J_\pi(X)$, we wish to minimize is:

$$J_\pi(X) = h(X_{i_1}|X_{i_2}) + h(X_{i_2}|X_{i_3}) + \ldots + h(X_{i_{n-1}}|X_{i_n}) + h(X_{i_n}). \quad (3)$$

The optimal π is the one that produces the lowest pairwise entropy with respect to the true distribution. By searching over all $n!$ permutations, it is possible to determine the optimal π. In the interests of computational efficiency, we employ a straightforward greedy algorithm to pick a permutation:

1. $i_n = arg\min_j \hat{h}(X_j)$.
2. $i_k = arg\min_j \hat{h}(X_j|X_{i_{k+1}})$, where $j \neq i_{k+1}\ldots i_n$ and $k = n-1, n-2, \ldots, 2, 1$.

where $\hat{h}()$ is the empirical entropy. Once a distribution is chosen, generating samples is also straightforward:

1. Choose a value for X_{i_n} based on its empirical probability $\hat{p}(X_{i_n})$.
2. for $k = n-1, n-2, \ldots, 2, 1$, choose element X_{i_k} based on the empirical conditional probability $\hat{p}(X_{i_k}|X_{i_{k+1}})$.

The first algorithm runs in time $\mathcal{O}(n^2)$ and the second in time $\mathcal{O}(n^2)$.

5 Experiments

To measure the performance of MIMIC, we performed three benchmark experiments and compared our results with those obtained using several standard optimization algorithms.

We will use four algorithms in our comparisons:

1. MIMIC - the algorithm above with 200 samples per iteration
2. PBIL - standard population based incremental learning
3. RHC - randomized hill climbing
4. GA - a standard genetic algorithm with single crossover and 10% mutation rate

5.1 Four Peaks

The Four Peaks problem is taken from (Baluja and Caruana, 1995). Given an N-dimensional input vector $\vec{X}$, the four peaks evaluation function is defined as:

$$f(\vec{X}, T) = \max[tail(0, \vec{X}), head(1, \vec{X})] + R(\vec{X}, T) \qquad (4)$$

where

$$tail(b, \vec{X}) = \text{number of trailing } b\text{'s in } \vec{X} \qquad (5)$$
$$head(b, \vec{X}) = \text{number of leading } b\text{'s in } \vec{X} \qquad (6)$$

$$R(\vec{X}, T) = \begin{cases} N & \text{if } tail(0, \vec{X}) > T \text{ and } head(1, \vec{X}) > T \\ 0 & \text{otherwise} \end{cases} \qquad (7)$$

There are two global maxima for this function. They are achieved either when there are $T+1$ leading 1's followed by all 0's or when there are $T+1$ trailing 0's preceded by all 1's. There are also two suboptimal local maxima that occur with a string of all 1's or all 0's. For large values of T, this problem becomes increasingly more difficult because the basin of attraction for the inferior local maxima become larger.

Results for running the algorithms are shown in figure 1. In all trials, T was set to be 10% of N, the total number of inputs. The MIMIC algorithm consistently maximizes the function with approximately one tenth the number of evaluations required by the second best algorithm.

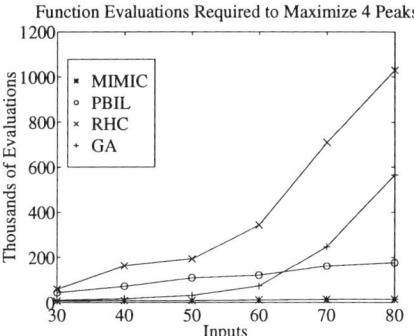

Figure 1: Number of evaluations of the Four-Peak cost function for different algorithms plotted for a variety of problems sizes.

5.2 Six Peaks

The Six Peaks problem is a slight variation on Four Peaks where

$$R(\vec{X}, T) = \begin{cases} N & \text{if } tail(0, x) > T \text{ and } head(1, x) > T \text{ or} \\ & \quad tail(1, x) > T \text{ and } head(0, x) > T \\ 0 & \text{otherwise} \end{cases} \quad (8)$$

This function has two additional global maxima where there are $T+1$ leading 0's followed by all 1's or when there are $T+1$ trailing 1's preceded by all 0's. In this case, it is not the values of the candidates that is important, but their structure: the first $T+1$ positions should take on the same value, the last $T+1$ positions should take on the same value, these two groups should take on different values, and the middle positions should take on all the same value.

Results for this problem are shown in figure 2. As might be expected, PBIL performed worse than on the Four Peak problem because it tends to oscillate in the middle of the space while contradictory signals pull it back and forth. The random crossover operation of the GA occasionally was able to capture some of the underlying structure, resulting in an improved relative performance of the GA. As we expected, the MIMIC algorithm was able to capture the underlying structure of the problem, and combine information from all the maxima. Thus MIMIC consistently maximizes the Six Peaks function with approximately one fiftieth the number of evaluations required by the other algorithms.

5.3 Max K-Coloring

A graph is K-Colorable if it is possible to assign one of k colors to each of the nodes of the graph such that no adjacent nodes have the same color. Determining whether a graph is K-Colorable is known to be NP-Complete. Here, we define Max K-Coloring to be the task of finding a coloring that minimizes the number of adjacent pairs colored the same.

Results for this problem are shown in figure 2. We used a subset of graphs with a single solution (up to permutations of color) so that the optimal solution is dependent *only* on the structure of the parameters. Because of this, PBIL performs poorly. GA's perform better because *any* crossover point is representative of some of the underlying structure of the graphs used. Finally, MIMIC performs best because

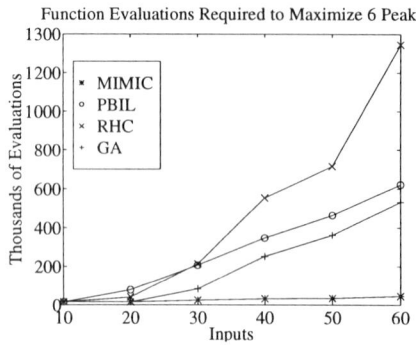 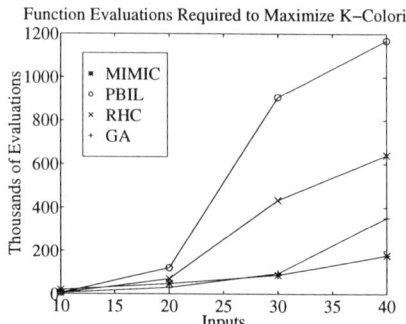

Figure 2: Number of evaluations of the Six-Peak cost function (left) and the K-Color cost function (right) for a variety of problem sizes.

it is able to capture all of the structural regularity within the inputs.

6 Conclusions

We have described MIMIC, a novel optimization algorithm that converges faster and more reliably than several other existing algorithms. MIMIC accomplishes this in two ways. First, it performs optimization by successively approximating the conditional distribution of the inputs given a bound on the cost function. Throughout this process, the optimum of the cost function becomes gradually more likely. As a result, MIMIC directly communicates information about the cost function from the early stages to the later stages of the search. Second, MIMIC attempts to discover common underlying structure about optima by computing second-order statistics and sampling from a distribution consistent with those statistics.

Acknowledgments

In this research, Jeremy De Bonet is supported by the DOD Multidisciplinary Research Program of the University Research Initiative, Charles Isbell by a fellowship granted by AT&T Labs-Research, and Paul Viola by Office of Naval Research Grant No. N00014-96-1-0311. Greg Galperin helped in the preparation of this paper.

References

Baluja, S. and Caruana, R. (1995). Removing the genetics from the standard genetic algorithm. Technical report, Carnegie Mellon Univerisity.

Baum, E. B., Boneh, D., and Garrett, C. (1995). Where genetic algorithms excel. In *Proceedings of the Conference on Computational Learning Theory*, New York. Association for Computing Machinery.

Holland, J. H. (1975). *Adaptation in Natural and Artificial Systems*. The Michigan University Press.

Kirkpatrick, S., Gelatt, C., and Vecchi, M. (1983). Optimization by Simulated Annealing. *Science*, 220(4598):671–680.

Lang, K. (1995). Hill climbing beats genetic search on a boolean circuit synthesis problem of koza's. In *Twelfth International Conference on Machine Learning*.

Sabes, P. N. and Jordan, M. I. (1995). Reinforcement learning by probability matching. In David S. Touretzky, M. M. and Perrone, M., editors, *Advances in Neural Information Processing*, volume 8, Denver 1995. MIT Press, Cambridge.

On a Modification to the Mean Field EM Algorithm in Factorial Learning

A. P. Dunmur D. M. Titterington
Department of Statistics
Maths Building
University of Glasgow
Glasgow G12 8QQ, UK

alan@stats.gla.ac.uk mike@stats.gla.ac.uk

Abstract

A modification is described to the use of mean field approximations in the E step of EM algorithms for analysing data from latent structure models, as described by Ghahramani (1995), among others. The modification involves second-order Taylor approximations to expectations computed in the E step. The potential benefits of the method are illustrated using very simple latent profile models.

1 Introduction

Ghahramani (1995) advocated the use of mean field methods as a means to avoid the heavy computation involved in the E step of the EM algorithm used for estimating parameters within a certain latent structure model, and Ghahramani & Jordan (1995) used the same ideas in a more complex situation. Dunmur & Titterington (1996a) identified Ghahramani's model as a so-called latent profile model, they observed that Zhang (1992, 1993) had used mean field methods for a similar purpose, and they showed, in a simulation study based on very simple examples, that the mean field version of the EM algorithm often performed very respectably. By this it is meant that, when data were generated from the model under analysis, the estimators of the underlying parameters were efficient, judging by empirical results, especially in comparison with estimators obtained by employing the 'correct' EM algorithm: the examples therefore had to be simple enough that the correct EM algorithm is numerically feasible, although any success reported for the mean field version is, one hopes, an indication that the method will also be adequate in more complex situations in which the correct EM algorithm is not implementable because of computational complexity.

In spite of the above positive remarks, there were circumstances in which there was a perceptible, if not dramatic, lack of efficiency in the simple (naive) mean field estimators, and the objective of this contribution is to propose and investigate ways of refining the method so as to improve performance without detracting from the appealing, and frequently essential, simplicity of the approach. The procedure used here is based on a second order correction to the naive mean field well known in statistical physics and sometimes called the cavity or TAP method (Mezard, Parisi & Virasoro, 1987). It has been applied recently in cluster analysis (Hofmann & Buhmann, 1996). In Section 2 we introduce the structure of our model, Section 3 explains the refined mean field approach, Section 4 provides numerical results, and Section 5 contains a statement of our conclusions.

2 The Model

The model under study is a latent profile model (Henry, 1983), which is a latent structure model involving continuous observables $\{x_r : r = 1\ldots p\}$ and discrete latent variables $\{y_i : i = 1\ldots d\}$. The y_i are represented by indicator vectors such that for each i there is a single j such that $y_{ij} = 1$ and $y_{ik} = 0$, for all $k \neq j$. The latent variables are connected to the observables by a set of weight matrices W_i in such a way that the distribution of the observations given the latent variables is a multivariate Gaussian with mean $\sum_i W_i y_i$ and covariance matrix Γ. To ease the notation, the covariance matrix is taken to be the identity matrix, although extension is quite easy to the case where Γ is a diagonal matrix whose elements have to be estimated (Dunmur & Titterington, 1996a). Also to simplify the notation, the marginal distributions of the latent variables are taken to be uniform, so that the totality of unknown parameters is made up of the set of weight matrices, to be denoted by $W = (W_1, W_2, \ldots, W_d)$.

3 Methodology

In order to learn about the model we have available a dataset $\mathcal{D} = \{x^\mu : \mu = 1\ldots N\}$ of N independent, p dimensional realizations of the model, and we adopt the Maximum Likelihood approach to the estimation of the weight matrices. As is typical of latent structure models, there is no explicit Maximum Likelihood estimate of the parameters of the model, but there is a version of the EM algorithm (Dempster, Laird & Rubin, 1977) that can be used to obtain the estimates numerically. The EM algorithm consists of a sequence of double steps, E steps and M steps.

At stage m the E step, based on a current estimate W^{m-1} of the parameters, calculates

$$\mathcal{Q}(W, W^{m-1}) = \langle \mathcal{L}_c(W) | \mathcal{D}, W^{m-1} \rangle,$$

where, the expectation $\langle \cdot \rangle$ is over the latent variables y, and is conditional on $\mathcal{D}$ and W^{m-1}, and $\mathcal{L}_c$ denotes the crucial part of the *complete-data* log-likelihood, given by

$$\mathcal{L}_c(W) = -\frac{1}{2}\sum_\mu \left(x^\mu - \sum_i W_i y_i^\mu\right)^T \left(x^\mu - \sum_j W_j y_j^\mu\right).$$

The M step then maximizes $\mathcal{Q}$ with respect to W and gives the new parameter estimate W^m.

For the simple model considered here, the M step gives

$$W^m = \left(\sum_\mu x^\mu \langle Y^{\mu T} \rangle\right) \left(\sum_\mu \langle Y^\mu Y^{\mu T} \rangle\right)^{-1}$$

where $W = (W_1, W_2, \ldots, W_d)$ and $Y^T = (y_1^T, y_2^T, \ldots, y_d^T)$ and, for brevity, explicit mention of the conditioned quantities in the expectations $\langle \cdot \rangle$ has been omitted. The above formula differs somewhat from that given by Ghahramani (1995).

Hence we need to evaluate the sets of expectations $\langle y_i \rangle$ and $\langle y_i y_j^T \rangle$ for each example in the dataset. (The superscript μ is omitted, for clarity.) As pointed out in Ghahramani (1995), it is possible to evaluate these expectations directly by summing over all possible latent states. This has the disadvantage of becoming exponentially more expensive as the size of the latent space increases.

The mean field approximation is well known in physics and can be used to reduce the computational complexity. At its simplest level, the mean field approximation replaces the joint expectations of the latent variables by the products of the individual expectations; this can be interpreted as bounding the likelihood from below (Saul, Jaakkola, Jordan, 1996). Here we consider a second order approximation, as outlined below.

Since the latent variables are categorical, it is simple to sum over the state space of a single latent variable. Hence, following Parisi (1988), the expectations of the latent variables are given by

$$\langle y_{ij} \rangle = \langle f_j(\epsilon_i) \rangle, \tag{1}$$

where $f_j(\epsilon_i)$ is the jth component of the softmax function; $\exp(\epsilon_{ij})/\sum_k \exp(\epsilon_{ik})$, and the expectation $\langle \cdot \rangle$ is taken over the remaining latent variables. The vector $\epsilon_i = \{\epsilon_{ij}\}$ contains the log probabilities (up to a constant) associated with each category of the latent variable for each example in the data set. For the simple model under study ϵ_{ij} is given by

$$\epsilon_{ij} = \left\{W_i^T(x - \sum_{k \neq i} W_k y_k)\right\}_j - \frac{1}{2}(W_i^T W_i)_{jj}. \tag{2}$$

The expectation in (1) can be expanded in a Taylor series about the average, $\langle \epsilon_i \rangle$, giving

$$\langle y_{ij} \rangle = f_j(\langle \epsilon_i \rangle) + \frac{1}{2}\sum_{kl} \langle \Delta\epsilon_{ik} \Delta\epsilon_{il} \rangle \frac{\partial^2 f_j(\langle \epsilon_i \rangle)}{\partial \epsilon_{ik} \partial \epsilon_{il}} + \mathcal{O}(\Delta\epsilon^3), \tag{3}$$

where $\Delta\epsilon_{ij} = \epsilon_{ij} - \langle \epsilon_{ij} \rangle$. The *naive* mean field approximation simply ignores all corrections. We can postulate that the second order fluctuations are taken care of

by a so called *cavity field*, (see, for instance, Mezard, Parisi & Virasoro , 1987, p.16), that is,
$$\langle y_{ij} \rangle = f_j(\langle \epsilon_i \rangle + h_i), \qquad (4)$$
where the vector of fields $h_i = \{h_{ik}\}$ has been introduced to take care of the correction terms. This equation may also be expanded in a Taylor series to give
$$\langle y_{ij} \rangle = f_j(\langle \epsilon_i \rangle) + \sum_k h_{ik} \frac{\partial f_j(\langle \epsilon_i \rangle)}{\partial \epsilon_{ik}} + \mathcal{O}(h^2).$$

Then, equating coefficients with (3) and after a little algebra, we get
$$h_{ij} = \frac{1}{2} \sum_k \langle \Delta \epsilon_{ij} \Delta \epsilon_{ik} \rangle (\delta_{jk} - 2 f_k(\langle \epsilon_i \rangle)), \qquad (5)$$
where δ_{jk} is the Kronecker delta and, for the model under consideration,
$$\langle \Delta \epsilon_{ij} \Delta \epsilon_{ik} \rangle = \left(W_i^T \sum_{mn \neq i} W_m (\langle y_m y_n^T \rangle - \langle y_m \rangle \langle y_n^T \rangle) W_n^T W_i \right)_{jk}. \qquad (6)$$

The naive mean field assumption may be used in (6), giving
$$(\langle y_i y_j^T \rangle - \langle y_i \rangle \langle y_j^T \rangle)_{kl} = \delta_{ij} \langle y_{ik} \rangle (\delta_{kl} - \langle y_{il} \rangle). \qquad (7)$$

Within the E step, for each realization in the data set, the mean fields (4), along with the cavity fields (5), can be evaluated by an iterative procedure which gives the individual expectations of the latent variables. The naive mean field approximation (7) is then used to evaluate the joint expectations $\langle y_i y_j^T \rangle$. In the next section we report, for a simple model, the effect on parameter estimation of the use of cavity fields.

4 Results

Simulations were carried out using latent variable models (i) with 5 observables and 4 binary hidden variables and (ii) with 5 observables and 3 3-state hidden variables. The weight matrices were generated from zero mean Gaussian variables with standard deviation w. In order to make the M step trivial it was assumed that the matrices were known up to the scale parameter w, and this is the parameter estimated by the algorithm. A data set was generated using the known parameter and this was then estimated using straight EM, naive mean field (MF) and mean field with cavity fields (MF$_{\text{cav}}$).

Although datasets of sizes 100 and 500 were generated, only the results for $N = 500$ are presented here since both scenarios showed the same qualitative behaviour. Also, the estimation algorithms were started from different initial positions; this too had no effect on the final estimates of the parameters. A representative selection of results follows; Table 1 shows the results for both the $5 \times 4 \times 2$ model and the $5 \times 3 \times 3$ model.

The results show that, when the true value, w_{tr}, of the parameter was small, there is little difference among the three methods. This is due to the fact that at these

A Modification to Mean Field EM

Table 1: Table of results N=500, results averaged over 50 simulations for 5 observables with 4 binary latent variables and for 5 observables with 3 3-state latent variables. The figures in brackets give the standard deviation of the estimates, w_{est}, in units according to the final decimal place. RMS is the root mean squared error of the estimate compared to the true value.

Method	w_{tr}	w_{init}	5 × 4 × 2		5 × 3 × 3	
			w_{est}	RMS	w_{est}	RMS
EM	0.1	0.05	0.09(1)	0.014	0.10(2)	0.024
MF	0.1	0.05	0.09(1)	0.014	0.10(2)	0.023
MF$_{cav}$	0.1	0.05	0.09(1)	0.014	0.10(2)	0.023
EM	0.5	0.1	0.49(2)	0.016	0.50(2)	0.019
MF	0.5	0.1	0.47(2)	0.029	0.46(2)	0.038
MF$_{cav}$	0.5	0.1	0.48(2)	0.026	0.47(2)	0.032
EM	1.0	0.1	0.99(2)	0.016	1.00(2)	0.018
MF	1.0	0.1	0.96(2)	0.040	0.98(2)	0.032
MF$_{cav}$	1.0	0.1	0.99(2)	0.018	1.00(2)	0.018
EM	2.0	0.2	1.99(1)	0.014	1.99(1)	0.015
MF	2.0	0.2	1.98(2)	0.021	1.98(2)	0.023
MF$_{cav}$	2.0	0.2	1.97(2)	0.027	1.97(2)	0.031
EM	5.0	0.1	4.99(1)	0.013	5.00(1)	0.013
MF	5.0	0.1	4.99(1)	0.016	4.96(2)	0.047
MF$_{cav}$	5.0	0.1	4.97(2)	0.032	4.88(3)	0.114

small values there is little separation among the mixtures that are used to generate the data and hence the methods are all equally good (or bad) at estimating the parameter. As the true parameter increases and becomes close to one, the cavity field method performs significantly better then naive mean field; in fact it performs as well as EM for $w_{tr}=1$.

For values of w_{tr} greater than one, the cavity field method performs less well than naive mean field. This suggests that the Taylor expansions (3) and (5) no longer provide reliable approximations. Since

$$\Delta \epsilon_{ij} = \left(\sum_{k \neq i} W_i^T W_k (\langle y_k \rangle - y_k) \right)_j , \qquad (8)$$

it is easy to see that if the elements in W_i are much less than one then the corrections to the Taylor expansion are small and hence the cavity fields are small, so the approximations hold. If w is much larger than one, then the mean field estimates become closer to zero and one since the energies ϵ_{ij} (equation 2) become more extreme. Hence if the mean fields correctly estimate the latent variables the corrections are indeed small, but if the mean fields incorrectly estimate the latent variable the error term is substantial, leading to a reduction in performance.

Another simulation, similar to that presented in Ghahramani (1995), was also studied to compare the modification to both the 'correct' EM and the naive mean field. The model has two latent variables that correspond to either horizontal or vertical lines in one of four positions. These are combined and zero mean Gaussian noise added to produce a 4 × 4 example image. A data set is created from many of these examples with the latent variables chosen at random. From the data set the weight matrices connecting the observables to the latent variables are estimated and compared to the true weights which consist of zeros and ones. Typical results for a sample size of 160 and Gaussian noise of variance 0.2 are presented in Figure 1. The number of iterations needed to converge were similar for all three methods.

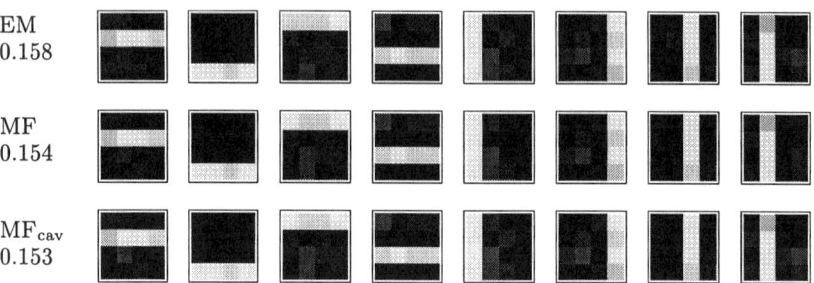

Figure 1: Estimated weights for a sample size of $N = 160$ and noise variance 0.2 added. The three rows correspond to EM, naive MF and MF_{cav} respectively. The number on the left hand end of the row is the mean squared error of the estimated weights compared with the true weights. The first four images are the estimates of the first latent vector and the remaining four images are the estimates of second latent vector.

As can be seen from Figure 1 there is very little difference between the estimates of the weights and the mean squared errors are all very close. The mean field method converged in approximately four iterations which means that for this simple model the MF E step is taking approximately 32 steps as compared to 16 steps for the straight EM. This is due to the simplicity of the latent structure for this model. For a more complicated model the MF algorithm should take fewer iterations. Again the results are encouraging for the MF method, but they do not show any obvious benefit from using the cavity field correction terms.

5 Conclusion

The cavity field method can be applied successfully to improve the performance of naive mean field estimates. However, care must be taken when the corrections become large and actually degrade the performance. Predicting the failure modes of the algorithm may become harder for larger (more realistic) models. The message seems to be that where the mean field does well the cavity fields will improve the situation, but where the mean field performs less well the cavity fields can degrade performance. This suggests that the cavity fields could be used as a check on the mean field method. Where the cavity fields are small we can be reasonably confident that the mean field is producing sensible answers. However where the cavity fields become large it is likely that the mean field is no longer producing accurate estimates.

Further work would consider larger simulations using more realistic models. It might no longer be feasible to compare these simulations with the 'correct' EM algorithm as the size of the model increases, though other techniques such as Gibbs sampling could be used instead. It would also be interesting to look at the next level of approximation where, instead of approximating the joint expectations by the product of the individual expectations in equation (6), the joint expectations are evaluated by summing over the joint state space (c.f. equation (1)) and possibly evaluating the corresponding cavity fields (Dunmur & Titterington, 1996b). This would perhaps improve the quality of the approximation without introducing the exponential complexity associated with the full E step.

Acknowledgements

This research was supported by a grant from the UK Engineering and Physical Sciences Research Council.

References

DEMPSTER, A. P., LAIRD, N. M. & RUBIN, D. B. (1977). Maximum likelihood estimation from incomplete data via the EM algorithm (with discussion). *J. R. Statist. Soc.* B **39**, 1-38.

DUNMUR, A. P. & TITTERINGTON, D. M. (1996a). Parameter estimation in latent structure models. *Tech. Report 96-2*, Dept. Statist., Univ. Glasgow.

DUNMUR, A. P. & TITTERINGTON, D. M. (1996b). Higher order mean field approximations. In preparation.

GHAHRAMANI, Z. (1995). Factorial learning and the EM algorithm. In *Advances in Neural Information Processing Systems 7*, Eds. G. Tesauro, D. S. Touretzky & T. K. Leen. Cambridge MA: MIT Press.

GHAHRAMANI, Z. & JORDAN, M. I. (1995). Factorial hidden Markov models. Computational Cognitive Science Technical Report 9502, MIT.

HENRY, N. W. (1983). Latent structure analysis. In *Encyclopedia of Statistical Sciences, Volume 4*, Eds. S. Kotz, N. L. Johnson & C. B. Read, pp.497-504. New York: Wiley.

HOFMANN, T. & BUHMANN, J. M. (1996) Pairwise Data Clustering by Deterministic Annealing. Tech. Rep. IAI-TR-95-7, Institut für Informatik III, Universität Bonn.

MEZARD, M., PARISI, G. & VIRASORO, M. A. (1987) *Spin Glass Theory and Beyond*. Lecture Notes in Physics, 9. Singapore: World Scientific.

PARISI, G. (1988). *Statistical Field Theory*. Redwood City CA: Addison-Wesley.

SAUL, L. K., JAAKKOLA, T. & JORDAN, M. I. (1996) Mean Field Theory for Sigmoid Belief Networks. *J. Artificial Intelligence Research* **4**, 61-76.

ZHANG, J. (1992). The Mean Field Theory in EM procedures for Markov random fields. *I. E. E. E. Trans. Signal Processing* **40**, 2570-83.

ZHANG, J. (1993). The Mean Field Theory in EM procedures for blind Markov random field image restoration. *I. E. E. E. Trans. Image Processing* **2**, 27-40.

Softening Discrete Relaxation

Andrew M. Finch, Richard C. Wilson and Edwin R. Hancock
Department of Computer Science,
University of York, York, Y01 5DD, UK

Abstract

This paper describes a new framework for relational graph matching. The starting point is a recently reported Bayesian consistency measure which gauges structural differences using Hamming distance. The main contributions of the work are threefold. Firstly, we demonstrate how the discrete components of the cost function can be softened. The second contribution is to show how the softened cost function can be used to locate matches using continuous non-linear optimisation. Finally, we show how the resulting graph matching algorithm relates to the standard quadratic assignment problem.

1 Introduction

Graph matching [6, 5, 7, 2, 3, 12, 11] is a topic of central importance in pattern perception. The main computational issues are how to compare inexact relational descriptions [7] and how to search efficiently for the best match [8]. These two issues have recently stimulated interest in the connectionist literature [9, 6, 5, 10]. For instance, Simic [9], Suganathan *et al.* [10] and Gold *et al.* [6, 5] have addressed the issue of how to expressively measure relational distance. Both Gold and Rangarajan [6] and Suganathan *et al* [10] have shown how non-linear optimisation techniques such as mean-field annealing [10] and graduated assignment [6] can be applied to find optimal matches.

In a recent series of papers we have developed a Bayesian framework for relational graph matching [2, 3, 11, 12]. The novelty resides in the fact that relational consistency is gauged by a probability distribution that uses Hamming distance to measure structural differences between the graphs under match. This new framework has not only been used to match complex infra-red [3] and radar imagery [11], it has also been used to successfully control a graph-edit process [12] of the sort originally proposed by Sanfeliu and Fu [7]. The optimisation of this relational consistency measure has hitherto been confined to the use of discrete update procedures [11, 2, 3]. Examples include discrete relaxation [7, 11], simulated annealing

[4, 3] and genetic search [2]. Our aim in this paper is to consider how the optimisation of the relational consistency measure can be realised by continuous means [6, 10]. Specifically we consider how the matching process can be effected using a non-linear technique similar to mean-field annealing [10] or graduated assignment [6]. In order to achieve this goal we must transform our discrete cost function [11] into a form suitable for optimisation by continuous techniques. The key idea is to exploit the apparatus of statistical physics [13] to compute the effective Gibbs potentials for our discrete relaxation process. The potentials are in-fact weighted sums of Hamming distance enumerated over the consistent relations of the model graph. The quantities of interest in the optimisation process are the derivatives of the global energy function computed from the Gibbs potentials. In the case of our weighted sum of Hamming distance, these derivatives take on a particularly interesting form which provides an intuitive insight into the dynamics of the update process. An experimental evaluation of the technique reveals not only that it is successful in matching noise corrupted graphs, but that it significantly outperforms the optimisation of the standard quadratic energy function.

2 Relational Consistency

Our overall goal in this paper is to formulate a non-linear optimisation technique for matching relational graphs. We use the notation $G = (V, E)$ to denote the graphs under match, where V is the set of nodes and E is the set of edges. Our aim in matching is to associate nodes in a graph $G_D = (V_D, E_D)$ representing data to be matched against those in a graph $G_M = (V_M, E_M)$ representing an available relational model. Formally, the matching is represented by a function $f : V_D \to V_M$ from the nodes in the data graph G_D to those in the model graph G_M. We represent the structure of the two graphs using a pair of connection matrices. The connection matrix for the data graph consists of the binary array

$$D_{ab} = \begin{cases} 1 & \text{if } (a,b) \in E_D \\ 0 & \text{otherwise} \end{cases} \quad (1)$$

while that for the model graph is

$$M_{\alpha\beta} = \begin{cases} 1 & \text{if } (\alpha,\beta) \in E_M \\ 0 & \text{otherwise} \end{cases} \quad (2)$$

The current state of match between the two graphs is represented by the function $f : V_D \to V_M$. In others words the statement $f(a) = \alpha$ means that the node $a \in V_D$ is matched to the node $\alpha \in V_M$. The binary representation of the current state of match is captured by a set of assignment variables which convey the following meaning

$$s_{a\alpha} = \begin{cases} 1 & \text{if } f(a) = \alpha \\ 0 & \text{otherwise} \end{cases} \quad (3)$$

The basic goal of the matching process is to optimise a consistency-measure which gauges the structural similarity of the matched data graph and the model graph. In a recent series of papers, Wilson and Hancock [11, 12] have shown how consistency of match can be modelled using a Bayesian framework. The basic idea is to construct a probability distribution which models the effect of memoryless matching errors in generating departures from consistency between the data and model graphs. Suppose that $S_\alpha = \alpha \cup \{\beta | (\alpha, \beta) \in E_M\}$ represents the set of nodes that form the immediate contextual neighbourhood of the node α in the model graph.

Further suppose that $\Gamma_a = f(a) \cup \{f(b)|(a,b) \in E_D\}$ represents the set of matches assigned to the contextual neighbourhood of the node $a \in V_D$ of the data graph. Basic to Wilson and Hancock's modelling of relational consistency is to regard the complete set of model-graph relations as mutually exclusive causes from which the potentially corrupt matched model-graph relations arise. As a result, the probability of the matched configuration Γ_a can be expressed as a mixture distribution over the corresponding space of model-graph configurations

$$P(\Gamma_a) = \sum_{\alpha \in V_M} P(\Gamma_a|S_\alpha)P(S_\alpha) \qquad (4)$$

The modelling of the match confusion probabilities $P(\Gamma_a|S_\alpha)$ draws on the assumption that the error process is independent of location. This allows $P(\Gamma_a|S_\alpha)$ to be factorised over its component matches. Individual label errors are further assumed to act with a memoryless probability P_e. With these ingredients the probability of the matched neighbourhood Γ_a reduces to [11, 12]

$$P(\Gamma_a) = \frac{K_a}{|V_M|} \sum_{\alpha \in V_M} \exp[-\mu H(a,\alpha)] \qquad (5)$$

where $K_a = (1 - P_e)^{|\Gamma_a|}$ and the exponential constant is related to the probability of label errors, i.e. $\mu = \ln \frac{(1-P_e)}{P_e}$. Consistency of match is gauged by the "Hamming distance", $H(a,\alpha)$ between the matched relation Γ_a and the set of consistent neighbourhood structures $S_\alpha, \forall \alpha \in V_M$ from the model graph. According to our binary representation of the matching process, the distance measure is computed using the connectivity matrices and the assignment variables in the following manner

$$H(a,\alpha) = \sum_{b \in V_D} \sum_{\beta \in V_M} M_{\alpha\beta} D_{ab}(1 - s_{b\beta}) \qquad (6)$$

The probability distribution $P(\Gamma_a)$ may be regarded as providing a natural way of modelling departures from consistency at the neighbourhood level. Matching consistency is graded by Hamming distance and controlled hardening may be induced by reducing the label-error probability P_e towards zero.

3 The Effective Potential for Discrete Relaxation

We commence the development of our graduated assignment approach to discrete relaxation by computing an effective Gibbs potential $U(\Gamma_a)$ for the matching configuration Γ_a. In other words, we aim to replace the compound exponential probability distribution appearing in equation (5) by the single Gibbs distribution

$$Q(\Gamma_a) = \frac{\exp\left[-\mu U(\Gamma_a)\right]}{\sum_\Upsilon \exp\left[-\mu U(\Upsilon)\right]} \qquad (7)$$

Our route to the effective potential is provided by statistical physics. If we represent $P(\Gamma_a)$ by an equivalent Gibbs distribution with an identical partition function, then the equilibrium configurational potential is related to the partial derivative of the log-probability with respect to the coupling constant μ in the following manner [13]

$$U(\Gamma_a) = -\frac{\partial \ln P(\Gamma_a)}{\partial \mu} \qquad (8)$$

Upon substituting for $P(\Gamma_a)$ from equation (5)

$$U(\Gamma_a) = \frac{\sum_{\alpha \in V_M} H(a,\alpha) \exp[-\mu H(a,\alpha)]}{\sum_{\alpha \in V_M} \exp[-\mu H(a,\alpha)]} \qquad (9)$$

In other words the neighbourhood Gibbs potentials are simply weighted sums of Hamming distance between the data and model graphs. In fact the local clique potentials display an interesting barrier property. The potential is concentrated at Hamming distance $H \simeq \frac{1}{\mu}$. Both very large and very small Hamming distances contribute insignificantly to the energy function, i.e. $\lim_{H \to 0} H \exp[-\mu H] = 0$ and $\lim_{H \to \infty} H \exp[-\mu H] = 0$.

With the neighbourhood matching potentials to hand, we construct a global "matching-energy" $\mathcal{E} = \sum_{a \in V_D} U(\Gamma_a)$ by summing the contributions over the nodes of the data graph.

4 Optimising the Global Cost Function

We are now in a position to develop a continuous update algorithm by softening the discrete ingredients of our graph matching potential. The idea is to compute the derivatives of the global energy given in equation (10) and to effect the softening process using the soft-max idea of Bridle [1].

4.1 Softassign

The energy function represented by equations (9) and (10) is defined over the discrete matching variables $s_{a\alpha}$. The basic idea underpinning this paper is to realise a continuous process for updating the assignment variables. The optimal step-size is determined by computing the partial derivatives of the global matching energy with respect to the assignment variables. We commence by computing the derivatives of the contributing neighbourhood Gibbs potentials, i.e.

$$\frac{\partial U(\Gamma_a)}{\partial s_{b\beta}} = \sum_{\alpha \in V_M} \left[1 - \mu\Big(H(a,\alpha) - U(\Gamma_a)\Big)\right] \xi_{a\alpha} \frac{\partial H(a,\alpha)}{\partial s_{b\beta}} \qquad (10)$$

where

$$\xi_{a\alpha} = \frac{\exp[-\mu H(a,\alpha)]}{\sum_{\alpha' \in V_M} \exp[-\mu H(a,\alpha')]} \qquad (11)$$

To further develop this result, we must compute the derivatives of the Hamming distances. From equation (6) it follows that

$$\frac{\partial H(a,\alpha)}{\partial s_{b\beta}} = -M_{\alpha\beta} D_{ab} \qquad (12)$$

It is now a straightforward matter to show that the derivative of the global matching energy is equal to

$$\frac{\partial \mathcal{E}}{\partial s_{b\beta}} = -\sum_{a \in V_D} \sum_{\alpha \in V_M} D_{ab} M_{\alpha\beta} \left[1 - \mu\Big(H(a,\alpha) - U(\Gamma_a)\Big)\right] \xi_{a\alpha} \qquad (13)$$

We would like our continuous matching variables to remain constrained to lie within the range $[0, 1]$. Rather than using a linear update rule, we exploit Bridle's soft-max ansatz [1]. In doing this we arrive at an update process which has many features in common with the well-known mean-field equations of statistical physics

$$s_{a\alpha} \leftarrow \frac{\exp\left[-\frac{1}{T}\frac{\partial \mathcal{E}}{\partial s_{a\alpha}}\right]}{\sum_{\alpha' \in V_M} \exp\left[-\frac{1}{T}\frac{\partial \mathcal{E}}{\partial s_{a\alpha'}}\right]} \quad (14)$$

The mathematical structure of this update process is important and deserves further comment. The quantity $\xi_{a\alpha}$ defined in equation (11) naturally plays the role of a matching probability. The first term appearing under the square bracket in equation (13) can therefore be thought of as analogous to the optimal update direction for the standard quadratic cost function [10, 6]; we will discus this relationship in more detail in Section 4.2. The second term modifies this principal update direction by taking into account the weighted fluctuations in the Hamming distance about the effective potential or average Hamming distance. If the average fluctuation is zero, then there is no net modification to the update direction. When the net fluctuation is non-zero, the direction of update is modified so as to compensate for the movement of the mean-value of the effective potential. This corrective tracking process provides an explicit mechanism for maintaining contact with the minimum of the effective potential under rescaling effects induced by changes in the value of the coupling constant μ. Moreover, since the fluctuation term is itself proportional to μ, this has an insignificant effect for $P_e \simeq \frac{1}{2}$ but dominates the update process when $P_e \to 0$.

4.2 Quadratic Assignment Problem

Before we proceed to experiment with the new graph matching process, it is interesting to briefly review the standard quadratic formulation of the matching problem investigated by Simic [9], Suganathan et al [10] and Gold and Rangarajan [6]. The common feature of these algorithms is to commence from the quadratic cost function

$$\mathcal{E}_H = -\frac{1}{2} \sum_{a \in V_D} \sum_{\alpha \in V_M} \sum_{b \in V_D} \sum_{\beta \in V_M} D_{ab} M_{\alpha\beta} s_{a\alpha} s_{b\beta} \quad (15)$$

In this case the derivative of the global cost function is linear in the assignment variables, i.e.

$$\frac{\partial \mathcal{E}_H}{\partial s_{b\beta}} = -\frac{1}{2} \sum_{a \in V_D} \sum_{\alpha \in V_M} D_{ab} M_{\alpha\beta} s_{a\alpha} \quad (16)$$

This step size is equivalent to that appearing in equation (14) provided that $\mu = 0$, i.e. $P_e \to \frac{1}{2}$. The update is realised by applying the soft-max ansatz of equation (14). In the next section, we will provide some experimental comparison with the resulting matching process. However, it is important to stress that the update process adopted here is very simplistic and leaves considerable scope for further refinement. For instance, Gold and Rangarajan [6] have exploited the doubly stochastic properties of Sinckhorn matrices to ensure two-way symmetry in the matching process.

5 Experiments and Conclusions

Our main aim in this Section is to compare the non-linear update equations with the optimisation of the quadratic matching criterion described in Section 4.2. The data for our study is provided by synthetic Delaunay graphs. These graphs are constructed by generating random dot patterns. Each random dot is used to seed a Voronoi cell. The Delaunay triangulation is the region adjacency graph for the Voronoi cells. In order to pose demanding tests of our matching technique, we have added controlled amounts of corruption to the synthetic graphs. This is effected by deleting and adding a specified fraction of the dots from the initial random patterns. The associated Delaunay graph is therefore subject to structural corruption. We measure the degree of corruption by the fraction of surviving nodes in the corrupted Delaunay graph.

Our experimental protocol has been as follows. For a series of different corruption levels, we have generated a sample of 100 random graphs. The graphs contain 50 nodes each. According to the specified corruption level, we have both added and deleted a predefined fraction of nodes at random locations in the initial graphs so as to maintain their overall size. For each graph we measure the quality of match by computing the fraction of the surviving nodes for which the assignment variables indicate the correct match. The value of the temperature T in the update process has been controlled using a logarithmic annealing schedule of the form suggested by Geman and Geman [4]. We initialise the assignment variables uniformly across the set of matches by setting $s_{a\alpha} = \frac{1}{V_M}$, $\forall a, \alpha$.

We have compared the results obtained with two different versions of the matching algorithm. The first of these involves updating the softened assignment variables by applying the non-linear update equation given in (14). The second matching algorithm involves applying the same optimisation apparatus to the quadratic cost function defined in equation (15) in a simplified form of the quadratic assignment algorithm [6, 10].

Figure 1 shows the final fraction of correct matches for both algorithms. The data curves show the correct matching fraction averaged over the graph samples as a function of the corruption fraction. The main conclusions that can be drawn from these plots is that the new matching technique described in this paper significantly outperforms its conventional quadratic counterpart described in Section 4.2. The main difference between the two techniques resides in the fact that our new method relies on updating with derivatives of the energy function that are non-linear in the assignment variables.

To conclude, our main contribution in this paper has been to demonstrate how the discrete Bayesian relational consistency measure of Wilson and Hancock [11] can be cast in a form that is amenable to continuous non-linear optimisation. We have shown how the method relates to the standard quadratic assignment algorithm extensively studied in the connectionist literature [6, 9, 10]. Moreover, an experimental analysis reveals that the method offers superior performance in terms of noise control.

References

[1] Bridle J.S. "Training stochastic model recognition algorithms can lead to maximum mutual information estimation of parameters" *NIPS2*, pp. 211-217, 1990.

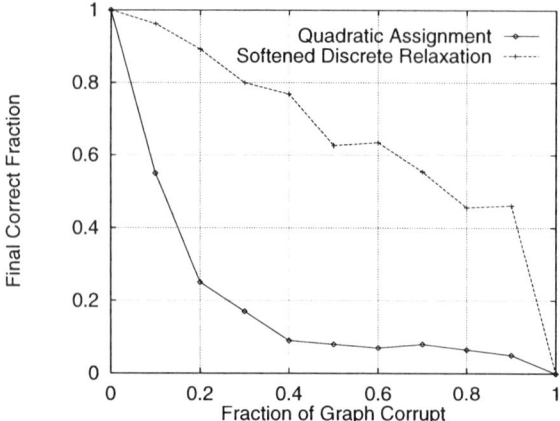

Figure 1: Experimental comparison: softened discrete relaxation (dotted curve); matching using the quadratic cost function (solid curve).

[2] Cross A.D.J., R.C.Wilson and E.R. Hancock, "Genetic search for structural matching", *Proceedings ECCV96*, **LNCS 1064**, pp. 514–525, 1996.

[3] Cross A.D.J. and E.R.Hancock, "Relational matching with stochastic optimisation" *IEEE Computer Society International Symposium on Computer Vision*, pp. 365–370, 1995.

[4] Geman S. and D. Geman, "Stochastic relaxation, Gibbs distributions and Bayesian restoration of images," *IEEE PAMI*, **PAMI-6** , pp.721–741, 1984.

[5] Gold S., A. Rangarajan and E. Mjolsness, "Learning with pre-knowledge: Clustering with point and graph-matching distance measures", *Neural Computation*, 8, pp. 787–804, 1996.

[6] Gold S. and A. Rangarajan, "A graduated assignment algorithm for graph matching", *IEEE PAMI*, 18, pp. 377–388, 1996.

[7] Sanfeliu A. and Fu K.S., "A distance measure between attributed relational graphs for pattern recognition", *IEEE SMC*, 13, pp 353–362, 1983.

[8] Shapiro L. and R.M.Haralick, "Structural description and inexact matching", *IEEE PAMI*, 3, pp 504–519, 1981.

[9] Simic P., "Constrained nets for graph matching and other quadratic assignment problems", *Neural Computation*, 3 , pp. 268–281, 1991.

[10] Suganathan P.N., E.K. Teoh and D.P. Mital, "Pattern recognition by graph matching using Potts MFT networks", *Pattern Recognition*, 28, pp. 997–1009, 1995.

[11] Wilson R.C., Evans A.N. and Hancock E.R., "Relational matching by discrete relaxation", *Image and Vision Computing*, 13, pp. 411–421, 1995.

[12] Wilson R.C and Hancock E.R., "Relational matching with dynamic graph structures", *Proceedings of the Fifth International Conference on Computer Vision*, pp. 450-456, 1995.

[13] Yuille A., "Generalised deformable models, statistical physics and matching problems", *Neural Computation*, 2, pp. 1-24, 1990.

Limitations of self-organizing maps for vector quantization and multidimensional scaling

Arthur Flexer
The Austrian Research Institute for Artificial Intelligence
Schottengasse 3, A-1010 Vienna, Austria
and
Department of Psychology, University of Vienna
Liebiggasse 5, A-1010 Vienna, Austria
arthur@ai.univie.ac.at

Abstract

The limitations of using self-organizing maps (SOM) for either clustering/vector quantization (VQ) or multidimensional scaling (MDS) are being discussed by reviewing recent empirical findings and the relevant theory. SOM's remaining ability of doing both VQ *and* MDS at the same time is challenged by a new combined technique of online K-means clustering plus Sammon mapping of the cluster centroids. SOM are shown to perform significantly worse in terms of quantization error, in recovering the structure of the clusters and in preserving the topology in a comprehensive empirical study using a series of multivariate normal clustering problems.

1 Introduction

Self-organizing maps (SOM) introduced by [Kohonen 84] are a very popular tool used for visualization of high dimensional data spaces. SOM can be said to do clustering/vector quantization (VQ) *and* at the same time to preserve the spatial ordering of the input data reflected by an ordering of the code book vectors (cluster centroids) in a one or two dimensional output space, where the latter property is closely related to multidimensional scaling (MDS) in statistics. Although the level of activity and research around the SOM algorithm is quite large (a recent overview by [Kohonen 95] contains more than 1000 citations), only little comparison among the numerous existing variants of the basic approach and also to more traditional statistical techniques of the larger frameworks of VQ and MDS is available. Additionally, there is only little advice in the literature about how to properly use

SOM in order to get optimal results in terms of either vector quantization (VQ) or multidimensional scaling or maybe even both of them. To make the notion of SOM being a tool for "data visualization" more precise, the following question has to be answered: Should SOM be used for doing VQ, MDS, both at the same time or none of them?

Two recent comprehensive studies comparing SOM either to traditional VQ *or* MDS techniques separately seem to indicate that SOM is not competitive when used for either VQ or MDS: [Balakrishnan et al. 94] compare SOM to K-means clustering on 108 multivariate normal clustering problems with known clustering solutions and show that SOM performs significantly worse in terms of data points misclassified[1], especially with higher numbers of clusters in the data sets. [Bezdek & Nikhil 95] compare SOM to principal component analysis and the MDS-technique Sammon mapping on seven artificial data sets with different numbers of points and dimensionality and different shapes of input distributions. The degree of preservation of the spatial ordering of the input data is measured via a Spearman rank correlation between the distances of points in the input space and the distances of their projections in the two dimensional output space. The traditional MDS-techniques preserve the distances much more effectively than SOM, the performance of which decreases rapidly with increasing dimensionality of the input data.

Despite these strong empirical findings that speak against the use of SOM for either VQ or MDS there remains the appealing ability of SOM to do both VQ *and* MDS at the same time. It is the aim of this work to find out, whether a combined technique of traditional vector quantization (clustering) *plus* MDS on the code book vectors (cluster centroids) can perform better than Kohonen's SOM on a series of multivariate normal clustering problems in terms of quantization error (mean squared error), recovering the cluster structure (Rand index) and preserving the topology (Pearson correlation). All the experiments were done in a rigoruos statistical design using multiple analysis of variance for evaluation of the results.

2 SOM and vector quantization/clustering

A vector quantizer (VQ) is a mapping, q, that assigns to each input vector x a reproduction (code book) vector $\hat{x} = q(x)$ drawn from a finite reproduction alphabet $\hat{A} = \{\hat{x}_i, i = 1, \ldots, N\}$. The quantizer q is completely described by the reproduction alphabet (or codebook) $\hat{A}$ together with the partition $S = \{S_i, i = 1, \ldots, N\}$, of the input vector space into the sets $S_i = \{x : q(x) = \hat{x}_i\}$ of input vectors mapping into the ith reproduction vector (or code word) [Linde et al. 80]. To be compareable to SOM, our VQ assigns to each of the input vectors $x = (x^0, x^1, \ldots, x^{k-1})$ a socalled code book vector $\hat{x} = (\hat{x}^0, \hat{x}^1, \ldots, \hat{x}^{k-1})$ of the same dimensionality k. For reasons of data compression, the number of code book vectors $N \ll n$, where n is the number of input vectors.

Demanded is a VQ that produces a mapping q for which the expected distortion caused by reproducing the input vectors x by code book vectors $q(x)$ is at least locally minimal. The expected distortion is usually esimated by using the average distortion D, where the most common distortion measure is the squared-error

---

[1] Although SOM is an unsupervised technique not built for classification, the number of points missclassified to a wrong cluster center *is* an appropriate and commonly used performance measure for cluster procedures if the true cluster structure is known.

distortion d:

$$D = \frac{1}{n}\sum_{i=0}^{n-1} d(x_i, q(x_i)) \quad (1) \qquad d(x, \hat{x}) = \sum_{i=0}^{k-1} |x_i - \hat{x}_i|^2 \quad (2)$$

The classical vector quantization technique to achieve such a mapping is the LBG-algorithm [Linde et al. 80], where a given quantizer is iteratively improved. Already [Linde et al. 80] noted that their proposed algorithm is almost similar to the k-means approach developed in the cluster analysis literature starting from [MacQueen 67]. Closely related to SOM is online K-means clustering (oKMC) consisting of the following steps:

1. Initialization: Given N = number of code book vectors, k = dimensionality of the vectors, n = number of input vectors, a training sequence $\{x_j; j = 0, \ldots, n-1\}$, an initial set $\hat{A}_0$ of N code book vectors $\hat{x}$ and a discrete-time coordinate $t = 0 \ldots, n-1$.

2. Given $\hat{A}_t = \{\hat{x}_i; i = 1, \ldots, N\}$, find the minimum distortion partition $P(\hat{A}_t) = \{S_i; i = 1, \ldots, N\}$. Compute $d(x_t, \hat{x}_i)$ for $i = 1, \ldots, N$. If $d(x_t, \hat{x}_i) \leq (x_t, \hat{x}_l)$ for all l, then $x_t \in S_i$.

3. Update the code book vector with the minimum distortion

$$\hat{x}_{(t)}(S_i) = \hat{x}_{(t-1)}(S_i) + \alpha[x_{(t)} - \hat{x}_{(t-1)}(S_i)] \quad (3)$$

where α is a learning parameter to be defined by the user. Define $\hat{A}_{t+1} = \hat{x}(P(\hat{A}_t))$, replace t by $t+1$, if $t = n-1$, halt. Else go to step 2.

The main difference between the SOM-algorithm and oKMC is the fact that the code book vectors are ordered either on a line or on a planar grid (i.e. in a one or two dimensional output space). The iterative procedure is the same as with oKMC where formula (3) is replaced by

$$\hat{x}_{(t)}(S_i) = \hat{x}_{(t-1)}(S_i) + h[x_{(t)} - \hat{x}_{(t-1)}(S_i)] \quad (4)$$

and this update is not only computed for the $\hat{x}_i$ that gives minimum distortion, but also for all the code book vectors which are in the neighbourhood of this $\hat{x}_i$ on the line or planar grid. The degree of neighbourhood and amount of code book vectors which are updated together with the $\hat{x}_i$ that gives minimum distortion is expressed by h, a function that decreases both with distance on the line or planar grid and with time and that also includes an additional learning parameter α. If the degree of neighbourhood is decreased to zero, the SOM-algorithm becomes equal to the oKMC-algorithm.

Whereas local convergence is guaranteed for oKMC (at least for decreasing α, [Bottou & Bengio 95]), no general proof for the convergence of SOM with nonzero neighbourhood is known. [Kohonen 95, p.128] notes that the last steps of the SOM algorithm should be computed with zero neighbourhood in order to guarantee "the most accurate density approximation of the input samples".

3 SOM and multidimensional scaling

Formally, a topology preserving algorithm is a transformation $\Phi : R^k \mapsto R^p$, that either preserves *similarities* or just *similarity orderings* of the points in the input space R^k when they are mapped into the outputspace R^p. For most algorithms it is the case that both the number of input vectors $\mid x \in R^k \mid$ and the number of output vectors $|\hat{x} \in R^p|$ are equal to n. A transformation $\Phi : \hat{x} = \Phi(x)$, that preserves *similarities* poses the strongest possible constraint since $d(x_i, x_j) = \hat{d}(\hat{x}_i, \hat{x}_j)$ for all $x_i, x_j \in R^k$, all $\hat{x}_i, \hat{x}_j \in R^p$, $i,j = 1,\ldots, n-1$ and d ($\hat{d}$) being a measure of distance in R^k (R^p). Such a transformation is said to produce an *isometric* image.

Techniques for finding such transformations Φ are, among others, various forms of *multidimensional scaling*[2] (MDS) like metric MDS [Torgerson 52], nonmetric MDS [Shepard 62] or Sammon mapping [Sammon 69], but also principal component analysis (PCA) (see e.g. [Jolliffe 86]) or SOM. Sammon mapping is doing MDS by minimizing the following via steepest descent:

$$\frac{1}{\sum_{i=0}^{n-1}\sum_{j<i} d(x_i, x_j)} \sum_{i=0}^{n-1}\sum_{j<i} \frac{(d(x_i, x_j) - \hat{d}(\hat{x}_i, \hat{x}_j))^2}{d(x_i, x_j)} \quad (5)$$

Since the SOM has been designed heuristically and not to find an extremum for a certain cost or energy function[3] and the theoretical connection to the other MDS algorithms remains unclear. It should be noted that for SOM the number of output vectors $|\hat{x} \in R^p|$ is limited to N, the number of cluster centroids $\hat{x}$ and that the $\hat{x}$ are further restricted to lie on a planar grid. This restriction entails a discretization of the outputspace R^p.

4 Online K-means clustering plus Sammon mapping of the cluster centroids

Our new combined approach consists of simply finding the set of $\hat{A} = \{\hat{x}_i, i = 1,\ldots, N\}$ code book vectors that give the minimum distortion partition $P(\hat{A}) = \{S_i; i = 1,\ldots, N\}$ via the oKMC algorithm and then using the $\hat{x}_i$ as input vectors to Sammon mapping and thereby obtaining a two dimensional representation of the $\hat{x}_i$ via minimizing formula (5). Contrary to SOM, this two dimensional representation is not restricted to any fixed form and the distances between the N mapped $\hat{x}_i$ directly correspond to those in the original higher dimension. This combined algorithm is abbreviated oKMC+.

5 Empirical comparison

The empirical comparison was done using a 3 factorial experimental design with 3 dependent variables. The multivariate normal distributions were generated using the procedure by [Milligan & Cooper 85], which since has been used for several comparisons of cluster algorithms (see e.g. [Balakrishnan et al. 94]). The marginal normal distributions gave internal cohesion of the clusters by warranting that more than 99% of the data lie within 3 standard deviations (σ). External isolation was defined as having the first dimension nonoverlapping by truncating the normal distributions in the first dimension to $\pm 2\sigma$ and defining the cluster centroids to be 4.5σ apart. In all other dimensions the clusters were allowed to overlap by setting the distance per dimension between two centroids randomly to lie between $\pm 6\sigma$. The data was normalized to zero mean and unit variance in all dimensions.

---

[2] Note that for MDS not the actual coordinates of the points in the input space but only their distances or the ordering of the latter are needed.

[3] [Erwin et al. 92] even showed that such an objective function cannot exist for SOM.

Limitations of Self-organizing Maps

algorithm	no. clusters	dimension	msqe	Rand	corr.
SOM	4	4	0.53	1.00	0.64
		6	1.53	0.91	0.72
		8	1.15	0.99	0.74
	9	4	0.33	0.97	0.48
		6	0.54	0.97	0.66
		8	0.81	0.96	0.74
	mean SOM		**0.81**	**0.97**	**0.67**
oKMC+	4	4	0.53	0.99	0.87
		6	1.06	0.99	0.87
		8	1.17	1.00	0.91
	9	4	0.29	0.98	0.89
		6	0.47	0.99	0.87
		8	0.56	0.98	0.86
	mean oKMC+		**0.68**	**0.99**	**0.88**

Factor 1, Type of algorithm: The number of code book vectors of both the SOM and the oKMC+ were set equal to the number of clusters known to be in the data. The SOMs were planar grids consisting of 2 × 2 (3 × 3) code book vectors. During the first phase (1000 code book updates) α was set to 0.05 and the radius of the neighbourhood to 2 (5). During the second phase (10000 code book updates) α was set to 0.02 and the radius of the neighbourhood to 0 to guarantee the most accurate vector quantization [Kohonen 95, p.128]. The oKMC+ algorithm had the parameter α fixed to 0.02 and was trained using each data set 20 times, the minimization of formula (5) was stopped after 100 iterations. Both SOM and oKMC+ were run 10 times on each data set and only the best solutions, in terms of mean squared error, were used for further analysis.

Factor 2, Number of clusters was set to 4 and 9.

Factor 3, Number of dimensions was set to 4, 6, or 8.

Dependent variable 1: mean squared error was computed using formula (1).

Dependent variable 2, Rand index (see [Hubert & Arabie 85]) is a measure of agreement between the true, known partition structure and the obtained clusters. Both the numerator and the denominator of the index reflect frequency counts. The numerator is the number of times a pair of data is either in the same or in different clusters in both known and obtained clusterings for all possible comparisons of data points. Since the denominator is the total number of all possible pairwise comparisons, an index value of 1.0 indicates an exact match of the clusterings.

Dependent variable 3, correlation is a measure of the topology preserving abilities of the algorithms. The Pearson correlation of the distances $d(x_1, x_2)$ in the input space and the distances $\hat{d}(\hat{x}_i, \hat{x}_j)$ in the output space for all possible pairwise comparisons of data points is computed. Note that for SOM the coordinates of the code book vectors on the planar grid were used to compute the $\hat{d}$. An algorithm that preserves all distances in every neighbourhood would produce an *isometric* image and yield a value of 1.0 (see [Bezdek & Nikhil 95] for a discussion of measures of topolgy preservation).

For each cell in the full-factorial 2 × 2 × 3 design 3 data sets with 25 points for each cluster were generated resulting in a total of 36 data sets. A multiple analysis of variance (MANOVA) yielded the following significant effects at the .05 error level:

The mean squared error is lower for oKMC+ than for SOM, it is lower for the 9-cluster problem than for the 4-cluster problem and is higher for higher dimensional data. There is also a combined effect of the number of clusters and dimensions on the mean squared error. The Rand index is higher for oKMC+ than for SOM, there is also a combined effect of the number of clusters and dimensions. The correlation index is higher for oKMC+ than for SOM. Since the main interest of this study is the effect of the type of algorithm on the dependent variables, the mean performances for SOM and oKMC+ are printed in bold letters in the table. Note that the overall differences in the performances of the two algorithms are blurred by the significant effects of the other factors and that therefore the differences of the grand means across the type of algorithms appear rather small. Only by applying a MANOVA, effects of the factor 'type of algorithms' that are masked by additional effects of the other two factors 'number of clusters' and 'number of dimensions' could still be detected.

6 Discussion and Conclusion

From the theoretical comparison of SOM to oKMC it should be clear that in terms of quantization error, SOM should only be possible to perform as good as oKMC if SOM's neighbourhood is set to zero. Additional experiments, not reported here in detail for brevity, with nonzero neighbourhood till the end of SOM training gave even worse results since the neighbourhood tends to pull the obtained cluster centroids away from the true ones. The Rand index is only slightly better for oKMC+. The high values indicate that both algorithms were able to recover the known cluster structure. Topology preserving is where SOM performs worst compared to oKMC+. This is a direct implication of the restriction to planar grids which allows only $\sum_{i=2}^{s} i, (s \geq 2)$ different distances in an $s \times s$ planar grid instead of $\frac{N(N-1)}{2}$ different distances for $N = s \times s$ cluster centroids mapped via Sammon mapping in the case of oKMC+. Using a nonzero neighbourhood at the end of SOM training did not warrant any significant improvements.

An argument that could be brought forward against our approach towards comparing SOM and oKMC+ is that it would be unfair or not correct to set the number of SOM's code book vectors equal to the number of clusters known to be in the data. In fact it seems to be common practice to apply SOM with numbers of code book vectors that are a multiple of the input vectors available for training (see e.g. [Kohonen 95, pp.113]). Two things have to be said against such an argumentation: First if one uses more or even only the same amount of code book vectors than input vectors during vector quantization, each code book vector will become identical to one of the input vectors in the limit of learning. So every x_i is replaced with an identical $\hat{x}_i$, which does not make any sense and runs counter to every notion of vector quantization. This means that SOMs employing numbers of code book vectors that are a multiple of the input vectors available can be used for MDS only. But even such big SOMs do MDS in a very crude way: We computed SOMs consisting of either 20×20 (for data sets consisting of 4 clusters and 100 points) or 30×30 (for data sets consisting of 9 clusters and 225 points) code book vectors for all 36 data sets which gave an average correlation of 0.77 between the distances d_i and $\hat{d}_i$. This is significantly worse at the .05 error level compared to the average correlation of 0.95 achieved by Sammon mapping applied to the input data directly.

Our data sets consisted of iid multivariate normal distributions which therefore have spherical shape. All VQ algorithms using squared distances as a distortion measure, including our versions of oKMC as well as SOM, are inherently designed for such distributions. Therefore, the clustering problems in this study, being also perfectly seperable in one dimension, were very simple and should be solveable with little or no error by any clustering or MDS algorithm.

In this work we examined the vague concept of using SOM as a "data visualization tool" both from a theoretical and empirical point of view. SOM cannot outperform traditional VQ techniques in terms of quantization error and should therefore not be used for doing VQ. From [Bezdek & Nikhil 95] as well as from our discussion of SOM's restriction to planar grids in the output space which allows only a restricted number of different distances to be represented, it should be evident that SOM is also a rather crude way of doing MDS. Our own empirical results show that if one wants to have an algorithm that does both VQ and MDS at the same time, there exists a very simple combination of traditional techniques (our oKMC+) with wellknown and established properties that clearly outperforms SOM.

Whether it is a good idea to combine clustering or vector quantization and multidimensional scaling at all and whether more principled approaches (see e.g. [Bishop et al. this volume], also for pointers to further related work) can yield even better results than our oKMC+ and last but not least what self-organizing maps *should* be used for under this new light remain questions to be answered by future investigations.

Acknowledgements: Thanks are due to James Pardey, University of Oxford, for the Sammon code. The SOM_PAK, Helsinki University of Technology, was used for all computations of self-organizing maps. This work has been started within the framework of the BIOMED-1 concerted action ANNDEE, sponsored by the European Commission, DG XII, and the Austrian Federal Ministry of Science, Transport, and the Arts, which is also supporting the Austrian Research Institute for Artificial Intelligence. The author is supported by a doctoral grant of the Austrian Academy of Sciences.

References

[Balakrishnan et al. 94] Balakrishnan P.V., Cooper M.C., Jacob V.S., Lewis P.A.: A study of the classification capabilities of neural networks using unsupervised learning: a comparison with k-means clustering, Psychometrika, Vol. 59, No. 4, 509-525, 1994.

[Bezdek & Nikhil 95] Bezdek J.C., Nikhil R.P.: An index of topological preservation for feature extraction, Pattern Recognition, Vol. 28, No. 3, pp.381-391, 1995.

[Bishop et al. this volume] Bishop C.M., Svensen M., Williams C.K.I.: GTM: A Principled Alternative to the Self-Organizing Map, this volume.

[Bottou & Bengio 95] Bottou L., Bengio Y.: Convergence Properties of the K-Means Algorithms, in Tesauro G., et al.(eds.), Advances in Neural Information Processing System 7, MIT Press, Cambridge, MA, pp.585-592, 1995.

[Erwin et al. 92] Erwin E., Obermayer K., Schulten K.: Self-organizing maps: ordering, convergence properties and energy functions, Biological Cybernetics, 67, 47- 55, 1992.

[Hubert & Arabie 85] Hubert L.J., Arabie P.: Comparing partitions, J. of Classification, 2, 63-76, 1985.

[Jolliffe 86] Jolliffe I.T.: Principal Component Analysis, Springer, 1986.

[Kohonen 84] Kohonen T.: Self-Organization and Associative Memory, Springer, 1984.

[Kohonen 95] Kohonen T.: Self-organizing maps, Springer, Berlin, 1995.

[Linde et al. 80] Linde Y., Buzo A., Gray R.M.: An Algorithm for Vector Quantizer Design, IEEE Transactions on Communications, Vol. COM-28, No. 1, January, 1980.

[MacQueen 67] MacQueen J.: Some Methods for Classification and Analysis of Multivariate Observations, Proc. of the Fifth Berkeley Symposium on Math., Stat. and Prob., Vol. 1, pp. 281-296, 1967.

[Milligan & Cooper 85] Milligan G.W., Cooper M.C.: An examination of procedures for determining the number of clusters in a data set, Psychometrika 50(2), 159-179, 1985.

[Sammon 69] Sammon J.W.: A Nonlinear Mapping for Data Structure Analysis, IEEE Transactions on Comp., Vol. C-18, No. 5, p.401-409, 1969.

[Shepard 62] Shepard R.N.: The analysis of proximities: multidimensional scaling with an unknown distance function. I., Psychometrika, Vol. 27, No. 2, p.125-140, 1962.

[Torgerson 52] Torgerson W.S.: Multidimensional Scaling, I: theory and method, Psychometrika, 17, 401-419, 1952.

Continuous sigmoidal belief networks trained using slice sampling

Brendan J. Frey
Department of Computer Science, University of Toronto
6 King's College Road, Toronto, Canada M5S 1A4

Abstract

Real-valued random hidden variables can be useful for modelling latent structure that explains correlations among observed variables. I propose a simple unit that adds zero-mean Gaussian noise to its input before passing it through a sigmoidal squashing function. Such units can produce a variety of useful behaviors, ranging from deterministic to binary stochastic to continuous stochastic. I show how "slice sampling" can be used for inference and learning in top-down networks of these units and demonstrate learning on two simple problems.

1 Introduction

A variety of unsupervised connectionist models containing discrete-valued hidden units have been developed. These include Boltzmann machines (Hinton and Sejnowski 1986), binary sigmoidal belief networks (Neal 1992) and Helmholtz machines (Hinton *et al.* 1995; Dayan *et al.* 1995). However, some hidden variables, such as translation or scaling in images of shapes, are best represented using continuous values. Continuous-valued Boltzmann machines have been developed (Movellan and McClelland 1993), but these suffer from long simulation settling times and the requirement of a "negative phase" during learning. Tibshirani (1992) and Bishop *et al.* (1996) consider learning mappings from a *continuous* latent variable space to a higher-dimensional input space. MacKay (1995) has developed "density networks" that can model both continuous and categorical latent spaces using stochasticity at the top-most network layer. In this paper I consider a new hierarchical top-down connectionist model that has stochastic hidden variables at all layers; moreover, these variables can *adapt* to be continuous or categorical.

The proposed top-down model can be viewed as a continuous-valued belief network, which can be simulated by performing a quick top-down pass (Pearl 1988). Work done on continuous-valued belief networks has focussed mainly on Gaussian random variables that are linked linearly such that the joint distribution over all

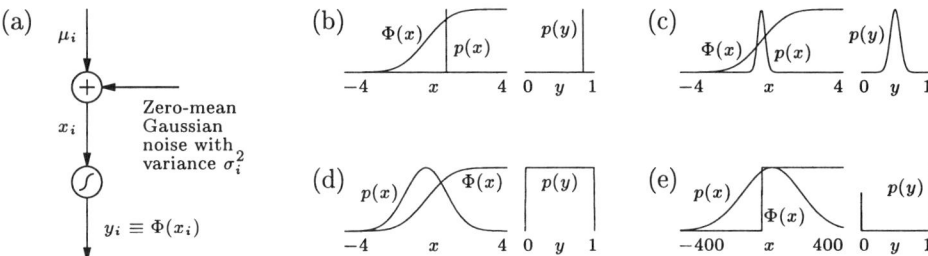

Figure 1: (a) shows the inner workings of the proposed unit. (b) to (e) illustrate four quite different modes of behavior: (b) deterministic mode; (c) stochastic linear mode; (d) stochastic nonlinear mode; and (e) stochastic binary mode (note the different horizontal scale). For the sake of graphical clarity, the density functions are normalized to have equal maxima and the subscripts are left off the variables.

variables is also Gaussian (Pearl 1988; Heckerman and Geiger 1995). Lauritzen et al. (1990) have included discrete random variables within the linear Gaussian framework. These approaches infer the distribution over unobserved unit activities given observed ones by "probability propagation" (Pearl 1988). However, this procedure is highly suboptimal for the richly connected networks that I am interested in. Also, these approaches tend to assume that all the conditional Gaussian distributions represented by the belief network can be easily derived using information elicited from experts. Hofmann and Tresp (1996) consider the case of inference and learning in continuous belief networks that may be richly connected. They use mixture models and Parzen windows to implement conditional densities.

My main contribution is a simple, but versatile, continuous random unit that can operate in several different modes ranging from deterministic to binary stochastic to continuous stochastic. This spectrum of behaviors is controlled by only two parameters. Whereas the above approaches assume a particular mode for each unit (Gaussian or discrete), the proposed units are capable of adapting in order to operate in whatever mode is most appropriate.

2 Description of the unit

The proposed unit is shown in Figure 1a. It is similar to the deterministic sigmoidal unit used in multilayer perceptrons, except that Gaussian noise is added to the total input, μ_i, before the sigmoidal squashing function is applied.[1] The probability density over *presigmoid* activity x_i for unit i is

$$p(x_i|\mu_i, \sigma_i^2) \equiv \exp[-(x_i - \mu_i)^2/2\sigma_i^2]/\sqrt{2\pi\sigma_i^2}, \quad (1)$$

where μ_i and σ_i^2 are the mean and variance for unit i. A *postsigmoid* activity, y_i, is obtained by passing the presigmoid activity through a sigmoidal squashing function:

$$y_i \equiv \Phi(x_i). \quad (2)$$

Including the transformation Jacobian, the postsigmoid distribution for unit i is

$$p(y_i|\mu_i, \sigma_i^2) = \frac{\exp[-(\Phi^{-1}(y_i) - \mu_i)^2/2\sigma_i^2]}{\Phi'(\Phi^{-1}(y_i))\sqrt{2\pi\sigma_i^2}}. \quad (3)$$

---
[1] Geoffrey Hinton suggested this unit as a way to make factor analysis nonlinear.

I use the cumulative Gaussian squashing function:

$$\Phi(x) \equiv \int_{-\infty}^{x} e^{-z^2/2}/\sqrt{2\pi}\, dz \qquad \Phi'(x) = \phi(x) \equiv e^{-x^2/2}/\sqrt{2\pi}. \tag{4}$$

Both $\Phi()$ and $\Phi^{-1}()$ are nonanalytic, so I use the C-library erf() function to implement $\Phi()$ and table lookup with quadratic interpolation to implement $\Phi^{-1}()$.

Networks of these units can *represent* a broad range of structures, including deterministic multilayer perceptrons, binary sigmoidal belief networks (*aka.* stochastic multilayer perceptrons), mixture models, mixture of expert models, hierarchical mixture of expert models, and factor analysis models. This versatility is brought about by a range of significantly different modes of behavior available to each unit. Figures 1b to 1e illustrate these modes.

Deterministic mode: If the noise variance of a unit is very small, the postsigmoid activity will be a practically deterministic sigmoidal function of the mean. This mode is useful for representing deterministic nonlinear mappings such as those found in deterministic multilayer perceptrons and mixture of expert models.

Stochastic linear mode: For a given mean, if the squashing function is approximately linear over the span of the added noise, the postsigmoid distribution will be approximately Gaussian with the mean and standard deviation linearly transformed. This mode is useful for representing Gaussian noise effects such as those found in mixture models, the outputs of mixture of expert models, and factor analysis models.

Stochastic nonlinear mode: If the variance of a unit in the stochastic linear mode is increased so that the squashing function is used in its nonlinear region, a variety of distributions are producible that range from skewed Gaussian to uniform to bimodal.

Stochastic binary mode: This is an extreme case of the stochastic nonlinear mode. If the variance of a unit is very large, then nearly all of the probability mass will lie near the ends of the interval $(0, 1)$ (see figure 1e). Using the cumulative Gaussian squashing function and a standard deviation of 150, less than 1% of the mass lies in $(0.1, 0.9)$. In this mode, the postsigmoid activity of unit i appears to be binary with probability of being "on" (ie., $y_i > 0.5$ or, equivalently, $x_i > 0$):

$$p(i \text{ on}|\mu_i, \sigma_i^2) = \int_0^\infty \frac{\exp[-(x-\mu_i)^2/2\sigma_i^2]}{\sqrt{2\pi\sigma_i^2}} dx = \int_{-\infty}^{\mu_i} \frac{\exp[-x^2/2\sigma_i^2]}{\sqrt{2\pi\sigma_i^2}} dx = \Phi\left(\frac{\mu_i}{\sigma_i}\right). \tag{5}$$

This sort of stochastic activation is found in binary sigmoidal belief networks (Jaakkola *et al.* 1996) and in the decision-making components of mixture of expert models and hierarchical mixture of expert models.

3 Continuous sigmoidal belief networks

If the mean of each unit depends on the activities of other units and there are feedback connections, it is difficult to relate the density in equation 3 to a joint distribution over all unit activities, and simulating the model would require a great deal of computational effort. However, when a top-down topology is imposed on the network (making it a directed acyclic graph), the densities given in equations 1 and 3 can be interpreted as conditional distributions and the joint distribution over all units can be expressed as

$$p(\{x_i\}) = \prod_{i=1}^{N} p(x_i|\{x_j\}_{j<i}) \quad \text{or} \quad p(\{y_i\}) = \prod_{i=1}^{N} p(y_i|\{y_j\}_{j<i}), \tag{6}$$

where N is the number of units. $p(x_i|\{x_j\}_{j<i})$ and $p(y_i|\{y_j\}_{j<i})$ are the presigmoid and postsigmoid densities of unit i conditioned on the activities of units with lower

indices. This ordered arrangement is the foundation of belief networks (Pearl, 1988). I let the mean of each unit be determined by a linear combination of the postsigmoid activities of preceding units:

$$\mu_i = \sum_{j<i} w_{ij} y_j, \qquad (7)$$

where $y_0 \equiv 1$ is used to implement biases. The variance for each unit is independent of unit activities. A single sample from the joint distribution can be obtained by using the bias as the mean for unit 1, randomly picking a noise value for unit 1, applying the squashing function, computing the mean for unit 2, picking a noise value for unit 2, and so on in a simple top-down pass.

Inference by slice sampling

Given the activities of a set of visible (observed) units, V, inferring the distribution over the remaining set of hidden (unobserved) units, H, is in general a difficult task. The brute force procedure proceeds by obtaining the posterior density using Bayes theorem:

$$p(\{y_i\}_{i\in H}|\{y_i\}_{i\in V}) = p(\{y_i\}_{i\in H},\{y_i\}_{i\in V})/\int_{\{y_i\}_{i\in H}} p(\{y_i\}_{i\in H},\{y_i\}_{i\in V}) \prod_{i\in H} dy_i. \qquad (8)$$

However, computing the integral in the denominator exactly is computationally intractable for any more than a few hidden units. The combinatorial explosion encountered in the corresponding sum for discrete-valued belief networks pales in comparison to this integral; not only is it combinatorial, but it is a continuous integral with a multimodal integrand whose peaks may be broad in some dimensions but narrow in others, depending on what modes the units are in.

An alternative to explicit integration is to sample from the posterior distribution using Markov chain Monte Carlo. Given a set of observed activities, this procedure produces a state sequence, $\{y_i\}_{i\in H}^{(0)}, \{y_i\}_{i\in H}^{(1)}, ..., \{y_i\}_{i\in H}^{(t)}, ...$, that is guaranteed to converge to the posterior distribution. Each successive state is randomly selected based on knowledge of only the previous state. To simplify these random choices, I consider changing only one unit at a time when making a state transition. Ideally, the new activity of unit i would be drawn from the conditional distribution $p(y_i|\{y_j\}_{j\neq i})$ (Gibbs sampling). However, it is difficult to sample from this distribution because it may have many peaks that range from broad to narrow.

I use a new Markov chain Monte Carlo method called "slice sampling" (Neal 1997) to pick a new activity for each unit. Consider the problem of drawing a value y from a univariate distribution $P(y)$ — in this application, $P(y)$ is the conditional distribution $p(y_i|\{y_j\}_{j\neq i})$. Slice sampling does not directly produce values distributed according to $P(y)$, but instead produces a sequence of values that is guaranteed to converge to $P(y)$. At each step in the sequence, the old value y_{old} is used as a guide for where to pick the new value y_{new}.

To perform slice sampling, all that is needed is an efficient way to evaluate a function $f(y)$ that is *proportional* to $P(y)$ — in this application, the easily computed value $p(y_i, \{y_j\}_{j\neq i})$ suffices, since $p(y_i, \{y_j\}_{j\neq i}) \propto p(y_i|\{y_j\}_{j\neq i})$. Figure 2a shows an example of a univariate distribution, $P(y)$. The version of slice sampling that I use requires that all of the density lies within a bounded *interval* as shown. To obtain y_{new} from y_{old}, $f(y_{\text{old}})$ is first computed and then a uniform random value is drawn from $[0, f(y_{\text{old}})]$. The distribution is then horizontally "sliced" at this value, as shown in figure 2a. Any y for which $f(y)$ is greater than this value is considered to be part of the slice, as indicated by the bold line segments in the picture shown at the top of figure 2b. Ideally, y_{new} would now be drawn uniformly from the slice. However, determining the line segments that comprise the slice is not easy, for although it is easy to determine whether a particular y is in the slice,

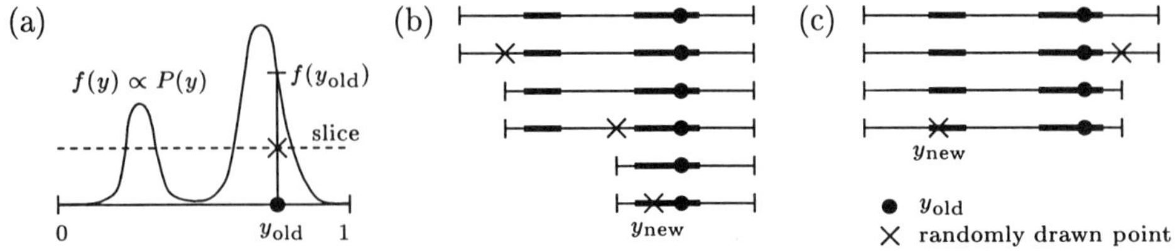

Figure 2: After obtaining a random slice from the density (a), random values are drawn until one is accepted. (b) and (c) show two such sequences.

it is much more difficult to determine the line segment boundaries, especially if the distribution is multimodal. Instead, a uniform value is drawn from the original interval as shown in the second picture of figure 2b. If this value is in the slice it is accepted as y_{new} (note that this decision requires an evaluation of $f(y)$). Otherwise either the left or the right interval boundary is moved to this new value, while keeping y_{old} in the interval. This procedure is repeated until a value is accepted. For the sequence in figure 2b, the new value is in the same mode as the old one, whereas for the sequence in figure 2c, the new value is in the other mode. Once y_{new} is obtained, it is used as y_{old} for the next step.

If the top-down influence causes there to be two very narrow peaks in $p(y_i|\{y_j\}_{j\neq i})$ (corresponding to a unit in the stochastic binary mode) the slices will almost always consist of two very short line segments and it will be very difficult for the above procedure to switch from one mode to another. To fix this problem, slice sampling is performed in a new domain, $z_i = \Phi(\{x_i - \mu_i\}/\sigma_i)$. In this domain the top-down distribution $p(z_i|\{y_j\}_{j<i})$ is uniform on $(0,1)$, so $p(z_i|\{y_j\}_{j\neq i}) = p(z_i|\{y_j\}_{j>i})$ and I use the following function for slice sampling:

$$f(z_i) = \exp\left[-\sum_{k=i+1}^{N}\{x_k - \mu_k^{-i} - w_{ki}\Phi(\sigma_i\Phi^{-1}(z_i) + \mu_i)\}^2/2\sigma_k^2\right], \quad (9)$$

where $\mu_k^{-i} = \sum_{j<k, j\neq i} w_{kj}y_j$. Since x_i, y_i and z_i are all deterministically related, sampling from the distribution of z_i will give appropriately distributed values for the other two. Many slice sampling steps could be performed to obtain a reliable sample from the conditional distribution for unit i, before moving on to the next unit. Instead, only one slice sampling step is performed for unit i before moving on. The latter procedure often converges to the correct distribution more quickly than the former. The Markov chain Monte Carlo procedure I use in the simulations below thus consists of sweeping a prespecified number of times through the set of hidden units, while updating each unit using slice sampling.

Learning

Given training examples indexed by τ, I use on-line stochastic gradient ascent to perform maximum likelihood learning — ie., maximize $\prod_\tau p(\{x_i^\tau\}_{i\in V})$. This consists of sweeping through the training set and for each case τ following the gradient of $\ln p(\{x_i\})$, while sampling hidden unit values from $p(\{x_i\}_{i\in H}|\{x_i^\tau\}_{i\in V})$ using the sampling algorithm described above. From equations 1, 6 and 7,

$$\Delta w_{jk} \equiv \eta\, \partial \ln p(\{x_i\})/\partial w_{jk} = \eta(x_j - \textstyle\sum_{l<j} w_{jl}y_l)y_k/\sigma_j^2, \quad (10)$$

$$\Delta \ln \sigma_j^2 \equiv \eta\, \partial \ln p(\{x_i\})/\partial \ln \sigma_j^2 = \eta[(x_j - \textstyle\sum_{l<j} w_{jl}y_l)^2/\sigma_j^2 - 1]/2, \quad (11)$$

where η is the learning rate.

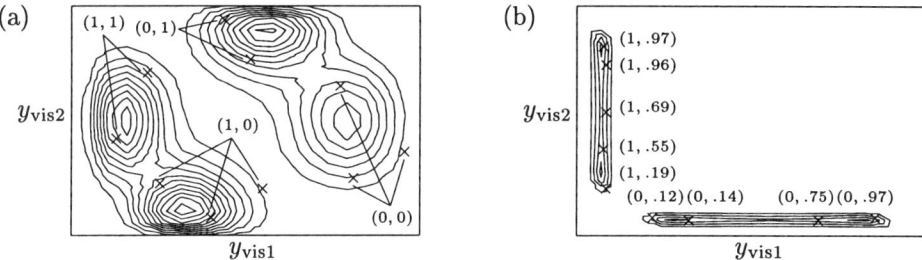

Figure 3: For each experiment (a) and (b), contours show the distribution of the 2-dimensional training cases. The inferred postsigmoid activities of the two hidden units after learning are shown in braces for several training cases, marked by ×.

4 Experiments

I designed two experiments meant to elicit the four modes of operation described in section 2. Both experiments were based on a simple network with one hidden layer containing two units and one visible layer containing two units. Training data was obtained by carefully selecting model parameters so as to induce various modes of operation and then generating 10,000 two-dimensional examples. Before training, the weights and biases were initialized to uniformly random values between -0.1 and 0.1; log-variances were initialized to 10.0. Training consisted of 100 epochs using a learning rate of 0.001 and 20 sweeps of slice sampling to complete each training case. Each task required roughly five minutes on a 200 MHz MIPS R4400 processor.

The distribution of the training cases in visible unit space ($y_{\text{vis1}} - y_{\text{vis2}}$) for the first experiment is shown by the contours in figure 3a. After training the network, I ran the inference algorithm for each of ten representative training cases. The postsigmoid activities of the two hidden units are shown beside the cases in figure 3a; clearly, the network has identified four classes that it labels $(0,0)...(1,1)$. Based on a 30x30 histogram, the Kullback-Leibler divergence between the training set and data generated from the trained network is 0.02 bits. Figure 3b shows a similar picture for the second experiment, using different training data. In this case, the network has identified two categories that it labels using the first postsigmoid activity. The second postsigmoid activity indicates how far along the respective "ridge" the data point lies. The Kullback-Leibler divergence in this case is 0.04 bits.

5 Discussion

The proposed continuous-valued nonlinear random unit is meant to be a useful atomic element for continuous belief networks in much the same way as the sigmoidal deterministic unit is a useful atomic element for multi-layer perceptrons. Four operational modes available to each unit allows small networks of these units to exhibit complex stochastic behaviors. The new "slice sampling" method that I employ for inference and learning in these networks uses easily computed local information.

The above experiments illustrate how the same network can be used to model two quite different types of data. In contrast, a Gaussian mixture model would require many more components for the second task as compared to the first. Although the methods due to Tibshirani and Bishop *et al.* would nicely model each submanifold in the second task, they would not properly distinguish between categories of data in either task. MacKay's method may be capable of extracting both the submanifolds and the categories, but I am not aware of any results on such a dual problem.

It is not difficult to conceive of models for which naive Markov chain Monte Carlo procedures will become fruitlessly slow. In particular, if two units have very highly correlated activities, the procedure of changing one activity at a time will converge extremely slowly. Also, the Markov chain method may be prohibitive for larger networks. One approach to avoiding these problems is to use the Helmholtz machine (Hinton *et al.* 1995) or mean field methods (Jaakkola *et al.* 1996).

Other variations on the theme presented in this paper include the use of other types of distributions for the hidden units (*e.g.*, Poisson variables may be more biologically plausible) and different ways of parameterizing the modes of behavior.

Acknowledgements

I thank Radford Neal and Geoffrey Hinton for several essential suggestions and I also thank Peter Dayan and Tommi Jaakkola for helpful discussions. This research was supported by grants from ITRC, IRIS, and NSERC.

References

Bishop, C. M, Svensen, M., and Williams, C.K.I. 1996. EM optimization of latent-variable density models. In D. Touretzky, M. Mozer, and M. Hasselmo (editors), *Advances in Neural Information Processing Systems 8*, MIT Press, Cambridge, MA.

Dayan, P., Hinton, G. E., Neal, R. M., and Zemel, R. S. 1995. The Helmholtz machine. *Neural Computation* **7**, 889-904.

Heckerman, D., and Geiger, D. 1994. Learning Bayesian networks: a unification for discrete and Gaussian domains. In P. Besnard and S. Hanks (editors), *Proceedings of the Eleventh Conference on Uncertainty in Artificial Intelligence*, Morgan Kaufmann, San Francisco, CA, 274-284.

Hinton, G. E., Dayan, P., Frey, B. J., and Neal, R. M. 1995. The wake-sleep algorithm for unsupervised neural networks. *Science* **268**, 1158-1161.

Hinton, G. E., and Sejnowski, T. J. 1986. Learning and relearning in Boltzmann machines. In D. E. Rumelhart and J. L. McClelland (editors), *Parallel Distributed Processing: Explorations in the Microstructure of Cognition. Volume 1: Foundations*. MIT Press, Cambridge, MA.

Hofmann, R., and Tresp, V. 1996. Discovering structure in continuous variables using Bayesian networks. In D. Touretzky, M. Mozer, and M. Hasselmo (editors), *Advances in Neural Information Processing Systems 8*, MIT Press, Cambridge, MA.

Jaakkola, T., Saul, L. K., and Jordan, M. I. 1996. Fast learning by bounding likelihoods in sigmoid type belief networks. In D. Touretzky, M. Mozer and M. Hasselmo (editors), *Advances in Neural Information Processing Systems 8*, MIT Press, Cambridge, MA.

Lauritzen, S. L., Dawid, A. P., Larsen, B. N., and Leimer, H. G. 1990. Independence properties of directed Markov Fields. *Networks* **20**, 491-505.

MacKay, D. J. C. 1995. Bayesian neural networks and density networks. *Nuclear Instruments and Methods in Physics Research, A* **354**, 73-80.

Movellan, J. R., and McClelland, J. L. 1992. Learning continuous probability distributions with symmetric diffusion networks. *Cognitive Science* **17**, 463-496.

Neal, R. M. 1992. Connectionist learning of belief networks. *Artificial Intelligence* **56**, 71-113.

Neal, R. M. 1997. Markov chain Monte Carlo methods based on "slicing" the density function. In preparation.

Pearl, J. 1988. *Probabilistic Reasoning in Intelligent Systems: Networks of Plausible Inference*. Morgan Kaufmann, San Mateo, CA.

Tibshirani, R. (1992). Principal curves revisited. *Statistics and Computing* **2**, 183-190.

Adaptively Growing Hierarchical Mixtures of Experts

Jürgen Fritsch, Michael Finke, Alex Waibel
{fritsch+,finkem,waibel}@cs.cmu.edu
Interactive Systems Laboratories
Carnegie Mellon University
Pittsburgh, PA 15213

Abstract

We propose a novel approach to automatically growing and pruning Hierarchical Mixtures of Experts. The constructive algorithm proposed here enables large hierarchies consisting of several hundred experts to be trained effectively. We show that HME's trained by our automatic growing procedure yield better generalization performance than traditional static and balanced hierarchies. Evaluation of the algorithm is performed (1) on vowel classification and (2) within a hybrid version of the JANUS [9] speech recognition system using a subset of the Switchboard large-vocabulary speaker-independent continuous speech recognition database.

INTRODUCTION

The Hierarchical Mixtures of Experts (HME) architecture [2,3,4] has proven useful for classification and regression tasks in small to medium sized applications with convergence times several orders of magnitude lower than comparable neural networks such as the multi-layer perceptron. The HME is best understood as a probabilistic decision tree, making use of soft splits of the input feature space at the internal nodes, to divide a given task into smaller, overlapping tasks that are solved by expert networks at the terminals of the tree. Training of the hierarchy is based on a generative model using the Expectation Maximisation (EM) [1,3] algorithm as a powerful and efficient tool for estimating the network parameters.

In [3], the architecture of the HME is considered pre-determined and remains fixed during training. This requires choice of structural parameters such as tree depth and branching factor in advance. As with other classification and regression techniques, it may be advantageous to have some sort of data-driven model-selection mechanism to (1) overcome false initialisations (2) speed-up training time and (3) adapt model size to task complexity for optimal generalization performance. In [11], a constructive algorithm for the HME is presented and evaluated on two small classification tasks: the two spirals and the 8-bit parity problems. However, this algorithm requires the evaluation of the increase in the overall log-likelihood for all potential splits (all terminal nodes) in an existing tree for each generation. This method is computationally too expensive when applied to the large HME's necessary in tasks with several million training vectors, as in speech recognition, where we can not afford to train all potential splits to eventually determine the single best split and discard all others. We have developed an alternative approach to growing HME trees which allows the fast training of even large HME's, when combined with a path pruning technique. Our algorithm monitors the performance of the hierarchy in terms of scaled log-likelihoods, assigning penalties to the expert networks, to determine the expert that performs worst in its local partition. This expert will then be expanded into a new subtree consisting of a new gating network and several new expert networks.

HIERARCHICAL MIXTURES OF EXPERTS

We restrict the presentation of the HME to the case of classification, although it was originally introduced in the context of regression. The architecture is a tree with gating networks at the non-terminal nodes and expert networks at the leaves. The gating networks receive the input vectors and divide the input space into a nested set of regions, that correspond to the leaves of the tree. The expert networks also receive the input vectors and produce estimates of the a-posteriori class probabilities which are then blended by the gating network outputs. All networks in the tree are linear, with a softmax non-linearity as their activation function. Such networks are known in statistics as multinomial logit models, a special case of Generalized Linear Models (GLIM) [5] in which the probabilistic component is the multinomial density. This allows for a probabilistic interpretation of the hierarchy in terms of a generative likelihood-based model. For each input vector $\mathbf{x}$, the outputs of the gating networks are interpreted as the input-dependent multinomial probabilities for the decisions about which child nodes are responsible for the generation of the actual target vector $\mathbf{y}$. After a sequence of these decisions, a particular expert network is chosen as the current classifier and computes multinomial probabilities for the output classes. The overall output of the hierarchy is

$$P(\mathbf{y}|\mathbf{x}, \Theta) = \sum_{i=1}^{N} g_i(\mathbf{x}, \mathbf{v}_i) \sum_{j=1}^{N} g_{j|i}(\mathbf{x}, \mathbf{v}_{ij}) P(\mathbf{y}|\mathbf{x}, \theta_{ij})$$

where the g_i and $g_{j|i}$ are the outputs of the gating networks.

The HME is trained using the EM algorithm [1] (see [3] for the application of EM to the HME architecture). The E-step requires the computation of posterior node probabilities as expected values for the unknown decision indicators:

$$h_i = \frac{g_i \sum_j g_{j|i} P_{ij}(\mathbf{y})}{\sum_i g_i \sum_j g_{j|i} P_{ij}(\mathbf{y})} \qquad h_{j|i} = \frac{g_{j|i} P_{ij}(\mathbf{y})}{\sum_j g_{j|i} P_{ij}(\mathbf{y})}$$

The M-step then leads to the following independent maximum-likelihood equations

$$\theta_{ij} = \arg\max_{\theta_{ij}} \sum_t h_{ij}^{(t)} \log P_{ij}(\mathbf{y}^{(t)})$$

$$\mathbf{v}_i = \arg\max_{\mathbf{V}_i} \sum_t \sum_k h_k^{(t)} \log g_k^{(t)}$$

$$\mathbf{v}_{ij} = \arg\max_{\mathbf{V}_{ij}} \sum_t \sum_k h_k^{(t)} \sum_l h_{l|k}^{(t)} \log g_{l|k}^{(t)}$$

where the θ_{ij} are the parameters of the expert networks and the v_i and v_{ij} are the parameters of the gating networks. In the case of a multinomial logit model, $P_{ij}(\mathbf{y}) = y_c$, where y_c is the output of the node associated with the correct class. The above maximum likelihood equations might be solved by gradient ascent, weighted least squares or Newton methods. In our implementation, we use a variant of Jordan & Jacobs' [3] least squares approach.

GROWING MIXTURES

In order to grow an HME, we have to define an evaluation criterion to score the experts performance on the training data. This in turn will allow us to select and split the worst expert into a new subtree, providing additional parameters which can help to overcome the errors made by this expert. Viewing the HME as a probabilistic model of the observed data, we partition the input dependent likelihood using expert selection probabilities provided by the gating networks

$$l(\Theta; \mathcal{X}) = \sum_t \log P(\mathbf{y}^{(t)}|\mathbf{x}^{(t)}, \Theta) = \sum_t \sum_k g_k \log P(\mathbf{y}^{(t)}|\mathbf{x}^{(t)}, \Theta)$$
$$= \sum_k \sum_t \log[P(\mathbf{y}^{(t)}|\mathbf{x}^{(t)}, \Theta)]^{g_k} = \sum_k l_k(\Theta; \mathcal{X})$$

where the g_k are the products of the gating probabilities along the path from the root node to the k-th expert. g_k is the probability that expert k is responsible for generating the observed data (note, that the g_k sum up to one). The expert-dependent scaled likelihoods $l_k(\Theta; \mathcal{X})$ can be used as a measure for the performance of an expert within its region of responsibility. We use this measure as the basis of our tree growing algorithm:

1. Initialize and train a simple HME consisting of only one gate and several experts.

2. Compute the expert-dependent scaled likelihoods $l_k(\Theta; \mathcal{X})$ for each expert in one additional pass through the training data.

3. Find the expert k with minimum l_k and expand the tree, replacing the expert by a new gate with random weights and new experts that copy the weights from the old expert with additional small random perturbations.

4. Train the architecture to a local minimum of the classification error using a cross-validation set.

5. Continue with step (2) until desired tree size is reached.

The number of tree growing phases may either be pre-determined, or based on difference in the likelihoods before and after splitting a node. In contrast to the growing algorithm in [11], our algorithm does not hypothesize all possible node splits, but determines the expansion node(s) directly, which is much faster, especially when dealing with large hierarchies. Furthermore, we implemented a path pruning technique similar to the one proposed in [11], which speeds up training and testing times significantly. During the recursive depth-first traversal of the tree (needed for forward evaluation, posterior probability computation and accumulation of node statistics) a path is pruned temporarily if the current node's probability of activation falls below a certain threshold. Additionally, we also prune subtrees permanently, if the sum of a node's activation probabilities over the whole training set falls below a certain threshold. This technique is consistent with the growing algorithm and also helps preventing instabilities and singularities in the parameter updates, since nodes that accumulate too little training information will not be considered for a parameter update because such nodes are automatically pruned by the algorithm.

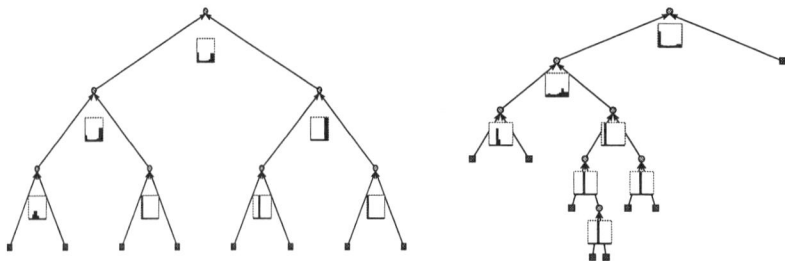

Figure 1: Histogram trees for a standard and a grown HME

VOWEL CLASSIFICATION

In initial experiments, we investigated the usefulness of the proposed tree growing algorithm on Peterson and Barney's [6] vowel classification data that uses formant frequencies as features. We chose this data set since it is small, non-artificial and low-dimensional, which allows for visualization and understanding of the way the growing HME tree performs classification tasks.

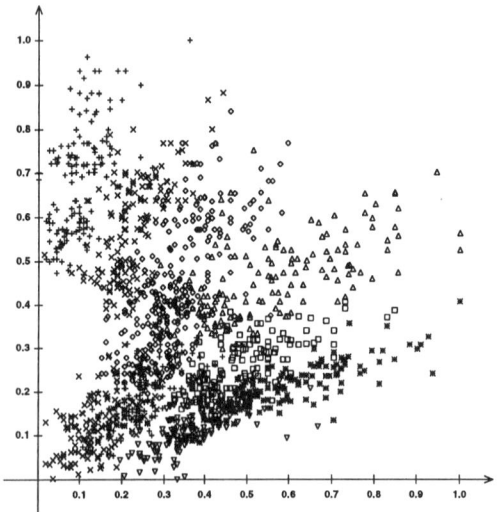

The vowel data set contains 1520 samples consisting of the formants F0, F1, F2 and F3 and a class label, indicating one of 10 different vowels. Experiments were carried out on the 4-dimensional feature space, however, in this paper graphical representations are restricted to the F1-F2 plane. The figure to the left shows the data set represented in this plane (The formant frequencies are normalized to the range [0,1]).

In the following experiments, we use binary branching HME's exclusively, but in general the growing algorithm poses no restrictions on the tree branching factor. We compare a standard, balanced HME of depth 3 with an HME that grows from a two expert tree to a tree with the same number of experts (eight) as the standard HME. The size of the standard HME was chosen based on a number of experiments with different sized HME's to find an optimal one. Fig. 1 shows the topology of the standard and the fully grown HME together with histograms of the gating probability distributions at the internal nodes.

Fig. 2 shows results on 4-dimensional feature vectors in terms of correct classification rate and log-likelihood. The growing HME achieved a slightly better (1.6% absolute) classification rate than the fixed HME. Note also, that the growing HME outperforms the fixed HME even before it reaches its full size. The growing HME was expanded every 4 iterations, which explains the bumpiness of the curves.

Fig. 3 shows the impact of path pruning during training on the final classification rate of the grown HME's. The pruning factor ranges from no pruning to full pruning (e.g. only the most likely path survives).

Fig. 4 shows how the gating networks partition the feature space. It contains plots

Adaptively Growing Hierarchical Mixtures of Experts 463

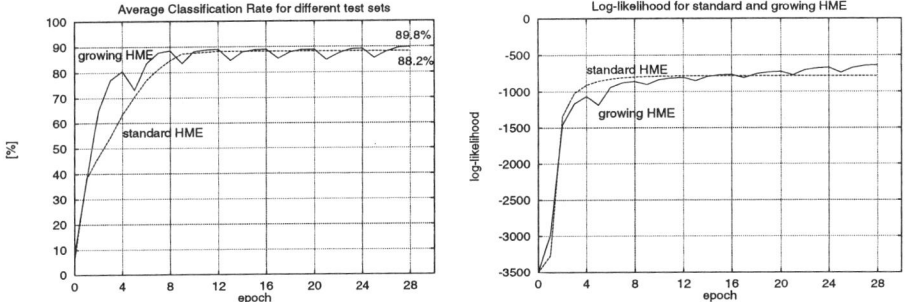

Figure 2: Classification rate and log-likelihood for standard and growing HME

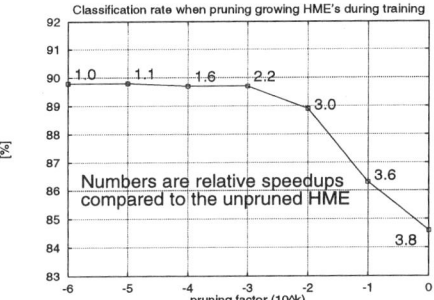

Figure 3: Impact of path pruning during training of growing HME's

of the activation regions of all 8 experts of the standard HME in the 2-dimensional range $[-0.1, 1.1]^2$. Activation probabilities (product of gating probabilities from root to expert) are colored in shades of gray from black to white. Fig. 5 shows the same kind of plot for all 8 experts of the grown HME. The plots in the upper right corner illustrate the class boundaries obtained by each HME.

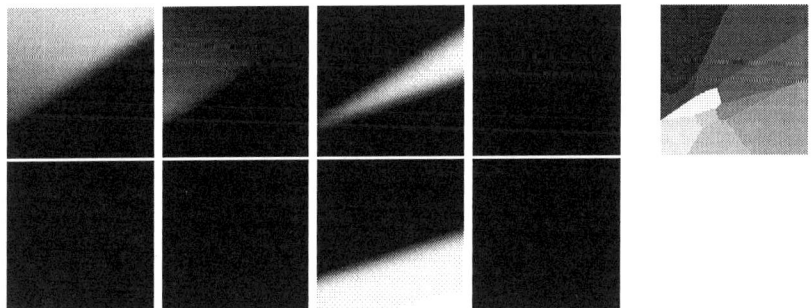

Figure 4: Expert activations for standard HME

Fig. 4 reveals a weakness of standard HME's: Gating networks at high levels in the tree can pinch off whole branches, rendering all the experts in the subtree useless. In our case, half of the experts of the standard HME do not contribute to the final decision at all (black boxes). The growing HME's are able to overcome this effect. All the experts of the grown HME (Fig. 5) have non-zero activation patterns and the overlap between experts is much higher in the growing case, which indicates a higher degree of cooperation among experts. This can also be seen in the histogram trees in Fig. 3, where gating networks in lower levels of the grown tree tend to

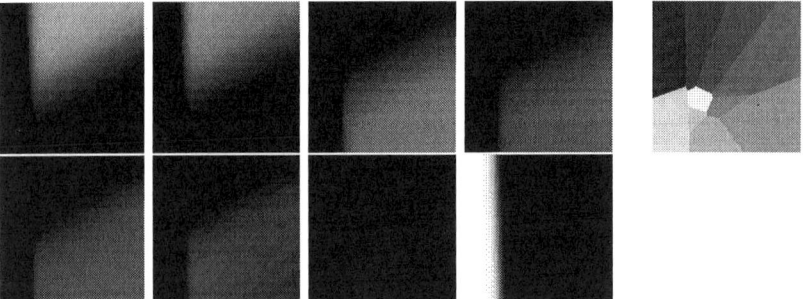

Figure 5: Expert activations for grown HME

average the experts outputs. The splits formed by the gating networks also have implications on the way class boundaries are formed by the HME. There are strong dependencies visible between the class boundaries and some of the experts activation regions.

EXPERIMENTS ON SWITCHBOARD

We recently started experiments using standard and growing HME's as estimators of posterior phone probabilities in a hybrid version of the JANUS [9] speech recognizer. Following the work in [12], we use different HME's for each state of a phonetic HMM. The posteriors for 52 phonemes computed by the HME's are converted into scaled likelihoods by dividing by prior probabilities to account for the likelihood based training and decoding of HMM's. During training, targets for the HME's are generated by forced-alignment using a baseline mixture of Gaussian HMM system. We evaluate the system on the Switchboard spontaneous telephone speech corpus. Our best current mixture of Gaussians based context-dependent HMM system achieves a word accuracy of 61.4% on this task, which is among the best current systems [7]. We started by using phonetic context-independent (CI) HME's for 3-state HMM's. We restricted the training set to all dialogues involving speakers from one dialect region (New York City), since the whole training set contains over 140 hours of speech. Our aim here was, to reduce training time (the subset contains only about 5% of the data) to be able to compare different HME architectures.

Context	♯ HME	branching	♯ experts	Word Acc.
CI	3	4	64	33.8%
CI growing	3	4	64	35.1%
CD/CI	3x52	8/4	8/64	42.1%
CD/CI growing	3x52	2/4	8/64	45.3%

Figure 6: Preliminary results on Switchboard telephone data

To improve performance, we then build context-dependent (CD) models consisting of a separate HME for each biphone context and state. The CD HME's output is smoothed with the CI models based on prior context probabilities. Current work focuses on improving context modeling (e.g. larger contexts and decision tree based clustering).

Fig. 6 summarizes the results so far, showing consistently that growing HME's outperform equally sized standard HME's. The results are not directly comparable with our best Gaussian mixture system, since we restricted context modeling to biphones and used only a small subset of the Switchboard database for training.

CONCLUSIONS

In this paper, we presented a method for adaptively growing Hierarchical Mixtures of Experts. We showed, that the algorithm allows the HME to use the resources (experts) more efficiently than a standard pre-determined HME architecture. The tree growing algorithm leads to better classification performance compared to standard HME's with equal numbers of parameters. Using growing instead of fixed HME's as continuous density estimators in a hybrid speech recognition system also improves performance.

References

[1] Dempster, A.P., Laird, N.M. & Rubin, D.B. (1977) Maximum likelihood from incomplete data via the EM algorithm. *J.R. Statist. Soc. B 39*, 1-38.

[2] Jacobs, R. A., Jordan, M. I., Nowlan, S. J., & Hinton, G. E. (1991) Adaptive mixtures of local experts. In *Neural Computation 3*, pp. 79-87, MIT press.

[3] Jordan, M.I. & Jacobs R.A. (1994) Hierarchical Mixtures of Experts and the EM Algorithm. In *Neural Computation 6*, pp. 181-214. MIT press.

[4] Jordan, M.I. & Jacobs, R.A. (1992) Hierarchies of adaptive experts. In *Advances in Neural Information Processing Systems 4*, J. Moody, S. Hanson, and R. Lippmann, eds., pp. 985-993. Morgan Kaufmann, San Mateo, CA.

[5] McCullagh, P. & Nelder, J.A. (1983) *Generalized Linear Models.* Chapman and Hall, London.

[6] Peterson, G. E. & Barney, H. L. (1952) Control measurements used in a study of the vowels. *Journal of the Acoustical Society of America 24*, 175-184.

[7] Proceedings of LVCSR Hub 5 workshop, Apr. 29 - May 1 (1996) MITAGS, Linthicum Heights, Maryland.

[8] Syrdal, A. K. & Gopal, H. S. (1986) A perceptual model of vowel recognition based on the auditory representation of American English vowels. *Journal of the Acoustical Society of America, 79* (4):1086-1100.

[9] Zeppenfeld T., Finke M., Ries K., Westphal M. & Waibel A. (1997) Recognition of Conversational Telephone Speech using the Janus Speech Engine. *Proceedings of ICASSP 97, Muenchen, Germany*

[10] Waterhouse, S.R., Robinson, A.J. (1994) Classification using Hierarchical Mixtures of Experts. In *Proc. 1994 IEEE Workshop on Neural Networks for Signal Processing IV*, pp. 177-186.

[11] Waterhouse, S.R., Robinson, A.J. (1995) Constructive Algorithms for Hierarchical Mixtures of Experts. In *Advances in Neural Information Processing Systems 8.*

[12] Zhao, Y., Schwartz, R., Sroka, J. & Makhoul, J. (1995) Hierarchical Mixtures of Experts Methodology Applied to Continuous Speech Recognition. In *ICASSP 1995*, volume 5, pp. 3443-6, May 1995.

Balancing between bagging and bumping

Tom Heskes
RWCP Novel Functions SNN Laboratory,[*] University of Nijmegen
Geert Grooteplein 21, 6525 EZ Nijmegen, The Netherlands
tom@mbfys.kun.nl

Abstract

We compare different methods to combine predictions from neural networks trained on different bootstrap samples of a regression problem. One of these methods, introduced in [6] and which we here call balancing, is based on the analysis of the ensemble generalization error into an ambiguity term and a term incorporating generalization performances of individual networks. We show how to estimate these individual errors from the residuals on validation patterns. Weighting factors for the different networks follow from a quadratic programming problem. On a real-world problem concerning the prediction of sales figures and on the well-known Boston housing data set, balancing clearly outperforms other recently proposed alternatives as bagging [1] and bumping [8].

1 EARLY STOPPING AND BOOTSTRAPPING

Stopped training is a popular strategy to prevent overfitting in neural networks. The complete data set is split up into a training and a validation set. Through learning the weights are adapted in order to minimize the error on the training data. Training is stopped when the error on the validation data starts increasing. The final network depends on the accidental subdivision in training and validation set, and often also on the, usually random, initial weight configuration and chosen minimization procedure. In other words, early stopped neural networks are highly unstable: small changes in the data or different initial conditions can produce large changes in the estimate. As argued in [1, 8], with unstable estimators it is advisable to resample, i.e., to apply the same procedure several times using different subdivisions in training and validation set and perhaps starting from different initial

---

[*]RWCP: Real World Computing Partnership; SNN: Foundation for Neural Networks.

configurations. In the neural network literature resampling is often referred to as training ensembles of neural networks [3, 6]. In this paper, we will discuss methods for combining the outputs of networks obtained through such a repetitive procedure.

First, however, we have to choose how to generate the subdivisions in training and validation sets. Options are, among others, k-fold cross-validation, subsampling and bootstrapping. In this paper we will consider bootstrapping [2] which is based on the idea that the available data set is nothing but a particular realization of some probability distribution. In principle, one would like to do inference on this "true" yet unknown probability distribution. A natural thing to do is then to define an empirical distribution. With so-called naive bootstrapping the empirical distribution is a sum of delta peaks on the available data points, each with probability content $1/p_{\text{data}}$ with p_{data} the number of patterns. A bootstrap sample is a collection of p_{data} patterns drawn with replacement from this empirical probability distribution. Some of the data points will occur once, some twice and some even more than twice in this bootstrap sample. The bootstrap sample is taken to be the training set, all patterns that do not occur in a particular bootstrap sample constitute the validation set. For large p_{data}, the probability that a pattern becomes part of the validation set is $(1 - 1/p_{\text{data}})^{p_{\text{data}}} \approx 1/e \approx 0.368$. An advantage of bootstrapping over other resampling techniques is that most statistical theory on resampling is nowadays based on the bootstrap.

Using naive bootstrapping we generate n_{run} training and validation sets out of our complete data set of p_{data} input-output combinations $\{\vec{x}^\mu, t^\mu\}$. In this paper we will restrict ourselves to regression problems with, for notational convenience, just one output variable. We keep track of a matrix with components q_i^μ indicating whether pattern μ is part of the validation set for run i ($q_i^\mu = 1$) or of the training set ($q_i^\mu = 0$). On each subdivision we train and stop a neural network with one layer of n_{hidden} hidden units. The output o_i^μ of network i with weight vector $\mathbf{w}(i)$ on input $\vec{x}^\mu$ reads

$$o_i^\mu = \sum_{j=1}^{n_{\text{hidden}}} w_j(i) \tanh \left[\sum_{k=0}^{n_{\text{input}}} w_{(k+1)n_{\text{hidden}}+j}(i) x_k^\mu \right] + w_0(i),$$

where we use the definition $x_0^\mu \equiv 1$. The validation error for run i can be written

$$E_{\text{validation}}(i) \equiv \frac{1}{p_i} \sum_{\mu=1}^{p_{\text{data}}} q_i^\mu r_i^\mu,$$

with $p_i \equiv \sum_\mu q_i^\mu \approx 0.368\, p_{\text{data}}$, the number of validation patterns in run i, and $r_i^\mu \equiv (o_i^\mu - t^\mu)^2/2$, the error of network i on pattern μ.

After training we are left with n_{run} networks, with, in practice, quite different performances on the complete data set. How should we combine all these outputs to get the best possible performance on new data?

2 COMBINING ESTIMATORS

Several methods have been proposed to combine estimators (see e.g. [5] for a review). In this paper we will only consider estimators with the same architecture but trained and stopped on different subdivisions of the data in training and validation sets. Recently, two such methods have been suggested for bootstrapped estimators: bagging [1], an acronym for bootstrap aggregating, and bumping [8], meaning bootstrap umbrella of model parameters. With bagging, the prediction on a newly arriving input vector is the average over all network predictions. Bagging completely disregards the performance of the individual networks on the data used for training and stopping. Bumping, on the other hand, throws away all networks except the one with the lowest error on the complete data set[1]. In the following we will describe an intermediate form due to [6], which we here call balancing. A theoretical analysis of the implications of this idea can be found in [7].

Suppose that after training we receive a new set of p_{test} test patterns for which we do not know the true targets $\tilde{t}^\nu$, but can calculate the network output $\tilde{o}_i$ for each network i. We give each network a weighting factor α_i and define the prediction of all networks on pattern ν as the weighted average

$$\tilde{m}^\nu \equiv \sum_{i=1}^{n_{\text{run}}} \alpha_i \tilde{o}_i^\nu .$$

The goal is to find the weighting factors α_i, subject to the constraints

$$\sum_{i=1}^{n_{\text{run}}} \alpha_i = 1 \text{ and } \alpha_i \geq 0 \; \forall i , \qquad (1)$$

yielding the smallest possible generalization error

$$E_{\text{test}} \equiv \frac{1}{p_{\text{test}}} \sum_{\nu=1}^{p_{\text{test}}} (\tilde{m}^\nu - \tilde{t}^\nu)^2 .$$

The problem, of course, is our ignorance about the targets $\tilde{t}^\nu$. Bagging simply takes $\alpha_i = 1/n_{\text{run}}$ for all networks, whereas bumping implies $\alpha_i = \delta_{i\kappa}$ with

$$\kappa = \underset{i}{\text{argmin}} \frac{1}{p_{\text{data}}} \sum_{\mu=1}^{p_{\text{data}}} (o_i^\mu - t^\mu)^2 .$$

As in [6, 7] we write the generalization error in the form

$$\begin{aligned} E_{\text{test}} &= \frac{1}{p_{\text{test}}} \sum_\nu \sum_{i,j} \alpha_i \alpha_j (\tilde{o}_i^\nu - \tilde{t}^\nu)(\tilde{o}_j^\nu - \tilde{t}^\nu) \\ &= \frac{1}{2p_{\text{test}}} \sum_\nu \sum_{i,j} \alpha_i \alpha_j \left[(\tilde{o}_i^\nu - \tilde{t}^\nu)^2 + (\tilde{o}_j^\nu - \tilde{t}^\nu)^2 - (\tilde{o}_i^\nu - \tilde{o}_j^\nu)^2 \right] \\ &= \sum_{i,j} \alpha_i \alpha_j \left[E_{\text{test}}(i) + E_{\text{test}}(j) - \frac{1}{2p_{\text{test}}} \sum_\nu (\tilde{o}_i^\nu - \tilde{o}_j^\nu)^2 \right] . \end{aligned} \qquad (2)$$

The last term depends only on the network outputs and can thus be calculated. This "ambiguity" term favors networks with conflicting outputs. The first part,

---
[1] The idea behind bumping is more general and involved than discussed here. The interested reader is referred to [8]. In this paper we will only consider its naive version.

containing the generalization errors $E_{\text{test}}(i)$ for individual networks, depends on the targets $\tilde{t}^\nu$ and is thus unknown. It favors networks that by themselves already have a low generalization error. In the next section we will find reasonable estimates for these generalization errors based on the network performances on validation data. Once we have obtained these estimates, finding the optimal weighting factors α_i under the constraints (1) is a straightforward quadratic programming problem.

3 ESTIMATING THE GENERALIZATION ERROR

At first sight, a good estimate for the generalization error of network i could be the performance on the validation data not included during training. However, the validation error $E_{\text{validation}}(i)$ strongly depends on the accidental subdivision in training and validation set. For example, if there are a few outliers which, by pure coincidence, are part of the validation set, the validation error will be relatively large and the training error relatively small. To correct for this bias as a result of the random subdivision, we introduce the "expected" validation error for run i. First we define n^μ as the number of runs in which pattern μ is part of the validation set and $E^\mu_{\text{validation}}$ as the error averaged over these runs:

$$n^\mu \equiv \sum_{i=1}^{n_{\text{run}}} q_i^\mu \quad \text{and} \quad E^\mu_{\text{validation}} \equiv \frac{1}{n^\mu} \sum_{i=1}^{n_{\text{run}}} q_i^\mu r_i^\mu ,$$

The expected validation error then follows from

$$\hat{E}_{\text{validation}}(i) \equiv \frac{1}{p_i} \sum_{\mu=1}^{p_{\text{data}}} q_i^\mu E^\mu_{\text{validation}} .$$

The ratio between the observed and the expected validation error indicates whether the validation error for network i is relatively high or low. Our estimate for the generalization error of network i is this ratio multiplied by an overall scaling factor being the estimated average generalization error:

$$E_{\text{test}}(i) \approx \frac{E_{\text{validation}}(i)}{\hat{E}_{\text{validation}}(i)} \frac{1}{p_{\text{data}}} \sum_{\mu=1}^{p_{\text{data}}} E^\mu_{\text{validation}} .$$

Note that we implicitly make the assumption that the bias introduced by stopping at the minimal error on the validation patterns is negligible, i.e., that the validation patterns used for stopping a network can be considered as new to this network as the completely independent test patterns.

4 SIMULATIONS

We compare the following methods for combining neural network outputs.

Individual: the average individual generalization error, i.e., the generalization error we will get on average when we decide to perform only one run. It serves as a reference with which the other methods will be compared.

Bumping: the generalization of the network with the lowest error on the data available for training and stopping.

	bumping	bagging	ambiguity	balancing	unfair bumping	unfair balancing
store 1	4 %	9 %	10 %	17 %	17 %	24 %
store 2	5 %	15 %	22 %	23 %	23 %	34 %
store 3	-7 %	11 %	18 %	25 %	25 %	36 %
store 4	6 %	11 %	17 %	26 %	26 %	31 %
store 5	6 %	10 %	22 %	19 %	22 %	26 %
store 6	1 %	8 %	14 %	19 %	16 %	26 %
mean	3 %	11 %	17 %	22 %	22 %	30 %

Table 1: Decrease in generalization error relative to the average individual generalization error as a result of several methods for combining neural networks trained to predict the sales figures for several stores.

Bagging: the generalization error when we take the average of all n_{run} network outputs as our prediction.

Ambiguity: the generalization error when the weighting factors are chosen to maximize the ambiguity, i.e., taking identical estimates for the individual generalization errors of all networks in expression (2).

Balancing: the generalization error when the weighting factors are chosen to minimize our estimate of the generalization error.

Unfair bumping: the smallest generalization error for an individual error, i.e., the result of bumping if we had indeed chosen the network with the smallest generalization error.

Unfair balancing: the lowest possible generalization error that we could obtain if we had perfect estimates of the individual generalization errors.

The last two methods, unfair bumping and unfair balancing, only serve as some kind of reference and can never be used in practice.

We applied these methods on a real-world problem concerning the prediction of sales figures for several department stores in the Netherlands. For each store, 100 networks with 4 hidden units were trained and stopped on bootstrap samples of about 500 patterns. The test set, on which the performances of the various methods for combination were measured, consists of about 100 patterns. Inputs include weather conditions, day of the week, previous sales figures, and season. The results are summarized in Table 1, where we give the decrease in the generalization error relative to the average individual generalization error.

As can be seen in Table 1, bumping hardly improves the performance. The reason is that the error on the data used for training and stopping is a lousy predictor of the generalization error, since some amount of overfitting is inevitable. The generalization performance obtained through bagging, i.e., first averaging over all outputs, can be proven to be always better than the average individual generalization error.

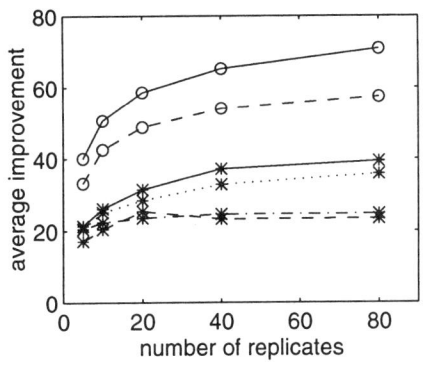 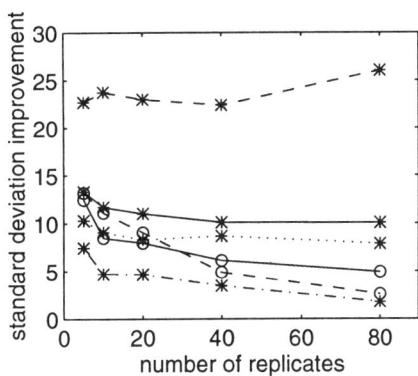

Figure 1: Decrease of generalization error relative to the average individual generalization error as a function of the number of bootstrap replicates for different combination methods: bagging (dashdot, star), ambiguity (dotted, star), bumping (dashed, star), balancing (solid, star), unfair bumping (dashed, circle), unfair balancing (solid, circle). Shown are the mean (left) and the standard deviation (right) of the decrease in percentages. Networks are trained and tested on the Boston housing database.

On these data bagging is definitely better than bumping, but also worse than maximizing the ambiguity. In all cases, except for store 5 where maximization of the ambiguity is slightly better, balancing is a clear winner among the "fair" methods. The last column in Table 1 shows how much better we can get if we could find more accurate estimates for the generalization errors of individual networks.

The method of balancing discards most of the networks, i.e., the solution to the quadratic programming problem (2) under constraints (1) yields just a few weighting factors different from zero (on average about 8 for this set of simulations). Balancing is thus indeed a compromise between bagging, taking all networks into acount, and bumping, keeping just one network.

We also compared these methods on the well-known Boston housing data set concerning the median housing price in several tracts based on 13 mainly socio-economic predictor variables (see e.g. [1] for more information). We left out 50 of the 506 available cases for assessment of the generalization performance. All other 456 cases were used for training and stopping neural networks with 4 hidden units. The average individual mean squared error over all 300 bootstrap runs is 16.2, which is comparable to the mean squared error reported in [1]. To study how the performance depends on the number of bootstrap replicates, we randomly drew sets of $n = 5, 10, 20, 40$ and 80 bootstrap replicates out of our ensemble of 300 replicates and applied the combination methods on these sets. For each n we did this 48 times. Figure 1 shows the mean decrease in the generalization error relative to the average individual generalization error and its standard deviation.

Again, balancing comes out best, especially for a larger number of bootstrap replicates. It seems that beyond say 20 replicates both bumping and bagging are hardly helped by more runs, whereas both maximization of the ambiguity and balancing still increase their performance. Bagging, fully taking into account all network predictions, yields the smallest variation, bumping, keeping just one of them, by far the largest. Balancing and maximization of the ambiguity combine several predictions and thus yield a variation that is somewhere in between.

5 CONCLUSION AND DISCUSSION

Balancing, a compromise between bagging and bumping, is an attempt to arrive at better performances on regression problems. The crux in all this is to obtain reasonable estimates for the quality of the different networks and to incorporate these estimates in the calculation of the proper weighting factors (see [5, 9] for similar ideas and related work in the context of stacked generalization).

Obtaining several estimators is computationally expensive. However, the notorious instability of feedforward neural networks hardly leaves us a choice. Furthermore, an ensemble of bootstrapped neural networks can also be used to deduce (approximate) confidence and prediction intervals (see e.g. [4]), to estimate the relevance of input fields and so on. It has also been argued that combination of several estimators destroys the structure that may be present in a single estimator [8]. Having hardly any interpretable structure, neural networks do not seem to have a lot they can lose. It is a challenge to show that an ensemble of neural networks does not only give more accurate predictions, but also reveals more information than a single network.

References

[1] L. Breiman. Bagging predictors. *Machine Learning*, 24:123–140, 1996.

[2] B. Efron and R. Tibshirani. *An Introduction to the Bootstrap*. Chapman & Hall, London, 1993.

[3] L. Hansen and P. Salomon. Neural network ensembles. *IEEE Transactions on Pattern Analysis and Machine Intelligence*, 12:993–1001, 1990.

[4] T. Heskes. Practical confidence and prediction intervals. *These proceedings*, 1997.

[5] R. Jacobs. Methods for combining experts' probability assessments. *Neural Computation*, 7:867–888, 1995.

[6] A. Krogh and J. Vedelsby. Neural network ensembles, cross validation, and active learning. In G. Tesauro, D. Touretzky, and T. Leen, editors, *Advances in Neural Information Processing Systems 7*, pages 231–238, Cambridge, 1995. MIT Press.

[7] P. Sollich and A. Krogh. Learning with ensembles: How over-fitting can be useful. In D. Touretzky, M. Mozer, and M. Hasselmo, editors, *Advances in Neural Information Processing Systems 8*, pages 190–196, San Mateo, 1996. Morgan Kaufmann.

[8] R. Tibshirani and K. Knight. Model search and inference by bootstrap "bumping". Technical report, University of Toronto, 1995.

[9] D. Wolpert and W. Macready. Combining stacking with bagging to improve a learning algorithm. Technical report, Santa Fe Institute, Santa Fe, 1996.

LSTM CAN SOLVE HARD LONG TIME LAG PROBLEMS

Sepp Hochreiter
Fakultät für Informatik
Technische Universität München
80290 München, Germany

Jürgen Schmidhuber
IDSIA
Corso Elvezia 36
6900 Lugano, Switzerland

Abstract

Standard recurrent nets cannot deal with long minimal time lags between relevant signals. Several recent NIPS papers propose alternative methods. We first show: problems used to promote various previous algorithms can be solved more quickly by random weight guessing than by the proposed algorithms. We then use LSTM, our own recent algorithm, to solve a hard problem that can neither be quickly solved by random search nor by any other recurrent net algorithm we are aware of.

1 TRIVIAL PREVIOUS LONG TIME LAG PROBLEMS

Traditional recurrent nets fail in case of long minimal time lags between input signals and corresponding error signals [7, 3]. Many recent papers propose alternative methods, e.g., [16, 12, 1, 5, 9]. For instance, Bengio et al. investigate methods such as simulated annealing, multi-grid random search, time-weighted pseudo-Newton optimization, and discrete error propagation [3]. They also propose an EM approach [1]. Quite a few papers use variants of the "2-sequence problem" (and "latch problem") to show the proposed algorithm's superiority, e.g. [3, 1, 5, 9]. Some papers also use the "parity problem", e.g., [3, 1]. Some of Tomita's [18] grammars are also often used as benchmark problems for recurrent nets [2, 19, 14, 11].

Trivial versus non-trivial tasks. By our definition, a "trivial" task is one that can be solved quickly by random search (RS) in weight space. RS works as follows: *REPEAT randomly initialize the weights and test the resulting net on a training set UNTIL solution found.*

Random search (RS) details. In all our RS experiments, we randomly initialize weights in [-100.0,100.0]. Binary inputs are -1.0 (for 0) and 1.0 (for 1). Targets are either 1.0 or 0.0. All activation functions are logistic sigmoid in [0.0,1.0]. We use two architectures (A1, A2) suitable for many widely used "benchmark" problems: A1 is a fully connected net with 1 input, 1 output, and n biased hidden units. A2 is like A1 with $n = 10$, but less densely connected: each hidden unit sees the input unit, the output unit, and itself; the output unit sees all other units; all units are biased. All activations are set to 0 at each sequence begin. We will indicate where we also use different architectures of other authors. All sequence lengths are randomly chosen between 500 and 600 (most other authors facilitate their problems by using much shorter training/test sequences). The "benchmark" problems always require to classify two types of sequences. Our training set consists of 100 sequences, 50 from class 1 (target 0) and 50 from class 2 (target 1). Correct sequence classification is defined as "absolute error at sequence end below 0.1". We stop the search once a random weight matrix correctly classifies all training sequences. Then we test on the test set (100 sequences). All results below are averages of 10 trials. **In all our simulations below, RS finally classified all test set sequences correctly; average final absolute test set errors were always below 0.001 — in most cases below 0.0001.**

"2-sequence problem" (and "latch problem") [3, 1, 9]. The task is to observe and classify input sequences. There are two classes. There is only one input unit or input line. Only the first N real-valued sequence elements convey relevant information about the class. Sequence elements at positions $t > N$ (we use $N = 1$) are generated by a Gaussian with mean zero and variance 0.2. The first sequence element is 1.0 (-1.0) for class 1 (2). Target at sequence end is 1.0 (0.0) for class 1 (2) (the latch problem is a simple version of the 2-sequence problem that allows for input tuning instead of weight tuning).

Bengio et al.'s results. For the 2-sequence problem, the best method among the six tested by Bengio et al. [3] was multigrid random search (sequence lengths 50 — 100; N and stopping criterion undefined), which solved the problem after 6,400 sequence presentations, with final classification error 0.06. In more recent work, Bengio and Frasconi reported that an EM-approach [1] solves the problem within 2,900 trials.

RS results. RS with architecture A2 (A1, $n = 1$) solves the problem within only 718 (1247) trials on average. Using an architecture with only 3 parameters (as in Bengio et al.'s architecture for the latch problem [3]), the problem was solved within only 22 trials on average, due to tiny parameter space. According to our definition above, the problem is trivial. RS outperforms Bengio et al.'s methods in every respect: (1) many fewer trials required, (2) much less computation time per trial. Also, in most cases (3) the solution quality is better (less error).

It should be mentioned, however, that different input representations and different types of noise may lead to worse RS performance (Yoshua Bengio, personal communication, 1996).

"Parity problem". The parity task [3, 1] requires to classify sequences with several 100 elements (only 1's or -1's) according to whether the number of 1's is even or odd. The target at sequence end is 1.0 for odd and 0.0 for even.

Bengio et al.'s results. For sequences with only 25-50 steps, among the six methods tested in [3] only simulated annealing was reported to achieve final classification error of 0.000 (within about 810,000 trials — the authors did not mention the precise stopping criterion). A method called "discrete error BP" took about 54,000 trials to achieve final classification error 0.05. In more recent work [1], for sequences with 250-500 steps, their EM-approach took about 3,400 trials to achieve final classification error 0.12.

RS results. RS with A1 ($n = 1$) solves the problem within only 2906 trials on average. RS with A2 solves it within 2797 trials. We also ran another experiment with architecture A2, but without self-connections for hidden units. RS solved the problem within 250 trials on average.

Again it should be mentioned that different input representations and noise types may lead to worse RS performance (Yoshua Bengio, personal communication, 1996).

Tomita grammars. Many authors also use Tomita's grammars [18] to test their algorithms. See, e.g., [2, 19, 14, 11, 10]. Since we already tested parity problems above, we now focus on a few "parity-free" Tomita grammars (nr.s #1, #2, #4). Previous work facilitated the problems by restricting sequence length. E.g., in [11], maximal test (training) sequence length is 15 (10). Reference [11] reports the number of sequences required for convergence (for various first and second order nets with 3 to 9 units): Tomita #1: 23,000 – 46,000; Tomita #2: 77,000 – 200,000; Tomita #4: 46,000 – 210,000. RS, however, clearly outperforms the methods in [11]. The average results are: Tomita #1: 182 (A1, $n = 1$) and 288 (A2), Tomita #2: 1,511 (A1, $n = 3$) and 17,953 (A2), Tomita #4: 13,833 (A1, $n = 2$) and 35,610 (A2).

Non-trivial tasks / Outline of remainder. Solutions of non-trivial tasks are sparse in weight space. They require either many free parameters (e.g., input weights) or high weight precision, such that RS becomes infeasible. To solve such tasks we need a novel method called "Long Short-Term Memory", or LSTM for short [8]. Section 2 will briefly review LSTM. Section 3 will show results on a task that cannot be solved at all by any other recurrent net learning algorithm we are aware of. The task involves distributed, high-precision, continuous-valued representations and long minimal time lags — there are no short time lag training exemplars facilitating learning.

2 LONG SHORT-TERM MEMORY

Memory cells and gate units: basic ideas. LSTM's basic unit is called a memory cell. Within each memory cell, there is a linear unit with a fixed-weight self-connection (compare Mozer's time constants [12]). This enforces constant, non-exploding, non-vanishing error flow within the memory cell. A multiplicative *input gate unit* learns to protect the constant error flow within the memory cell from perturbation by irrelevant inputs. Likewise, a multiplicative *output gate unit* learns to protect other units from perturbation by currently irrelevant memory contents stored in the memory cell. The gates learn to open and close access to constant error flow. *Why is constant error flow important?* For instance, with conventional "backprop through time" (BPTT, e.g., [20]) or RTRL (e.g., [15]), error signals "flowing backwards in time" tend to vanish: the temporal evolution of the backpropagated error exponentially depends on the size of the weights. For the first theoretical error flow analysis see [7]. See [3] for a more recent, independent, essentially identical analysis.

LSTM details. In what follows, w_{uv} denotes the weight on the connection from unit v to unit u. $net_u(t), y^u(t)$ are net input and activation of unit u (with activation function f_u) at time t. For all non-input units that aren't memory cells (e.g. output units), we have $y^u(t) = f_u(net_u(t))$, where $net_u(t) = \sum_v w_{uv} y^v(t-1)$. The j-th memory cell is denoted c_j. Each memory cell is built around a central linear unit with a fixed self-connection (weight 1.0) and identity function as activation function (see definition of s_{c_j} below). In addition to $net_{c_j}(t) = \sum_u w_{c_j u} y^u(t-1)$, c_j also gets input from a special unit out_j (the "output gate"), and from another special unit in_j (the "input gate"). in_j's activation at time t is denoted by $y^{in_j}(t)$. out_j's activation at time t is denoted by $y^{out_j}(t)$. in_j, out_j are viewed as ordinary hidden units. We have $y^{out_j}(t) = f_{out_j}(net_{out_j}(t))$, $y^{in_j}(t) = f_{in_j}(net_{in_j}(t))$, where $net_{out_j}(t) = \sum_u w_{out_j u} y^u(t-1)$, $net_{in_j}(t) = \sum_u w_{in_j u} y^u(t-1)$. The summation indices u may stand for input units, gate units, memory cells, or even conventional hidden units if there are any (see also paragraph on "network topology" below). All these different types of units may convey useful information about the current state of the net. For instance, an input gate (output gate) may use inputs from other memory cells to decide whether to store (access) certain information in its memory cell. There even may be recurrent self-connections like $w_{c_j c_j}$. It is up to the user to define the network topology. At time t, c_j's output $y^{c_j}(t)$ is computed in a sigma-pi-like fashion: $y^{c_j}(t) = y^{out_j}(t) h(s_{c_j}(t))$, where

$$s_{c_j}(0) = 0, s_{c_j}(t) = s_{c_j}(t-1) + y^{in_j}(t) g\left(net_{c_j}(t)\right) \text{ for } t > 0.$$

The differentiable function g scales net_{c_j}. The differentiable function h scales memory cell outputs computed from the internal state s_{c_j}.

Why gate units? in_j controls the error flow to memory cell c_j's input connections $w_{c_j u}$. out_j controls the error flow from unit j's output connections. Error signals trapped within a memory cell *cannot* change – but different error signals flowing into the cell (at different times) via its output gate may get superimposed. The output gate will have to learn *which* errors to trap in its memory cell, by appropriately scaling them. Likewise, the input gate will have to learn when to release errors. Gates open and close access to constant error flow.

Network topology. There is one input, one hidden, and one output layer. The fully self-connected hidden layer contains memory cells and corresponding gate units (for convenience, we refer to both memory cells and gate units as hidden units located in the hidden layer). The hidden layer may also contain "conventional" hidden units providing inputs to gate units and memory cells. All units (except for gate units) in all layers have directed connections (serve as inputs) to all units in higher layers.

Memory cell blocks. S memory cells sharing one input gate and one output gate form a "memory cell block of size S". They can facilitate information storage.

Learning with excellent computational complexity — see details in appendix of [8]. We use a variant of RTRL which properly takes into account the altered (sigma-pi-like) dynamics caused by input and output gates. However, to ensure constant error backprop, like with truncated BPTT [20], errors arriving at "memory cell net inputs" (for cell c_j, this includes net_{c_j}, net_{in_j}, net_{out_j}) do not get propagated back further in time (although they *do* serve to change the incoming weights). Only within memory cells, errors are propagated back through previous internal states s_{c_j}. This enforces constant error flow within memory cells. Thus only the derivatives $\frac{\partial s_{c_j}}{\partial w_{il}}$ need to be stored and updated. Hence, **the algorithm is very efficient**, and LSTM's update complexity per time step is excellent in comparison to other approaches such as RTRL: given n units and a fixed number of output units, LSTM's update complexity per time step is at most $O(n^2)$, just like BPTT's.

3 EXPERIMENT: ADDING PROBLEM

Our previous experimental comparisons (on widely used benchmark problems) with RTRL (e.g., [15]; results compared to the ones in [17]), Recurrent Cascade-Correlation [6], Elman nets (results compared to the ones in [4]), and Neural Sequence Chunking [16], demonstrated that LSTM leads to many more successful runs than its competitors, and learns much faster [8]. The following task, though, is more difficult than the above benchmark problems: it cannot be solved at all in reasonable time by RS (we tried various architectures) nor any other recurrent net learning algorithm we are aware of (see [13] for an overview). The experiment will show that LSTM can solve non-trivial, complex long time lag problems involving distributed, high-precision, continuous-valued representations.

Task. Each element of each input sequence is a pair consisting of two components. The first component is a real value randomly chosen from the interval $[-1, 1]$. The second component is either 1.0, 0.0, or -1.0, and is used as a marker: at the end of each sequence, the task is to output the sum of the first components of those pairs that are *marked* by second components equal to 1.0. The value T is used to determine average sequence length, which is a randomly chosen integer between T and $T + \frac{T}{10}$. With a given sequence, exactly two pairs are marked as follows: we first randomly select and mark one of the first ten pairs (whose first component is called X_1). Then we randomly select and mark one of the first $\frac{T}{2} - 1$ still unmarked pairs (whose first component is called X_2). The second components of the remaining pairs are zero except for the first and final pair, whose second components are -1 (X_1 is set to zero in the rare case where the *first* pair of the sequence got marked). An error signal is generated only at the sequence end: the target is $0.5 + \frac{X_1+X_2}{4.0}$ (the sum $X_1 + X_2$ scaled to the interval $[0, 1]$). A sequence was processed correctly if the absolute error at the sequence end is below 0.04.

Architecture. We use a 3-layer net with 2 input units, 1 output unit, and 2 memory cell blocks of size 2 (a cell block size of 1 works well, too). The output layer receives connections only from memory cells. Memory cells/ gate units receive inputs from memory cells/gate units (fully connected hidden layer). Gate units (f_{in_j}, f_{out_j}) and output units are sigmoid in $[0, 1]$. h is sigmoid in $[-1, 1]$, and g is sigmoid in $[-2, 2]$.

State drift versus initial bias. Note that the task requires to store the precise values of real numbers for long durations — the system must learn to protect memory cell contents against even minor "internal state drifts". Our simple but highly effective way of solving drift problems at the beginning of learning is to initially bias the input gate in_j towards zero. *There is no need for fine tuning initial bias:* with sigmoid logistic activation functions, the precise initial bias hardly matters because vastly different initial bias values produce almost the same near-zero activations. In fact, the system itself learns to generate the most appropriate input gate bias. To study the significance of the drift problem, we bias all non-input units, thus artificially inducing internal state drifts. Weights (including bias weights) are randomly initialized in the range $[-0.1, 0.1]$. The first (second) input gate bias is initialized with -3.0 (-6.0) (recall that the precise initialization values hardly matters, as confirmed by additional experiments).

Training / Testing. The learning rate is 0.5. Training examples are generated on-line. Training is stopped if the average training error is below 0.01, and the 2000 most recent sequences were processed correctly (see definition above).

Results. With a test set consisting of 2560 randomly chosen sequences, the average test set error was always below 0.01, and there were never more than 3 incorrectly processed sequences. The following results are means of 10 trials: For $T = 100$ ($T = 500$, $T = 1000$), training was stopped after 74,000 (209,000; 853,000) training sequences, and then only 1 (0, 1) of the test sequences was not processed correctly. For $T = 1000$, the number of required training examples varied between 370,000 and 2,020,000, exceeding 700,000 in only 3 cases.

The experiment demonstrates even for very long minimal time lags: (1) LSTM is able to work well with distributed representations. (2) LSTM is able to perform calculations involving *high-precision, continuous* values. Such tasks are impossible to solve within reasonable time by other algorithms: the main problem of gradient-based approaches (including TDNN, pseudo Newton) is their inability to deal with very long minimal time lags (vanishing gradient). A main problem of "global" and "discrete" approaches (RS, Bengio's and Frasconi's EM-approach, discrete error propagation) is their inability to deal with high-precision, continuous values.

Other experiments. In [8] LSTM is used to solve numerous additional tasks that cannot be solved by other recurrent net learning algorithm we are aware of. For instance, LSTM can extract information conveyed by the temporal order of widely separated inputs. LSTM also can learn real-valued, conditional expectations of strongly delayed, noisy targets, given the inputs.

Conclusion. For non-trivial tasks (where RS is infeasible), we recommend LSTM.

4 ACKNOWLEDGMENTS

This work was supported by *DFG grant SCHM 942/3-1* from "Deutsche Forschungsgemeinschaft".

References

[1] Y. Bengio and P. Frasconi. Credit assignment through time: Alternatives to backpropagation. In J. D. Cowan, G. Tesauro, and J. Alspector, editors, *Advances in Neural Information Processing Systems 6*, pages 75–82. San Mateo, CA: Morgan Kaufmann, 1994.

[2] Y. Bengio and P. Frasconi. An input output HMM architecture. In G. Tesauro, D. S. Touretzky, and T. K. Leen, editors, *Advances in Neural Information Processing Systems 7*, pages 427–434. MIT Press, Cambridge MA, 1995.

[3] Y. Bengio, P. Simard, and P. Frasconi. Learning long-term dependencies with gradient descent is difficult. *IEEE Transactions on Neural Networks*, 5(2):157–166, 1994.

[4] A. Cleeremans, D. Servan-Schreiber, and J. L. McClelland. Finite-state automata and simple recurrent networks. *Neural Computation*, 1:372–381, 1989.

[5] S. El Hihi and Y. Bengio. Hierarchical recurrent neural networks for long-term dependencies. In *Advances in Neural Information Processing Systems 8*, 1995. to appear.

[6] S. E. Fahlman. The recurrent cascade-correlation learning algorithm. In R. P. Lippmann, J. E. Moody, and D. S. Touretzky, editors, *Advances in Neural Information Processing Systems 3*, pages 190–196. San Mateo, CA: Morgan Kaufmann, 1991.

[7] J. Hochreiter. Untersuchungen zu dynamischen neuronalen Netzen. Diploma thesis, Institut für Informatik, Lehrstuhl Prof. Brauer, Technische Universität München, 1991. See www7.informatik.tu-muenchen.de/~hochreit.

[8] S. Hochreiter and J. Schmidhuber. Long short-term memory. Technical Report FKI-207-95, Fakultät für Informatik, Technische Universität München, 1995. Revised 1996 (see www.idsia.ch/~juergen, www7.informatik.tu-muenchen.de/~hochreit).

[9] T. Lin, B. G. Horne, P. Tino, and C. L. Giles. Learning long-term dependencies is not as difficult with NARX recurrent neural networks. Technical Report UMIACS-TR-95-78 and CS-TR-3500, Institute for Advanced Computer Studies, University of Maryland, College Park, MD 20742, 1995.

[10] P. Manolios and R. Fanelli. First-order recurrent neural networks and deterministic finite state automata. *Neural Computation*, 6:1155–1173, 1994.

[11] C. B. Miller and C. L. Giles. Experimental comparison of the effect of order in recurrent neural networks. *International Journal of Pattern Recognition and Artificial Intelligence*, 7(4):849–872, 1993.

[12] M. C. Mozer. Induction of multiscale temporal structure. In J. E. Moody, S. J. Hanson, and R. P. Lippman, editors, *Advances in Neural Information Processing Systems 4*, pages 275–282. San Mateo, CA: Morgan Kaufmann, 1992.

[13] B. A. Pearlmutter. Gradient calculations for dynamic recurrent neural networks: A survey. *IEEE Transactions on Neural Networks*, 6(5):1212–1228, 1995.

[14] J. B. Pollack. The induction of dynamical recognizers. *Machine Learning*, 7:227–252, 1991.

[15] A. J. Robinson and F. Fallside. The utility driven dynamic error propagation network. Technical Report CUED/F-INFENG/TR.1, Cambridge University Engineering Department, 1987.

[16] J. H. Schmidhuber. Learning complex, extended sequences using the principle of history compression. *Neural Computation*, 4(2):234–242, 1992.

[17] A. W. Smith and D. Zipser. Learning sequential structures with the real-time recurrent learning algorithm. *International Journal of Neural Systems*, 1(2):125–131, 1989.

[18] M. Tomita. Dynamic construction of finite automata from examples using hill-climbing. In *Proceedings of the Fourth Annual Cognitive Science Conference*, pages 105–108. Ann Arbor, MI, 1982.

[19] R. L. Watrous and G. M. Kuhn. Induction of finite-state automata using second-order recurrent networks. In J. E. Moody, S. J. Hanson, and R. P. Lippman, editors, *Advances in Neural Information Processing Systems 4*, pages 309–316. San Mateo, CA: Morgan Kaufmann, 1992.

[20] R. J. Williams and J. Peng. An efficient gradient-based algorithm for on-line training of recurrent network trajectories. *Neural Computation*, 4:491–501, 1990.

One-unit Learning Rules for Independent Component Analysis

Aapo Hyvärinen and Erkki Oja
Helsinki University of Technology
Laboratory of Computer and Information Science
Rakentajanaukio 2 C, FIN-02150 Espoo, Finland
email: {Aapo.Hyvarinen,Erkki.Oja}@hut.fi

Abstract

Neural one-unit learning rules for the problem of Independent Component Analysis (ICA) and blind source separation are introduced. In these new algorithms, every ICA neuron develops into a separator that finds one of the independent components. The learning rules use very simple constrained Hebbian/anti-Hebbian learning in which decorrelating feedback may be added. To speed up the convergence of these stochastic gradient descent rules, a novel computationally efficient fixed-point algorithm is introduced.

1 Introduction

Independent Component Analysis (ICA) (Comon, 1994; Jutten and Herault, 1991) is a signal processing technique whose goal is to express a set of random variables as linear combinations of statistically independent component variables. The main applications of ICA are in blind source separation, feature extraction, and blind deconvolution. In the simplest form of ICA (Comon, 1994), we observe m scalar random variables $x_1, ..., x_m$ which are assumed to be linear combinations of n unknown components $s_1, ...s_n$ that are zero-mean and *mutually statistically independent*. In addition, we must assume $n \leq m$. If we arrange the observed variables x_i into a vector $\mathbf{x} = (x_1, x_2, ..., x_m)^T$ and the component variables s_j into a vector $\mathbf{s}$, the linear relationship can be expressed as

$$\mathbf{x} = \mathbf{As} \tag{1}$$

Here, $\mathbf{A}$ is an *unknown* $m \times n$ matrix of full rank, called the mixing matrix. Noise may also be added to the model, but it is omitted here for simplicity. The basic problem of ICA is then to estimate (separate) the realizations of the original independent components s_j, or a subset of them, using only the mixtures x_i. This is roughly equivalent to estimating the rows, or a subset of the rows, of the pseudoinverse of the mixing matrix $\mathbf{A}$. The fundamental restriction of the model is that *we can only estimate non-Gaussian independent components*, or ICs (except if just one of the ICs is Gaussian). Moreover, the ICs and the columns of $\mathbf{A}$ can only be estimated up to a multiplicative constant, because any constant multiplying an IC in eq. (1) could be cancelled by dividing the corresponding column of the mixing matrix $\mathbf{A}$ by the same constant. For mathematical convenience, we define here that the ICs s_j have unit variance. This makes the (non-Gaussian) ICs unique, up to their signs. Note the assumption of zero mean of the ICs is in fact no restriction, as this can always be accomplished by subtracting the mean from the random vector $\mathbf{x}$. Note also that no order is defined between the ICs.

In *blind source separation* (Jutten and Herault, 1991), the observed values of $\mathbf{x}$ correspond to a realization of an m-dimensional discrete-time signal $\mathbf{x}(t)$, $t = 1, 2, \ldots$. Then the components $s_j(t)$ are called source signals. The source signals are usually original, uncorrupted signals or noise sources. Another application of ICA is *feature extraction* (Bell and Sejnowski, 1996; Hurri et al., 1996), where the columns of the mixing matrix $\mathbf{A}$ define features, and the s_j signal the presence and the amplitude of a feature. A closely related problem is *blind deconvolution*, in which a convolved version $x(t)$ of a scalar i.i.d. signal $s(t)$ is observed. The goal is then to recover the original signal $s(t)$ without knowing the convolution kernel (Donoho, 1981). This problem can be represented in a way similar to eq. (1), replacing the matrix $\mathbf{A}$ by a filter.

The current neural algorithms for Independent Component Analysis, e.g. (Bell and Sejnowski, 1995; Cardoso and Laheld, 1996; Jutten and Herault, 1991; Karhunen et al., 1997; Oja, 1995) try to estimate simultaneously all the components. This is often not necessary, nor feasible, and it is often desired to estimate only a subset of the ICs. This is the starting point of our paper. We introduce *learning rules for a single neuron*, by which the neuron learns to estimate one of the ICs. A network of several such neurons can then estimate several (1 to n) ICs. Both learning rules for the 'raw' data (Section 3) and for whitened data (Section 4) are introduced. If the data is whitened, the convergence is speeded up, and some interesting simplifications and approximations are made possible. Feedback mechanisms (Section 5) are also mentioned. Finally, we introduce a novel approach for performing the computations needed in the ICA learning rules, which uses a very simple, yet highly efficient, *fixed-point iteration scheme* (Section 6). An important generalization of our learning rules is discussed in Section 7, and an illustrative experiment is shown in Section 8.

2 Using Kurtosis for ICA Estimation

We begin by introducing the basic mathematical framework of ICA. Most suggested solutions for ICA use the fourth-order cumulant or *kurtosis* of the signals, defined for a zero-mean random variable v as $\mathrm{kurt}(v) = E\{v^4\} - 3(E\{v^2\})^2$. For a Gaussian random variable, kurtosis is zero. Therefore, random variables of positive kurtosis are sometimes called super-Gaussian, and variables of negative kurtosis sub-Gaussian. Note that for two independent random variables v_1 and v_2 and for a scalar α, it holds $\mathrm{kurt}(v_1 + v_2) = \mathrm{kurt}(v_1) + \mathrm{kurt}(v_2)$ and $\mathrm{kurt}(\alpha v_1) = \alpha^4 \mathrm{kurt}(v_1)$.

Let us search for a linear combination of the observations x_i, say, $\mathbf{w}^T\mathbf{x}$, such that it has maximal or minimal kurtosis. Obviously, this is meaningful only if $\mathbf{w}$ is somehow bounded; let us assume that the variance of the linear combination is constant: $E\{(\mathbf{w}^T\mathbf{x})^2\} = 1$. Using the mixing matrix $\mathbf{A}$ in eq. (1), let us define $\mathbf{z} = \mathbf{A}^T\mathbf{w}$. Then also $\|\mathbf{z}\|^2 = \mathbf{w}^T\mathbf{A}\,\mathbf{A}^T\mathbf{w} = \mathbf{w}^T E\{\mathbf{x}\mathbf{x}^T\}\mathbf{w} = E\{(\mathbf{w}^T\mathbf{x})^2\} = 1$. Using eq. (1) and the properties of the kurtosis, we have

$$\text{kurt}(\mathbf{w}^T\mathbf{x}) = \text{kurt}(\mathbf{w}^T\mathbf{A}\mathbf{s}) = \text{kurt}(\mathbf{z}^T\mathbf{s}) = \sum_{j=1}^{n} z_j^4 \, \text{kurt}(s_j) \qquad (2)$$

Under the constraint $E\{(\mathbf{w}^T\mathbf{x})^2\} = \|\mathbf{z}\|^2 = 1$, the function in (2) has a number of local minima and maxima. To make the argument clearer, let us assume for the moment that the mixture contains at least one IC whose kurtosis is negative, and at least one whose kurtosis is positive. Then, as may be obvious, and was rigorously proven by Delfosse and Loubaton (1995), the extremal points of (2) are obtained when all the components z_j of $\mathbf{z}$ are zero except one component which equals ± 1. In particular, the function in (2) is maximized (resp. minimized) exactly when the linear combination $\mathbf{w}^T\mathbf{x} = \mathbf{z}^T\mathbf{s}$ equals, up to the sign, one of the ICs s_j of positive (resp. negative) kurtosis. Thus, *finding the extrema of kurtosis of $\mathbf{w}^T\mathbf{x}$ enables estimation of the independent components.* Equation (2) also shows that Gaussian components, or other components whose kurtosis is zero, cannot be estimated by this method.

To actually minimize or maximize $\text{kurt}(\mathbf{w}^T\mathbf{x})$, a neural algorithm based on gradient descent or ascent can be used. Then $\mathbf{w}$ is interpreted as the weight vector of a neuron with input vector $\mathbf{x}$ and linear output $\mathbf{w}^T\mathbf{x}$. The objective function can be simplified because of the constraint $E\{(\mathbf{w}^T\mathbf{x})^2\} = 1$: it holds $\text{kurt}(\mathbf{w}^T\mathbf{x}) = E\{(\mathbf{w}^T\mathbf{x})^4\} - 3$. The constraint $E\{(\mathbf{w}^T\mathbf{x})^2\} = 1$ itself can be taken into account by a penalty term. The final objective function is then of the form

$$J(\mathbf{w}) = \alpha E\{(\mathbf{w}^T\mathbf{x})^4\} + \beta F(E\{(\mathbf{w}^T\mathbf{x})^2\}) \qquad (3)$$

where $\alpha, \beta > 0$ are arbitrary scaling constants, and F is a suitable penalty function. Our basic ICA learning rules are stochastic gradient descents or ascents for an objective function of this form. In the next two sections, we present learning rules resulting from adequate choices of the penalty function F. Preprocessing of the data (whitening) is also used to simplify J in Section 4. An alternative method for finding the extrema of kurtosis is the fixed-point algorithm; see Section 6.

3 Basic One-Unit ICA Learning Rules

In this section, we introduce learning rules for a single neural unit. These basic learning rules require *no preprocessing of the data*, except that the data must be made zero-mean. Our learning rules are divided into two categories. As explained in Section 2, the learning rules either minimize the kurtosis of the output to separate ICs of negative kurtosis, or maximize it for components of positive kurtosis.

Let us assume that we observe a sample sequence $\mathbf{x}(t)$ of a vector $\mathbf{x}$ that is a linear combination of independent components $s_1, ..., s_n$ according to eq. (1). For separating one of the ICs of *negative kurtosis*, we use the following learning rule for the weight vector $\mathbf{w}$ of a neuron:

$$\Delta \mathbf{w}(t) \propto \mathbf{x}(t) g^-(\mathbf{w}(t)^T \mathbf{x}(t)) \tag{4}$$

Here, the non-linear learning function g^- is a simple polynomial: $g^-(u) = au - bu^3$ with arbitrary scaling constants $a, b > 0$. This learning rule is clearly a stochastic gradient descent for a function of the form (3), with $F(u) = -u$. To separate an IC of *positive kurtosis*, we use the following learning rule:

$$\Delta \mathbf{w}(t) \propto \mathbf{x}(t) g^+_{\mathbf{w}(t)}(\mathbf{w}(t)^T \mathbf{x}(t)) \tag{5}$$

where the learning function $g^+_{\mathbf{w}(t)}$ is defined as follows: $g^+_{\mathbf{w}}(u) = -au(\mathbf{w}(t)^T \mathbf{C} \mathbf{w}(t))^2 + bu^3$ where $\mathbf{C}$ is the covariance matrix of $\mathbf{x}(t)$, i.e. $\mathbf{C} = E\{\mathbf{x}(t)\mathbf{x}(t)^T\}$, and $a, b > 0$ are arbitrary constants. This learning rule is a stochastic gradient ascent for a function of the form (3), with $F(u) = -u^2$. Note that $\mathbf{w}(t)^T \mathbf{C} \mathbf{w}(t)$ in g^+ might also be replaced by $(E\{(\mathbf{w}(t)^T \mathbf{x}(t))^2\})^2$ or by $\|\mathbf{w}(t)\|^4$ to enable a simpler implementation.

It can be proven (Hyvärinen and Oja, 1996b) that using the learning rules (4) and (5), the linear output converges to $cs_j(t)$ where $s_j(t)$ is one of the ICs, and c is a scalar constant. This multiplication of the source signal by the constant c is in fact not a restriction, as the variance and the sign of the sources cannot be estimated. The only condition for convergence is that one of the ICs must be of negative (resp. positive) kurtosis, when learning rule (4) (resp. learning rule (5)) is used. Thus we can say that *the neuron learns to separate (estimate) one of the independent components*. It is also possible to combine these two learning rules into a single rule that separates an IC of any kurtosis; see (Hyvärinen and Oja, 1996b).

4 One-Unit ICA Learning Rules for Whitened Data

Whitening, also called sphering, is a very useful preprocessing technique. It *speeds up the convergence* considerably, makes the learning more stable numerically, and allows some interesting modifications of the learning rules. Whitening means that the observed vector $\mathbf{x}$ is linearly transformed to a vector $\mathbf{v} = \mathbf{U}\mathbf{x}$ such that its elements v_i are mutually uncorrelated and all have unit variance (Comon, 1994). Thus the correlation matrix of $\mathbf{v}$ equals unity: $E\{\mathbf{v}\mathbf{v}^T\} = \mathbf{I}$. This transformation is always possible and can be accomplished by classical Principal Component Analysis. At the same time, the dimensionality of the data should be reduced so that the dimension of the transformed data vector $\mathbf{v}$ equals n, the number of independent components. This also has the effect of reducing noise.

Let us thus suppose that the observed signal $\mathbf{v}(t)$ is whitened (sphered). Then, in order to separate one of the components of *negative kurtosis*, we can modify the learning rule (4) so as to get the following learning rule for the weight vector $\mathbf{w}$:

$$\Delta \mathbf{w}(t) \propto \mathbf{v}(t) g^-(\mathbf{w}(t)^T \mathbf{v}(t)) - \mathbf{w}(t) \tag{6}$$

Here, the function g^- is the same polynomial as above: $g^-(u) = au - bu^3$ with $a > 1$ and $b > 0$. This modification is valid because we now have $E\mathbf{v}(\mathbf{w}^T \mathbf{v}) = \mathbf{w}$ and thus we can add $+\mathbf{w}(t)$ in the linear part of g^- and subtract $\mathbf{w}(t)$ explicitly afterwards. The modification is useful because it allows us to approximate g^- with the 'tanh' function, as $\mathbf{w}(t)^T\mathbf{v}(t)$ then stays in the range where this approximation is valid. Thus we get what is perhaps the simplest possible stable Hebbian learning rule for a nonlinear Perceptron.

To separate one of the components of *positive kurtosis*, rule (5) simplifies to:

$$\Delta \mathbf{w}(t) \propto b\mathbf{v}(t)(\mathbf{w}(t)^T\mathbf{v}(t))^3 - a\|\mathbf{w}(t)\|^4\mathbf{w}(t). \qquad (7)$$

5 Multi-Unit ICA Learning Rules

If estimation of several independent components is desired, it is possible to construct a neural network by combining N ($1 \leq N \leq n$) neurons that learn according to the learning rules given above, and *adding a feedback* term to each of those learning rules. A discussion of such networks can be found in (Hyvärinen and Oja, 1996b).

6 Fixed-Point Algorithm for ICA

The advantage of neural on-line learning rules like those introduced above is that the inputs $\mathbf{v}(t)$ can be used in the algorithm at once, thus enabling faster adaptation in a non-stationary environment. A resulting trade-off, however, is that the convergence is slow, and depends on a good choice of the learning rate sequence, i.e. the step size at each iteration. A bad choice of the learning rate can, in practice, destroy convergence. Therefore, some ways to *make the learning radically faster and more reliable* may be needed. The fixed-point iteration algorithms are such an alternative. Based on the learning rules introduced above, we introduce here a fixed-point algorithm, whose convergence is proven and analyzed in detail in (Hyvärinen and Oja, 1997). For simplicity, we only consider the case of whitened data here.

Consider the general neural learning rule trying to find the extrema of kurtosis. In a fixed point of such a learning rule, the sum of the gradient of kurtosis and the penalty term must equal zero: $E\{\mathbf{v}(\mathbf{w}^T\mathbf{v})^3\} - 3\|\mathbf{w}\|^2\mathbf{w} + f(\|\mathbf{w}\|^2)\mathbf{w} = 0$. The solutions of this equation must satisfy

$$\mathbf{w} = \text{scalar} \times (E\{\mathbf{v}(\mathbf{w}^T\mathbf{v})^3\} - 3\mathbf{w}\|\mathbf{w}\|^2) \qquad (8)$$

Actually, because the norm of $\mathbf{w}$ is irrelevant, it is the direction of the right hand side that is important. Therefore the scalar in eq. (8) is not significant and its effect can be replaced by explicit normalization.

Assume now that we have collected a sample of the random vector $\mathbf{v}$, which is a whitened (or sphered) version of the vector $\mathbf{x}$ in eq. (1). Using (8), we obtain the following *fixed-point algorithm for ICA*:

   1. Take a random initial vector $\mathbf{w}(0)$ of norm 1. Let $k = 1$.

   2. Let $\mathbf{w}(k) = E\{\mathbf{v}(\mathbf{w}(k-1)^T\mathbf{v})^3\} - 3\mathbf{w}(k-1)$. The expectation can be estimated using a large sample of $\mathbf{v}$ vectors (say, 1,000 points).

   3. Divide $\mathbf{w}(k)$ by its norm.

   4. If $|\mathbf{w}(k)^T\mathbf{w}(k-1)|$ is not close enough to 1, let $k = k+1$ and go back to step 2. Otherwise, output the vector $\mathbf{w}(k)$.

The final vector $\mathbf{w}^* = \lim_k \mathbf{w}(k)$ given by the algorithm separates one of the non-Gaussian ICs in the sense that $\mathbf{w}^{*T}\mathbf{v}$ equals one of the ICs s_j. No distinction between components of positive or negative kurtosis is needed here. A remarkable property of our algorithm is that a very small number of iterations, usually 5-10, seems to be enough to obtain the maximal accuracy allowed by the sample data. This is due to the fact that the convergence of the fixed point algorithm is in fact *cubic*, as shown in (Hyvärinen and Oja, 1997).

To estimate N ICs, we run this algorithm N times. To ensure that we estimate each time a different IC, we only need to add a simple projection inside the loop, which forces the solution vector $\mathbf{w}(k)$ to be orthogonal to the previously found solutions. This is possible because the desired weight vectors are orthonormal for whitened data (Hyvärinen and Oja, 1996b; Karhunen et al., 1997). Symmetric methods of orthogonalization may also be used (Hyvärinen, 1997).

This fixed-point algorithm has several advantages when compared to other suggested ICA methods. First, the convergence of our algorithm is cubic. This means very fast convergence and is rather unique among the ICA algorithms. Second, contrary to gradient-based algorithms, there is no learning rate or other adjustable parameters in the algorithm, which makes it easy to use and more reliable. Third, components of both positive and negative kurtosis can be directly estimated by the same fixed-point algorithm.

7 Generalizations of Kurtosis

In the learning rules introduced above, we used kurtosis as an optimization criterion for ICA estimation. This approach can be generalized to a large class of such optimizaton criteria, called contrast functions. For the case of on-line learning rules, this approach is developed in (Hyvärinen and Oja, 1996a), in which it is shown that the function g in the learning rules in section 4 can be, in fact, replaced by practically any non-linear function (provided that $\mathbf{w}$ is normalized properly). Whether one must use Hebbian or anti-Hebbian learning is then determined by the sign of certain 'non-polynomial cumulants'. The utility of such a generalization is that one can then choose the non-linearity according to some statistical optimality criteria, such as *robustness against outliers*.

The fixed-point algorithm may also be generalized for an arbitrary non-linearity, say g. Step 2 in the fixed-point algorithm then becomes (for whitened data) (Hyvärinen, 1997): $\mathbf{w}(k) = E\{\mathbf{v}g(\mathbf{w}(k-1)^T\mathbf{v})\} - E\{g'(\mathbf{w}(k-1)^T\mathbf{v})\}\mathbf{w}(k-1)$.

8 Experiments

A visually appealing way of demonstrating how ICA algorithms work is to use them to separate images from their linear mixtures. On the left in Fig. 1, four superimposed mixtures of 4 unknown images are depicted. Defining the j-th IC s_j to be the gray-level value of the j-th image in a given position, and scanning the 4 images simultaneously pixel by pixel, we can use the ICA model and recover the original images. For example, we ran the fixed-point algorithm four times, estimating the four images shown on the right in Fig. 1. The algorithm needed on the average 7 iterations for each IC.

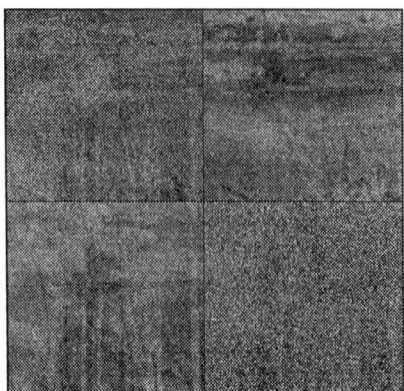
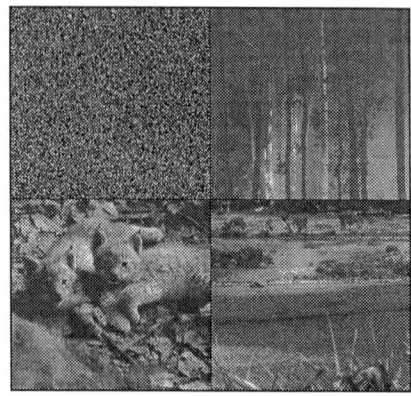

Figure 1: Three photographs of natural scenes and a noise image were linearly mixed to illustrate our algorithms. The mixtures are depicted on the left. On the right, the images recovered by the fixed-point algorithm are shown.

References

Bell, A. and Sejnowski, T. (1995). An information-maximization approach to blind separation and blind deconvolution. *Neural Computation*, 7:1129–1159.

Bell, A. and Sejnowski, T. J. (1996). Edges are the independent components of natural scenes. In *NIPS*96*, Denver, Colorado.

Cardoso, J.-F. and Laheld, B. H. (1996). Equivariant adaptive source separation. *IEEE Trans. on Signal Processing*, 44(12).

Comon, P. (1994). Independent component analysis – a new concept? *Signal Processing*, 36:287–314.

Delfosse, N. and Loubaton, P. (1995). Adaptive blind separation of independent sources: a deflation approach. *Signal Processing*, 45:59–83.

Donoho, D. (1981). On minimum entropy deconvolution. In *Applied Time Series Analysis II*. Academic Press.

Hurri, J., Hyvärinen, A., Karhunen, J., and Oja, E. (1996). Image feature extraction using independent component analysis. In *Proc. NORSIG'96*, Espoo, Finland.

Hyvärinen, A. (1997). A family of fixed-point algorithms for independent component analysis. In *Proc. ICASSP'97*, Munich, Germany.

Hyvärinen, A. and Oja, E. (1996a). Independent component analysis by general nonlinear hebbian-like learning rules. Technical Report A41, Helsinki University of Technology, Laboratory of Computer and Information Science.

Hyvärinen, A. and Oja, E. (1996b). Simple neuron models for independent component analysis. Technical Report A37, Helsinki University of Technology, Laboratory of Computer and Information Science.

Hyvärinen, A. and Oja, E. (1997). A fast fixed-point algorithm for independent component analysis. *Neural Computation*. To appear.

Jutten, C. and Herault, J. (1991). Blind separation of sources, part I: An adaptive algorithm based on neuromimetic architecture. *Signal Processing*, 24:1–10.

Karhunen, J., Oja, E., Wang, L., Vigario, R., and Joutsensalo, J. (1997). A class of neural networks for independent component analysis. *IEEE Trans. on Neural Networks*. To appear.

Oja, E. (1995). The nonlinear PCA learning rule and signal separation – mathematical analysis. Technical Report A 26, Helsinki University of Technology, Laboratory of Computer and Information Science. Submitted to a journal.

Recursive algorithms for approximating probabilities in graphical models

Tommi S. Jaakkola and Michael I. Jordan
{tommi,jordan}@psyche.mit.edu
Department of Brain and Cognitive Sciences
Massachusetts Institute of Technology
Cambridge, MA 02139

Abstract

We develop a recursive node-elimination formalism for efficiently approximating large probabilistic networks. No constraints are set on the network topologies. Yet the formalism can be straightforwardly integrated with exact methods whenever they are/become applicable. The approximations we use are controlled: they maintain consistently upper and lower bounds on the desired quantities at all times. We show that Boltzmann machines, sigmoid belief networks, or any combination (i.e., chain graphs) can be handled within the same framework. The accuracy of the methods is verified experimentally.

1 Introduction

Graphical models (see, e.g., Lauritzen 1996) provide a medium for rigorously embedding domain knowledge into network models. The structure in these graphical models embodies the qualitative assumptions about the independence relationships in the domain while the probability model attached to the graph permits a consistent computation of belief (or uncertainty) about the values of the variables in the network. The feasibility of performing this computation determines the ability to make inferences or to learn on the basis of observations. The standard framework for carrying out this computation consists of exact probabilistic methods (Lauritzen 1996). Such methods are nevertheless restricted to fairly small or sparsely connected networks and the use of approximate techniques is likely to be the rule for highly interconnected graphs of the kind studied in the neural network literature.

There are several desiderata for methods that calculate approximations to posterior probabilities on graphs. Besides having to be (1) reasonably accurate and fast to compute, such techniques should yield (2) rigorous estimates of confidence about the attained results; this is especially important in many real-world applications (e.g., in medicine). Furthermore, a considerable gain in accuracy could be obtained from (3) the ability to use the techniques in conjunction with exact calculations whenever feasible. These goals have been addressed in the literature with varying degrees of success. For inference and learning in Boltzmann machines, for example, classical mean field approximations (Peterson & Anderson, 1987) address only the first goal. In the case of sigmoid belief networks (Neal 1992), partial solutions have been provided to the first two goals (Dayan et al. 1995; Saul et al. 1996; Jaakkola & Jordan 1996). The goal of integrating approximations with exact techniques has been introduced in the context of Boltzmann machines (Saul & Jordan 1996) but nevertheless leaving the solution to our second goal unattained. In this paper, we develop a recursive node-elimination formalism that meets all three objectives for a powerful class of networks known as chain graphs (see, e.g., Lauritzen 1996); the chain graphs we consider are of a restricted type but they nevertheless include Boltzmann machines and sigmoid belief networks as special cases.

We start by deriving the recursive formalism for Boltzmann machines. The results are then generalized to sigmoid belief networks and the chain graphs.

2 Boltzmann machines

We begin by considering Boltzmann machines with binary (0/1) variables. We assume the joint probability distribution for the variables $S = \{S_1, \ldots, S_n\}$ to be given by

$$P_n(S|h, J) = \frac{1}{Z_n(h, J)} B_n(S|h, J) \tag{1}$$

where h and J are the vector of biases and weights respectively, and the Boltzmann factor B has the form

$$B_n(S|h, J) = \exp\left\{ \sum_{i=1}^n h_i S_i + \frac{1}{2} \sum_{i,j=1}^n J_{ij} S_i S_j \right\} \tag{2}$$

The partition function $Z_n(h, J) = \sum_S B_n(S|h, J)$ normalizes the distribution. The Boltzmann distribution defined in this manner is tractable insofar as we are able to compute the partition function; indeed, all marginal distributions can be reduced to ratios of partition functions in different settings.

We now turn to methods for computing the partition function. In special cases (e.g., trees or chains) the structure of the weight matrix J_{ij} may allow us to employ exact methods for calculating Z. Although exact methods are not feasible in more generic networks, selective approximations may nevertheless restore their utility. The recursive framework we develop provides a general and straightforward methodology for combining approximate and exact techniques.

The crux of our approach lies in obtaining variational bounds that allow the creation of recursive node-elimination formulas of the form[1]:

$$Z_n(h, J) \lessgtr C(h, J) Z_{n-1}(\tilde{h}, \tilde{J}) \tag{3}$$

Such formulas are attractive for three main reasons: (1) a variable (or many at the same time) can be eliminated by merely transforming the model parameters (h and J); (2) the approximations involved in the elimination are controlled, i.e., they

---

[1] Related schemes in the physics literature (renormalization group) are unsuitable here as they generally don't provide strict upper/lower bounds.

consistently yield upper or lower bounds at each stage of the recursion; (3) most importantly, if the remaining (simplified) partition function $Z_{n-1}(\tilde{h}, \tilde{J})$ allow the use of exact methods, the corresponding model parameters $\tilde{h}$ and $\tilde{J}$ can simply be passed on to such routines.

Next we will consider how to obtain the bounds and outline their implications. Note that since the quantities of interest are predominantly ratios of partition functions, it is the combination of upper and lower bounds that is necessary to rigorously bound the target quantities. This applies to parameter estimation as well even if only a lower bound on likelihood of examples is used; such likelihood bound relies on both upper and lower bounds on partition functions.

2.1 Simple recursive factorizations

We start by developing a lower bound recursion. Consider eliminating the variable S_i:

$$Z_n(h, J) = \sum_S B_n(S|h, J) = \sum_{S \setminus S_i} \sum_{S_i} B_n(S|h, J) \qquad (4)$$

$$= \sum_{S \setminus S_i} (1 + e^{h_i + \sum_j J_{ij} S_j}) B_{n-1}(S \setminus S_i | h, J) \qquad (5)$$

$$\geq \sum_{S \setminus S_i} e^{\mu_i(h_i + \sum_j J_{ij} S_j) + H(\mu_i)} B_{n-1}(S \setminus S_i | h, J) \qquad (6)$$

$$= e^{\mu_i h_i + H(\mu_i)} \sum_{S \setminus S_i} B_{n-1}(S \setminus S_i | \tilde{h}, J) \qquad (7)$$

$$= e^{\mu_i h_i + H(\mu_i)} Z_{n-1}(\tilde{h}, J) \qquad (8)$$

where $\tilde{h}_j = h_j + \mu_i J_{ij}$ for $j \neq i$, $H(\cdot)$ is the binary entropy function and μ_i are free parameters that we will refer to as "variational parameters." The variational bound introduced in eq. (6) can be verified by a direct maximization which recovers the original expression. This lower bound recursion bears a connection to mean field approximation and in particular to the structured mean field approximation studied by Saul and Jordan (1996).[2]

Each recursive elimination translates into an additional bound and therefore the approximation (lower bound) deteriorates with the number of such iterations. It is necessary, however, to continue with the recursion only to the extent that the prevailing partition function remains unwieldy to exact methods. Consequently, the problem becomes that of finding the variables the elimination of which would render the rest of the graph tractable. Figure 1 illustrates this objective. Note that the simple recursion does not change the connection matrix J for the remaining variables; thus, graphically, the operation translates into merely removing the variable.

The above recursive procedure maintains a lower bound on the partition function that results from the variational representation introduced in eq. (6). For rigorous

---

[2] Each lower bound recursion can be shown to be equivalent to a mean field approximation of the eliminated variable(s). The structured mean field approach of Saul and Jordan (1996) suggests using exact methods for tractable substructures while mean field for the variables mediating these structures. Translated into our framework this amounts to eliminating the mediating variables through the recursive lower bound formula with a subsequent appeal to exact methods. The connection is limited to the lower bound.

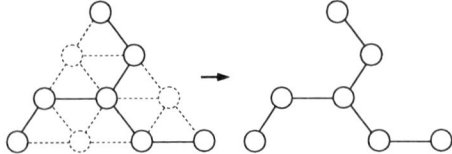

Figure 1: Enforcing tractable networks. Each variable in the graph can be removed (in any order) by adding the appropriate biases for the existing adjacent variables. The elimination of the dotted nodes reveals a simplified graph underneath.

bounds we need an upper bound as well. In order to preserve the graphical interpretation of the lower bound, the upper bound should also be factorized. With this in mind, the bound of eq. (6) can be replaced with

$$1 + e^{h_i + \sum_j J_{ij} S_j} \leq e^{\hat{h}_0 + \sum_j S_j \hat{h}_j} \tag{9}$$

where

$$\hat{h}_j = q_j \left[f\left(J_{ij}/q_j + h_i\right) - f(h_i) \right] \tag{10}$$

for $j > 0$, $\hat{h}_0 = f(h_i)$, $f(x) = \log(1 + e^x)$, and q_j are variational parameters such that $\sum_j q_j = 1$. The derivation of this bound can be found in appendix A.

2.2 Refined recursive bound

If the (sub)network is densely or fully connected the simple recursive methods presented earlier can hardly uncover any useful structure. Thus a large number of recursive steps are needed before relying on exact methods and the accuracy of the overall bound is compromised. To improve the accuracy, we introduce a more sophisticated variational (upper) bound to replace the one in eq. (6). By denoting $X_i = h_i + \sum_j J_{ij} S_j$ we have:

$$1 + e^{X_i} \leq e^{X_i/2 + \lambda(x_i) X_i^2 - F(\lambda, x_i)} \tag{11}$$

The derivation and the functional forms of $\lambda(x_i)$ and $F(\lambda, x_i)$ are presented in appendix B. We note here, however, that the bound is exact whenever $x_i = X_i$. In terms of the recursion we obtain

$$Z_n(h, J) \leq e^{h_i/2 + \lambda(x_i) h_i^2 - F(\lambda, x_i)} Z_{n-1}(\tilde{h}, \tilde{J}) \tag{12}$$

where

$$\tilde{h}_j = h_j + 2h_i \lambda(x_i) J_{ij} + J_{ij}/2 + \lambda(x_i) J_{ij}^2 \tag{13}$$

$$\tilde{J}_{jk} = J_{jk} + 2\lambda(x_i) J_{ji} J_{ik} \tag{14}$$

for $j \neq k \neq i$. Importantly and as shown in figure 2a, this refined recursion imposes (qualitatively) the proper structural changes on the remaining network: the variables adjacent to the eliminated (or marginalized) variable become connected. In other words, if $J_{ij} \neq 0$ and $J_{ik} \neq 0$ then $\tilde{J}_{jk} \neq 0$ after the recursion.

To substantiate the claim of improved accuracy we tested the refined upper bound recursion against the factorized lower bound recursion in random fully connected networks with 8 variables[3]. The weights in these networks were chosen uniformly in the range $[-d, d]$ and all the initial biases were set to zero. Figure 3a plots the relative errors in the log-partition function estimates for the two recursions as a

---
[3] The small network size was chosen to facilitate comparisons with exact results.

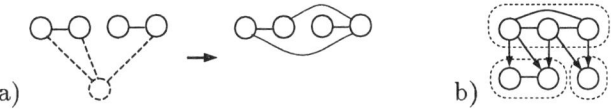

Figure 2: a) The graphical changes in the network following the refined recursion match those of proper marginalization. b) Example of a chain graph. The dotted ovals indicate the undirected clusters.

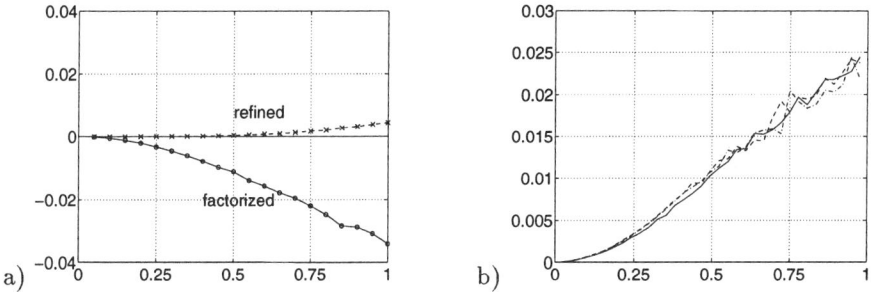

Figure 3: a) The mean relative errors in the log-partition function as a function of the scale of the random weights (uniform in $[-d, d]$). Solid line: factorized lower bound recursion; dashed line: refined upper bound. b) Mean relative difference between the upper and lower bound recursions as a function of $d\sqrt{n/8}$, where n is the network size. Solid: $n = 8$; dashed: $n = 64$; dotdashed: $n = 128$.

function of the scale d. Figure 3b reveals how the relative difference between the two bounds is affected by the network size. In the illustrated scale the size has little effect on the difference. We note that the difference is mainly due to the factorized lower bound recursion as is evident from Figure 3a.

3 Chain graphs and sigmoid belief networks

The recursive bounds presented earlier can be carried over to chain graphs[4]. An example of a chain graph is given in figure 2b. The joint distribution for a chain graph can written as a product of conditional distributions for clusters of variables:

$$P_n(S|J) = \prod_k P(S^k|\text{pa}[k], h^k, J^k) \tag{15}$$

where $S^k = \{S_i\}_{i \in C_k}$ is the set of variables in cluster k. In our case, the conditional probabilities for each cluster are conditional Boltzmann distributions given by

$$P(S^k|\text{pa}[k], h^k, J^k) = \frac{B(S^k|h_S^k, J^k)}{Z(h_S^k, J^k)} \tag{16}$$

where the added complexity beyond that of ordinary Boltzmann machines is that the Boltzmann factors now include also outside cluster biases:

$$[h_S^k]_i = h_i^k + \sum_{j \notin C_k} J_{ij}^{k,out} S_j \tag{17}$$

---

[4] While Boltzmann machines are undirected networks (interactions defined through potentials), sigmoid networks are directed models (constructed from conditional probabilities). Chain graphs contain both directed and undirected interactions.

where the index i stays within the kth cluster. We note that sigmoid belief networks correspond to the special case where there is only single binary variable in each cluster; Boltzmann machines, on the other hand, have only one cluster.

We now show that the recursive formalism can be extended to chain graphs. This is achieved by rewriting or bounding the conditional probabilities in terms of variational Boltzmann factors. Consequently, the joint distribution – being a product of the conditionals – will also be a Boltzmann factor. Computing likelihoods (marginals) from such a joint distribution amounts to calculating the value of a particular partition function and therefore reduces to the case considered earlier.

It suffices to find variational Boltzmann factors that bound (or rerepresent in some cases) the cluster partition functions in the conditional probabilities. We observe first that in the factorized lower bound or in the refined upper bound recursions, the initial biases will appear in the resulting expressions either linearly or quadratically in the exponent[5]. Since the initial biases for the clusters are of the form of eq. (17), the resulting expressions must be Boltzmann factors with respect to the variables outside the cluster. Thus, applying the recursive approximations to each cluster partition function yields an upper/lower bound in the form of a Boltzmann factor. Combining such bounds from each cluster finally gives upper/lower bounds for the joint distribution in terms of variational Boltzmann factors.

We note that for sigmoid belief networks the Boltzmann factors bounding the joint distribution are in fact exact variational translations of the true joint distribution. To see this, let us denote $X_i = \sum J_{ij} S_j + h_i$ and use the variational forms, for example, from eq. (6) and (11):

$$\sigma(X_i) = (1 + e^{-X_i})^{-1} \leq e^{\mu_i X_i - H(\mu_i)} \tag{18}$$
$$\geq e^{X_i/2 - \lambda(x_i) X_i^2 + F(\lambda, x_i)} \tag{19}$$

where the sigmoid function $\sigma(\cdot)$ is the inverse cluster partition function in this case. Both the variational forms are Boltzmann factors (at most quadratic in X_i in the exponent) and are exact if minimized/maximized with respect to the variational parameters.

In sum, we have shown how the joint distribution for chain graphs can be bounded by (translated into) Boltzmann factors to which the recursive approximation formalism is again applicable.

4 Conclusion

To reap the benefits of probabilistic formulations of network architectures, approximate methods are often unavoidable in real-world problems. We have developed a recursive node-elimination formalism for rigorously approximating intractable networks. The formalism applies to a large class of networks known as chain graphs and can be straightforwardly integrated with exact probabilistic calculations whenever they are applicable. Furthermore, the formalism provides rigorous upper and lower bounds on any desired quantity (e.g., the variable means) which is crucial in high risk application domains such as medicine.

---

[5]This follows from the linearity of the propagation rules for the biases, and the fact that the emerging prefactors are either linear or quadratic in the exponent.

References

P. Dayan, G. Hinton, R. Neal, and R. Zemel (1995). The Helmholtz machine. *Neural Computation* **7**: 889-904.

S. L. Lauritzen (1996). *Graphical Models.* Oxford: Oxford University Press.

T. Jaakkola and M. Jordan (1996). Computing upper and lower bounds on likelihoods in intractable networks. To appear in *Proceedings of the twelfth Conference on Uncertainty in Artificial Intelligence.*

R. Neal. Connectionist learning of belief networks (1992). *Artificial Intelligence* **56**: 71-113.

C. Peterson and J. R. Anderson (1987). A mean field theory learning algorithm for neural networks. *Complex Systems* **1**: 995-1019.

L. K. Saul, T. Jaakkola, and M. I. Jordan (1996). Mean field theory for sigmoid belief networks. *JAIR* **4**: 61-76.

L. Saul and M. Jordan (1996). Exploiting tractable substructures in intractable networks. To appear in *Advances of Neural Information Processing Systems 8.* MIT Press.

A Factorized upper bound

The bound follows from the convexity of $f(x) = \log(1+e^x)$ and from an application of Jensen's inequality. Let $f_k(x) = f(x + h_k)$ and note that $f_k(x)$ has the same convexity properties as f. For any convex function f_k then we have (by Jensen's inequality)

$$f_k\left(\sum_j J_{kj}S_j\right) = f_k\left(\sum_j q_j \frac{J_{kj}S_j}{q_j}\right) \le \sum_j q_j f_k\left(\frac{J_{kj}S_j}{q_j}\right) \qquad (20)$$

By rewriting $f_k\left(\frac{J_{kj}S_j}{q_j}\right) = S_j\left[f_k\left(\frac{J_{kj}}{q_j}\right) - f_k(0)\right] + f_k(0)$ we get the desired result.

B Refined upper bound

To derive the upper bound consider first

$$1 + e^x = e^{x/2} + \log(e^{-x/2} + e^{x/2}) \qquad (21)$$

Now, $g(x) = \log(e^{-x/2} + e^{x/2})$ is a symmetric function of x and also a concave function of x^2. Any tangent line for a concave function always remains above the function and so it also serves as an upper bound. Therefore we may bound $g(x)$ by the tangents of $g(\sqrt{y})$ (due to the concavity in x^2). Thus

$$\log(e^{-x/2} + e^{x/2}) \le \frac{\partial g(\sqrt{y})}{\partial y}(x^2 - y) + g(\sqrt{y}) \qquad (22)$$
$$= \lambda(y)x^2 - F(\lambda, y) \qquad (23)$$

where

$$\lambda(y) = \frac{\partial}{\partial y}g(\sqrt{y}) \qquad (24)$$
$$F(\lambda, y) = \lambda(y)\, y - g(\sqrt{y}) \qquad (25)$$

The desired result now follows the change of variables: $y = x_i^2$. Note that the tangent bound is exact whenever $x_i = x$ (a tangent defined at that point).

Combined Weak Classifiers

Chuanyi Ji and Sheng Ma
Department of Electrical, Computer and System Engineering
Rensselaer Polytechnic Institute, Troy, NY 12180
chuanyi@ecse.rpi.edu, shengm@ecse.rpi.edu

Abstract

To obtain classification systems with both good generalization performance and efficiency in space and time, we propose a learning method based on combinations of weak classifiers, where weak classifiers are linear classifiers (perceptrons) which can do a little better than making random guesses. A randomized algorithm is proposed to find the weak classifiers. They are then combined through a majority vote. As demonstrated through systematic experiments, the method developed is able to obtain combinations of weak classifiers with good generalization performance and a fast training time on a variety of test problems and real applications.

1 Introduction

The problem we will investigate in this work is how to develop a classifier with both good generalization performance and efficiency in space and time in a supervised learning environment. The generalization performance is measured by the probability of classification error of a classifier. A classifier is said to be efficient if its size and the (average) time needed to develop such a classifier scale nicely (polynomially) with the dimension of the feature vectors, and other parameters in the training algorithm.

The method we propose to tackle this problem is based on combinations of weak classifiers[8][6], where the weak classifiers are the classifiers which can do a little better than random guessing. It has been shown by Schapire and Freund [8][4] that the computational power of weak classifiers is equivalent to that of a well-trained classifier, and an algorithm has been given to boost the performance of weak classifiers. What has not been investigated is the type of weak classifiers that can be used and how to find them. In practice, the ideas have been applied with success in hand-written character recognition to boost the performance of an already well-trained classifier. But the original idea on combining a large number of weak classifiers has not been used in solving real problems. An independent work by Kleinberg[6] suggests that in addition to a good generalization performance, combinations of weak classifiers also provide advantages in computation time, since weak classifiers are computationally easier to obtain than well-trained classifiers. However, since the proposed method is based on an assumption which is difficult to realize, discrepancies have been found between the theory and the experimental results[7]. The recent work by Breiman[1][2] also suggests that combinations of classifiers can be computationally efficient, especially when used to learn large data sets.

The focus of this work is to investigate the following problems: (1) how to find weak classifiers, (2) what are the performance and efficiency of combinations of weak classifiers, and (3) what are the advantages of using combined weak classifiers compared with other pattern classification methods?

We will develop a randomized algorithm to obtain weak classifiers. We will then provide simulation results on both synthetic real problems to show capabilities and efficiency of combined weak classifiers. The extended version of this work with some of the theoretical analysis can be found in [5].

2 Weak Classifiers

In the present work, we choose linear classifiers (perceptrons) as weak classifiers. Let $\frac{1}{2} - \frac{1}{\nu}$ be the required generalization error of a classifier, where $\nu \geq 2$, is called the weakness factor which is used to characterize the strength of a classifier. The larger the ν, the weaker the weak classifier. A set of weak classifiers are combined through a simple majority vote.

3 Algorithm

Our algorithm for combinations of weak classifiers consists of two steps: (1) generating individual weak classifiers through a simple randomized algorithm; and (2) combining a collection of weak classifiers through a simple majority vote.

Three parameters need to be chosen a priori for the algorithm: a weakness factor ν, a number θ ($\frac{1}{2} \leq \theta < 1$) which will be used as a threshold to partition the training set, and the number of weak classifiers $2L+1$ to be generated, where L is a positive integer.

3.1 Partitioning the Training Set

The method we use to partition a training set is motivated by what given in [4]. Suppose a combined classifier consists of K ($K \geq 1$) weak classifiers already. In order to generate a (new) weak classifier, the entire training set of N training samples is partitioned into two subsets: a set of M_1 samples which contain all the misclassified samples and a small fraction of samples correctly-classified by the existing combined classifier; and the remaining $N - M_1$ training samples. The set of M_1 samples are called "cares", since they will be used to select a new weak classifier, while the rest of the samples are the "don't-cares".

The threshold θ is used to determine which samples should be assigned as cares. For instance, for the n-th training sample ($1 \leq n \leq N$), the performance index $a(n)$ is recorded, where $a(n)$ is the fraction of the weak classifiers in the existing combined classifier which classify the n-th sample correctly. If $a(n) < \theta$, this sample is assigned to the cares. Otherwise, it is a don't-care. This is done for all N samples.

Through partitioning a training set in this way, a newly-generated weak classifier is forced to learn the samples which have not been learned by the existing weak classifiers. In the meantime, a properly-chosen θ can ensure that enough samples are used to obtain each weak classifier.

3.2 Random Sampling

To achieve a fast training time, we obtain a weak classifier by randomly sampling the classifier-space of all possible linear classifiers.

Assume that a feature vector $x \in R^d$ is distributed over a compact region D. The direction of a hyperplane characterized by a linear classifier with a weight vector, is first generated by randomly selecting the elements of the weight vector based on a uniform distribution over $(-1, 1)^d$. Then the threshold of the hyperplane is determined by randomly picking an $x \in D$, and letting the hyperplane pass through x. This will generate random hyperplanes which pass through the region D, and whose directions are randomly distributed in all directions. Such a randomly selected classifier will then be tested on all the cares. If it misclassifies a fraction of cares no more than $\frac{1}{2} - \frac{1}{\nu} - \epsilon$ ($\epsilon > 0$ and small), the classifier is kept and will be used in the combination. Otherwise, it is discarded. This process is repeated until a weak classifier is finally obtained.

A newly-generated weak classifier is then combined with the existing ones through a simple majority vote. The entire training set will then be tested on the combined classifier to result in a new set of cares, and don't-cares. The whole process will be repeated until the total number $2L + 1$ of weak classifiers are generated. The algorithm can be easily extended to multiple classes. Details can be found in [5].

4 Experimental Results

Extensive simulations have been carried out on both synthetic and real problems using our algorithm. One synthetic problem is chosen to test the efficiency of our method. Real applications from standard data bases are selected to compare the generalization performance of combinations of weak classifiers (CW) with that of other methods such as K-Nearest-Neighbor classifiers (K-NN)[1], artificial neural networks (ANN), combinations of neural networks (CNN), and stochastic discriminations (SD).

4.1 A Synthetic Problem: Two Overlapping Gaussians

To test the scaling properties of combinations of weak classifiers, a non-linearly separable problem is chosen from a standard database called ELENA [2]. The problem is a two-class classification problem, where the distributions of samples in both classes are multi-variate Gaussians with the same mean but different variances for each independent variable. There is a considerable amount of overlap between the samples in two classes, and the problem is non-linearly separable. The average generalization error and the standard deviations are given in Figure 1 for our algorithm based on 20 runs, and for other classifiers. The Bayes error is also given to show the theoretical limit. The results show that the performance of kNN degrades very quickly. The performance of ANN is better than that of kNN but still deviates more and more from the Bayes error as d gets large. The combination of weak classifiers

---

[1] The best result of different k is reported.
[2] /pub/neural-nets/ELENA/databases/Benchmarks.ps.Z on ftp.dice.ucl.ac.be

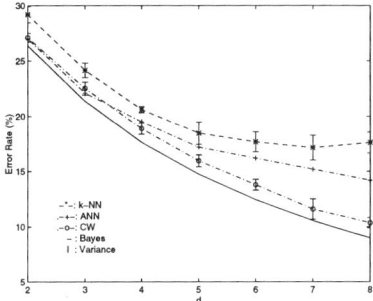

Figure 1: Performance versus the dimension of the feature vectors

Algorithms	Card1	Diabetes1	Gene1
	(%) Error /σ	(%) Error /σ	(%) Error /σ
Combined Weak Classifiers	11.3/ 0.85	22.70 / 0.70	11.80 / 0.52
k Nearest Neighbor	15.67	25.8	22.87
Neural Networks	13.64/ 0.85	23.52/ 0.72	13.47/ 0.44
Combined Neural Networks	13.02/0.33	22.79 /0.57	12.08 / 0.23

Table 1: Performance on Card1, Diabetes1 and Gene1. σ: standard deviation

continues to follow the trend of the Bayes error.

4.2 Proben1 Data Sets

Three data sets, Card1, Diabetes1 and Gene1 were selected to test our algorithm from Proben1 databases which contain data sets from real applications[3].

Card1 data set is for a problem on determining whether a credit-card application from a customer can be approved based on information given in 51-dimensional feature vectors. 345 out of 690 examples are used for training and the rest for testing. Diabetes1 data set is for determining whether diabetes is present based on 8-dimensional input patterns. 384 examples are used for training and the same number of samples for testing. Gene1 data set is for deciding whether a DNA sequence is from a donor, an acceptor or neither from 120 dimensional binary feature vectors. 1588 samples out of total of 3175 were used for training, and the rest for testing.

The average generalization error as well as the standard deviations are reported in Table 1. The results from combinations of weak classifiers are based on 25 runs. The results of neural networks and combinations of well-trained neural networks are from the database. As demonstrated by the results, combinations of weak classifiers have been able to achieve the generalization performance comparable to or better than that of combinations of well-trained neural networks.

4.3 Hand-written Digit Recognition

Hand-written digit recognition is chosen to test our algorithm, since one of the previously developed method on combinations of weak classifiers (stochastic discrimination[6]) was applied to this problem. For the purpose of comparison, the

---

[3] Available by anonymous ftp from ftp.ira.uka.de, as /pub/papers/techreports/1994/1994-21.ps.z.

Algorithms	(%) Error/σ
Combined Weak Classifiers	4.23 / 0.1
k Nearest Neighbor	4.84
Neural Networks	5.33
Stochastic Discriminations	3.92

Table 2: Performance on handwritten digit recognition.

Parameters	Gaussians	Card1	Diabetes1	Gene1	Digits
$1/2 + 1/\nu$	0.51	0.51	0.51	0.55	0.54
θ	0.51	0.51	0.54	0.54	0.53
2L+1	2000	1000	1000	4000	20000
Average Tries	2	3	7	4	2

Table 3: Parameters used in our experiments.

same set of data as used in [6](from the NIST data base) is utilized to train and to test our algorithm. The data set contains 10000 digits written by different people. Each digit is represented by 16 by 16 black and white pixels. The first 4997 digits are used to form a training set, and the rest are for testing. Performance of our algorithm, k-NN, neural networks, and stochastic discriminations are given in Table 2. The results for our methods are based on 5 runs, while the results for the other methods are from [6]. The results show that the performance of our algorithm is slightly worse (by 0.3%) than that of stochastic discriminations, which uses a different method for multi-class classification[6].

4.4 Effects of The Weakness Factor

Experiments are done to test the effects of ν on the problem of two 8-dimensional overlapping Gaussians. The performance and the average training time (CPU-time on Sun Spac-10) of combined weak classifiers based on 10 runs are given for different ν's in Figures 2 and 3, respectively. The results indicate as ν increases an individual weak classifier is obtained more quickly, but more weak classifiers are needed to achieve good performance. When a proper ν is chosen, a nice scaling property can be observed in training time.

A record of the parameters used in all the experiments on real applications are provided in Table 3. The average tries, which are the average number of times needed to sample the classifier space to obtain an acceptable weak classifier, are also given in the table to characterize the training time for these problems.

4.5 Training Time

To compare learning time with off-line BackPropagation (BP), feedforward two layer neural network with 10 sigmoidal hidden units are trained by gradient-descent to learn the problem on the two 8-dimensional overlapping Gaussians. 2500 training samples are used. The performance versus CPU time[4] are plotted for both our algorithm and BP in Figure 4. For our algorithm, 2000 weak classifiers are combined. For BP, 1000 epoches are used. The figure shows that our algorithm is much faster than the BP algorithm. Moreover, when several well-trained neural networks are combined to achieve a better performance, the cost on training time will be

---
[4] Both algorithms are run on a Sun Sparc-10 sun workstation

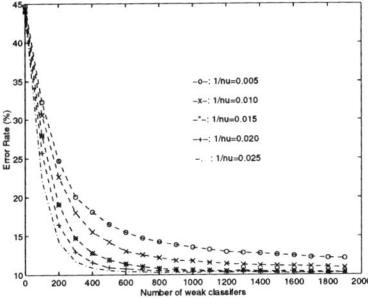

Figure 2: Performance versus the number of weak classifiers for different ν. nu: ν.

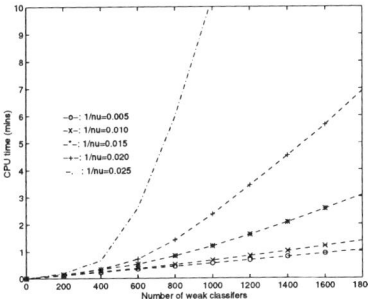

Figure 3: Training time versus the number of weak classifiers for different ν.

even higher. Therefore, compared to combinations of well-trained neural networks, combining weak classifiers is computationally much cheaper.

5 Discussions

From the experimental results, we observe that the performance of the combined weak classifiers is comparable or even better than combinations of well-trained classifiers, and out-performs individual neural network classifiers and k-Nearest Neighbor classifiers. In the meantime whereas the k-nearest neighbor classifiers suffer from the curse of dimensionality, a nice scaling property in terms of the dimension of feature vectors has been observed for combined weak classifiers. Another

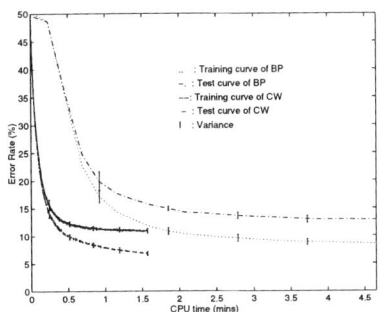

Figure 4: Performance versus CPU time

important observation obtained from the experiments is that the weakness factor directly impacts the size of a combined classifier and the training time. Therefore, the choice of the weakness factor is important to obtain efficient combined weak classifiers. It has been shown in our theoretical analysis on learning an underlying perceptron [5] that ν should be at least large as $O(dlnd)$ to obtain a polynomial training time, and the price paid to accomplish this is a space-complexity which is polynomial in d as well. This cost can be observed from our experimental results for the need of a large number of weak classifiers.

Acknowledgement

Specials thanks are due to Tin Kan Ho for providing NIST data, related references and helpful discussions. Support from the National Science Foundation (ECS-9312594 and (CAREER) IRI-9502518) is gratefully acknowledged.

References

[1] L. Breiman, "Bias, Variance and Arcing Classifiers," *Technical Report, TR-460, Department of Statistics, University of California, Berkeley*, April, 1996.

[2] L. Breiman, "Pasting, Bites Together for Prediction in Large Data sets and On-Line," ftp.stat.berkeley.edu/users/breiman, 1996.

[3] H. Drucker, R. Schapire and P. Simard, "Improving Performance in Neural Networks Using a Boosting Algorithm," *Neural Information Processing Symposium*, 42-49, 1993.

[4] Y. Freund and R. Schapire, "A Decision-Theoretic Generalization of On-Line Learning and An Application to Boosting," http://www.research.att.com/orgs/ssr/people/yoav or schapire.

[5] C. Ji and S. Ma, "Combinations of Weak Classifiers," *IEEE Trans. Neural Networks, Special Issue on Neural Networks and Pattern Recognition*, vol. 8, 32-42, Jan., 1997.

[6] E.M. Kleinberg, "Stochastic Discrimination," *Annals of Mathematics and Artificial Intelligence*, vol.1, 207-239, 1990.

[7] E.M. Kleinberg and T. Ho, "Pattern Recognition by Stochastic Modeling," *Proceedings of the Third International Workshop on Frontiers in Handwriting Recognition*, 175-183, Buffalo, May 1993.

[8] R.E. Schapire, "The Strength of Weak Learnability," *Machine Learning*, vol. 5, 197-227, 1990.

Hidden Markov decision trees

Michael I. Jordan*, Zoubin Ghahramani†, and Lawrence K. Saul*
{jordan,zoubin,lksaul}@psyche.mit.edu

*Center for Biological and Computational Learning
Massachusetts Institute of Technology
Cambridge, MA USA 02139

†Department of Computer Science
University of Toronto
Toronto, ON Canada M5S 1A4

Abstract

We study a time series model that can be viewed as a decision tree with Markov temporal structure. The model is intractable for exact calculations, thus we utilize variational approximations. We consider three different distributions for the approximation: one in which the Markov calculations are performed exactly and the layers of the decision tree are decoupled, one in which the decision tree calculations are performed exactly and the time steps of the Markov chain are decoupled, and one in which a Viterbi-like assumption is made to pick out a single most likely state sequence. We present simulation results for artificial data and the Bach chorales.

1 Introduction

Decision trees are regression or classification models that are based on a nested decomposition of the input space. An input vector **x** is classified recursively by a set of "decisions" at the nonterminal nodes of a tree, resulting in the choice of a terminal node at which an output **y** is generated. A statistical approach to decision tree modeling was presented by Jordan and Jacobs (1994), where the decisions were treated as hidden multinomial random variables and a likelihood was computed by summing over these hidden variables. This approach, as well as earlier statistical analyses of decision trees, was restricted to independently, identically distributed data. The goal of the current paper is to remove this restriction; we describe a generalization of the decision tree statistical model which is appropriate for time series.

The basic idea is straightforward—we assume that each decision in the decision tree is dependent on the decision taken at that node at the previous time step. Thus we augment the decision tree model to include Markovian dynamics for the decisions.

For simplicity we restrict ourselves to the case in which the decision variable at a given nonterminal is dependent only on the same decision variable at the same nonterminal at the previous time step. It is of interest, however, to consider more complex models in which inter-nonterminal pathways allow for the possibility of various kinds of synchronization.

Why should the decision tree model provide a useful starting point for time series modeling? The key feature of decision trees is the nested decomposition. If we view each nonterminal node as a basis function, with support given by the subset of possible input vectors $\mathbf{x}$ that arrive at the node, then the support of each node is the union of the support associated with its children. This is reminiscent of wavelets, although without the strict condition of multiplicative scaling. Moreover, the regions associated with the decision tree are polygons, which would seem to provide a useful generalization of wavelet-like decompositions in the case of a high-dimensional input space.

The architecture that we describe in the current paper is fully probabilistic. We view the decisions in the decision tree as multinomial random variables, and we are concerned with calculating the posterior probabilities of the time sequence of hidden decisions given a time sequence of input and output vectors. Although such calculations are tractable for decision trees and for hidden Markov models separately, the calculation is intractable for our model. Thus we must make use of approximations. We utilize the partially factorized variational approximations described by Saul and Jordan (1996), which allow tractable substructures (e.g., the decision tree and Markov chain substructures) to be handled via exact methods, within an overall approximation that guarantees a lower bound on the log likelihood.

2 Architectures

2.1 Probabilistic decision trees

The "hierarchical mixture of experts" (HME) model (Jordan & Jacobs, 1994) is a decision tree in which the decisions are modeled probabilistically, as are the outputs. The total probability of an output given an input is the sum over all paths in the tree from the input to the output. The HME model is shown in the graphical model formalism in Figure 2.1. Here a node represents a random variable, and the links represent probabilistic dependencies. A conditional probability distribution is associated with each node in the graph, where the conditioning variables are the node's parents.

Let $\mathbf{z}^1$, $\mathbf{z}^2$, and $\mathbf{z}^3$ denote the (multinomial) random variables corresponding to the first, second and third levels of the decision tree.[1] We associate multinomial probabilities $P(\mathbf{z}^1|\mathbf{x}, \eta^1)$, $P(\mathbf{z}^2|\mathbf{x}, \mathbf{z}^1, \eta^2)$, and $P(\mathbf{z}^3|\mathbf{x}, \mathbf{z}^1, \mathbf{z}^2, \eta^3)$ with the decision nodes, where η^1, η^2, and η^3 are parameters (e.g., Jordan and Jacobs utilized softmax transformations of linear functions of $\mathbf{x}$ for these probabilities). The leaf probabilities $P(\mathbf{y}|\mathbf{x}, \mathbf{z}^1, \mathbf{z}^2, \mathbf{z}^3, \theta)$ are arbitrary conditional probability models; e.g., linear/Gaussian models for regression problems.

The key calculation in the fitting of the HME model to data is the calculation of the posterior probabilities of the hidden decisions given the clamped values of $\mathbf{x}$ and $\mathbf{y}$. This calculation is a recursion extending upward and downward in the tree, in which the posterior probability at a given nonterminal is the sum of posterior probabilities associated with its children. The recursion can be viewed as a special

---

[1] Throughout the paper we restrict ourselves to three levels for simplicity of presentation.

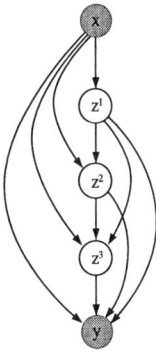

Figure 1: The hierarchical mixture of experts as a graphical model. The E step of the learning algorithm for HME's involves calculating the posterior probabilities of the hidden (unshaded) variables given the observed (shaded) variables.

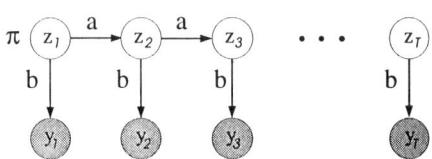

Figure 2: An HMM as a graphical model. The transition matrix appears on the horizontal links and the output probability distribution on the vertical links. The E step of the learning algorithm for HMM's involves calculating the posterior probabilities of the hidden (unshaded) variables given the observed (shaded) variables.

case of generic algorithms for calculating posterior probabilities on directed graphs (see, e.g., Shachter, 1990).

2.2 Hidden Markov models

In the graphical model formalism a hidden Markov model (HMM; Rabiner, 1989) is represented as a chain structure as shown in Figure 2.1. Each state node is a multinomial random variable z_t. The links between the state nodes are parameterized by the transition matrix $a(z_t|z_{t-1})$, assumed homogeneous in time. The links between the state nodes z_t and output nodes y_t are parameterized by the output probability distribution $b(y_t|z_t)$, which in the current paper we assume to be Gaussian with (tied) covariance matrix Σ.

As in the HME model, the key calculation in the fitting of the HMM to observed data is the calculation of the posterior probabilities of the hidden state nodes given the sequence of output vectors. This calculation—the E step of the Baum-Welch algorithm—is a recursion which proceeds forward or backward in the chain.

2.3 Hidden Markov decision trees

We now marry the HME and the HMM to produce the hidden Markov decision tree (HMDT) shown in Figure 3. This architecture can be viewed in one of two ways: (a) as a time sequence of decision trees in which the decisions in a given decision tree depend probabilistically on the decisions in the decision tree at the preceding moment in time; (b) as an HMM in which the state variable at each moment in time is factorized (cf. Ghahramani & Jordan, 1996) and the factors are coupled vertically to form a decision tree structure.

Let the state of the Markov process defining the HMDT be given by the values of hidden multinomial decisions z_t^1, z_t^2, and z_t^3, where the superscripts denote the level of the decision tree (the vertical dimension) and the subscripts denote the time (the horizontal dimension). Given our assumption that the state transition matrix has only intra-level Markovian dependencies, we obtain the following expression for the

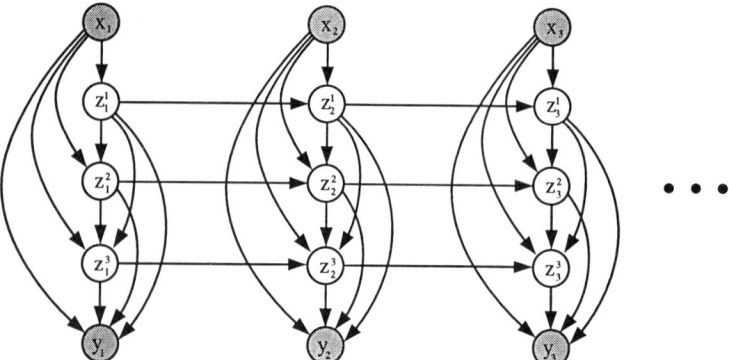

Figure 3: The HMDT model is an HME decision tree (in the vertical dimension) with Markov time dependencies (in the horizontal dimension).

HMDT probability model:

$$P(\{z_t^1, z_t^2, z_t^3\}, \{y_t\}|\{x_t\}) = \pi^1(z_1^1|x_1)\pi^2(z_1^2|x_1, z_1^1)\pi^3(z_1^3|x_1, z_1^1, z_1^2)$$
$$\prod_{t=2}^{T} a^1(z_t^1|x_t, z_{t-1}^1)a^2(z_t^2|x_t, z_{t-1}^2, z_t^1)a^3(z_t^3|x_t, z_{t-1}^3, z_t^1, z_t^2) \prod_{t=1}^{T} b(y_t|x_t, z_t^1, z_t^2, z_t^3)$$

Summing this probability over the hidden values z_t^1, z_t^2, and z_t^3 yields the HMDT likelihood.

The HMDT is a 2-D lattice with inhomogeneous field terms (the observed data). It is well-known that such lattice structures are intractable for exact probabilistic calculations. Thus, although it is straightforward to write down the EM algorithm for the HMDT and to write recursions for the calculations of posterior probabilities in the E step, these calculations are likely to be too time-consuming for practical use (for T time steps, K values per node and M levels, the algorithm scales as $O(K^{M+1}T)$). Thus we turn to methods that allow us to approximate the posterior probabilities of interest.

3 Algorithms

3.1 Partially factorized variational approximations

Completely factorized approximations to probability distributions on graphs can often be obtained variationally as mean field theories in physics (Parisi, 1988). For the HMDT in Figure 3, the completely factorized mean field approximation would delink all of the nodes, replacing the interactions with constant fields acting at each of the nodes. This approximation, although useful, neglects to take into account the existence of efficient algorithms for tractable substructures in the graph.

Saul and Jordan (1996) proposed a refined mean field approximation to allow interactions associated with tractable substructures to be taken into account. The basic idea is to associate with the intractable distribution P a simplified distribution Q that retains certain of the terms in P and neglects others, replacing them with parameters μ_i that we will refer to as "variational parameters." Graphically the method can be viewed as deleting arcs from the original graph until a forest of tractable substructures is obtained. Arcs that remain in the simplified graph correspond to terms that are retained in Q; arcs that are deleted correspond to variational parameters.

To obtain the best possible approximation of P we minimize the Kullback-Liebler divergence $KL(Q||P)$ with respect to the parameters μ_i. The result is a coupled set of equations that are solved iteratively. These equations make reference to the values of expectations of nodes in the tractable substructures; thus the (efficient) algorithms that provide such expectations are run as subroutines. Based on the posterior expectations computed under Q, the parameters defining P are adjusted. The algorithm as a whole is guaranteed to increase a lower bound on the log likelihood.

3.2 A forest of chains

The HMDT can be viewed as a coupled set of chains, with couplings induced directly via the decision tree structure and indirectly via the common coupling to the output vector. If these couplings are removed in the variational approximation, we obtain a Q distribution whose graph is a forest of chains. There are several ways to parameterize this graph; in the current paper we investigate a parameterization with time-varying transition matrices and time-varying fields. Thus the Q distribution is given by

$$Q(\{z_t^1, z_t^2, z_t^3\} \mid \{y_t\}, \{x_t\}) = \frac{1}{Z_Q} \prod_{t=2}^{T} \tilde{a}_t^1(z_t^1|z_{t-1}^1) \tilde{a}_t^2(z_t^2|z_{t-1}^2) \tilde{a}_t^3(z_t^3|z_{t-1}^3)$$

$$\prod_{t=1}^{T} \tilde{q}_t^1(z_t^1) \tilde{q}_t^2(z_t^2) \tilde{q}_t^3(z_t^3)$$

where $\tilde{a}_t^i(z_t^i|z_{t-1}^i)$ and $\tilde{q}_t^i(z_t^i)$ are potentials that provide the variational parameterization.

3.3 A forest of decision trees

Alternatively we can drop the horizontal couplings in the HMDT and obtain a variational approximation in which the decision tree structure is handled exactly and the Markov structure is approximated. The Q distribution in this case is

$$Q(\{z_t^1, z_t^2, z_t^3\} \mid \{y_t\}, \{x_t\}) = \prod_{t=1}^{T} \tilde{r}_t^1(z_1^1) \tilde{r}_t^2(z_1^2|z_1^1) \tilde{r}_t^3(z_1^3|z_1^1, z_1^2)$$

Note that a decision tree is a fully coupled graphical model; thus we can view the partially factorized approximation in this case as a completely factorized mean field approximation on "super-nodes" whose configurations include all possible configurations of the decision tree.

3.4 A Viterbi-like approximation

In hidden Markov modeling it is often found that a particular sequence of states has significantly higher probability than any other sequence. In such cases the Viterbi algorithm, which calculates only the most probable path, provides a useful computational alternative.

We can develop a Viterbi-like algorithm by utilizing an approximation Q that assigns probability one to a single path $\{\bar{z}_t^1, \bar{z}_t^2, \bar{z}_t^3\}$:

$$Q(\{z_t^1, z_t^2, z_t^3\} \mid \{y_t\}, \{x_t\}) = \begin{cases} 1 & \text{if } z_t^i = \bar{z}_t^i, \ \forall t, i \\ 0 & \text{otherwise} \end{cases} \quad (1)$$

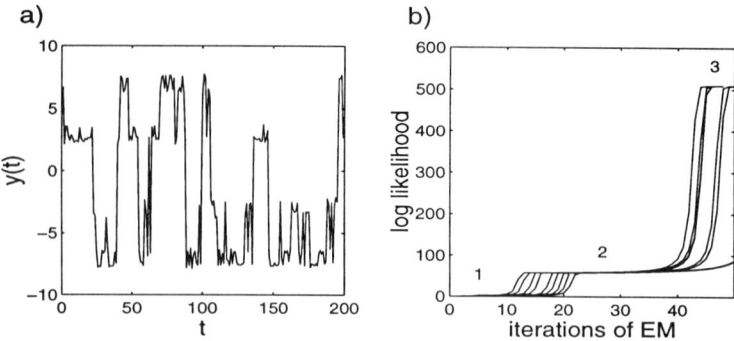

Figure 4: a) Artificial time series data. b) Learning curves for the HMDT.

Note that the entropy $Q \ln Q$ is zero, moreover the evaluation of the energy $Q \ln P$ reduces to substituting $\bar{z}_t^i$ for z_t^i in P. Thus the variational approximation is particularly simple in this case. The resulting algorithm involves a subroutine in which a standard Viterbi algorithm is run on a single chain, with the other (fixed) chains providing field terms.

4 Results

We illustrate the HMDT on (1) an artificial time series generated to exhibit spatial and temporal structure at multiple scales, and (2) a domain which is likely to exhibit such structure naturally—the melody lines from J.S. Bach's chorales.

The artificial data was generated from a three level binary HMDT with no inputs, in which the root node determined coarse-scale shifts (± 5) in the time series, the middle node determined medium-scale shifts (± 2), and the bottom node determined fine-scale shifts (± 0.5) (Figure 4a). The temporal scales at these three nodes—as measured by the rate of convergence (second eigenvalue) of the transition matrices, with 0 (1) signifying immediate (no) convergence—were 0.85, 0.5, and 0.3, respectively.

We implemented forest-of-chains, forest-of-trees and Viterbi-like approximations. The learning curves for ten runs of the forest-of-chains approximation are shown in Figure 4b. Three plateau regions are apparent, corresponding to having extracted the coarse, medium, and fine scale structures of the time series. Five runs captured all three spatio-temporal scales at their correct level in the hierarchy; three runs captured the scales but placed them at incorrect nodes in the decision tree; and two captured only the coarse-scale structure.[2] Similar results were obtained with the Viterbi-like approximation. We found that the forest-of-trees approximation was not sufficiently accurate for these data.

The Bach chorales dataset consists of 30 melody lines with 40 events each.[3] Each discrete event encoded 6 attributes—start time of the event (st), pitch (pitch), duration (dur), key signature (key), time signature (time), and whether the event was under a fermata (ferm).

The chorales dataset was modeled with 3-level HMDTs with branching factors (K)

---

[2] Note that it is possible to bias the ordering of the time scales by ordering the initial random values for the nodes of the tree; we did not utilize such a bias in this simulation.

[3] This dataset was obtained from the UCI Repository of Machine Learning Datasets.

	Percent variance explained						Temporal scale		
K	st	pitch	dur	key	time	ferm	level 1	level 2	level 3
2	3	6	6	84	95	0	1.00	1.00	0.51
3	22	38	7	93	99	0	1.00	0.96	0.85
4	55	48	36	96	99	5	1.00	1.00	0.69
5	57	41	41	97	99	61	1.00	0.95	0.75
6	70	40	58	94	99	10	1.00	0.93	0.76

Table 1: Hidden Markov decision tree models of the Bach chorales dataset: mean percentage of variance explained for each attribute and mean temporal scales at the different nodes.

2, 3, 4, 5, and 6 (3 runs at each size, summarized in Table 1). Thirteen out of 15 runs resulted in a coarse-to-fine progression of temporal scales from root to leaves of the tree. A typical run at branching factor 4, for example, dedicated the top level node to modeling the time and key signatures—attributes that are constant throughout any single chorale—the middle node to modeling start times, and the bottom node to modeling pitch or duration.

5 Conclusions

Viewed in the context of the burgeoning literature on adaptive graphical probabilistic models—which includes HMM's, HME's, CVQ's, IOHMM's (Bengio & Frasconi, 1995), and factorial HMM's—the HMDT would appear to be a natural next step. The HMDT includes as special cases all of these architectures, moreover it arguably combines their best features: factorized state spaces, conditional densities, representation at multiple levels of resolution and recursive estimation algorithms. Our work on the HMDT is in its early stages, but the earlier literature provides a reasonably secure foundation for its development.

References

Bengio, Y., & Frasconi, P. (1995). An input output HMM architecture. In G. Tesauro, D. S. Touretzky & T. K. Leen, (Eds.), *Advances in Neural Information Processing Systems 7*, MIT Press, Cambridge MA.

Ghahramani, Z., & Jordan, M. I. (1996). Factorial hidden Markov models. In D. S. Touretzky, M. C. Mozer, & M. E. Hasselmo (Eds.), *Advances in Neural Information Processing Systems 8*, MIT Press, Cambridge MA.

Jordan, M. I., & Jacobs, R. A. (1994). Hierarchical mixtures of experts and the EM algorithm. *Neural Computation, 6*, 181–214.

Parisi, G. (1988). *Statistical Field Theory*. Redwood City, CA: Addison-Wesley.

Rabiner, L. (1989). A tutorial on hidden Markov models and selected application s in speech recognition. *Proceedings of the IEEE, 77*, 257–285.

Saul, L. K., & Jordan, M. I. (1996). Exploiting tractable substructures in intractable networks. In D. S. Touretzky, M. C. Mozer, & M. E. Hasselmo (Eds.), *Advances in Neural Information Processing Systems 8*, MIT Press, Cambridge MA.

Shachter, R. (1990). An ordered examination of influence diagrams. *Networks, 20*, 535–563.

Unification of Information Maximization and Minimization

Ryotaro Kamimura
Information Science Laboratory
Tokai University
1117 Kitakaname Hiratsuka Kanagawa 259-12, Japan
E-mail: ryo@cc.u-tokai.ac.jp

Abstract

In the present paper, we propose a method to unify information maximization and minimization in hidden units. The information maximization and minimization are performed on two different levels: collective and individual level. Thus, two kinds of information: collective and individual information are defined. By maximizing collective information and by minimizing individual information, simple networks can be generated in terms of the number of connections and the number of hidden units. Obtained networks are expected to give better generalization and improved interpretation of internal representations. This method was applied to the inference of the maximum onset principle of an artificial language. In this problem, it was shown that the individual information minimization is not contradictory to the collective information maximization. In addition, experimental results confirmed improved generalization performance, because over-training can significantly be suppressed.

1 Introduction

There have been many attempts to interpret neural networks from the information theoretical point of view [2], [4], [5]. Applied to the supervised learning, information has been maximized and minimized, depending on problems. In these methods, information is defined by the outputs of hidden units. Thus, the methods aim to control hidden unit activity patterns in an optimal manner. Information maximization methods have been used to interpret explicitly internal representations and simultaneously to reduce the number of necessary hidden units [5]. On the other hand, information minimization methods have been especially used to improve generalization performance [2], [4] and to speed up learning. Thus, if it is possible to maximize and minimize information simultaneously, information theoretic methods are expected to be applied to a wide range of problems.

In this paper, we unify the above mentioned two methods, namely, information maximization and minimization methods, into one framework to improve generalization performance and to interpret explicitly internal representations. However, it is apparently impossible to maximize and minimize simultaneously the information defined by the hidden unit activity. Our goal is to maximize and to minimize information on two different levels, namely, collective and individual levels. This means that information can be maximized in collective ways and information is minimized for individual input-hidden connections. The seeming contradictory proposition of the simultaneous information maximization and minimization can be overcome by assuming the existence of the two levels for the information control.

Information is supposed to be controlled by an information controller located outside neural networks and used exclusively to control information. By assuming the information controller, we can clearly see how information appropriately defined can be maximized or minimized. In addition, the actual implementation of information methods is much easier by introducing a concept of the information controller.

2 Concept of Information

In this section, we explain a concept of information in a general framework of an information theory. Let Y take on a finite number of possible values $y_1, y_2, ..., y_M$ with probabilities $p(y_1), p(y_2), ..., p(y_M)$, respectively. Then, initial uncertainty $H(Y)$ of a random variable Y is defined by

$$H(Y) = -\sum_{j=1}^{M} p(y_j) \log p(y_j). \tag{1}$$

Now, consider conditional uncertainty after the observation of another random variable X, taking possible values $x_1, x_2, ..., x_S$ with probabilities $p(x_1), p(x_2), ..., p(x_M)$, respectively. Conditional uncertainty $H(Y \mid X)$ can be defined as

$$H(Y \mid X) = \sum_{s=1}^{S} p(x_s) \sum_{j=1}^{M} p(y_j \mid x_s) \log p(x_j \mid y_s). \tag{2}$$

We can easily verify that conditional uncertainty is always less than or equal to initial uncertainty. Information is usually defined as the decrease of this uncertainty [1].

$$\begin{aligned}
I(Y \mid X) &= H(Y) - H(Y \mid X) \\
&= -\sum_{j=1}^{M} p(y_j) \log p(y_j) + \sum_{s=1}^{S} p(x_s) \sum_{j=1}^{M} p(y_j \mid x_s) \log p(y_j \mid x_s) \\
&= \sum_{s} \sum_{j} p(x_s) p(y_j \mid x_s) \log \frac{p(y_j \mid x_s)}{p(y_j)} \\
&= \sum_{s} p(x_s) I(Y \mid x_s)
\end{aligned} \tag{3}$$

where

$$I(Y \mid x_s) = \sum_{j} p(y_j \mid x_s) \log \frac{p(y_j \mid x_s)}{p(y_j)}$$

$$= -\sum_j p(y_j \mid x_s) \log p(y_j) + \sum_j p(y_j \mid x_s) \log p(y_j \mid x_s), \quad (4)$$

which is referred to as conditional information. Especially, when prior uncertainty is maximum, that is, a prior probability is equi-probable $(1/M)$, then information is

$$I(Y \mid X) = \log M + \sum_{s=1}^{S} p(x_s) \sum_{j=1}^{M} p(y_j \mid x_s) \log p(y_j \mid x_s) \quad (5)$$

where $\log M$ is maximum uncertainty concering A.

3 Formulation of Information Controller

In this section, we apply a concept of information to actual network architectures and define collective information and individual information. The notation in the above section is changed into ordinary notation used in the neural network.

3.1 Unification by Information Controller

Two kinds of information, collective information and individual information, are controlled by using an information controller. The information controller is devised to interpret the mechanism of the information maximization and minimization more explicitly. As shown in Figure 1, the information controller is composed of two subcomponents, that is, an individual information minimizer and collective information maximizer. A collective information maximizer is used to increase collective information as much as possible. An individual information minimizer is used to decrease individual information. By this minimization, the majority of connections are pushed toward zero. Eventually, all the hidden units tend to be intermediately activated. Thus, when the collective information maximizer and individual information maximizer are simultaneously applied, a hidden unit activity pattern is a pattern of the maximum information in which only one hidden unit is on, while all the other hidden units are off. However, multiple strongly negative connections to produce a maximum information state, are replaced by extremely weak input-hidden connections. Strongly negative connections are inhibited by the individual information minimization. This means that by the information controller, information can be maximized and at the same time one of the most important properties of the information minimization, namely, weight decay or weight elimination, can approximately be realized. Consequently, the information controller can generate much simplified networks in terms of hidden units and in terms of input-hidden connections.

3.2 Collective Information Maximizer

A neural network to be controlled is composed of input, hidden and output units with bias, as shown in Figure 1. The jth hidden unit receives a net input from input units and at the same time from a collective information maximizer:

$$u_j^s = x_j + \sum_{k=0}^{L} w_{jk} \xi_k^s \quad (6)$$

where x_j is an information maximizer from the jth collective information maximizer to the jth hidden unit, L is the number of input units, w_{jk} is a connection from the kth input unit to the jth hidden unit and ξ_k^s is the kth element of the sth input

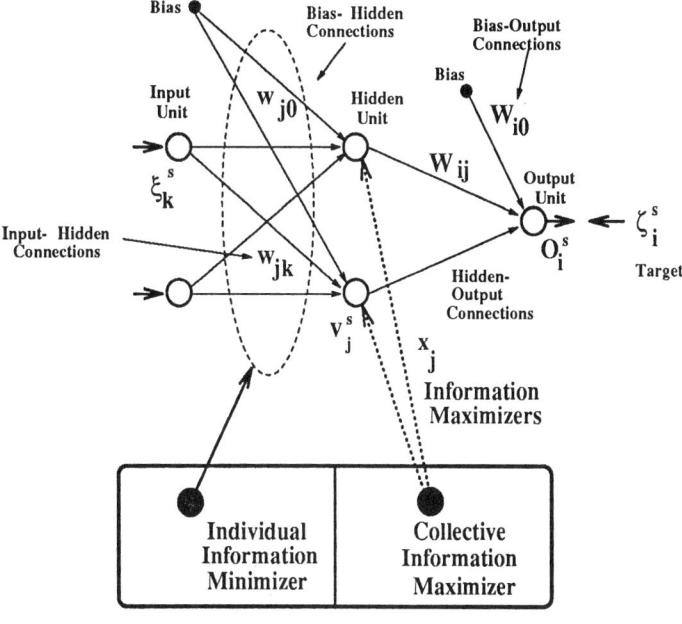

Figure 1: A network architecture, realizing the information controller.

pattern. The jth hidden unit produces an activity or an output by a sigmoidal activation function:

$$v_j^s = f(u_j^s)$$
$$= \frac{1}{1+\exp(-u_j^s)}. \quad (7)$$

The collective information maximizer is used to maximize the information contained in hidden units. For this purpose, we should define collective information. Now, suppose that in the previous formulation in information, a symbol X and Y represent a set of input patterns and hidden units respectively. Then, let us approximate a probability $p(y_j \mid x_s)$ by a normalized output p_j^s of the jth hidden unit computed by

$$p_j^s = \frac{v_j^s}{\sum_{m=1}^{M} v_m^s} \quad (8)$$

where the summation is over all the hidden units. Then, it is reasonable to suppose that at an initial stage all the hidden units are activated randomly or uniformly and all the input patterns are also randomly given to networks. Thus, a probability $p(y_j)$ of the activation of hidden units at the initial stage is equi-probable, that is, $1/M$. A probability $p(x_s)$ of input patterns is also supposed to be equi-probable, namely, $1/S$. Thus, information in the equation (3) is rewritten as

$$I(Y \mid X) \approx -\sum_{j=1}^{M} \frac{1}{M} \log \frac{1}{M} + \frac{1}{S}\sum_{s=1}^{S}\sum_{j=1}^{M} p_j^s \log p_j^s$$

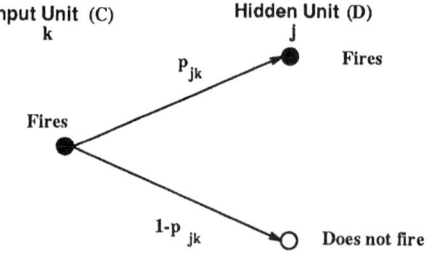

Figure 2: An interpretation of an input-hidden connection for defining the individual information.

$$= \log M + \frac{1}{S}\sum_{s=1}^{S}\sum_{j=1}^{M} p_j^s \log p_j^s \qquad (9)$$

where $\log M$ is maximum uncertainty. This information is considered to be the information acquired in a course of learning. Information maximizers are updated to increase collective information. For obtaining update rules, we should differentiate the information function with respect to information maximizers x_j:

$$\Delta x_j = \beta S \frac{\partial I(Y\mid X)}{\partial x_j}$$

$$= \beta \sum_{s=1}^{S}\left(\log p_j^s - \sum_{m=1}^{M} p_m^s \log p_m^s\right) p_j^s (1 - v_j^s) \qquad (10)$$

where β is a parameter.

3.3 Individual Information Minimization

For representing individual information by a concept of information discussed in the previous section, we consider an output p_{jk} from the jth hidden unit only with a connection from the kth input unit to the jth output unit:

$$p_{jk} = f(w_{jk}) \qquad (11)$$

which is supposed to be a probability of the firing of the jth hidden unit, given the firing of the kth input unit, as shown in Figure 2. Since this probability is considered to be a probability, given the firing of the kth input unit, conditional information is appropriate for measuring the information. In addition, it is reasonable to suppose that a probability of the firing of the jth hidden unit is $1/2$ at an initial stage of learning, because we have no knowledge on hidden units. Thus, conditional information for a pair of the kth unit and the jth hidden unit is formulated as

$$I_{jk}(D\mid fires) \approx -p_{jk}\log\frac{1}{2} - (1-p_{jk})\log\left(1-\frac{1}{2}\right)$$
$$+ p_{jk}\log p_{jk} + (1-p_{jk})\log(1-p_{jk})$$
$$= \log 2 + p_{jk}\log p_{jk} + (1-p_{jk})\log(1-p_{jk}) \qquad (12)$$

If connections are close to zero, this function is close to minimum information, meaning that it is impossible to estimate the firing of the kth hidden unit. If

Table 1: An example of obtained input-hidden connections w_{jk} by the information controller. The parameter β, μ and η were 0.015, 0.0008, and 0.01.

Hidden Units v_j^s	Input Units ξ_k^s				Bias w_{j0}	Information Maximizer x_j
	1	2	3	4		
1	3.09	10.77	26.48	13.82	22.07	-60.88
2	-3.35	0.11	0.33	-3.08	-0.95	1.63
3	-0.01	0.00	0.00	-0.01	0.00	-10.93
4	0.00	0.00	0.00	0.00	0.00	-10.94
5	0.00	0.00	-0.01	0.00	0.00	-10.97
6	0.02	0.01	-0.04	0.01	0.06	-12.01
7	0.00	0.00	-0.01	0.00	0.00	-11.01
8	0.00	0.00	-0.01	0.00	0.00	-11.00
9	0.02	0.01	-0.03	0.01	0.03	-11.61
10	0.01	0.00	-0.02	0.00	0.07	-11.67

connections are larger, the information is larger and correlation between input and hidden units is larger. Total individual information is the sum of all the individual individual information, namely,

$$I(D \mid fires) = \sum_{j=1}^{M} \sum_{k=0}^{L} I_{jk}(D \mid fires), \qquad (13)$$

because each connection is treated separately or independently. The individual information minimization directly controls the input-hidden connections. By differentiating the individual information function and a cross entropy cost function with respect to input-hidden connections w_{jk}, we have rules for updating concerning input-hidden connections:

$$\begin{aligned} \Delta w_{jk} &= -\mu \frac{\partial I(D \mid fires)}{\partial w_{jk}} - \eta \frac{\partial G}{\partial w_{jk}} \\ &= -\mu\, w_{jk}\, p_{jk}(1 - p_{jk}) + \eta \sum_{s=1}^{S} \delta_j^s \xi_k^s \end{aligned} \qquad (14)$$

where δ_j^s is an ordinary delta for the cross entropy function and η and μ are parameters. Thus, rules for updating with respect to input-hidden connections are closely related to the weight decay method. Clearly, as the individual information minimization corresponds to diminishing the strength of input-hidden connections.

4 Results and Discussion

The information controller was applied to the segmentation of strings of an artificial language into appropriate minimal elements, that is, syllables. Table 1 shows input-hidden connections with the bias and the information maximizers. Hidden units were ordered by the magnitude of the relevance of each hidden unit [6]. Collective information and individual information could sufficiently be maximized and minimized. Relative collective and individual information were 0.94 and 0.13. In this state, all the input-hidden connections except connections into the first two hidden units are almost zero. Information maximizers x_j are all strongly negative for these cases. These negative information maximizers make eight hidden units (from the third to tenth hidden unit) inactive, that is, close to zero. By carefully

Table 2: Generalization performance comparison for 200 and 200 training patterns. Averages in the table are average generalization errors over seven errors of ten errors with ten different initial values.

(a) 200 patterns

Methods	Generalization Errors			
	RMS		Error Rates	
	Averages	Std. Dev.	Averages	Std. Dev.
Standard	0.188	0.010	0.087	0.015
Weight Decay	0.183	0.004	0.082	0.009
Weight Elimination	0.172	0.014	0.064	0.015
Information Controller	0.167	0.011	0.052	0.008

(b) 300 patterns

Methods	Generalization Errors			
	RMS		Error Rates	
	Averages	Std. Dev.	Averages	Std. Dev.
Standard	0.108	0.009	0.024	0.009
Weight Decay	0.110	0.003	0.012	0.004
Weight Elimination	0.083	0.005	0.009	0.006
Information Controller	0.072	0.006	0.008	0.004

examing the first two hidden units, we could see that the first hidden unit and the second hidden unit are concerned with rules for syllabification and a exceptional case.

Then, networks were trained to infer the well-formedness of strings in addition to the segmentation to examine generalization performance. Table 2 shows generalization errors for 200 and 300 training patterns. As clearly shown in the figure, the best generalization performance in terms of RMS and error rates is obtained by the information controller. Thus, experimental results confirmed that in all cases the generalization performance of the information controller is well over the other methods. In addition, experimental results explicitly confirmed that better generalization performance is due to the suppression of over-training by the information controller.

References

[1] R. Ash, *Information Theory*, John Wiley & Sons: New York, 1965.

[2] G. Deco, W. Finnof and H. G. Zimmermann, "Unsupervised mutual information criterion for elimination of overtraining in Supervised Multilayer Networks," *Neural Computation*, Vol. 7, pp.86-107, 1995.

[3] R. Kamimura "Entropy minimization to increase the selectivity: selection and competition in neural networks," *Intelligent Engineering Systems through Artificial Neural Networks*, ASME Press, pp.227-232, 1992.

[4] R. Kamimura, T. Takagi and S. Nakanishi, "Improving generalization performance by information minimization," *IEICE Transactions on Information and Systems*, Vol. E78-D, No.2, pp.163-173, 1995.

[5] R. Kamimura and S. Nakanishi, "Hidden information maximization for feature detection and rule discovery," *Network: Computation in Neural Systems*, Vol.6, pp.577-602, 1995.

[6] M. C. Mozer and P. Smolensky, "Using relevance to reduce network size automatically," *Connection Science*, Vo.1, No.1, pp.3-16, 1989.

Unsupervised Learning by Convex and Conic Coding

D. D. Lee and H. S. Seung
Bell Laboratories, Lucent Technologies
Murray Hill, NJ 07974
{ddlee|seung}@bell-labs.com

Abstract

Unsupervised learning algorithms based on convex and conic encoders are proposed. The encoders find the closest convex or conic combination of basis vectors to the input. The learning algorithms produce basis vectors that minimize the reconstruction error of the encoders. The convex algorithm develops locally linear models of the input, while the conic algorithm discovers features. Both algorithms are used to model handwritten digits and compared with vector quantization and principal component analysis. The neural network implementations involve feedback connections that project a reconstruction back to the input layer.

1 Introduction

Vector quantization (VQ) and principal component analysis (PCA) are two widely used unsupervised learning algorithms, based on two fundamentally different ways of encoding data. In VQ, the input is encoded as the index of the closest prototype stored in memory. In PCA, the input is encoded as the coefficients of a linear superposition of a set of basis vectors. VQ can capture nonlinear structure in input data, but is weak because of its highly localized or "grandmother neuron" representation. Many prototypes are typically required to adequately represent the input data when the number of dimensions is large. On the other hand, PCA uses a distributed representation so it needs only a small number of basis vectors to model the input. Unfortunately, it can only model linear structures.

Learning algorithms based on convex and conic encoders are introduced here. These encoders are less constrained than VQ but more constrained than PCA. As a result,

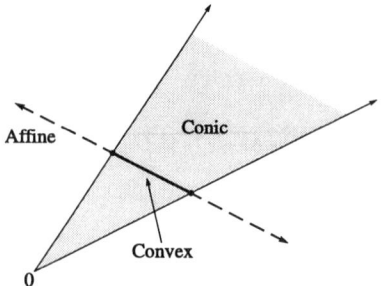

Figure 1: The affine, convex, and conic hulls for two basis vectors.

they are able to produce sparse distributed representations that are efficient to compute. The resulting learning algorithms can be understood as approximate matrix factorizations and can also be implemented as neural networks with feedforward and feedback connections between neurons.

2 Affine, convex, conic, and point encoding

Given a set of basis vectors $\{\vec{w}_a\}$, the linear combination $\sum_{a=1}^{r} v_a \vec{w}_a$ is called

$$\left.\begin{array}{l}\text{affine}\\\text{convex}\\\text{conic}\end{array}\right\} \text{ if } \left\{\begin{array}{l}\sum_a v_a = 1,\\ v_a \geq 0, \quad \sum_a v_a = 1,\\ v_a \geq 0.\end{array}\right.$$

The complete set of affine, convex, and conic combinations are called respectively the affine, convex, and conic hulls of the basis. These hulls are geometrically depicted in Figure 1. The convex hull contains only interpolations of the basis vectors, whereas the affine hull contains not only the convex hull but also linear extrapolations. The conic hull also contains the convex hull but is not constrained to stay within the set $\sum_a v_a = 1$. It extends to any nonnegative combination of the basis vectors and forms a cone in the vector space.

Four encoders are considered in this paper. The convex and conic encoders are novel, and find the nearest point to the input $\vec{x}$ in the convex and conic hull of the basis vectors. These encoders are compared with the well-known affine and point encoders. The affine encoder finds the nearest point to $\vec{x}$ in the affine hull and is equivalent to the encoding in PCA, while the point encoder or VQ finds the nearest basis vector to the input. All of these encoders minimize the *reconstruction error*:

$$\min_{v_a} \left\| \vec{x} - \sum_{a=1}^{r} v_a \vec{w}_a \right\|^2. \tag{1}$$

The constraints on v_a for the convex, conic, and affine encoders were described above. Point encoding can be thought of as a heavily constrained optimization of Eq. (1): a single v_a must equal unity while all the rest vanish.

Efficient algorithms exist for computing all of these encodings. The affine and point encoders are the fastest. Affine encoding is simply a linear transformation of the input vector. Point encoding is a nonlinear operation, but is computationally simple since it involves only a minimum distance computation. The convex and conic encoders require solving a quadratic programming problem. These encodings are more computationally demanding than the affine and point encodings; nevertheless, polynomial time algorithms do exist. The tractability of these problems is related to the fact that the cost function in Eq. (1) has no local minima on the convex domains in question. These encodings should be contrasted with computationally inefficient ones. A natural modification of the point encoder with combinatorial expressiveness can be obtained by allowing $\vec{v}$ to be any vector of zeros and ones [1, 2]. Unfortunately, with this constraint the optimization of Eq. (1) becomes an integer programming problem and is quite inefficient to solve.

The convex and conic encodings of an input generally contain coefficients v_a that vanish, due to the nonnegativity constraints in the optimization of Eq. (1). This method of obtaining sparse encodings is distinct from the method of simply truncating a linear combination by discarding small coefficients [3].

3 Learning

There correspond learning algorithms for each of the encoders described above that minimize the average reconstruction error over an ensemble of inputs. If a training set of m examples is arranged as the columns of a $N \times m$ matrix X, then the learning and encoding minimization can be expressed as:

$$\min_{W,V} \|X - WV\|^2 \qquad (2)$$

where $\|X\|^2$ is the summed squares of the elements of X. Learning and encoding can thus be described as the approximate factorization of the data matrix X into a $N \times r$ matrix W of r basis vectors and a $r \times m$ matrix V of m code vectors.

Assuming that the input vectors in X have been scaled to the range $[0, 1]$, the constraints on the optimizations in Eq. (2) are given by:

Affine: $\quad 0 \leq W_{ia} \leq 1, \qquad\qquad\qquad\quad \sum_a V_{a\mu} = 1$
Convex: $\ 0 \leq W_{ia} \leq 1, \quad V_{a\mu} \geq 0, \quad \sum_a V_{a\mu} = 1$
Conic: $\quad 0 \leq W_{ia} \leq 1, \quad V_{a\mu} \geq 0.$

The nonnegativity constraints on W and V prevent cancellations from occurring in the linear combinations, and their importance will be seen shortly. The upper bound on W is chosen such that the basis vectors are normalized in the same range as the inputs X. We noted earlier that the computation for encoding is tractable since the cost function Eq. (2) is a quadratic function of V. However, when considered as a function of both W and V, the cost function is quartic and finding its global minimum for learning can be very difficult. The issue of local minima is discussed in the following example.

4 Example: modeling handwritten digits

We applied **Affine, Convex, Conic,** and VQ learning to the USPS database [4], which consists of examples of handwritten digits segmented from actual zip codes. Each of the 7291 training and 2007 test images were normalized to a 16×16 grid

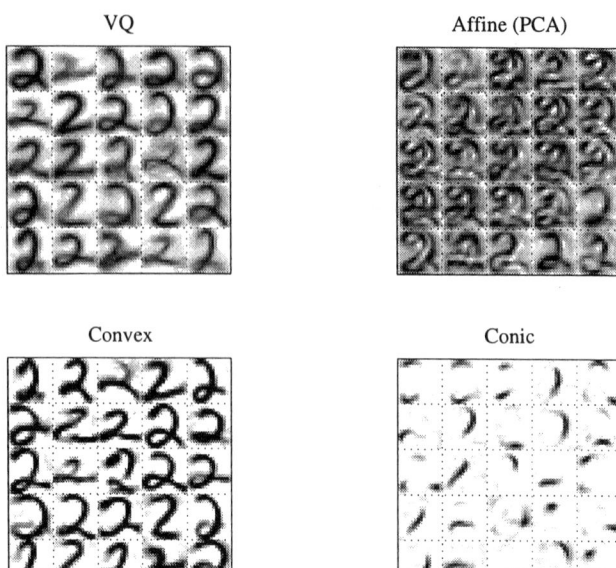

Figure 2: Basis vectors for "2" found by VQ, **Affine**, **Convex**, and **Conic** learning.

with pixel intensities in the range $[0, 1]$. There were noticeable segmentation errors resulting in unrecognizable digits, but these images were left in both the training and test sets. The training examples were segregated by digit class and separate basis vectors were trained for each of the classes using the four encodings. Figure 2 shows our results for the digit class "2" with $r = 25$ basis vectors.

The k-means algorithm was used to find the VQ basis vectors shown in Figure 2. Because the encoding is over a discontinuous and highly constrained space, there exist many local minima to Eq. (2). In order to deal with this problem, the algorithm was restarted with various initial conditions and the best solution was chosen. The resulting basis vectors look like "2" templates and are blurry because each basis vector is the mean of a large number of input images.

Affine determines the affine space that best models the input data. As can be seen in the figure, the individual basis vectors have no obvious interpretation. Although the space found by **Affine** is unique, its representation by basis vectors is degenerate. Any set of r linearly independent vectors drawn from the affine space can be used to represent it. This is due to the fact that the product WV is invariant under the transformation $W \to WS$ and $V \to S^{-1}V$.[1]

Convex finds the r basis vectors whose convex hull best fits the input data. The optimization was performed by alternating between projected gradient steps of W and V. The constraint that the column sums of V equal unity was implemented

---

[1] **Affine** is essentially equivalent to PCA, except that they represent the affine space in different ways. **Affine** represents it with r points chosen from the space. PCA represents the affine space with a single point from the space and $r-1$ orthonormal directions. This is still a degenerate representation, but PCA fixes it by taking the point to be the sample mean and the $r-1$ directions to be the eigenvectors of the covariance matrix of X with the largest eigenvalues.

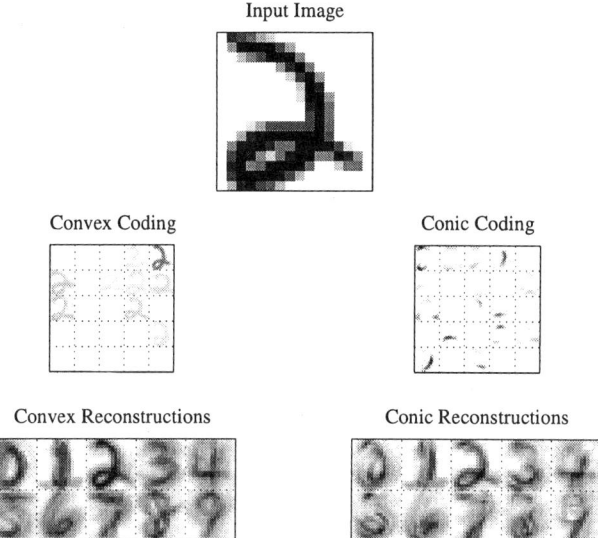

Figure 3: Activities and reconstructions of a "2" using conic and convex coding.

by adding a quadratic penalty term. In contrast to **Affine**, the basis vectors are interpretable as templates and are less blurred than those found by VQ. Many of the elements of W and also of V are zero at the minimum. This eliminates many invariant transformations S, because they would violate the nonnegativity constraints on W and V. From our simulations, it appears that most of the degeneracy seen in **Affine** is lifted by the nonnegativity constraints.

Conic finds basis vectors whose conic hull best models the input images. The learning algorithm is similar to **Convex** except there is no penalty term on the sum of the activities. The **Conic** representation allows combinations of basis vectors, not just interpolations between them. As a result, the basis vectors found are features rather than templates, as seen in Figure 2. In contrast to **Affine**, the nonnegativity constraint leads to features that are interpretable as correlated strokes. As the number of basis vectors r increases, these features decrease in size until they become individual pixels.

These models were used to classify novel test images. Recognition was accomplished by separately reconstructing the test images with the different digit models and associating the image with the model having the smallest reconstruction error. Figure 3 illustrates an example of classifying a "2" using the conic and convex encodings. The basis vectors are displayed weighted by their activites v_a and the sparsity in the representations can be clearly seen. The bottom part of the figure shows the different reconstructions generated by the various digit models.

With $r = 25$ patterns per digit class, **Convex** incorrectly classified 113 digits out of the 2007 test examples for an overall error rate of 5.6%. This is virtually identical to the performance of $k = 1$ nearest neighbor (112 errors) and linear $r = 25$ PCA models (111 errors). However, scaling up the convex models to $r = 100$ patterns results in an error rate of 4.4% (89 errors). This improvement arises because the larger convex hulls can better represent the overall nonlinear nature of the input distributions. This is good performance relative to other methods that do not use prior knowledge of invariances, such as the support vector machine (4.0% [5]). However, it is not as good as methods that do use prior knowledge, such as nearest neighbor with tangent distance (2.6% [6]).

On the other hand, **Conic** coding with $r = 25$ results in an error rate of 6.8% (138 errors). With larger basis sets $r > 50$, **Conic** shows worse performance as the features shrink to small spots. These results indicate that by itself, **Conic** does not yield good models; non-trivial correlations still remain in the v_a and also need to be taken into account. For instance, while the conic basis for "9" can fit some "7"'s quite well with little reconstruction error, the codes v_a are distinct from when it fits "9"'s.

5 Neural network implementation

Conic and **Convex** were described above as matrix factorizations. Alternatively, the encoding can be performed by a neural network dynamics [7] and the learning by a synaptic update rule. We describe here the implementation for the **Conic** network; the **Convex** network is similar. The **Conic** network has a layer of N error neurons e_i and a layer of r encoding neurons v_a. The fixed point of the encoding dynamics

$$\frac{dv_a}{dt} + v_a = \left[\sum_{i=1}^{N} e_i W_{ia} + v_a \right]^+ , \qquad (3)$$

$$\frac{de_i}{dt} + e_i = x_i - \sum_{a=1}^{r} W_{ia} v_a , \qquad (4)$$

optimizes Eq. (1), finding the best convex encoding of the input x_i. The rectification nonlinearity $[x]^+ = \max(x, 0)$ enforces the nonnegativity constraint. The error neurons subtract the reconstruction from the input x_i. The excitatory connection from e_i to v_a is equal and opposite to the inhibitory connection from v_a back to e_i. The Hebbian synaptic weight update

$$\Delta W_{ia} = \eta \, e_i v_a \qquad (5)$$

is made following convergence of the encoding dynamics for each input, while respecting the bound constraints on W_{ia}. This performs stochastic gradient descent on the ensemble reconstruction error with learning rate η.

6 Discussion

Convex coding is similar to other locally linear models [8, 9, 10, 11]. Distance to a convex hull was previously used in nearest neighbor classification [12], though no learning algorithm was proposed. **Conic** coding is similar to the noisy OR [13, 14] and harmonium [15] models. The main difference is that these previous models contain discrete binary variables, whereas **Conic** uses continuous ones. The use of analog rather than binary variables makes the encoding computationally tractable and allows for interpolation between basis vectors.

Here we have emphasized the geometrical interpretation of **Convex** and **Conic** coding. They can also be viewed as probabilistic hidden variable models. The inputs x_i are visible while the v_a are hidden variables, and the reconstruction error in Eq. (1) is related to the log likelihood, $\log P(x_i|v_a)$. No explicit model $P(v_a)$ for the hidden variables was used, which limited the quality of the **Conic** models in particular. The feature discovery capabilities of **Conic**, however, make it a promising tool for building hierarchical representations. We are currently working on extending these new coding schemes and learning algorithms to multilayer networks.

We acknowledge the support of Bell Laboratories. We thank C. Burges, C. Cortes, and Y. LeCun for providing us with the USPS database. We are also grateful to K. Clarkson, R. Freund, L. Kaufman, L. Saul, and M. Wright for helpful discussions.

References

[1] Hinton, GE & Zemel, RS (1994). Autoencoders, minimum description length and Helmholtz free energy. *Advances in Neural Information Processing Systems 6*, 3–10.

[2] Ghahramani, Z (1995). Factorial learning and the EM algorithm. *Advances in Neural Information Processing Systems 7*, 617–624.

[3] Olshausen, BA & Field, DJ (1996). Emergence of simple-cell receptive field properties by learning a sparse code for natural images. *Nature 381*, 607–609.

[4] Le Cun, Y et al. (1989). Backpropagation applied to handwritten zip code recognition. *Neural Comput.* **1**, 541–551.

[5] Scholkopf, B, Burges, C, & Vapnik, V (1995). Extracting support data for a given task. *KDD-95 Proceedings*, 252–257.

[6] Simard, P, Le Cun Y & Denker J (1993). Efficient pattern recognition using a new transformation distance. *Advances in Neural Information Processing Systems 5*, 50–58.

[7] Tank, DW & Hopfield, JJ (1986). Simple neural optimization networks: an A/D converter, signal decision circuit, and a linear programming circuit. *IEEE Trans. Circ. Syst.* **CAS-33**, 533–541.

[8] Bezdek, JC, Coray, C, Gunderson, R & Watson J (1981). Detection and characterization of cluster substructure. *SIAM J. Appl. Math.* **40**, 339–357; 358–372.

[9] Bregler, C & Omohundro, SM (1995). Nonlinear image interpolation using manifold learning. *Advances in Neural Information Processing Systems 7*, 973–980.

[10] Hinton, GE, Dayan, P & Revow M (1996). Modeling the manifolds of images of handwritten digits. *IEEE Trans. Neural Networks*, submitted.

[11] Hastie, T, Simard, P & Säckinger E (1995). Learning prototype models for tangent distance. *Advances in Neural Information Processing Systems 7*, 999–1006.

[12] Haas, HPA, Backer, E & Boxma, I (1980). Convex hull nearest neighbor rule. *Fifth Intl. Conf. on Pattern Recognition Proceedings*, 87–90.

[13] Dayan, P & Zemel, RS (1995). Competition and multiple cause models. *Neural Comput.* **7**, 565–579.

[14] Saund, E (1995). A multiple cause mixture model for unsupervised learning. *Neural Comput.* **7**, 51–71.

[15] Freund, Y & Haussler, D (1992). Unsupervised learning of distributions on binary vectors using two layer networks. *Advances in Neural Information Processing Systems 4*, 912–919.

ARC-LH: A New Adaptive Resampling Algorithm for Improving ANN Classifiers

Friedrich Leisch
Friedrich.Leisch@ci.tuwien.ac.at

Kurt Hornik
Kurt.Hornik@ci.tuwien.ac.at

Institut für Statistik und Wahrscheinlichkeitstheorie
Technische Universität Wien
A-1040 Wien, Austria

Abstract

We introduce arc-lh, a new algorithm for improvement of ANN classifier performance, which measures the importance of patterns by aggregated network output errors. On several artificial benchmark problems, this algorithm compares favorably with other resample and combine techniques.

1 Introduction

The training of artificial neural networks (ANNs) is usually a stochastic and unstable process. As the weights of the network are initialized at random and training patterns are presented in random order, ANNs trained on the same data will typically be different in value and performance. In addition, small changes in the training set can lead to two completely different trained networks with different performance even if the nets had the same initial weights.

Roughly speaking, ANNs have a low bias because of their approximation capabilities, but a rather high variance because of the instability. Recently, several resample and combine techniques for improving ANN performance have been proposed. In this paper we introduce an new arcing ("adaptive resample and combine") method called arc-lh. Contrary to the arc-fs method by Freund & Schapire (1995), which uses misclassification rates for adapting the resampling probabilities, arc-lh uses the aggregated network output error. The performance of arc-lh is compared with other techniques on several popular artificial benchmark problems.

2 Bias-Variance Decomposition of 0-1 Loss

Consider the task of classifying a random vector ξ taking values in $\mathcal{X}$ into one of c classes $C_1, \ldots, C_c$, and let $g(\cdot)$ be a classification function mapping the input space on the finite set $\{1, \ldots, c\}$.

The classification task is to find an optimal function g minimizing the risk

$$Rg = \mathbb{E}Lg(\xi) = \int_{\mathcal{X}} Lg(x)\, dF(x) \qquad (1)$$

where F denotes the (typically unknown) distribution function of ξ, and L is a loss function. In this paper, we consider 0-1 loss only, i.e., the loss is 1 for all misclassified patterns and zero otherwise.

It is well known that the optimal classifier, i.e., the classifier with minimum risk, is the Bayes classifier $g^\star$ assigning to each input x the class with maximum posterior probability $\mathbb{P}(C_n|x)$. These posterior probabilities are typically unknown, hence the Bayes classifier cannot be used directly. Note that $Rg^\star = 0$ for disjoint classes and $Rg^\star > 0$ otherwise.

Let $X_N = \{x_1, \ldots, x_N\}$ be a set of independent input vectors for which the true class is known, available for training the classifier. Further, let $g_{X_N}(\cdot)$ denote a classifier trained using set X_N. The risk $Rg_{X_N} \geq Rg^\star$ of classifier g_{X_N} is a random variable depending on the training sample X_N. In the case of ANN classifiers it also depends on the network training, i.e., even for fixed X_N the performance of a trained ANN is a random variable depending on the initialization of weights and the (often random) presentation of the patterns $[x_n]$ during training.

Following Breiman (1996a) we decompose the risk of a classifier into the (minimum possible) Bayes error, a systematic bias term of the model class and the variance of the classifier within its model class. We call a classifier model *unbiased* for input x if, over replications of all possible training sets X_N of size N, network initializations and pattern presentations, g picks the correct class more often than any other class. Let $\mathcal{U} = \mathcal{U}(g)$ denote the set of all $x \in \mathcal{X}$ where g is unbiased; and $\mathcal{B} = \mathcal{B}(g) = \mathcal{X} \setminus \mathcal{U}$ the set of all points where g is biased. The risk of classifier g can be decomposed as

$$Rg = Rg^\star + \text{Bias}(g) + \text{Var}(g) \qquad (2)$$

where $Rg^\star$ is the risk of the Bayes classifier,

$$\begin{aligned} \text{Bias}(g) &= R_\mathcal{B} g - R_\mathcal{B} g^\star \\ \text{Var}(g) &= R_\mathcal{U} g - R_\mathcal{U} g^\star \end{aligned}$$

and $R_\mathcal{B}$ and $R_\mathcal{U}$ denote the risk on set $\mathcal{B}$ and $\mathcal{U}$, respectively, i.e., the integration in Equation 1 is over $\mathcal{B}$ or $\mathcal{U}$ instead of $\mathcal{X}$, repectively.

A simpler bias-variance decomposition has been proposed by Kong & Dietterich (1995):

$$\begin{aligned} \text{Bias}(g) &= \mathbb{P}\{\mathcal{B}\} \\ \text{Var}(g) &= Rg - \text{Bias}(g) \end{aligned}$$

The size of the bias set is seen as the bias of the model (i.e., the error the model class "typically" makes). The variance is simply the difference between the actual risk and this bias term. This decompostion yields negative variance if the current classifier performs better than the average classifier.

In both decompositions, the bias gives the systematic risk of the model, whereas the variance measures how good the current realization is compared to the best possible realization of the model. Neural networks are very powerful but rather unstable approximators, hence their bias should be low, but the variance may be high.

3 Resample and Combine

Suppose we had k independent training sets $X_{N_1}, \ldots, X_{N_k}$ and corresponding classifiers $g_1, \ldots, g_k$ trained using these sets, respectively. We can then combine these single classifiers into a joint voting classifier g_k^v by assigning to each input x the class the majority of the g_i votes for. If the g_i have low bias, then g_k^v should have low bias, too. If the model is unbiased for an input x, then the variance of g_k^v vanishes as $k \to \infty$, and $g^v = \lim_{k \to \infty} g_k^v$ is optimal for x. Hence, by resampling training sets from the original training set and combining the resulting classifiers into a voting classifier it might be possible to reduce the high variance of unstable classification algorithms.

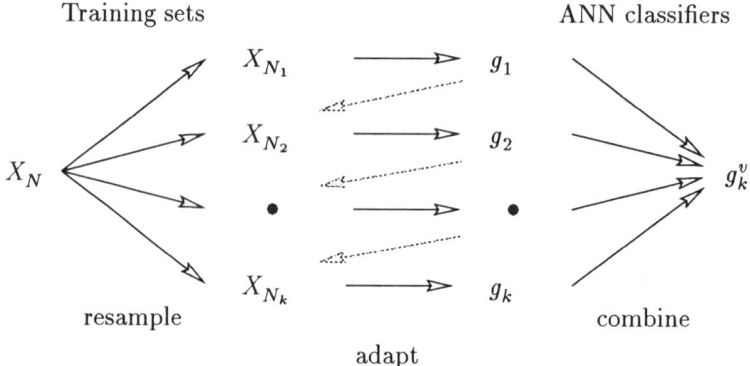

3.1 Bagging

Breiman (1994, 1996a) introduced a procedure called bagging ("<u>b</u>ootstrap <u>agg</u>regating") for tree classifiers that may also be used for ANNs. The bagging algorithm starts with a training set X_N of size N. Several bootstrap replica $X_N^1, \ldots, X_N^k$ are constructed and a neural network is trained on each. These networks are finally combined by majority voting. The bootstrap sets X_N^i consist of N patterns drawn with replacement from the original training set (see Efron & Tibshirani (1993) for more information on the bootstrap).

3.2 Arcing

3.2.1 Arcing Based on Misclassification Rates

Arcing, which is a more sophisticated version of bagging, was first introduced by Freund & Schapire (1995) and called *boosting*. The new training sets are not constructed by uniformly sampling from the empirical distribution of the training set X_N, but from a distribution over X_N that includes information about previous misclassifications.

Let p_n^i denote the probability that pattern x_n is included into the i-th training set X_N^i and initialize with $p_n^1 = 1/N$. Freund and Schapire's arcing algorithm, called arc-fs as in Breiman (1996a), works as follows:

1. Construct a pattern set X_N^i by sampling with replacement with probabilities p_n^i from X_N and train a classifier g_i using set X_N^i.

2. Set $d_n = 1$ for all patterns that are misclassified by g_i and zero otherwise. With $\epsilon_i = \sum_{n=1}^N p_n^i d_n$ and $\beta_i = (1 - \epsilon_i)/\epsilon_i$ update the probabilities by

$$p_n^{i+1} = \frac{p_n^i \beta_i^{d_n}}{\sum_{n=1}^N p_n^i \beta_i^{d_n}}$$

3. Set $i := i + 1$ and repeat.

After k steps, $g_1, \ldots, g_k$ are combined with weighted voting were each g_i's vote has weight $\log \beta_i$. Breiman (1996a) and Quinlan (1996) compare bagging and arcing for CART and C4.5 classifiers, respectively. Both bagging and arc-fs are very effective in reducing the high variance component of tree classifiers, with adaptive resampling being a bit better than simple bagging.

3.2.2 Arcing Based on Network Error

Independently from the arcing and bagging procedures described above, adaptive resampling has been introduced for active pattern selection in leave-k-out cross-validation CV/APS (Leisch & Jain, 1996; Leisch et al., 1995). Whereas arc-fs (or Breiman's arc-x4) uses only the information whether a pattern is misclassified or not, in CV/APS the fact that MLPs approximate the posterior probabilities of the classes (Kanaya & Miyake, 1991) is utilized, too. We introduce a simple new arcing method based on the main idea of CV/APS that the "importance" of a pattern for the learning process can be measured by the aggregated output error of an MLP for the pattern over several training runs.

Let the classifier g be an ANN using 1-of-c coding, i.e., one output node per class, the target $t(x)$ for each input x is one at the node corresponding to the class of x and zero at the remaining output nodes. Let $e(x) = |t(x) - g(x)|^2$ be the squared error of the network for input x. Patterns that repeatedly have high output errors are somewhat harder to learn for the network and therefore their resampling probabilities are increased proportionally to the error. Error-dependent resampling introduces a "grey-scale" of pattern-importance as opposed to the "black and white" paradigm of misclassification dependent resampling.

Again let p_n^i denote the probability that pattern x_n is included into the i-th training set X_N^i and initialize with $p_n^1 = 1/N$. Our new arcing algorithm, called arc-lh, works as follows:

1. Construct a pattern set X_N^i by sampling with replacement with probabilities p_n^i from X_N and train a classifier g_i using set X_N^i.

2. Add the network output error of each pattern to the resampling probabilities:
$$p_n^{i+1} = \frac{p_n^i + e_i(x_n)}{\sum_{n=1}^{N} p_n^i + e_i(x_n)}, \qquad e_i(x_n) = |t(x_n) - g_i(x_n))|^2$$

3. Set $i := i + 1$ and repeat.

After k steps, $g_1, \ldots, g_k$ are combined by majority voting.

3.3 Jittering

In our experiments, we also compare the above resample and combine methods with jittering, which resamples the training set by contaminating the inputs by artificial noise. No voting is done, but the size of the training set is increased by creation of artificial inputs "around" the original inputs, see Koistinen & Holmström (1992).

4 Experiments

We demonstrate the effects of bagging and arcing on several well known artificial benchmark problems. For all problems, $i - h - c$ single hidden layer perceptrons (SHLPs) with i input, h hidden and c output nodes were used. The number of hidden nodes h was chosen in a way that the corresponding networks have reasonably low bias.

2 Spirals with noise: 2-dimensional input, 2 classes. Inputs with uniform noise around two spirals. $N = 300$. $Rg^\star = 0\%$. 2-14-2 SHLP.

Continuous XOR: 2-dimensional input, 2 classes. Uniform inputs on the 2-dimensional square $-1 \leq x, y \leq 1$ classified in the two classes $x * y \geq 0$ and $x * y < 0$. $N = 300$. $Rg^\star = 0\%$. 2-4-2 SHLP.

Ringnorm: 20-dimensional input, 2 classes. Class 1 is normal wit mean zero and covariance 4 times the identity matrix. Class 2 is a unit normal with mean $(a, a, \ldots, a)$. $a = 2/\sqrt{20}$. $N = 300$. $Rg^\star = 1.2\%$. 20-4-2 SHLP.

The first two problems are standard benchmark problems (note however that we use a noisy variant of the standard spirals problem); the last one is, e.g., used in Breiman (1994, 1996a).

All experiments were replicated 50 times, in each bagging and arcing replication 10 classifiers were combined to build a voting classifier. Generalization errors were computed using Monte Carlo techniques on test sets of size 10000.

Table 1 gives the average risk over the 50 replications for a standard single SHLP, an SHLP trained on a jittered training set and for voting classifiers using ten votes constructed with bagging, arc-lh and arc-fs, respectively. The Bayes risk of the spiral and xor example is zero, hence the risk of a network equals the sum of its bias and variance. The Bayes risk of the ringnorm example is 1.2%.

	Rg	Breiman		Kong & Dietterich	
		Bias(g)	Var(g)	Bias(g)	Var(g)
2 Spirals					
standard	7.75	0.32	7.43	0.82	6.93
jitter	6.53	0.26	6.27	0.52	6.02
bagging	4.39	0.35	4.04	0.68	3.71
arc-fs	4.31	0.35	3.96	0.60	3.71
arc-lh	4.32	0.31	4.01	0.72	3.60
XOR					
standard	6.54	0.53	6.01	1.32	5.22
jitter	6.29	0.37	5.92	1.08	5.21
bagging	3.69	0.59	3.09	1.22	2.47
arc-fs	3.73	0.58	3.15	1.12	2.61
arc-lh	3.58	0.50	3.08	1.20	2.38
Ringnorm					
standard	18.64	9.19	8.26	13.84	4.80
jitter	18.56	9.03	8.34	13.72	4.84
bagging	15.72	9.61	4.91	13.54	2.18
arc-fs	15.71	9.70	4.81	13.58	2.13
arc-lh	15.63	9.30	5.13	13.20	2.43

Table 1: Bias-variance decompositions.

The variance part was drastically reduced by the resample & combine methods, with only a negligible change in bias. Note the low bias in the spiral and xor problems. ANNs obviously can solve these classification tasks (one could create appropriate nets by hand), but of course training cannot find the exact boundaries between the classes. Averaging over several nets helps to overcome this problem. The bias in the ringnorm example is rather high, indicating that a change of network topology (bigger net, etc.) or training algorithm (learning rate, etc.) may lower the overall risk.

5 Summary

Comparison of of the resample and combine algorithms shows slight advantages for adaptive resampling, but no algorithm dominates the other two. Further improvements should be possible based on a better understanding of the theoretical properties of resample and combine techniques. These issues are currently being investigated.

References

Breiman, L. (1994). *Bagging predictors*. Tech. Rep. 421, Department of Statistics, University of California, Berkeley, California, USA.

Breiman, L. (1996a). *Bias, variance, and arcing classifiers*. Tech. Rep. 460, Statistics Department, University of California, Berkeley, CA, USA.

Breiman, L. (1996b). Stacked regressions. *Machine Learning*, **24**, 49.

Drucker, H. & Cortes, C. (1996). Boosting decision trees. In Touretzky, S., Mozer, M. C., & Hasselmo, M. E. (eds.), *Advances in Neural Information Processing Systems*, vol. 8. MIT Press.

Efron, B. & Tibshirani, R. J. (1993). *An introduction to the bootstrap*. Monographs on Statistics and Applied Probability. New York: Chapman & Hall.

Freund, Y. & Schapire, R. E. (1995). *A decision-theoretic generalization of on-line learning and an application to boosting*. Tech. rep., AT&T Bell Laboratories, 600 Mountain Ave, Murray Hill, NJ, USA.

Kanaya, F. & Miyake, S. (1991). Bayes statistical behavior and valid generalization of pattern classifying neural networks. *IEEE Transactions on Neural Networks*, **2**(4), 471–475.

Kohavi, R. & Wolpert, D. H. (1996). Bias plus variance decomposition for zero-one loss. In *Machine Learning: Proceedings of the 13th International Conference*.

Koistinen, P. & Holmström, L. (1992). Kernel regression and backpropagation training with noise. In Moody, J. E., Hanson, S. J., & Lippmann, R. P. (eds.), *Advances in Neural Information Processing Systems*, vol. 4, pp. 1033–1039. Morgan Kaufmann Publishers, Inc.

Kong, E. B. & Dietterich, T. G. (1995). Error-correcting output coding corrects bias and variance. In *Machine Learning: Proceedings of the 12th International Conference*, pp. 313–321. Morgan-Kaufmann.

Leisch, F. & Jain, L. C. (1996). Cross-validation with active pattern selection for neural network classifiers. Submitted to IEEE Transactions on Neural Networks, in Review.

Leisch, F., Jain, L. C., & Hornik, K. (1995). NN classifiers: Reducing the computational cost of cross-validation by active pattern selection. In *Artificial Neural Networks and Expert Systems*, vol. 2. Los Alamitos, CA, USA: IEEE Computer Society Press.

Quinlan, J. R. (1996). Bagging, boosting and C4.5. University of Sydney, Australia.

Ripley, B. D. (1996). *Pattern recognition and neural networks*. Cambridge, UK: Cambridge University Press.

Tibshirani, R. (1996a). Bias, variance and prediction error for classification rules. University of Toronto, Canada.

Tibshirani, R. (1996b). A comparison of some error estimates for neural network models. *Neural Computation*, **8**(1), 152–163.

Bayesian Unsupervised Learning of Higher Order Structure

Michael S. Lewicki
lewicki@salk.edu

Terrence J. Sejnowski
terry@salk.edu

The Salk Institute
Howard Hughes Medical Institute
Computational Neurobiology Lab
10010 N. Torrey Pines Rd.
La Jolla, CA 92037

Abstract

Multilayer architectures such as those used in Bayesian belief networks and Helmholtz machines provide a powerful framework for representing and learning higher order statistical relations among inputs. Because exact probability calculations with these models are often intractable, there is much interest in finding approximate algorithms. We present an algorithm that efficiently discovers higher order structure using EM and Gibbs sampling. The model can be interpreted as a stochastic recurrent network in which ambiguity in lower-level states is resolved through feedback from higher levels. We demonstrate the performance of the algorithm on benchmark problems.

1 Introduction

Discovering high order structure in patterns is one of the keys to performing complex recognition and discrimination tasks. Many real world patterns have a hierarchical underlying structure in which simple features have a higher order structure among themselves. Because these relationships are often statistical in nature, it is natural to view the process of discovering such structures as a statistical inference problem in which a hierarchical model is fit to data.

Hierarchical statistical structure can be conveniently represented with Bayesian belief networks (Pearl, 1988; Lauritzen and Spiegelhalter, 1988; Neal, 1992). These models are powerful, because they can capture complex statistical relationships among the data variables, and also mathematically convenient, because they allow efficient computation of the joint probability for any given set of model parameters. The joint probability density of a network of binary states is given by a product of conditional probabilities

$$P(S_1 \ldots S_n | \mathbf{W}) = \prod_i P(S_i | \text{pa}[S_i], \mathbf{W}) \tag{1}$$

where $\mathbf{W}$ is the weight matrix that parameterizes the model. Note that the probability of an individual state S_i depends only on its parents. This probability is given by

$$P(S_i = 1 | \text{pa}[S_i], \mathbf{W}) = h(\sum_j S_j w_{ji}) \tag{2}$$

where w_{ji} is the weight from S_j to S_i ($w_{ji} = 0$ for $j < i$).

The weights specify a hierarchical prior on the input states, which are the fixed subset of states at the lowest layer of units. The active parents of state S_i represent the underlying causes of that state. The function h specifies how these causes are combined to give the probability of S_i. We assume h to be the "noisy OR" function, $h(u) = 1 - \exp(-u)$, $u >= 0$.

2 Learning Objective

The learning objective is to adapt $\mathbf{W}$ to find the most probable explanation of the input patterns. The probability of the input data is

$$P(\mathbf{D}_{1:N} | \mathbf{W}) = \prod_n P(\mathbf{D}_n | \mathbf{W}) \tag{3}$$

$P(\mathbf{D}_n | \mathbf{W})$ is computed by marginalizing over all states of the network

$$P(\mathbf{D}_n | \mathbf{W}) = \sum_k P(\mathbf{D}_n | S_k, \mathbf{W}) P(S_k | \mathbf{W}) \tag{4}$$

Because the number of different states, S_k, is exponential in the number of units, computing the sum exactly is intractable and must be approximated. The nature of the learning tasks discussed here, however, allow us to make accurate approximations. A desirable property for representations is that most patterns have just one or a few possible explanations. In this case, all but a few terms $P(\mathbf{D}_n | S_k, \mathbf{W})$ will be zero, and, as described below, it becomes feasible to use sampling based methods which select S_k according to $P(S_k | \mathbf{D}_n, \mathbf{W})$.

3 Inferring the Internal Representation

Given the input data, finding its most likely explanation is an *inference* process. Although it is simple to calculate the probability of any particular network state, there is no simple way to determine the most probable state given input D. A general approach to this problem is Gibbs sampling (Pearl, 1988; Neal, 1992).

In Gibbs sampling, each state S_i of the network is updated iteratively according to the probability of S_i given the remaining states in the network. This conditional probability can be computed using

$$P(S_i|S_j : j \neq i, \mathbf{W}) \propto P(S_i|\text{pa}[S_i], \mathbf{W}) \prod_{j \in \text{ch}[S_i]} P(S_j|\text{pa}[S_j], S_i, \mathbf{W}) \quad (5)$$

where ch$[S_i]$ indicates the children of state S_i. In the limit, the ensemble of states obtained by this procedure will be typical samples from $P(\mathbf{S}|\mathbf{D}, \mathbf{W})$. More generally, any subset of states can be fixed and the rest sampled.

The Gibbs equations have an interpretation in terms of a stochastic recurrent neural network in which feedback from higher levels influences the states at lower levels. For the models defined here, the probability of S_i changing state given the remaining states is

$$P(S_i = 1 - S_i|S_j : j \neq i, \mathbf{W}) = \frac{1}{1 + \exp(-\Delta x_i)} \quad (6)$$

The variable Δx_i indicates how much changing the state S_i changes the probability of the network state

$$\Delta x_i = \log h(u_i; 1 - S_i) - \log h(u_i; S_i) + \sum_{j \in \text{ch}[S_i]} \log h(u_j + \delta_{ij}; S_j) - \log h(u_j; S_j) \quad (7)$$

where $h(u; a) = h(u)$ if $a = 1$ and $1 - h(u)$ if $a = 0$. The variable u_i is the causal input to S_i, given by $\sum_k S_k w_{ki}$. The variable δ_j specifies the change in u_j for a change in S_i: $\delta_{ij} = +S_j w_{ij}$ if $S_i = 0$ and $-S_j w_{ij}$ if $S_i = 1$.

The first two terms in (7) can be interpreted as the feedback from higher levels. The sum can be interpreted as the feedforward input from the children of S_i. Feedback allows the lower level units to use information only computable at higher levels. The feedforward terms typically dominate the expression, but the feedback becomes the determining factor when the feedforward input is ambiguous.

For general distributions, Gibbs sampling can require many samples to achieve a representative samples. But if there is little ambiguity in the internal representation, as is the goal, Gibbs sampling can be as efficient as a single feedforward pass. One potential problem is that Gibbs sampling will not work before the weights have adapted, when the representations are highly ambiguous. We show below, however, that it is not necessary to sample for long periods in order for good representations to be learned. As learning proceeds, the internal representations obtained with limited Gibbs sampling become increasingly accurate.

4 Adapting the Weights

The complexity of the model is controlled by placing a prior on the weights. For the form of the noisy OR function in which all weights are constrained to be positive, we assume the prior to be the product of independent gamma distributions parameterized by α and β. The objective function becomes

$$\mathcal{L} = P(\mathbf{D}_{1:N}|\mathbf{W})P(\mathbf{W}|\alpha, \beta) \quad (8)$$

A simple and efficient EM-type formula for adapt the weights can be derived by setting $\partial \mathcal{L}/\partial w_{ij}$ to zero and solving for w_{ij}. Using the transformations $f_{ij} = 1 -$

$\exp(-w_{ij})$ and $g_i = 1 - \exp(-u_i)$ we obtain

$$f_{ij} = \frac{\alpha - 1 + 2f_{ij} + \sum_n S_i^{(n)} S_j^{(n)} f_{ij}/g_j^{(n)}}{\alpha + \beta + \sum_n S_i^{(n)}} \tag{9}$$

where $S^{(n)}$ is the state obtained with Gibbs sampling for the nth input pattern. The variable f_{ij} can be interpreted as the frequency of state S_j given cause S_i. The sum in the above expression is a weighted average of the number of times S_j was active when S_i was active. The ratio f_{ij}/g_j weights each term in the sum inversely according to the number of different causes for S_j. If S_i is the unique cause of S_j then $f_{ij} = g_j$ and the term would have full weight.

A straightforward application of the learning algorithm would adapt all the weights at the same time. This does not produce good results, however, because there is nothing to prevent the model from learning overly strong priors. This can be prevented by adapting the weights in the upper levels after the weights in the lower levels have stabilized. This allows the higher levels to adapt to structure that is actually present in the data. We have obtained good results from both the naive method of adapting the lowest layers first and from more sophisticated methods where stability was based on how often a unit changed during the Gibbs sampling.

5 Examples

In the following examples, the weight prior was specified with $\alpha = 1.0$ and $\beta = 1.5$. Weights were set to random values between 0.05 and 0.15. Gibbs sampling was stopped if the maximum state change probability was less than 0.05 or after 15 sweeps through the units. Weights were reestimated after blocks of 200 patterns. Each layer of weights was adapted for 10 epochs before adapting the next layer.

A High Order Lines Problem. The first example illustrates that the algorithm can discover the underlying features in complicated patterns and that the higher layers can capture interesting higher order structure. The first dataset is a variant of the lines problem proposed by Földiák (1989). The patterns in the dataset are composed of horizontal and vertical lines as illustrated in figure 1. Note that, although

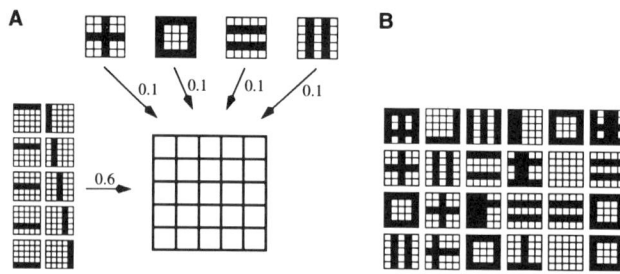

Figure 1: Dataset for the high order lines problem. (**A**) Patterns are generated by selecting one of the pattern types according to the probabilities next to the arrows. Top patterns are copied to the input. The horizontal and vertical lines on the left are selected with probability 0.3. (**B**) Typical input patterns.

the datasets are displayed on a 2-D grid, the network makes no assumptions about topography. Because the network is fully connected, all spatial arrangements of the inputs are identical. The weights learned by the network are shown in figure 2.

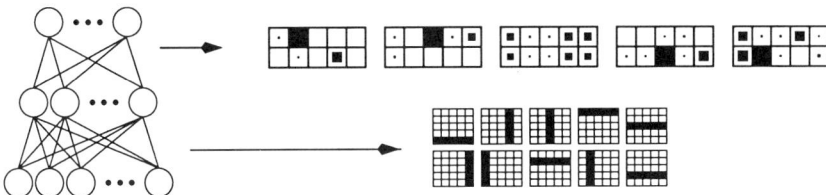

Figure 2: The weights in a 25-10-5 network after training. Blocks indicate the weights to each unit. Square size is proportional to the weight values. Second layer units capture the structure of the horizontal and vertical lines. Third layer units capture the correlations among the lines. The first unit in the third layer is active when the '|||' is present. The second, fourth, and fifth units have learned to represent the '+', '=', and '☐' respectively, with the remaining unit acting as a bias.

The Shifter Problem. The shifter problem (Hinton and Sejnowski, 1986), explained in figure 3, is important because the structure that must be discovered is in the higher order input correlations. This example also illustrates the importance of allowing high level states to influence low level states to determine the most probable internal representation. The units in the second layer can only capture second order statistics and cannot determine the direction of the shift. The only way these units can be disambiguated is to use the feedback from the units in the third layer which detect the direction of the shift by integrating the output of the units in the second layer. This allows the representation in the second layer to be "cleaned up" and makes it easier to discover the higher order structure of the global shift. The speed and reliability of the learning was tested by learning from random initial conditions. The results are shown in figure 4. Note that the best solutions have a cost of about one bit higher than the optimal cost of less than 9 bits, because top units cannot capture the fact that they are mutually exclusive.

6 Discussion

The methods we have described work well on these simple benchmark problems and scale well to larger problems such as the handwritten digits example used in (Hinton et al., 1995). We believe there are two main reasons why the algorithm described here runs considerably faster than other Gibbs sampling based methods. The first is that there is no need to collect state statistics for each pattern. The weight values are reestimated using just one sampled internal state per pattern. The second is that weights that are not connected to informative units are not updated. This prevents the model from learning what are effectively overly strong priors and allows the weights in upper layers to adapt to structure actually in the data.

Gibbs sampling allows internal representations to be selected according to their true posterior probability. This was shown to be effective in cases where the resulting

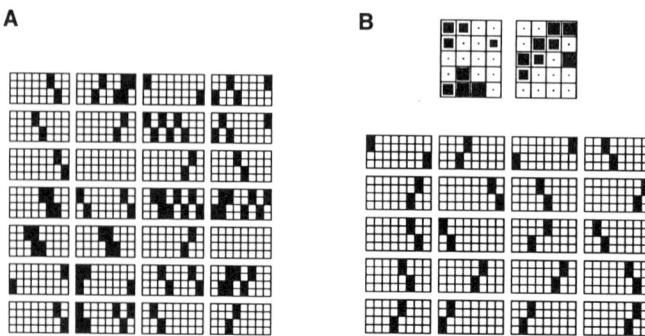

Figure 3: The shifter problem. (**A**) Input patterns are generated by generating a random binary vector in the bottom row. This pattern is shifted either left or right (with wrap around) with equal probability and copied to the top row. The input rows are duplicated to add redundancy as in Dayan et al. (1995). (**B**) The weights of a 32-20-2 after learning. The second layer of units learn to detect either local left shifts or right shifts in the data. These units cannot determine the shift direction alone, however, and require feedback from third layer units which integrate the outputs of all the units that represent a common shift (note that there is no overlap in the weights for the two third-layer units). This feedback turns off units that are inconsistent with the direction of shift. The weights that are close to zero for both third layer units effectively remove redundant second layer units that are not required to represent the input patterns.

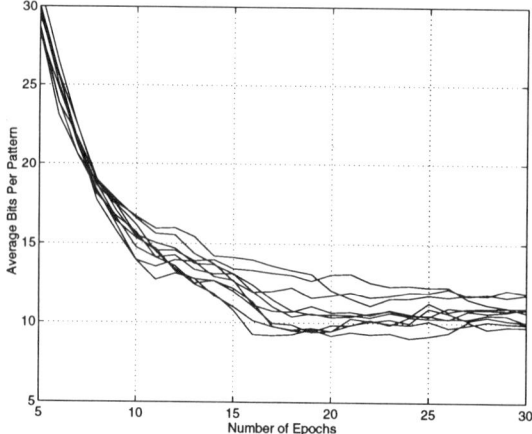

Figure 4: The graph shows 10 runs on the shifter problem from random initial conditions. The average bits per pattern is computed by $-\log(\mathcal{L})/(N \log 2)$. Each epoch used 200 input randomly generated input patterns. Two additional epochs were performed with 1000 random patterns to obtain accurate estimates of the average bits per pattern. The network converges rapidly and reliably. The best solutions, like the one shown in figure 3b, were found in 4/10 runs and had costs of approximately 10 bits at epoch 30. In this example, the network can get caught in local minima if too many units learn to represent the same local shifts.

representation has little ambiguity, *i.e.* each pattern has only a small number of probable explanations. If the causal structure to be learned is inherently ambiguous, *e.g.* in modeling the causal structure of medical symptoms, Gibbs sampling will be slow and better performance can be obtained with wake-sleep learning (Hinton et al., 1995; Frey et al., 1995) or mean field approximations (Saul et al., 1996).

There are many natural situations when there is ambiguity in low level features. This ambiguity can only be resolved by integrating the contextual information which itself is derived from the ambiguous simple features. This problem is common in the case of noisy input patterns and in feature grouping problems such as figure-ground separation. Feedback is crucial for ensuring that low-level representations are consistent within the larger context.

Some systems, such as the Helmholtz machine (Dayan et al., 1995; Hinton et al., 1995), arrive at the internal state through a feedforward process. It possible that this ambiguity in lower-level representations could be resolved by circuitry in the higher-level representations, but if multiple higher-level modules make use of the same low-level representations, the additional circuitry would have to be duplicated in each module. It seems more parsimonious to use feedback to influence the formation of the lower-level representations.

References

Dayan, P., Hinton, G. E., Neal, R. M., and Zemel, R. S. (1995). The Helmholtz machine. *Neural Computation*, 7:889–904.

Földiák, P. (1989). Adaptive network for optimal linear feature extraction. In *Proceedings of the International Joint Conference on Neural Networks*, volume I, pages 401–405, Washington, D. C.

Frey, B. J., Hinton, G. E., and Dayan, P. (1995). Does the wake-sleep algorithm produce good density estimators? In Touretzky, D. S., Mozer, M., and Hasselmo, M., editors, *Advances in Neural Information Processing Systems*, volume 8, pages 661–667, San Mateo. Morgan Kaufmann.

Hinton, G. E., Dayan, P., Frey, B. J., and Neal, R. M. (1995). The wake-sleep algorithm for unsupervised neural networks. *Science*, 268(5214):1158–1161.

Hinton, G. E. and Sejnowski, T. J. (1986). Learning and relearning in Boltzmann machines. In Rumelhart, D. E. and McClelland, J. L., editors, *Parallel Distributed Processing*, volume 1, chapter 7, pages 282–317. MIT Press, Cambridge.

Lauritzen, S. L. and Spiegelhalter, D. J. (1988). Local computations with probabilities on graphical structures and their application to expert systems. *J. Royal Statistical Soc. Series B Methodological*, 50(2):157–224.

Neal, R. M. (1992). Connectionist learning of belief networks. *Artificial Intelligence*, 56(1):71–113.

Pearl, J. (1988). *Probabilistic Reasoning in Intelligent Systems*. Morgan Kaufmann, San Mateo.

Saul, L. K., Jaakkola, T., and Jordan, M. I. (1996). Mean field theory for sigmoid belief networks. *J. Artificial Intelligence Research*, 4:61–76.

Source Separation and Density Estimation by Faithful Equivariant SOM

Juan K. Lin
Department of Physics
University of Chicago
Chicago, IL 60637
jk-lin@uchicago.edu

David G. Grier
Department of Physics
University of Chicago
Chicago, IL 60637
d-grier@uchicago.edu

Jack D. Cowan
Department of Math
University of Chicago
Chicago, IL 60637
j-cowan@uchicago.edu

Abstract

We couple the tasks of source separation and density estimation by extracting the local geometrical structure of distributions obtained from mixtures of statistically independent sources. Our modifications of the self–organizing map (SOM) algorithm results in purely digital learning rules which perform non–parametric histogram density estimation. The non–parametric nature of the separation allows for source separation of non–linear mixtures. An anisotropic coupling is introduced into our SOM with the role of aligning the network locally with the independent component contours. This approach provides an exact verification condition for source separation with no prior on the source distributions.

1 INTRODUCTION

Much of the current work on visual cortex modeling has focused on the generation of coding which captures statistical independence and sparseness (Bell and Sejnowski 1996, Olshausen and Field 1996). The Bell and Sejnowski model suffers from the parametric and intrinsically non–local nature of their source separation algorithm, while the Olshausen and Field model does not achieve true sparse–distributed coding where each cell has the same response probability (Field 1994). In this paper, we construct an extensively modified SOM with equipartition of activity as a steady–state for the task of local statistical independence processing and sparse–distributed coding.

Ritter and Schulten (1986) demonstrated that the density of the Kohonen SOM units is not proportional to the input density in the steady–state. In one dimension the Kohonen net under–represents high density and over–represents low density regions. Thus SOM's are generally not used for density estimation. Several modifications for controlling the magnification of the representation have appeared. Recently, Bauer et. al. (1996) used an "adaptive step size" , and Lin and Cowan (1996) used an L_p-norm weighting to control the magnification. Here we concentrate on the later's "faithful representation" algorithms for source separation and density estimation.

2 SHARPLY PEAKED DISTRIBUTIONS

Mixtures of sharply peaked source distributions will contain high density contours which correspond to the independent component contours. Blind separation can be performed rapidly for this case in a net with one dimensional branched topology. A digital learning rule where the updates only take on discrete values was used: [1]

$$\Delta \vec{w}_i = \kappa \Lambda(\epsilon) \cdot sgn(\vec{\xi} - \vec{w}_i), \tag{1}$$

where κ is the learning rate, $\Lambda(\epsilon)$ the neighborhood function, $\{\vec{w}\}$ the SOM unit positions, and $\vec{\xi}$ the input.

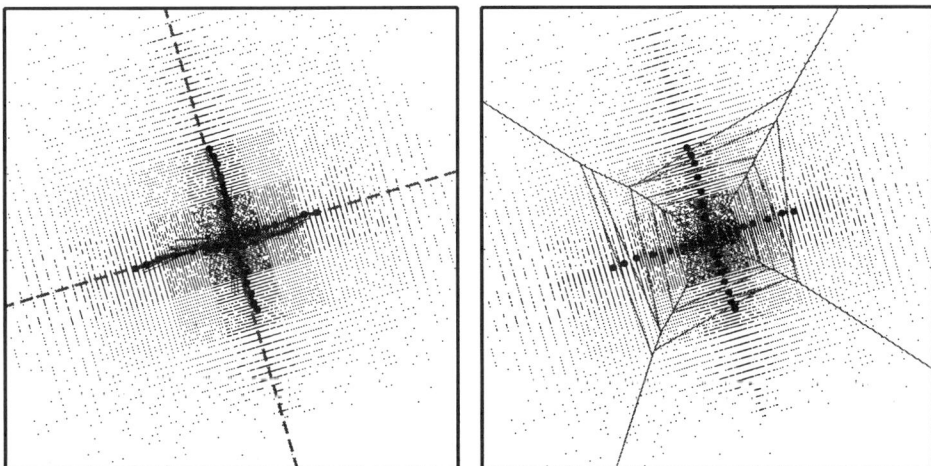

Figure 1: Left: linear source separation by branched net. Dashed lines correspond to the independent component axes. Net configuration is shown every 200 points. Dots denote the unit positions after 4000 points. Right: Voronoi partition of the vector space by the SOM units.

We performed source separation and coding of two mixed signals in a net with the topology of two cross-linked branches (see Fig. (1)). The neighborhood function

---

[1] The sign function $sgn(i)$ takes on a value of 1 for $i > 0$, 0 for $i = 0$ and -1 for $i < 0$. Here the sign function acts component-wise on the vector.

$\Lambda(\epsilon)$ is taken to be Gaussian where ϵ is the distance to the winning unit along the branch structure. Two speech audio files were randomly mixed and pre–whitened first to decorrelate the two mixtures. Since pre–whitening tends to orthogonalize the independent component axes, much of the processing that remains is rotation to find the independent component coordinate system. A typical simulation is shown in Fig. (1). The branches of the net quickly zero in on the high density directions. As seen from the nearest–neighbor Voronoi partition of the distribution (Fig. 1b), the branched SOM essentially performs a one dimensional equipartition of the mixture. The learning rule Eqn. 1 attempts to place each unit at the component-wise median of the distribution encompassed by its Voronoi partition. For sharply peaked sources, the algorithm will place the units directly on top of the high density ridges.

To demonstrate the generality of our non–parametric approach, we perform source separation and density coding of a non-linear mixture. Because our network has local dynamics, with enough units, the network can follow the curved "independent component contours" of the input distribution. The result is shown in Fig. (2).

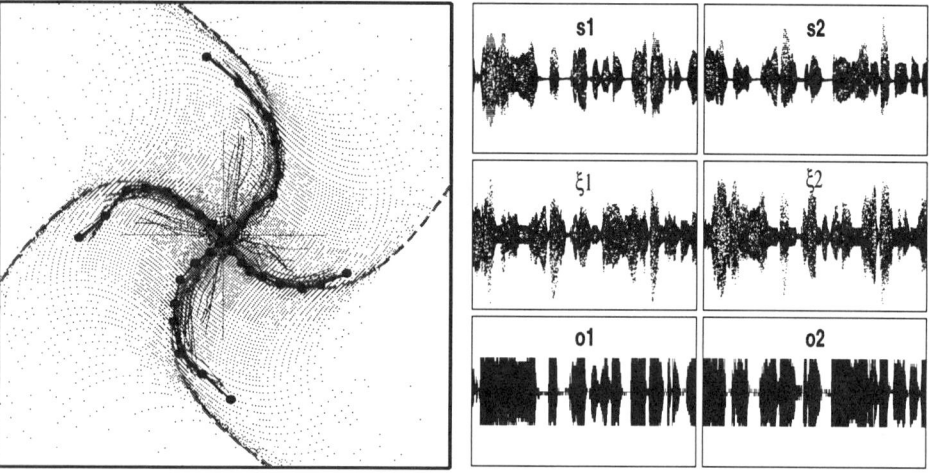

Figure 2: Source separation of non–linear mixture. The mixture is given by $\xi_1 = -2sgn(s_1) \cdot s_1^2 + 1.1s_1 - s_2$, $\xi_2 = -2sgn(s_2) \cdot s_2^2 + s_1 + 1.1s_2$. Left: the SOM configuration is shown periodically in the figure, with the configuration after 12000 points indicated by the dots. Dashed lines denote two independent component contours. Right: the sources (s_1, s_2), mixtures (ξ_1, ξ_2) and pseudo–histogram–equalized representations (o_1, o_2).

To unmix the input, a parametric separation approach can be taken where least squares fit to the branch contours is used. For the source separation in Fig. (1a), assuming linear mixing and inserting the branch coordinate system into an unmixing matrix, we find a reduction of the amplitudes of the mixtures to less than one percent of the signal. This is typical of the quality of separation obtained in our simulations. For the non–linear source separation in Fig. (2), parametric unmixing can similarly be accomplished by least squares fit to polynomial contours with quadratic terms. Alternatively, taking full advantage of the non–parametric nature of the SOM approach, an approximation of the independent sources can be constructed from the positions $\vec{w}_{i^*}$ of the winning unit. Or as we show in Fig. (2b), the cell labels i^* can be used to give a pseudo–histogram–equalized source representation. This non–parametric approach is thus much more general in the sense that no model is needed of the mixing transformation. Since there is only one winning unit along one branch, only one output channel is active at any given time. For sharply peaked source distributions such as speech, this does not significantly hinder the fidelity of the source representation since the input sources hover around zero most of the time. This property also has the potential for utilization in compression. However, for a full rigorous histogram–equalized source representation, we must turn to a network with a topology that matches the dimensionality of the input.

3 ARBITRARY DISTRIBUTIONS

For mixtures of sources with arbitrary distributions, we seek a full N dimensional equipartition. We define an (M, N) partition of $\Re^N$ to be a partition of $\Re^N$ into $(M+1)^N$ regions by M parallel cuts normal to each of N distinct directions. The simplest equipartition of a source mixtures is the trivial equipartition along the independent component axes (ICA). Our goal is to achieve this trivial ICA aligned equipartition using a hypercube architecture SOM with $M+1$ units per dimension. For an (M, N) equipartition, since the number of degrees of freedom to define the MN hyperplanes grows quadratically in N, while the number of constraints grows exponentially in N, for large enough M the desired trivial equipartition will the unique (M, N) equipartition. We postulate that $M = 2$ suffices for uniqueness. Complementary to this claim, it is known that a $(1, N)$ equipartition does not exist for *arbitrary* distributions for $N \geq 5$ (Ramos 1996). The uniqueness of the (M, N) equipartition of source mixtures thus provides an exact verification condition for noiseless source separation.

With $\vec{\epsilon} = \vec{i^*} - \vec{i}$, the digital equipartition learning rule is given by:

$$\Delta \vec{w}_{\vec{i}} = \kappa \Lambda(\vec{\epsilon}) \cdot sgn(\vec{\epsilon}) \qquad (2)$$

$$\Delta \vec{w}_{\vec{i^*}} = \sum_{\vec{i}} \Delta \vec{w}_{\vec{i}}, \qquad (3)$$

where

$$\Lambda(\vec{\epsilon}) = \Lambda(-\vec{\epsilon}). \qquad (4)$$

Equipartion of the input distribution can easily be shown to be a steady–state of the dynamics. Let $q_{\vec{k}}$ be the probability measure of unit $\vec{k}$. For the steady–state:

$$<\Delta \vec{w}_{\vec{k}}> = 0$$
$$= \sum_{\vec{i}} q_{\vec{i}} \cdot \Lambda(\vec{i} - \vec{k}) \cdot sgn(\vec{i} - \vec{k}) + q_{\vec{k}} \sum_{\vec{i}} \Lambda(\vec{k} - \vec{i}) \cdot sgn(\vec{k} - \vec{i})$$
$$= \sum_{\vec{i}} (q_{\vec{i}} - q_{\vec{k}}) \cdot \Lambda(\vec{i} - \vec{k}) \cdot sgn(\vec{i} - \vec{k}),$$

for all units $\vec{k}$. By inspection, equipartition, where $q_{\vec{i}} = q_{\vec{k_0}}$ for all units $\vec{i}$ is a solution to the equation above. It has been shown that equipartition is the only steady–state of the learning rule in two dimensional rectangular SOM's (Lin and Cowan 1996), though with the highly overconstrained steady–state equations, the result should be much more general.

One further modification of the SOM is required. The desired trivial ICA equipartition is not a proper Voronoi partition except when the independent component axes are orthogonal. To obtain the desired equipartition, it is necessary to change the definition of the winning unit $\vec{i}^*$. Let

$$\Omega(\vec{w_i}) = \{\vec{\xi} \in \Re^N : \vec{i}^* = \vec{i}\} \tag{5}$$

be the winning region of the unit at $\vec{w_i}$. Since a histogram–equalized representation independent of the mixing transformation A is desired, we require that

$$\{A\Omega(\vec{w})\} = \{\Omega(A\vec{w})\}, \tag{6}$$

i.e., Ω is *equivariant* under the action of A (see e.g. Golubitsky 1988).

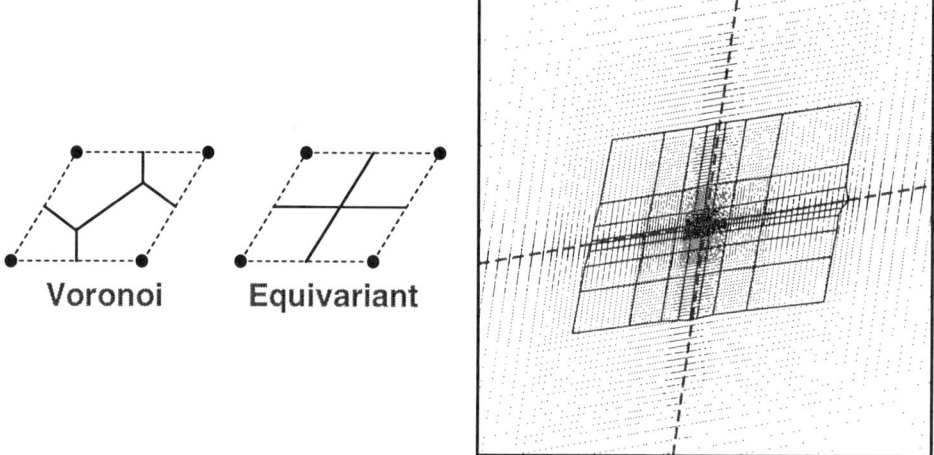

Figure 3: Left: Voronoi and equivariant partitions of the a primitive cell. Right: configuration of the SOM after 4000 points. Initially the units of the SOM were equally spaced and aligned along the two mixture coordinate directions.

In two dimensions, we modify the tessellation by dividing up a primitive cell amongst its constituent units along lines joining the midpoints of the sides. For a primitive cell composed of units at $\vec{a}$, $\vec{b}$, $\vec{c}$ and $\vec{d}$, the region of the primitive cell represented by $\vec{a}$ is the simply connected polygon defined by vertices at $\vec{a}$, $(\vec{a}+\vec{b})/2$, $(\vec{a}+\vec{d})/2$ and $(\vec{a}+\vec{b}+\vec{c}+\vec{d})/4$. The two partitions are contrasted in Fig. (3a). Our modified equivariant partition satisfies Eqn. (6) for all non–singular linear transformations.

The learning rule given above was shown to have an equipartition steady state. It remains, however, to align the partitions so that it becomes a valid (M, N) partition. The addition of a local anisotropic coupling which physically, in analogy to elastic nets, might correspond to a bending modulus along the network's axes, will tend to align the partitions and enhance convergence to the desired steady state. We supplemented the digital learning rule (Eqs. (2)-(3)) with a movement of the units towards the intersections of least squares line fits to the SOM grid.

Numerics are shown in Fig. 3b, where alignment with the independent component coordinate system and density estimation in the form of equipartition can be seen. The aligned equipartition representation formed by the network gives histogram–equalized representations of the independent sources, which, because of the equivariant nature of the SOM, will be independent of the mixing matrix.

4 DISCUSSION

Most source separation algorithms are parametric density estimation approaches (e.g. Bell and Sejnowski 1995, Pearlmutter and Parra 1996). Alternatively in parallel with this work, the standard SOM was used for the separation of both discrete and uniform sources (Herrmann and Yang 1996, Pajunen et. al. 1996). The source separation approach taken here is very general in the sense that no *a priori* assumptions about the individual source distributions and mixing transformation are made. Our approach's local non–parametric nature allows for source separation of non–linear mixtures and also possibly the separation of more sharply peaked sources from fewer mixtures. The low to high dimensional map required for the later task will be prohibitively difficult for parametric unmixing approaches.

For density estimation in the form of equipartition, we point out the importance of a digital scale–invariant algorithm. Direct dependence on $\vec{\xi}$ and $\vec{w}_i$ has been extracted out of the learning rule. Because the update depends only upon the partition, the network learns from its own coarse response to stimuli. This along with the equivariant partition modification underscore the dynamic partition nature of the our algorithm. More direct computational geometry partitioning algorithms are currently being pursued. It is also clear that a hybrid local parametric density estimation approach will work for the separation of sharply peaked sources (Bishop et. al. 1996, Utsugi 1996).

5 CONCLUSIONS

We have extracted the local geometrical structure of transformations of product distributions. By modifying the SOM algorithm we developed a network with the capability of non–parametrically separating out non–linear source mixtures. Sharply peaked sources allow for quick separation via a branched SOM network. For arbitrary source distributions, we introduce the (M,N) equipartition, the uniqueness of which provides an exact verification condition for source separation.

Fundamentally, equipartition of activity is a very sensible resource allocation principle. In this work, the local equipartition coding and source separation processing proceed in tandem, resulting in optimal coding and processing of source mixtures. We believe the digital "counting" aspect of the learning rule, the learning based on the network's own coarse response to stimuli, the local nature of the dynamics, and the coupling of coding and processing make this an attractive approach from both computational and neural modeling perspectives.

References

Bauer, H.-U., Der, R., and Herrmann, M. 1996. Controlling the magnification factor of self–organizing feature maps. *Neural Comp.* **8**, 757-771.

Bell, A. J., and Sejnowski, T. J. 1995. An information-maximization approach to blind separation and blind deconvolution. *Neural Comp.* **7**,1129-1159.

Bell, A. J., and Sejnowski, T. J. 1996. Edges are the "independent components" of natural scenes. *NIPS*9*.

Bishop, C. M. and Williams, C. 1996. GTM: A principled alternative to the self–organizing map. *NIPS*9*.

Field, D. J. 1994. What is the goal of sensory coding? *Neural Comp.* **6**, 559-601.

Golubitsky, M., Stewart, I., and Schaeffer, D. G. 1988. *Singularities and Groups in Bifurcation Theory.* Springer-Verlag, Berlin.

Herrmann, M. and Yang, H. H. 1996. Perspectives and limitations of self–organizing maps in blind separation of source signals. Proc. ICONIP'96.

Hertz, J., Krogh A., and Palmer, R. G. 1991. *Introduction to the Theory of Neural Computation.* Addison-Wesley, Redwood City.

Kohonen, T. 1995. *Self-Organizing Maps.* Springer-Verlag, Berlin.

Lin, J. K. and Cowan, J. D. 1996. Faithful representation of separable input distributions. To appear in *Neural Computation.*

Olshausen, B. A. and D. J. Field 1996. Emergence of simple–cell receptive field properties by learning a sparse code for natural images. *Nature* **381**, 607-609.

Pajunen, P., Hyvarinen, A. and Karhunen, J. 1996. Nonlinear blind source separation by self–organizing maps. Proc. ICONIP'96.

Pearlmutter, B. A. and Parra, L. 1996. Maximum likelihood blind source separation: a context–sensitive generalization of ICA. *NIPS*9*.

Ramos, E. A. 1996. Equipartition of mass distributions by hyperplanes. *Discrete Comput. Geom.* **15**, 147-167.

Ritter, H., and Schulten, K. 1986. On the stationary state of Kohonen's self-organizing sensory mapping. *Biol. Cybern.*, **54**, 99-106.

Utsugi, A. 1996. Hyperparameter selection for self-organizing maps. To appear in *Neural Computation.*

NeuroScale: Novel Topographic Feature Extraction using RBF Networks

David Lowe
D.Lowe@aston.ac.uk

Michael E. Tipping
M.E.Tipping@aston.ac.uk

Neural Computing Research Group
Aston University, Aston Triangle, Birmingham B4 7ET, UK
http://www.ncrg.aston.ac.uk/

Abstract

Dimension-reducing feature extraction neural network techniques which also preserve neighbourhood relationships in data have traditionally been the exclusive domain of Kohonen self organising maps. Recently, we introduced a novel dimension-reducing feature extraction process, which is also topographic, based upon a Radial Basis Function architecture. It has been observed that the generalisation performance of the system is broadly insensitive to model order complexity and other smoothing factors such as the kernel widths, contrary to intuition derived from supervised neural network models. In this paper we provide an effective demonstration of this property and give a theoretical justification for the apparent 'self-regularising' behaviour of the 'NEUROSCALE' architecture.

1 'NeuroScale': A Feed-forward Neural Network Topographic Transformation

Recently an important class of topographic neural network based feature extraction approaches, which can be related to the traditional statistical methods of Sammon Mappings (Sammon, 1969) and Multidimensional Scaling (Kruskal, 1964), have been introduced (Mao and Jain, 1995; Lowe, 1993; Webb, 1995; Lowe and Tipping, 1996). These novel alternatives to Kohonen-like approaches for topographic feature extraction possess several interesting properties. For instance, the NEUROSCALE architecture has the empirically observed property that the generalisation performance does not seem to depend critically on model order complexity, contrary to intuition based upon knowledge of its supervised counterparts. This paper presents evidence for their 'self-regularising' behaviour and provides an explanation in terms of the curvature of the trained models.

We now provide a brief introduction to the NEUROSCALE philosophy of nonlinear topographic feature extraction. Further details may be found in (Lowe, 1993; Lowe and Tipping, 1996). We seek a dimension-reducing, *topographic* transformation of data for the purposes of visualisation and analysis. By 'topographic', we imply that the geometric structure of the data be optimally preserved in the transformation, and the embodiment of this constraint is that the inter-point distances in the feature space should correspond as closely as possible to those distances in the data space. The implementation of this principle by a neural network is very simple. A Radial Basis Function (RBF) neural network is utilised to predict the coordinates of the data point in the transformed feature space. The locations of the feature points are indirectly determined by adjusting the weights of the network. The transformation is determined by optimising the network parameters in order to minimise a suitable error measure that embodies the topographic principle.

The specific details of this alternative approach are as follows. Given an m-dimensional input space of N data points $\mathbf{x}_q$, an n-dimensional feature space of points $\mathbf{y}_q$ is generated such that the relative positions of the feature space points minimise the error, or 'STRESS', term:

$$E = \sum_p \sum_{q>p}^{N} (d_{qp}^* - d_{qp})^2, \qquad (1)$$

where the d_{qp}^* are the inter-point Euclidean distances in the data space: $d_{qp}^* = \sqrt{(\mathbf{x}_q - \mathbf{x}_p)^T(\mathbf{x}_q - \mathbf{x}_p)}$, and the d_{qp} are the corresponding distances in the feature space: $d_{qp} = \sqrt{(\mathbf{y}_q - \mathbf{y}_p)^T(\mathbf{y}_q - \mathbf{y}_p)}$.

The points $\mathbf{y}$ are generated by the RBF, given the data points as input. That is, $\mathbf{y}_q = \mathbf{f}(\mathbf{x}_q; \mathbf{W})$, where $\mathbf{f}$ is the nonlinear transformation effected by the RBF with parameters (weights and any kernel smoothing factors) $\mathbf{W}$. The distances in the feature space may thus be given by $d_{qp} = \| \mathbf{f}(\mathbf{x}_q) - \mathbf{f}(\mathbf{x}_p) \|$ and so more explicitly by

$$d_{qp}^2 = \sum_{l=1}^{n} \left(\sum_k w_{lk} \left[\phi_k(\| \mathbf{x}_q - \boldsymbol{\mu}_k \|) - \phi_k(\| \mathbf{x}_p - \boldsymbol{\mu}_k \|) \right] \right)^2, \qquad (2)$$

where $\phi_k()$ are the basis functions, $\boldsymbol{\mu}_k$ are the centres of those functions, which are fixed, and w_{lk} are the weights from the basis functions to the output.

The topographic nature of the transformation is imposed by the STRESS term which attempts to match the inter-point Euclidean distances in the feature space with those in the input space. This mapping is *relatively supervised* because there is no specific target for each $\mathbf{y}_q$; only a relative measure of target separation between each $\mathbf{y}_q, \mathbf{y}_p$ pair is provided. In this form it does not take account of any additional information (for example, class labels) that might be associated with the data points, but is determined strictly by their spatial distribution. However, the approach may be extended to incorporate the use of extra 'subjective' information which may be used to influence the transformation and permits the extraction of 'enhanced', more informative, feature spaces (Lowe and Tipping, 1996).

Combining equations (1) and (2) and differentiating with respect to the weights in the network allows the partial derivatives of the STRESS $\partial E/\partial w_{lk}$ to be derived for each pattern pair. These may be accumulated over the entire pattern set and the weights adjusted by an iterative procedure to minimise the STRESS term E. Note that the objective function for the RBF is no longer quadratic, and so a standard analytic matrix-inversion method for fixing the final layer weights cannot be employed.

We refer to this overall procedure as 'NEUROSCALE'. Although any universal approximator may be exploited within NEUROSCALE, using a Radial Basis Function network allows more theoretical analysis of the resulting behaviour, despite the fact that we have lost the usual linearity advantages of the RBF because of the STRESS measure. A schematic of the NEUROSCALE model is given in figure 1, and illustrates the rôle of the RBF in transforming the data space to the feature space.

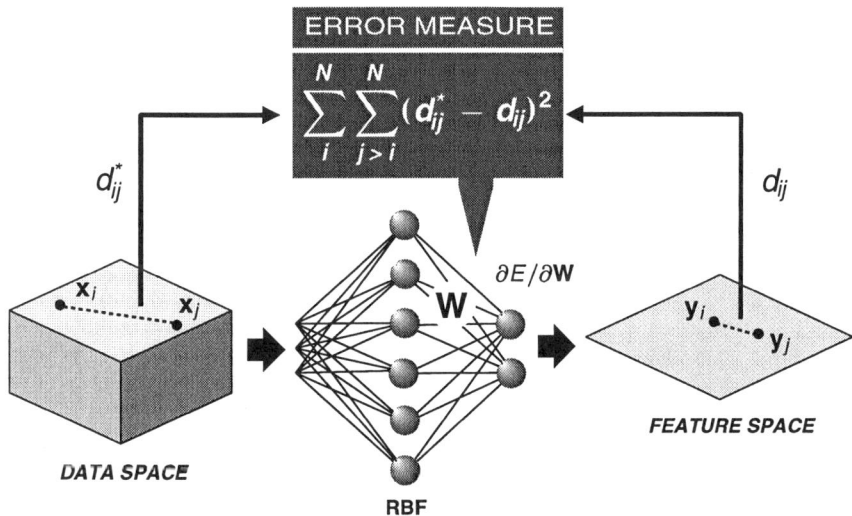

Figure 1: The NEUROSCALE architecture.

2 Generalisation

In a supervised learning context, generalisation performance deteriorates for over-complex networks as 'overfitting' occurs. By contrast, it is an interesting empirical observation that the generalisation performance of NEUROSCALE, and related models, is largely insensitive to excessive model complexity. This applies both to the number of centres used in the RBF and in the kernel smoothing factors which themselves may be viewed as regularising hyperparameters in a feed-forward supervised situation.

This insensitivity may be illustrated by Figure 2, which shows the training and test set performances on the IRIS data (for 5-45 basis functions trained and tested on 45 separate samples). To within acceptable deviations, the training and test set

STRESS values are approximately constant. This behaviour is counter-intuitive when compared with research on feed forward networks trained according to supervised approaches. We have observed this general trend on a variety of diverse real world problems, and it is not peculiar to the IRIS data.

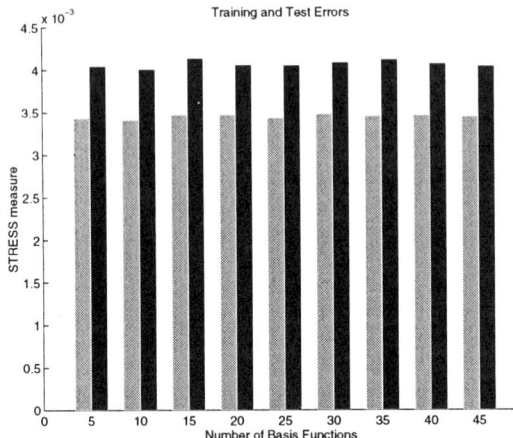

Figure 2: Training and test errors for NEUROSCALE Radial Basis Functions with various numbers of basis functions. Training errors are on the left, test errors are on the right.

There are two fundamental causes of this observed behaviour. Firstly, we may derive significant insight into the necessary form of the functional transformation independent of the data. Secondly, given this prior functional knowledge, there is an appropriate regularising component implicitly incorporated in the training algorithm outlined in the previous section.

2.1 Smoothness and Topographic Transformations

For a supervised problem, in the absence of any explicit prior information, the smoothness of the network function must be determined by the data, typically necessitating the setting of regularising hyperparameters to counter overfitting behaviour. In the case of the distance-preserving transformation effected by NEUROSCALE, an understanding of the necessary smoothness may be deduced *a priori*.

Consider a point $\mathbf{x}_q$ in input space and a nearby test point $\mathbf{x}_p = \mathbf{x}_q + \epsilon_{pq}$, where ϵ_{pq} is an arbitrary displacement vector. Optimum generalisation demands that the distance between the corresponding image points $\mathbf{y}_q$ and $\mathbf{y}_p$ should thus be $\|\epsilon_{pq}\|$. Considering the Taylor expansions around the point $\mathbf{y}_q$ we find

$$\|\mathbf{y}_p - \mathbf{y}_q\|^2 = \sum_{l=1}^{n}(\epsilon_{pq}^{\mathrm{T}}\mathbf{g}_{ql})^2 + O(\epsilon^4),$$

$$= \epsilon_{pq}^{\mathrm{T}}\left(\sum_{l=1}^{n}\mathbf{g}_{ql}\mathbf{g}_{ql}^{T}\right)\epsilon_{pq} + O(\epsilon^4), \quad (3)$$

$$= \epsilon_{pq}^{\mathrm{T}}\mathbf{G}_q\epsilon_{pq} + O(\epsilon^4),$$

where the matrix $\mathbf{G}_q = \sum_{l=1}^{n} \mathbf{g}_{ql} \mathbf{g}_{ql}^T$ and $\mathbf{g}_{ql}$ is the gradient vector $(\partial y_l(q)/\partial x_1, \ldots, \partial y_l(q)/\partial x_n)^T$ evaluated at $\mathbf{x} = \mathbf{x}_q$. For structure preservation the corresponding distances in input and output spaces need to be retained for all values of ϵ_{pq}: $\|\mathbf{y}_p - \mathbf{y}_q\|^2 = \epsilon^T \epsilon$, and so $\mathbf{G}_q = \mathbf{I}$ with the requirement that second- and higher-order terms must vanish. In particular note that measures of curvature proportional to $\left(\partial^2 y_l(q)/\partial x_i^2\right)^2$ should vanish. In general, for dimension reduction, we cannot ensure that exact structure preservation is obtained since the rank of $\mathbf{G}_q$ is necessarily less than n and hence can never equate to the identity matrix. However, when minimising STRESS we are locally attempting to minimise the residual $\|\mathbf{I} - \mathbf{G}_q\|$, which is achieved when all the vectors ϵ_{pq} of interest lie within the range of $\mathbf{G}_q$.

2.2 The Training Mechanism

An important feature of this class of topographic transformations is that the STRESS measure is invariant under arbitrary rotations and transformations of the output configuration. The algorithm outlined previously tends towards those configurations that generally reduce the sum-of-squared weight values (Tipping, 1996). This is achieved without any explicit addition of regularisation, but rather it is a feature of the relative supervision algorithm.

The effect of this reduction in weight magnitudes on the smoothness of the network transformation may be observed by monitoring an explicit quantitative measure of *total* curvature:

$$C = \sum_{q}^{N} \sum_{l}^{n} \sum_{i}^{m} \left(\frac{\partial^2 y_l(q)}{\partial x_i^2}\right)^2, \qquad (4)$$

where q ranges over the patterns, i over the input dimensions and l over the output dimensions.

Figure 3 depicts the total curvature of NEUROSCALE as a function of the training iterations on the IRIS subset data for a variety of model complexities. As predicted, curvature generally decreases during the training process, with the final value independent of the model complexity. Theoretical insight into this phenomenon is given in (Tipping, 1996).

This behaviour is highly relevant, given the analysis of the previous subsection. That the training algorithm implicitly reduces the sum-of-squares weight values implies that there is a *weight decay* process occurring with an associated smoothing effect. While there is no control over the magnitude of this element, it was shown that for good generalisation, the optimal transformation should be maximally smooth. This self-regularisation operates differently to regularisers normally introduced to stabilise the ill-posed problems of supervised neural network models. In the latter case the regulariser acts to oppose the effect of reducing the error on the training set. In NEUROSCALE the implicit weight decay operates *with* the minimisation of STRESS since the aim is to 'fit' the *relative* input positions exactly.

That there are many RBF networks which satisfy a given STRESS level may be seen by training a network *a posteriori* on a predetermined Sammon mapping of a data set by a supervised approach (since then the targets *are* known explicitly). In general, such *a posteriori* trained networks do not have a low curvature and hence

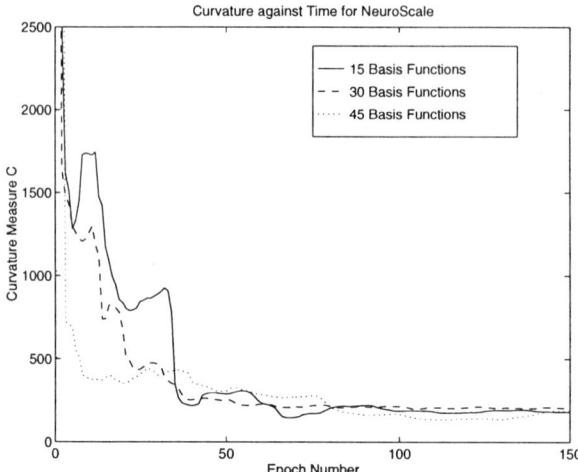

Figure 3: Curvature against time during the training of a NEUROSCALE mapping on the Iris data, for networks with 15, 30 and 45 basis functions.

do not show as good a generalisation behaviour as networks trained according to the relative supervision approach. The method by which NEUROSCALE reduces curvature, is to select, automatically, RBF networks with minimum norm weights. This is an inherent property of the training algorithm to reduce the STRESS criterion.

2.3 An example

An effective example of the ease of production of good generalising transformations is given by the following experiment. A synthetic data set comprised four Gaussian clusters, each with spherical variance of 0.5, located in four dimensions with centres at $(x_c, 0, 0, 0) : x_c \in \{1, 2, 3, 4\}$. A NEUROSCALE transformation to two dimensions was trained using the relative supervision approach, using the three clusters at $x_c = 1, 3$ and 4. The network was then tested on the entire dataset, with the fourth cluster included, and the projections are given in Figure 4 below.

The apparently excellent generalisation to test data not sampled from the same distribution as the training data is a function of the inherent smoothing within the training process and also reflects the fact that the test data lay approximately within the range of the matrices $\mathbf{G_q}$ determined during training.

3 Conclusion

We have described NEUROSCALE, a parameterised RBF Sammon mapping approach for topographic feature extraction. The NEUROSCALE method may be viewed as a technique which is closely related to Sammon mappings and nonlinear metric MDS, with the added flexibility of producing a generalising transformation.

A theoretical justification has been provided for the empirical observation that the generalisation performance is not affected by model order complexity issues. This counter-intuitive result is based on arguments of necessary transformation smooth-

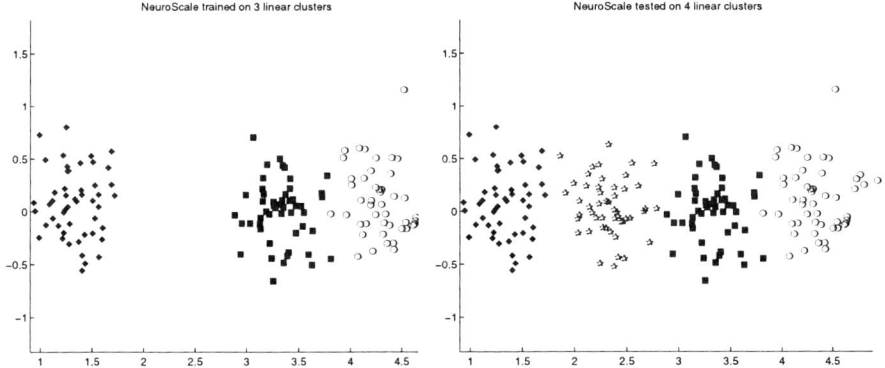

Figure 4: Training and test projections of the four clusters. Training STRESS was 0.00515 and test STRESS 0.00532.

ness coupled with the apparent self-regularising aspects of NEUROSCALE. The relative supervision training algorithm implicitly minimises a measure of curvature by incorporating an automatic 'weight decay' effect which favours solutions generated by networks with small overall weights.

Acknowledgements

This work was supported in part under the EPSRC contract GR/J75425, *"Novel Developments in Learning Theory for Neural Networks"*.

References

Kruskal, J. B. (1964). Multidimensional scaling by optimising goodness of fit to a nonmetric hypothesis. *Psychometrika*, 29(1):1–27.

Lowe, D. (1993). Novel 'topographic' nonlinear feature extraction using radial basis functions for concentration coding in the 'artificial nose'. In *3rd IEE International Conference on Artificial Neural Networks*. London: IEE.

Lowe, D. and Tipping, M. E. (1996). Feed-forward neural networks and topographic mappings for exploratory data analysis. *Neural Computing and Applications*, 4:83–95.

Mao, J. and Jain, A. K. (1995). Artificial neural networks for feature extraction and multivariate data projection. *IEEE Transactions on Neural Networks*, 6(2):296–317.

Sammon, J. W. (1969). A nonlinear mapping for data structure analysis. *IEEE Transactions on Computers*, C-18(5):401–409.

Tipping, M. E. (1996). *Topographic Mappings and Feed-Forward Neural Networks*. PhD thesis, Aston University, Aston Street, Birmingham B4 7ET, UK. Available from http://www.ncrg.aston.ac.uk/.

Webb, A. R. (1995). Multidimensional scaling by iterative majorisation using radial basis functions. *Pattern Recognition*, 28(5):753–759.

Ordered Classes and Incomplete Examples in Classification

Mark Mathieson
Department of Statistics, University of Oxford
1 South Parks Road, Oxford OX1 3TG, UK
E-mail: mathies@stats.ox.ac.uk

Abstract

The classes in classification tasks often have a natural ordering, and the training and testing examples are often incomplete. We propose a non-linear ordinal model for classification into ordered classes. Predictive, simulation-based approaches are used to learn from past and classify future incomplete examples. These techniques are illustrated by making prognoses for patients who have suffered severe head injuries.

1 Motivation

Jennett *et al.* (1979) reported data on patients with severe head injuries. For each patient some of the information in Table 1 was available shortly after injury. The objective is to predict the degree of recovery attained within six months as measured by outcome. This problem exhibits two characteristics that are common in classification tasks: allocation of examples into classes which have a natural ordering, and learning from past and classifying future incomplete examples.

2 A Flexible Model for Ordered Classes

The Bayes decision rule (see, for example, Ripley, 1996) depends on the loss $L(j,k)$ incurred in assigning to class k an object belonging to class j. When better information is unavailable, for unordered or *nominal* classes we treat every mis-classification as equally serious: $L(j,k)$ is 0 when $j = k$ and 1 otherwise. For ordered classes, when the K classes are numbered from 1 to K in their natural order, a better default choice is $L(j,k) = |j-k|$. A class is then given support by its position in the ordering, and the Bayes rule will sometimes assign patterns to classes that do not have maximum posterior probability to avoid making a serious error.

Table 1: Definition of variables with proportion missing.

Variable	Definition	Missing %
age	Age in decades (1=0–9, 2=10–19, ..., 8=70+).	0
emv	Measure of eye, motor and verbal response to stimulation (1–7).	41
motor	Motor response patterns for all limbs (1–7).	33
change	Change in neurological function over the first 24 hours (–1,0,+1).	78
eye	Eye indicant. 1 (bad), 2 (impaired), 3 (good).	65
pupils	Pupil reaction to light. 1 (non-reacting), 2 (reacting).	30
outcome	Recovery after six months based on Glasgow Outcome Scale. 1 (dead/vegetative), 2 (severe disability), 3 (moderate/good recovery).	0

If the classes in a classification problem are ordered the ordering should also be reflected in the probability model. Methods for nominal tasks can certainly be used for ordinal problems, but an ordinal model should have a simpler parameterization than comparable nominal models, and interpretation will be easier. Suppose that an example represented by a row vector X belongs to class $C = C(X)$. To make the Bayes-optimal classification it is sufficient to know the posterior probabilities $p(C = k \mid X = x)$. The *ordinal logistic regression* (OLR) model for K ordered classes models the cumulative posterior class probabilities $p(C \leqslant k \mid X = x)$ by

$$\log\left[\frac{p(C \leqslant k \mid X = x)}{1 - p(C \leqslant k \mid X = x)}\right] = \phi_k - \eta(x) \qquad k = 1, \ldots, K-1, \qquad (1)$$

for some function η. We impose the constraints $\phi_1 \leqslant \ldots \leqslant \phi_{K-1}$ on the *cut-points* to ensure that $p(C \leqslant k \mid X = x)$ increases with k. If $\phi_0 = -\infty$ and $\phi_K = \infty$ then (1) gives

$$p(C = k \mid X = x) = \sigma(\phi_k - \eta(x)) - \sigma(\phi_{k-1} - \eta(x)) \qquad k = 1, \ldots, K$$

where $\sigma(x) = 1/(1 + e^{-x})$. McCullagh (1980) proposed linear OLR where $\eta(x) = x\beta$.

The posterior probabilities depend on the patterns x only through η, and high values of $\eta(x)$ correspond to higher predicted classes (Figure 1a). This can be useful for interpreting the fitted model. However, linear OLR is rather inflexible since the decision boundaries are always parallel hyperplanes. Departures from linearity can be accommodated by allowing η to be a non-linear function of the feature space. We extend OLR to non-linear ordinal logistic regression (NOLR) by letting $\eta(x)$ be the single linear output of a feed-forward neural network with input vector x, having skip-layer connections and sigmoid transfer functions in the hidden layer (Figure 1b). Then for weights w_{ij} and biases b_j we have

$$\eta(x) = \sum_{i \to o} w_{io} x_{(i)} + \sum_{j \to o} w_{jo} \sigma(b_j + \sum_{i \to j} w_{ij} x_{(i)}),$$

where $\sum_{i \to j}$ denotes the sum over i such that node i is connected to node j, and node o is the single output node. The usual output-unit bias is incorporated in the cut-points. Observe that OLR is the special case of NOLR with no hidden nodes. Although the network component of NOLR is a universal approximator the NOLR model cannot approximate all probability densities arbitrarily well (unlike 'softmax', the most similar nominal method).

The likelihood for the cut-points $\phi = (\phi_1, \ldots, \phi_{K-1})$ and network parameters $\mathbf{w}$ given a training set $\mathcal{T} = \{(x_i, c_i) \mid i = 1, \ldots, n\}$ of n correctly classified examples is

$$\ell(\mathbf{w}, \phi) = \prod_{i=1}^{n} p(c_i \mid x_i) = \prod_{i=1}^{n} \left[\sigma(\phi_{c_i} - \eta(x_i; \mathbf{w})) - \sigma(\phi_{c_i-1} - \eta(x_i; \mathbf{w}))\right]. \qquad (2)$$

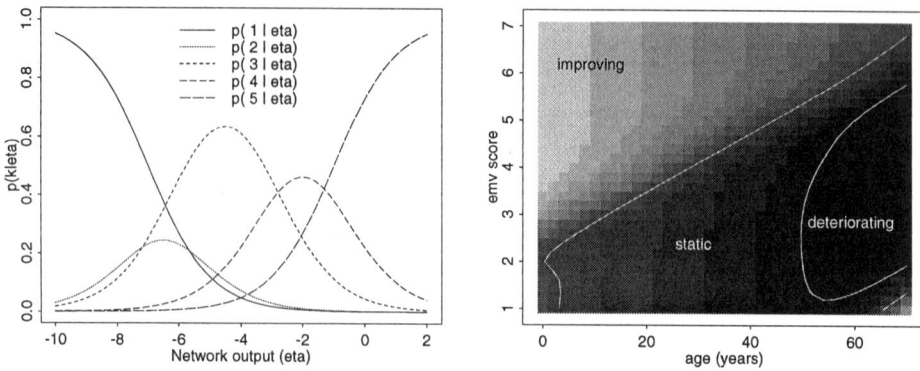

Figure 1: **(a)** $p(k \mid \eta)$ plotted against η for an OLR model with $K = 5$ classes and $\phi = (-7, -6, -3, -1)$. **(b)** The network output $\eta(x)$ from a NOLR model used to predict change given all other variables (except outcome) predicts that young patients with high emv score are likely to improve over first 24 hours. While age and emv are varied, other variables are fixed. Dark shading denotes low values of $\eta(x)$. The Bayes decision boundaries are shown for loss $L(j, k) = \mid j - k \mid$.

If we estimate the classifier by substituting the maximum likelihood estimates we must maximize (2) whilst constraining the cut-points to be increasing (Mathieson, 1996). To avoid over-fitting we regularize both by weight decay (which is equivalent to putting independent Gaussian priors on the network weights) and by imposing independent Gamma priors on the differences between adjacent cut-points. The minimand is now $-\log \ell(\mathbf{w}, \phi) + \lambda D(\mathbf{w}) + E(\phi; t, \alpha)$ with hyperparameters $\lambda > 0, t, \alpha$ (to be chosen by cross-validation, for example, or averaged over under a Bayesian scheme) where $D(\mathbf{w}) = \sum_{i,j} w_{ij}^2$ and

$$E(\phi) = \sum_{i=2}^{K-1} \left[t(\phi_i - \phi_{i-1}) + (1 - \alpha) \log(\phi_i - \phi_{i-1}) \right].$$

3 Classification and Incomplete Examples

We now consider simulation-based methods for training diagnostic paradigm classifiers from incomplete examples, and classifying future incomplete examples. To avoid modelling the missing data we assume that the missing data mechanism is independent of the missing values given the observed values (*missing at random*) and that the missing data and data generation mechanisms are independent (*ignorable*) (Little & Rubin, 1987). This assumption is rarely true but is usually less damaging than adopting crude *ad hoc* approaches to missing values.

3.1 Learning from Incomplete Examples

The training set is $\mathcal{T} = \{(x_i^o, c_i) \mid i = 1, \ldots, n\}$ where x_i^o, x_i^u are the observed and unobserved parts of the ith example, which belongs to class c_i. Define $\mathcal{X}^o = \{x_i^o \mid i = 1, \ldots, n\}$ and $\mathcal{X}^u = \{x_i^u \mid i = 1, \ldots, n\}$, and use $\mathcal{C}$ to denote all the classes, so $\mathcal{T} = (\mathcal{X}^o, \mathcal{C})$. We assume that $\mathcal{C}$ is fully observed. Under the diagnostic paradigm (which includes logistic regression and its non-linear and ordinal variants such as 'softmax' and

Ordered Classes and Incomplete Examples in Classification

NOLR) we model $p(c \mid x)$ by $p(c \mid x; \theta)$ giving the conditional likelihood

$$\ell(\theta) = \prod_{i=1}^{n} p(c_i \mid x_i^o; \theta) = \prod_{i=1}^{n} \mathbb{E}_{X_i^u \mid x_i^o} p(c_i \mid x_i^o, X_i^u; \theta) = \mathbb{E}_{\mathcal{X}^u \mid \mathcal{X}^o} \prod_{i=1}^{n} p(c_i \mid x_i^o, X_i^u; \theta) \quad (3)$$

when the examples are independent. The model for $p(c \mid x)$ contains no information about $p(x)$ and so we construct a model for $p(x^u \mid x^o)$ separately using $\mathcal{T}$ (Section 3.2). Once we can sample $x_{i1}^u, \ldots, x_{im}^u$ from $p(x_i^u \mid x_i^o, c_i)$ a Monte Carlo approximation for $\ell(\theta)$ based on the last expression of (3) by averaging over repeated imputations of the missing values in the training set (Little & Rubin, 1987, and earlier):

$$\log \ell(\theta) \approx \log\left(\frac{1}{m}\sum_{j=1}^{m}\prod_{i=1}^{n} p(c_i \mid x_i^o, x_{ij}^u; \theta)\right). \quad (4)$$

Existing algorithms for finding maximum likelihood estimates for θ allow maximization of the individual summands in (4) with respect to θ, but in general the software will require extensive modification in order to maximize the average. This problem can be avoided if we approximate the arithmetic average over the imputations by a geometric one so that $\ell(\theta) \approx \left(\prod_j \prod_i p(c_i \mid x_i^o, x_{ij}^u; \theta)\right)^{1/m}$. Now the log-posterior averages over the *log* of the likelihoods of the completed training sets, so standard estimation algorithms can be used on a training set formed by pooling all completions of the training set, giving each weight $1/m$. The approximation $\log \frac{1}{m}\sum_j p_j \approx \frac{1}{m}\sum_j \log p_j$ has been made, where we define $p_j(\theta) = \prod_i p(c_i \mid x_i^o, x_{ij}^u; \theta)$, although in fact $\log \frac{1}{m}\sum_j p_j \geq \frac{1}{m}\sum_j \log p_j$ everywhere. Suppose that the p_j are well approximated by some function p for the region of interest in the parameter space. Then in this region

$$\log \frac{1}{m}\sum_j p_j - \frac{1}{m}\sum_j \log p_j \approx \frac{1}{2m}\sum_i \left(\frac{p_i - p}{p}\right)^2 - \frac{1}{2m^2}\sum_{i,j} \frac{(p_i - p)(p_j - p)}{p^2} \quad (5)$$

and so the approximation will be reasonable when the imputed values have little effect on the likelihood of the completed training sets. Note that the approximation cannot be improved by increasing m; (5) does not tend to zero as $m \to \infty$. The relative effects on the likelihood of making this approximation and the Monte Carlo approximation (4) will be problem specific and dependent on m.

The predictive approach (Ripley, 1996, for example) incorporates uncertainty in θ by estimating $p(c \mid x)$ as $\tilde{p}(c \mid x) = \mathbb{E}_{\theta \mid \mathcal{T}} p(c \mid x; \theta)$. Changing the order of integration gives

$$\tilde{p}(c \mid x) = \int p(c \mid x; \theta) p(\theta \mid \mathcal{T}) \, d\theta \propto \int p(c \mid x; \theta) p(\theta) \prod_{i=1}^{n} \mathbb{E}_{X_i^u \mid x_i^o} p(c_i \mid x_i^o, X_i^u; \theta) \, d\theta$$

$$= \mathbb{E}_{\mathcal{X}^u \mid \mathcal{X}^o} \int p(c \mid x; \theta) p(\theta) \prod_{i=1}^{n} p(c_i \mid x_i^o, X_i^u; \theta) \, d\theta \quad (6)$$

This justifies applying standard techniques for complete data to build a separate classifier using each completed training set, and then averaging the posterior class probabilities that they predict. The integral over θ in (6) will usually require approximation; in particular we could average over plug-in estimates to obtain $\tilde{p}(c \mid x) \approx \frac{1}{m}\sum_{j=1}^{m} p(c \mid x; \hat{\theta}_j)$, where $\hat{\theta}_j$ is the MAP estimate of θ based only on the jth imputed training set. A more subtle approach

Table 2: Classifier performance on 301 complete test examples. See Section 4.

Training set	Test set loss
40 complete training examples only	132
40 complete + 206 incomplete training examples:	
• Median imputation (In each variable, substitute the median for missing values whenever they occur.)	149
• Averaging predicted probabilities over 1000 completions of $\mathcal{T}$ generated by:	
▷ Unconditional imputation (Sample missing values from the empirical distribution of each variable in the training set.)	133
▷ Gibbs sampling from $p(\mathcal{X}^u \mid \mathcal{X}^o, \hat{\psi})$	118
Pool the 1000 completions from the line above to form a single training set	117

(Ripley, 1994) approximates each posterior by a mixture of Gaussians centred at the local maxima $\hat{\theta}_{j1}, \ldots, \hat{\theta}_{jR_j}$ of $p(\theta \mid \mathcal{T}, \mathcal{X}_j^u)$ to give

$$p(\theta \mid \mathcal{T}, \mathcal{X}_j^u) \approx \frac{1}{\sum_r w_{jr}} \sum_{r=1}^{R_j} w_{jr} \mathrm{N}(\theta; \hat{\theta}_{jr}, H_{jr}^{-1}) \tag{7}$$

where: $\mathrm{N}(\cdot; \mu, \Sigma)$ is the Gaussian density function with mean μ and covariance matrix Σ, the Hessian $H_{jr} = \frac{\partial^2}{\partial \theta^T \partial \theta} \log p(\theta \mid \mathcal{T}, \mathcal{X}_j^u)$ is evaluated at $\hat{\theta}_{jr}$ and, using Laplace's approximation, $w_{jr} = p(\hat{\theta}_{jr} \mid \mathcal{T}, \mathcal{X}_j^u) \mid H_{jr} \mid^{-1/2}$. We can average over the maxima to get $\tilde{p}(c \mid x) \approx (m \sum_{j,r} w_{jr})^{-1} \sum_{j,r} p(c \mid x; \hat{\theta}_{jr})$, but the full-blooded approach samples from the 'mixture of mixtures' approximation to $p(\theta \mid \mathcal{T})$ and also uses importance sampling to compute the predictive estimates $\tilde{p}$.

3.2 The Imputation Model

We need samples from $p(x_i^u \mid x_i^o, c_i)$ for each i. When many patterns of missing values occur it is not practical to model $p(x^u \mid x^o, c)$ for each pattern, but Markov chain Monte Carlo methods can be employed. The Gibbs sampler is convenient and in its most basic form requires models for the distribution of each element of x given the others, that is $p(x^{(j)} \mid x^{(-j)}, c)$ where $x^{(-j)} = (x^{(1)}, \ldots, x^{(j-1)}, x^{(j+1)}, \ldots, x^{(p)})$. We model these *full conditionals* parametrically as $p(x^{(j)} \mid x^{(-j)}, c; \psi)$ and assume here that the parameters for each of the full conditionals are disjoint, so $p(x^{(j)} \mid x^{(-j)}, c; \psi^{(j)})$ where $\psi = (\psi^{(1)}, \ldots, \psi^{(p)})$. When $x^{(j)}$ takes discrete values this is a classification task, and for continuous values a regression problem. Under certain conditions the chain of dependent samples of X^u converges in distribution to $p(x^u \mid x^o, \psi)$ and the ergodic average of $p(c \mid x^o, X^u)$ converges as required to the predictive estimate $\tilde{p}(c \mid x^o)$. We usually take every wth sample to provide a cover of the space in fewer samples, reducing the computation required to learn the classifier. It is essential to check convergence of the Gibbs sampler although we do not give details here.

If we have sufficient complete examples we might use them to estimate ψ to be $\hat{\psi}$ and Gibbs sample from $p(\mathcal{X}^u \mid \mathcal{X}^o; \hat{\psi})$. Otherwise, in the Bayesian framework, incorporate ψ into the sampling scheme by Gibbs sampling from $p(\psi, \mathcal{X}^u \mid \mathcal{X}^o)$ (the solution suggested by Li, 1988). In the head injury example we report results using the former approach. (The latter was found to make little improvement and requires considerably more computation time.)

Table 3: Predictive approximations for a NOLR model fitted to a single completion $\mathcal{T}, \mathcal{X}^u$ of the training set. The likelihood maxima at $\hat{\theta}_1$ and $\hat{\theta}_2$ account for over 0.99 of the posterior probability.

	$\hat{\theta}_1$	$\hat{\theta}_2$	
Posterior probability	0.929	0.071	
$-\log p(\hat{\theta}_i \mid \mathcal{T}, \mathcal{X}^u)$	176.10	174.65	
Test set loss:			Predictive:
• using the plug-in classifier $p(c \mid x; \hat{\theta}_i)$	128	149	126
• averaging over 10,000 samples from Gaussian	120	137	119

3.3 Classifying Incomplete Examples

We could build a separate classifier for each pattern of missing data that occurs, but this can be computationally expensive, will lose information and the classifiers need not make consistent predictions. We know that $p(c \mid x^o) = \mathbb{E}_{X^u \mid x^o} p(c \mid x^o, X^u)$ so it seems better to classify x^o by averaging over repeated imputations of x^u from the imputation model.

4 Prognosis After Head Injury

We now return to the head injury prognosis example to learn a NOLR classifier from a training set containing 40 complete and 206 incomplete examples. The NOLR architecture (4 nodes, skip-layer connections and $\lambda = 0.01$) was selected by cross-validation on a single imputation of the training set, and we use a predictive approximation.[1] Table 2 shows the performance of this classifier on a test set of 301 complete examples and loss $L(j, k) = \mid j - k \mid$ for different strategies for dealing with the missing values. For imputation by Gibbs sampling we modelled each of the full conditionals using NOLR because all variables in this dataset are ordinal. Categorical inputs to models are put in as level indicators, so change corresponds to two indicators taking values (0,0), (1,0) and (1,1). Throughout this example we predict age, emv and motor as categorical variables but treat them as continuous inputs to models. Models were selected by cross-validation based on the complete training examples only and used the predictive approximation described above. Several full conditionals benefited from a non linear model.

We now classify 199 incomplete test examples using the classifier found in the last line of Table 2. Median imputation of missing values in the test set incurs loss 132 whereas unconditional imputation incurs loss 106. The Gibbs sampling imputation model incurs loss 91 and is predicting probabilities accurately (Figure 2). Michie *et al.* (1994) and references therein give alternative analyses of the head injury data.

NOLR has provided an interpretable network model for ordered classes, the missing data strategy successfully learns from incomplete training examples and classifies incomplete future examples, and the predictive approach is beneficial.

---

[1] For each completion $\mathcal{T}, \mathcal{X}_j^u$ of the training set we form a mixture approximation (7) to $p(\theta \mid \mathcal{T}, \mathcal{X}_j^u)$, sample from this 10,000 times and average the predicted probabilities. These predictions are averaged over completions. Maxima were found by running the optimizer 50 times from randomized starting weights. Up to 26 distinct maxima were found and approximately 5 generally accounted for over 95% of the posterior probability in most cases. Table 3 gives an example: averaging over maxima has greater effect than sampling around them, although both are useful. The cut-points ϕ in the NOLR model must satisfy order constraints, so we rejected samples of θ where these did not hold. However, the parameters were sufficiently well determined that this occurred in less than 0.5% of samples.

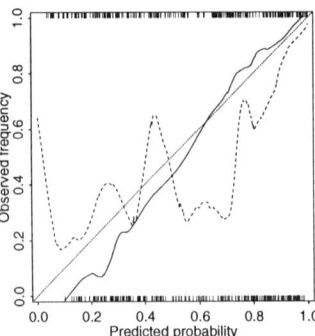 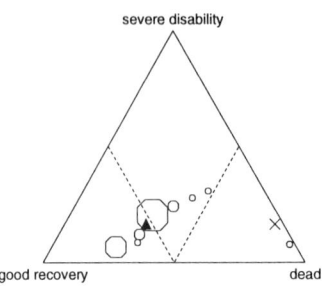

Figure 2: (a) Test set calibration for median imputation (dashed) and conditional imputation (solid). For predictions by conditional imputation we average $p(c \mid x^o, X^u)$ over 100 pseudo-independent samples from $p(x^u \mid x^o)$. Ticks on the lower (upper) axis denote predicted probabilities for the test examples using median (conditional) imputation. (b) In 100 pseudo-independent conditional imputations of the missing parts x^u of a particular incomplete test example eight distinct values x_i^u ($i = 1, \ldots, 8$) occur. (Recall that all components of x are discrete.) For each distinct imputation we plot a circle with centre corresponding to $(p(1 \mid x^o, x_i^u), p(2 \mid x^o, x_i^u), p(3 \mid x^o, x_i^u))$ and area proportional to the number of occurrences of x_i^u in the 100 imputations. The prediction by median imputation is located by ×; the average prediction over conditional imputations is located by ▲. Actual outcome is 'good recovery'. The conditional method correctly classifies the example and shows that the example is close to the Bayes decision boundary under loss $L(j, k) = \mid j - k \mid$ (dashed). Median imputation results in a confident and incorrect classification.

Software: A software library for fitting NOLR models in S-Plus is available at URL http://www.stats.ox.ac.uk/~mathies

Acknowledgements: The author thanks Brian Ripley for productive discussions of this work and Gordon Murray for permission to use the head injury dataset. This research was funded by the UK EPSRC and investment managers GMO Woolley Ltd.

References

Jennett, B., Teasdale, G., Braakman, R., Minderhoud, J., Heiden, J. & Kurze, T. (1979) Prognosis of patients with severe head injury. *Neurosurgery,* **4** 782–790.

Li, K.-H. (1988) Imputation using Markov chains. *Journal of Statistical Computation and Simulation,* **30** 57–79.

Little, R. & Rubin, D. B. (1987) Statistical Analysis with Missing Data. (Wiley, New York).

Mathieson, M. J. (1996) Ordinal models for neural networks. In *Neural Networks in Financial Engineering,* eds A.-P. Refenes, Y. Abu-Mostafa, J. Moody and A. S. Weigend (World Scientific, Singapore) 523–536.

McCullagh, P. (1980) Regression models for ordinal data. *Journal of the Royal Statistical Society Series B,* **42** 109–142.

Michie, D., Spiegelhalter, D. J. & Taylor, C. C. (eds) (1994) Machine Learning, Neural and Statistical Classification. (Ellis Horwood, New York).

Ripley, B. D. (1994) Flexible non-linear approaches to classification. In *From Statistics to Neural Networks. Theory and Pattern Recognition Applications,* eds V. Cherkassky, J. H. Friedman and H. Wechsler (Springer Verlag, New York) 108–126.

Ripley, B. D. (1996) *Pattern Recognition and Neural Networks.* (Cambridge University Press, Cambridge).

Triangulation by Continuous Embedding

Marina Meilă and Michael I. Jordan
{mmp, jordan}@ai.mit.edu
Center for Biological & Computational Learning
Massachusetts Institute of Technology
45 Carleton St. E25-201
Cambridge, MA 02142

Abstract

When triangulating a belief network we aim to obtain a junction tree of minimum state space. According to (Rose, 1970), searching for the optimal triangulation can be cast as a search over all the permutations of the graph's vertices. Our approach is to embed the discrete set of permutations in a convex continuous domain D. By suitably extending the cost function over D and solving the continous nonlinear optimization task we hope to obtain a good triangulation with respect to the aforementioned cost. This paper presents two ways of embedding the triangulation problem into continuous domain and shows that they perform well compared to the best known heuristic.

1 INTRODUCTION. WHAT IS TRIANGULATION ?

Belief networks are graphical representations of probability distributions over a set of variables. In what follows it will be always assumed that the variables take values in a finite set and that they correspond to the vertices of a graph. The graph's arcs will represent the dependencies among variables. There are two kinds of representations that have gained wide use: one is the directed acyclic graph model, also called a *Bayes net*, which represents the joint distribution as a product of the probabilities of each vertex conditioned on the values of its parents; the other is the undirected graph model, also called a *Markov field*, where the joint distribution is factorized over the *cliques*[1] of an undirected graph. This factorization is called a *junction tree* and optimizing it is the subject of the present paper. The power of both models lies in their ability to display and exploit existent marginal and conditional independencies among subsets of variables. Emphasizing independencies is useful

---

[1] A *clique* is a fully connected set of vertices and a maximal clique is a clique that is not contained in any other clique.

from both a qualitative point of view (it reveals something about the domain under study) and a quantitative one (it makes computations tractable). The two models differ in the kinds of independencies they are able to represent and often times in their naturalness in particular tasks. Directed graphs are more convenient for learning a model from data; on the other hand, the clique structure of undirected graphs organizes the information in a way that makes it immediately available to inference algorithms. Therefore it is a standard procedure to construct the model of a domain as a Bayes net and then to convert it to a Markov field for the purpose of querying it.

This process is known as *decomposition* and it consists of the following stages: first, the directed graph is transformed into an undirected graph by an operation called *moralization*. Second, the moralized graph is triangulated. A graph is called *triangulated* if any cycle of length > 3 has a *chord* (i.e. an edge connecting two nonconsecutive vertices). If a graph is not triangulated it is always possible to add new edges so that the resulting graph is triangulated. We shall call this procedure *triangulation* and the added edges the *fill-in*. In the final stage, the junction tree (Kjærulff, 1991) is constructed from the maximal cliques of the triangulated graph. We define the state space of a clique to be the cartesian product of the state spaces of the variables associated to the vertices in the clique and we call *weight* of the clique the size of this state space. The *weight of the junction tree* is the sum of the weights of its component cliques. All further exact inference in the net takes place in the junction tree representation. The number of computations required by an inference operation is proportional to the weight of the tree.

For each graph there are several and usually a large number of possible triangulations, with widely varying state space sizes. Moreover, triangulation is the only stage where the cost of inference can be influenced. It is therefore critical that the triangulation procedure produces a graph that is optimal or at least "good" in this respect.

Unfortunately, this is a hard problem. No optimal triangulation algorithm is known to date. However, a number of heuristic algorithms like *maximum cardinality search* (Tarjan and Yannakakis, 1984), *lexicographic search* (Rose et al., 1976) and the *minimum weight heuristic* (MW) (Kjærulff, 1990) are known. An optimization method based on simulated annealing which performs better than the heuristics on large graphs has been proposed in (Kjærulff, 1991) and recently a "divide and conquer" algorithm which bounds the maximum clique size of the triangulated graph has been published (Becker and Geiger, 1996). All but the last algorithm are based on Rose's (Rose, 1970) *elimination procedure*: choose a node v of the graph, connect all its neighbors to form a clique, then eliminate v and all the edges incident to it and proceed recursively. The resulting filled-in graph is triangulated.

It can be proven that the optimal triangulation can always be obtained by applying Rose's elimination procedure with an appropriate ordering of the nodes. It follows then that searching for an optimal triangulation can be cast as a search in the space of all node permutations. The idea of the present work is the following: embed the discrete search space of permutations of n objects (where n is the number of vertices) into a suitably chosen continuous space. Then extend the cost to a smooth function over the continuous domain and thus transform the discrete optimization problem into a continuous nonlinear optimization task. This allows one to take advantage of the thesaurus of optimization methods that exist for continuous cost functions. The rest of the paper will present this procedure in the following sequence: the next section introduces and discusses the objective function; section 3 states the continuous version of the problem; section 4 discusses further aspects of the optimization procedure and presents experimental results and section 5 concludes

2 THE OBJECTIVE

In this section we introduce the objective function that we used and we discuss its relationship to the junction tree weight. First, some notation. Let $G = (V, E)$ be a graph, its vertex set and its edge set respectively. Denote by n the cardinality of the vertex set, by r_v the number of values of the (discrete) variable associated to vertex $v \in V$, by $\#$ the elimination ordering of the nodes, such that $\#v = i$ means that node v is the i-th node to be eliminated according to ordering $\#$, by $n(v)$ the set of neighbors of $v \in V$ in the triangulated graph and by $C_v = \{v\} \cup \{u \in n(v) \mid \#u > \#v\}$.[2] Then, a result in (Golumbic, 1980) allows us to express the total weight of the junction tree obtained with elimination ordering $\#$ as

$$J^*_{(\#)} = \sum_{v \in V} \mathrm{ismax}(C_v) \prod_{u \in C_v} r_u \qquad (1)$$

where $\mathrm{ismax}(C_v)$ is a variable which is 1 when C_v is a maximal clique and 0 otherwise. As stated, this is the objective of interest for belief net triangulation. Any reference to optimality henceforth will be made with respect to J^*.

This result implies that there are no more than n maximal cliques in a junction tree and provides a method to enumerate them. This suggests defining a cost function that we call the *raw weight* J as the sum over all the cliques C_v (thus possibly including some non-maximal cliques):

$$J_{(\#)} = \sum_{v \in V} \prod_{u \in C_v} r_u \qquad (2)$$

J is the cost function that will be used throughout this paper. A reason to use it instead of J^* in our algorithm is that the former is easier to compute and to approximate. How to do this will be the object of the next section. But it is natural to ask first how well do the two agree?

Obviously, J is an upper bound for J^*. Moreover, it can be proved that if $r = \min r_v$

$$J^*_{(\#)} \leq J_{(\#)} \leq J^*_{(\#)} \frac{r}{r-1}\left(1 - \frac{1}{r^n}\right) \qquad (3)$$

and therefore that J is less than a fraction $1/(r-1)$ away from J^*. The upper bound is attained when the triangulated graph is fully connected and all r_v are equal.

In other words, the differece between J and J^* is largest for the highest cost triangulation. We also expect this difference to be low for the low cost triangulation. An intuitive argument for this is that good triangulations are associated with a large number of smaller cliques rather than with a few large ones. But the former situation means that there will be only a small number of small size non-maximal cliques to contribute to the difference $J - J^*$, and therefore that the agreement with J^* is usually closer than (3) implies. This conclusion is supported by simulations (Meilă and Jordan, 1997).

---

[2] Both $n(v)$ and C_v depend on $\#$ but we chose not to emphasize this in the notation for the sake of readability.

3 THE CONTINUOUS OPTIMIZATION PROBLEM

This section shows two ways of defining J over continuous domains. Both rely on a formulation of J that eliminates explicit reference to the cliques C_v; we describe this formulation here.

Let us first define new variables μ_{uv} and e_{uv}, $u, v = 1, .., n$. For any permutation #

$$\mu_{uv} = \begin{cases} 1 & \text{if } \#u \leq \#v \\ 0 & \text{otherwise} \end{cases} \qquad e_{uv} = \begin{cases} 1 & \text{if the edge } (u,v) \in E \cup F_\# \\ 0 & \text{otherwise} \end{cases}$$

where $F_\#$ is the set of fill-in edges.

In other words, μ represent precedence relationships and e represent the edges between the n vertices. Therefore, they will be called *precedence* variables and *edge* variables respectively. With these variables, J can be expressed as

$$J_{(\#)} = \sum_{v \in V} \prod_{u \in V} r_u^{\mu_{vu} e_{vu}} \qquad (4)$$

In (4), the product $\mu_{vu} e_{vu}$ acts as an indicator variable being 1 iff "$u \in C_v$" is true. For any given permutation, finding the μ variables is straightforward. Computing the edge variables is possible thanks to a result in (Rose et al., 1976). It states that an edge (u,v) is contained in $F_\#$ iff there is a path in G between u and v containing only nodes w for which $\#w < \min(\#u, \#v)$. Formally, $e_{uv} = e_{vu} = 1$ iff there exists a path $P = (u, w_1, w_2, \ldots v)$ such that

$$\prod_{w_i \in P} \mu_{w_i u} \mu_{w_i v} = 1$$

So far, we have succeeded in defining the cost J associated with any permutation in terms of the variables μ and e. In the following, the set of permutations will be embedded in a continuous domain. As a consequence, μ and e will take values in the interval $[0, 1]$ but the form of J in (4) will stay the same.

The first method, called μ-continuous embedding (μ-CE) assumes that the variables $\mu_{uv} \in [0,1]$ represent independent probabilities that $\#u < \#v$. For any permutation, the precedence variables have to satisfy the transitivity condition. Transitivity means that if $\#u < \#v$ and $\#v < \#w$, then $\#u < \#w$, or, that for any triple $(\mu_{uv}, \mu_{vw}, \mu_{wu})$ the assignments $(0,0,0)$ and $(1,1,1)$ are forbidden. According to the probabilistic interpretation of μ we introduce a term that penalizes the probability of a transitivity violation:

$$R(\mu) = \sum_{u<v<w} P[(u,v,w) \text{ nontransitive}] \qquad (5)$$

$$= \sum_{u<v<w} [\mu_{uv}\mu_{vw}\mu_{wu} + (1-\mu_{uv})(1-\mu_{vw})(1-\mu_{wu})] \qquad (6)$$

$$\geq P[\text{assignment non transitive}] \qquad (7)$$

In the second approach, called θ-continuous embedding (θ-CE), the permutations are directly embedded into the set of doubly stochastic matrices. A *doubly stochastic matrix* θ is a matrix for which the elements in a row or column sum to one.

$$\sum_i \theta_{ij} = \sum_j \theta_{ij} = 1 \quad \theta_{ij} \geq 0 \quad \text{for } i,j = 1,..n. \qquad (8)$$

When θ_{ij} are either 0 or 1, implying that there is exactly one nonzero element in each row or column, the matrix is called a *permutation matrix*. $\theta_{ij} = 1$ and $\#i = j$ both mean that the position of object i is j in the given permutation. The set of doubly stochastic matrices Θ is a convex polytope of dimension $(n-1)^2$ whose extreme points are the permutation matrices (Balinski and Russakoff, 1974). Thus, every doubly stochastic matrix can be represented as a convex combination of permutation matrices. To constrain the optimum to be a an extreme point, we use the penalty term

$$R(\theta) = \sum_{ij} \theta_{ij}(1 - \theta_{ij}) \tag{9}$$

The precedence variables are defined over Θ as

$$\mu_{uv} = 1 - \mu_{vu} = \frac{1}{1 - \sum_i \theta_{ui}\theta_{vi}} \sum_{j<i} \theta_{uj}\theta_{vi} \quad u,v,i,j = 1,..n \text{ and } v \neq u$$
$$\mu_{vv} = 1$$

Now, for both embeddings, the edge variables can be computed from μ as follows

$$e_{uv} = e_{vu} = \begin{cases} 1 & \text{for } (u,v) \in E \text{ or } u = v \\ \max_{P \in \{paths\ u \to v\}} \prod_{w \in P} \mu_{wu}\mu_{wv} & \text{otherwise} \end{cases}$$

The above assignments give the correct values for μ and e for any point representing a permutation. Over the interior of the domain, e is a continuous, piecewise differentiable function. Each e_{uv}, $(u,v) \notin E$ can be computed by a shortest path algorithm between u and v, with the length of $(w_1, w_2) \in E$ defined as $(-\log \mu_{w_1 u}\mu_{w_2 v})$.

θ-CE is an interior point method whereas in μ-CE the current point, although inside $[0,1]^{n(n-1)/2}$, isn't necessarily in the convex hull of the hypercube's corners that represent permutations. The number of operation required for one evaluation of J and its gradient is as follows: $\mathcal{O}(n^4)$ operations to compute μ from θ, $\mathcal{O}(n^3 \log n)$ to compute e, $\mathcal{O}(n^3)$ for $\frac{\partial J}{\partial e}$ and $\mathcal{O}(n^2)$ for $\frac{\partial J}{\partial \mu}$ and $\frac{\partial J}{\partial \theta}$ afterwards. Since computing μ is the most computationally intensive step, μ-CE is a clear win in terms of computation cost. In addition, by operating directly in the μ domain, one level of approximation is eliminated, which makes one expect μ-CE to perform better than θ-CE. The results in the following section will confirm this.

4 EXPERIMENTAL RESULTS

To assess the performance of our algorithms we compared their results with the results of the minimum weight heuristic (MW), the heuristic that scored best in empirical tests (Kjærulff, 1990). The lowest junction tree weight obtained in 200 runs of MW was retained and denoted by J^*_{MW}. Tests were run on 6 graphs of different sizes and densities:

graph	h9	h12	d10	m20	a20	d20
$n = \|V\|$	9	12	10	20	20	20
density	.33	.25	.6	.25	.45	.6
$r_{min}/r_{max}/r_{avg}$	2/2/2/	3/3/3	6/15/10	2/8/5	6/15/10	6/15/10
$\log_{10} J^*_{MW}$	2.43	2.71	7.44	5.47	12.75	13.94

The last row of the table shows the $\log_{10} J^*_{MW}$. We ran 11 or more trials of each of our two algorithms on each graph. To enforce the variables to converge to a permutation, we minimized the objective $J + \lambda R$, where $\lambda > 0$ is a parameter

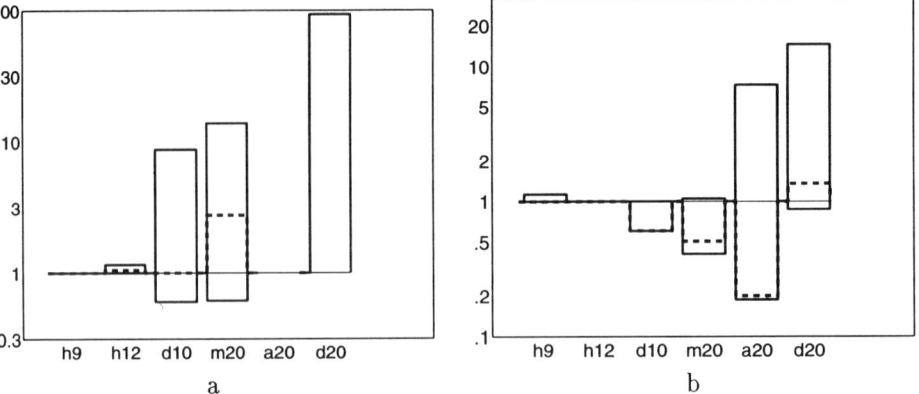

Figure 1: Minimum, maximum (solid line) and median (dashed line) values of $\frac{J^*}{J^*_{MW}}$ obtained by θ-CE (a) and μ-CE (b).

that was progressively increased following a deterministic annealing schedule and R is one of the aforementioned penalty terms. The algorithms were run for 50-150 optimization cycles, usually enough to reach convergence. However, for the μ-embedding on graph **d20**, there were several cases where many μ values did not converge to 0 or 1. In those cases we picked the most plausible permutation to be the answer.

The results are shown in figure 1 in terms of the ratio of the true cost obtained by the continuous embedding algorithm (denoted by J^*) and J^*_{MW}. For the first two graphs, **h9** and **h12**, J^*_{MW} is the optimal cost; the embedding algorithms reach it most trials. On the remaining graphs, μ-CE clearly outperforms θ-CE, which also performs poorer than MW on average. On **d10**, **a20** and **m20** it also outperforms the MW heuristic, attaining junction tree weights that are 1.6 to 5 times lower on average than those obtained by MW. On **d20**, a denser graph, the results are similar for MW and μ-CE in half of the cases and worse for μ-CE otherwise. The plots also show that the variability of the results is much larger for CE than for MW. This behaviour is not surprising, given that the search space for CE, although continuous, comprises a large number of local minima. This induces dependence on the initial point and, as a consequence, nondeterministic behaviour of the algorithm. Moreover, while the number of choices that MW has is much lower than the upper limit of $n!$, the "choices" that CE algorithms consider, although soft, span the space of all possible permutations.

5 CONCLUSION

The idea of continuous embedding is not new in the field of applied mathematics. The large body of literature dealing with smooth (sygmoidal) functions instead of hard nonlinearities (step functions) is only one example. The present paper shows a nontrivial way of applying a similar treatment to a new problem in a new field. The results obtained by μ-embedding are on average better than the standard MW heuristic. Although not directly comparable, the best results reported on triangulation (Kjærulff, 1991; Becker and Geiger, 1996) are only by little better than ours. Therefore the significance of the latter goes beyond the scope of the present problem. They are obtained on a hard problem, whose cost function has no feature to ease its minimization (J is neither linear, nor quadratic, nor is it additive w.r.t. the vertices or the edges) and therefore they demonstrate the potential of continuous embedding as a general tool.

Colaterally, we have introduced the cost function J, which is directly amenable to continuous approximations and is in good agreement with the true cost J^*. Since minimizing J may not be NP-hard, this opens a way for investigating new triangulation methods.

Acknowledgements

The authors are grateful to Tommi Jaakkola for many discussions and to Ellie Bonsaint for her invaluable help in typing the paper.

References

Balinski, M. and Russakoff, R. (1974). On the assignment polytope. *SIAM Rev.*

Becker, A. and Geiger, D. (1996). A sufficiently fast algorithm for finding close to optimal junction trees. In *UAI 96 Proceedings*.

Golumbic, M. (1980). *Algorithmic Graph Theory and Perfect Graphs*. Academic Press, New York.

Kjærulff, U. (1990). Triangulation of graphs–algorithms giving small total state space. Technical Report R 90-09, Department of Mathematics and Computer Science, Aalborg University, Denmark.

Kjærulff, U. (1991). Optimal decomposition of probabilistic networks by simulated annealing. *Statistics and Computing*.

Meilă, M. and Jordan, M. I. (1997). An objective function for belief net triangulation. In Madigan, D., editor, *AI and Statistics*, number 7. (to appear).

Rose, D. J. (1970). Triangulated graphs and the elimination process. *Journal of Mathematical Analysis and Applications*.

Rose, D. J., Tarjan, R. E., and Lueker, E. (1976). Algorithmic aspects of vertex elimination on graphs. *SIAM J. Comput.*

Tarjan, R. and Yannakakis, M. (1984). Simple linear-time algorithms to test chordality of graphs, test acyclicity of hypergraphs, and select reduced acyclic hypergraphs. *SIAM J. Comput.*

Combining Neural Network Regression Estimates with Regularized Linear Weights

Christopher J. Merz and Michael J. Pazzani

Dept. of Information and Computer Science
University of California, Irvine, CA 92717-3425 U.S.A.
{cmerz,pazzani}@ics.uci.edu

Category: Algorithms and Architectures.

Abstract

When combining a set of learned models to form an improved estimator, the issue of redundancy or multicollinearity in the set of models must be addressed. A progression of existing approaches and their limitations with respect to the redundancy is discussed. A new approach, PCR*, based on principal components regression is proposed to address these limitations. An evaluation of the new approach on a collection of domains reveals that: 1) PCR* was the most robust combination method as the redundancy of the learned models increased, 2) redundancy could be handled without eliminating any of the learned models, and 3) the principal components of the learned models provided a continuum of "regularized" weights from which PCR* could choose.

1 INTRODUCTION

Combining a set of learned models[1] to improve classification and regression estimates has been an area of much research in machine learning and neural networks [Wolpert, 1992, Merz, 1995, Perrone and Cooper, 1992, Leblanc and Tibshirani, 1993, Breiman, 1992, Meir, 1995, Krogh and Vedelsby, 1995, Tresp, 1995, Chan and Stolfo, 1995]. The challenge of this problem is to decide which models to rely on for prediction and how much weight to give each.

---

[1] A learned model may be anything from a decision/regression tree to a neural network.

The goal of combining learned models is to obtain a more accurate prediction than can be obtained from any single source alone. One major issue in combining a set of learned models is redundancy. *Redundancy* refers to the amount of agreement or linear dependence between models when making a set of predictions. The more the set agrees, the more redundancy is present. In statistical terms, this is referred to as the multicollinearity problem.

The focus of this paper is to explore and evaluate the properties of existing methods for combining regression estimates (Section 2), and to motivate the need for more advanced methods which deal with multicollinearity in the set of learned models (Section 3). In particular, a method based on principal components regression (PCR, [Draper and Smith, 1981]) is described, and is evaluated emperically demonstrating the it is a robust and efficient method for finding a set of combining weights with low prediction error (Section 4). Finally, Section 5 draws some conclusions.

2 MOTIVATION

The problem of combining a set of learned models is defined using the terminology of [Perrone and Cooper, 1992]. Suppose two sets of data are given: a training set $\mathcal{D}_{Train} = (x_m, y_m)$ and a test set $\mathcal{D}_{Test} = (x_l, y_l)$. Now suppose $\mathcal{D}_{Train}$ is used to build a set of functions, $\mathcal{F} = f_i(x)$, each element of which approximates $f(x)$. The goal is to find the best approximation of $f(x)$ using $\mathcal{F}$.

To date, most approaches to this problem limit the space of approximations of $f(x)$ to linear combinations of the elements of $\mathcal{F}$, i.e.,

$$\hat{f}(x) = \sum_{i=1}^{N} \alpha_i f_i(x)$$

where α_i is the coefficient or weight of $f_i(x)$.

The focus of this paper is to evaluate and address the limitations of these approaches. To do so, a brief summary of these approaches is now provided progressing from simpler to more complex methods pointing out their limitations along the way.

The simplest method for combining the members of $\mathcal{F}$ is by taking the unweighted average, (i.e., $\alpha_i = 1/N$). Perrone and Cooper refer to this as the Basic Ensemble Method (BEM), written as

$$f_{BEM} = 1/N \sum_{i=1}^{N} f_i(x)$$

This equation can also be written in terms of the *misfit function* for each $f_i(x)$. These functions describe the deviations of the elements of $\mathcal{F}$ from the true solution and are written as

$$m_i(x) = f(x) - f_i(x).$$

Thus,

$$f_{BEM} = f(x) - 1/N \sum_{i=1}^{N} m_i(x).$$

Perrone and Cooper show that as long as the $m_i(x)$ are mutually independent with zero mean, the error in estimating $f(x)$ can be made arbitrarily small by increasing the population size of $\mathcal{F}$. Since these assumptions break down in practice, they developed a more general approach which finds the "optimal"[2] weights while allowing the $m_i(x)$'s to be correlated and have non-zero means. This Generalized Ensemble Method (GEM) is written as

$$f_{GEM} = \sum_{i=1}^{N} \alpha_i f_i(x) = f(x) - \sum_{i=1}^{N} \alpha_i m_i(x)$$

where

$$\alpha_i = \frac{\sum_{j=1}^{N} C_{ij}^{-1}}{\sum_{k=1}^{N} \sum_{j=1}^{N} C_{kj}^{-1}} \text{ and } C_{ij} = E[m_i(x)m_j(x)].$$

C is the symmetric sample covariance matrix for the misfit function and the goal is to minimize $\sum_{i,j}^{N} \alpha_i \alpha_j C_{ij}$. Note that the misfit functions are calculated on the training data and $f(x)$ is not required. The main disadvantage to this approach is that it involves taking the inverse of C which can be "unstable". That is, redundancy in the members of $\mathcal{F}$ leads to linear dependence in the rows and columns of C which in turn leads to unreliable estimates of C^{-1}.

To circumvent this sensitivity redundancy, Perrone and Cooper propose a method for discarding member(s) of $\mathcal{F}$ when the strength of its agreement with another member exceeds a certain threshold. Unfortunately, this approach only checks for linear dependence (or redundancy) between pairs of $f_i(x)$ and two $f_i(x)$ for $i \neq j$. In fact, $f_i(x)$ could be a linear combination of several other members of $\mathcal{F}$ and the instability problem would be manifest. Also, depending on how high the threshold is set, a member of $\mathcal{F}$ could be discarded while still having some degree of uniqueness and utility. An ideal method for weighting the members of $\mathcal{F}$ would neither discard any models nor suffer when there is redundancy in the model set.

The next approach reviewed is linear regression (LR)[3] which also finds the "optimal" weights for the $f_i(x)$ with respect to the training data. In fact, GEM and LR are both considered "optimal" because they are closely related in that GEM is a form of linear regression with the added constraint that $\sum_{i=1}^{N} \alpha_i = 1$. The weights for LR are found as follows[4],

$$f_{LR} = \sum_{i=1}^{N} \alpha_i f_i(x)$$

where

$$\alpha = (f^T f)^{-1} f^T F \; f_{ji} = f_i(x_j) 1 \leq j \leq M \text{ and } F_j = f(x_j).$$

Like GEM, LR and LRC are subject to the multicollinearity problem because finding the α_i's involves taking the inverse of a matrix. That is, if the f matrix is composed of $f_i(x)$ which strongly agree with other members of $\mathcal{F}$, some linear dependence will be present.

---

[2] Optimal here refers to weights which minimize mean square error for the training data.

[3] Actually, it is a form of linear regression without the intercept term. The more general form, denote by LRC, would be formulated the same way but with member, f_0 which always predicts 1. According to [Leblanc and Tibshirani, 1993] having the extra constant term will not be necessary (i.e., it will equal zero) because in practice, $E[f_i(x)] = E[f(x)]$.

[4] Note that the constraint, $\sum_{i=1}^{N} \alpha_i = 1$, for GEM is a form of *regularization* [Leblanc and Tibshirani, 1993]. The purpose of regularizing the weights is to provide an estimate which is less biased by the training sample. Thus, one would not expect GEM and LR to produce identical weights.

Given the limitations of these methods, the goal of this research was to find a method which finds weights for the learned models with low prediction error without discarding any of the original models, and without being subject to the multicollinearity problem.

3 METHODS FOR HANDLING MULTICOLLINEARITY

In the abovementioned methods, multicollinearity leads to inflation of the variance of the estimated weights, α. Consequently, the weights obtained from fitting the model to a particular sample may be far from their true values. To circumvent this problem, approaches have been developed which: 1) constrain the estimated regression coefficients so as to improve prediction performance (i.e., ridge regression, RIDGE [Montgomery and Friedman 1993], and principal components regression), 2) search for the coefficients via gradient descent procedures (i.e., Widrow-Hoff learning, GD and EG+- [Kivinen and Warmuth, 1994]), or build models which make decorrelated errors by adjusting the bias of the learning algorithm [Opitz and Shavlik, 1995] or the data which it sees [Meir, 1995]. The third approach ameliorates, but does not solve, the problem because redundancy is an inherent part of the task of combining estimators.

The focus of this paper is on the first approach. Leblanc and Tibshirani [Leblanc and Tibshirani, 1993] have proposed several ways of constraining or *regularizing* the weights to help produce estimators with lower prediction error:

1. Shrink $\hat{\alpha}$ towards $(1/K, 1/K, \ldots, 1/K)^T$ where K is the number of learned models.
2. $\sum_{i=1}^{N} \alpha_i = 1$
3. $\alpha_i \geq 0, i = 1, 2 \ldots K$

Breiman [Breiman, 1992] provides an intuitive justification for these constraints by pointing out that the more strongly they are satisfied, the more interpolative the weighting scheme is. In the extreme case, a uniformly weighted set of learned models is likely to produce a prediction *between* the maximum and minimum predicted values of the learned models. Without these constraints, there is no guarantee that the resulting predictor will stay near that range and generalization may be poor. The next subsection describes a variant of principal components regression and explains how it provides a continuum of regularized weights for the original learned models.

3.1 PRINCIPAL COMPONENTS REGRESSION

When dealing with the above mentioned multicollinearity problem, principal components regression [Draper and Smith, 1981] may be used to summarize and extract the "relevant" information from the learned models. The main idea of PCR is to map the original learned models to a set of (independent) principal components in which each component is a linear combination of the original learned models, and then to build a regression equation using the best subset of the principal components to predict $f(x)$.

The advantage of this representation is that the components are sorted according to how much information (or variance) from the original learned models for which they account. Given this representation, the goal is to choose the number of principal components to include in the final regression by retaining the first k which meet a preselected stopping criteria. The basic approach is summarized as follows:

1. Do a principal components analysis (PCA) on the covariance matrix of the learned models' predictions on the training data (i.e., do a PCA on the covariance matrix of M, where $M_{i,j}$ is the j-th model's reponse for the i-th training example) to produce a set of principal components, $PC = \{PC_1, ..., PC_N\}$.

2. Use a stopping criteria to decide on k, the number of principal components to use.

3. Do a least squares regression on the selected components (i.e., include PC_i for $i \leq k$).

4. Derive the weights, α_i, for the original learned models by expanding

$$f_{PCR*} = \beta_1 PC_1 + ... + \beta_k PC_k$$

according to

$$PC_i = \gamma_{i,0} f_0 + ... + \gamma_{i,N} f_N,$$

and simplifying for the coefficients of f_i. Note that $\gamma_{i,j}$ is the j-th coefficient of the i-th principal component.

The second step is very important because choosing too few or too many principal components may result in underfitting or overfitting, respectively. Ten-fold cross-validation is used to select k here.

Examining the spectrum of (N) weight sets derived in step four reveals that PCR* provides a continuum of weight sets spanning from highly constrained (i.e., weights generated from PCR_1 satisfy all three regularization constraints) to completely unconstrained (i.e., PCR_N is equivalent to unconstrained linear regression). To see that the weights, α, derived from PCR_1 are (nearly) uniform, recall that the first principal component accounts for where the learned models agree. Because the learned models are all fairly accurate they agree quite often so their first principal component weights, $\gamma_{1,*}$ will be similar. The γ-weights are in turn multiplied by a constant when PCR_1 is regressed upon. Thus, the resulting α_i's will be fairly uniform. The later principal components serve as refinements to those already included producing less constrained weight sets until finally PCR_N is included resulting in an unconstrained estimator much like LR, LRC and GEM.

4 EXPERIMENTAL RESULTS

The set of learned models, $\mathcal{F}$, were generated using Backpropagation [Rumelhart, 1986]. For each dataset, a network topology was developed which gave good performance. The collection of networks built differed only in their initial weights[5].

Three data sets were chosen: *cpu* and *housing* (from the UCI repository), and *bodyfat* (from the Statistics Library at Carnegie Mellon University). Due to space limitation, the data sets reported on were chosen because they were representative of the basic trends found in a larger collection of datasets. The combining methods evaluated consist of all the methods discussed in Sections 2 and 3, as well as PCR_1 and PCR_N (to demonstrate PCR*'s most and least regularized weight sets,

---

[5] There was no extreme effort to produce networks with more decorrelated errors. Even with such networks, the issue of extreme multicollinearity would still exist because $E[f_i(x)] = E[f_j(x)]$ for all i and j.

Table 1: Results

Data	bodyfat		cpu		housing	
N	10	50	10	50	10	50
BEM	1.03	1.04	**38.57**	**38.62**	2.79	2.77
GEM	**1.02**	**0.86**	46.59	227.54	**2.72**	**2.57**
LR	**1.02**	3.09	44.9	238.0	**2.72**	6.44
RIDGE	**1.02**	**0.826**	44.8	191.0	**2.72**	**2.55**
GD	1.03	1.04	38.9	38.8	2.79	2.77
EGPM	1.03	1.07	**38.4**	**38.0**	2.77	2.75
PCR$_1$	1.04	1.05	39.0	39.0	2.78	2.76
PCR$_N$	**1.02**	**0.848**	44.8	249.9	**2.72**	**2.57**
PCR*	**0.99**	**0.786**	40.3	40.8	**2.70**	**2.56**

respectively). The more computationally intense procedures based on stacking and bootstrapping proposed by [Leblanc and Tibshirani, 1993, Breiman, 1992] were not evaluated here because they required many more models (i.e., neural networks) to be generated for each of the elements of $\mathcal{F}$.

There were 20 trials run for each of the datasets. On each trial the data was randomly divided into 70% training data and 30% test data. These trials were rerun for varying sizes of $\mathcal{F}$ (i.e., 10 and 50, respectively). As more models are included the linear dependence amongst them goes up showing how well the multicollinearity problem is handled[6]. Table 1 shows the average residual errors for the each of the methods on the three data sets. Each row is a particular method and each column is the size of $\mathcal{F}$ for a given data set. Bold-faced entries indicate methods which were *not* significantly different from the method with the lowest error (via two-tailed paired t-tests with $p \leq 0.05$).

PCR* is the only approach which is among the leaders for all three data sets. For the *bodyfat* and *housing* data sets the weights produced by BEM, PCR$_1$, GD, and EG+- tended to be too constrained, while the weights for LR tended to be too unconstrained for the larger collection of models. The less constrained weights of GEM, LR, RIDGE, and PCR$_N$ severely harmed performance in the *cpu* domain where uniform weighting performed better.

The biggest demonstration of PCR*'s robustness is its ability to gravitate towards the more constrained weights produced by the earlier principal components when appropriate (i.e., in the *cpu* dataset). Similarly, it uses the less constrained principal components closer to PCR$_n$ when it is preferable as in the *bodyfat* and *housing* domains.

5 CONCLUSION

This investigation suggests that the principal components of a set of learned models can be useful when combining the models to form an improved estimator. It was demonstrated that the principal components provide a continuum of weight sets from highly regularized to unconstrained. An algorithm, PCR*, was developed which attempts to automatically select the subset of these components which provides the lowest prediction error. Experiments on a collection of domains demonstrated PCR*'s ability to robustly handle redundancy in the set of learned models. Future work will be to improve upon PCR* and expand it to the classification task.

---

[6]This is verified by observing the eigenvalues of the principal components and values in the covariance matrix of the models in $\mathcal{F}$

References

[Breiman et al, 1984] Breiman, L., Friedman, J.H., Olshen, R.A. & Stone, C.J. (1984). *Classification and Regression Trees*. Belmont, CA: Wadsworth.

[Breiman, 1992] Breiman, L. (1992). Stacked Regression. Dept of Statistics, Berkeley, TR No. 367.

[Chan and Stolfo, 1995] Chan, P.K., Stolfo, S.J. (1995). A Comparative Evaluation of Voting and Meta-Learning on Partitioned Data *Proceedings of the Twelvth International Machine Learning Conference* (90-98). San Mateo, CA: Morgan Kaufmann.

[Draper and Smith, 1981] Draper, N.R., Smith, H. (1981). *Applied Regression Analysis*. New York, NY: John Wiley and Sons.

[Kivinen and Warmuth, 1994] Kivinen, J., and Warmuth, M. (1994). Exponentiated Gradient Descent Versus Gradient Descent for Linear Predictors. Dept. of Computer Science, UC-Santa Cruz, TR No. ucsc-crl-94-16.

[Krogh and Vedelsby, 1995] Krogh, A., and Vedelsby, J. (1995). Neural Network Ensembles, Cross Validation, and Active Learning. In *Advances in Neural Information Processing Systems 7*. San Mateo, CA: Morgan Kaufmann.

[Hansen and Salamon, 1990] Hansen, L.K., and Salamon, P. (1990). Neural Network Ensembles. *IEEE Transactions on Pattern Analysis and Machine Intelligence, 12* (993-1001).

[Leblanc and Tibshirani, 1993] Leblanc, M., Tibshirani, R. (1993) Combining estimates in regression and classification Dept. of Statistics, University of Toronto, TR.

[Meir, 1995] Meir, R. (1995). Bias, variance and the combination of estimators. In *Advances in Neural Information Processing Systems 7*. San Mateo, CA: Morgan Kaufmann.

[Merz, 1995] Merz, C.J. (1995) Dynamical Selection of Learning Algorithms. In Fisher, C. and Lenz, H. (Eds.) Learning from Data: Artificial Intelligence and Statistics, 5). Springer Verlag

[Montgomery and Friedman 1993] Mongomery, D.C., and Friedman, D.J. (1993). Prediction Using Regression Models with Multicollinear Predictor Variables. IIE Transactions, vol. 25, no. 3 73–85.

[Opitz and Shavlik, 1995] Opitz, D.W., Shavlik, J.W. (1996). Generating Accurate and Diverse Members of a Neural-Network Ensemble. Advances in Neural and Information Processing Systems 8. Touretzky, D.S., Mozer, M.C., and Hasselmo, M.E., eds. Cambridge MA: MIT Press.

[Perrone and Cooper, 1992] Perrone, M. P., Cooper, L. N., (1993). When Networks Disagree: Ensemble Methods for Hybrid Neural Networks. *Neural Networks for Speech and Image Processing*, edited by Mammone, R. J.. New York: Chapman and Hall.

[Rumelhart, 1986] Rumelhart, D. E., Hinton, G. E., & Williams, R. J. (1986). Learning Interior Representation by Error Propagation. *Parallel Distributed Processing, 1* 318–362. Cambridge, MASS.: MIT Press.

[Tresp, 1995] Tresp, V., Taniguchi, M. (1995). Combining Estimators Using Non-Constant Weighting Functions. In *Advances in Neural Information Processing Systems 7*. San Mateo, CA: Morgan Kaufmann.

[Wolpert, 1992] Wolpert, D. H. (1992). Stacked Generalization. *Neural Networks, 5*, 241–259.

A Mixture of Experts Classifier with Learning Based on Both Labelled and Unlabelled Data

David J. Miller and Hasan S. Uyar
Department of Electrical Engineering
The Pennsylvania State University
University Park, Pa. 16802
miller@perseus.ee.psu.edu

Abstract

We address statistical classifier design given a mixed training set consisting of a small labelled feature set and a (generally larger) set of *unlabelled* features. This situation arises, e.g., for medical images, where although training features may be plentiful, expensive expertise is required to extract their class labels. We propose a classifier structure and learning algorithm that make effective use of unlabelled data to improve performance. The learning is based on maximization of the total data likelihood, i.e. over both the labelled and unlabelled data subsets. Two *distinct* EM learning algorithms are proposed, differing in the EM formalism applied for unlabelled data. The classifier, based on a joint probability model for features and labels, is a "mixture of experts" structure that is equivalent to the radial basis function (RBF) classifier, but unlike RBFs, is amenable to likelihood-based training. The scope of application for the new method is greatly extended by the observation that test data, or any new data to classify, is in fact additional, *unlabelled data* – thus, a combined learning/classification operation – much akin to what is done in image segmentation – can be invoked whenever there is new data to classify. Experiments with data sets from the UC Irvine database demonstrate that the new learning algorithms and structure achieve substantial performance gains over alternative approaches.

1 Introduction

Statistical classifier design is fundamentally a supervised learning problem, wherein a decision function, mapping an input feature vector to an output class label, is learned based on representative (feature,class label) training pairs. While a variety of classifier structures and associated learning algorithms have been developed, a common element of nearly all approaches is the assumption that class labels are known for each feature vector used for training. This is certainly true of neural networks such as multilayer perceptrons and radial basis functions (RBFs), for which classification is usually viewed as function approximation, with the networks trained to minimize the squared distance to target class values. Knowledge of class labels is also required for parametric classifiers such as mixture of Gaussian classifiers, for which learning typically involves dividing the training data into subsets by class and then using maximum likelihood estimation (MLE) to separately learn each class density. While labelled training data may be plentiful for some applications, for others, such as remote sensing and medical imaging, the training set is in principle vast but the size of the labelled subset may be inadequate. The difficulty in obtaining class labels may arise due to limited knowledge or limited resources, as expensive expertise is often required to derive class labels for features. In this work, we address classifier design under these conditions, i.e. the training set $\mathcal{X}$ is assumed to consist of two subsets, $\mathcal{X} = \{\mathcal{X}_l, \mathcal{X}_u\}$, where $\mathcal{X}_l = \{(x_1, c_1), (x_2, c_2), \ldots, (x_{N_l}, c_{N_l})\}$ is the labelled subset and $\mathcal{X}_u = \{x_{N_l+1}, \ldots, x_N\}$ is the unlabelled subset[1]. Here, $x_i \in \mathcal{R}^k$ is the feature vector and $c_i \in \mathcal{I}$ is the class label from the label set $\mathcal{I} = \{1, 2, \ldots, N_c\}$.

The practical significance of this mixed training problem was recognized in (Lippmann 1989). However, despite this realization, there has been surprisingly little work done on this problem. One likely reason is that it does not appear possible to incorporate unlabelled data directly within conventional supervised learning methods such as back propagation. For these methods, unlabelled features must either be discarded or preprocessed in a suboptimal, heuristic fashion to obtain class label estimates. We also note the existence of work which is less than optimistic concerning the value of unlabelled data for classification (Castelli and Cover 1994). However, (Shashahani and Landgrebe 1994) found that unlabelled data could be used effectively in label-deficient situations. While we build on their work, as well as on our own previous work (Miller and Uyar 1996), our approach differs from (Shashahani and Landgrebe 1994) in several important respects. First, we suggest a more powerful mixture-based probability model with an associated classifier structure that has been shown to be equivalent to the RBF classifier (Miller 1996). The practical significance of this equivalence is that unlike RBFs, which are trained in a conventional supervised fashion, the RBF-equivalent mixture model is naturally suited for statistical training (MLE). The statistical framework is the key to incorporating unlabelled data in the learning. A second departure from prior work is the choice of learning criterion. We maximize the joint data likelihood and suggest two *distinct* EM algorithms for this purpose, whereas the conditional likelihood was considered in (Shashahani and Landgrebe 1994). We have found that our approach achieves superior results. A final novel contribution is a considerable expansion of the range of situations for which the mixed training paradigm can be applied. This is made possible by the realization that test data or new data to classify can *also* be viewed as an unlabelled set, available for "training". This notion will be clarified in the sequel.

2 Unlabelled Data and Classification

Here we briefly provide some intuitive motivation for the use of unlabelled data. Suppose, not very restrictively, that the data is well-modelled by a mixture density,

---

[1]This problem can be viewed as a type of "missing data" problem, wherein the missing items are class labels. As such, it is related to, albeit distinct from supervised learning involving missing and/or noisy *feature* components, addressed in (Ghahramani and Jordan 1995),(Tresp et al. 1995).

in the following way. The feature vectors are generated according to the density $f(x/\theta) = \sum_{l=1}^{L} \alpha_l f(x/\theta_l)$, where $f(x/\theta_l)$ is one of L component densities, with non-negative mixing parameters α_l, such that $\sum_{l=1}^{L} \alpha_l = 1$. Here, θ_l is the set of parameters specifying the component density, with $\theta = \{\theta_l\}$. The class labels are also viewed as *random* quantities and are assumed chosen conditioned on the selected mixture component $m_i \in \{1, 2, \ldots, L\}$ and possibly on the feature value, i.e. according to the probabilities $P[c_i/x_i, m_i]$ [2]. Thus, the data pairs are assumed generated by selecting, in order, the mixture component, the feature value, and the class label, with each selection depending in general on preceding ones. The optimal classification rule for this model is the maximum a posteriori rule:

$$S(x) = \arg\max_k \sum_j P[c_i = k/m_i = j, x_i] P[m_i = j/x_i], \qquad (1)$$

where $P[m_i = j/x_i] = \frac{\alpha_j f(x_i/\theta_j)}{\sum_{l=1}^{L} \alpha_l f(x_i/\theta_l)}$, and where $S(x)$ is a selector function with range in $\mathcal{I}$. Since this rule is based on the a posteriori class probabilities, one can argue that learning should focus solely on estimating these probabilities. However, if the classifier truly implements (1), then implicitly it has been assumed that the estimated mixture density accurately models the feature vectors. If this is not true, then presumably estimates of the a posteriori probabilities will also be affected. This suggests that *even in the absence of class labels*, the feature vectors can be used to better learn a posteriori probabilities via improved estimation of the mixture-based feature density. A commonly used measure of mixture density accuracy is the data *likelihood*.

3 Joint Likelihood Maximization for a Mixtures of Experts Classifier

The previous section basically argues for a learning approach that uses labelled data to directly estimate a posteriori probabilities and unlabelled data to estimate the feature density. A criterion which essentially fulfills these objectives is the joint data likelihood, computed over both the labelled and unlabelled data subsets. Given our model, the joint data log-likelihood is written in the form

$$\log L = \sum_{x_i \in \mathcal{X}_u} \log \sum_{l=1}^{L} \alpha_l f(x_i/\theta_l) + \sum_{x_i \in \mathcal{X}_l} \log \sum_{l=1}^{L} \alpha_l P[c_i/x_i, m_i = l] f(x_i/\theta_l). \qquad (2)$$

This objective function consists of a "supervised" term based on $\mathcal{X}_l$ and an "unsupervised" term based on $\mathcal{X}_u$. The joint data likelihood was previously considered in a learning context in (Xu et al. 1995). However, there the primary justification was simplification of the learning algorithm in order to allow parameter estimation based on fixed point iterations rather than gradient descent. Here, the joint likelihood allows the inclusion of unlabelled samples in the learning. We next consider two special cases of the probability model described until now.

---

[2] The usual assumption made is that components are "hard-partitioned", in a deterministic fashion, to classes. Our random model includes the "partitioned" one as a special case. We have generally found this model to be more powerful than the "partitioned" one (Miller Uyar 1996).

The "partitioned" mixture (PM) model: This is the previously mentioned case where mixture components are "hard-partitioned" to classes (Shashahani and Landgrebe 1994). This is written $M_j \in C_k$, where M_j denotes mixture component j and C_k is the subset of components owned by class k. The posterior probabilities have the form

$$P[c_i = k/x] = \frac{\sum\limits_{j:M_j \in C_k} \alpha_j f(x/\theta_j)}{\sum\limits_{l=1}^{L} \alpha_l f(x/\theta_l)}. \tag{3}$$

The generalized mixture (GM) model: The form of the posterior for each mixture component is now $P[c_i/m_j, x_i] = P[c_i/m_j] \equiv \beta_{c_i/m_j}$, i.e., it is independent of the feature value. The overall posterior probability takes the form

$$P[c_i/x_i] = \sum_j \left(\frac{\alpha_j f(x_i/\theta_j)}{\sum_l \alpha_l f(x_i/\theta_l)} \right) \beta_{c_i|j}. \tag{4}$$

This model was introduced in (Miller and Uyar 1996) and was shown there to lead to performance improvement over the PM model. Note that the probabilities have a "mixture of experts" structure, where the "gating units" are the probabilities $P[m_i = j|x_i]$ (in parentheses), and with the "expert" for component j just the probability $\beta_{c_i|j}$. Elsewhere (Miller 1996), it has been shown that the associated classifier decision function is in fact equivalent to that of an RBF classifier (Moody and Darken 1989). Thus, we suggest a probability model equivalent to a widely used neural network classifier, but with the advantage that, unlike the standard RBF, the RBF-equivalent probability model is amenable to statistical training, and hence to the incorporation of unlabelled data in the learning. Note that more powerful models $P[c_i|m_i, x_i]$ that do condition on x_i are also possible. However, such models will require many more parameters which will likely hurt generalization performance, especially in a label-deficient learning context. Interestingly, for the mixed training problem, there are two Expectation-Maximization (EM) (Dempster et al. 1977) formulations that can be applied to maximize the likelihood associated with a given probability model. These two formulations lead to *distinct* methods that take different learning "trajectories", although both ascend in the data likelihood. The difference between the formulations lies in how the *"incomplete"* and *"complete"* data elements are defined within the EM framework. We will develop these two approaches for the suggested GM model.

EM-I (No class labels assumed): Distinct data interpretations are given for $\mathcal{X}_l$ and $\mathcal{X}_u$. In this case, for $\mathcal{X}_u$, the *incomplete data* consists of the features $\{x_i\}$ and the *complete data* consists of $\{(x_i, m_i)\}$. For $\mathcal{X}_l$, the *incomplete data* consists of $\{(x_i, c_i)\}$, with the *complete data* now the triple $\{(x_i, c_i, m_i)\}$. To clarify, in this case *mixture* labels are viewed as the sole missing data elements, for $\mathcal{X}_u$ as well as for $\mathcal{X}_l$. Thus, in effect class labels are not even postulated to exist for $\mathcal{X}_u$.

EM-II (Class labels assumed): The definitions for $\mathcal{X}_l$ are the same as before. However, for $\mathcal{X}_u$, the *complete data* now consists of the triple $\{(x_i, c_i, m_i)\}$, i.e. class labels are also assumed missing for $\mathcal{X}_u$.

For Gaussian components, we have $\theta_l = \{\mu_l, \Sigma_l\}$, with μ_l the mean vector and Σ_l the covariance matrix. For EM-I, the resulting fixed point iterations for updating the parameters are:

$$\mu_j^{(t+1)} = \frac{1}{N\alpha_j^{(t)}} \left(\sum_{x_i \in \mathcal{X}_l} x_i P[m_i = j/x_i, c_i, \theta^{(t)}] + \sum_{x_i \in \mathcal{X}_u} x_i P[m_i = j/x_i, \theta^{(t)}] \right)$$

$$\Sigma_j^{(t+1)} = \frac{1}{N\alpha_j^{(t)}} \left(\sum_{x_i \in \mathcal{X}_l} S_{ij}^{(t)} P[m_i = j/x_i, c_i, \theta^{(t)}] + \sum_{x_i \in \mathcal{X}_u} S_{ij}^{(t)} P[m_i = j/x_i, \theta^{(t)}] \right)$$

$$\alpha_j^{(t+1)} = \frac{1}{N} \left(\sum_{x_i \in \mathcal{X}_l} P[m_i = j/x_i, c_i, \theta^{(t)}] + \sum_{x_i \in \mathcal{X}_u} P[m_i = j/x_i, \theta^{(t)}] \right) \quad \forall j$$

$$\beta_{k/j}^{(t+1)} = \frac{\sum_{x_i \in \mathcal{X}_l \cap c_i = k} P[m_i = j/x_i, c_i, \theta^{(t)}]}{\sum_{x_i \in \mathcal{X}_l} P[m_i = j/x_i, c_i, \theta^{(t)}]} \quad \forall k, j \qquad (5)$$

Here, $S_{ij}^{(t)} \equiv (x_i - \mu_j^{(t)})(x_i - \mu_j^{(t)})^T$. New parameters are computed at iteration $t+1$ based on their values at iteration t. In these equations, $P[m_i = j/x_i, c_i, \theta^{(t)}] = \frac{\alpha_j^{(t)} \beta_{c_i/j}^{(t)} f(x_i/\theta_j^{(t)})}{\sum_m \alpha_m^{(t)} \beta_{c_i/m}^{(t)} f(x_i/\theta_m^{(t)})}$ and $P[m_i = j/x_i, \theta^{(t)}] = \frac{\alpha_j^{(t)} f(x_i/\theta_j^{(t)})}{\sum_{n=1}^{M} \alpha_n^{(t)} f(x_i/\theta_n^{(t)})}$. For EM-II, it can be shown that the resulting re-estimation equations are identical to those in (5) *except* regarding the parameters $\{\beta_{k/j}\}$. The updates for these parameters now take the form

$$\beta_{k/j}^{(t+1)} = \frac{1}{N\alpha_j^{(t)}} \left(\sum_{x_i \in \mathcal{X}_l \cap c_i = k} P[m_i = j/x_i, c_i, \theta^{(t)}] + \sum_{x_i \in \mathcal{X}_u} P[m_i = j, c_i = k/x_i, \theta^{(t)}] \right)$$

Here, we identify $P[m_i = j, c_i = k/x_i, \theta^{(t)}] = \frac{\alpha_j^{(t)} \beta_{k/j}^{(t)} f(x_i/\theta_j^{(t)})}{\sum_m \alpha_m^{(t)} f(x_i/\theta_m^{(t)})}$. In this formulation, joint probabilities for class and mixture labels are computed for data in $\mathcal{X}_u$ and used in the estimation of $\{\beta_{k/j}\}$, whereas in the previous formulation $\{\beta_{k/j}\}$ are updated solely on the basis of $\mathcal{X}_l$. While this does appear to be a significant qualitative difference between the two methods, both do ascend in $\log L$, and in practice we have found that they achieve comparable performance.

4 Combined Learning and Classification

The range of application for mixed training is greatly extended by the following observation: *test data (with labels withheld), or for that matter, any new batch of data to be classified, can be viewed as a new, unlabelled data set.* Hence, this new data can be taken to be $\mathcal{X}_u$ and used for learning (based on EM-I or EM-II) prior to its classification. What we are suggesting is a combined learning/classification operation that can be applied whenever there is a new batch of data to classify. In the usual supervised learning setting, there is a clear division between the learning and classification (use) phases. In this setting, modification of the classifier for *new* data is not possible (because the data is unlabelled), while for test data such modification is a form of "cheating". However, in our suggested scheme, this learning for unlabelled data is viewed simply as part of the classification operation. This is analogous to image segmentation, wherein we have a common energy function that is minimized for each new image to be segmented. Each such minimization determines a model local to the image *and* a segmentation for the image. Our "segmentation" is just classification, with $\log L$ playing the role of the energy function. It may consist of one term which is always fixed (based on a given labelled training set) and one term which is modified based on each new batch of unlabelled data to classify. We can envision several distinct learning contexts where this scheme can be used, as well as different ways of realizing the combined learning/classification operation[3] One use is in classification of an image/speech archive, where each image/speaker segment is a separate data "batch". Each batch to classify can be used as an unlabelled "training" set, either in concert with a representative labelled data set, or to modify a design based on such a set[4]. Effectively, this scheme would adapt the classifier to each new data batch. A second application is supervised learning wherein the *total* amount of data is fixed. Here, we need to divide the data into training and test sets with the conflicting goals of i) achieving a good design and ii) accurately measuring generalization performance. Combined learning and classification can be used here to mitigate the loss in performance associated with the choice of a large test set. More generally, our scheme can be used effectively in any setting where the new data to classify is either a) sizable or b) innovative relative to the existing training set.

5 Experimental Results

Figure 1a shows results for the 40-dimensional, 3-class *waveform-+noise* data set from the UC Irvine database. The 5000 data pairs were split into equal-size training and test sets. Performance curves were obtained by varying the amount of labelled training data. For each choice of N_l, various learning approaches produced 6 solutions based on random parameter initialization, for each of 7 different labelled subset realizations. The test set performance was then averaged over these 42 "trials". All schemes used $L = 12$ components. DA-RBF (Miller et al. 1996) is a deterministic annealing method for RBF classifiers that has been found to achieve very good results, when given adequate training data[5]. However, this supervised learning method is forced to discard unlabelled data, which severely handicaps its performance relative to EM-I, especially for small N_l, where the difference is substantial. TEM-I and TEM-II are results for the EM methods (both I and II) in combined learning and classification mode, i.e., where the 2500 test vectors were also used as part of $\mathcal{X}_u$. As seen in the figure, this leads to additional, significant performance gains for small N_l. Note also that performance of the two EM methods is comparable. Figure 1b shows results of similar experiments performed on 6-class satellite imagery data (*sat*), also from the UC Irvine database. For this set, the feature dimension is 36, and we chose $L = 18$ components. Here we compared EM-I with the method suggested in (Shashahani and Landgrebe 1994) (SL), based on the PM model. EM-I is seen to achieve substantial performance gains over this alternative learning approach. Note also that the EM-I performance is nearly constant, over the entire range of N_l.

Future work will investigate practical applications of combined learning and classification, as well as variations on this scheme which we have only briefly outlined. Moreover, we will investigate possible extensions of the methods described here for the regression problem.

---

[3]The image segmentation analogy in fact suggests an alternative scheme where we perform joint likelihood maximization over both the model parameters *and the "hard", missing class labels*. This approach, which is analogous to segmentation methods such as ICM, would encapsulate the classification operation directly within the learning. Such a scheme will be investigated in future work.

[4]Note that if the classifier is simply modified based on $\mathcal{X}_u$, EM-I will not need to update $\{\beta_{k|j}\}$, while EM-II must update the entire model.

[5]We assumed the same number of basis functions as mixture components. Also, for the DA design, there was only one initialization, since DA is roughly insensitive to this choice.

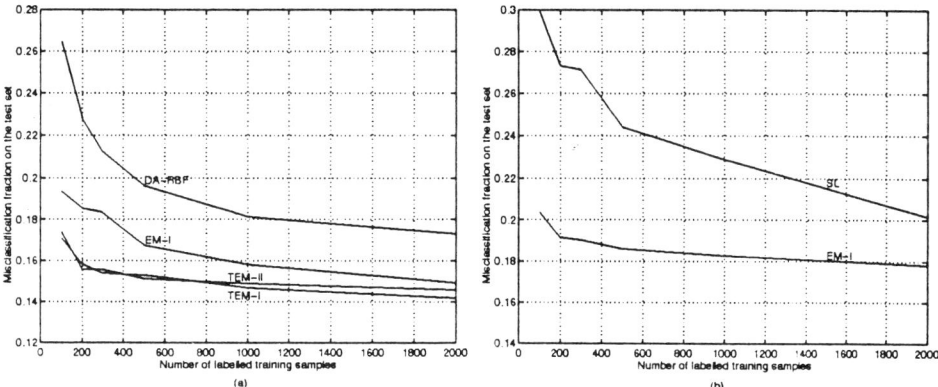

Acknowledgements

This work was supported in part by National Science Foundation Career Award IRI-9624870.

References

V. Castelli and T. M. Cover. On the exponential value of labeled samples. *Pattern Recognition Letters*, 16:105–111, 1995.

A.P. Dempster, N.M. Laird, and D.B. Rubin. Maximum-likelihood from incomplete data via the EM algorithm. *Journal of the Roy. Stat. Soc., Ser. B*, 39:1–38, 1977.

Z. Ghahramani and M. I. Jordan. Supervised learning from incomplete data via an EM approach. In *Neural Information Processing Systems 6*, 120-127, 1994.

M. I. Jordan and R. A. Jacobs. Hierarchical mixtures of experts and the EM algorithm. *Neural Computation*, 6:181–214, 1994.

R. P. Lippmann. Pattern classification using neural networks. *IEEE Communications Magazine*, 27, 47-64, 1989.

D. J. Miller, A. Rao, K. Rose, and A. Gersho. A global optimization method for statistical classifier design. *IEEE Transactions on Signal Processing*, Dec. 1996.

D. J. Miller and H. S. Uyar. A generalized Gaussian mixture classifier with learning based on both labelled and unlabelled data. *Conf. on Info. Sci. and Sys.*, 1996.

D. J. Miller. A mixture model equivalent to the radial basis function classifier. Submitted to *Neural Computation*, 1996.

J. Moody and C. J. Darken. Fast learning in locally-tuned processing units. *Neural Computation*, 1:281–294, 1989.

B. Shashahani and D. Landgrebe. The effect of unlabeled samples in reducing the small sample size problem and mitigating the Hughes phenomenon. *IEEE Transactions on Geoscience and Remote Sensing*, 32:1087–1095, 1994.

V. Tresp, R. Neuneier, and S. Ahmad. Efficient methods for dealing with missing data in supervised learning. In *Neural Information Processing Systems 7*, 689-696, 1995.

L. Xu, M. I. Jordan, and G. E. Hinton. An alternative model for mixtures of experts. In *Neural Information Processing Systems 7*, 633-640, 1995.

Learning Bayesian belief networks with neural network estimators

Stefano Monti*
*Intelligent Systems Program
University of Pittsburgh
901M CL, Pittsburgh, PA – 15260
smonti@isp.pitt.edu

Gregory F. Cooper*,**
**Center for Biomedical Informatics
University of Pittsburgh
8084 Forbes Tower, Pittsburgh, PA – 15261
gfc@cbmi.upmc.edu

Abstract

In this paper we propose a method for learning Bayesian belief networks from data. The method uses artificial neural networks as probability estimators, thus avoiding the need for making prior assumptions on the nature of the probability distributions governing the relationships among the participating variables. This new method has the potential for being applied to domains containing both discrete and continuous variables arbitrarily distributed. We compare the learning performance of this new method with the performance of the method proposed by Cooper and Herskovits in [7]. The experimental results show that, although the learning scheme based on the use of ANN estimators is slower, the learning accuracy of the two methods is comparable.
Category: Algorithms and Architectures.

1 Introduction

Bayesian belief networks (BBN) are a powerful formalism for representing and reasoning under uncertainty. This representation has a solid theoretical foundation [13], and its practical value is suggested by the rapidly growing number of areas to which it is being applied. BBNs concisely represent the joint probability distribution over a set of random variables, by explicitly identifying the probabilistic dependencies and independencies between these variables. Their clear semantics make BBNs particularly suitable for being used in tasks such as diagnosis, planning, and control.

The task of learning a BBN from data can usually be formulated as a search over the space of network structures, and as the subsequent search for an optimal parametrization of the discovered structure or structures. The task can be further complicated by extending the search to account for hidden variables and for the presence of data points with missing values. Different approaches have been successfully applied to the task of learning probabilistic networks from data [5]. In all these approaches, simplifying assumptions are made to circumvent practical problems in the implementation of the theory. One common assumption that is made is that all variables are discrete, or that all variables are continuous and normally distributed.

In this paper, we propose a novel method for learning BBNs from data that makes use of artificial neural networks (ANN) as probability distribution estimators, thus avoiding the need for making prior assumptions on the nature of the probability distribution governing the relationships among the participating variables. The use of ANNs as probability distribution estimators is not new [3], and its application to the task of learning Bayesian belief networks from data has been recently explored in [11]. However, in [11] the ANN estimators were used in the parametrization of the BBN structure only, and cross validation was the method of choice for comparing different network structures. In our approach, the ANN estimators are an essential component of the scoring metric used to search over the BBN structure space. We ran several simulations to compare the performance of this new method with the learning method described in [7]. The results show that, although the learning scheme based on the use of ANN estimators is slower, the learning accuracy of the two methods is comparable.

The rest of the paper is organized as follows. In Section 2 we briefly introduce the Bayesian belief network formalism and some basics of how to learn BBNs from data. In Section 3, we describe our learning method, and detail the use of artificial neural networks as probability distribution estimators. In Section 4 we present some experimental results comparing the performance of this new method with the one proposed in [7]. We conclude the paper with some suggestions for further research.

2   Background

A Bayesian belief network is defined by a triple (G, Ω, P), where $G = (\mathcal{X}, E)$ is a directed acyclic graph with a set of nodes $\mathcal{X} = \{x_1, \ldots, x_n\}$ representing domain variables, and with a set of arcs E representing probabilistic dependencies among domain variables; Ω is the space of possible instantiations of the domain variables[1]; and P is a probability distribution over the instantiations in Ω. Given a node $x \in \mathcal{X}$, we use π_x to denote the set of parents of x in $\mathcal{X}$. The essential property of BBNs is summarized by the *Markov condition*, which asserts that each variable is independent of its non-descendants given its parents. This property allows for the representation of the multivariate joint probability distribution over $\mathcal{X}$ in terms of the univariate conditional distributions $P(x_i \mid \pi_i, \theta_i)$ of each variable x_i given its parents π_i, with θ_i the set of parameters needed to fully characterize the conditional probability. Application of the chain rule, together with the Markov condition, yields the following factorization of the joint probability of any particular instantiation of all n variables:

$$P(x'_1, \ldots, x'_n) = \prod_{i=1}^{n} P(x'_i \mid \pi'_{x_i}, \theta_i) . \tag{1}$$

---

[1] An instantiation ω of all n variables in $\mathcal{X}$ is an n-uple of values $\{x'_1, \ldots, x'_n\}$ such that $x_i = x'_i$ for $i = 1 \ldots n$.

2.1 Learning Bayesian belief networks

The task of learning BBNs involves learning the network structure and learning the parameters of the conditional probability distributions. A well established set of learning methods is based on the definition of a scoring metric measuring the fitness of a network structure to the data, and on the search for high-scoring network structures based on the defined scoring metric [7, 10]. We focus on these methods, and in particular on the definition of Bayesian scoring metrics.

In a Bayesian framework, ideally classification and prediction would be performed by taking a weighted average over the inferences of every possible belief network containing the domain variables. Since this approach is in general computationally infeasible, often an attempt has been made to use a high scoring belief network for classification. We will assume this approach in the remainder of this paper.

The basic idea of the Bayesian approach is to maximize the probability $P(B_S \mid \mathcal{D}) = P(B_S, \mathcal{D})/P(\mathcal{D})$ of a network structure B_S given a database of cases $\mathcal{D}$. Because for all network structures the term $P(\mathcal{D})$ is the same, for the purpose of model selection it suffices to calculate $P(B_S, \mathcal{D})$ for all B_S. The Bayesian metrics developed so far all rely on the following assumptions: 1) given a BBN structure, all cases in $\mathcal{D}$ are drawn independently from the same distribution (multinomial sample); 2) there are no cases with missing values (complete database); 3) the parameters of the conditional probability distribution of each variable are independent (*global parameter independence*); and 4) the parameters associated with each instantiation of the parents of a variable are independent (*local parameter independence*).

The application of these assumptions allows for the following factorization of the probability $P(B_S, \mathcal{D})$

$$P(B_S, \mathcal{D}) = P(B_S)P(\mathcal{D} \mid B_S) = P(B_S) \prod_{i=1}^{n} s(x_i, \pi_i, \mathcal{D}) , \qquad (2)$$

where n is the number of nodes in the network, and each $s(x_i, \pi_i, \mathcal{D})$ is a term measuring the contribution of x_i and its parents π_i to the overall score of the network B_S. The exact form of the terms $s(x_i, \pi_i, \mathcal{D})$ slightly differs in the Bayesian scoring metrics defined so far, and for lack of space we refer the interested reader to the relevant literature [7, 10].

By looking at Equation (2), it is clear that if we assume a uniform prior distribution over all network structures, the scoring metric is decomposable, in that it is just the product of the $s(x_i, \pi_i, \mathcal{D})$ over all x_i times a constant $P(B_S)$. Suppose that two network structures B_S and $B_{S'}$ differ only for the presence or absence of a given arc into x_i. To compare their metrics, it suffices to compute $s(x_i, \pi_i, \mathcal{D})$ for both structures, since the other terms are the same. Likewise, if we assume a decomposable prior distribution over network structures, of the form $P(B_S) = \prod_i p_i$, as suggested in [10], the scoring metric is still decomposable, since we can include each p_i into the corresponding $s(x_i, \pi_i, \mathcal{D})$.

Once a scoring metric is defined, a search for a high-scoring network structure can be carried out. This search task (in several forms) has been shown to be NP-hard [4, 6]. Various heuristics have been proposed to find network structures with a high score. One such heuristic is known as K2 [7], and it implements a greedy search over the space of network structures. The algorithm assumes a given ordering on the variables. For simplicity, it also assumes that no prior information on the network is available, so the prior probability distribution over the network structures is uniform and can be ignored in comparing network structures.

The Bayesian scoring metrics developed so far either assume discrete variables [7, 10], or continuous variables normally distributed [9]. In the next section, we propose a possible generalization which allows for the inclusion of both discrete and continuous variables with arbitrary probability distributions.

3 An ANN-based scoring metric

The main idea of this work is to use artificial neural networks as probability estimators, to define a decomposable scoring metric for which no informative priors on the class, or classes, of the probability distributions of the participating variables are needed. The first three of the four assumptions described in the previous section are still needed, namely, the assumption of a multinomial sample, the assumption of a complete database, and the assumption of global parameter independence. However, the use of ANN estimators allows for the elimination of the assumption of local parameter independence. In fact, the conditional probabilities corresponding to the different instantiations of the parents of a variable are represented by the same ANN, and they share the same network weights and the same training data.

Let us denote with $\mathcal{D}_l \equiv \{C_1, \ldots, C_{l-1}\}$ the set of the first l cases in the database, and with $x_i^{(l)}$ and $\pi_i^{(l)}$ the instantiations of x_i and π_i in the l-th case respectively. The joint probability $P(B_S, \mathcal{D})$ can be written as:

$$P(B_S, \mathcal{D}) = P(B_S) P(\mathcal{D} | B_S) = P(B_S) \prod_{l=1}^{m} P(C_l | \mathcal{D}_l, B_S) =$$

$$= P(B_S) \prod_{l=1}^{m} \prod_{i=1}^{n} P(x_i^{(l)} | \pi_i^{(l)}, \mathcal{D}_l, B_S). \quad (3)$$

If we assume uninformative priors, or decomposable priors on network structures, of the form $P(B_S) = \prod_i p_i$, the probability $P(B_S, \mathcal{D})$ is decomposable. In fact, we can interchange the two products in Equation 3, so as to obtain

$$P(B_S, \mathcal{D}) = \prod_{i=1}^{n} [\, p_i \prod_{l=1}^{m} P(x_i^{(l)} | \pi_i^{(l)}, \mathcal{D}_l, B_S) \,] = \prod_{i=1}^{n} s(x_i, \pi_i, \mathcal{D}), \quad (4)$$

where $s(x_i, \pi_i, \mathcal{D})$ is the term between square brackets, and it is only a function of x_i and its parents in the network structure B_S (p_i can be neglected if we assume a uniform prior over the network structures). The computation of Equation 4 corresponds to the application of the prequential method discussed by Dawid [8].

The estimation of each term $P(x_i | \pi_i, \mathcal{D}_l, B_S)$ can be done by means of neural network. Several schemes are available for training a neural network to approximate a given probability distribution, or density. Notice that the calculation of each term $s(x_i, \pi_i, \mathcal{D})$ can be computationally very expensive. For each node x_i, computing $s(x_i, \pi_i, \mathcal{D})$ requires the training of m ANNs, where m is the size of the database. To reduce this computational cost, we use the following approximation, which we call the t-invariance approximation: for any $l \in \{1, \ldots, m-1\}$, given the probability $P(x_i | \pi_i, \mathcal{D}_l, B_S)$, at least t ($1 \leq t \leq m - l$) new cases are needed in order to alter such probability. That is, for each positive integer h, such that $h < t$, we assume $P(x_i | \pi_i, \mathcal{D}_{l+h}, B_S) = P(x_i | \pi_i, \mathcal{D}_l, B_S)$. Intuitively, this approximation implies the assumption that, given our present belief about the value of each $P(x_i | \pi_i, \mathcal{D}_l, B_S)$, at least t new cases are needed to revise this belief. By making this approximation, we achieve a t-fold reduction in the computation needed, since we now need to build and train only m/t ANNs for each x_i, instead of the original m. In fact, application of the t-invariance approximatioin to the computation of a given $s(x_i, \pi_i, \mathcal{D})$ yields:

$$s(x_i, \pi_i, \mathcal{D}) = \prod_{l=1}^{m} P(x_i^{(l)} \mid \pi_i^{(l)}, \mathcal{D}_l, B_S) = \prod_{k=0}^{m/t-1} \prod_{l=tk+1}^{t(k+1)} P(x_i^{(l)} \mid \pi_i^{(l)}, \mathcal{D}_{tk}, B_S). \quad (5)$$

Rather than selecting a constant value for t, we can choose to increment t as the size of the training database $\mathcal{D}_l$ increases. This approach seems preferable. When estimating $P(x_i \mid \pi_i, \mathcal{D}_l, B_S)$, this estimate will be very sensitive to the addition of new cases when l is small, but will become increasingly insensitive to the addition of new cases as l grows. A scheme for the incremental updating of t can be summarized in the equation $t = \lceil \lambda l \rceil$, where l is the number of cases already seen (i.e., the cardinality of $\mathcal{D}_l$), and $0 < \lambda \leq 1$. For example, given a data set of 50 cases, the updating scheme $t = \lceil 0.5 l \rceil$ would require the training of the ANN estimators $P(x_i \mid \pi_i, \mathcal{D}_l, B_S)$ for $l = 1, 2, 3, 5, 8, 12, 18, 27, 41$.

4 Evaluation

In this section, we describe the experimental evaluation we conducted to test the feasibility of use of the ANN-based scoring metric developed in the previous section. All the experiments are performed on the belief network Alarm, a multiply-connected network originally developed to model anesthesiology problems that may occur during surgery [2]. It contains 37 nodes/variables and 46 arcs. The variables are all discrete, and take between 2 and 4 distinct values. The database used in the experiments was generated from Alarm, and it is the same database used in [7].

In the experiments, we use a modification of the algorithm K2 [7]. The modified algorithm, which we call ANN-K2, replaces the closed-form scoring metric developed in [7] with the ANN-based scoring metric of Equation (5). The performance of ANN-K2 is measured in terms of accuracy of the recovered network structure, by counting the number of edges added and omitted with respect to the Alarm network; and in terms of the accuracy of the learned joint probability distribution, by computing its cross entropy with respect to the joint probability distribution of Alarm. The learning performance of ANN-K2 is also compared with the performance of K2. To train the ANNs, we used the conjugate-gradient search algorithm [12].

Since all the variables in the Alarm network are discrete, the ANN estimators are defined based on the softmax model, with normalized exponential output units, and with cross entropy as cost function. As a regularization technique, we augment the training set so as to induce a uniform conditional probability over the unseen instantiations of the ANN input. Given the probability $P(x_i \mid \pi_i, \mathcal{D}_l)$ to be estimated, and assuming x_i is a k-valued variable, for each instantiation π'_i that does not appear in the database D_l, we generate k new cases, with π_i instantiated to π'_i, and x_i taking each of its k values. As a result, the neural network estimates $P(x_i \mid \pi'_i, \mathcal{D}_l)$ to be uniform, with $P(x_i \mid \pi'_i, \mathcal{D}_l) = 1/k$ for each of x_i's values $x_{11}, \ldots, x_{1k}$.

We ran simulations where we varied the size of the training data set (100, 500, 1000, 2000, and 3000 cases), and the value of λ in the updating scheme $t = \lceil \lambda l \rceil$ described in Section 3. We used the settings $\lambda = 0.35$, and $\lambda = 0.5$. For each run, we measured the number of arcs added, the number of arcs omitted, the cross entropy, and the computation time, for each variable in the network. That is, we considered each node, together with its parents, as a simple BBN, and collected the measures of interest for each of these BBNs. Table 1 reports mean and standard deviation of each measure over the 37 variables of Alarm, for both ANN-K2 and K2. The results for ANN-K2 shown in Table 1 correspond to the setting $\lambda = 0.5$,

Data set	Algo.	arcs +		arcs −		cross entropy			time (secs)		
		m	s.d.	m	s.d.	m	med	s.d.	m	med	s.d.
100	ANN-K2	0.19	0.40	0.62	0.86	0.23	.051	0.52	130	88	159
	K2	0.75	1.28	0.22	0.48	0.08	.070	0.10	0.44	.06	1.48
500	ANN-K2	0.19	0.40	0.22	0.48	0.04	.010	0.11	1077	480	1312
	K2	0.22	0.42	0.11	0.31	0.02	.010	0.02	0.13	.06	0.22
1000	ANN-K2	0.24	0.49	0.22	0.48	0.05	.005	0.15	6909	4866	6718
	K2	0.11	0.31	0.03	0.16	0.01	.006	0.01	0.34	.23	0.46
2000	ANN-K2	0.19	0.40	0.11	0.31	0.02	.002	0.06	6458	4155	7864
	K2	0.05	0.23	0.03	0.16	0.005	.002	0.007	0.46	.44	0.65
3000	ANN-K2	0.16	0.37	0.05	0.23	0.01	.001	0.017	11155	4672	2136
	K2	0.00	0.00	0.03	0.16	0.004	.001	0.005	1.02	.84	1.11

Table 1: Comparison of the performance of ANN-K2 and of K2 in terms of number of arcs wrongly added (+), number of arcs wrongly omitted (−), cross entropy, and computation time. Each column reports the mean m, the median med, and the standard deviation $s.d.$ of the corresponding measure over the 37 nodes/variables of Alarm. The median for the number of arcs added and omitted is always 0, and is not reported.

since their difference from the results corresponding to the setting $\lambda = 0.35$ was not statistically significant.

Standard t-tests were performed to assess the significance of the difference between the measures for K2 and the measures for ANN-K2, for each data set cardinality. No technique to correct for multiple-testing was applied. Most measures show no statistically significant difference, either at the 0.05 level or at the 0.01 level (most p values are well above 0.2). In the simulation with 100 cases, both the difference between the mean number of arcs added and the difference between the mean number of arcs omitted are statistically significant ($p \simeq 0.01$). However, these differences cancel out, in that ANN-K2 adds fewer extra arcs than K2, and K2 omits fewer arcs than ANN-K2. This is reflected in the corresponding cross entropies, whose difference is not statistically significant ($p = 0.08$). In the simulation with 1000 cases, only the difference in the number of arcs omitted is statistically significant ($p \simeq .03$). Finally, in the simulation with 3000 cases, only the difference in the number of arcs added is statistically significant ($p \simeq .02$). K2 misses a single arc, and does not add any extra arc, and this is the best result to date. By comparison, ANN-K2 omits 2 arcs, and adds 5 extra arcs. For the simulation with 3000 cases, we also computed Wilcoxon rank sum tests. The results were consistent with the t-test results, showing a statistically significant difference only in the number of arcs added. Finally, as it can be noted in Table 1, the difference in computation time is of several order of magnitude, thus making a statistical analysis superfluous.

A natural question to ask is how sensitive is the learning procedure to the order of the cases in the training set. Ideally, the procedure would be insensitive to this order. Since we are using ANN estimators, however, which perform a greedy search in the solution space, particular permutations of the training cases might cause the ANN estimators to be more susceptible to getting stuck in local maxima. We performed some preliminary experiments to test the sensitivity of the learning procedure to the order of the cases in the training set. We ran few simulations in which we randomly changed the order of the cases. The recovered structure was identical in all simulations. Morevoer, the difference in cross entropy for different orderings of the cases in the training set showed not to be statistically significant.

5 Conclusions

In this paper we presented a novel method for learning BBNs from data based on the use of artificial neural networks as probability distribution estimators. As a preliminary evaluation, we have compared the performance of the new algorithm with the performance of K2, a well established learning algorithm for discrete domains, for which extensive empirical evaluation is available [1, 7]. With regard to the learning accuracy of the new method, the results are encouraging, being comparable to state-of-the-art results for the chosen domain. The next step is the application of this method to domains where current techniques for learning BBNs from data are not applicable, namely domains with continuous variables not normally distributed, and domains with mixtures of continuous and discrete variables. The main drawback of the new algorithm is its time requirements. However, in this preliminary evaluation, our main concern was the learning accuracy of the algorithm, and little effort was spent in trying to optimize its time requirements. We believe there is ample room for improvement in the time performance of the algorithm. More importantly, the scoring metric of Section 3 provides a general framework for experimenting with different classes of probability estimators. In this paper we used ANN estimators, but more efficient estimators can easily be adopted, especially if we assume the availability of prior information on the class of probability distributions to be used.

Acknowledgments

This work was funded by grant IRI-9509792 from the National Science Foundation.

References

[1] C. Aliferis and G. F. Cooper. An evaluation of an algorithm for inductive learning of Bayesian belief networks using simulated data sets. In *Proceedings of the 10th Conference of Uncertainty in AI*, pages 8–14, San Francisco, California, 1994.

[2] I. Beinlich, H. Suermondt, H. Chavez, and G. Cooper. The ALARM monitoring system: A case study with two probabilistic inference techniques for belief networks. In *2nd Conference of AI in Medicine Europe*, pages 247–256, London, England, 1989.

[3] C. Bishop. *Neural Networks for Pattern Recognition*. Oxford University Press, 1995.

[4] R. Bouckaert. Properties of learning algorithms for Bayesian belief networks. In *Proceedings of the 10th Conference of Uncertainty in AI*, pages 102–109, 1994.

[5] W. Buntine. A guide to the literature on learning probabilistic networks from data. *IEEE Transactions on Knowledge and Data Engineering*, 1996. To appear.

[6] D. Chickering, D. Geiger, and D. Heckerman. Learning Bayesian networks: search methods and experimental results. *Proc. 5th Workshop on AI and Statistics*, 1995.

[7] G. Cooper and E. Herskovits. A Bayesian method for the induction of probabilistic networks from data. *Machine Learning*, 9:309–347, 1992.

[8] A. Dawid. Present position and potential developments: Some personal views. Statistical theory. The prequential approach. *Journal of Royal Statistical Society A*, 147:278–292, 1984.

[9] D. Geiger and D. Heckerman. Learning Gaussian networks. Technical Report MSR-TR-94-10, Microsoft Research, One Microsoft Way, Redmond, WA 98052, 1994.

[10] D. Heckerman, D. Geiger, and D. Chickering. Learning Bayesian networks: the combination of knowledge and statistical data. *Machine Learning*, 1995.

[11] R. Hofmann and V. Tresp. Discovering structure in continuous variables using Bayesian networks. In *Advances in NIPS 8*. MIT Press, 1995.

[12] M. Moller. A scaled conjugate gradient algorithm for fast supervised learning. *Neural Networks*, 6:525–533, 1993.

[13] J. Pearl. *Probabilistic Reasoning in Intelligent Systems: networks of plausible inference*. Morgan Kaufman Publishers, Inc., 1988.

Smoothing Regularizers for Projective Basis Function Networks

John E. Moody and Thorsteinn S. Rögnvaldsson [*]
Department of Computer Science, Oregon Graduate Institute
PO Box 91000, Portland, OR 97291
moody@cse.ogi.edu denni@cca.hh.se

Abstract

Smoothing regularizers for radial basis functions have been studied extensively, but no general smoothing regularizers for *projective basis functions* (PBFs), such as the widely-used sigmoidal PBFs, have heretofore been proposed. We derive new classes of algebraically-simple m^{th}-order smoothing regularizers for networks of the form $f(W, x) = \sum_{j=1}^{N} u_j g\left[x^T v_j + v_{j0}\right] + u_0$, with general projective basis functions $g[\cdot]$. These regularizers are:

$$R_G(W, m) = \sum_{j=1}^{N} u_j^2 \|v_j\|^{2m-1} \quad \text{Global Form}$$

$$R_L(W, m) = \sum_{j=1}^{N} u_j^2 \|v_j\|^{2m} \quad \text{Local Form}$$

These regularizers bound the corresponding m^{th}-order smoothing integral

$$S(W, m) = \int d^D x\, \Omega(x) \left\|\frac{\partial^m f(W, x)}{\partial x^m}\right\|^2 ,$$

where W denotes all the network weights $\{u_j, u_0, v_j, v_0\}$, and $\Omega(x)$ is a weighting function on the D-dimensional input space. The global and local cases are distinguished by different choices of $\Omega(x)$.

The simple algebraic forms $R(W, m)$ enable the direct enforcement of smoothness without the need for costly Monte-Carlo integrations of $S(W, m)$. The new regularizers are shown to yield better generalization errors than weight decay when the implicit assumptions in the latter are wrong. Unlike weight decay, the new regularizers distinguish between the roles of the input and output weights and capture the interactions between them.

---

[*] Address as of September 1, 1996: Centre for Computer Architecture, University of Halmstad, P.O.Box 823, S-301 18 Halmstad, Sweden

1 Introduction: What are the right biases?

Regularization is a technique for reducing prediction risk by balancing model bias and model variance. A regularizer $R(W)$ imposes prior constraints on the network parameters W. Using squared error as the most common example, the objective functional that is minimized during training is

$$E = \frac{1}{2M}\sum_{i=1}^{M}[y^{(i)} - f(W, x^{(i)})]^2 + \lambda R(W) ,\quad (1)$$

where $y^{(i)}$ are target values corresponding to the inputs $x^{(i)}$, M is the number of training patterns, and the regularization parameter λ controls the importance of the prior constraints relative to the fit to the data. Several approaches can be applied to estimate λ (e.g. Eubank (1988) or Wahba (1990)).

Regularization reduces model variance at the cost of some model bias. An important question arises: What are the right biases? (Geman, Bienenstock & Doursat 1992). A good choice of $R(W)$ will result in lower expected prediction error than will a poor choice.

Weight decay is often used effectively, but it is an *ad hoc* technique that controls weight values without regard to the function $f(\cdot)$. It is thus not necessarily optimal and not appropriate for arbitrary function parameterizations. It will give very different results, depending upon whether a function is parameterized, for example, as $f(w, x)$ or as $f(w^{-1}, x)$.

Since many real world problems are intrinsically smooth, we propose that in many cases, an appropriate bias to impose is to favor solutions with low m^{th}-order curvature. Direct penalization of curvature is a parametrization-independent approach. The desired regularizer is the standard D dimensional curvature functional of order m:

$$S(W, m) = \int d^D x \, \Omega(x) \left\| \frac{\partial^m f(W, x)}{\partial x^m} \right\|^2 . \quad (2)$$

Here $\| \ \|$ denotes the ordinary euclidean tensor norm and $\partial^m/\partial x^m$ denotes the mth order differential operator. The weighting function $\Omega(x)$ ensures that the integral converges and determines the region over which we require the function to be smooth. $\Omega(x)$ is not required to be equal to the input density $p(x)$, and will most often be different.

The use of smoothing functionals like (2) has been extensively studied for smoothing splines (Eubank 1988, Hastie & Tibshirani 1990, Wahba 1990) and for radial basis function (RBF) networks (Powell 1987, Poggio & Girosi 1990, Girosi, Jones & Poggio 1995). However, no general class of smoothing regularizers that directly enforce smoothness $S(W, m)$ for *projective basis functions* (PBFs), such as the widely used sigmoidal PBFs, has been previously proposed.

Since explicit enforcement of smoothness using (2) requires costly, impractical Monte-Carlo integrations,[1] we derive algebraically-simple regularizers $R(W, m)$ that tightly bound $S(W, m)$.

2 Derivation of Simple Regularizers from Smoothing Functionals

We consider single hidden layer networks with D input variables, N_h nonlinear hidden units, and N_o linear output units. For clarity, we set $N_o = 1$, and drop the subscript on N_h

---

[1] Note that (2) is not just one integral, but actually $\mathcal{O}(D^m)$ integrals, since the norm of the operator $\partial^m/\partial x^m$ has $\mathcal{O}(D^m)$ terms. This is extremely expensive to compute for large D or large m.

(the derivation is trivially extended to the case $N_o > 1$). Thus, our network function is

$$f(x) = \sum_{j=1}^{N} u_j g[\theta_j, x] + u_0 \qquad (3)$$

where $g[\cdot]$ are the nonlinear transfer functions of the internal hidden units, $x \in R^D$ is the input vector[2], θ_j are the parameters associated with internal unit j, and W denotes all parameters in the network.

For regularizers $R(W)$, we will derive *strict upper bounds* for $S(W, m)$. We desire the regularizers to be as general as possible so that they can easily be applied to different network models. Without making any assumptions about $\Omega(x)$ or $g(\cdot)$, we have the upper bound

$$S(W, m) \leq N \sum_{j=1}^{N} u_j^2 \int d^D x \, \Omega(x) \left\| \frac{\partial^m g[\theta_j, x]}{\partial x^m} \right\|^2, \qquad (4)$$

which follows from the inequality $\left(\sum_{i=1}^{N} a_i\right)^2 \leq N \sum_{i=1}^{N} a_i^2$. We consider two possible options for the weighting function $\Omega(x)$. One is to require *global* smoothness, in which case $\Omega(x)$ is a very wide function that covers all relevant parts of the input space (e.g. a very wide gaussian distribution or a constant distribution). The other option is to require *local* smoothness, in which case $\Omega(x)$ approaches zero outside small regions around some reference points (e.g. the training data).

2.1 Projective Basis Representations

Projective basis functions (PBFs) are of the form $g[\theta_j, x] = g[x^T v_j + v_{j0}]$, where $\theta_j = \{v_j, v_{j0}\}$, $v_j = (v_{j1}, v_{j2}, \ldots, v_{jD})$ is the vector of weights connecting hidden unit j to the inputs, and v_{j0} is the bias, offset, or threshold. For PBFs, expression (4) simplifies to

$$S(W, m) \leq N \sum_{j=1}^{N} u_j^2 \|v_j\|^{2m} I_j(W, m), \qquad (5)$$

with

$$I_j(W, m) \equiv \int d^D x \, \Omega(x) \left(\frac{d^m g[z_j(x)]}{dz_j^m}\right)^2 \qquad (6)$$

where $z_j(x) \equiv x^T v_j + v_{j0}$.

Although the most commonly used $g[\cdot]$'s are sigmoids, our analysis applies to many other forms, for example flexible fourier units, polynomials, and rational functions.[3] The classes of PBF transfer functions $g[\cdot]$ that are applicable (as determined by $\Omega(x)$) are those for which the integral (8) is finite and well-defined.

2.2 Global weighting

For the global case, we select a gaussian form for the weighting function

$$\Omega_G(x) = (\sqrt{2\pi}\sigma)^{-D} \exp\left[\frac{-\|x\|^2}{2\sigma^2}\right] \qquad (7)$$

---
[2] Throughout, we use small letter boldface to denote vector quantities.
[3] See for example Moody & Yarvin (1992).

and require σ to be large. Integrating out all dimensions, except the one associated with the projection vector v_j, we are left with

$$I_j(W,m) = \frac{1}{\sigma\sqrt{2\pi}} \int_{-\infty}^{\infty} dx\, e^{-x^2/2\sigma^2} \left(\frac{d^m g[z_j(x)]}{dz_j^m}\right)^2. \tag{8}$$

If $(d^m g[z]/dz^m)^2$ is integrable and approaches zero outside a region that is small compared to σ, we can bound (8) by setting the exponential equal to unity. This implies

$$I_j(W,m) \leq \frac{I(m)}{\|v_j\|} \quad \text{with} \quad I(m) \equiv \frac{1}{\sigma\sqrt{2\pi}} \int_{-\infty}^{\infty} dz \left(\frac{d^m g[z]}{dz^m}\right)^2. \tag{9}$$

The bound of equation (5) then becomes

$$S(W,m) \leq NI(m) \sum_{j=1}^{N} u_j^2 \|v_j\|^{2m-1} = NI(m)R_G(W,m), \tag{10}$$

where the subscript G stands for *global*. Since λ absorbs all constant multiplicative factors, we need only weigh $R_G(W,m)$ into the training objective function.

2.2.1 Local weighting

For the local case, we consider weighting functions of the general form

$$\Omega_L(x) = \frac{1}{M} \sum_{i=1}^{M} \Omega(x^{(i)}, \sigma) \tag{11}$$

where $x^{(i)}$ are a set of points, and $\Omega(x^{(i)}, \sigma)$ is a function that decays rapidly for large $\|x - x^{(i)}\|$. We require that $\lim_{\sigma \to 0} \Omega(x^{(i)}, \sigma) = \delta(x - x^{(i)})$. Thus, when the $x^{(i)}$ are the training data points, the limiting distribution of (11) is the *empirical distribution*.

In the limit $\sigma \to 0$, equation (5) becomes

$$S(W,m) \leq \frac{N}{M} \sum_{j=1}^{N} u_j^2 \|v_j\|^{2m} \sum_{i=1}^{M} \left(\frac{d^m g[z_j(x^{(i)})]}{dz_j^m}\right)^2. \tag{12}$$

For the empirical distribution, we could compute the expression within parentheses in (12) for each input pattern $x^{(i)}$ during training and use it as our regularization cost. This is done by Bishop (1993) for the special case $m = 2$. However, this requires explicit design for each transfer function and becomes increasingly complicated as we go to higher m. To construct a simpler and more general form, we instead assume that the mth derivative of $g[\cdot]$ is bounded from above by $C_L(m) \equiv \max_z \left(\frac{d^m g[z]}{dz^m}\right)^2$.

This gives the bound

$$S(W,m) \leq NC_L(m) \sum_{j=1}^{N} u_j^2 \|v_j\|^{2m} = NC_L(m) R_L(W,m) \tag{13}$$

for the maximum local curvature of the function (the subscript L denotes *local* limit).

3 Empirical Example

We have done extensive simulation studies that demonstrate the efficacy of our new regularizers for PBF networks on a variety of problems. An account is given in Moody & Rögnvaldsson (1996). Here, we demonstrate the value of using smoothing regularizers on a simple problem which illustrates a key difference between smoothing and quadratic weight decay, the two dimensional bilinear function

$$t(x_1, x_2) = x_1 x_2. \tag{14}$$

This example was used by Friedman & Stuetzle (1981) to demonstrate projection pursuit regression. It is the simplest function with interactions between input variables.

We fit this function with one hidden layer networks using the $m = \{1, 2, 3\}$ smoothing regularizers, comparing the results with using weight decay. In a large set of experiments, we find that both the global and local smoothing regularizers with $m = 2$ and $m = 3$ outperform weight decay. An example is shown in figure 1. The local $m = 1$ case performs poorly, which is unsurprising, given that the target function is quadratic. Weight decay performs poorly because it lacks any form of interaction between the input layer and output layer weights v_j and u_j.

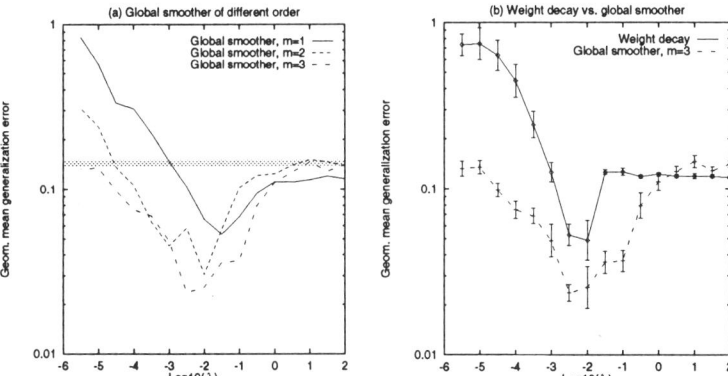

Figure 1: (a) Generalization errors on the $x_1 x_2$ problem, with 40 training data points and a signal-to-noise ratio of 2/3, for different values of the regularization parameter and different orders of the smoothing regularizer. For each value of λ, 10 networks with 8 hidden units have been trained and averaged (geometric average). The shaded area shows the 95% confidence bands for the average performance of a linear model on the same problem. (b) Similar plot for the $m = 3$ smoother compared to the standard weight decay method. Error bars mark the estimated standard deviation of the mean generalization error of the 10 networks. The $m = 3$ regularizer performs significantly better than weight decay.

4 Quality of the Regularizers: Approximations *vs* Bounds

Equations (10) and (13) are strict upper bounds to the smoothness functional $S(W, m)$, eq. (2), in the global and local limits, $\sigma \to \infty$ and $\sigma \to 0$. However, if the bounds are not sufficiently tight, then penalizing $R(W, m)$ may not have the effect of penalizing $S(W, m)$[4].

---

[4]For the proposed regularizers $R(W, m)$ to be effective in penalizing $S(W, m)$, we need only have an approximate monotonic relationship between them.

The bound (4) is tighter the more uncorrelated the mth derivatives of the internal unit activities are. If they are uncorrelated, then the bounds of equations (10) and (13) can be replaced by the approximations:

$$S_G(W,m) \approx I_G(m) R_G(W,m) \tag{15}$$
$$S_L(W,m) \approx C_L(m) R_L(W,m) , \tag{16}$$

using $\left(\sum_{i=1}^N a_i\right)^2 \approx \sum_{i=1}^N a_i^2$. The right hand sides differ from those in equations (10) and (13) only by a factor of N, so these approximations are actually proportional to the bounds.

For our regularizers, the constant factor N doesn't matter, since it can be absorbed into the regularization parameter λ (along with the values of the factors $I_G(m)$ or $C_L(m)$). In practical terms, there is no difference between using the upper bounds (10) and (13) or the uncorrelated approximations (15) and (16). Our empirical results (see figure 2) indicate that an approximate linear relationship holds between $S(W,m)$ and $R(W,m)$ for both the global and the local cases. This suggests that the uncorrelated hidden unit assumption yields a good approximation. This approximation also improves with the dimensionality of the input space. Extensive results and discussion are presented in (Moody & Rögnvaldsson 1996).

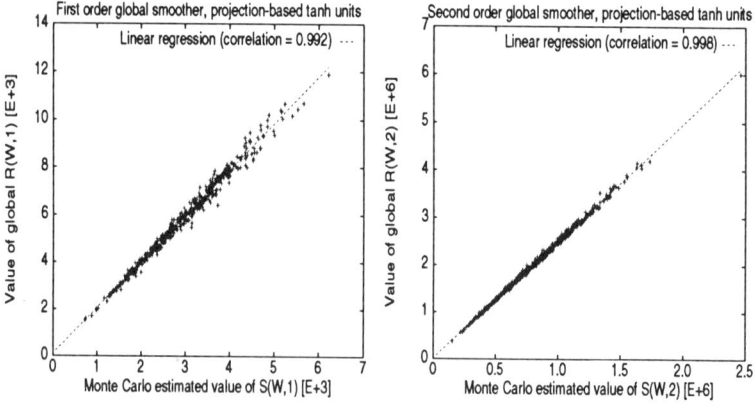

Figure 2: Linear correlation between $S(W,m)$ and the global $R_G(W,m)$ for neural networks with 10 input units, 10 internal tanh[·] PBF units, and one linear output. The values of $S(W,m)$ are computed through Monte Carlo integration. The left graph shows $m = 1$ and the right graph shows $m = 2$. Results are similar for the local form $R_L(W,m)$.

5 Summary

Our regularizers $R(W,m)$ are the first general class of mth-order smoothing regularizers to be proposed for projective basis function (PBF) networks. They apply to large classes of transfer functions $g[\cdot]$, including sigmoids. They differ fundamentally from quadratic weight decay in that they distinguish the roles of the input and output weights and capture the interactions between them.

Our approach is quite different from that developed for smoothing splines and smoothing radial basis functions (RBFs), since we derive smoothing regularizers for given classes of units $g[\theta, x]$, rather than derive the forms of the units $g[\cdot]$ by requiring them to be Greens functions of the smoothing operator $S(\cdot)$. Our approach thus has the advantage that it can be applied to the types of networks most often used in practice, namely PBFs.

In Moody & Rögnvaldsson (1996), we present further analysis and simulation results for PBFs. We have also extended our work to RBFs (Moody & Rögnvaldsson 1997).

Acknowledgements

Both authors thank Steve Rehfuss and Lizhong Wu for stimulating input. John Moody thanks Volker Tresp for a provocative discussion at a 1991 Neural Networks Workshop sponsored by the Deutsche Informatik Akademie. We gratefully acknowledge support for this work from ARPA and ONR (grant N00014-92-J-4062), NSF (grant CDA-9503968), the Swedish Institute, and the Swedish Research Council for Engineering Sciences (contract TFR-282-95-847).

References

Bishop, C. (1993), 'Curvature-driven smoothing: A learning algorithm for feedforward networks', *IEEE Trans. Neural Networks* **4**, 882–884.

Eubank, R. L. (1988), *Spline Smoothing and Nonparametric Regression*, Marcel Dekker, Inc.

Friedman, J. H. & Stuetzle, W. (1981), 'Projection pursuit regression', *J. Amer. Stat. Assoc.* **76**(376), 817–823.

Geman, S., Bienenstock, E. & Doursat, R. (1992), 'Neural networks and the bias/variance dilemma', *Neural Computation* **4**(1), 1–58.

Girosi, F., Jones, M. & Poggio, T. (1995), 'Regularization theory and neural network architectures', *Neural Computation* **7**, 219–269.

Hastie, T. J. & Tibshirani, R. J. (1990), *Generalized Additive Models*, Vol. 43 of *Monographs on Statistics and Applied Probability*, Chapman and Hall.

Moody, J. E. & Yarvin, N. (1992), Networks with learned unit response functions, *in* J. E. Moody, S. J. Hanson & R. P. Lippmann, eds, 'Advances in Neural Information Processing Systems 4', Morgan Kaufmann Publishers, San Mateo, CA, pp. 1048–55.

Moody, J. & Rögnvaldsson, T. (1996), Smoothing regularizers for projective basis function networks, Submitted to *Neural Computation*.

Moody, J. & Rögnvaldsson, T. (1997), Smoothing regularizers for radial basis function networks, Manuscript in preparation.

Poggio, T. & Girosi, F. (1990), 'Networks for approximation and learning', *IEEE Proceedings* **78**(9).

Powell, M. (1987), Radial basis functions for multivariable interpolation: a review., *in* J. Mason & M. Cox, eds, 'Algorithms for Approximation', Clarendon Press, Oxford.

Wahba, G. (1990), *Spline models for observational data*, CBMS-NSF Regional Conference Series in Applied Mathematics.

Competition Among Networks Improves Committee Performance

Paul W. Munro
Department of Information Science
and Telecommunications
University of Pittsburgh
Pittsburgh PA 15260
munro@sis.pitt.edu

Bambang Parmanto
Department of Health Information
Management
University of Pittsburgh
Pittsburgh PA 15260
parmanto+@pitt.edu

ABSTRACT

The separation of generalization error into two types, bias and variance (Geman, Bienenstock, Doursat, 1992), leads to the notion of error reduction by averaging over a "committee" of classifiers (Perrone, 1993). Committee performance decreases with both the average error of the constituent classifiers and increases with the degree to which the misclassifications are correlated across the committee. Here, a method for reducing correlations is introduced, that uses a winner-take-all procedure similar to competitive learning to drive the individual networks to different minima in weight space with respect to the training set, such that correlations in generalization performance will be reduced, thereby reducing committee error.

1 INTRODUCTION

The problem of constructing a predictor can generally be viewed as finding the right combination of bias and variance (Geman, Bienenstock, Doursat, 1992) to reduce the expected error. Since a neural network predictor inherently has an excessive number of parameters, reducing the prediction error is usually done by reducing variance. Methods for reducing neural network complexity can be viewed as a regularization technique to reduce this variance. Examples of such methods are Optimal Brain Damage (Le Cun et. al., 1991), weight decay (Chauvin, 1989), and early stopping (Morgan & Boulard, 1990).

The idea of combining several predictors to form a single, better predictor (Bates & Granger, 1969) has been applied using neural networks in recent years (Wolpert, 1992; Perrone, 1993; Hashem, 1994).

2 REDUCING MISCLASSIFICATION CORRELATION

Since committee errors occur when too many individual predictors are in error, committee performance improves as the correlation of network misclassifications decreases. Error correlations can be handled by using a weighted sum to generate a committee prediction; the weights can be estimated by using ordinary least squares (OLS) estimators (Hashem, 1994) or by using Lagrange multipliers (Perrone, 1993).

Another approach (Parmanto et al., 1994) is to reduce error correlation directly by attempting to drive the networks to different minima in weight space, that will presumably have different generalization *syndromes*, or patterns of error with respect to a test set (or better yet, the entire stimulus space).

2.1 Data Manipulations

Training the networks using nonidentical data has been shown to improve committee performance, both when the data sets are from mutually exclusive continuous regions (eg, Jacobs et al.,1991), or when the training subsets are arbitrarily chosen (Breiman, 1992; Parmanto, Munro, and Doyle, 1995). Networks tend to converge to different weight states, because the error surface itself depends on the training set; hence changing the data changes the error surface.

2.2 Auxiliary tasks

Another way to influence the networks to disagree is to introduce a second output unit with a different task to each network in the committee. Thus, each network has two outputs, a *primary unit* which is trained to predict the class of the input, and a *secondary unit*, with some other task that is *different* than the tasks assigned to the secondary units of the other committee members. *The success of this approach rests on the assumption that the decorrelation of the network errors will more than compensate for any degradation of performance induced on the primary task by the auxiliary task.* The presence of a hidden layer in each network guarantees that the two output response functions share some weight parameters (i.e., the input-hidden weights), and so the learning of the secondary task influences the function learned by the primary output unit.

Parmanto et al. (1994) acheived significant decorrelation and improved performance on a varoety of tasks using one of the input variables as the training signal for the secondary unit. Interestingly, the secondary task does not necessarily degrade performance on the primary task. Our studies, as well as those of Caruana (1995), show that extra tasks can facilitate learning time and generalization performance on an individual network. On the other hand, certain auxiliary tasks interfere with the primary task. We have found however, that even when the individual performance is degraded, committee performance is nevertheless enahnced (relative to a committee of single output networks) due to the magnitude of error decorrelation.

3 THE COMPETITIVE COMMITTEE

An alternative to using a stationary task per se, such as replicating an input variable or projecting onto principal components (as was done in Parmanto et al, 1994), is to use a signal that depends on the other networks, in such a manner that the functions computed by the secondary units are negatively correlated after training. This notion is reminiscent of competitive learning (Rumelhart and Zipser, 1986); that is, the functions computed by the secondary units will partition the stimulus space.

Thus, a Competitive Committee Machine (CCM) is defined as a committee of neural network classifiers, each with two output units: a *primary* unit trained according to the classification task, and a *secondary* unit participating in a competitive process with secondary units of the other networks in the committee; let the outputs of network i be denoted P_i and S_i, respectively (see Figure 1). The network weights are modified according to the following variant of the back propagation procedure.

When data item α from the training set is presented to the committee during training, with input vector x^α and known output classification value y^α (binary), the networks each process x^α simultaneously, and the P and S output units of each network respond. Each P-unit receives the identical training signal, y^α, that corresponds to the input item; the training signal to the S-units is zero for all networks except the network with the greatest S-unit response among the committee; the maximum S_i among the networks in the committee receives a training signal of 1, and the others receive a training signal of 0.

$$\delta_i^P = y^\alpha - P_i$$

$$\delta_i^S = \begin{cases} 1 - S_i & \text{if } S_i = \max_j S_j \\ -S_i & \text{otherwise} \end{cases}$$

where δ_i^P and δ_i^S are the errors attributed to the primary and secondary units respectively to adjust network weights with back propagation[1]. During the course of training, the S-unit's response is explicitly trained to become sensitive to a unique region (relative to the other networks' S-units) of the stimulus space. This training signal is different from typical "tasks" that are used to train neural networks in that it is not a static function of the input; instead, since it depends on the other networks in the committee, it has a dynamic quality.

4 RESULTS

Some experiments have been run using the sine wave classification task (Figure 2) of Geman and Bienenstock (1992).

Comparisons of CCM performance versus the baseline performance of a committee with a simple average over a range of architectures (as indicated by the number of hidden units) are favorable (Figure 3). Also, note that the improvement is primarily attributable to descreased correlation, since the average individual performance is not significantly affected.

Visualization of the response of the individual networks to the entire stimulus space gives a complete picture of how the networks generalize and shows the effect of the competition (Figure 4). For this particular data set, the classes are easily separated in the central region (note that all the networks do well here). But at the edges, there is much more variance in the networks trained with competitive secondary units (Figure 5).

5 DISCUSSION

Caruana (1995) has demontrated significant improvement on "target" classification tasks in individual networks by adding one or more supplementary output units trained to compute tasks related to the target task. The additional output unit added to each network

---

[1] For notational convenience, the derivative factor sometimes included in the definition of δ is not included in this description of δ^P and δ^S.

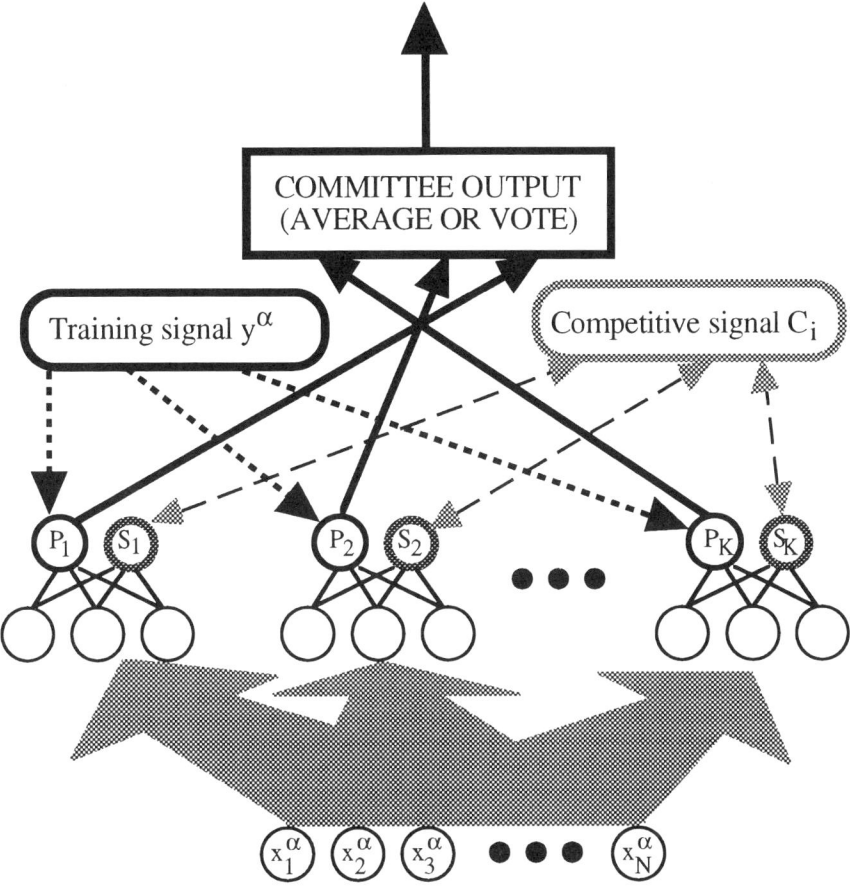

Input Variables (simultaneously presented to all networks)

Figure 1: *A Competitive Committee Machine.* Each of the K networks receives the same input and produces two outputs, P and S. The P responses of all the networks are compared to a common training signal to compute an error value for backpropagation (dark dashed arrows); the P responses are combined (by vote or by sum) to determine the committee response. The S-unit responses are compared with each other, with the "winner" (highest response) receiving a training signal of 1, and the others receiving a training signal of 0. Thus the training signal for network i is computed by comparing all S-unit responses, and then fed back to the S-units, hence the two-way arrows (gray).

in the CCM merges a variant of Rumelhart and Zipser's (1986) competitive learning procedure with backpropagation, to form a novel hybrid of a supervised training technique with an unsupervised method. The training signal delivered to the secondary unit under CCM is more *direct* than an arbitrary task, in that it is *defined* explicitly in terms of dissociating response properties.

Note that the training signals for the S-units differ from the P-unit training signals in two important respects:
1. Not static: The signal *depends on the S-unit responses from the other networks* and hence changes during the course of training.
2. Not uniform: It is not constant across the committee (whereas the P-unit training signal is.)

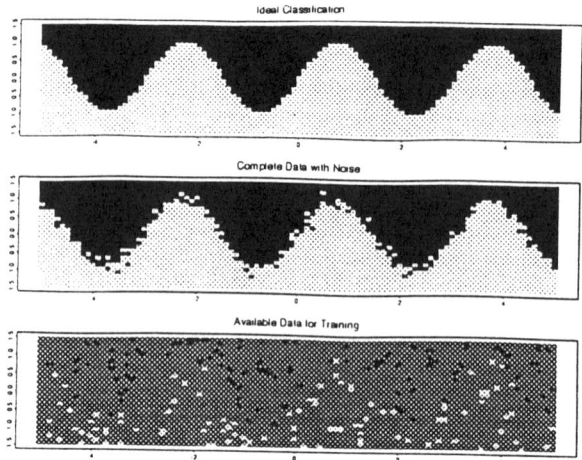

Figure 2. *A classification task.* Training data (bottom) is sampled from a classification task defined by a sinusoid (top) corrupted by noise (middle).

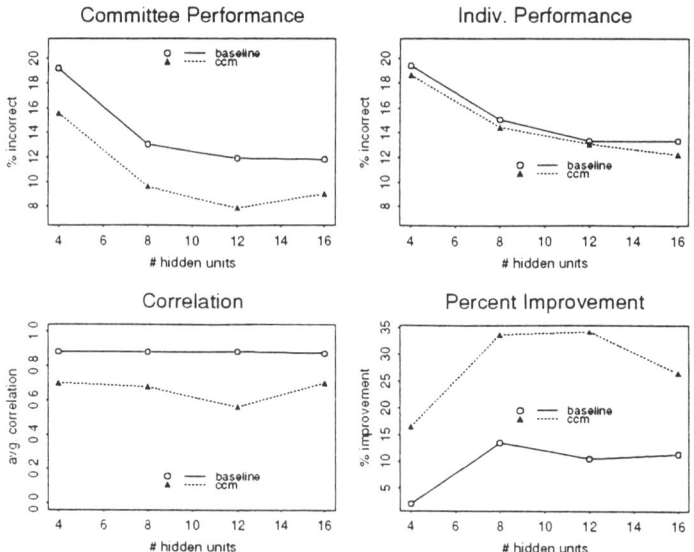

Figure 3. *Performance of CCM.* Committees of 5 networks were trained with competitive learning (CCM) and without (baseline). Each data point is an average over 5 simulations with different initial weights.

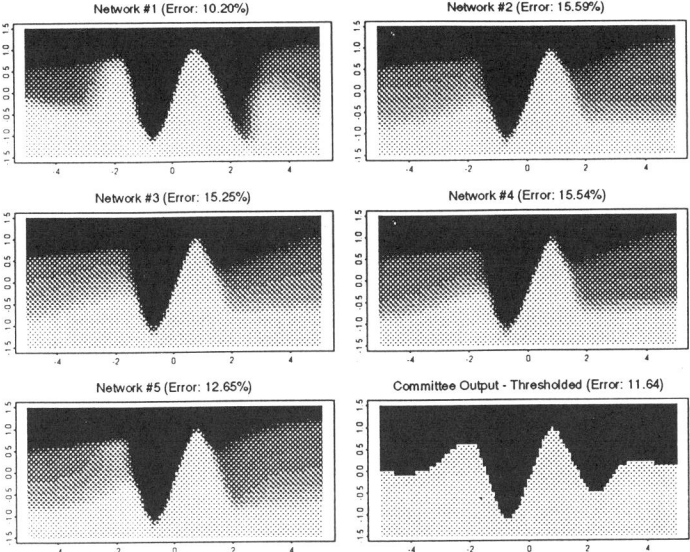

Figure 4. *Generalization plots for a committee.* The level of gray indicates the response for each network of a committee trained without competition. The panel on the lower right shows the (thresholded) committee output. The average pairwise correlation of the committee is 0.91.

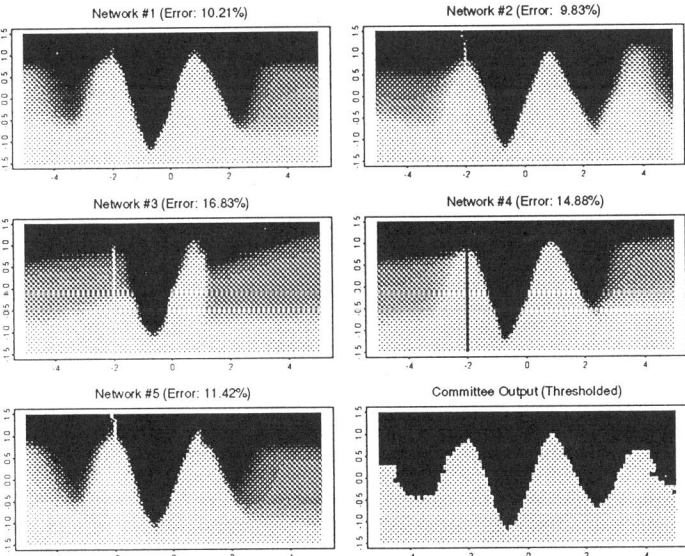

Figure 5. *Generalization plots for a CCM committee.* Comparison with Figure 4 shows much more variance among the committee at the edges. Note that the committee performs much better near the right and left ends of the stimulus space than does any individual network. This committee had an error rate of 8.11% (cf 11.64% in the baseline case).

The weighting of δ^S relative to δ^P is an important consideration; in the simulations above, the signal from the secondary unit was arbitrarily multiplied by a factor of 0.1. While we have not yet examined this systematically, it is assumed that this factor will modulate the tradeoff between degradation of the primary task and reduction of error correlation.

References

Bates, J.M., and Granger, C.W. (1969) "The combination of forecasts," Operation Research Quarterly, 20(4), 451-468.

Breiman, L, (1992) "Stacked Regressions", TR 367, Dept. of Statistics, Univ. of Cal. Berkeley.

Caruana, R (1995) "Learning many related tasks at the same time with backpropagation," In: *Advances in Neural Information Processing Systems 7.* D. S. Touretsky, ed. Morgan Kaufmann.

Chauvin, Y. (1989) "A backpropagation algorithm with optimal use of hidden units." In Touretzky D., (ed.), *Advances in Neural Information Processing 1*, Denver, 1988, Morgan Kaufmann.

Geman, S., Bienenstock, E., and Doursat, R. (1992) "Neural networks and the bias/variance dilemma," *Neural Computation 4*, 1-58.

Hashem, S. (1994). Optimal Linear Combinations of Neural Networks., PhD Thesis, Purdue University.

Jacobs, R.A., Jordan, M.I., Nowlan, S.J., and Hinton, G.E. (1991) "Adaptive mixtures of local experts," *Neural Computation, 3*, 79-87

Le Cun, Y., Denker J. and Solla, S. (1990). Optimal Brain Damage. In D. Touretzky (Ed.) *Advances in Neural Information Processing Systems 2*, San Mateo: Morgan Kaufmann. 598-605.

Morgan, N. & Boulard, H. (1990) Generalization and parameter estimation in feedforward nets: some experiments. In D. Touretzky (Ed.) *Advances in Neural Information Processing Systems 2* San Mateo: Morgan Kaufmann.

Parmanto, B., Munro, P.W., Doyle, H.R., Doria, C., Aldrighetti, L., Marino, I.R., Mitchel, S., and Fung, J.J. (1994) "Neural network classifier for hepatoma detection," *Proceedings of the World Congress of Neural Networks*

Parmanto, B., Munro, P.W., Doyle, H.R. (1996) "Improving committee diagnosis with resampling techniques," In: D. S. Touretzky, M. C. Mozer, M. E. Hasselmo, eds. *Advances in Neural Information Processing Systems 8.* MIT Press: Cambridge, MA.

Perrone, M.P. (1993) "Improving Regression Estimation: Averaging Methods for Variance Reduction with Extension to General Convex Measure Optimization," PhD Thesis, Department of Physics, Brown University.

Rumelhart. D.E and Zipser, D. (1986) "Feature discovery by competitive learning," In: Rumelhart, D.E.and McClelland, J.E. (Eds.), *Parallel Distributed Processing: Explorations in the Microstructure of Cognition.* MIT Press, Cambridge, MA.

Wolpert, D. (1992). Stacked generalization, *Neural Networks, 5*, 241-259.

Adaptive On-line Learning in Changing Environments

Noboru Murata, Klaus-Robert Müller, Andreas Ziehe
GMD-First, Rudower Chaussee 5, 12489 Berlin, Germany
{mura,klaus,ziehe}@first.gmd.de

Shun-ichi Amari
Laboratory for Information Representation, RIKEN
Hirosawa 2–1, Wako–shi, Saitama 351–01, Japan
amari@zoo.riken.go.jp

Abstract

An adaptive on-line algorithm extending the learning of learning idea is proposed and theoretically motivated. Relying only on gradient flow information it can be applied to learning continuous functions or distributions, even when no explicit loss function is given and the Hessian is not available. Its efficiency is demonstrated for a non-stationary blind separation task of acoustic signals.

1 Introduction

Neural networks provide powerful tools to capture the structure in data by learning. Often the batch learning paradigm is assumed, where the learner is given all training examples simultaneously and allowed to use them as often as desired. In large practical applications batch learning is often experienced to be rather infeasible and instead on-line learning is employed.
In the on-line learning scenario only one example is given at a time and then discarded after learning. So it is less memory consuming and at the same time it fits well into more natural learning, where the learner receives new information and should adapt to it, without having a large memory for storing old data. On-line learning has been analyzed extensively within the framework of statistics (Robbins & Monro [1951], Amari [1967] and others) and statistical mechanics (see eg. Saad & Solla [1995]). It was shown that on-line learning is asymptotically as effective as batch

learning (cf. Robbins & Monro [1951]). However this only holds, if the appropriate learning rate η is chosen. A too large η spoils the convergence of learning. In earlier work on dichotomies Sompolinsky et al. [1995] showed the effect on the rate of convergence of the generalization error of a constant, annealed and adaptive learning rate. In particular, the annealed learning rate provides an optimal convergence rate, however it cannot follow changes in the environment. Since on-line learning aims to follow the change of the rule which generated the data, Sompolinsky et al. [1995], Darken & Moody [1991] and Sutton [1992] proposed adaptive learning rates, which learn how to learn. Recently Cichoki et al. [1996] proposed an adaptive on-line learning algorithm for blind separation based on low pass filtering to stabilize learning.

We will extend the reasoning of Sompolinsky et al. in several points: (1) we give an adaptive learning rule for learning continuous functions (section 3) and (2) we consider the case, where no explicit loss function is given and the Hessian cannot be accessed (section 4). This will help us to apply our idea to the problem of on-line blind separation in a changing environment (section 5).

2 On-line Learning

Let us consider an infinite sequence of independent examples $(x_1, y_1), (x_2, y_2), \ldots$. The purpose of learning is to obtain a network with parameter $\hat{w}$ which can simulate the rule inherent to this data. To this end, the neural network modifies its parameter $\hat{w}_t$ at time t into $\hat{w}_{t+1}$ by using only the next example (x_{t+1}, y_{t+1}) given by the rule. We introduce a loss function $l(x, y; w)$ to evaluate the performance of the network with parameter w. Let $R(w) = \langle l(x, y; w) \rangle$ be the expected loss or the generalization error of the network having parameter w, where $\langle\ \rangle$ denotes the average over the distribution of examples (x, y). The parameter w^* of the best machine is given by $w^* = \arg\min R(w)$. We use the following stochastic gradient descent algorithm (see Amari [1967] and Rumelhart et al. [1986]):

$$\hat{w}_{t+1} = \hat{w}_t - \eta_t C(\hat{w}_t) \frac{\partial}{\partial w} l(x_{t+1}, y_{t+1}; \hat{w}_t), \qquad (1)$$

where η_t is the learning rate which may depend on t and $C(\hat{w}_t)$ is a positive-definite matrix which may depend on $\hat{w}_t$. The matrix C plays the role of the Riemannian metric tensor of the underlying parameter space $\{w\}$.

When η_t is fixed to be equal to a small constant η, $E[\hat{w}_t]$ converges to w^* and $\text{Var}[\hat{w}_t]$ converges to a non-zero matrix which is order $O(\eta)$. It means that $\hat{w}_t$ fluctuates around w^* (see Amari [1967], Heskes & Kappen [1991]). If $\eta_t = c/t$ (annealed learning rate) $\hat{w}_t$ converges to w^* locally (Sompolinsky et al. [1995]). However when the rule changes over time, an annealed learning rate cannot follow the changes fast enough since $\eta_t = c/t$ is too small.

3 Adaptive Learning Rate

The idea of an adaptively changing η_t was called learning of the learning rule (Sompolinsky et al. [1995]). In this section we investigate an extension of this idea to differentiable loss functions. Following their algorithm, we consider

$$\hat{w}_{t+1} = \hat{w}_t - \eta_t K^{-1}(\hat{w}_t) \frac{\partial}{\partial w} l(x_{t+1}, y_{t+1}; \hat{w}_t), \qquad (2)$$

$$\eta_{t+1} = \eta_t + \alpha \eta_t \left(\beta \left(l(\boldsymbol{x}_{t+1}, \boldsymbol{y}_{t+1}; \hat{\boldsymbol{w}}_t) - \hat{R} \right) - \eta_t \right), \tag{3}$$

where α and β are constants, $K(\hat{\boldsymbol{w}}_t)$ is a Hessian matrix of the expected loss function $\partial^2 R(\hat{\boldsymbol{w}}_t)/\partial \boldsymbol{w} \partial \boldsymbol{w}$ and $\hat{R}$ is an estimator of $R(\boldsymbol{w}^*)$. Intuitively speaking, the coefficient η in Eq.(3) is controlled by the remaining error. When the error is large, η takes a relatively large value. When the error is small, it means that the estimated parameter is close to the optimal parameter; η approaches to 0 automatically. However, for the above algorithm all quantities $(K, l, \hat{R})$ have to be accessible which they are certainly not in general. Furthermore $l(\boldsymbol{x}_{t+1}, \boldsymbol{y}_{t+1}; \hat{\boldsymbol{w}}_t) - \hat{R}$ could take negative values. Nevertheless in order to still get an intuition of the learning behaviour, we use the continuous versions of (2) and (3), averaged with respect to the current input-output pair $(\boldsymbol{x}_t, \boldsymbol{y}_t)$ and we omit correlations and variances between the quantities $(\eta_t, \boldsymbol{w}_t, l)$ for the sake of simplicity

$$\frac{d}{dt} \boldsymbol{w}_t = -\eta_t K(\boldsymbol{w}_t)^{-1} \left\langle \frac{\partial}{\partial \boldsymbol{w}} l(\boldsymbol{x}, \boldsymbol{y}; \boldsymbol{w}_t) \right\rangle \text{ and } \frac{d}{dt} \eta_t = \alpha \eta_t \left(\beta \langle l(\boldsymbol{x}, \boldsymbol{y}; \boldsymbol{w}_t) - \hat{R} \rangle - \eta_t \right).$$

Noting that $\langle \partial l(\boldsymbol{x}, \boldsymbol{y}; \boldsymbol{w}^*)/\partial \boldsymbol{w} \rangle = 0$, we have the asymptotic evaluations

$$\left\langle \frac{\partial}{\partial \boldsymbol{w}} l(\boldsymbol{x}, \boldsymbol{y}; \boldsymbol{w}_t) \right\rangle \simeq K^*(\boldsymbol{w}_t - \boldsymbol{w}^*),$$

$$\langle l(\boldsymbol{x}, \boldsymbol{y}; \boldsymbol{w}_t) - \hat{R} \rangle \simeq R(\boldsymbol{w}^*) - \hat{R} + \frac{1}{2}(\boldsymbol{w}_t - \boldsymbol{w}^*)^T K^*(\boldsymbol{w}_t - \boldsymbol{w}^*),$$

with $K^* = \partial^2 R(\boldsymbol{w}^*)/\partial \boldsymbol{w} \partial \boldsymbol{w}$. Assuming $R(\boldsymbol{w}^*) - \hat{R}$ is small and $K(\boldsymbol{w}_t) \simeq K^*$ yields

$$\frac{d}{dt} \boldsymbol{w}_t = -\eta_t (\boldsymbol{w}_t - \boldsymbol{w}^*), \quad \frac{d}{dt} \eta_t = \alpha \eta_t \left(\frac{\beta}{2}(\boldsymbol{w}_t - \boldsymbol{w}^*)^T K^*(\boldsymbol{w}_t - \boldsymbol{w}^*) - \eta_t \right). \tag{4}$$

Introducing the squared error $e_t = \frac{1}{2}(\boldsymbol{w}_t - \boldsymbol{w}^*)^T K^*(\boldsymbol{w}_t - \boldsymbol{w}^*)$, gives rise to

$$\dot{e}_t = -2\eta_t e_t, \quad \dot{\eta}_t = \alpha \beta \eta_t e_t - \alpha \eta_t^2. \tag{5}$$

The behavior of the above equation system is interesting: The origin $(0, 0)$ is its attractor and the basin of attraction has a fractal boundary. Starting from an adequate initial value, it has the solution of the form

$$e_t = \frac{1}{\beta} \left(\frac{1}{2} - \frac{1}{\alpha} \right) \cdot \frac{1}{t} \quad (\alpha > 2), \quad \text{and} \quad \eta_t = \frac{1}{2} \cdot \frac{1}{t}. \tag{6}$$

It is important to note that this $1/t$-convergence rate of the generalization error e_t is the optimal order of any estimator $\hat{\boldsymbol{w}}_t$ converging to $\boldsymbol{w}^*$. So we find that Eq.(4) gives us an on-line learning algorithm which converges with a fast rate. This holds also if the target rule is slowly fluctuating or suddenly changing. The technique to prove convergence was to use the scalar distance in weight space e_t. Note also that Eq.(6) holds only within an appropriate parameter range; for small η and $\boldsymbol{w}_t - \boldsymbol{w}^*$ correlations and variances between $(\eta_t, \boldsymbol{w}_t, l)$ can no longer be neglected.

4 Modification

From the practical point of view **(1)** the Hessian K^* of the expected loss or **(2)** the minimum value of the expected loss $\hat{R}$ are in general not known or **(3)** in some applications we cannot access the explicit loss function (e.g. blind separation). Let us therefore consider a generalized learning algorithm:

$$\hat{w}_{t+1} = \hat{w}_t - \eta_t f(x_{t+1}, y_{t+1}; \hat{w}_t), \tag{7}$$

where f is a flow which determines the modification when an example (x_{t+1}, y_{t+1}) is given. Here we do not assume the existence of a loss function and we only assume that the averaged flow vanishes at the optimal parameter, i.e. $\langle f(x, y; w^*) \rangle = 0$. With a loss function, the flow corresponds to the gradient of the loss. We consider the averaged continuous equation and expand it around the optimal parameter:

$$\frac{d}{dt} w_t = -\eta_t \langle f(x, y; w_t) \rangle \simeq -\eta_t K^*(w_t - w^*), \tag{8}$$

where $K^* = \langle \partial f(x, y; w^*)/\partial w \rangle$. Suppose that we have an eigenvector of the Hessian K^* vector v satisfying $v^T K^* = \lambda v^T$ and let us define

$$\xi_t = \langle v^T f(x, y; w_t) \rangle \simeq v^T K^*(w_t - w^*), \tag{9}$$

then the dynamics of ξ can be approximately represented as

$$\frac{d}{dt} \xi_t = -\lambda \eta_t \xi_t. \tag{10}$$

By using ξ, we define a discrete and continuous modification of the rule for η:

$$\eta_{t+1} = \eta_t + \alpha \eta_t (\beta |\xi_t| - \eta_t) \quad \text{and} \quad \frac{d}{dt} \eta_t = \alpha \eta_t (\beta |\xi_t| - \eta_t). \tag{11}$$

Intuitively ξ corresponds to a 1-dimensional pseudo distance, where the average flow f is projected down to a single direction v. The idea is to choose a clever direction such that it is sufficient to observe all dynamics of the flow only along this projection. In this sense the scalar ξ is the simplest obtainable value to observe learning. Noting that ξ is always positive or negative depending on its initial value and η can be positive, these two equations (10) and (11) are equivalent to the equation system (5). Therefore their asymptotic solutions are

$$\xi_t = \frac{1}{\beta} \left(\frac{1}{\lambda} - \frac{1}{\alpha} \right) \cdot \frac{1}{t}, \quad \text{and} \quad \eta_t = \frac{1}{\lambda} \cdot \frac{1}{t}. \tag{12}$$

Again similar to the last section we have shown that the algorithm converges properly, however this time without using loss or Hessian. In this algorithm, an important problem is how to get a good projection v. Here we assume the following facts and approximate the previous algorithm: **(1)** the minimum eigenvalue of matrix K^* is sufficiently smaller than the second minimum eigenvalue and **(2)** therefore after a large number of iterations, the parameter vector $\hat{w}_t$ will approach from the direction of the minimum eigenvector of K^*. Since under these conditions the evolution of the estimated parameter can be thought of as a one-dimensional process, any vector can be used as v except for the vectors which are orthogonal to the minimum eigenvector. The most efficient vector will be the minimum eigenvector itself which can be approximated (for a large number of iterations) by

$$v = \langle f \rangle / \| \langle f \rangle \|,$$

where $\| \ \|$ denotes the L^2 norm. Hence we can adopt $\xi = \|\langle \boldsymbol{f} \rangle\|$. Substituting the instantaneous average of the flow by a leaky average, we arrive at

$$\hat{w}_{t+1} = \hat{w}_t - \eta_t \boldsymbol{f}(x_{t+1}, y_{t+1}; \hat{w}_t), \tag{13}$$
$$r_{t+1} = (1-\delta) r_t + \delta \boldsymbol{f}(x_{t+1}, y_{t+1}; \hat{w}_t), \quad (0 < \delta < 1) \tag{14}$$
$$\eta_{t+1} = \eta_t + \alpha \eta_t \left(\beta \| r_{t+1} \| - \eta_t \right), \tag{15}$$

where δ controls the leakiness of the average and r is used as auxiliary variable to calculate the leaky average of the flow $\boldsymbol{f}$. This set of rules is easy to compute. However η will now approach a small value because of fluctuations in the estimation of r which depend on the choice of α, β, γ. In practice, to assure the stability of the algorithm, the learning rate in Eq.(13) should be limited to a maximum value $\eta_{\max}$ and a cut-off $\eta_{\min}$ should be imposed.

5 Numerical Experiment: an application to blind separation

In the following we will describe the blind separation experiment that we conducted (see eg. Bell & Sejnowski [1995], Jutten & Herault [1991], Molgedey & Schuster [1994] for more details on blind separation). As an example we use the two sun audio files (sampling rate 8kHz): "rooster" (s_t^1) and "space music" (s_t^2) (see Fig. 1). Both sources are mixed on the computer via $\vec{I}_t = (\mathbb{1} + A)\vec{s}_t$ where $0s < t < 1.25s$ and $3.75s \leq t \leq 5s$ and $\vec{I}_t = (\mathbb{1} + B)\vec{s}_t$ for $1.25s \leq t < 3.75s$, using $A = (0\ 0.9; 0.7\ 0)$ and $B = (0\ 0.8; 0.6\ 0)$ as mixing matrices. So the rule *switches* twice in the given data. The goal is to obtain the sources $\vec{s}_t$ by estimating $\hat{A}$ and $\hat{B}$, given *only* the measured mixed signals $\vec{I}_t$. A change of the mixing is a scenario often encountered in real blind separation tasks, e.g. a speaker turns his head or moves during his utterances. Our on-line algorithm is especially suited to this non-stationary separation task, since adaptation is not limited by the above-discussed generic drawbacks of a constant learning rate as in Bell & Sejnowski [1995], Jutten & Herault [1991], Molgedey & Schuster [1994]. Let $\vec{u}_t$ be the unmixed signals

$$\vec{u}_t = (\mathbb{1} + T_t)^{-1} \vec{I}_t, \tag{16}$$

where T is the estimated mixing matrix. Along the lines of Molgedey & Schuster [1994] we use as modification rule for T_t

$$\Delta T_t^{ij} \propto \eta_t \boldsymbol{f}\left(\langle I_t^j u_t^j \rangle, \langle u_t^i u_t^j \rangle, \langle I_t^j u_{t-1}^j \rangle, \langle u_t^i u_{t-1}^j \rangle \right) \propto \eta_t \langle I_t^j u_t^j \rangle \langle u_t^i u_t^j \rangle + \langle I_t^j u_{t-1}^j \rangle \langle u_t^i u_{t-1}^j \rangle,$$

$(i, j = 1, 2, i \neq j)$, where we substitute instantaneous averages with leaky averages

$$\langle I_t^j u_t^j \rangle_{\text{leaky}} = (1 - \epsilon) \langle I_{t-1}^j u_{t-1}^j \rangle_{\text{leaky}} + \epsilon I_t^j u_t^j.$$

Note that the necessary ingredients for the flow $\boldsymbol{f}$ in Eq.(13)-(14) are in this case simply the correlations at equal or different times; η_t is computed according to Eq.(15). In Fig.2 we observe the results of the simulation (for parameter details, see figure caption). After a short time (t=0.4s) of large η and strong fluctuations in η the mixing matrix is estimated correctly. Until t=1.25s the learning rate adapts cooling down approximately similar to $1/t$ (cf. Fig. 2c), which was predicted in Eq.(12) in the previous section, i.e. it finds the optimal rate for annealing. At the point of the switch where simple annealed learning would have failed to adapt to the sudden change, our adaptive rule increases η drastically and is able to follow the switch within another 0.4s rsp. 0.1s. Then again, the learning rate is cooled down automatically as intended. Comparing the mixed, original and unmixed signals in Fig.1 confirms the accurate and fast estimate that we already observed in the mixing matrix elements. The same also holds for an acoustic cross check: for a small part of a second both signals are audible, then as time proceeds only one signal, and again after the switches both signals are audible but only for a very short moment. The fading away of the signal is so fast to the listener that it seems that one signal is simply "switched off" by the separation algorithm.

Altogether we found an excellent adaptation behavior of the proposed on-line algorithm, which was also reproduced in other simulation examples omitted here.

6 Conclusion

We gave a theoretically motivated adaptive on-line algorithm extending the work of Sompolinsky et al. [1995]. Our algorithm applies to general feed-forward networks and can be used to accelerate learning by the learning about learning strategy in the difficult setting where (a) continuous functions or distributions are to be learned, (b) the Hessian K is not available and (c) no explicit loss function is given. Note, that if an explicit loss function or K is given, this additional information can be incorporated easily, e.g. we can make use of the real gradient otherwise we only rely on the *flow*. Non-stationary blind separation is a typical implementation of the setting (a)-(c) and we use it as an application of the adaptive on-line algorithm in a changing environment. Note that we can apply the learning rate adaptation to most existing blind separation algorithms and thus make them feasible for a non-stationary environment. However, we would like to emphasize that blind separation is just an example for the general adaptive on-line strategy proposed and applications of our algorithm are by no means limited to this scenario. Future work will also consider applications where the rules change more gradually (e.g. *drift*).

References

Amari, S. (1967) *IEEE Trans. EC* **16**(3):299-307.
Bell, T., Sejnowski, T. (1995) *Neural Comp.* **7**:1129-1159.
Cichocki A., Amari S., Adachi M., Kasprzak W. (1996) Self-Adaptive Neural Networks for Blind Separation of Sources, ISCAS'96 (IEEE), Vol. 2, 157-160.
Darken, C., Moody, J. (1991) in NIPS 3, Morgan Kaufmann, Palo Alto.
Heskes, T.M., Kappen, B. (1991) *Phys. Rev. A* **440**:2718-2726.
Jutten, C., Herault, J. (1991) *Signal Processing* **24**:1-10.
Molgedey, L., Schuster, H.G. (1994) *Phys. Rev. Lett.* **72**(23):3634-3637.
Robbins, H., Monro, S. (1951) *Ann. Math. Statist.*, **22**:400-407.
Rumelhart, D., McClelland, J.L and the PDP Research Group (eds.) (1986), PDP Vol. 1, pp. 318-362, Cambridge, MA: MIT Press.
Saad D., and Solla S. (1995), *Workshop at NIPS'95*, see World–Wide–Web page: http://neural-server.aston.ac.uk/nips95/workshop.html and references therein.
Sompolinsky, H., Barkai, N., Seung, H.S. (1995) in *Neural Networks: The Statistical Mechanics Perspective*, pp. 105-130. Singapore: World Scientific.
Sutton, R.S. (1992) in Proc. 10th nat. conf. on AI, 171-176, MIT Press.

Adaptive On-line Learning in Changing Environments

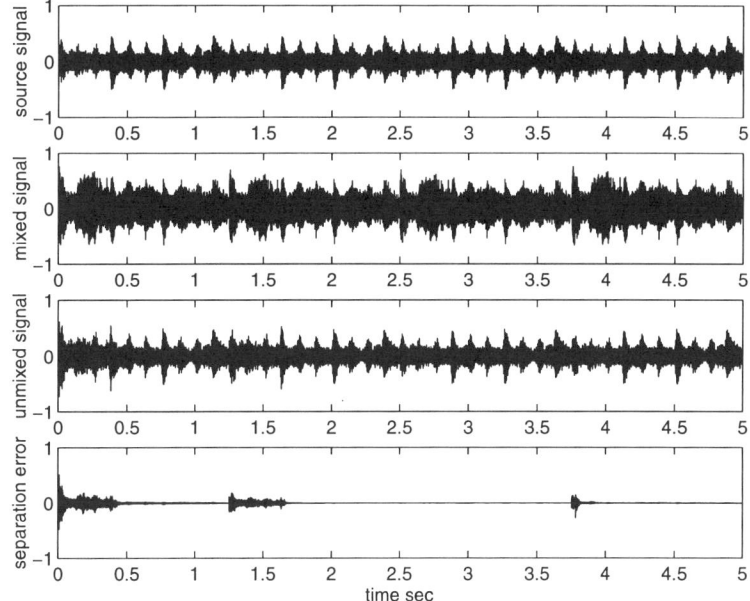

Figure 1: s_t^2 "space music", the mixture signal I_t^2, the unmixed signal u_t^2 and the separation error $u_t^2 - s_t^2$ as functions of time in seconds.

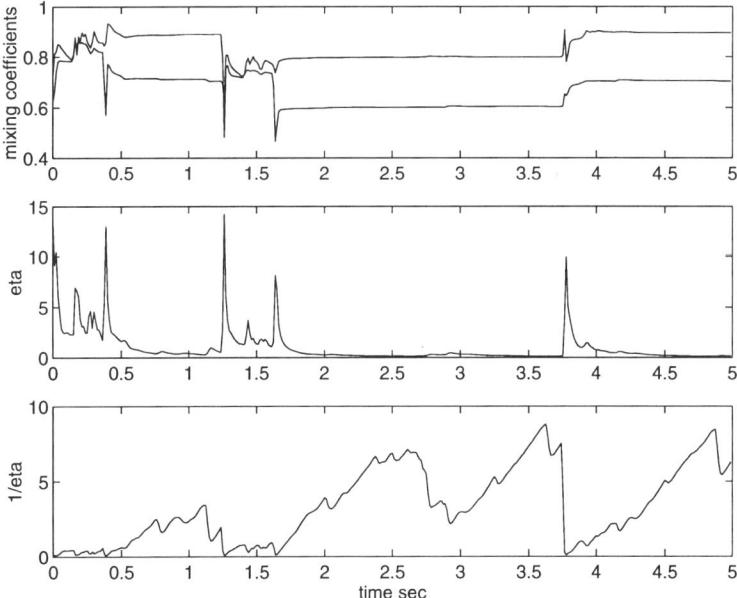

Figure 2: Estimated mixing matrix T_t, evolution of the learning rate η_t and inverse learning rate $1/\eta_t$ over time. Rule switches (t=1.25s, 3.75s) are clearly observed as drastic changes in η_t. Asymptotic $1/t$ scaling in η amounts to a straight line in $1/\eta_t$. Simulation parameters are $\alpha = 0.002, \beta = 20/\max\|\langle r \rangle\|, \epsilon = \delta = 0.01$. $\max\|\langle r \rangle\|$ denotes the maximal value of the past observations.

Using Curvature Information for Fast Stochastic Search

Genevieve B. Orr
Dept of Computer Science
Willamette University
900 State Street
Salem, OR 97301
gorr@willamette.edu

Todd K. Leen
Dept of Computer Science and Engineering
Oregon Graduate Institute of
Science and Technology
P.O.Box 91000, Portland, Oregon 97291-1000
tleen@cse.ogi.edu

Abstract

We present an algorithm for fast stochastic gradient descent that uses a nonlinear adaptive momentum scheme to optimize the late time convergence rate. The algorithm makes effective use of curvature information, requires only $\mathcal{O}(n)$ storage and computation, and delivers convergence rates close to the theoretical optimum. We demonstrate the technique on linear and large nonlinear backprop networks.

Improving Stochastic Search

Learning algorithms that perform gradient descent on a cost function can be formulated in either stochastic (on-line) or batch form. The stochastic version takes the form

$$\omega_{t+1} = \omega_t + \mu_t \, G(\omega_t, x_t) \tag{1}$$

where ω_t is the current weight estimate, μ_t is the learning rate, G is minus the instantaneous gradient estimate, and x_t is the input at time t[1]. One obtains the corresponding batch mode learning rule by taking μ constant and averaging G over all x.

Stochastic learning provides several advantages over batch learning. For large datasets the batch average is expensive to compute. Stochastic learning eliminates the averaging. The stochastic update can be regarded as a noisy estimate of the batch update, and this intrinsic noise can reduce the likelihood of becoming trapped in poor local optima [1, 2].

---
[1]We assume that the inputs are i.i.d. This is achieved by random sampling with replacement from the training data.

The noise must be reduced late in the training to allow weights to converge. After settling within the basin of a local optimum w_*, learning rate annealing allows convergence of the weight error $v \equiv w - w_*$. It is well-known that the expected squared weight error, $E[|v|^2]$ decays at its maximal rate $\propto 1/t$ with the annealing schedule μ_0/t. Furthermore to achieve this rate one must have $\mu_0 > \mu_{crit} = 1/(2\lambda_{min})$ where λ_{min} is the smallest eigenvalue of the Hessian at w_* [3, 4, 5, and references therein]. Finally the *optimal* μ_0, which gives the lowest possible value of $E[|v|^2]$ is $\mu_0 = 1/\lambda$. In multiple dimensions the optimal *learning rate matrix* is $\mu(t) = (1/t)\mathcal{H}^{-1}$, where $\mathcal{H}$ is the Hessian at the local optimum.

Incorporating this curvature information into stochastic learning is difficult for two reasons. First, the Hessian is not available since the point of stochastic learning is *not* to perform averages over the training data. Second, even if the Hessian were available, optimal learning requires its *inverse* – which is prohibitively expensive to compute [2].

The primary result of this paper is that one can achieve an algorithm that behaves optimally, i.e. as if one had incorporated the inverse of the full Hessian, without the storage or computational burden. The algorithm, which requires only $\mathcal{O}(n)$ storage and computation (n = number of weights in the network), uses an adaptive momentum parameter, extending our earlier work [7] to fully non-linear problems. We demonstrate the performance on several large back-prop networks trained with large datasets.

Implementations of stochastic learning typically use a constant learning rate during the early part of training (what Darken and Moody [4] call the search phase) to obtain exponential convergence towards a local optimum, and then switch to annealed learning (called the converge phase). We use Darken and Moody's adaptive search then converge (ASTC) algorithm to determine the point at which to switch to $1/t$ annealing. ASTC was originally conceived as a means to insure $\mu_0 > \mu_{crit}$ during the annealed phase, and we compare its performance with adaptive momentum as well. We also provide a comparison with conjugate gradient optimization.

1 Momentum in Stochastic Gradient Descent

The adaptive momentum algorithm we propose was suggested by earlier work on convergence rates for annealed learning with constant momentum. In this section we summarize the relevant results of that work.

Extending (1) to include momentum leaves the learning rule

$$w_{t+1} = w_t + \mu_t G(w_t, x_t) + \beta (w_t - w_{t-1}) \qquad (2)$$

where β is the momentum parameter constrained so that $0 < \beta < 1$. Analysis of the dynamics of the expected squared weight error $E[|v|^2]$ with $\mu_t = \mu_0/t$ learning rate annealing [7, 8] shows that at late times, learning proceeds as for the algorithm without momentum, but with a scaled or *effective* learning rate

$$\mu_{eff} \equiv \frac{\mu_0}{1-\beta} \qquad (3)$$

This result is consistent with earlier work on momentum learning with small, *constant* μ, where the same result holds [9, 10, 11]

---

[2] Venter [6] proposed a 1-D algorithm for optimizing the convergence rate that estimates the Hessian by time averaging finite differences of the gradient and scaling the learning rate by the inverse. Its extension to multiple dimensions would require $\mathcal{O}(n^2)$ storage and $\mathcal{O}(n^3)$ time for inversion. Both are prohibitive for large models.

If we allow the effective learning rate to be a matrix, then, following our comments in the introduction, the *lowest value* of the misadjustment is achieved when $\mu_{eff} = \mathcal{H}^{-1}$ [7, 8]. Combining this result with (3) suggests that we adopt the heuristic[3]

$$\beta_{opt} = I - \mu_0 \mathcal{H}. \qquad (4)$$

where β_{opt} is a *matrix* of momentum parameters, I is the identity matrix, and μ_0 is a scalar.

We started with a scalar momentum parameter constrained by $0 < \beta < 1$. The equivalent constraint for our matrix β_{opt} is that its eigenvalues lie between 0 and 1. Thus we require $\mu_0 < 1/\lambda_{max}$ where λ_{max} is the largest eigenvalue of $\mathcal{H}$.

A scalar annealed learning rate μ_0/t combined with the momentum parameter β_{opt} ought to provide an effective learning rate asymptotically equal to the optimal learning rate $\mathcal{H}^{-1}$. This rate 1) is achieved *without* ever performing a matrix inversion on $\mathcal{H}$ and 2) is independent of the choice of μ_0, subject to the restriction in the previous paragraph.

We have dispensed with the need to invert the Hessian, and we next dispense with the need to store it. First notice that, unlike its inverse, stochastic estimates of $\mathcal{H}$ are readily available, so we use a stochastic estimate in (4). Secondly according to (2) we do not require the matrix β_{opt}, but rather β_{opt} times the last weight update. For both linear and non-linear networks this dispenses with the $\mathcal{O}(n^2)$ storage requirements. This algorithm, which we refer to as adaptive momentum, does not require explicit knowledge or inversion of the Hessian, and can be implemented very efficiently as is shown in the next section.

2 Implementation

The algorithm we propose is

$$\omega_{t+1} = \omega_t + \mu_t G(\omega_t, x_t) + (I - \mu_0 \hat{\mathcal{H}}_t) \Delta \omega_t \qquad (5)$$

where $\Delta \omega_t \equiv \omega_t - \omega_{t-1}$ and $\hat{\mathcal{H}}_t$ is a stochastic estimate of the Hessian at time t.

We first consider a single layer feedforward linear network. Since the weights connecting the inputs to different outputs are independent of each other we need only discuss the case for one output node. Each output node is then treated identically.

For one output node and N inputs, the Hessian is $\mathcal{H} = \langle xx^T \rangle_x \in \mathbb{R}^{N \times N}$ where $\langle \cdot \rangle_x$ indicates expectation over the inputs x and where x^T is the transpose of x. The *single*-step estimate of the hessian is then just $\hat{\mathcal{H}}_t = x_t x_t^T$. The momentum term becomes

$$(I - \mu_0 \hat{\mathcal{H}}_t) \Delta \omega_t = (I - \mu_0 (x_t x_t^T)) \Delta \omega_t = \Delta \omega_t - \mu_0 x_t (x_t^T \Delta \omega_t). \qquad (6)$$

Written in this way, we note that there is no matrix multiplication, just the vector dot product $x_t^T \Delta \omega_t$ and vector addition that are both $\mathcal{O}(n)$. For M output nodes, the algorithm is then $\mathcal{O}(N_\omega)$ where $N_\omega = NM$ is the total number weights in the network.

For nonlinear networks the problem is somewhat more complicated. To compute $\hat{\mathcal{H}}_t \Delta \omega_t$ we use the algorithm developed by Pearlmutter [12] for computing the product of the hessian times an arbitrary vector.[4] The equivalent of one forward-back

---

[3]We refer to (4) as a heuristic since we have no theoretical results on the dynamics of the squared weight error for learning with this matrix of momentum parameters.

[4]We actually use a slight modification that calculates the *linearized* Hessian times a vector: $Df \otimes Df \Delta \omega_t$ where Df is the Jacobian of the network output (vector) with respect to the weights, and $\otimes$ indicates a tensor product.

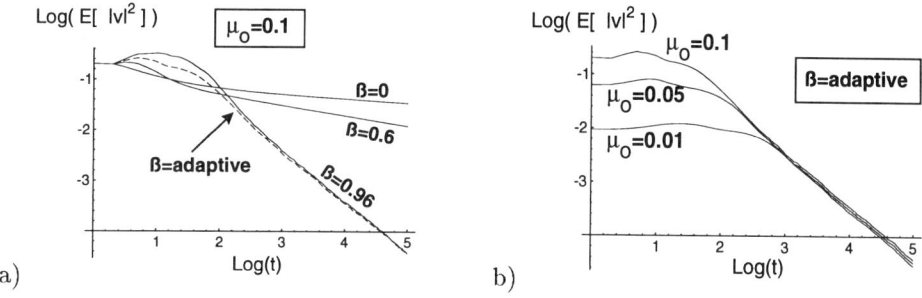

Figure 1: 2-D LMS Simulations: Behavior of $\log(E[|v|^2])$ over an ensemble of 1000 networks with $\lambda_1 = .4$ and $\lambda_1 = 4$, $\sigma_\epsilon^2 = 1$. a) $\mu_0 = 0.1$ with various β. Dashed curve corresponds to adaptive momentum. b) β adaptive for various μ_0.

propagation is required for this calculation. Thus, to compute the entire weight update requires two forward-backward propagations, one for the gradient calculation and one for computing $\hat{\mathcal{H}}_t \Delta w_t$.

The only constraint on μ_0 is that $\mu_0 < 1/\lambda_{max}$. We use the on-line algorithm developed by LeCun, Simard, and Pearlmutter [13] to find the largest eigenvalue prior to the start of training.

3 Examples

In the following two subsections we examine the behavior of annealed learning with adaptive momentum on networks previously trained to a point close to an optimum, where the noise dominates. We look at very simple linear nets, large linear nets, and a large nonlinear net. In section 3.3 we couple adaptive momentum with automatic switching from constant to annealed learning.

3.1 Linear Networks

We begin with a simple 2-D LMS network. Inputs x_t are gaussian distributed with zero mean and the targets d at each timestep t are $d_t = w_*^T x_t + \epsilon_t$ where ϵ_t is zero mean gaussian noise, and w_* is the optimal weight vector. The weight error at time t is just $v \equiv w_t - w_*$.

Figure 1 displays results for both constant and adaptive momentum with averages computed over an ensemble of 1000 networks. Figure (1a) shows the decay of $E[|v|^2]$ for $\mu_0 = 0.1$ and various values of β. As momentum is increased, the convergence rate increases. The optimal *scalar* momentum parameter is $\beta \equiv (1 - \mu_0 \lambda_{min}) = .96$. Adaptive momentum achieves essentially the same rate of convergence *without* prior knowledge of the Hessian.

Figure 1b shows the behavior of $E[|v|^2]$ for various μ_0 when adaptive momentum is used. One can see that after a few hundred iterations the value of $E[|v|^2]$ is independent of μ_0 (in all cases $\mu_0 < 1/\lambda_{max} < \mu_{\text{crit}}$).

Figure 2 shows the behavior of the misadjustment (mean squared error in excess of the optimum) for a 4-D LMS problem with a large condition number $\rho \equiv \lambda_{max}/\lambda_{min} = 10^5$. We compare 3 cases: 1) the *optimal learning rate matrix* $\mu_0 = \mathcal{H}^{-1}$ without momentum, 2) $\mu_0 = .5$ with the *optimal constant momentum matrix* $\beta = I - \mu_0 \mathcal{H}$, and 3) $\mu_0 = .5$ with the *adaptive momentum*. All three cases show similar behavior, showing the efficacy with which the *matrix* momentum

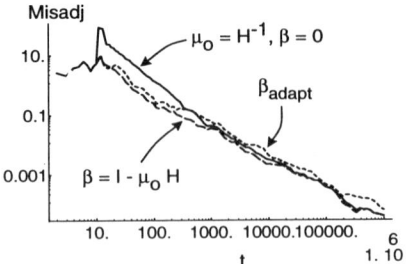
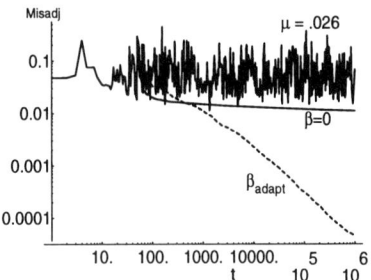

Figure 2: 4-D LMS with $\rho = 10^5$: Plot displays misadjustment. Annealing starts at $t = 10$. For β_{adapt} and $\beta = I - \mu_0 \mathcal{H}$, we use $\mu_0 = .5$. Each curve is an average of 10 runs.

Figure 3: Linear Prediction: $\mu_0 = 0.26$. Curves show constant learning rate, annealing started at $t = 50$ without momentum, and with adaptive momentum.

mocks up the optimal learning rate matrix $\mu_0 = \mathcal{H}^{-1}$, and lending credence to the stochastic estimate of the Hessian used in adaptive momentum.

We next consider a large linear prediction problem (128 inputs, 16 outputs and eigenvalues ranging from 1.06×10^{-5} to 19.98 – condition number $\rho = 1.9 \times 10^6$)[5]. Figure 3 displays the misadjustment for 1) annealed learning with $\beta = \beta_{adapt}$, 2) annealed learning with $\beta = 0$, and 3) constant learning rate (for comparison purposes). As before, we have first trained (not shown completely) at constant learning rate $\mu_0 = .026$ until the MSE and the weight error have leveled out. As can be seen β_{adapt} does much better than annealing without momentum.

3.2 Phoneme Classification

We next use phoneme classification as an example of a large nonlinear problem. The database consists of 9000 phoneme vectors taken from 48 50-second speech monologues. Each input vector consists of 70 PLP coefficients. There are 39 target classes. The architecture was a standard fully connected feedforward network with 71 (includes bias) input nodes, 70 hidden nodes, and 39 output nodes for a total of 7700 weights.

We first trained the network with constant learning rate until the MSE flattened out. At that point we either annealed without momentum, annealed with adaptive momentum, or used ASTC (which attempts to adjust μ_0 to be above μ_{crit} – see next section). When annealing was used without momentum, we found that the noise went away, but the percent of correctly classified phonemes did not improve. Both the adaptive momentum and ASTC resulted in significant increases in the percent correct, however, adaptive momentum was significantly better than ASTC. In the next section, we examine this problem in more detail.

3.3 Switching on Annealing

A complete algorithm must choose an appropriate point to change from constant μ search to annealed learning. We use Moody and Darken's ASTC algorithm [4, 14] to accomplish this. ASTC measures the roughness of trajectories, switching to $1/t$ annealing when the trajectories become very rough – an indication that the noise in the updates is dominating the algorithm's behavior. In an attempt to satisfy

---

[5] Prediction of a 4 × 4 block of image pixels from the surrounding 8 blocks.

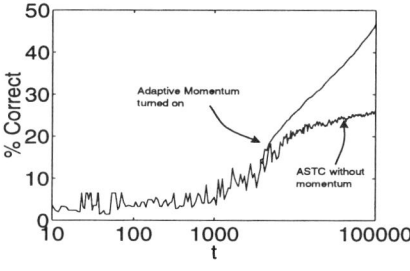 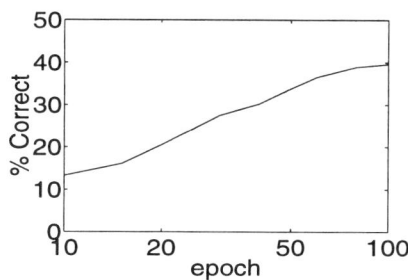

Figure 4: Phoneme Classification: Percent Correct a) ASTC without momentum (bottom curve) and adaptive momentum (top) as function of the number of input presentations. b) Conjugate Gradient Descent – one epoch equals one pass through the data, i.e. 9000 input presentations.

$\mu_0 > \mu_{crit}$, ASTC can also switch back to constant learning when trajectories become too smooth.

We return to the phoneme problem using three different training methods: 1) ASTC without momentum (with switching back and forth between annealed and constant learning), 2) adaptive momentum with annealing turned on when ASTC first suggests the transition (but no subsequent return to constant learning rate), and 3) standard conjugate gradient descent.

Figure 4a compares ASTC (no momentum) with adaptive momentum (using ASTC to turn on annealing). After annealing is turned on, the classification accuracy improves far more quickly with adaptive momentum.

Figure 4b displays the classification performance as a function of epoch using conjugate gradient descent (CGD). After 100 passes through the 9000 example dataset (900,000 presentations), the classification accuracy is 39.6%, or 7% below adaptive momentum's performance at 100,000 presentations. Note also that adaptive momentum is continuing to improve the optimization, while the ASTC and conjugate gradient descent curves have flattened out.

The cpu time used for the optimization was about the same for the CGD and adaptive momentum algorithms. It thus appears that our implementation of adaptive momentum costs about 9 times as much per pattern as CGD. We believe that the performance can be improved. Our complexity analysis [8] predicts a 3:1 cost ratio, rather than 9:1, and optimization comparable to that applied to the CGD code[6] should enhance the run-time performance of CGD.

For this problem, the performance of the two algorityms on the test set (no shown on graph) is not much different (31.7% for CGD versus 33.4% for adaptive momentum. Howver we are concerned here with the efficiency of the optimization, not generalization performance. The latter depends on dataset size and regularization techniques, which can easily be combined with any optimizer.

4 Summary

We have presented an efficient $\mathcal{O}(n)$ stochastic algorithm with few adjustable parameters that achieves fast convergence during the converge phase for both linear and nonlinear problems. It does this by incorporating curvature information without

---

[6]CGD was performed using *nopt* written by Etienne Barnard and made available through the Center for Spoken Language Understanding at the Oregon Graduate Institute.

explicit computation of the Hessian. We also combined it with a method (ASTC) for detecting when to make the transition between search and converge regimes.

Acknowledgments

The authors thank Yann LeCun for his helpful critique. This work was supported by EPRI under grant RP8015-2 and AFOSR under grant FF4962-93-1-0253.

References

[1] Genevieve B. Orr and Todd K. Leen. Weight space probability densities in stochastic learning: II. Transients and basin hopping times. In Giles, Hanson, and Cowan, editors, *Advances in Neural Information Processing Systems, vol. 5*, San Mateo, CA, 1993. Morgan Kaufmann.

[2] William Finnoff. Diffusion approximations for the constant learning rate backpropagation algorithm and resistence to local minima. In Giles, Hanson, and Cowan, editors, *Advances in Neural Information Processing Systems, vol. 5*, San Mateo, CA, 1993. Morgan Kaufmann.

[3] Larry Goldstein. Mean square optimality in the continuous time Robbins Monro procedure. Technical Report DRB-306, Dept. of Mathematics, University of Southern California, LA, 1987.

[4] Christian Darken and John Moody. Towards faster stochastic gradient search. In J.E. Moody, S.J. Hanson, and R.P. Lipmann, editors, *Advances in Neural Information Processing Systems 4*. Morgan Kaufmann Publishers, San Mateo, CA, 1992.

[5] Halbert White. Learning in artificial neural networks: A statistical perspective. *Neural Computation*, 1:425–464, 1989.

[6] J. H. Venter. An extension of the robbins-monro procedure. *Annals of Mathematical Statistics*, 38:117–127, 1967.

[7] Todd K. Leen and Genevieve B. Orr. Optimal stochastic search and adaptive momentum. In J.D. Cowan, G. Tesauro, and J. Alspector, editors, *Advances in Neural Information Processing Systems 6*, San Francisco, CA., 1994. Morgan Kaufmann Publishers.

[8] Genevieve B. Orr. *Dynamics and Algorithms for Stochastic Search*. PhD thesis, Oregon Graduate Institute, 1996.

[9] Mehmet Ali Tugay and Yalcin Tanik. Properties of the momentum LMS algorithm. *Signal Processing*, 18:117–127, 1989.

[10] John J. Shynk and Sumit Roy. Analysis of the momentum LMS algorithm. *IEEE Transactions on Acoustics, Speech, and Signal Processing*, 38(12):2088–2098, 1990.

[11] W. Wiegerinck, A. Komoda, and T. Heskes. Stochastic dynamics of learning with momentum in neural networks. *Journal of Physics A*, 27:4425–4437, 1994.

[12] Barak A. Pearlmutter. Fast exact multiplication by the hessian. *Neural Computation*, 6:147–160, 1994.

[13] Yann LeCun, Patrice Y. Simard, and Barak Pearlmutter. Automatic learning rate maximization by on-line estimation of the hessian's eigenvectors. In Giles, Hanson, and Cowan, editors, *Advances in Neural Information Processing Systems, vol. 5*, San Mateo, CA, 1993. Morgan Kaufmann.

[14] Christian Darken. *Learning Rate Schedules for Stochastic Gradient Algorithms*. PhD thesis, Yale University, 1993.

Maximum Likelihood Blind Source Separation: A Context-Sensitive Generalization of ICA

Barak A. Pearlmutter
Computer Science Dept, FEC 313
University of New Mexico
Albuquerque, NM 87131
bap@cs.unm.edu

Lucas C. Parra
Siemens Corporate Research
755 College Road East
Princeton, NJ 08540-6632
lucas@scr.siemens.com

Abstract

In the square linear blind source separation problem, one must find a linear unmixing operator which can detangle the result $x_i(t)$ of mixing n unknown independent sources $s_i(t)$ through an unknown $n \times n$ mixing matrix $\mathbf{A}(t)$ of causal linear filters: $x_i = \sum_j a_{ij} * s_j$. We cast the problem as one of maximum likelihood density estimation, and in that framework introduce an algorithm that searches for independent components using both temporal and spatial cues. We call the resulting algorithm "Contextual ICA," after the (Bell and Sejnowski 1995) Infomax algorithm, which we show to be a special case of cICA. Because cICA can make use of the temporal structure of its input, it is able separate in a number of situations where standard methods cannot, including sources with low kurtosis, colored Gaussian sources, and sources which have Gaussian histograms.

1 The Blind Source Separation Problem

Consider a set of n indepent sources $s_1(t), \ldots, s_n(t)$. We are given n linearly distorted sensor reading which combine these sources, $x_i = \sum_j a_{ij} s_j$, where a_{ij} is a filter between source j and sensor i, as shown in figure 1a. This can be expressed as

$$x_i(t) = \sum_j \sum_{\tau=0}^{\infty} a_{ji}(\tau) s_j(t-\tau) = \sum_j a_{ji} * s_j$$

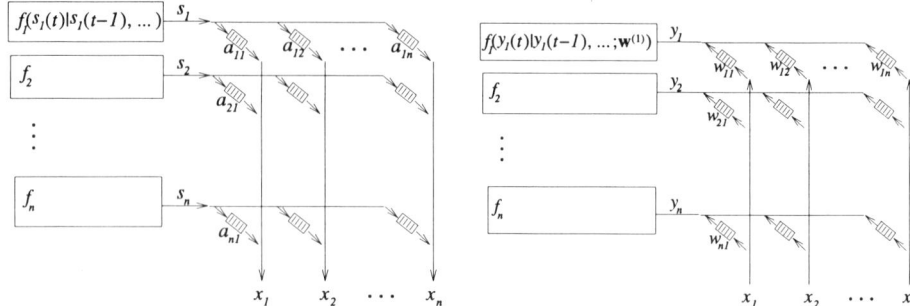

Figure 1: The left diagram shows a generative model of data production for blind source separation problem. The cICA algorithm fits the reparametrized generative model on the right to the data. Since (unless the mixing process is singular) both diagrams give linear maps between the sources and the sensors, they are mathematically equivalent. However, (a) makes the transformation from s to x explicit, while (b) makes the transformation from x to y, the estimated sources, explicit.

or, in matrix notation, $\mathbf{x}(t) = \sum_{\tau=0}^{\infty} A(\tau) \mathbf{s}(t - \tau) = A * \mathbf{s}$. The square linear blind source separation problem is to recover s from x. There is an inherent ambiguity in this, for if we define a new set of sources s' by $s'_i = b_i * s_i$ where $b_i(\tau)$ is some invertable filter, then the various s'_i are independent, and constitute just as good a solution to the problem as the true s_i, since $x_i = \sum_j (a_{ij} * b_j^{-1}) * s'_j$. Similarly the sources could be arbitrarily permuted.

Surprisingly, up to permutation of the sources and linear filtering of the individual sources, the problem is well posed—assuming that the sources s_j are *not* Gaussian. The reason for this is that only with a correct separation are the recovered sources truly statistically independent, and this fact serves as a sufficient constraint. Under the assumptions we have made,[1] and further assuming that the linear transformation A is invertible, we will speak of recovering $y_i(t) = \sum_j w_{ji} * x_j$ where these y_i are a filtered and permuted version of the original unknown s_i. For clarity of exposition, will often refer to "the" solution and refer to the y_i as "the" recovered sources, rather than refering to an point in the manifold of solutions and a set of consistent recovered sources.

2 Maximum likelihood density estimation

Following Pham, Garrat, and Jutten (1992) and Belouchrani and Cardoso (1995), we cast the BSS problem as one of maximum likelihood density estimation. In the MLE framework, one begins with a probabilistic model of the data production process. This probabilistic model is parametrized by a vector of modifiable parameters $\mathbf{w}$, and it therefore assigns a $\mathbf{w}$-dependent probability density $p(\mathbf{x}_0, \mathbf{x}_1, \ldots; \mathbf{w})$ to a each possible dataset $\mathbf{x}_0, \mathbf{x}_1, \ldots$. The task is then to find a $\mathbf{w}$ which maximizes this probability.

There are a number of approaches to performing this maximization. Here we apply

---

[1]Without these assumptions, for instance in the presence of noise, even a linear mixing process leads to an optimal unmixing process that is highly nonlinear.

the stochastic gradient method, in which a single stochastic sample x is chosen from the dataset and $-dlogp(\mathbf{x};\mathbf{w})/d\mathbf{w}$ is used as a stochastic estimate of the gradient of the negative likelihood $\sum_t -dlogp(\mathbf{x}(t);\mathbf{w})/d\mathbf{w}$.

2.1 The likelihood of the data

The model of data production we consider is shown in figure 1a. In that model, the sensor readings x are an explicit linear function of the underlying sources s.

In this model of the data production, there are two stages. In the first stage, the sources independently produce signals. These signals are time-dependent, and the probability density of source i producing value $s_j(t)$ at time t is $f_j(s_j(t)|s_j(t-1), s_j(t-2), \ldots)$. Although this source model could be of almost any differentiable form, we used a generalized autoregressive model described in appendix A. For expository purposes, we can consider using a simple AR model, so we model $s_j(t) = b_j(1)s_j(t-1) + b_j(2)s_j(t-2) + \cdots + b_j(T)s_j(t-T) + r_j$, where r_j is an iid random variable, perhaps with a complicated density.

It is important to distinguish two different, although related, linear filters. When the source models are simple AR models, there are two types of linear convolutions being performed. The first is in the way each source produces its signal: as a linear function of its recent history plus a white driving term, which could be expressed as a moving average model, a convolution with a white driving term, $s_j = b'_j * r_j$. The second is in the way the sources are mixed: linear functions of the output of each source are added, $x_i = \sum_j a_{ji} * s_j = \sum_j (a_{ji} * b'_j) * r_j$. Thus, with AR sources, the source convolution could be folded into the convolutions of the linear mixing process.

If we were to estimate values for the free parameters of this model, *i.e.* to estimate the filters, then the task of recovering the estimated sources from the sensor output would require inverting the linear $A = (a_{ij})$, as well as some technique to guarantee its non-singularity. Such a model is shown in figure 1a. Instead, we parameterize the model by $W = A^{-1}$, an estimated unmixing matrix, as shown in figure 1b. In this indirect representation, s is an explicit linear function of x, and therefore x is only an *implicit* linear function of s. This parameterization of the model is equally convenient for assigning probabilities to samples x, and is therefore suitable for MLE. Its advantage is that because the transformation from sensors to sources is estimated explicitly, the sources can be recovered directly from the data and the estimated model, without invertion. Note that in this inverse parameterization, the estimated mixture process is stored in inverse form. The source-specific models f_i are kept in forward form. Each source-specific model i has a vector of parameters, which we denote $\mathbf{w}^{(i)}$.

We are now in a position to calculate the likelihood of the data. For simplicity we use a matrix W of real numbers rather than FIR filters. Generalizing this derivation to a matrix of filters is straightforward, following the same techniques used by Lambert (1996), Torkkola (1996), A. Bell (1997), but space precludes a derivation here.

The individual generative source models give

$$p(\mathbf{y}(t)|\mathbf{y}(t-1), \mathbf{y}(t-2), \ldots) = \prod_i f_i(y_i(t)|y_i(t-1), y_i(t-2), \ldots) \qquad (1)$$

where the probability densities f_i are each parameterized by vectors $\mathbf{w}^{(i)}$. Using these equations, we would like to express the likelihood of $\mathbf{x}(t)$ in closed form, given the history $\mathbf{x}(t-1), \mathbf{x}(t-2), \ldots$. Since the history is known, we therefore also know the history of the recovered sources, $\mathbf{y}(t-1), \mathbf{y}(t-2), \ldots$. This means that we can calculate the density $p(\mathbf{y}(t)|\mathbf{y}(t-1), \ldots)$. Using this, we can express the density of $\mathbf{x}(t)$ and expand $\widehat{G} = \log \hat{p}(\mathbf{x}; \mathbf{w}) = \log|\mathbf{W}| + \sum_j \log f_j(y_j(t)|y_j(t-1), y_j(t-2), \ldots; \mathbf{w}^{(j)})$ There are two sorts of parameters which we must take the derivative with respect to: the matrix W and the source parameters $\mathbf{w}^{(j)}$. The source parameters do not influence our recovered sources, and therefore have a simple form

$$\frac{d\widehat{G}}{d\mathbf{w}_j} = -\frac{df_j(y_j; \mathbf{w}_j)/d\mathbf{w}_j}{f_j(y_j; \mathbf{w}_j)}$$

However, a change to the matrix W changes $\mathbf{y}$, which introduces a few extra terms. Note that $d\log|W|/dW = W^{-T}$, the transpose inverse. Next, since $\mathbf{y} = W\mathbf{x}$, we see that $dy_j/dW = (0|\mathbf{x}|0)^T$, a matrix of zeros except for the vector $\mathbf{x}$ in row j. Now we note that $df_j(\cdot)/dW$ term has two logical components: the first from the effect of changing W upon $y_j(t)$, and the second from the effect of changing W upon $y_j(t-1), y_j(t-2), \ldots$. (This second is called the "recurrent term", and such terms are frequently dropped for convenience. As shown in figure 3, dropping this term here is not a reasonable approximation.)

$$\frac{df_j(y_j(t)|y_j(t-1), \ldots; \mathbf{w}_j)}{dW} = \frac{\partial f_j}{\partial y_j(t)} \frac{dy_j(t)}{dW} + \sum_\tau \frac{\partial f_j}{\partial y_j(t-\tau)} \frac{dy_j(t-\tau)}{dW}$$

Note that the expression $\frac{dy_j(t-\tau)}{dW}$ is the only matrix, and it is zero except for the jth row, which is $\mathbf{x}(t-\tau)$. The expression $\partial f_j/\partial y_j(t)$ we shall denote $f'_j(\cdot)$, and the expression $\partial f_j \partial y_j(t-\tau)$ we shall denote $f^{(\tau)}(\cdot)$. We then have

$$\frac{d\widehat{G}}{d\mathbf{W}} = -\mathbf{W}^{-T} - \left(\frac{f'_j(\cdot)}{f_j(\cdot)}\right)_j \mathbf{x}(t)^T - \sum_{\tau=1}^{\infty} \left(\frac{f_j^{(\tau)}(\cdot)}{f_j(\cdot)}\right)_j \mathbf{x}(t-\tau)^T \qquad (2)$$

where $(expr(j))_j$ denotes the column vector whose elements are $expr(1), \ldots, expr(n)$.

2.2 The natural gradient

Following Amari, Cichocki, and Yang (1996), we follow a pseudogradient. Instead of using equation 2, we post-multiply this quantity by $W^T W$. Since this is a positive-definite matrix, it does not affect the stochastic gradient convergence criteria, and the resulting quantity simplifies in a fashion that neatly eliminates the costly matrix inversion otherwise required. Convergence is also accelerated.

3 Experiments

We conducted a number of experiments to test the efficacy of the cICA algorithm. The first, shown in figure 2, was a toy problem involving a set of processed deliberately constructed to be difficult for conventional source separation algorithms. In the second experiment, shown in figure 3, ten real sources were digitally mixed with an instantaneous matrix and separation performance was measured as a funciton of varying model complexity parameters. These sources have are available for benchmarking purposes in http://www.cs.unm.edu/~bap/demos.html.

Maximum Likelihood Blind Source Separation: Contextual ICA

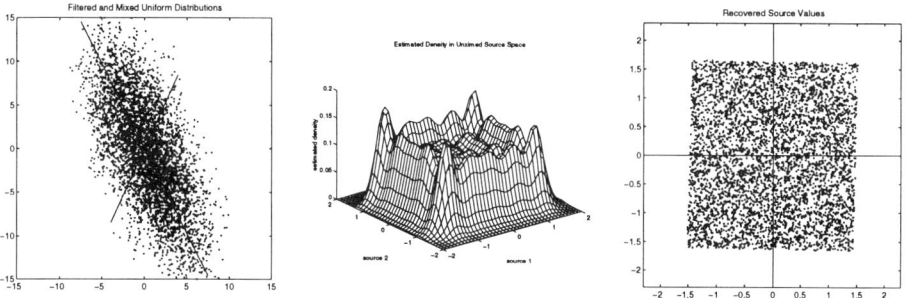

Figure 2: cICA using a history of one time step and a mixture of five logistic densities for each source was applied to 5,000 samples of a mixture of two one-dimensional uniform distributions each filtered by convolution with a decaying exponential of time constant of 99.5. Shown is a scatterplot of the data input to the algorithm, along with the true source axes (left), the estimated residual probability density (center), and a scatterplot of the residuals of the data transformed into the estimated source space coordinates (right). The product of the true mixing matrix and the estimated unmixing matrix deviates from a scaling and permutation matrix by about 3%.

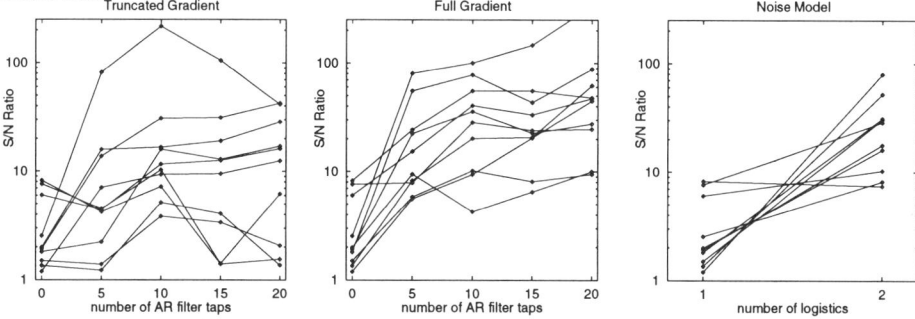

Figure 3: The performance of cICA as a function of model complexity and gradient accuracy. In all simulations, ten five-second clips taken digitally from ten audio CD were digitally mixed through a random ten by ten instantanious mixing matrix. The signal to noise ratio of each original source as expressed in the recovered sources is plotted. In (a) and (b), AR source models with a logistic noise term were used, and the number of taps of the AR model was varied. (This reduces to Bell-Sejnowski infomax when the number of taps is zero.) Is (a), the recurrent term of the gradient was left out, while in (b) the recurrent term was included. Clearly the recurrent term is important. In (c), a degenerate AR model with zero taps was used, but the noise term was a mixture of logistics, and the number of logistics was varied.

4 Discussion

The Infomax algorithm (Baram and Roth 1994) used for source separation (Bell and Sejnowski 1995) is a special case of the above algorithm in which (a) the mixing is not convolutional, so $W(1) = W(2) = \ldots = 0$, and (b) the sources are assumed to be iid, and therefore the distributions $f_i(y(t))$ are not history sensitive. Further, the form of the f_i is restricted to a very special distribution: the logistic density, the derivative of the sigmoidal function $1/(1+\exp-\xi)$. Although ICA has enjoyed a variety of applications (Makeig *et al.* 1996; Bell and Sejnowski 1996b; Baram and Roth 1995; Bell and Sejnowski 1996a), there are a number of sources which it cannot separate. These include all sources with Gaussian histograms (*e.g.* colored gaussian sources, or even speech to run through the right sort of slight nonlinearity), and sources with low kurtosis. As shown in the experiments above, these are of more than theoretical interest.

If we simplify our model to use ordinary AR models for the sources, with gaussian noise terms of fixed variance, it is possible to derive a closed-form expression for W (Hagai Attias, personal communication). It may be that for many sources of practical interest, trading away this model accuracy for speed will be fruitful.

4.1 Weakened assumptions

It seems clear that, in general, separating when there are fewer microphones than sources requires a strong bayesian prior, and even given perfect knowledge of the mixture process and perfect source models, inverting the mixing process will be computationally burdensome. However, when there are more microphones than sources, there is an opportunity to improve the performance of the system in the presence of noise. This seems straightforward to integrate into our framework. Similarly, fast-timescale microphone nonlinearities are easily incorporated into this maximum likelihood approach.

The structure of this problem would seem to lend itself to EM. Certainly the individual source models can be easily optimized using EM, assuming that they themselves are of suitable form.

References

A. Bell, T.-W. L. (1997). Blind separation of delayed and convolved sources. In *Advances in Neural Information Processing Systems 9*. MIT Press. In this volume.

Amari, S., Cichocki, A., and Yang, H. H. (1996). A new learning algorithm for blind signal separation. In *Advances in Neural Information Processing Systems 8*. MIT Press.

Baram, Y. and Roth, Z. (1994). Density Shaping by Neural Networks with Application to Classification, Estimation and Forecasting. Tech. rep. CIS-94-20, Center for Intelligent Systems, Technion, Israel Institute for Technology, Haifa.

Baram, Y. and Roth, Z. (1995). Forecasting by Density Shaping Using Neural Networks. In *Computational Intelligence for Financial Engineering* New York City. IEEE Press.

Bell, A. J. and Sejnowski, T. J. (1995). An Information-Maximization Approach to Blind Separation and Blind Deconvolution. *Neural Computation*, 7(6), 1129–1159.

Bell, A. J. and Sejnowski, T. J. (1996a). The Independent Components of Natural Scenes. *Vision Research*. Submitted.

Bell, A. J. and Sejnowski, T. J. (1996b). Learning the higher-order structure of a natural sound. *Network: Computation in Neural Systems*. In press.

Belouchrani, A. and Cardoso, J.-F. (1995). Maximum likelihood source separation by the expectation-maximization technique: Deterministic and stochastic implementation. In *Proceedings of 1995 International Symposium on Non-Linear Theory and Applications*, pp. 49–53 Las Vegas, NV. In press.

Lambert, R. H. (1996). *Multichannel Blind Deconvolution: FIR Matrix Algebra and Separation of Multipath Mixtures*. Ph.D. thesis, USC.

Makeig, S., Anllo-Vento, L., Jung, T.-P., Bell, A. J., Sejnowski, T. J., and Hillyard, S. A. (1996). Independent component analysis of event-related potentials during selective attention. *Society for Neuroscience Abstracts, 22*.

Pearlmutter, B. A. and Parra, L. C. (1996). A Context-Sensitive Generalization of ICA. In *International Conference on Neural Information Processing* Hong Kong. Springer-Verlag. Url ftp://ftp.cnl.salk.edu/pub/bap/iconip-96-cica.ps.gz.

Pham, D., Garrat, P., and Jutten, C. (1992). Separation of a mixture of independent sources through a maximum likelihood approach. In *European Signal Processing Conference*, pp. 771–774.

Torkkola, K. (1996). Blind separation of convolved sources based on information maximization. In *Neural Networks for Signal Processing VI* Kyoto, Japan. IEEE Press. In press.

A Fixed mixture AR models

The $f_j(u_j; \mathbf{w}_j)$ we used were a mixture AR processes driven by logistic noise terms, as in Pearlmutter and Parra (1996). Each source model was

$$f_j(u_j(t)|u_j(t-1), u_j(t-2), \ldots; \mathbf{w}_j) = \sum_k m_{jk} \, h((u_j(t) - \bar{u}_{jk})/\sigma_{jk})/\sigma_{jk} \quad (3)$$

where σ_{jk} is a scale parameter for logistic density k of source j and is an element of $\mathbf{w}_j$, and the mixing coefficients m_{jk} are elements of $\mathbf{w}_j$ and are constrained by $\sum_k m_{jk} = 1$. The component means $\bar{u}_{jk}$ are taken to be linear functions of the recent values of that source,

$$\bar{u}_{jk} = \sum_{\tau=1} a_{jk}(\tau) \, u_j(t-\tau) + b_{jk} \quad (4)$$

where the linear prediction coefficients $a_{jk}(\tau)$ and bias b_{jk} are elements of $\mathbf{w}_j$. The derivatives of these are straightforward; see Pearlmutter and Parra (1996) for details. One complication is to note that, after each weight update, the mixing coefficients must be normalized, $m_{jk} \leftarrow m_{jk}/\sum_{k'} m_{jk'}$.

A Convergence Proof for the Softassign Quadratic Assignment Algorithm

Anand Rangarajan
Department of Diagnostic Radiology
Yale University School of Medicine
New Haven, CT 06520-8042
e-mail: anand@noodle.med.yale.edu

Alan Yuille
Smith-Kettlewell Eye Institute
2232 Webster Street
San Francisco, CA 94115
e-mail: yuille@skivs.ski.org

Steven Gold
CuraGen Corporation
322 East Main Street
Branford, CT 06405
e-mail: gold-steven@cs.yale.edu

Eric Mjolsness
Dept. of Comp. Sci. and Engg.
Univ. of California San Diego (UCSD)
La Jolla, CA 92093-0114
e-mail: emj@cs.ucsd.edu

Abstract

The softassign quadratic assignment algorithm has recently emerged as an effective strategy for a variety of optimization problems in pattern recognition and combinatorial optimization. While the effectiveness of the algorithm was demonstrated in thousands of simulations, there was no known proof of convergence. Here, we provide a proof of convergence for the most general form of the algorithm.

1 Introduction

Recently, a new neural optimization algorithm has emerged for solving quadratic assignment like problems [4, 2]. Quadratic assignment problems (QAP) are characterized by quadratic objectives with the variables obeying permutation matrix constraints. Problems that roughly fall into this class are TSP, graph partitioning (GP) and graph matching. The new algorithm is based on the softassign procedure which guarantees the satisfaction of the doubly stochastic matrix constraints (resulting from a "neural" style relaxation of the permutation matrix constraints). While the effectiveness of the softassign procedure has been demonstrated via thousands of simulations, no proof of convergence was ever shown.

Here, we show a proof of convergence for the softassign quadratic assignment algorithm. The proof is based on algebraic transformations of the original objective and on the non-negativity of the Kullback-Leibler measure. A central requirement of the proof is that the softassign procedure always returns a doubly stochastic matrix. After providing a general criterion for convergence, we separately analyze the cases of TSP and graph matching.

2 Convergence proof

The deterministic annealing quadratic assignment objective function is written as [4, 5]:

$$E_{\text{qap}}(M, \mu, \nu) = -\frac{1}{2} \sum_{aibj} C_{ai;bj} M_{ai} M_{bj} + \sum_{a} \mu_a (\sum_{i} M_{ai} - 1) + \sum_{i} \nu_i (\sum_{a} M_{ai} - 1)$$
$$- \frac{\gamma}{2} \sum_{ai} M_{ai}^2 + \frac{1}{\beta} \sum_{ai} M_{ai} \log M_{ai} \quad (1)$$

Here M is the desired $N \times N$ permutation matrix. This form of the energy function has a *self-amplification* term with a parameter γ, two Lagrange parameters μ and ν for constraint satisfaction, an $x \log x$ barrier function which ensures positivity of M_{ai} and a deterministic annealing control parameter β. The QAP benefit matrix $C_{ai;bj}$ is preset based on the chosen problem, for example, graph matching or TSP. In the following deterministic annealing pseudocode β_0 and β_f are the initial and final values of β, β_r is the rate at which β is increased, I_B is an iteration cap and ξ is an $N \times N$ matrix of small positive-valued random numbers.

Initialize β to β_0, M_{ai} to $\frac{1}{N} + \xi_{ai}$

Begin A: Deterministic annealing. Do A until $\beta \geq \beta_f$

    Begin B: Relaxation. Do B until all M_{ai} converge or number of iterations $> I_B$
    $Q_{ai} \leftarrow \sum_{bj} C_{ai;bj} M_{bj} + \gamma M_{ai}$
    Begin Softassign:
    $M_{ai} \leftarrow \exp(\beta Q_{ai})$
        Begin C: Sinkhorn. Do C until all M_{ai} converge
        Update M_{ai} by normalizing the rows:
        $M_{ai} \leftarrow \frac{M_{ai}}{\sum_i M_{ai}}$
        Update M_{ai} by normalizing the columns:
        $M_{ai} \leftarrow \frac{M_{ai}}{\sum_a M_{ai}}$
        End C
    End Softassign
    End B

$\beta \leftarrow \beta_r \beta$

End A

The softassign is used for constraint satisfaction. The softassign is based on Sinkhorn's theorem [4] but can be independently derived as coordinate ascent on the Lagrange parameters μ and ν. Sinkhorn's theorem ensures that we obtain a doubly stochastic matrix by the simple process of alternating row and column normalizations. The QAP algorithm above was developed using the graduated assignment heuristic [1] with no proof of convergence until now.

We simplify the objective function in (1) by collecting together all terms quadratic in M_{ai}. This is achieved by defining

$$C_{ai;ai}^{(\gamma)} = C_{ai;ai} + \gamma. \tag{2}$$

Then we use an *algebraic transformation* [3] to transform the quadratic form into a more manageable linear form:

$$-\frac{X^2}{2} \to \min_{\sigma}\left(-X\sigma + \frac{1}{2}\sigma^2\right) \tag{3}$$

Application of the algebraic transformation (in a vectorized form) to the quadratic term in (1) yields:

$$E_{\text{qap}}(M,\sigma,\mu,\nu) = -\sum_{aibj} C_{ai;bj}^{(\gamma)} M_{ai}\sigma_{bj} + \frac{1}{2}\sum_{aibj} C_{ai;bj}^{(\gamma)} \sigma_{ai}\sigma_{bj}$$

$$+ \sum_a \mu_a\left(\sum_i M_{ai} - 1\right) + \sum_i \nu_i\left(\sum_a M_{ai} - 1\right) + \frac{1}{\beta}\sum_{ai} M_{ai} \log M_{ai} \tag{4}$$

Extremizing (4) w.r.t. σ, we get

$$\sum_{bj} C_{ai;bj}^{(\gamma)} M_{bj} = \sum_{bj} C_{ai;bj}^{(\gamma)} \sigma_{bj} \Rightarrow \sigma_{ai} = M_{ai} \tag{5}$$

is a minimum, provided certain conditions hold which we specify below.

In the first part of the proof, we show that setting $\sigma_{ai} = M_{ai}$ is guaranteed to decrease the energy function. Restated, we require that

$$\sigma_{ai} = M_{ai} = \arg\min_{\sigma}\left(-\sum_{aibj} C_{ai;bj}^{(\gamma)} M_{ai}\sigma_{bj} + \frac{1}{2}\sum_{aibj} C_{ai;bj}^{(\gamma)} \sigma_{ai}\sigma_{bj}\right) \tag{6}$$

If $C_{ai;bj}^{(\gamma)}$ is positive definite in the subspace spanned by M, then $\sigma_{ai} = M_{ai}$ is a minimum of the energy function $-\sum_{aibj} C_{ai;bj}^{(\gamma)} M_{ai}\sigma_{bj} + \frac{1}{2}\sum_{aibj} C_{ai;bj}^{(\gamma)} \sigma_{ai}\sigma_{bj}$.

At this juncture, we make a crucial assumption that considerably simplifies the proof. Since this assumption is central, we formally state it here: "*M is always constrained to be a doubly stochastic matrix.*" In other words, for our proof of convergence, we require the softassign algorithm to return a doubly stochastic matrix (as Sinkhorn's theorem guarantees that it will) instead of a matrix which is merely close to being doubly stochastic (based on some reasonable metric). We also require the variable σ to be a doubly stochastic matrix.

Since M is always constrained to be a doubly stochastic matrix, $C_{ai;bj}^{(\gamma)}$ is required to be positive definite in the linear subspace of rows and columns of M summing to one. The value of γ should be set high enough such that $C^{(\gamma)}_{ai;bj}$ does not have any negative eigenvalues in the subspace spanned by the row and column constraints. This is the same requirement imposed in [5] to ensure that we obtain a permutation matrix at zero temperature.

To derive a more explicit criterion for γ, we first define a matrix r in the following manner:

$$r \stackrel{\text{def}}{=} I_N - \frac{1}{N}ee' \tag{7}$$

where I_N is the $N \times N$ identity matrix, e is the vector of all ones and the "prime" indicates a transpose operation. The matrix r has the property that any vector rs with s arbitrary will sum to zero. We would like to extend such a property to cover matrices whose row and column sums stay fixed. To achieve this, take the Kronecker product of r with itself:

$$R \stackrel{\text{def}}{=} r \otimes r \tag{8}$$

R has the property that it will annihilate all row and column sums. Form a vector m by concatenating all the columns of the matrix M together into a single column [$m = \text{vec}(M)$]. Then the vector Rm has the equivalent property of the "rows" and "columns" summing to zero. Hence the matrix $RC^{(\gamma)}R$ (where $C^{(\gamma)}$ is the matrix equivalent of $C^{(\gamma)}_{ai;bj}$) satisfies the criterion of annihilated row and column sums in any quadratic form; $m'RC^{(\gamma)}Rm = (Rm)'C^{(\gamma)}(Rm)$.

The parameter γ is chosen such that all eigenvalues of $RC^{(\gamma)}R$ are positive:

$$\gamma = -\min_\lambda \lambda(RCR) + \epsilon \tag{9}$$

where $\epsilon > 0$ is a small quantity. Note that C is the original QAP benefit matrix whereas $C^{(\gamma)}$ is the augmented matrix of (2). We cannot always efficiently compute the largest negative eigenvalue of the matrix RCR. Since the original $C_{ai;bj}$ is four dimensional, the dimensions of RCR are $N^2 \times N^2$ where N is the number of elements in one set. Fortunately, as we show later, for specific problems it's possible to break up RCR into its constituents thereby making the calculation of the largest negative eigenvalue of RCR more efficient. We return to this point in Section 3.

The second part of the proof involves demonstrating that the softassign operation also decreases the objective in (4). (Note that the two Lagrange parameters μ and ν are specified by the softassign algorithm [4]).

$$M = \text{Softassign}(Q, \beta) \text{ where } Q_{ai} = \sum_{bj} C^{(\gamma)}_{ai;bj} \sigma_{bj} \tag{10}$$

Recall that the step immediately preceding the softassign operation sets $\sigma_{ai} = M_{ai}$. We are therefore justified in referring to σ_{ai} as the "old" value of M_{ai}. For convergence, we have to show that $E_{\text{qap}}(\sigma, \sigma) \geq E_{\text{qap}}(M, \sigma)$ in (4).

Minimizing (4) w.r.t. M_{ai}, we get

$$\frac{1}{\beta} \log M_{ai} = \sum_{bj} C^{(\gamma)}_{ai;bj} \sigma_{bj} - (\mu_a + \nu_i) - \frac{1}{\beta} \tag{11}$$

From (11), we see that

$$\frac{1}{\beta}\sum_{ai} M_{ai}\log M_{ai} = \sum_{aibj} C_{ai;bj}^{(\gamma)} M_{ai}\sigma_{bj} - \sum_{a}\mu_a \sum_i M_{ai} - \sum_i \nu_i \sum_a M_{ai} - \frac{1}{\beta}\sum_{ai} M_{ai} \quad (12)$$

and

$$\frac{1}{\beta}\sum_{ai} \sigma_{ai}\log M_{ai} = \sum_{aibj} C_{ai;bj}^{(\gamma)} \sigma_{ai}\sigma_{bj} - \sum_{a}\mu_a \sum_i \sigma_{ai} - \sum_i \nu_i \sum_a \sigma_{ai} - \frac{1}{\beta}\sum_{ai} \sigma_{ai} \quad (13)$$

From (12) and (13), we get (after some algebraic manipulations)

$$E_{\text{qap}}(\sigma,\sigma) - E_{\text{qap}}(M,\sigma) =$$

$$-\sum_{aibj} C_{ai;bj}^{(\gamma)} \sigma_{ai}\sigma_{bj} - \left(-\sum_{aibj} C_{ai;bj}^{(\gamma)} M_{ai}\sigma_{bj}\right) + \frac{1}{\beta}\sum_{ai} \sigma_{ai}\log\sigma_{ai} - \frac{1}{\beta}\sum_{ai} M_{ai}\log M_{ai}$$

$$= \frac{1}{\beta}\sum_{ai} \sigma_{ai}\log\frac{\sigma_{ai}}{M_{ai}} \geq 0$$

by the non-negativity of the Kullback-Leibler measure. We have shown that the change in energy *after σ has been initialized with the "old" value of M* is non-negative. We require that σ and M are always doubly stochastic via the action of the softassign operation. Consequently, the terms involving the Lagrange parameters μ and ν can be eliminated from the energy function (4). Setting $\sigma = M$ followed by the softassign operation decreases the objective in (4) after excluding the terms involving the Lagrange parameters.

We summarize the essence of the proof to bring out the salient points. At each temperature, the quadratic assignment algorithm executes the following steps until convergence is established.

Step 1: $\sigma_{ai} \leftarrow M_{ai}$.

Step 2:

Step 2a: $Q_{ai} \leftarrow \sum_{bj} C_{ai;bj}^{(\gamma)} \sigma_{bj}$.
Step 2b: $M \leftarrow \text{Softassign}(Q,\beta)$.

Return to Step 1 until convergence.

Our proof is based on demonstrating that an appropriately designed energy function decreases in both Step 1 and Step 2 (at fixed temperature). This energy function is Equation (4) after excluding the Lagrange parameter terms.

Step 1: Energy decreases due to the positive definiteness of $C_{ai;bj}^{(\gamma)}$ in the *linear* subspace spanned by the row and column constraints. γ has to be set high enough for this statement to be true.

Step 2: Energy decreases due to the non-negativity of the Kullback-Leibler measure and due to the restriction that M (and σ) are doubly stochastic.

3 Applications

3.1 Quadratic Assignment

The QAP benefit matrix is chosen such that the softassign algorithm will not converge without adding the γ term in (1). To achieve this, we randomly picked a unit vector v of dimension N^2. The benefit matrix C is set to $-vv'$. Since C has only one negative eigenvalue, the softassign algorithm cannot possibly converge. We ran the softassign algorithm with $\beta_0 = 1$, $\beta_r = 0.9$ and $\gamma = 0$. The energy difference plot on the left in Figure 1 shows the energy never decreasing with increasing iteration number. Next, we followed the recipe for setting γ exactly as in Section 2. After projecting C into the subspace of the row and column constraints, we calculated the largest negative eigenvalue of the matrix RCR which turned out to be -0.8152. We set γ to 0.8162 ($\epsilon = 0.001$) and reran the softassign algorithm. The energy difference plot shows (Figure 1) that the energy never increases. We have shown that a proper choice of γ leads to a convergent algorithm.

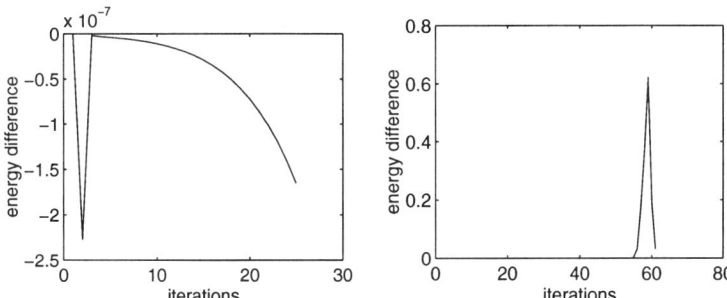

Figure 1: **Energy difference plot.** Left: $\gamma = 0$ and Right: $\gamma = 0.8162$. While the change in energy is always negative when $\gamma = 0$, it is always non-negative when $\gamma = 0.8162$. The negative energy difference (on the left) implies that the energy function increases whereas the non-negative energy difference (on the right) implies that the energy function never increases.

3.2 TSP

The TSP objective function is written as follows: Given N cities,

$$E_{\text{tsp}}(M) = \sum_{aij} d_{ij} M_{ai} M_{(a\oplus 1)j} = \text{trace}(DM'TM) \tag{14}$$

where the symbol $\oplus$ is used to indicate that the summation in (14) is taken modulo N, d_{ij} (D) is the inter-city distance matrix and M is the desired permutation matrix. T is a matrix whose $(i,j)^{\text{th}}$ entry is $\delta_{(i\oplus 1)j}$ (δ_{ij} is the Kronecker delta function). Equation (14) is transformed into the $m'Cm$ form:

$$E_{\text{tsp}}(m) = \text{trace}(m'(D \otimes T)m) \tag{15}$$

where $m = \text{vec}(M)$. We identify our general matrix C with $-2D \otimes T$.

For convergence, we require the largest eigenvalue of

$$-RCR = 2(r \otimes r)(D \otimes T)(r \otimes r) = 2(rDr) \otimes (rTr) = 2(rDr) \otimes (rT) \qquad (16)$$

The eigenvalues of rT are bounded by unity. The eigenvalues of rDr will depend on the form of D. Even in Euclidean TSP the values will depend on whether the Euclidean distance or the distance squared between the cities is used.

3.3 Graph Matching

The graph matching objective function is written as follows: Given N_1 and N_2 node graphs with adjacency matrices G and g respectively,

$$E_{\text{gm}}(M) = -\frac{1}{2} \sum_{aibj} C_{ai;bj} M_{ai} M_{bj} \qquad (17)$$

where $C_{ai;bj} = 1 - 3|G_{ab} - g_{ij}|$ is the compatibility matrix [1]. The matching constraints are somewhat different from TSP due to the presence of slack variables [1]. This makes no difference however to our projection operators. We add an extra row and column of zeros to g and G in order to handle the slack variable case. Now G is $(N_1 + 1) \times (N_1 + 1)$ and g is $(N_2 + 1) \times (N_2 + 1)$. Equation (17) can be readily transformed into the $m'Cm$ form. Our projection apparatus remains unchanged. For convergence, we require the largest negative eigenvalue of RCR.

4 Conclusion

We have derived a convergence proof for the softassign quadratic assignment algorithm and specialized to the cases of TSP and graph matching. An extension to graph partitioning follows along the same lines as graph matching. Central to our proof is the requirement that the QAP matrix M is always doubly stochastic. As a by-product, the convergence proof yields a criterion by which the free self-amplification parameter γ is set. We believe that the combination of good theoretical properties and experimental success of the softassign algorithm make it the technique of choice for quadratic assignment neural optimization.

References

[1] S. Gold and A. Rangarajan. A graduated assignment algorithm for graph matching. *IEEE Transactions on Pattern Analysis and Machine Intelligence*, 18(4):377–388, 1996.

[2] S. Gold and A. Rangarajan. Softassign versus softmax: Benchmarks in combinatorial optimization. In *Advances in Neural Information Processing Systems 8*, pages 626–632. MIT Press, 1996.

[3] E. Mjolsness and C. Garrett. Algebraic transformations of objective functions. *Neural Networks*, 3:651–669, 1990.

[4] A. Rangarajan, S. Gold, and E. Mjolsness. A novel optimizing network architecture with applications. *Neural Computation*, 8(5):1041–1060, 1996.

[5] A. L. Yuille and J. J. Kosowsky. Statistical physics algorithms that converge. *Neural Computation*, 6(3):341–356, May 1994.

Second-order Learning Algorithm with Squared Penalty Term

Kazumi Saito   Ryohei Nakano
NTT Communication Science Laboratories
2 Hikaridai, Seika-cho, Soraku-gun, Kyoto 619-02 Japan
{saito,nakano}@cslab.kecl.ntt.jp

Abstract

This paper compares three penalty terms with respect to the efficiency of supervised learning, by using first- and second-order learning algorithms. Our experiments showed that for a reasonably adequate penalty factor, the combination of the squared penalty term and the second-order learning algorithm drastically improves the convergence performance more than 20 times over the other combinations, at the same time bringing about a better generalization performance.

1 INTRODUCTION

It has been found empirically that adding some penalty term to an objective function in the learning of neural networks can lead to significant improvements in network generalization. Such terms have been proposed on the basis of several viewpoints such as weight-decay (Hinton, 1987), regularization (Poggio & Girosi, 1990), function-smoothing (Bishop, 1995), weight-pruning (Hanson & Pratt, 1989; Ishikawa, 1990), and Bayesian priors (MacKay, 1992; Williams, 1995). Some are calculated by using simple arithmetic operations, while others utilize higher-order derivatives. The most important evaluation criterion for these terms is how the generalization performance improves, but the learning efficiency is also an important criterion in large-scale practical problems; i.e., computationally demanding terms are hardly applicable to such problems. Here, it is naturally conceivable that the effects of penalty terms depend on learning algorithms; thus, we need comparative evaluations.

This paper evaluates the efficiency of first- and second-order learning algorithms with three penalty terms. Section 2 explains the framework of the present learning and shows a second-order algorithm with the penalty terms. Section 3 shows experimental results for a regression problem, a graphical evaluation, and a penalty factor determination using cross-validation.

2 LEARNING WITH PENALTY TERM

2.1 Framework

Let $\{(\mathbf{x}_1, y_1), \cdots, (\mathbf{x}_m, y_m)\}$ be a set of examples, where $\mathbf{x}_t$ denotes an n-dimensional input vector and y_t a target value corresponding to $\mathbf{x}_t$. In a three-layer neural network, let h be the number of hidden units, $\mathbf{w}_j$ ($j = 1, \cdots, h$) be the weight vector between all the input units and the hidden unit j, and $\mathbf{w}_0 = (w_{00}, \cdots, w_{0h})^T$ be the weight vector between all the hidden units and the output unit; w_{j0} means a bias term and x_{t0} is set to 1. Note that $\mathbf{a}^T$ denotes the transposed vector of $\mathbf{a}$. Hereafter, a vector consisting of all parameters, $(\mathbf{w}_0^T, \cdots, \mathbf{w}_h^T)^T$, is simply expressed as $\mathbf{\Phi} = (\phi_1, \cdots, \phi_N)^T$, where $N(= nh + 2h + 1)$ denotes the dimension of $\mathbf{\Phi}$. Then, the training error in the three-layer neural network can be defined as follows:

$$f(\mathbf{\Phi}) = \frac{1}{2} \sum_{t=1}^{m} \left\{ y_t - \left(w_{00} + \sum_{j=1}^{h} w_{0j} \sigma(\mathbf{w}_j^T \mathbf{x}_t) \right) \right\}^2, \quad (1)$$

where $\sigma(u)$ represents a sigmoidal function, $\sigma(u) = 1/(1 + e^{-u})$.

In this paper, we consider the following three penalty terms:

$$\Omega_1(\mathbf{\Phi}) = \frac{1}{2} \sum_{k=1}^{N} \phi_k^2, \quad \Omega_2(\mathbf{\Phi}) = \sum_{k=1}^{N} |\phi_k|, \quad \Omega_3(\mathbf{\Phi}) = \frac{1}{2} \sum_{k=1}^{N} \frac{\phi_k^2}{1 + \phi_k^2}. \quad (2)$$

Hereafter, Ω_1, Ω_2, and Ω_3 are referred to as the squared (Hinton, 1987; MacKay, 1992), absolute (Ishikawa, 1990; Williams, 1995), and normalized (Hanson & Pratt, 1989) penalty terms, respectively. Then, learning with one of these terms can be defined as the problem of minimizing the following objective function

$$F_i(\mathbf{\Phi}) = f(\mathbf{\Phi}) + \mu \Omega_i(\mathbf{\Phi}), \quad (3)$$

where μ is a penalty factor.

2.2 Second-order Algorithm with Penalty Term

In order to minimize the objective function, we employ a newly invented second-order learning algorithm based on a quasi-Newton method, called BPQ (Saito & Nakano, 1997), where the descent direction, $\Delta\mathbf{\Phi}$, is calculated on the basis of a partial BFGS update and a reasonably accurate step-length, λ, is efficiently calculated as the minimal point of a second-order approximation. Here, the partial BFGS update can be directly applied, while the step-length λ is evaluated as follows:

$$\lambda = \frac{-\nabla F_i(\mathbf{\Phi}) \Delta\mathbf{\Phi}^T}{\Delta\mathbf{\Phi}^T \nabla^2 F_i(\mathbf{\Phi}) \Delta\mathbf{\Phi}} = \frac{-\nabla F_i(\mathbf{\Phi}) \Delta\mathbf{\Phi}^T}{\Delta\mathbf{\Phi}^T \nabla^2 f(\mathbf{\Phi}) \Delta\mathbf{\Phi} + \mu \Delta\mathbf{\Phi}^T \nabla^2 \Omega_i(\mathbf{\Phi}) \Delta\mathbf{\Phi}}. \quad (4)$$

The quadratic form for the training error term, $\Delta\Phi^T\nabla^2 f(\Phi)\Delta\Phi$, can be calculated efficiently with the computational complexity of $Nm + O(hm)$ by using the procedure of BPQ, while those for penalty terms are calculated as follows:

$$\Delta\Phi^T\nabla^2\Omega_1(\Phi)\Delta\Phi = \sum_{k=1}^{N}\Delta\phi_k^2, \quad \Delta\Phi^T\nabla^2\Omega_2(\Phi)\Delta\Phi = 0,$$

$$\Delta\Phi^T\nabla^2\Omega_3(\Phi)\Delta\Phi = \sum_{k=1}^{N}\frac{(1-3\phi_k^2)\Delta\phi_k^2}{(1+\phi_k^2)^3}. \tag{5}$$

Note that, in the step-length calculation, $\Delta\Phi^T\nabla^2 F_i(\Phi)\Delta\Phi$ is basically assumed to be positive. The three terms have a different effect on it, i.e., the squared penalty term always adds a non-negative value; the absolute penalty term has no effect; the normalized penalty term may add a negative value if many weight values are larger than $\sqrt{1/3}$. This indicates that the squared penalty term has a desirable feature. Incidentally, we can employ other second-order learning algorithms such as SCG (Møller, 1993) or OSS (Battiti, 1992), but BPQ worked the most efficiently among them in our own experience (Saito & Nakano, 1997).

3 EVALUATION BY EXPERIMENTS

3.1 Regression Problem

By using a regression problem for a function $y = (1 - x + 2x^2)e^{-0.5x^2}$, the learning performance of adding a penalty term was evaluated. In the experiment, a value of x was randomly generated in the range of $[-4, 4]$, and the corresponding value of y was calculated from x; each value of y was corrupted by adding Gaussian noise with a mean of 0 and a standard deviation of 0.2. The total number of training examples was set to 30. The number of hidden units was set to 5, where the initial values for the weights between the input and hidden units were independently generated according to a normal distribution with a mean of 0 and a standard deviation of 1; the initial values for the weights between the hidden and output units were set to 0, but the bias value at the output unit was initially set to the average output value of all training examples. The iteration was terminated when the gradient vector was sufficiently small (i.e., $\|\nabla F_i(\Phi)\|^2/N < 10^{-12}$) or the total processing time exceeded 100 seconds. The penalty factor μ was changed from 2^0 to 2^{-19} by multiplying by 2^{-1}; trials were performed 20 times for each penalty factor.

Figure 1 shows the training examples, the true function, and a function obtained after learning without a penalty term. We can see that such a learning over-fitted the training examples to some degree.

3.2 Evaluation using Second-order Algorithm

By using BPQ, an evaluation was made after adding each penalty term. Figure 2(a) compares the generalization performance, which was evaluated by using the average RMSE (root mean squared error) for a set of 5,000 test examples. The best possible RMSE level is 0.2 because each test example includes the same amount of Gaussian noise given to each training example. For each penalty term, the generalization performance was improved when μ was set adequately, but the normalized

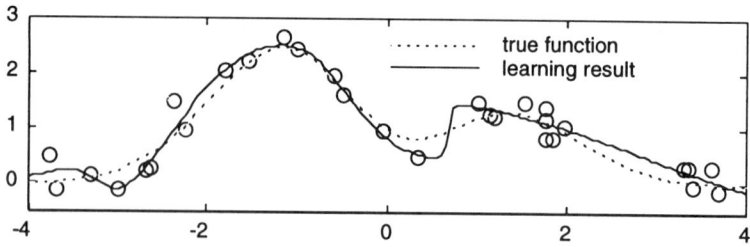

Figure 1: Learning problem

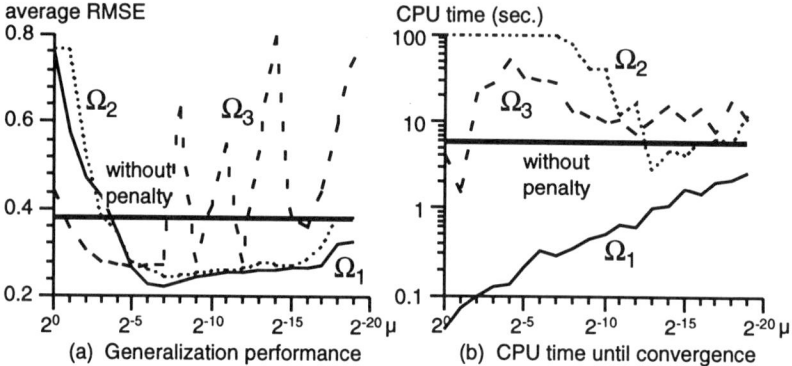

Figure 2: Comparison using second-order algorithm BPQ

penalty term was the most unstable among the three, because it frequently got stuck in undesirable local minima. Figure 2(b) compares the processing time[1] until convergence. In comparison to the learning without a penalty term, the squared penalty term drastically decreased the processing time especially when μ was large, while the absolute penalty term did not converge when μ was large; the normalized penalty term generally required a larger processing time. Thus, only the squared penalty term improved the convergence performance more than 2 ∼ 100 times, keeping a better generalization performance for an adequate penalty factor.

3.3 Evaluation using First-order Algorithm

By using BP, a similar evaluation was made after adding each penalty term. Here, we adopted Silva and Almeida's learning rate adaptation rule (Silva & Almeida, 1990), i.e., learning rate η_k for each weight ϕ_k is adjusted by the signs of two successive gradient values[2]. Figure 3(a) compares the generalization performance and Figure 3(b) compares the processing time until convergence, where the average processing time for the trials without a penalty term is not displayed because all trials did not converge within 100 seconds. For each penalty term, the generalization

---

[1] Our experiments were done on SUN S-4/20 computers.
[2] The increasing and decreasing parameters were set to 1.1 and 1/1.1, respectively, as recommended by (Silva & Almeida, 1990); if the value of the objective function increases, all learning rates are halved until the value decreases.

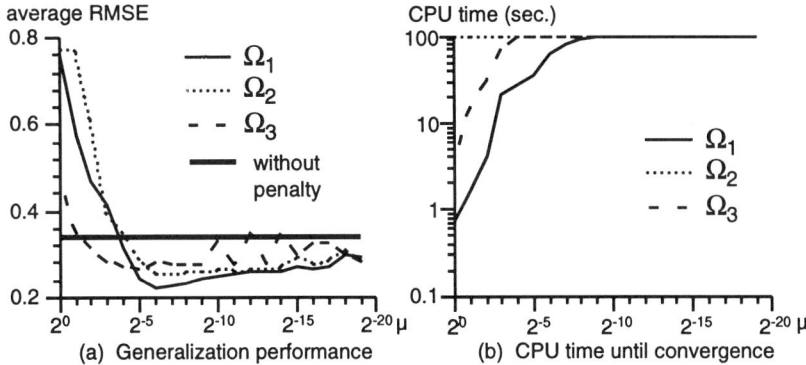

Figure 3: Comparison using first-order algorithm BP

performance was improved when μ was set adequately. Note that BP with the squared penalty term Ω_1 required more processing time than BPQ with Ω_1. As for the normalized penalty term Ω_3, BP with Ω_3 worked more stably than BPQ with Ω_3. Incidentally, the generalization performance of BP without a penalty term was better than that of BPQ without it; we predict that this is because the effect of early stopping (Bishop, 1995) worked for BP. Actually, for the training examples, the average RMSE of BP without a penalty term was 0.138, while that of BPQ without it was 0.133.

3.4 Graphical Evaluation

In order to graphically examine the reasons why the effect of the addition of each penalty term differed, we designed a simple problem; that is, learning a function $y = \sigma(w_1 x) + \sigma(w_2 x)$, where only two weights, w_1 and w_2, are adjustable. In the three-layer network, the input and output layers consist of only one unit, while the hidden layer consists of two units. Note that the weights between the hidden units and the output unit are fixed at 1, there is no bias, and the activation function of hidden units is assumed to be $\sigma(x) = 1/(1 + \exp(-x))$. Each target value y_t was calculated from the corresponding input value $x_t \in \{-0.2, -0.1, 0, 0.1, 0.2\}$ by setting $(w_1, w_2) = (1, 3)$.

Figure 4 shows the learning trajectories on error contour maps with respect to w_1 and w_2 during 100 iterations starting at $(w_1, w_2) = (-1, -3)$, where the penalty factor μ was set to 0.1 or 0.01. Here, BPQ was used as a learning algorithm. The contours for the squared penalty term form ovals, making BPQ learn easily. When $\mu = 0.1$, the contours for the absolute penalty term form an almost square-like shape, and the learning trajectories oscillate near the origin ($w_1 = w_2 = 0$), due to the discontinuity of the gradient function. The contours for the normalized penalty term form a valley, making BPQ's learning more difficult.

3.5 Determining Penalty Factor

In general, for a given problem, we cannot know an adequate penalty factor in advance. Given a limited number of examples, we must find a reasonably adequate

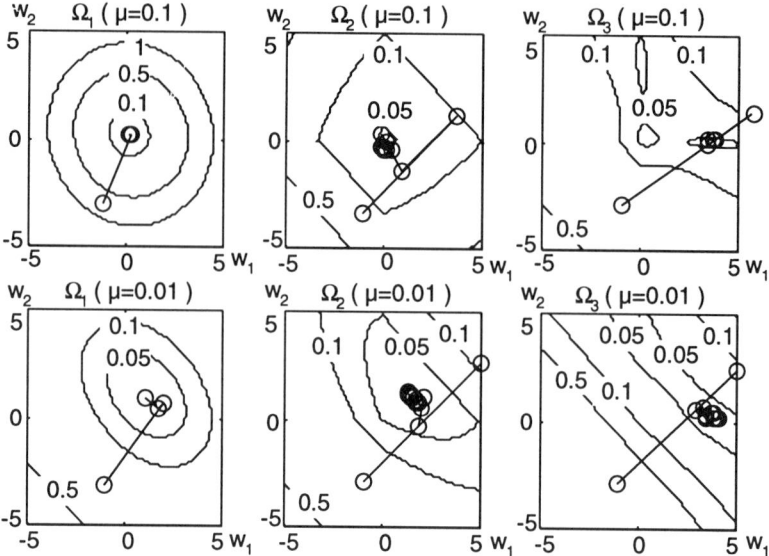

Figure 4: Graphical evaluation

penalty factor. The procedure of cross-validation (Stone, 1978) is adopted for this purpose. Since we knew the combination of the squared penalty term Ω_1 and the second-order algorithm BPQ works very efficiently, we performed experiments using the above regression problem with exactly the same experimental conditions.

Figure 5 shows the experimental results, where the procedure of cross-validation was implemented as a leave-one-out method, and the initial weight values for evaluating the cross-validation error were set as the learning results of the entire training examples. Figure 5(a) compares the average generalization error and the average cross-validation error. Although the cross-validation error was a pessimistic estimator of the generalization error, it showed the same tendency and was minimized at almost the same penalty factor. Figure 5(b) shows the average processing time and its standard deviation; although the processing time includes the cross-validation evaluation, we can see that the learning was performed quite efficiently.

4 CONCLUSION

This paper investigated the efficiency of supervised learning with each of three penalty terms, by using first- and second-order learning algorithms, BP and BPQ. Our experiments showed that for a reasonably adequate penalty factor, the combination of the squared penalty term and the second-order algorithm drastically improves the convergence performance about 20 times over the other combinations, together with an improvement in the generalization performance. In the case of other second-order learning algorithms such as SCG or OSS, similar results are possible because the main difference between BPQ and those other algorithms involves only the learning efficiency. In the future, we plan to do further evaluations using larger-scale problems.

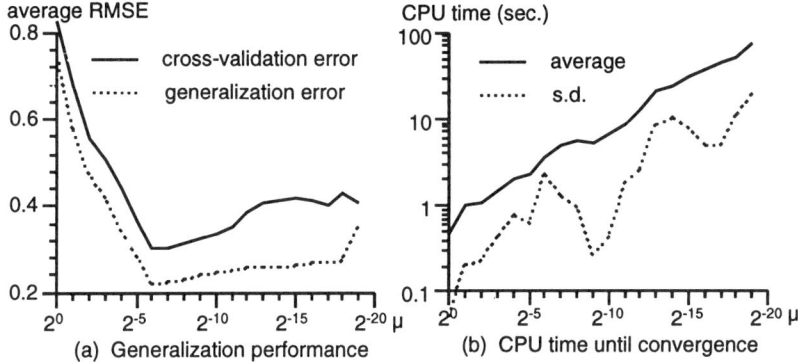

Figure 5: Learning result

References

Battiti, R. (1992) First- and second-order methods for learning between steepest descent and Newton's method. *Neural Computation* **4**(2):141–166.

Bishop, C.M. (1995) *Neural networks for pattern recognition*. Clarendon Press.

Hanson, S.J. & Pratt, L. Y. (1989) Comparing biases for minimal network construction with back-propagation. In D. S. Touretzky (ed.), *Advances in Neural Processing Systems*, Volume 1, pp. 177–185. San Mateo, CA: Morgan Kaufmann.

Hinton, G.E. (1987) Learning translation invariant recognition in massively parallel networks. In J. W. de Bakker, A. J. Nijman and P. C. Treleaven (eds.), *Proceedings PARLE Conference on Parallel Architectures and Languages Europe*, pp. 1–13. Berlin: Springer-Verlag.

Ishikawa, M. (1990) A structural learning algorithm with forgetting of link weight. Tech. Rep. TR-90-7, Electrotechnical Lab. Tsukuba-City, Japan.

MacKay, D.J.C. (1992) Bayesian interpolation. *Neural Computation* **4**(3):415–447.

Møller, M.F. (1993) A scaled conjugate gradient algorithm for fast supervised learning. *Neural Networks* **6**(4):525–533.

Poggio, T. & Girosi, F. (1990) Regularization algorithms for learning that are equivalent to multilayer networks. *Science* **247**:978–982.

Saito, K. & Nakano, R. (1997) Partial BFGS update and efficient step-length calculation for three-layer neural networks. *Neural Computation* **9**(1):239–257 (in press).

Silva, F.M. & Almeida, L.B. (1990) Speeding up backpropagation. In R. Eckmiller (ed.), *Advanced Neural Computers*, pp. 151–160. Amsterdam: North–Holland.

Stone, M. (1978) Cross-validation: A review. *Operationsforsch. Statist. Ser. Statistics B* **9**(1):111–147.

Williams, P.M. (1995) Bayesian regularization and pruning using a Laplace prior. *Neural Computation* **7**(1):117–143.

Monotonicity Hints

Joseph Sill
Computation and Neural Systems program
California Institute of Technology
email: joe@cs.caltech.edu

Yaser S. Abu-Mostafa
EE and CS Deptartments
California Institute of Technology
email: yaser@cs.caltech.edu

Abstract

A hint is any piece of side information about the target function to be learned. We consider the monotonicity hint, which states that the function to be learned is monotonic in some or all of the input variables. The application of monotonicity hints is demonstrated on two real-world problems- a credit card application task, and a problem in medical diagnosis. A measure of the monotonicity error of a candidate function is defined and an objective function for the enforcement of monotonicity is derived from Bayesian principles. We report experimental results which show that using monotonicity hints leads to a statistically significant improvement in performance on both problems.

1 Introduction

Researchers in pattern recognition, statistics, and machine learning often draw a contrast between linear models and nonlinear models such as neural networks. Linear models make very strong assumptions about the function to be modelled, whereas neural networks are said to make no such assumptions and can in principle approximate any smooth function given enough hidden units. Between these two extremes, there exists a frequently neglected middle ground of nonlinear models which incorporate strong prior information and obey powerful constraints.

A monotonic model is one example which might occupy this middle area. Monotonic models would be more flexible than linear models but still highly constrained. Many applications arise in which there is good reason to believe the target function is monotonic in some or all input variables. In screening credit card applicants, for instance, one would expect that the probability of default decreases monotonically with the applicant's salary. It would be very useful, therefore, to be able to constrain a nonlinear model to obey monotonicity.

The general framework for incorporating prior information into learning is well established and is known as learning from hints[1]. A hint is any piece of information about the target function beyond the available input-output examples. Hints can improve the performance of learning models by reducing capacity without sacrificing approximation ability [2]. Invariances in character recognition [3] and symmetries in financial-market forecasting [4] are some of the hints which have proven beneficial in real-world learning applications. This paper describes the first practical applications of monotonicity hints. The method is tested on two noisy real-world problems: a classification task concerned with credit card applications and a regression problem in medical diagnosis.

Section II derives, from Bayesian principles, an appropriate objective function for simultaneously enforcing monotonicity and fitting the data. Section III describes the details and results of the experiments. Section IV analyzes the results and discusses possible future work.

2 Bayesian Interpretation of Objective Function

Let **x** be a vector drawn from the input distribution and **x**' be such that

$$\forall j \neq i, x'_j = x_j \tag{1}$$

$$x'_i > x_i \tag{2}$$

The statement that f is monotonically increasing in input variable x_i means that for all such **x**, **x**' defined as above

$$f(\mathbf{x}') \geq f(\mathbf{x}) \tag{3}$$

Decreasing monotonicity is defined similarly.

We wish to define a single scalar measure of the degree to which a particular candidate function y obeys monotonicity in a set of input variables.

One such natural measure, the one used in the experiments in Section IV, is defined in the following way: Let **x** be an input vector drawn from the input distribution. Let i be the index of an input variable randomly chosen from a uniform distribution over those variables for which monotonicity holds. Define a perturbation distribution, e.g., U[0,1], and draw δx_i from this distribution. Define **x**' such that

$$\forall j \neq i, x'_j = x_j \tag{4}$$

$$x'_i = x_i + sgn(i)\delta x_i \tag{5}$$

where $sgn(i) = 1$ or -1 depending on whether f is monotonically increasing or decreasing in variable i. We will call E_h the *monotonicity error* of y on the input pair $(\mathbf{x}, \mathbf{x}')$.

$$E_h = \begin{cases} 0 & y(\mathbf{x}') \geq y(\mathbf{x}) \\ (y(\mathbf{x}) - y(\mathbf{x}'))^2 & y(\mathbf{x}') < y(\mathbf{x}) \end{cases} \qquad (6)$$

Our measure of y's violation of monotonicity is $\mathcal{E}[E_h]$, where the expectation is taken with respect to random variables $\mathbf{x}$, i and δx_i.

We believe that the best possible approximation to f given the architecture used is probably approximately monotonic. This belief may be quantified in a prior distribution over the candidate functions implementable by the architecture:

$$Pr(y) \propto e^{-\lambda \mathcal{E}[E_h]} \qquad (7)$$

This distribution represents the *a priori* probability density, or likelihood, assigned to a candidate function with a given level of monotonicity error. The probability that a function is the best possible approximation to f decreases exponentially with the increase in monotonicity error. λ is a positive constant which indicates how strong our bias is towards monotonic functions.

In addition to obeying prior information, the model should fit the data well. For classification problems, we take the network output y to represent the probability of class $c = 1$ conditioned on the observation of the input vector (the two possible classes are denoted by 0 and 1). We wish to pick the most probable model given the data. Equivalently, we may choose to maximize $log(P(model|data))$. Using Bayes' Theorem,

$$log(P(model|data)) \propto log(P(data|model)) + log(P(model)) \qquad (8)$$

$$= \sum_{m=1}^{M} c_m log(y_m) + (1 - c_m) log(1 - y_m) - \lambda \mathcal{E}[E_h] \qquad (9)$$

For continuous-output regression problems, we interpret y as the conditional mean of the observed output t given the observation of $\mathbf{x}$. If we assume constant-variance gaussian noise, then by the same reasoning as in the classification case, the objective function to be maximized is :

$$-\sum_{m=1}^{M} (y_m - t_m)^2 - \lambda \mathcal{E}[E_h] \qquad (10)$$

The Bayesian prior leads to a familiar form of objective function, with the first term reflecting the desire to fit the data and a second term penalizing deviation from monotonicity.

3 Experimental Results

Both databases were obtained via FTP from the machine learning database repository maintained by UC-Irvine [1].

The credit card task is to predict whether or not an applicant will default. For each of 690 applicant case histories, the database contains 15 features describing the applicant plus the class label indicating whether or not a default ultimately occurred. The meaning of the features is confidential for proprietary reasons. Only the 6 continuous features were used in the experiments reported here. 24 of the case histories had at least one feature missing. These examples were omitted, leaving 666 which were used in the experiments. The two classes occur with almost equal frequency; the split is 55%-45%.

Intuition suggests that the classification should be monotonic in the features. Although the specific meanings of the continuous features are not known, we assume here that they represent various quantities such as salary, assets, debt, number of years at current job, etc. Common sense dictates that the higher the salary or the lower the debt, the less likely a default is, all else being equal. Monotonicity in all features was therefore asserted.

The motivation in the medical diagnosis problem is to determine the extent to which various blood tests are sensitive to disorders related to excessive drinking. Specifically, the task is to predict the number of drinks a particular patient consumes per day given the results of 5 blood tests. 345 patient histories were collected, each consisting of the 5 test results and the daily number of drinks. The "number of drinks" variable was normalized to have variance 1. This normalization makes the results easier to interpret, since a trivial mean-squared-error performance of 1.0 may be obtained by simply predicting for mean number of drinks for each patient, irrespective of the blood tests.

The justification for monotonicity in this case is based on the idea that an abnormal result for each test is indicative of excessive drinking, where abnormal means either abnormally high or abnormally low.

In all experiments, batch-mode backpropagation with a simple adaptive learning rate scheme was used [2]. Several methods were tested. The performance of a linear perceptron was observed for benchmark purposes. For the experiments using nonlinear methods, a single hidden layer neural network with 6 hidden units and direct input-output connections was used on the credit data; 3 hidden units and direct input-output connections were used for the liver task. The most basic method tested was simply to train the network on all the training data and optimize the objective function as much as possible. Another technique tried was to use a validation set to avoid overfitting. Training for all of the above models was performed by maximizing only the first term in the objective function, i.e., by maximizing the log-likelihood of the data (minimizing training error). Finally, training the networks with the monotonicity constraints was performed, using an approximation to (9)

---

[1] They may be obtained as follows: ftp ics.uci.edu. cd pub/machine-learning-databases. The credit data is in the subdirectory /credit-screening, while the liver data is in the subdirectory /liver-disorders.

[2] If the previous iteration resulted in a increase in likelihood, the learning rate was increased by 3%. If the likelihood decreased, the learning rate was cut in half

and (10).

A leave-k-out procedure was used in order to get statistically significant comparisons of the difference in performance. For each method, the data was randomly partitioned 200 different ways (The split was 550 training, 116 test for the credit data; 270 training and 75 test for the liver data). The results shown in Table 1 are averages over the 200 different partitions.

In the early stopping experiments, the training set was further subdivided into a set (450 for the credit data, 200 for the liver data) used for direct training and a second validation set (100 for the credit data, 70 for the liver data). The classification error on the validation set was monitored over the entire course of training, and the values of the network weights at the point of lowest validation error were chosen as the final values.

The process of training the networks with the monotonicity hints was divided into two stages. Since the meanings of the features were unaccessible, the directions of monotonicity were not known *a priori*. These directions were determined by training a linear perceptron on the training data for 300 iterations and observing the resulting weights. A positive weight was taken to imply increasing monotonicity, while a negative weight meant decreasing monotonicity.

Once the directions of monotonicity were determined, the networks were trained with the monotonicity hints. For the credit problem, an approximation to the theoretical objective function (10) was maximized:

$$\frac{1}{M} \sum_{m=1}^{M} c_m log(y_m) + (1 - c_m)log(1 - y_m) - \frac{\lambda}{N} \sum_{n=1}^{N} E_{h,n} \qquad (13)$$

For the liver problem, objective function (12) was approximated by

$$-\frac{1}{M} \sum_{m=1}^{M} (y_m - t_m)^2 - \frac{\lambda}{N} \sum_{n=1}^{N} E_{h,n} \qquad (14)$$

$E_{h,n}$ represents the network's monotonicity error on a particular pair of input vectors x, x'. Each pair was generated according to the method described in Section II. The input distribution was modelled as a joint gaussian with a covariance matrix estimated from the training data.

For each input variable, 500 pairs of vectors representing monotonicity in that variable were generated. This yielded a total of N=3000 hint example pairs for the credit problem and N=2500 pairs for the liver problem. λ was chosen to be 5000. No optimization of λ was attempted; 5000 was chosen somewhat arbitrarily as simply a high value which would greatly penalize non-monotonicity. Hint generalization, i.e. monotonicity test error, was measured by using 100 pairs of vectors for each variable which were not trained on but whose monotonicity error was calculated. For contrast, monotonicity test error was also monitored for the two-layer networks trained only on the input-output examples. Figure 1 shows test error and monotonicity error vs. training time for the credit data for the networks trained only on the training data (i.e, no hints), averaged over the 200 different data splits.

Monotonicity Hints

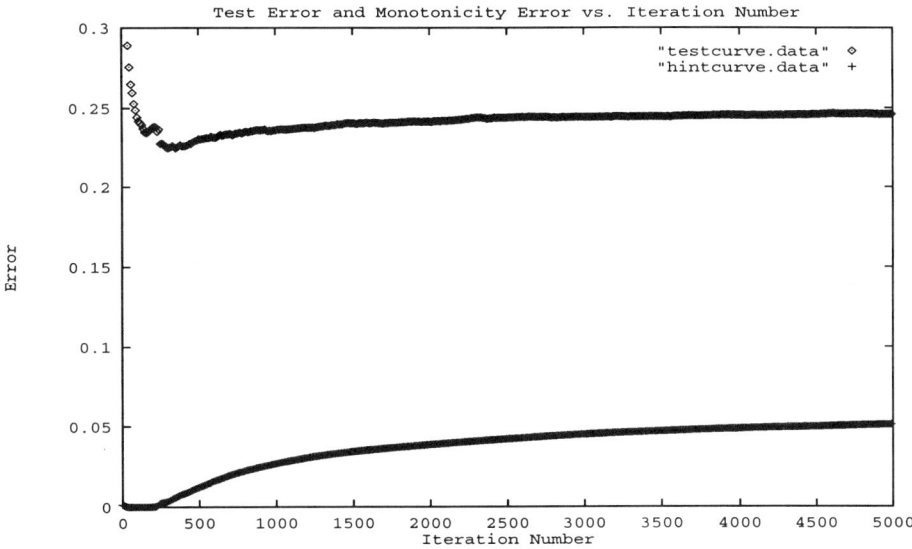

Figure 1: The violation of monotonicity tracks the overfitting occurring during training

The monotonicity error is multiplied by a factor of 10 in the figure to make it more easily visible. The figure indicates a substantial correlation between overfitting and monotonicity error during the course of training. The curves for the liver data look similar but are omitted due to space considerations.

Method	training error	test error	hint test error
Linear	22.7% ± 0.1%	23.7% ± 0.2%	-
6-6-1 net	15.2% ± 0.1%	24.6% ± 0.3%	.005115
6-6-1 net, w/val.	18.8% ± 0.2%	23.4% ± 0.3%	-
6-6-1 net, w/hint	18.7% ± 0.1%	21.8% ± 0.2%	.000020

Table 1: Performance of methods on credit problem

The performance of each method is shown in tables 1 and 2. Without early stopping, the two-layer network overfits and performs worse than a linear model. Even with early stopping, the performance of the linear model and the two-layer network are almost the same; the difference is not statistically significant. This similarity in performance is consistent with the thesis of a monotonic target function. A monotonic classifier may be thought of as a mildly nonlinear generalization of a linear classifier. The two-layer network does have the advantage of being able to implement some of this nonlinearity. However, this advantage is cancelled out (and in other cases could be outweighed) by the overfitting resulting from excessive and unnecessary degrees of freedom. When monotonicity hints are introduced, much of this unnecessary freedom is eliminated, although the network is still allowed to implement monotonic nonlinearities. Accordingly, a modest but clearly statistically significant improvement on the credit problem (nearly 2%) results from the introduction of

Method	training error	test error	hint test error
Linear	.802 ± .005	.873 ± .013	-
5-3-1 net	.640 ± .003	.920 ± .014	.004967
5-3-1 net, w/val.	.758 ± .008	.871 ± .013	-
5-3-1 net, w/hint	.758 ± .003	.830 ± .013	.000002

Table 2: Performance of methods on liver problem

monotonicity hints. Such an improvement could translate into a substantial increase in profit for a bank. Monotonicity hints also significantly improve test error on the liver problem; 4% more of the target variance is explained.

4 Conclusion

This paper has shown that monotonicity hints can significantly improve the performance of a neural network on two noisy real-world tasks. It is worthwhile to note that the beneficial effect of imposing monotonicity does not necessarily imply that the target function is entirely monotonic. If there exist some non-monotonicities in the target function, then monotonicity hints may result in some decrease in the model's ability to implement this function. It may be, though, that this penalty is outweighed by the improved estimation of model parameters due to the decrease in model complexity. Therefore, the use of monotonicity hints probably should be considered in cases where the target function is thought to be at least roughly monotonic and the training examples are limited in number and noisy.

Future work may include the application of monotonicity hints to other real world problems and further investigations into techniques for enforcing the hints.

Acknowledgements

The authors thank Eric Bax, Zehra Cataltepe, Malik Magdon-Ismail, and Xubo Song for many useful discussions.

References

[1] Y. Abu-Mostafa (1990). Learning from Hints in Neural Networks *Journal of Complexity* **6**, 192-198.

[2] Y. Abu-Mostafa (1993) Hints and the VC Dimension *Neural Computation* **4**, 278-288

[3] P. Simard, Y. LeCun & J Denker (1993) Efficient Pattern Recognition Using a New Transformation Distance *NIPS5*, 50-58.

[4] Y. Abu-Mostafa (1995) Financial Market Applications of Learning from Hints *Neural Networks in the Capital Markets*, A. Refenes, ed., 221-232. Wiley, London, UK.

Training Algorithms for Hidden Markov Models Using Entropy Based Distance Functions

Yoram Singer
AT&T Laboratories
600 Mountain Avenue
Murray Hill, NJ 07974
singer@research.att.com

Manfred K. Warmuth
Computer Science Department
University of California
Santa Cruz, CA 95064
manfred@cse.ucsc.edu

Abstract

We present new algorithms for parameter estimation of HMMs. By adapting a framework used for supervised learning, we construct iterative algorithms that maximize the likelihood of the observations while also attempting to stay "close" to the current estimated parameters. We use a bound on the relative entropy between the two HMMs as a distance measure between them. The result is new iterative training algorithms which are similar to the EM (Baum-Welch) algorithm for training HMMs. The proposed algorithms are composed of a step *similar* to the expectation step of Baum-Welch and a new update of the parameters which replaces the maximization (re-estimation) step. The algorithm takes only negligibly more time per iteration and an approximated version uses the same expectation step as Baum-Welch. We evaluate experimentally the new algorithms on synthetic and natural speech pronunciation data. For sparse models, i.e. models with relatively small number of non-zero parameters, the proposed algorithms require significantly fewer iterations.

1 Preliminaries

We use the numbers from 0 to N to name the states of an HMM. State 0 is a special initial state and state N is a special final state. Any state sequence, denoted by s, starts with the initial state but never returns to it and ends in the final state. Observations symbols are also numbers in $\{1, \ldots, M\}$ and observation sequences are denoted by x. A discrete output hidden Markov model (HMM) is parameterized by two matrices $\mathbf{A}$ and $\mathbf{B}$. The first matrix is of dimension $[N, N]$ and $a_{i,j}$ ($0 \leq i \leq N-1, 1 \leq j \leq N$) denotes the probability of moving from state i to state j. The second matrix is of dimension $[N+1, M]$ and $b_{i,k}$ is the probability of outputting symbol k at state i. The set of parameters of an HMM is denoted by $\theta = (\mathbf{A}, \mathbf{B})$. (The initial state distribution vector is represented by the first row of $\mathbf{A}$.)

An HMM is a probabilistic generator of sequences. It starts in the initial state 0. It then iteratively does the following until the final state is reached. If i is the current state then a next state j is chosen according to the transition probabilities out of the current state (row i of matrix $\mathbf{A}$). After arriving at state j a symbol is output according to the output probabilities of that state (row j of matrix $\mathbf{B}$). Let $P(\mathbf{x}, \mathbf{s}|\theta)$ denote the probability (likelihood) that an HMM θ generates the observation sequence $\mathbf{x}$ on the path s starting at state 0 and ending at state N: $P(\mathbf{x}, \mathbf{s} | |\mathbf{s}| = |\mathbf{x}| + 1, s_0 = 0, s_{|\mathbf{s}|} = N, \theta) \stackrel{\text{def}}{=} \prod_{t=1}^{|\mathbf{x}|} a_{s_{t-1}, s_t} b_{s_t, x_t}$. For the sake of brevity we omit the conditions on s and x. Throughout the paper we assume that the HMMs are *absorbing*, that is from every state there is a path to the final state with a non-zero probability. Similar parameter estimation algorithms can be derived for ergodic HMMs. Absorbing HMMs induce a probability over all state-observation sequences, i.e. $\sum_{\mathbf{x},\mathbf{s}} P(\mathbf{x},\mathbf{s}|\theta) = 1$. The likelihood of an observation sequence $\mathbf{x}$ is obtained by summing over all possible hidden paths (state sequences), $P(\mathbf{x}|\theta) = \sum_{\mathbf{s}} P(\mathbf{x},\mathbf{s}|\theta)$. To obtain the likelihood for a set $\mathcal{X}$ of observations we simply multiply the likelihood values for the individual sequences. We seek an HMM θ that maximizes the likelihood for a given set of observations $\mathcal{X}$, or equivalently, maximizes the log-likelihood, $LL(\mathcal{X}|\theta) = \frac{1}{|\mathcal{X}|} \sum_{\mathbf{x} \in \mathcal{X}} \ln P(\mathbf{x}|\theta)$.

To simplify our notation we denote the generic parameter in θ by θ_i, where i ranges from 1 to the total number of parameters in $\mathbf{A}$ and $\mathbf{B}$ (There might be less if some are clamped to zero). We denote the total number of parameters of θ by $\mathcal{I}$ and leave the (fixed) correspondence between the θ_i and the entries of $\mathbf{A}$ and $\mathbf{B}$ unspecified. The indices are naturally partitioned into classes corresponding to the rows of the matrices. We denote by $[i]$ the class of parameters to which θ_i belongs and by $\theta_{[i]}$ the vector of all θ_j s.t. $j \in [i]$. If $j \in [i]$ then both θ_i and θ_j are parameters from the same row of one of the two matrices. Whenever it is clear from the context, we will use $[i]$ to denote both a class of parameters and the row number (i.e. state) associated with the class. We now can rewrite $P(\mathbf{x},\mathbf{s}|\theta)$ as $\prod_{i=1}^{\mathcal{I}} \theta_i^{n_i(\mathbf{x},\mathbf{s})}$, where $n_i(\mathbf{x},\mathbf{s})$ is the number of times parameter i is used along the path $\mathbf{s}$ with observation sequence $\mathbf{x}$. (Note that this value does not depend on the actual parameters θ.) We next compute partial derivatives of the likelihood and the log-likelihood using this notation.

$$\frac{\partial}{\partial \theta_i} P(\mathbf{x},\mathbf{s}|\theta) = \theta_1^{n_1(\mathbf{x},\mathbf{s})} \cdots \theta_{i-1}^{n_{i-1}(\mathbf{x},\mathbf{s})} n_i(\mathbf{x},\mathbf{s}) \theta_i^{n_i(\mathbf{x},\mathbf{s})-1} \cdots \theta_{\mathcal{I}}^{n_{\mathcal{I}}(\mathbf{x},\mathbf{s})}$$

$$= \frac{n_i(\mathbf{x},\mathbf{s})}{\theta_i} \prod_{i=1}^{\mathcal{I}} \theta_i^{n_i(\mathbf{x},\mathbf{s})} = \frac{n_i(\mathbf{x},\mathbf{s})}{\theta_i} P(\mathbf{x},\mathbf{s}|\theta). \quad (1)$$

$$\frac{\partial LL(\mathcal{X}|\theta)}{\partial \theta_i} = \frac{1}{|\mathcal{X}|} \sum_{\mathbf{x} \in \mathcal{X}} \sum_{\mathbf{s}} \frac{\frac{\partial}{\partial \theta_i} P(\mathbf{x},\mathbf{s}|\theta)}{P(\mathbf{x}|\theta)} = \frac{1}{|\mathcal{X}|} \sum_{\mathbf{x} \in \mathcal{X}} \sum_{\mathbf{s}} \frac{n_i(\mathbf{x},\mathbf{s})}{\theta_i} \frac{P(\mathbf{x},\mathbf{s}|\theta)}{P(\mathbf{x}|\theta)}$$

$$= \frac{1}{|\mathcal{X}|} \sum_{\mathbf{x} \in \mathcal{X}} \sum_{\mathbf{s}} \frac{n_i(\mathbf{x},\mathbf{s})}{\theta_i} P(\mathbf{s}|\mathbf{x},\theta) = \frac{\sum_{\mathbf{x} \in \mathcal{X}} \hat{n}_i(\mathbf{x}|\theta)}{|\mathcal{X}|\theta_i}. \quad (2)$$

Here $\hat{n}_i(\mathbf{x}|\theta) \stackrel{\text{def}}{=} \sum_{\mathbf{s}} n_i(\mathbf{x},\mathbf{s}) P(\mathbf{s}|\mathbf{x},\theta)$ is the expected number of occurrences of the transition/output that corresponds to θ_i over all paths that produce $\mathbf{x}$ in θ. These values are calculated in the expectation step of the Expectation-Maximization (EM) training algorithm for HMMs [7], also known as the Baum-Welch [2] or the Forward-Backward algorithm. In the next sections we use the additional following expectations, $\hat{n}_i(\theta) \stackrel{\text{def}}{=} \sum_{\mathbf{x},\mathbf{s}} n_i(\mathbf{x},\mathbf{s}) P(\mathbf{x},\mathbf{s}|\theta)$ and $\hat{n}_{[i]}(\theta) \stackrel{\text{def}}{=} \sum_{j \in [i]} \hat{n}_j(\theta)$. Note that the summation here is over all legal $\mathbf{x}$ and $\mathbf{s}$ of arbitrary length and $\hat{n}_{[i]}(\theta)$ is the expected number of times the state $[i]$ was visited.

2 Entropic distance functions for HMMs

Our training algorithms are based on the following framework of Kivinen and Warmuth for motivating iterative updates [6]. Assume we have already done a number of iterations and our current parameters are θ. Assume further that $\mathcal{X}$ is the set of observations to be processed in the current iteration. In the batch case this set never changes and in the on-line case $\mathcal{X}$ is typically a single observation. The new parameters $\tilde{\theta}$ should stay close to θ, which incorporates all the knowledge obtained in past iterations, but it should also maximize the log-likelihood on the current date set $\mathcal{X}$. Thus, instead of maximizing the log-likelihood we maximize, $U(\tilde{\theta}) = \eta LL(\mathcal{X}|\tilde{\theta}) - d(\tilde{\theta},\theta)$ (see [6, 5] for further motivation).

Training Algorithms for Hidden Markov Models

Here d measures the distance between the old and new parameters and $\eta > 0$ is a trade-off factor. Maximizing $U(\tilde{\theta})$ is usually difficult since both the distance function and the log-likelihood depend on $\tilde{\theta}$. As in [6, 5], we approximate the log-likelihood by a first order Taylor expansion around $\tilde{\theta} = \theta$ and add Lagrange multipliers for the constraints that the parameters of each class must sum to one:

$$U(\tilde{\theta}) \approx \eta \left(LL(\mathcal{X}|\theta) + (\tilde{\theta} - \theta)\nabla_\theta LL(\mathcal{X}|\theta) \right) - d(\tilde{\theta}, \theta) + \sum_{[i]} \lambda_{[i]} \sum_{j \in [i]} \tilde{\theta}_j \ . \quad (3)$$

A commonly used distance function is the relative entropy. To calculate the relative entropy between two HMMs we need to sum over all possible hidden state sequence which leads to the following definition,

$$d_{RE}(\tilde{\theta}, \theta) \stackrel{\text{def}}{=} \sum_{\mathbf{x}} P(\mathbf{x}|\tilde{\theta}) \ln \frac{P(\mathbf{x}|\tilde{\theta})}{P(\mathbf{x}|\theta)} = \sum_{\mathbf{x}} \left(\sum_{\mathbf{s}} P(\mathbf{x},\mathbf{s}|\tilde{\theta}) \right) \ln \frac{\sum_{\mathbf{s}} P(\mathbf{x},\mathbf{s}|\tilde{\theta})}{\sum_{\mathbf{s}} P(\mathbf{x},\mathbf{s}|\theta)}$$

However, the above divergence is very difficult to calculate and is not a convex function in θ. To avoid the computational difficulties and the non-convexity of d_{RE} we upper bound the relative entropy using the *log sum inequality* [3]:

$$d_{RE}(\tilde{\theta}, \theta) \leq \hat{d}_{RE}(\tilde{\theta}, \theta) \stackrel{\text{def}}{=} \sum_{\mathbf{x},\mathbf{s}} P(\mathbf{x},\mathbf{s}|\tilde{\theta}) \ln \frac{P(\mathbf{x},\mathbf{s}|\tilde{\theta})}{P(\mathbf{x},\mathbf{s}|\theta)}$$

$$= \sum_{\mathbf{x},\mathbf{s}} P(\mathbf{x},\mathbf{s}|\tilde{\theta}) \ln \left(\frac{\prod_{i=1}^{\mathcal{I}} \tilde{\theta}_i^{n_i(\mathbf{x},\mathbf{s})}}{\prod_{i=1}^{\mathcal{I}} \theta_i^{n_i(\mathbf{x},\mathbf{s})}} \right) = \sum_{\mathbf{x},\mathbf{s}} P(\mathbf{x},\mathbf{s}|\tilde{\theta}) \sum_{i=1}^{\mathcal{I}} n_i(\mathbf{x},\mathbf{s}) \ln \frac{\tilde{\theta}_i}{\theta_i}$$

$$= \sum_{i=1}^{\mathcal{I}} \ln \frac{\tilde{\theta}_i}{\theta_i} \sum_{\mathbf{x},\mathbf{s}} P(\mathbf{x},\mathbf{s}|\tilde{\theta}) \, n_i(\mathbf{x},\mathbf{s}) = \sum_{i=1}^{\mathcal{I}} \hat{n}_i(\tilde{\theta}) \ln \frac{\tilde{\theta}_i}{\theta_i}$$

Note that for the distance function $\hat{d}_{RE}(\tilde{\theta}, \theta)$ an HMM is viewed as a joint distribution between observation sequences and hidden state sequences. We can further simplify the bound on the relative entropy using the following lemma (proof omitted).

Lemma 1 *For any absorbing HMM, θ, and any parameter $\theta_i \in \theta$, $\hat{n}_i(\theta) = \theta_i \hat{n}_{[i]}(\theta)$.*

This gives the following new formula, $\hat{d}_{RE}(\tilde{\theta}, \theta) = \sum_{i=1}^{\mathcal{I}} \hat{n}_{[i]}(\tilde{\theta}) \left[\tilde{\theta}_i \ln \frac{\tilde{\theta}_i}{\theta_i} \right]$, which can be rewritten as, $\hat{d}_{RE}(\tilde{\theta}, \theta) = \sum_{[i]} \hat{n}_{[i]}(\tilde{\theta}) \, d_{RE}(\tilde{\theta}_{[i]}, \theta_{[i]}) = \sum_{[i]} \hat{n}_{[i]}(\tilde{\theta}) \sum_{j \in [i]} \tilde{\theta}_j \ln \frac{\tilde{\theta}_j}{\theta_j}$.
Equation (3) is still difficult to solve since the variables $\hat{n}_{[i]}(\tilde{\theta})$ depend on the new set of parameters (which are not known). We therefore further approximate $\hat{d}_{RE}(\tilde{\theta}, \theta)$ by the distance function, $\widehat{\hat{d}}_{RE}(\tilde{\theta}, \theta) = \sum_{[i]} \hat{n}_{[i]}(\theta) \sum_{j \in [i]} \tilde{\theta}_j \ln \frac{\tilde{\theta}_j}{\theta_j}$.

3 New Parameter Updates

We now would like to use the distance functions discussed in previous section in $U(\tilde{\theta})$. We first derive our main update using this distance function. This is done by replacing $d(\tilde{\theta}, \theta)$ in $U(\tilde{\theta})$ with $\widehat{\hat{d}}_{RE}(\tilde{\theta}, \theta)$ and setting the derivatives of the resulting $U(\tilde{\theta})$ w.r.t $\tilde{\theta}_i$ to 0. This gives the following set of equations ($i \in \{1, \ldots, \mathcal{I}\}$),

$$\eta \frac{\sum_{\mathbf{x} \in \mathcal{X}} \hat{n}_i(\mathbf{x}|\theta)}{|\mathcal{X}|\theta_i} - \hat{n}_{[i]}(\theta) \left(\ln \frac{\tilde{\theta}_i}{\theta_i} - 1 \right) + \lambda_{[i]} = 0 \ ,$$

which are equivalent to

$$\frac{\eta}{\hat{n}_{[i]}(\theta)} \frac{\sum_{\mathbf{x} \in \mathcal{X}} \hat{n}_i(\mathbf{x}|\theta)}{|\mathcal{X}|\theta_i} - \ln \frac{\tilde{\theta}_i}{\theta_i} + \lambda'_{[i]} = 0 \ .$$

We now can solve for $\tilde{\theta}_i$ and replace $\lambda'_{[i]}$ by a normalization factor which ensures that the sum of the parameters in $[i]$ is 1:

$$\tilde{\theta}_i = \frac{\theta_i \exp\left(\frac{\eta}{\hat{n}_{[i]}(\theta)} \frac{\sum_{\mathbf{x} \in \mathcal{X}} \hat{n}_i(\mathbf{x}|\theta)}{|\mathcal{X}| \theta_i}\right)}{\sum_{j \in [i]} \theta_j \exp\left(\frac{\eta}{\hat{n}_{[i]}(\theta)} \frac{\sum_{\mathbf{x} \in \mathcal{X}} \hat{n}_j(\mathbf{x}|\theta)}{|\mathcal{X}| \theta_j}\right)} . \tag{4}$$

The above re-estimation rule is the *entropic update* for HMMs.[1]

We now derive an alternate to the update of (4). The mixture weights $\hat{n}_{[i]}(\theta)$ (which approximate the original mixture weights $\hat{n}_{[i]}(\tilde{\theta})$ in $\widehat{d}_{RE}(\tilde{\theta}, \theta)$) lead to a state dependent learning rate of $\frac{\eta}{\hat{n}_{[i]}(\theta)}$ for the parameters of class $[i]$. If computation time is limited (see discussion below) then the expectations $\hat{n}_{[i]}(\theta)$ can be approximated by values that are readily available. One possible choice is to use the sample based expectations $\sum_{j \in [i]} \sum_{\mathbf{x} \in \mathcal{X}} \hat{n}_j(\mathbf{x}|\theta)/|\mathcal{X}|$ as an approximation for $\hat{n}_{[i]}(\theta)$. These weights are needed for calculating the gradient and are evaluated in the expectation step of Baum-Welch. Let, $\hat{n}_{[i]}(\mathbf{x}|\theta) \stackrel{\text{def}}{=} \sum_{j \in [i]} \hat{n}_j(\mathbf{x}|\theta)$, then this approximation leads to the following distance function

$$\sum_{[i]} \frac{\sum_{\mathbf{x} \in \mathcal{X}} \hat{n}_{[i]}(\mathbf{x}|\theta)}{|\mathcal{X}|} d_{RE}(\tilde{\theta}_{[i]}, \theta_{[i]}) = \sum_{[i]} \frac{\sum_{\mathbf{x} \in \mathcal{X}} \hat{n}_{[i]}(\mathbf{x}|\theta)}{|\mathcal{X}|} \sum_{j \in [i]} \tilde{\theta}_j \ln \frac{\tilde{\theta}_j}{\theta_j} , \tag{5}$$

which results in an update which we call the *approximated entropic update* for HMMs:

$$\tilde{\theta}_i = \frac{\theta_i \exp\left(\frac{\eta}{\sum_{\mathbf{x} \in \mathcal{X}} \hat{n}_{[i]}(\mathbf{x}|\theta)} \frac{\sum_{\mathbf{x} \in \mathcal{X}} \hat{n}_i(\mathbf{x}|\theta)}{\theta_i}\right)}{\sum_{j \in [i]} \theta_j \exp\left(\frac{\eta}{\sum_{\mathbf{x} \in \mathcal{X}} \hat{n}_{[i]}(\mathbf{x}|\theta)} \frac{\sum_{\mathbf{x} \in \mathcal{X}} \hat{n}_j(\mathbf{x}|\theta)}{\theta_j}\right)} . \tag{6}$$

Given a current set of parameters θ and a learning rate η we obtain a new set of parameters $\tilde{\theta}$ by iteratively evaluating the right-hand-side of the entropic update or the approximated entropic update. We calculate the expectations $\hat{n}_i(\mathbf{x}|\theta)$ as done in the expectation step of Baum-Welch. The weights $\hat{n}_{[i]}(\mathbf{x}|\theta)$ are obtained by averaging $\hat{n}_j(\mathbf{x}|\theta)$ for $j \in [i]$. This lets us evaluate the right-hand-side of the approximated entropic update. The entropic update is slightly more involved and requires an additional calculation of $\hat{n}_{[i]}(\theta)$. (Recall that $\hat{n}_{[i]}(\theta)$ is the expected number of times state $[i]$ is visited, *unconditioned* on the data). To compute these expectations we need to sum over all possible sequences of state-observation pairs. Since the probability of outputting the possible symbols at a given state sum to one, calculating $\hat{n}_{[i]}(\theta)$ reduces to evaluating the probability of reaching a state for each possible time and sequence length. For absorbing HMMs $\hat{n}_{[i]}(\theta)$ can be approximated efficiently using dynamic programming; we compute $\hat{n}_{[i]}(\theta)$ by summing the probabilities of all legal state sequences s of up to length CN (typically $C = 3$ proved to be sufficient to obtain very accurate approximations of $\hat{n}_{[i]}(\theta)$). Therefore, the time complexity of calculating $\hat{n}_{[i]}(\theta)$ depends only on the number of states, regardless of the dimension of the output vector M and the training data $\mathcal{X}$.

---

[1] A subtle improvement is possible over the update (4) by treating the transition probabilities and output probabilities differently. First the transition probabilities are updated based on (4). Then the state probabilities $\hat{n}_{[i]}(\tilde{\theta}) = \hat{n}_{[i]}(\tilde{\mathbf{A}})$ are recomputed based on the new parameters $\tilde{\mathbf{A}}$. This is possible since the state probabilities depend only on the transition probabilities and not on the output probabilities. Finally the output probabilities are updated with (4) where the $\hat{n}_{[i]}(\tilde{\theta})$ are used in place of the $\hat{n}_{[i]}(\theta)$.

4 The relation to EM and convergence properties

We first show that the EM algorithm for HMMs can be derived using our framework. To do so, we approximate the relative entropy by the χ^2 distance (see [3]), $d_{RE}(\tilde{p}, p) \approx d_{\chi^2}(\tilde{p}, p) \stackrel{\text{def}}{=} \frac{1}{2}\sum_i \frac{(\tilde{p}_i - p_i)^2}{p_i}$, and use this distance to approximate $\hat{d}_{RE}(\tilde{\theta}, \theta)$:

$$\hat{d}_{RE}(\tilde{\theta}, \theta) \approx \hat{d}_{\chi^2}(\tilde{\theta}, \theta) \stackrel{\text{def}}{=} \sum_{[i]} \hat{n}_{[i]}(\theta) \; d_{\chi^2}(\tilde{\theta}_{[i]}, \theta_{[i]})$$

$$\approx \sum_{[i]} \hat{n}_{[i]}(\theta) \; d_{\chi^2}(\tilde{\theta}_{[i]}, \theta_{[i]}) \approx \sum_{[i]} \frac{\sum_{\mathbf{x} \in \mathcal{X}} \hat{n}_{[i]}(\mathbf{x}|\theta)}{|\mathcal{X}|} \; d_{\chi^2}(\tilde{\theta}_{[i]}, \theta_{[i]}) \;.$$

Here $d_{\chi^2}(\tilde{\theta}_{[i]}, \theta_{[i]}) = \frac{1}{2}\sum_{j \in [i]} \frac{(\tilde{\theta}_i - \theta_i)^2}{\theta_i}$. By minimizing $U(\tilde{\theta})$ with the last version of the χ^2 distance function and following the same derivation steps as for the approximated entropic update we arrive at what we call the *approximated χ^2 update* for HMMs:

$$\tilde{\theta}_i = (1 - \eta)\theta_i + \eta \sum_{\mathbf{x} \in \mathcal{X}} \hat{n}_i(\mathbf{x}|\theta) \;/\; \sum_{\mathbf{x} \in \mathcal{X}} \hat{n}_{[i]}(\mathbf{x}|\theta) \;. \quad (7)$$

Setting $\eta = 1$ results in the update, $\tilde{\theta}_i = \sum_{\mathbf{x} \in \mathcal{X}} \hat{n}_i(\mathbf{x}|\theta) / \sum_{\mathbf{x} \in \mathcal{X}} \hat{n}_{[i]}(\mathbf{x}|\theta)$, which is the maximization (re-estimation) step of the EM algorithm.

Although omitted from this paper due to the lack of space, it is can be shown that for $\eta \in (0, 1]$ the entropic updates and the χ^2 update improve the likelihood on each iteration. Therefore, these updates belong to the family of Generalized EM (GEM) algorithms which are guaranteed to converge to a local maximum given some additional conditions [4]. Furthermore, using infinitesimal analysis and second order approximation of the likelihood function at the (local) maximum similar to [10], it can be shown that the approximated χ^2 update is a contraction mapping and close to the local maximum there exists a learning rate $\eta > 1$ which results in a faster rate of convergence than when using $\eta = 1$.

5 Experiments with Artificial and Natural Data

In order to test the actual convergence rate of the algorithms and to compare them to Baum-Welch we created synthetic data using HMMs. In our experiments we mainly used sparse models, that is, models with many parameters clamped to zero. Previous work (e.g., [5, 6]) might suggest that the entropic updates will perform better on sparse models. (Indeed, when we used dense models to generate the data, the algorithms showed almost the same performance). The training algorithms, however, were started from a randomly chosen *dense* model. When comparing the algorithms we used the same initial model. Due to different trajectories in parameter space, each algorithm may converge to a different (local) maximum. For the clarity of presentation we show here results for cases where all updates converged to the same maximum, which often occur when the HMM generating the data is sparse and there are enough examples (typically tens of observations per non-zero parameter). We tested both the entropic updates and the χ^2 updates. Learning rates greater than one speed up convergence. The two entropic updates converge almost equally fast on synthetic data generated by an HMM. For natural data the entropic update converges slightly faster than the approximated version. The χ^2 update also benefits from learning rates larger than one. However, the χ^2-update need to be used carefully since it does not necessarily ensure non-negativeness of the new parameters for $\eta > 1$. This problems is exaggerated when the data is not generated by an HMM. We therefore used the entropic updates in our experiments with natural data. In order to have a fair comparison, we did *not* tune the learning rate η and set it to 1.5. In Figure 1 we give a comparison of the entropic update, the approximated entropic update, and Baum-Welch (left figure), using an HMM to generate the random observation sequences, where $N = M = 40$ but only 25% (10 parameters on the average for each transition/observation vector) of the parameters of the

HMM are non-zero. The performance of the entropic update and the approximated entropic update are practically the same and both updates clearly outperform Baum-Welch. One reason the performance of the two entropic updates is the same is that the observations were indeed generated by an HMM. In this case, approximating the expectations $\hat{n}_{[i]}(\theta)$ by the sample based expectations seems reasonable. These results suggest a valuable alternative to using Baum-Welch with a *predetermined* sparse, potentially biased, HMM where a large number of parameters is clamped to zero. Instead, we suggest starting with a full model and let one of the entropic updates find the relevant parameters. This approach is demonstrated on the right part of Figure 1. In this example the data was generated by a sparse HMM with 100 states and 100 possible output symbols. Only 10% of the HMM's parameters were non-zero. Three log-likelihood curves are given in the figure. One is the log-likelihood achieved by Baum-Welch when only those parameters that are non-zero in the HMM generating the data are initialized to random non-zero values. The other two are the log-likelihood of the entropic update and Baum-Welch when *all* the parameters are initialized randomly. The curves show that the entropic update compensates for its inferior initialization in less than 10 iterations (see horizontal line in Figure 1) and from this point on it requires only 23 more iterations to converge compared to Baum-Welch which is given prior knowledge of the non-zero parameters. In contrast, when Baum-Welch is started with a full model then its convergence is much slower than the entropic update.

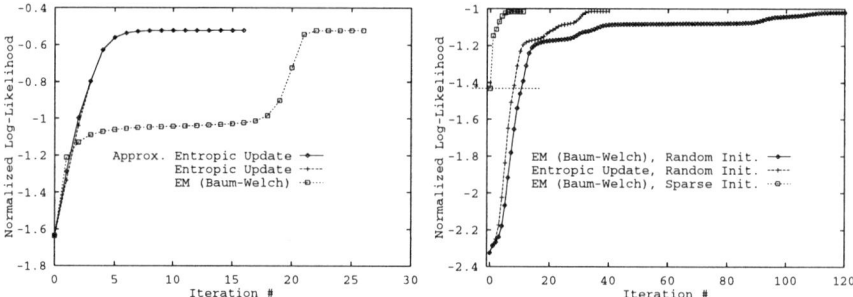

Figure 1: Comparison of the entropic updates and Baum-Welch.

We next tested the updates on speech pronunciation data. In natural speech, a word might be pronounced differently by different speakers. A common practice is to construct a set of stochastic models in order to capture the variability of the possible pronunciations. alternative pronunciations of a given word. This problem was studied previously in [9] using a state merging algorithm for HMMs and in [8] using a subclass of probabilistic finite automata. The purpose of the experiments discussed here is not to compare the above algorithms to the entropic updates but rather compare the entropic updates to Baum-Welch. Nevertheless, the resulting HMM pronunciation models are usually sparse. Typically, only two or three phonemes have a non zero output probability at a given state and the average number of states that in practice can follow a states is about 2. Therefore, the entropic updates may provide a good alternative to the algorithms presented in [8, 9].

We used the TIMIT (Texas Instruments-MIT) database as in [8, 9]. This database contains the acoustic waveforms of continuous speech with phone labels from an alphabet of 62 phones which constitute a temporally aligned phonetic transcription to the uttered words. For the purpose of building pronunciation models, the acoustic data was ignored and we partitioned the phonetic labels according to the words that appeared in the data. The data was filtered and partitioned so that words occurring between 20 and 100 times in the dataset were used for training and evaluation according to the following partition. 75% of the occurrences of each word were used as training data for the learning algorithm and the remaining 25% were used for evaluation. We then built for each word three pronunciation models by training a fully connected HMM whose number of states was set to 1, 1.5 and 1.75 times the longest sample (denoted by N_m). The models were evaluated by calculating the log-likelihood (averaged over 10 different random parameter initializations) of each HMM on the phonetic transcription of each word in the test set. In Table 1 we give the negative log-likelihood achieved on the test data together with the average number of iterations needed for training. Overall the differences in the log-likelihood are small which means that the results should be interpreted with some caution. Nevertheless, the entropic update obtained the highest likelihood on the test data while needing the least number of iterations. The approximated entropic update and Baum-Welch achieve similar results on the test data but the latter requires more iterations. Checking the resulting models reveals one reason why the entropic update achieves higher likelihood values, namely, it does a better job in setting the irrelevant parameters to zero (and it does it faster).

# States	Negative Log-Likelihood			# Iterations		
	$1.0N_m$	$1.5N_m$	$1.75N_m$	$1.0N_m$	$1.5N_m$	$1.75N_m$
Baum-Welch	2448	2388	2425	27.4	36.1	41.1
Approx. EU	2440	2389	2426	25.5	35.0	37.0
Entropic Update	2418	2352	2405	23.1	30.9	32.6

Table 1: Comparison of the entropic updates and Baum-Welch on speech pronunciation data.

6 Conclusions and future research

In this paper we have showed how the framework of Kivinen and Warmuth [6] can be used to derive parameter updates algorithms for HMMs. We view an HMM as a joint distribution between the observation sequences and hidden state sequences and use a bound on relative entropy as a distance between the new and old parameter settings. If we approximate of the relative entropy by the χ^2 distance, replace the exact state expectations by a sample based approximation, and fix the learning rate to one then the framework yields an alternative derivation of the EM algorithm for HMMs. Since the EM update uses sample based estimates of the state expectations it is hard to use it in an on-line setting. In contrast, the on-line versions of our updates can be easily derived using only one observation sequence at a time. Also, there are alternative gradient descent based methods for estimating the parameters of HMMs. Such methods usually employ an exponential parameterization (such as soft-max) of the parameters (see [1]). For the case of learning one set of mixture coefficients an exponential parameterization led to an algorithm with a slower convergence rate compared to algorithms derived using entropic distances [5]. However, it is not clear whether this is still the case for HMMs. Our future goals is to perform a comparative study of the different updates with emphasis on the on-line versions.

Acknowledgments
We thank Anders Krogh for showing us the simple derivative calculations used in this paper and thank Fernando Pereira and Yasubumi Sakakibara for interesting discussions.

References

[1] P. Baldi and Y. Chauvin. Smooth on-line learning algorithms for Hidden Markov Models. *Neural Computation*, 6(2), 1994.

[2] L.E. Baum and T. Petrie. Statistical inference for probabilistic functions of finite state markov chains. *Annals of Mathematical Statisitics*, 37, 1966.

[3] T. Cover and J. Thomas. *Elements of Information Theory*. Wiley, 1991.

[4] A. P. Dempster, N. M. Laird, and D. B. Rubin. Maximum-likelihood from incomplete data via the EM algorithm. *Journal of the Royal Statistical Society*, B39:1–38, 1977.

[5] D. P. Helmbold, R. E. Schapire, Y. Singer, and M. K. Warmuth. A comparison of new and old algorithms for a mixture estimation problem. In *Proceedings of the Eighth Annual Workshop on Computational Learning Theory*, pages 69–78, 1995.

[6] J. Kivinen and M. K. Warmuth. Exponentiated gradient versus gradient descent for linear predictors. *Informationa and Computation*, 1997. To appear.

[7] L.R. Rabiner and B. H. Juang. An introduction to hidden markov models. *IEEE ASSP Magazine*, 3(1):4–16, 1986.

[8] D. Ron, Y. Singer, and N. Tishby. On the learnability and usage of acyclic probabilistic finite automata. In *Proc. of the Eighth Annual Workshop on Computational Learning Theory*, 1995.

[9] A. Stolcke and S. Omohundro. Hidden Markov model induction by Bayesian model merging. In *Advances in Neural Information Processing Systems*, volume 5. Morgan Kaufmann, 1993.

[10] L. Xu and M.I. Jordan. On convergence properties of the EM algorithm for Gaussian mixtures. *Neural Computation*, 8:129–151, 1996.

Clustering Sequences with Hidden Markov Models

Padhraic Smyth
Information and Computer Science
University of California, Irvine
CA 92697-3425
smyth@ics.uci.edu

Abstract

This paper discusses a probabilistic model-based approach to clustering *sequences*, using hidden Markov models (HMMs). The problem can be framed as a generalization of the standard mixture model approach to clustering in feature space. Two primary issues are addressed. First, a novel parameter initialization procedure is proposed, and second, the more difficult problem of determining the number of clusters K, from the data, is investigated. Experimental results indicate that the proposed techniques are useful for revealing hidden cluster structure in data sets of sequences.

1 Introduction

Consider a data set D consisting of N sequences, $D = \{S_1, \ldots, S_N\}$. $S_i = (\underline{x}_1^i, \ldots \underline{x}_{L_i}^i)$ is a sequence of length L_i composed of potentially multivariate feature vectors $\underline{x}$. The problem addressed in this paper is the discovery from data of a natural grouping of the sequences into K clusters. This is analagous to clustering in multivariate feature space which is normally handled by methods such as k-means and Gaussian mixtures. Here, however, one is trying to cluster the sequences S rather than the feature vectors $\underline{x}$. As an example Figure 1 shows four sequences which were generated by two different models (hidden Markov models in this case). The first and third came from a model with "slower" dynamics than the second and fourth (details will be provided later). The sequence clustering problem consists of being given sample sequences such as those in Figure 1 and inferring from the data what the underlying clusters are. This is non-trivial since the sequences can be of different lengths and it is not clear what a meaningful distance metric is for sequence comparison.

The use of hidden Markov models for clustering sequences appears to have first

Clustering Sequences with Hidden Markov Models

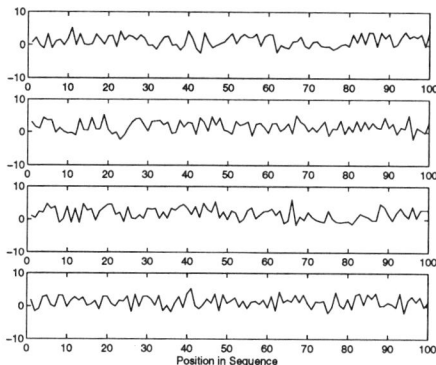

Figure 1: Which sequences came from which hidden Markov model ?

been mentioned in Juang and Rabiner (1985) and subsequently used in the context of discovering subfamilies of protein sequences in Krogh et al. (1994). This present paper contains two new contributions in this context: a cluster-based method for initializing the model parameters and a novel method based on cross-validated likelihood for determining automatically how many clusters to fit to the data.

A natural probabilistic model for this problem is that of a finite mixture model:

$$f_K(S) = \sum_{j=1}^{K} f_j(S|\theta_j) p_j \qquad (1)$$

where S denotes a sequence, p_j is the weight of the jth model, and $f_j(S|\theta_j)$ is the density function for the sequence data S given the component model f_j with parameters θ_j. Here we will assume that the f_j's are HMMs: thus, the θ_j's are the transition matrices, observation density parameters, and initial state probabilities, all for the jth component. $f_j(S|\theta_j)$ can be computed via the forward part of the forward backward procedure. More generally, the component models could be any probabilistic model for S such as linear autoregressive models, graphical models, non-linear networks with probabilistic semantics, and so forth.

It is important to note that the motivation for this problem comes from the goal of building a *descriptive* model for the data, rather than *prediction* per se. For the prediction problem there is a clearly defined metric for performance, namely average prediction error on out-of-sample data (cf. Rabiner et al. (1989) in a speech context with clusters of HMMs and Zeevi, Meir, and Adler (1997) in a general time-series context). In contrast, for descriptive modeling it is not always clear what the appropriate metric for evaluation is, particularly when K, the number of clusters, is unknown. In this paper a density estimation viewpoint is taken and the likelihood of out-of-sample data is used as the measure of the quality of a particular model.

2 An Algorithm for Clustering Sequences into K Clusters

Assume first that K, the number of clusters, is known. Our model is that of a mixture of HMMs as in Equation 1. We can immediately observe that this mixture can itself be viewed as a single "composite" HMM where the transition matrix A of the model is block-diagonal, e.g., if the mixture model consists of two components with transition matrices A_1 and A_2 we can represent the overall mixture model as a single HMM (in effect, a hierarchical mixture) with transition matrix

$$A = \begin{pmatrix} A_1 & 0 \\ 0 & A_2 \end{pmatrix} \qquad (2)$$

where the initial state probabilities are chosen appropriately to reflect the relative weights of the mixture components (the p_k in Equation 1). Intuitively, a sequence is generated from this model by initially randomly choosing either the "upper" matrix A_1 (with probability p_1) or the "lower" matrix with probability A_2 (with probability $1 - p_1$) and then generating data according to the appropriate A_i. There is no "crossover" in this mixture model: data are assumed to come from one component or the other. Given this composite HMM a natural approach is to try to learn the parameters of the model using standard HMM estimation techniques, i.e., some form of initialization followed by Baum-Welch to maximize the likelihood. Note that unlike predictive modelling (where likelihood is not necessarily an appropriate metric to evaluate model quality), likelihood maximization is exactly what we want to do here since we seek a generative (descriptive) model for the data. We will assume throughout that the *number of states per component* is known a priori, i.e., that we are looking for K HMM components each of which has m states and m is known. An obvious extension is to address the problem of learning K and m simultaneously but this is not dealt with here.

2.1 Initialization using Clustering in "Log-Likelihood Space"

Since the EM algorithm is effectively hill-climbing the likelihood surface, the quality of the final solution can depend critically on the initial conditions. Thus, using as much prior information as possible about the problem to seed the initialization is potentially worthwhile. This motivates the following scheme for initializing the A matrix of the composite HMM:

1. Fit N m-state HMMs, one to *each* individual sequence $S_i, 1 \leq i \leq N$. These HMMs can be initialized in a "default" manner: set the transition matrices uniformly and set the means and covariances using the k-means algorithm, where here $k = m$, not to be confused with K, the number of HMM components. For discrete observation alphabets modify accordingly.

2. For each fitted model M_i, evaluate the log-likelihood of each of the N sequences given model M_i, i.e., calculate $L_{ij} = \log L(S_j|M_i), 1 \leq i, j \leq N$.

3. Use the log-likelihood distance matrix to cluster the sequences into K groups (details of the clustering are discussed below).

4. Having pooled the sequences into K groups, fit K HMMs, one to each group, using the default initialization described above. From the K HMMs we get K sets of parameters: initialize the composite HMM in the obvious way, i.e., the $m \times m$ "block-diagonal" component A_j of A (where A is $mK \times mK$) is set to the estimated transition matrix from the jth group and the means and covariances of the jth set of states are set accordingly. Initialize the p_j in Equation 1 to N_j/N where N_j is the number of sequences which belong to cluster j.

After this initialization step is complete, learning proceeds directly on the composite HMM (with matrix A) in the usual Baum-Welch fashion using all of the sequences. The intuition behind this initialization procedure is as follows. The hypothesis is that the data are being generated by K models. Thus, if we fit models to each individual sequence, we will get noisier estimates of the model parameters (than if we used all of the sequences from that cluster) but the parameters should be

Clustering Sequences with Hidden Markov Models

clustered in some manner into K groups about their true values (assuming the model is correct). Clustering directly in parameter space would be inappropriate (how does one define distance?): however, the log-likelihoods are a natural way to define pairwise distances.

Note that step 1 above requires the training of N sequences individually and step 2 requires the evaluation of N^2 distances. For large N this may be impractical. Suitable modifications which train only on a small random sample of the N sequences and randomly sample the distance matrix could help reduce the computational burden, but this is not pursued here. A variety of possible clustering methods can be used in step 3 above. The "symmetrized distance" $L_{ij} = 1/2(L(S_i|M_j)+L(S_j|M_i))$ can be shown to be an appropriate measure of dissimilarity between models M_i and M_j (Juang and Rabiner 1985). For the results described in this paper, hierarchical clustering was used to generate K clusters from the symmetrized distance matrix. The "furthest-neighbor" merging heuristic was used to encourage compact clusters and worked well empirically, although there is no particular reason to use only this method.

We will refer to the above clustering-based initialization followed by Baum-Welch training on the composite model as the "HMM-Clustering" algorithm in the rest of the paper.

2.2 Experimental Results

Consider a deceptively simple "toy" problem. 1-dimensional feature data are generated from a 2-component HMM mixture ($K = 2$), each with 2 states. We have

$$A_1 = \begin{pmatrix} 0.6 & 0.4 \\ 0.4 & 0.6 \end{pmatrix} \qquad A_2 = \begin{pmatrix} 0.4 & 0.6 \\ 0.6 & 0.4 \end{pmatrix}$$

and the observable feature data obey a Gaussian density in each state with $\sigma_1 = \sigma_2 = 1$ for each state in each component, and $\mu_1 = 0, \mu_2 = 3$ for the respective mean of each state of each component. 4 sample sequences are shown in Figure 1. The top, and third from top, sequences are from the "slower" component A_1 (is more likely to stay in any state than switch). In total the training data contain 20 sample sequences from each component of length 200. The problem is non-trivial both because the data have exactly the same marginal statistics if the temporal sequence information is removed and because the Markov dynamics (as governed by A_1 and A_2) are relatively similar for each component making identification somewhat difficult.

The HMM clustering algorithm was applied to these sequences. The symmetrized likelihood distance matrix is shown as a grey-scale image in Figure 2. The axes have been ordered so that the sequences from the same clusters are adjacent. The difference in distances between the two clusters is apparent and the hierarchical clustering algorithm (with $K = 2$) easily separates the two groups. This initial clustering, followed by training separately the two clusters on the set of sequences assigned to each cluster, yielded:

$$\hat{A}_1 = \begin{pmatrix} 0.580 & 0.402 \\ 0.420 & 0.598 \end{pmatrix} \qquad \hat{\mu}_1 = \begin{pmatrix} 2.892 \\ 0.040 \end{pmatrix} \qquad \hat{\sigma}_1 = \begin{pmatrix} 1.353 \\ 1.219 \end{pmatrix}$$

$$\hat{A}_2 = \begin{pmatrix} 0.392 & 0.611 \\ 0.608 & 0.389 \end{pmatrix} \qquad \hat{\mu}_2 = \begin{pmatrix} 2.911 \\ 0.138 \end{pmatrix} \qquad \hat{\sigma}_2 = \begin{pmatrix} 1.239 \\ 1.339 \end{pmatrix}$$

Subsequent training of the composite model on all of the sequences produced more refined parameter estimates, although the basic cluster structure of the model remained the same (i.e., the initial clustering was robust).

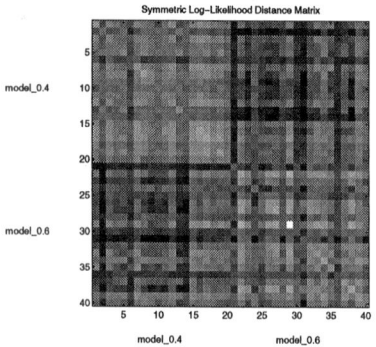

Figure 2: Symmetrized log-likelihood distance matrix.

For comparative purposes two alternative initialization procedures were used to initialize the training of the composite HMM. The "unstructured" method uniformly initializes the A matrix without any knowledge of the fact that the off-block-diagonal terms are zero (this is the "standard" way of fitting a HMM). The "block-uniform" method uniformly initializes the K block-diagonal matrices within A and sets the off-block-diagonal terms to zero. Random initialization gave poorer results overall compared to uniform.

Table 1: Differences in log-likelihood for different initialization methods.

Initialization Method	Maximum Log-Likelihood Value	Mean Log-Likelihood Value	Standard Deviation of Log-Likelihoods
Unstructured	7.6	0.0	1.3
Block-Uniform	44.8	8.1	28.7
HMM-Clustering	55.1	50.4	0.9

The three alternatives were run 20 times on the data above, where for each run the seeds for the k-means component of the initialization were changed. The maximum, mean and standard deviations of log-likelihoods on test data are reported in Table 1 (the log-likelihoods were offset so that the mean unstructured log-likelihood is zero). The unstructured approach is substantially inferior to the others on this problem: this is not surprising since it is not given the block-diagonal structure of the true model. The Block-Uniform method is closer in performance to HMM-Clustering but is still inferior. In particular, its log-likelihood is consistently lower than that of the HMM-Clustering solution and has much greater variability across different initial seeds. The same qualitative behavior was observed across a variety of simulated data sets (results are not presented here due to lack of space).

3 Learning K, the Number of Sequence Components

3.1 Background

Above we have assumed that K, the number of clusters, is known. The problem of learning the "best" value for K in a mixture model is a difficult one in practice even for the simpler (non-dynamic) case of Gaussian mixtures. There has been considerable prior work on this problem. Penalized likelihood approaches are popular, where the log-likelihood on the training data is penalized by the subtraction of a complexity term. A more general approach is the full Bayesian solution where the posterior probability of each value of K is calculated given the data, priors on the mixture parameters, and priors on K itself. A potential difficulty here is the the computational complexity of integrating over the parameter space to get the posterior probabilities on K. Various analytic and sampling approximations are used in practice. In theory, the full Bayesian approach is fully optimal and probably the most useful. However, in practice the ideal Bayesian solution must be approximated and it is not always obvious how the approximation affects the quality of the final answer. Thus, there is room to explore alternative methods for determining K.

3.2 A Monte-Carlo Cross-Validation Approach

Imagine that we had a large test data set D^{test} which is not used in fitting any of the models. Let $L_K(D^{\text{test}})$ be the log-likelihood where the model with K components is fit to the training data D but the likelihood is evaluated on D^{test}. We can view this likelihood as a function of the "parameter" K, keeping all other parameters and D fixed. Intuitively, this "test likelihood" should be a much more useful estimator than the training data likelihood for comparing mixture models with different numbers of components. In fact, the test likelihood can be shown to be an unbiased estimator of the Kullback-Leibler distance between the true (but unknown) density and the model. Thus, maximizing out-of-sample likelihood over K is a reasonable model selection strategy. In practice, one does not usually want to reserve a large fraction of one's data for test purposes: thus, a cross-validated estimate of log-likelihood can be used instead.

In Smyth (1996) it was found that for standard multivariate Gaussian mixture modeling, the standard v-fold cross-validation techniques (with say $v = 10$) performed poorly in terms of selecting the correct model on simulated data. Instead Monte-Carlo cross-validation (Shao, 1993) was found to be much more stable: the data are partitioned into a fraction β for testing and $1 - \beta$ for training, and this procedure is repeated M times where the partitions are randomly chosen on each run (i.e., need not be disjoint). In choosing β one must tradeoff the variability of the performance estimate on the test set with the variability in model fitting on the training set. In general, as the total amount of data increases relative to the model complexity, the optimal β becomes larger. For the mixture clustering problem $\beta = 0.5$ was found empirically to work well (Smyth, 1996) and is used in the results reported here.

3.3 Experimental Results

The same data set as described earlier was used where now K is not known a priori. The 40 sequences were randomly partitioned 20 times into training and test cross-validation sets. For each train/test partition the value of K was varied between 1 and 6, and for each value of K the HMM-Clustering algorithm was fit to the training data, and the likelihood was evaluated on the test data. The mean cross-validated likelihood was evaluated as the average over the 20 runs. Assuming the models are equally likely a priori, one can generate an approximate posterior distribution $p(K|D)$ by Bayes rule: these posterior probabilities are shown in Figure 3. The cross-validation procedure produces a clear peak at $K = 2$ which is the true model size. In general, the cross-validation method has been tested on a variety of other simulated sequence clustering data sets and typically converges as a function of the number of training samples to the true value of K (from below). As the number of

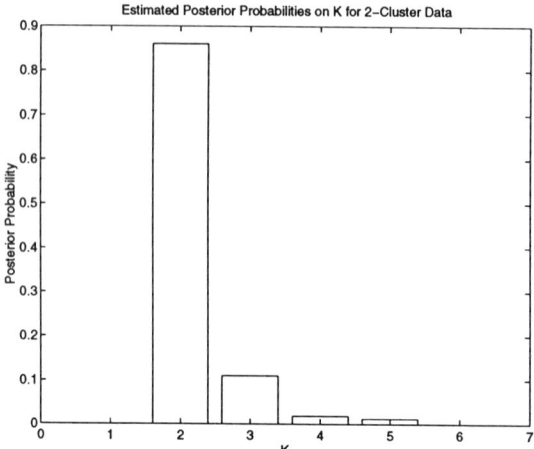

Figure 3: Posterior probability distribution on K as estimated by cross-validation.

data points grow, the posterior distribution on K narrows about the true value of K. If the data were not generated by the assumed form of the model, the posterior distribution on K will tend to be peaked about the model size which is closest (in K-L distance) to the true model. Results in the context of Gaussian mixture clustering(Smyth 1996) have shown that the Monte Carlo cross-validation technique performs as well as the better Bayesian approximation methods and is more robust then penalized likelihood methods such as BIC.

In conclusion, we have shown that model-based probabilistic clustering can be generalized from feature-space clustering to sequence clustering. Log-likelihood between sequence models and sequences was found useful for detecting cluster structure and cross-validated likelihood was shown to be able to detect the true number of clusters.

References

Baldi, P. and Y. Chauvin, 'Hierarchical hybrid modeling, HMM/NN architectures, and protein applications,' *Neural Computation*, 8(6), 1541–1565, 1996.

Krogh, A. et al., 'Hidden Markov models in computational biology: applications to protein modeling,' it J. Mol. Bio., 235:1501–1531, 1994.

Juang, B. H., and L. R. Rabiner, 'A probabilistic distance measure for hidden Markov models,' *AT&T Technical Journal*, vol.64, no.2, February 1985.

Rabiner, L. R., C. H. Lee, B. H. Juang, and J. G. Wilpon, 'HMM clustering for connected word recognition,' *Proc. Int. Conf. Ac. Speech. Sig. Proc*, IEEE Press, 405–408, 1989.

Shao, J., 'Linear model selection by cross-validation,' *J. Am. Stat. Assoc.*, 88(422), 486–494, 1993.

Smyth, P., 'Clustering using Monte-Carlo cross validation,' in *Proceedings of the Second International Conference on Knowledge Discovery and Data Mining*, Menlo Park, CA: AAAI Press, pp.126–133, 1996.

Zeevi, A. J., Meir, R., Adler, R., 'Time series prediction using mixtures of experts,' in this volume, 1997.

Fast Network Pruning and Feature Extraction Using the Unit-OBS Algorithm

Achim Stahlberger and Martin Riedmiller
Institut für Logik, Komplexität und Deduktionssysteme
Universität Karlsruhe, 76128 Karlsruhe, Germany
email: stahlb@ira.uka.de, riedml@ira.uka.de

Abstract

The algorithm described in this article is based on the OBS algorithm by Hassibi, Stork and Wolff ([1] and [2]). The main disadvantage of OBS is its high complexity. OBS needs to calculate the inverse Hessian to delete only one weight (thus needing much time to prune a big net). A better algorithm should use this matrix to remove more than only one weight, because calculating the inverse Hessian takes the most time in the OBS algorithm.

The algorithm, called Unit–OBS, described in this article is a method to overcome this disadvantage. This algorithm only needs to calculate the inverse Hessian once to remove one whole unit thus drastically reducing the time to prune big nets.

A further advantage of Unit–OBS is that it can be used to do a feature extraction on the input data. This can be helpful on the understanding of unknown problems.

1 Introduction

This article is based on the technical report [3] about speeding up the OBS algorithm. The main target of this work was to reduce the high complexity $O(n^2 p)$ of the OBS algorithm in order to use it for big nets in a reasonable time. Two "exact" algorithms were developed which lead to exactly the same results as OBS but using less time. The first with time $O(n^{1.8} p)$ makes use of Strassens' fast matrix multiplication algorithm. The second algorithm uses algebraic transformations to speed up calculation and needs time $O(np^2)$. This algorithm is faster than OBS in the special case of $p < n$.

To get a much higher speedup than these exact algorithms can do, an improved OBS algorithm was developed which reduces the runtime needed to prune a big network drastically. The basic idea is to use the inverse Hessian to remove a group of weights instead of only one, because the calculation of this matrix takes the most time in the OBS algorithm. This idea leads to an algorithm called Unit–OBS that is able to remove whole units.

Unit–OBS has two main advantages: First it is a fast algorithm to prune big nets, because whole units are removed in every step instead of slow pruning weight by weight. On the other side it can be used to do a feature extraction on the input data by removing unimportant input units. This is helpful for the understanding of unknown problems.

2 Optimal Brain Surgeon

This section gives a small summary of the OBS algorithm described by Hassibi, Stork and Wolff in [1] and [2]. As they showed the increase in error (when changing weights by Δw) is

$$\Delta E = \frac{1}{2} \Delta w^T H \Delta w \tag{1}$$

where H is the Hessian matrix. The goal is to eliminate weight w_q and minimize the increase in error given by Eq. 1. Eliminating w_q can be expressed by $w_q + \Delta w_q = 0$ which is equivalent to $(w + \Delta w)^T e_q = 0$ where e_q is the unit vector corresponding to weight w_q ($w^T e_q = w_q$). Solving this extremum problem with side condition using Lagrange's method leads to the solution

$$\Delta E = \frac{w_q^2}{2 H^{-1}{}_{qq}} \tag{2}$$

$$\Delta w = -\frac{w_q}{H^{-1}{}_{qq}} H^{-1} e_q \tag{3}$$

$H^{-1}{}_{qq}$ denotes the element (q, q) of matrix H^{-1}. For every weight w_q the minimal increase in error $\Delta E(w_q)$ is calculated and the weight which leads to overall minimum will be removed and all other weights be adapted referring to Eq. 3. Hassibi, Stork and Wolff also showed how to calculate H^{-1} using time $O(n^2 p)$ where n is the number of weights and p the number of pattern.

The main disadvantage of the OBS algorithm is that it needs time $O(n^2 p)$ to remove only one weight thus needing much time to prune big nets. The basic idea to soften this disadvantage is to use H^{-1} to remove more than only one weight! This generalized OBS algorithm is described in the next section.

3 Generalized OBS (G–OBS)

This section shows a generalized OBS algorithm (G–OBS) which can be used to delete m weights in one step with minimal increase in error. Like in the OBS algorithm the increase in error is given by $\Delta E = \frac{1}{2} \Delta w^T H \Delta w$. But the condition $w_q + \Delta w_q = 0$ is replaced by the generalized condition

$$(w + \Delta w)^T M = 0 \quad \text{with} \quad M = (e_{q_1}\ e_{q_2}\ \ldots\ e_{q_m}) \tag{4}$$

where M is the selection matrix (selecting the weights to be removed) and $q_1, q_2, \ldots, q_m$ are the indices of the weights that will be removed. Solving this extremum problem with side condition using Lagrange's method leads to the solution

$$\Delta E = \frac{1}{2} w^T M (M^T H^{-1} M)^{-1} M^T w \tag{5}$$

$$\Delta w = -H^{-1} M (M^T H^{-1} M)^{-1} M^T w \tag{6}$$

Choosing $M = e_q$ Eq. 5 and 6 reduce to Eq. 2 and 3. This shows that OBS is (as expected) a special case of G–OBS. The problem of calculating H^{-1} was already solved by Hassibi, Stork and Wolff ([1] and [2]).

4 Analysis of G–OBS

Hassibi, Stork and Wolff ([1] and [2]) showed that the time to calculate H^{-1} is in $O(n^2 p)$. The calculation of ΔE referring to Eq. 5 needs time $O(m^3)^\dagger$ where m is the number of weights to be removed. The calculation of Δw (Eq. 6) needs time $O(nm + m^3)$.

The problem within this solution consists of not knowing which weights should be deleted and thus ΔE has to be calculated for *all* possible combinations to find the global minimum in error increase. Choosing m weights out of n can be done with $\binom{n}{m}$ possible combinations. This takes time $\binom{n}{m} O(m^3)$ to find the minimum. Therefore the total runtime of the generalized OBS algorithm to remove m weights (with minimal increase in error) is

$$T_{\text{G–OBS}} = O(n^2 p + \binom{n}{m} m^3).$$

The problem is that for $m > 3$ the term $\binom{n}{m} m^3$ dominates and $T_{\text{G–OBS}}$ is in $\Omega(n^4)$. In other words G–OBS can be used only to remove a maximum of three weights in one step. But this means little advantage over OBS.

To overcome this problem the set of possible combinations has to be restricted to a small subset of combinations that seem to be "good" combinations. This reduces the term $\binom{n}{m} m^3$ to a reasonable amount. One way to do this is that a good combination exists of all outgoing connections of a unit. This reduces the number of combinations to the number of units! The basic idea for that subset is: If all outgoing connections of a unit can be removed then the whole unit can be deleted because it can not influence the net output anymore. Therefore choosing this subset leads to an algorithm called Unit–OBS that is able to remove whole units without the need to recalculate H^{-1}.

5 Special Case of G–OBS: Unit–OBS

With the results of the last sections we can now describe an algorithm called Unit–OBS to remove whole units.

1. Train a network to minimum error.

$^\dagger M$ is a matrix of special type and thus the calculation of $(M^T H^{-1} M)$ needs only $O(m^2)$ operations!

2. Compute H^{-1}.

3. For each unit u

   (a) Compute the indices $q_1, q_2, \ldots, q_{m(u)}$ of the outgoing connections of unit u where $m(u)$ is the number of outgoing connections of unit u.

   (b) $M := (e_{q_1}\ e_{q_2}\ \ldots\ e_{q_{m(u)}})$

   (c) $\Delta E(u) := \frac{1}{2} w^T M (M^T H^{-1} M)^{-1} M^T w$

4. Find the u_0 that gives the smallest increase in error $\Delta E(u_0)$.

5. $M := M(u_0)$ (refer to steps 3.(a) and 3.(b))

6. $\Delta w := -H^{-1} M (M^T H^{-1} M)^{-1} M^T w$

7. Remove unit u_0 and use Δw to update all weights.

8. Repeat steps 2 to 7 until a break criteria is reached.

Following the analysis of G–OBS the time to remove one unit is

$$T_{\text{Unit-OBS}} = O(n^2 p + u m^3) \tag{7}$$

where u is the number of units in the network and m is the maximum number of outgoing connections. If m is much smaller than n we can neglect the term um^3 and the main problem is to calculate H^{-1}. Therefore, if m is small, we can say that Unit–OBS needs the same time to remove a whole unit as OBS needs to remove a single weight. The speedup when removing units with an average of s outgoing connections should then be s.

6 Simulation results

6.1 The Monk–1 benchmark

Unit–OBS was applied to the MONK's problems because the underlying logical rules are well known and it is easy to say which input units are important to the problem and which input units can be removed. The simulations showed that in no case Unit–OBS removed a wrong unit and that it has the ability to remove all unimportant input units.

Figure 1 shows a MONK–1–net pruned with Unit–OBS. This net is the minimal network that can be found by Unit–OBS. Table 1 shows the speedup of Unit-OBS compared to OBS to find an equal–size network for the MONK–1 problem.

The network shown in Fig. 1 is only minimal in the number of units but not minimal with respect to the number of weights. Hassibi, Stork and Wolff ([1] and [2]) found a network with only 14 weights by applying OBS (Fig. 3). In the framework of Unit–OBS, OBS can be used to do further pruning on the network after all possible units have been pruned. The advantage lies in the fact that now the time consuming OBS–algorithm is applied to a much smaller network (22 weights instead of 58). The result of this combination of Unit–OBS and OBS is a network with only 14 weights (Fig. 2) which has also 100 % accuracy like the minimal net found by OBS (see Table 1).

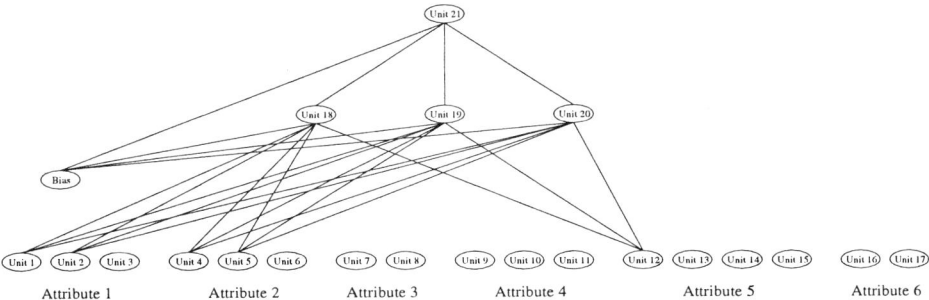

Figure 1: MONK–1–net pruned with Unit–OBS, 22 weights. All unimportant units are removed and this net needs less units than the minimal network found by OBS!

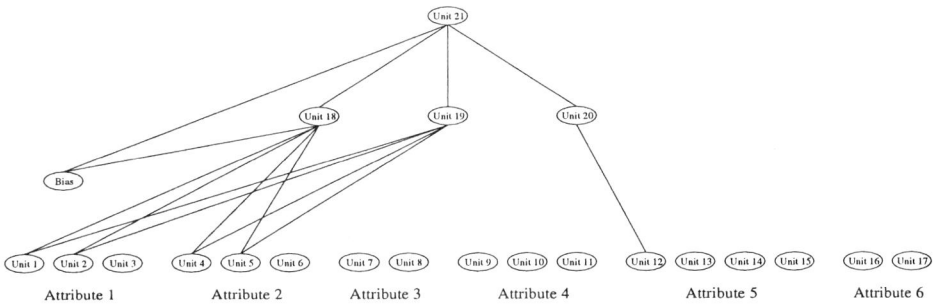

Figure 2: Minimal network (14 weights) for the MONK–1 problem found by the combination of Unit–OBS with OBS. The logical rule for the MONK–1 problem is more evident in this network than in the minimal network found by OBS (comp. Fig. 3).

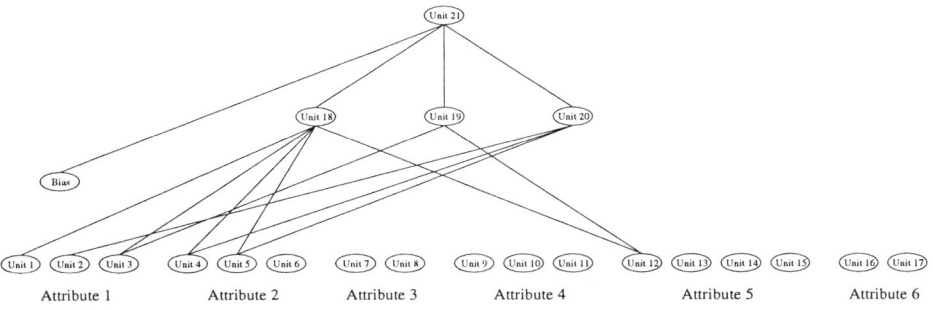

Figure 3: Minimal network (14 weights) for the MONK–1 problem found by OBS (see [1] and [2]).

algorithm	# weights	topology	speedup‡	perf. train	perf. test
no pruning	58	17-3-1	–	100 %	100 %
OBS	14	6-3-1	1.0	100 %	100 %
Unit-OBS	22	5-3-1	2.8	100 %	100 %
Unit-OBS + OBS	14	5-3-1	2.6	100 %	100 %

Table 1: The Monk–1 problem

For the initial Monk–1 network the maximum number of outgoing connections (m in Eq. 7) is 3 and this is much smaller than the number of weights. The average number of outgoing connections of the removed units is 3 and therefore we expect a speedup by factor 3 (compare Table 1).

By comparing the two minimal nets found by Unit–OBS/OBS (Fig. 2) and OBS (Fig. 3) it can be seen that the underlying logical rule (out=1 ⇔ Attribut_1=Attribut_2 or Attribut_5=1) is more evident in the network found by Unit–OBS/OBS. The other advantage of Unit–OBS is that it needs only 38 % of the time OBS needs to find this minimal network. This advantage makes it possible to apply Unit–OBS to big nets for which OBS is not useful because of its long computation time.

6.2 The Thyroid Benchmark

The following describes the application of pruning on a medical classification problem. The task is to classify measured data values of patients into three categories. The output of the three layered feedforward network therefore consists of three neurons indicating the corresponding class. The input consists of 21 both continuos and binary signals.

The task was first described in [4]. The results obtained there are shown in the first row of Table 2. The initially used network has 21 input neurons, 10 hidden and 3 output neurons, which are fully connected using shortcut connections.

When applying OBS to prune the network weights, more than 90 % of the weights can be pruned. However, over 8 hours of cpu-time on a sparc workstation are used to do so (row 2 in Table 2). The solution finally found by OBS uses only 8 of the originally 21 input features. The pruned network shows a slightly improved classification rate on the test set.

Unit–OBS finds a solution with 41 weights in only 76 minutes of cpu-time. In comparison to the original OBS algorithm, Unit–OBS is about 8 times as fast when deleting the same number of weights. Also another important fact can be seen from the result: The Unit–OBS network considers only 7 of the originally 21 inputs, 1 less than the weight-focused OBS–algorithm. The number of hidden units is reduced to 2 units, 5 units less than the OBS network uses.

When further looking for an absolute minimum in the number of used weights, the Unit–OBS network can be additionally pruned using OBS. This finally leeds to an optimized network with only 24 weights. The classification performance of this very

---

‡Compared to OBS deleting the same number of weights.

small network is 98.5% which is even slightly better than obtained by the much bigger initial net.

algorithm	# weights	topology	speedup	cpu-time	perf. test
no pruning	316	21-10-3	-	-	98.4%
OBS	28	8-7-3	1.0	511 min.	98.5%
Unit-OBS	41	7-2-3	7.8	76 min.	98.4%
Unit-OBS + OBS	24	7-2-3	-	137 min.	98.5%

Table 2: The thyroid benchmark

7 Conclusion

The article describes an improvement of the OBS–algorithm introduced in [1] called Generalized OBS (G–OBS). The underlying idea is to exploit second order information to delete *mutliple* weights at once. The aim to reduce the number of different weight groups leads to the formulation of the Unit-OBS algorithm, which considers the outgoing weights of one unit as a group of candidate weights: When all the weights of a unit can be deleted, the unit itself can be pruned. The new Unit-OBS algorithm has two major advantages: First, it considerably accelerates pruning by a speedup factor which lies in the range of the average number of outgoing weights of each unit. Second, deleting complete units is especially interesting to determine the input features which *really* contribute to the computation of the output. This information can be used to get more insight in the underlying problem structure, e.g. to facilitate the process of rule extraction.

References

[1] B. Hassibi, D. G. Storck: *Second Order Derivatives for Network Pruning: Optimal Brain Surgeon.* Advances in Neural Information Processing Systems 5, Morgan Kaufmann, 1993, pages 164–171.

[2] B. Hassibi, D. G. Stork, G. J. Wolff: *Optimal Brain Surgeon and general Network Pruning.* IEEE International Conference on Neural Networks, 1993 Volume 1, pages 293–299.

[3] A. Stahlberger: *OBS – Verbesserungen und neue Ansätze.* Diplomarbeit, Universität Karlsruhe, Institut für Logik, Komplexität und Deduktionssysteme, 1996.

[4] W. Schiffmann, M. Joost, R. Werner: *Optimization of the Backpropagation Algorithm for Training Multilayer Perceptrons.* Technical Report, University of Koblenz, Institute of Physics, 1993.

Separating Style and Content

Joshua B. Tenenbaum
Dept. of Brain and Cognitive Sciences
Massachusetts Institute of Technology
Cambridge, MA 02139
jbt@psyche.mit.edu

William T. Freeman
MERL, Mitsubishi Electric Res. Lab.
201 Broadway
Cambridge, MA 02139
freeman@merl.com

Abstract

We seek to analyze and manipulate two factors, which we call style and content, underlying a set of observations. We fit training data with bilinear models which explicitly represent the two-factor structure. These models can adapt easily during testing to new styles or content, allowing us to solve three general tasks: *extrapolation* of a new style to unobserved content; *classification* of content observed in a new style; and *translation* of new content observed in a new style. For classification, we embed bilinear models in a probabilistic framework, *Separable Mixture Models (SMMs)*, which generalizes earlier work on factorial mixture models [7, 3]. Significant performance improvement on a benchmark speech dataset shows the benefits of our approach.

1 Introduction

In many pattern analysis or synthesis tasks, the observed data are generated from the interaction of two underlying factors which we will generically call "style" and "content." For example, in a character recognition task, we might observe different letters in different fonts (see Fig. 1); with handwriting, different words in different writing styles; with speech, different phonemes in different accents; with visual images, the faces of different people under different lighting conditions.

Such data raises a number of learning problems. Extracting a hidden two-factor structure given only the raw observations has received significant attention [7, 3], but unsupervised *factorial* learning of this kind has yet to prove tractable for our focus: real-world data with subtly interacting factors. We work in a more supervised setting, where labels for style or content may be available during training or testing. Figure 1 shows three problems we want to solve. Given a labelled training set of observations in multiple styles, we want to *extrapolate* a new style to unobserved content classes (Fig. 1a), *classify* content observed in a new style (Fig. 1b), and *translate* new content observed in a new style (Fig. 1c).

This paper treats these problems in a common framework, by fitting the training data with a separable model that can easily adapt during testing to new styles or content classes. We write an observation vector in style s and content class c as $\mathbf{y}^{sc}$. We seek to fit these observations with some model

$$\mathbf{y}^{sc} = f(\mathbf{a}^s, \mathbf{b}^c; W), \qquad (1)$$

where a particular functional form of f is assumed. We must estimate parameter vectors $\mathbf{a}^s$ and $\mathbf{b}^c$ describing style s and content c, respectively, and W, parameters

Separating Style and Content

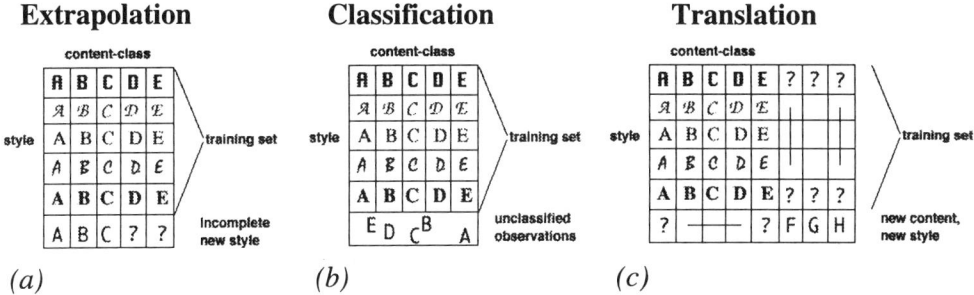

Figure 1: Given observations of content (letters) in different styles (fonts), we want to extrapolate, classify, and translate observations from a new style or content class.

for f that are independent of style and content but govern their interaction. In terms of Fig. 1 (and in the spirit of [8]), the model represents what the elements of each row have in common independent of column ($\mathbf{a}^s$), what the elements of each column have in common independent of row ($\mathbf{b}^c$), and what all elements have in common independent of row and column (W). With these three modular components, we can solve problems like those illustrated in Fig. 1. For example, we can extrapolate a new style to unobserved content classes (Fig. 1a) by combining content and interaction parameters learned during training with style parameters estimated from available data in the new style.

2 Bilinear models

We propose to separate style and content using bilinear models – two-factor models that are linear in either factor when the other is held constant. These simple models are still complex enough to model subtle interactions of style and content. The empirical success of linear models in many pattern recognition applications with single-factor data (e.g. "eigenface" models of faces under varying identity but constant illumination and pose [15], or under varying illumination but constant identity and pose [5]), makes bilinear models a natural choice when two such factors vary independently across the data set. Also, many of the computationally desirable properties of linear models extend to bilinear models. Model fitting (discussed in Section 3 below) is easy, based on efficient and well-known techniques such as the singular value decomposition (SVD) and the expectation-maximization (EM) algorithm. Model complexity can be controlled by varying model dimensionality to achieve a compromise between reproduction of the training data and generalization during testing. Finally, the approach extends to multilinear models [10], for data generated by three or more interacting factors.

We have explored two bilinear models for Eq. 1. In the *symmetric* model (so called because it treats the two factors symmetrically), we assume f is a bilinear mapping given by

$$y_k^{sc} = {\mathbf{a}^s}^T \mathbf{W}_k \mathbf{b}^c = \sum_{ij} a_i^s b_j^c W_{ijk}. \qquad (2)$$

The W_{ijk} parameters represent a set of basis functions independent of style and content, which characterize the interaction between these two factors. Observations in style s and content c are generated by mixing these basis functions with coefficients given by the tensor product of $\mathbf{a}^s$ and $\mathbf{b}^c$ vectors. The model exactly reproduces the observations when the dimensionalities of $\mathbf{a}^s$ and $\mathbf{b}^c$ equal the number of styles N_s and content classes N_c observed. It finds coarser but more compact representations as these dimensionalities are decreased.

Sometimes it may not be practical to represent both style and content with low-dimensional vectors. For example, a linear combination of a few basis styles learned during training may not describe new styles well. We can obtain more flexible, *asymmetric* bilinear models by letting the basis functions W_{ijk} themselves depend on style or content. For example, if the basis functions are allowed to depend on style, the bilinear model from Eq. 2 becomes $y_k^{sc} = \sum_{ij} a_i^s b_j^c W_{ijk}^s$. This simplifies to $y_k^{sc} = \sum_j A_{jk}^s b_j^c$, by summing out the i index and identifying $A_{jk}^s \equiv \sum_i a_i^s W_{ijk}^s$. In vector notation, we have

$$\mathbf{y}^{sc} = \mathbf{A}^s \mathbf{b}^c, \qquad (3)$$

where $\mathbf{A}^s$ is a matrix of basis functions specific to style s (independent of content), and $\mathbf{b}^c$ is a vector of coefficients specific to content c (independent of style). Alternatively, the basis functions may depend on content, which gives

$$\mathbf{y}^{sc} = \mathbf{B}^c \mathbf{a}^s. \qquad (4)$$

Asymmetric models do not parameterize the rendering function f independently of style and content, and so cannot translate across both factors simultaneously (Fig. 1c). Further, a matrix representation of style or content may be *too* flexible and overfit the training data. But if overfitting is not a problem or can be controlled by some additional constraint, asymmetric models may solve extrapolation and classification tasks using less training data than symmetric models.

Figure 2 illustrates an example of an asymmetric model used to separate style and content. We have collected a small database of face images, with 11 different people (content classes) in 15 different head poses (styles). The images are 22 × 32 pixels, which we treat as 704-dimensional vectors. A subset of the data is shown in Fig. 2a. Fig. 2b schematically depicts an asymmetric bilinear model of the data, with each pose represented by a set of basis vectors $\mathbf{A}^{pose}$ (shown as images) and each person represented by a set of coefficients $\mathbf{b}^{person}$. To render an image of a particular person in a particular pose, the pose-specific basis vectors are mixed according to the person-specific coefficients. Note that the basis vectors for each pose look like eigenfaces [15] in the appropriate style of each pose. However, the bilinear structure of the model ensures that corresponding basis vectors play corresponding roles across poses (e.g. the first vector holds (roughly) the mean face for that pose, the second may modulate overall head size, the third may modulate head thickness, etc.), which is crucial for adapting to new styles or content classes.

3 Model fitting

All the tasks shown in Fig. 1 break down into a training phase and a testing phase; both involve some model fitting. In the training phase (corresponding to the first 5 rows and columns of Figs. 1a-c), we learn all the parameters of a bilinear model from a complete matrix of observations of N_c content classes in N_s styles. In the testing phase (corresponding to the final rows of Figs. 1a,b and the final row and last 3 columns of Fig. 1c), we adapt the same model to data in a new style or content class (or both), estimating new parameters for the new style or content, clamping the other parameters. Then new and old parameters are combined to accomplish the desired classification, extrapolation, or translation task. This section focuses on the asymmetric model and its use in extrapolation and classification. Training and

Separating Style and Content

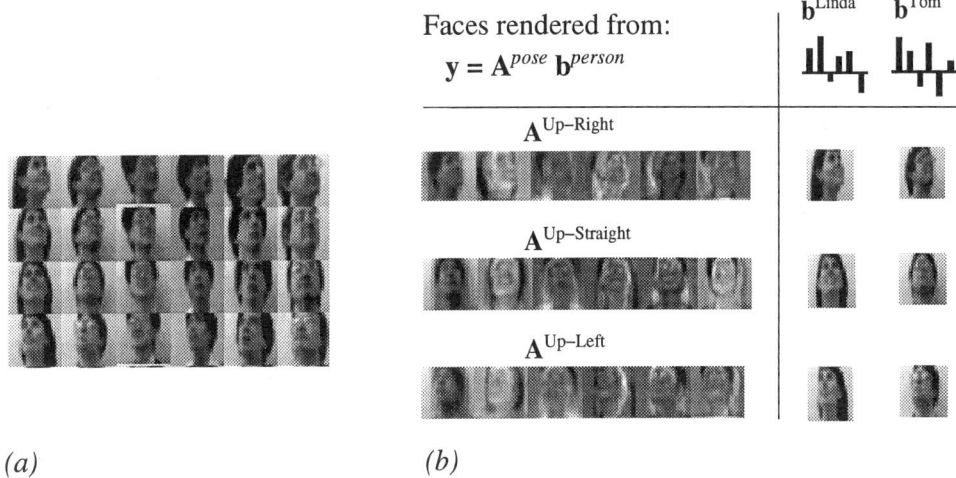

(a) (b)

Figure 2: An illustraton of the asymmetric model, with faces varying in identity and head pose.

adaptation procedures for the symmetric model are similar and based on algorithms in [10, 11]. In [2], we describe these procedures and their application to extrapolation and translation tasks.

3.1 Training

Let n_{sc} be the number of observations in style s and content c, and let $\mathbf{m}^{sc} = \sum \mathbf{y}^{sc}$ be the sum of these observations. Then estimates of $\mathbf{A}^s$ and $\mathbf{b}^c$ that minimize the sum-of-squared-errors for the asymmetric model in Eq. 3 can be found by iterating the fixed point equations

$$\hat{\mathbf{A}}^s = \left[\sum_c \mathbf{m}^{sc}\mathbf{b}^{c^T}\right]\left[\sum_c n_{sc}\mathbf{b}^c\mathbf{b}^{c^T}\right]^{-1}, \quad \hat{\mathbf{b}}^c = \left[\sum_s n_{sc}\mathbf{A}^{s^T}\mathbf{A}^s\right]^{-1}\left[\sum_s \mathbf{A}^{s^T}\mathbf{m}^{sc}\right] \quad (5)$$

obtained by setting derivatives of the error equal to 0. To ensure stability, we update the parameters according to $\mathbf{A}^s = (1-\eta)\mathbf{A}^s + \eta\hat{\mathbf{A}}^s$ and $\mathbf{b}^c = (1-\eta)\mathbf{b}^c + \eta\hat{\mathbf{b}}^c$, typically using a stepsize $0.2 < \eta < 0.5$. Replacing $\mathbf{A}^s$ with $\mathbf{B}^c$ and $\mathbf{b}^c$ with $\mathbf{a}^s$ yields the analogous procedure for training the model in Eq. 4.

If the same number of observations are available for all style-content pairs, there exists a closed-form procedure to fit the asymmetric model using the SVD. Let the K-dimensional vector $\bar{\mathbf{y}}^{sc}$ denote the mean of the observed data generated by style s and content c, and stack these vectors into a single $(K \times N_s) \times N_c$ matrix

$$\mathbf{Y} = \begin{bmatrix} \bar{\mathbf{y}}^{11} & \cdots & \bar{\mathbf{y}}^{1N_c} \\ \vdots & \ddots & \\ \bar{\mathbf{y}}^{N_s 1} & & \bar{\mathbf{y}}^{N_s N_c} \end{bmatrix}. \quad (6)$$

We compute the SVD of $\mathbf{Y} = \mathbf{U}\mathbf{S}\mathbf{V}^T$, and define the $(K \times N_s) \times J$ matrix $\mathbf{A}$ to be the first J columns of $\mathbf{U}$, and the $J \times N_c$ matrix $\mathbf{B}$ to be the first J rows of $\mathbf{S}\mathbf{V}^T$. Finally, we identify $\mathbf{A}$ and $\mathbf{B}$ as the desired parameter estimates in stacked form (see also [9, 14]),

$$A = \begin{bmatrix} A^1 \\ \vdots \\ A^{N_s} \end{bmatrix}, \quad B = [b^1 \cdots b^{N_c}]. \tag{7}$$

The model dimensionality J can be chosen in various standard ways: by a priori considerations, by requiring a sufficiently good approximation to the data (as measured by mean squared error or some more subjective metric), or by looking for a gap in the singular value spectrum.

3.2 Testing

It is straightforward to adapt the asymmetric model to an incomplete new style s^*, in order to extrapolate that style to unseen content. We simply estimate A^{s^*} from Eq. 5, using b^c values learned during training and restricting the sums over c to those content classes observed in the new style. Then data in content c and style s^* can be synthesized from $A^{s^*}b^c$. Extrapolating incomplete new content to unseen styles is done similarly.

Adapting the asymmetric model for classification in new styles is more involved, because the content class of the new data (and possibly its style as well) is unlabeled. To deal with this uncertainty, we embed the bilinear model within a gaussian mixture model to yield a *separable mixture model (SMM)*, which can then be fit efficiently to data in new styles using the EM algorithm. Specifically, we assume that the probability of a new, unlabeled observation y being generated by style s and content c is given by a spherical gaussian centered at the prediction of the asymmetric bilinear model: $p(y|s,c) \propto \exp\{-\|y - A^s b^c\|^2/(2\sigma^2)\}$. The total probability of y is then $p(y) = \sum_{s,c} p(y|s,c)p(s,c)$; we use equal priors $p(s,c)$. We assume that the content vectors b^c are known from training, but that new style matrices A^s must be found to explain the test data. The EM algorithm alternates between computing soft style and content-class assignments $p(s,c|y) = p(y|s,c)p(s,c)/p(y)$ for each test vector y given the current style matrix estimates (E-step), and estimating new style matrices by setting A^s to maximize $\sum_y \log p(y)$ (M-step). The M-step is solved in closed form using the update rule for A^s from Eq. 5, with $m^{sc} = \sum_y p(s,c|y) y$ and $n_{sc} = \sum_y p(s,c|y)$. Test vectors in new styles can now be classified by grouping each vector y with the content class c that maximizes $p(c|y) = \sum_s p(s,c|y)$.

4 Application: speaker-adaptive speech recognition

This example illustrates our approach to style-adaptive classification on a real-world data set that is a benchmark for many connectionist learning algorithms. The data consist of 6 samples of each of 11 vowels uttered by 15 speakers of British English (originally collected by David Deterding, from the CMU neural-bench ftp archive). Each data vector consists of 10 parameters computed from a linear predictive analysis of the digitized speech. Robinson [13] compared many learning algorithms trained to categorize vowels from the first 8 speakers (4 male and 4 female) and tested on samples from the remaining 7 speakers (4 male and 3 female).

Using the SVD-based procedure described above, we fit an asymmetric bilinear model to the training data, labeled by style (speaker) and content (vowel). We then used the learned vowel parameters b^c in an SMM and tested classification performance with varying degrees of style information for the 7 new speakers' data:

both style and content labels missing for each test vector (SMM1), style labels present (indicating a change of speaker) but content labels missing (SMM2), and both labels missing but with the test data loglikelihood $\sum_\mathbf{y} \log p(\mathbf{y})$ augmented by a prior favoring temporal continuity of style assignments (SMM3).

The few training styles makes this problem difficult and a good showcase for our approach. Robinson [13] obtained 51% correct vowel classification on the test set with a multi-layer perceptron and 56% with a 1-nearest neighbor (1-NN) classifier, the best performance of the many standard techniques he tried. Hastie and Tibshirani [6] recently obtained 62% correct using their discriminant adaptive nearest neighbor algorithm, the best result we know of for an approach that does not model speaker style. We obtained 69% correct for SMM1, 77% for SMM2, and 76% for SMM3, using a model dimensionality of $J = 4$, model variance of $\sigma^2 = .5$, and using the vowel class assignments of 1-NN to initialize the E-step of EM. While good initial conditions were important for the EM algorithm, a range of model dimensionality and variance settings gave reasonable performance.

We also applied these methods to the head pose data of Fig. 2a. We trained on 10 subjects in the 15 poses, and used SMM2 to learn a style model for a new person while simultaneously classifying the head poses. We obtained 81% correct pose categorization (averaged over all 11 test subjects), compared with 53% correct performance for 1-NN matching.

These results demonstrate that modeling style and content can substantially improve content classification in new styles even when no style information is available during testing (SMM1), and dramatically so when some style demarkation is available explicitly (SMM2) or implicitly (SMM3). Bilinear models offer an easy way to improve performance using style labels which are frequently available for many classification tasks.

5   Pointers to other work and conclusions

We discuss the extrapolation and translation problems in [2]. Here we summarize results. Figure 3 shows extrapolation of a partially observed font (Monaco) to the unseen letters (see also the gridfont work of [8, 4]). During training, we presented all letters of the five fonts shown at the left. To accomodate many shape topologies, we described letters by the warps of black particles from a reference shape into the letter shape. During testing, we fit an asymmetric model style matrix to all the letters of the Monaco font *except* those shown in the figure. We used the best fitting linear combination of training fonts as a prior for the style matrix, in order to control model complexity. Using the fit style, we then synthesized the unseen letters of the Monaco font. These compare well with the actual letters in that style.

Because the W weights of the symmetric model are independent of any particular style and content class, they allow translation of observations from unknown styles *and* content-classes to known ones. During training, we fit the symmetric model to the observations. For a test observation under a new style and content class, we find $\mathbf{a}^s$ and $\mathbf{b}^c$ values using the known W numbers, iterating least squares fits of the two parameters. Typically, the resulting $\mathbf{a}^s$ and $\mathbf{b}^c$ vectors are unique up to an uncertainty in scale. We have used this approach to translate across shape or lighting conditions for images of faces, and to translate across illumination color for color measurements (assuming small specular reflections).

Our work naturally combines two current themes in the connectionist learning literature: factorial learning [7, 3] and learning a family of many related tasks [1, 12]

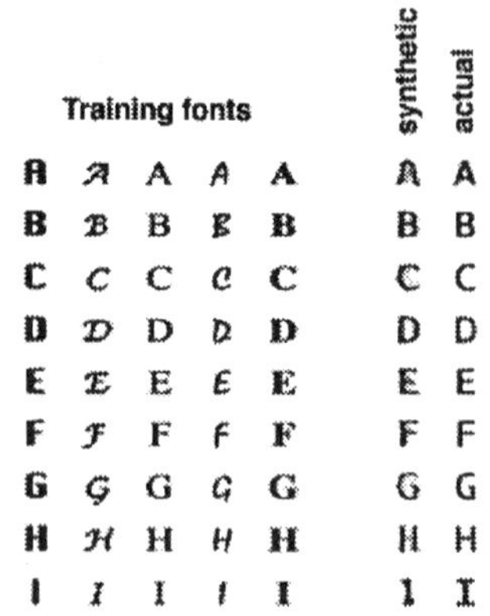

Training fonts					synthetic	actual
A	A	A	A	A	A	A
B	B	B	B	B	B	B
C	C	C	C	C	C	C
D	D	D	D	D	D	D
E	E	E	E	E	E	E
F	F	F	F	F	F	F
G	G	G	G	G	G	G
H	H	H	H	H	H	H
I	I	I	I	I	I	I

Figure 3: Style extrapolation in typography. The training data were all letters of the 5 fonts at left. The test data were all the Monaco letters except those shown at right. The synthesized Monaco letters compare well with the missing ones.

to facilitate task transfer. Separable bilinear models provide a powerful framework for separating style and content by combining explicit representation of each factor with the computational efficiency of linear models.

Acknowledgements

We thank W. Richards, Y. Weiss, and M. Bernstein for helpful discussions. Joshua Tenenbaum is a Howard Hughes Medical Institute Predoctoral Fellow.

References

[1] R. Caruana. Learning many related tasks at the same time with backpropagation. In *Adv. in Neural Info. Proc. Systems*, volume 7, pages 657–674, 1995.

[2] W. T. Freeman and J. B. Tenenbaum. Learning bilinear models for two-factor problems in vision. TR 96-37, MERL, 201 Broadway, Cambridge, MA 02139, 1996.

[3] Z. Ghahramani. Factorial learning and the EM algorithm. In *Adv. in Neural Info. Proc. Systems*, volume 7, pages 617–624, 1995.

[4] I. Grebert, D. G. Stork, R. Keesing, and S. Mims. Connectionist generalization for production: An example from gridfont. *Neural Networks*, 5:699–710, 1992.

[5] P. W. Hallinan. A low-dimensional representation of human faces for arbitrary lighting conditions. In *Proc. IEEE CVPR*, pages 995–999, 1994.

[6] T. Hastie and R. Tibshirani. Discriminant adaptive nearest neighbor classification. *IEEE Pat. Anal. Mach. Intell.*, (18):607–616, 1996.

[7] G. E. Hinton and R. Zemel. Autoencoders, minimum description length, and Helmholtz free energy. In *Adv. in Neural Info. Proc. Systems*, volume 6, 1994.

[8] D. Hofstadter. *Fluid Concepts and Creative Analogies*. Basic Books, 1995.

[9] J. J. Koenderink and A. J. van Doorn. The generic bilinear calibration–estimation problem. *Intl. J. Comp. Vis.*, 1997. in press.

[10] J. R. Magnus and H. Neudecker. *Matrix differential calculus with applications in statistics and econometrics*. Wiley, 1988.

[11] D. H. Marimont and B. A. Wandell. Linear models of surface and illuminant spectra. *J. Opt. Soc. Am. A*, 9(11):1905–1913, 1992.

[12] S. M. Omohundro. Family discovery. In *Adv. in Neural Info. Proc. Sys.*, vol. 8, 1995.

[13] A. Robinson. *Dynamic error propagation networks*. PhD thesis, Cambridge University Engineering Dept., 1989.

[14] C. Tomasi and T. Kanade. Shape and motion from image streams under orthography: a factorization method. *Intl. J. Comp. Vis.*, 9(2):137–154, 1992.

[15] M. Turk and A. Pentland. Eigenfaces for recognition. *J. Cog. Neurosci.*, 3(1), 1991.

Early Brain Damage

Volker Tresp, Ralph Neuneier and Hans Georg Zimmermann*
Siemens AG, Corporate Technologies
Otto-Hahn-Ring 6
81730 München, Germany

Abstract

Optimal Brain Damage (OBD) is a method for reducing the number of weights in a neural network. OBD estimates the increase in cost function if weights are pruned and is a valid approximation if the learning algorithm has converged into a local minimum. On the other hand it is often desirable to terminate the learning process before a local minimum is reached (early stopping). In this paper we show that OBD estimates the increase in cost function incorrectly if the network is not in a local minimum. We also show how OBD can be extended such that it can be used in connection with early stopping. We call this new approach *Early Brain Damage*, EBD. EBD also allows to revive already pruned weights. We demonstrate the improvements achieved by EBD using three publicly available data sets.

1 Introduction

Optimal Brain Damage (OBD) was introduced by Le Cun *et al.* (1990) as a method to significantly reduce the number of weights in a neural network. By reducing the number of free parameters, the variance in the prediction of the network is often reduced considerably which —in some cases— leads to an improvement in generalization performance of the neural network. OBD might be considered a realization of the principle of Occam's razor which states that the simplest explanation (of the training data) should be preferred to more complex explanations (requiring more weights).

If E is the cost function which is minimized during training, OBD calculates the

---

{Volker.Tresp, Ralph.Neuneier, Georg.Zimmermann}@mchp.siemens.de.

saliency of each parameter w_i defined as

$$OBD(w_i) = A(w_i) = \frac{1}{2}\frac{\partial^2 E}{\partial w_i^2}w_i^2.$$

Weights with a small $OBD(w_i)$ are candidates for removal. $OBD(w_i)$ has the intuitive meaning of being the increase in cost function if weight w_i is set to zero under the assumptions

- that the cost function is quadratic,

  - that the cost function is "diagonal" which means it can be written as $E = Bias + 1/2 \sum_i h_i(w_i - w_i^*)^2$ where where $\{w_i^*\}_{i=1}^W$ are the weights in a (local) optimum of the cost function (Figure 1) and the h_i and $BIAS$ are parameters which are dependent on the training data set.

- and that $w_i \approx w_i^*$.

In practice, all three assumptions are often violated but experiments have demonstrated that OBD is a useful method for weight removal.

In this paper we want to take a closer look at the third assumption, i. e. the assumption that weights are close to optimum. The motivation is that theory and practice have shown that it is often advantageous to perform *early stopping* which means that training is terminated before convergence. Early stopping can be thought of as a form of regularization: since training typically starts with small weights, with early stopping weights are biased towards small weights analogously to other regularization methods such as ridge regression and weight decay. According to the assumptions in OBD we might be able to apply OBD only in heavily overtrained networks where we loose the benefits of early stopping. In this paper we show that OBD can be extended such that it can work together with early stopping. We call the new criterion *Early Brain Damage* (EBD). As in OBD, EBD contains a number of simplifying assumptions which are typically invalid in practice. Therefore, experimental results have to demonstrate that EBD has benefits. We validate EBD using three publicly available data sets.

2 Theory

As in OBD we approximate the cost function locally by a quadratic function and assume a "diagonal" form. Figure 1 illustrates that $OBD(w_i)$ for $w_i = w_i^*$ calculates the increase in cost function if w_i is set to zero. In early stopping where $w_i \neq w_i^*$, $OBD(w_i)$ calculates the quantity denoted as A_i in Figure 1. Consider

$$B_i = -\frac{\partial E}{\partial w_i}w_i.$$

The saliency of weights w_i in *Early Stopping Pruning*

$$ESP(w_i) = A_i + B_i$$

is an estimate of how much the cost function increases if the *current* w_i (i. e. w_i in early stopping) is set to zero. Finally, consider

$$C_i = \frac{1}{2}\left(\frac{\partial^2 E}{\partial w_i^2}\right)^{-1}\left(\frac{\partial E}{\partial w_i}\right)^2.$$

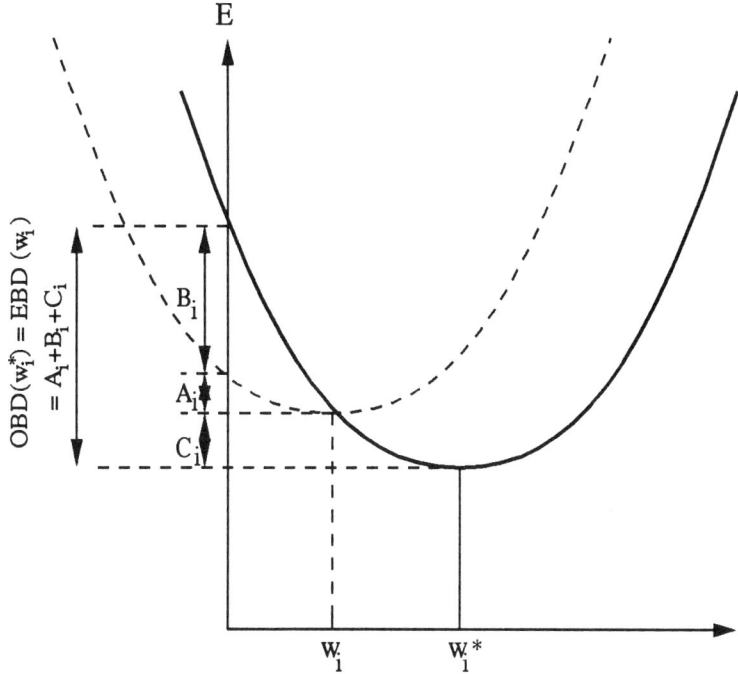

Figure 1: The figure shows the cost function E as a function of one weight w_i in the network. w_i^* is the optimal weight. w_i is the weight at an early stopping point. If OBD is applied at w_i, it estimates the quantity A_i. $ESP(w_i) = A_i + B_i = E(w_i) - E(w_i = 0)$ estimate the increase in cost function if w_i is pruned. $EBD(w_i) = A_i + B_i + C_i = E(w_i^*) - E(w_i = 0)$ is the difference in cost function if we would train to convergence and if we would set $w_i = 0$. In other words $EBD(w_i) = OBD(w_i^*)$.

The saliency of weight w_i in EBD is

$$EBD(w_i) = OBD(w_i^*) = A_i + B_i + C_i$$

which estimates the increase in cost function if w_i is pruned after convergence (i.e. $EBD(w_i) = OBD(w_i^*)$) but based on local information around the current value of w_i. In this sense EBD evaluates the "potential" of w_i. Weights with a small $EBD(w_i)$ are candidates for pruning.

Note, that all terms required for EBD are easily calculated. With a quadratic cost function $E = \sum_{k=1}^{K}(y^k - NN(x^k))^2$ OBD approximates (OBD-approximation)

$$\frac{\partial^2 E}{\partial w_i^2} \approx 2\sum_{k=1}^{K}\left(\frac{\partial NN(x^k)}{\partial w_i}\right)^2 \quad (1)$$

where $(x^k, y^k)_{k=1}^{K}$ are the training data and $NN(x^k)$ is the network response.

3 Extensions

3.1 Revival of Weights

In some cases, it is beneficial to revive weights which are already pruned. Note, that C_i exactly estimate the decrease in cost function if weight w_i is "revived". Weights with a large $C_i(w_i = 0)$ are candidates for revival.

3.2 Early Brain Surgeon (EBS)

After OBD or EBD is performed, the network needs to be retrained since the "diagonal" approximation is typically violated and there are dependencies between weights. *Optimal Brain Surgeon* (OBS, Hassibi and Storck, 1993) does not use the "diagonal" approximation and recalculates the new weights without explicit retraining. OBS still assumes a quadratic approximation of the cost function. The saliency in OBS is

$$L_i = \frac{w_i^2}{2[H^{-1}]_{ii}}$$

where $[H^{-1}]_{ii}$ is i-th diagonal element of the inverse of the Hessian. L_i estimates the increase in cost if the i-th weight is set to zero and all other weights are retrained. To recalculate all weights after weight w_i is removed apply

$$w_{new} = w_{old} - \frac{w_i}{[H^{-1}]_{ii}} H^{-1} e_i$$

where e_i is the unit vector in the i-th direction.

Analogously to OBS, *Early Brain Surgeon* EBS would first calculate the optimal weight vector using a second order approximation of the cost function

$$\hat{w}^* = w - H^{-1}\frac{\partial E}{\partial w}$$

and then apply OBS using $\hat{w}^*$. We did not pursue this idea any further since our initial experiments indicated that w^* was not estimated very accurately in praxis. Hassibi et al. (1994) achieved good performance with OBS even when weights were far from optimal.

Early Brain Damage

3.3 Approximations to the Hessian and the Gradient

Finnoff et al. (1993) have introduced the interesting idea that the relevant quantities for OBD can be estimated from the statistics of the weight changes.

Consider the update in pattern by pattern gradient descent learning and a quadratic cost function

$$\Delta w_i = -\eta \frac{\partial E_k}{\partial w} = 2\eta (y^k - NN(x^k))\frac{\partial NN(x^k)}{\partial w_i}$$

with $E_k = (y_k - NN(x_k))^2$ where η is the learning rate.

We assume that x^k and y^k are drawn online from a fixed distribution (which is strictly not true since in pattern by pattern learning we draw samples from a fixed training data set). Then, using the quadratic and "diagonal" approximation of the cost function and assuming that the noise ϵ in the model

$$y^k = NN(x^k) + \epsilon^k$$

is additive uncorrelated with variance σ^2 [1]

$$\mathcal{E}(\Delta w_i) \approx \frac{1}{K}\eta\frac{\partial E}{\partial w} \qquad (2)$$

and

$$VAR(\Delta w_i) = VAR\left(2\eta(y^k - NN(x^k))\frac{\partial NN(x^k)}{\partial w_i}\right)$$

$$= 4\eta^2 VAR\left((y^k - NN^*(x^k))\frac{\partial NN(x^k)}{\partial w_i}\right) + 4\eta^2 VAR\left((w_i^* - w_i)\left(\frac{\partial NN(x^k)}{\partial w_i}\right)^2\right)$$

$$= 4\sigma^2\eta^2 \mathcal{E}\left(\frac{\partial NN(x^k)}{\partial w_i}\right)^2 + 4\eta^2 (w_i^* - w_i)^2 VAR\left(\left(\frac{\partial NN(x^k)}{\partial w_i}\right)^2\right)$$

where $NN^*(x^k)$ is the network output with optimal weights $\{w_i^*\}_{i=1}^W$. Note, that in the OBD approximation (Equation 1)

$$\mathcal{E}\left(\frac{\partial NN(x^k)}{\partial w_i}\right)^2 \approx \frac{1}{2K}\frac{\partial^2 E}{\partial w_i^2}$$

and

$$w - w* \approx \frac{1/\eta\, \mathcal{E}(\Delta w_i)}{2\, \mathcal{E}\left(\frac{\partial NN(x^k)}{\partial w_i}\right)^2}.$$

If we make the further assumption that $\partial NN(x^k)/\partial w_i$ is Gaussian distributed with zero mean [2]

$$VAR\left(\left(\frac{\partial NN(x^k)}{\partial w_i}\right)^2\right) = 2\left(\mathcal{E}\left(\frac{\partial NN(x^k)}{\partial w_i}\right)^2\right)^2$$

---

[1] $\mathcal{E}$ stands for the expected value. With w_i kept at a fixed value.
[2] The zero mean assumption is typically violated but might be enforced by renormalization.

we obtain

$$VAR(\Delta w_i) = \frac{2}{K}\sigma^2\eta^2\frac{\partial^2 E}{\partial w_i^2} + 2*(\mathcal{E}(\Delta w_i))^2. \tag{3}$$

The first term in Equation 3 is a result of the residual error which is translated into weight fluctuations. But note, that weights with a small variance with a large $\partial^2 E/\partial w_i^2$ fluctuate the most. The first term is only active when there is a residual error, i.e. $\sigma^2 > 0$. The second term is non-zero independent of σ^2 and is due to the fact that in sample-by-sample learning, weight updates have a random component. From Equation 2 and Equation 3 all terms needed in EBD (i. e. $\partial E/\partial w$, and $\partial^2 E/\partial w_i^2$) are easily estimated.

4 Experimental Results

In our experiments we studied the performance of OBD, ESP and EBD in connection with early stopping. Although theory tells us that EBD should provide the best estimate of the the increase in cost function by the removal of weight w_i, it is not obvious how reliable that estimate is when the assumptions ("diagonal" quadratic cost function) are violated. Also we are not really interested in the correct estimate of the increase in cost function but in a ranking of the weights. Since the assumptions which go into OBD, EBD, ESP (and also OBS and EBS) are questionable, the usefulness of the new methods have to be demonstrated using practical experiments.

We used three different data sets: Breast Cancer Data, Diabetes Data, and Boston Housing Data. All three data sets can be obtained from the UCI repository (ftp:ics.uci.edu/pub/machine-learning-databases). The Breast Cancer Data contains 699 samples with 9 input variables consisting of cellular characteristics and one binary output with 458 benign and 241 malignant cases. The Diabetes Data contains 768 samples with 8 input variables and one binary output. The Boston Housing Data consist of 506 samples with 13 input variables which potentially influence the housing price (output variable) in a Boston neighborhood (Harrison & Rubinfeld, 1978).

Our procedure is as follows. The data set is divided into training data, validation data and test data. A neural network (MLP) is trained until the error on the validation data set starts to increase. At this point OBD, ESP and EBD are employed and 50% of all weights are removed. After pruning the networks are retrained until again the error on the validation set starts to increase. At this point the results are compared. Each experiment was repeated 5-times with different divisions of the data into training data, validation data and test data and we report averages over those 5 experiments.

Table 1 sums up the results. The first row shows the number of data in training set, validation set and test set. The second row displays the test set error at the (first) early stopping point. Rows 3 to 5 show test set performance of OBD, ESP and EBD at the stopping point after pruning and retraining (absolute / relative to early stopping). In all three experiments, EBD performed best and OBD was second best in two experiments (Breast Cancer Data and Diabetes Data). In two experiments (Breast Cancer Data and Boston Housing Data) the performance after pruning improved.

Table 1: Comparing OBD, ESP, and EBD.

	Breast Cancer	Diabetes	Boston Housing Data
Train/V/Test	233/233/233	256/256/256	168/169/169
Hidden units	10	5	3
MSE (Stopp)	0.0340	0.1625	0.2283
OBD	0.0328 / 0.965	0.1652 / 1.017	0.2275 /0.997
ESP	0.0331 / 0.973	0.1657 /1.020	0.2178 / 0.954
EBD	0.0326 / 0.959	0.1647 /1.014	0.2160 / 0.946

5 Conclusions

In our experiments, EBD showed better performance than OBD if used in conjunction with early stopping. The improvement in performance is not dramatic which indicates that the rankings of the weights in OBD are reasonable as well.

References

Finnoff, W., Hergert, F., and Zimmermann, H. (1993). Improving model selection by nonconvergent methods, *Neural Networks*, Vol. 6, No. 6.

Hassibi, B. and Storck, D. G. (1993). Second order derivatives for network pruning: Optimal Brain Surgeon. In: Hanson, S. J., Cowan, J. D., and Giles, C. L. (Eds.). *Advances in Neural Information Processing Systems 5,* San Mateo, CA, Morgan Kaufman.

Hassibi, B., Storck, D. G., and Wolff, G. (1994). Optimal Brain Surgeon: Extensions and performance comparisons. In: Cowan, J. D., Tesauro, G., and Alspector, J. (Eds.). *Advances in Neural Information Processing Systems 6,* San Mateo, CA, Morgan Kaufman.

Le Cun, Y., Denker, J. S., and Solla, S. A. (1990). Optimal brain damage. In: D. S. Tourctzky (Ed.). *Advances in Neural Information Processing Systems 2,* San Mateo, CA, Morgan Kaufman.

Probabilistic Interpretation of Population Codes

Richard S. Zemel
zemel@u.arizona.edu

Peter Dayan
dayan@ai.mit.edu

Alexandre Pouget
alex@salk.edu

Abstract

We present a theoretical framework for population codes which generalizes naturally to the important case where the population provides information about a whole probability distribution over an underlying quantity rather than just a single value. We use the framework to analyze two existing models, and to suggest and evaluate a third model for encoding such probability distributions.

1 Introduction

Population codes, where information is represented in the activities of whole populations of units, are ubiquitous in the brain. There has been substantial work on how animals should and/or actually do extract information about the underlying encoded quantity.[5,3,11,9,12] With the exception of Anderson,[1] this work has concentrated on the case of extracting a *single value* for this quantity. We study ways of characterizing the joint activity of a population as coding a whole *probability distribution* over the underlying quantity.

Two examples motivate this paper: place cells in the hippocampus of freely moving rats that fire when the animal is at a particular part of an environment,[8] and cells in area MT of monkeys firing to a random moving dot stimulus.[7] Treating the activity of such populations of cells as reporting a single value of their underlying variables is inadequate if there is (a) insufficient information to be sure (*eg* if a rat can be uncertain as to whether it is in place x_A or x_B then perhaps place cells for both locations should fire; or (b) if multiple values underlie the input, as in the whole distribution of moving random dots in the motion display. Our aim is to capture the computational power of representing a probability distribution over the underlying parameters.[6]

RSZ is at University of Arizona, Tucson, AZ 85721; PD is at MIT, Cambridge, MA 02139; AP is at Georgetown University, Washington, DC 20007. This work was funded by McDonnell-Pew, NIH, AFOSR and startup funds from all three institutions.

In this paper, we provide a general statistical framework for population codes, use it to understand existing methods for coding probability distributions and also to generate a novel method. We evaluate the methods on some example tasks.

2 Population Code Interpretations

The starting point for almost all work on neural population codes is the neurophysiological finding that many neurons respond to particular variable(s) underlying a stimulus according to a unimodal tuning function such as a Gaussian. This characterizes cells near the sensory periphery and also cells that report the results of more complex processing, including receiving information from groups of cells that themselves have these tuning properties (in MT, for instance). Following Zemel & Hinton's[13] analysis, we distinguish two spaces: the *explicit* space which consists of the activities $\mathbf{r} = \{r_i\}$ of the cells in the population, and a (typically low dimensional) *implicit* space which contains the underlying information $\mathcal{X}$ that the population encodes in which they are tuned. All processing on the basis of the activities $\mathbf{r}$ has to be referred to the implicit space, but it itself plays no explicit role in determining activities.

Figure 1 illustrates our framework. At the top is the measured activities of a population of cells. There are two key operations. **Encoding:** What is the relationship between the activities $\mathbf{r}$ of the cells and the underlying quantity in the world $\mathcal{X}$ that is represented? **Decoding:** What information about the quantity $\mathcal{X}$ can be extracted from the activities? Since neurons are generally noisy, it is often convenient to characterize encoding (operations A and B) in a probabilistic way, by specifying $\mathcal{P}[\mathbf{r}|\mathcal{X}]$. The simplest models make a further assumption of conditional independence of the different units given the underlying quantity $\mathcal{P}[\mathbf{r}|\mathcal{X}] = \prod_i \mathcal{P}[r_i|\mathcal{X}]$ although others characterize the degree of correlation between the units. If the encoding model is true, then a Bayesian decoding model specifies that the information $\mathbf{r}$ carries about $\mathcal{X}$ can be characterized precisely as: $\mathcal{P}[\mathcal{X}|\mathbf{r}] \propto \mathcal{P}[\mathbf{r}|\mathcal{X}]\mathcal{P}[\mathcal{X}]$, where $\mathcal{P}[\mathcal{X}]$ is the prior distribution about $\mathcal{X}$ and the constant of proportionality is set so that $\int_\mathcal{X} \mathcal{P}[\mathcal{X}|\mathbf{r}]d\mathcal{X} = 1$. Note that starting with a deterministic quantity $\mathcal{X}$ in the world, encoding in the firing rates $\mathbf{r}$, and decoding it (operation C) results in a probability distribution over $\mathcal{X}$. This uncertainty arises from the stochasticity represented by $\mathcal{P}[\mathbf{r}|\mathcal{X}]$. Given a loss function, we could then go on to extract a single value from this distribution (operation D).

We attack the common assumption that $\mathcal{X}$ is a single value of some variable $\mathbf{x}$, *eg* the single position of a rat in an environment, or the single coherent direction of motion of a set of dots in a direction discrimination task. This does not capture the subtleties of certain experiments, such as those in which rats can be made to be uncertain about their position, or in which one direction of motion predominates yet there are several simultaneous motion directions.[7] Here, the natural characterization of $\mathcal{X}$ is actually a whole probability distribution $\mathcal{P}[\mathbf{x}|\omega]$ over the value of the variable $\mathbf{x}$ (perhaps plus extra information about the number of dots), where ω represents all the available information. We can now cast two existing classes of proposals for population codes in terms of this framework.

The Poisson Model

Under the Poisson encoding model, the quantity $\mathcal{X}$ encoded is indeed one particular value which we will call $\mathbf{x}$, and the activities of the individual units are independent,

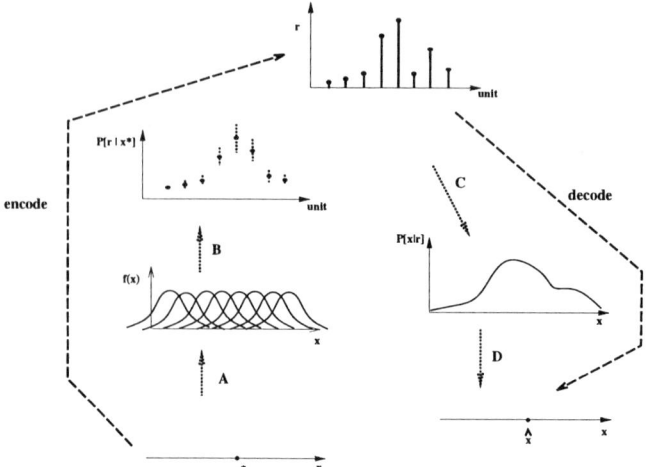

Figure 1: *Left:* encoding maps $\mathcal{X}$ from the world through tuning functions (A) into mean activities (B), leading to *Top:* observed activities **r**. We assume complete knowledge of the variables governing systematic changes to the activities of the cells. Here $\mathcal{X}$ is a single value $\mathbf{x}^*$ in the space of underlying variables. *Right:* decoding extracts $\mathcal{P}[\mathcal{X}|\mathbf{r}]$ (C); a single value can be picked (D) from this distribution given a loss function.

with the terms $\mathcal{P}[r_i|\mathbf{x}] = e^{-f_i(\mathbf{x})}(f_i(\mathbf{x}))^{r_i}/r_i!$. The activity r_i could, for example, be the number of spikes the cell emits in a fixed time interval following the stimulus onset. A typical form for the tuning function $f_i(\mathbf{x})$ is Gaussian $f_i(\mathbf{x}) \propto e^{-(\mathbf{x}-\mathbf{x}_i)^2/2\sigma^2}$ about a preferred value $\mathbf{x}_i$ for cell i. The Poisson decoding model is:[3, 11, 9, 12]

$$\log \mathcal{P}[\mathbf{x}|\mathbf{r}] = \mathcal{K} - \sum_i f_i(\mathbf{x}) + \sum_i r_i \log f_i(\mathbf{x}) \quad (1)$$

where $\mathcal{K}$ is a constant with respect to $\mathbf{x}$.

Although simple, the Poisson model makes the the assumption criticized above, that $\mathcal{X}$ is just a single value $\mathbf{x}$. We argued for a characterization of the quantity $\mathcal{X}$ in the world that the activities of the cells encode as now $\mathcal{P}[\mathbf{x}|\omega]$. We describe below a method of encoding that takes exactly this definition of $\mathcal{X}$. However, wouldn't $\mathcal{P}[\mathbf{x}|\mathbf{r}]$ from Equation 1 be good enough? Not if $f_i(\mathbf{x})$ are Gaussian, since

$$\log \mathcal{P}[\mathbf{x}|\mathbf{r}] = \mathcal{K}' - \frac{1}{2}\left(\frac{\sum_i r_i}{\sigma^2}\right)\left(\mathbf{x} - \frac{\sum_i r_i \mathbf{x}_i}{\sum_i r_i}\right)^2,$$

completing the square, implying that $\mathcal{P}[\mathbf{x}|\mathbf{r}]$ is Gaussian, and therefore inevitably unimodal. Worse, the width of this distribution goes down with $\sum_i r_i$, making it, in most practical cases, a close approximation to a delta function.

The KDE Model

Anderson[1, 2] set out to represent whole probability distributions over $\mathbf{x}$ rather than just single values. Activities $\mathbf{r}$ represent distribution $\hat{\mathcal{P}}^\mathbf{r}(\mathbf{x})$ through a linear combination of basis functions $\psi_i(\mathbf{x})$, ie $\hat{\mathcal{P}}^\mathbf{r}(\mathbf{x}) = \sum_i r'_i \psi_i(\mathbf{x})$ where r'_i are normalized such that $\hat{\mathcal{P}}^\mathbf{r}(\mathbf{x})$ is a probability distribution. The kernel functions $\psi_i(\mathbf{x})$ are *not* the tuning functions $f_i(\mathbf{x})$ of the cells that would commonly be measured in an experiment. They need have *no* neural instantiation; instead, they form part of the interpretive structure for the population code. If the $\psi_i(\mathbf{x})$ are probability distributions, and so are positive, then the range of spatial frequencies in $\mathcal{P}[\mathbf{x}|\omega]$ that they can reproduce in $\hat{\mathcal{P}}^{\mathbf{r}}(\mathbf{x})$ is likely to be severely limited.

In terms of our framework, the KDE model specifies the method of decoding, and makes encoding its corollary. Evaluating KDE requires some choice of encoding – representing $\mathcal{P}[\mathbf{x}|\omega]$ by $\hat{\mathcal{P}}^{\mathbf{r}}(\mathbf{x})$ through appropriate $\mathbf{r}$. One way to encode is to use the Kullback-Leibler divergence as a measure of the discrepancy between $\mathcal{P}[\mathbf{x}|\omega]$ and $\sum_i r'_i \psi_i(\mathbf{x})$ and use the expectation-maximization (EM) algorithm to fit the $\{r'_i\}$, treating them as mixing proportions in a mixture model.[4] This relies on $\{\psi_i(\mathbf{x})\}$ being probability distributions themselves. The *projection method*[1] is a one-shot linear filtering based alternative using the $\mathcal{L}_2$ distance. r_i are computed as a projection of $\mathcal{P}[\mathbf{x}|\omega]$ onto tuning functions $f_i(\mathbf{x})$ that are calculated from $\psi_j(\mathbf{x})$.

$$r_i = \int_{\mathbf{x}} \mathcal{P}[\mathbf{x}|\omega] f_i(\mathbf{x}) d\mathbf{x} \quad \mathbf{f_i(x)} = \sum_j A_{ij}^{-1} \psi_j(\mathbf{x}) \quad A_{ij} = \int_{\mathbf{x}} \psi_i(\mathbf{x}) \psi_j(\mathbf{x}) d\mathbf{x} \quad (2)$$

$f_i(\mathbf{x})$ are likely to need regularizing,[1] particularly if the $\psi_i(\mathbf{x})$ overlap substantially.

3 The Extended Poisson Model

The KDE model is likely to have difficulty capturing in $\hat{\mathcal{P}}^{\mathbf{r}}(\mathbf{x})$ probability distributions $\mathcal{P}[\mathbf{x}|\omega]$ that include high frequencies, such as delta functions. Conversely, the standard Poisson model decodes almost *any* pattern of activities $\mathbf{r}$ into something that rapidly approaches a delta function as the activities increase. Is there any middle ground?

We extend the standard Poisson encoding model to allow the recorded activities $\mathbf{r}$ to depend on general $\mathcal{P}[\mathbf{x}|\omega]$, having Poisson statistics with mean:

$$\langle r_i \rangle = \int_{\mathbf{x}} \mathcal{P}[\mathbf{x}|\omega] f_i(\mathbf{x}) d\mathbf{x}. \quad (3)$$

This equation is identical to that for the KDE model (Equation 2), except that variability is built into the Poisson statistics, and decoding is now required to be the Bayesian inverse of encoding. Note that since r_i depends stochastically on $\mathcal{P}[\mathbf{x}|\omega]$, the full Bayesian inverse will specify a distribution $\mathcal{P}[\mathcal{P}[\mathbf{x}|\omega]|\mathbf{r}]$ over possible distributions. We summarize this by an approximation to its most likely member— we perform an approximate form of maximum likelihood, not in the value of $\mathbf{x}$, but in distributions over $\mathbf{x}$. We approximate $\mathcal{P}[\mathbf{x}|\omega]$ as a piece-wise constant histogram which takes the value ϕ_j in $(\mathbf{x}_j, \mathbf{x}_{j+1}]$, and $f_i(\mathbf{x})$ by a piece-wise constant histogram that take the values f_{ij} in $(\mathbf{x}_j, \mathbf{x}_{j+1}]$. Generally, the maximum *a posteriori* estimate for $\{\phi_j\}$ can be shown to be derived by maximizing:

$$L(\{\hat{\phi}_j\}) = \sum_i r_i \log \left[\sum_j \hat{\phi}_j f_{ij} \right] - \epsilon \sum_j \left(\hat{\phi}_j - \hat{\phi}_{j+1} \right)^2 \quad (4)$$

where ϵ is the variance of a smoothness prior. We use a form of EM to maximize the likelihood and adopt the crude approximation of averaging neighboring values

Operation	Extended Poisson	KDE (Projection)	KDE (EM)
Encode $\langle r_i \rangle$	$\langle r_i \rangle = h \left[\int_x \mathcal{P}[x\|\omega] f_i(x) dx \right]$ $f_i(x) = R_{max} \mathcal{N}(x_i, \sigma)$	$\langle r_i \rangle = h \left[R_{max} \int_x \mathcal{P}[x\|\omega] f_i(x) dx \right]$ $f_i(x) = \sum_j A_{ij}^{-1} \psi_j(x)$ $A_{ij} = \int_x \psi_i(x) \psi_j(x) dx$	$\langle r_i \rangle = h [R_{max} r_i']$ r_i' to max. L
Decode $\hat{\mathcal{P}}^r(x)$	$\hat{\mathcal{P}}^r(x)$ to max. L $\hat{r}_i = \int_x \hat{\mathcal{P}}^r(x) f_i(x) dx \approx \sum_j \phi_j f_{ij}$	$\hat{\mathcal{P}}^r(x) = \sum_i r_i' \psi_i(x)$ $r_i' = r_i / \sum_j r_j$	$\hat{\mathcal{P}}^r(x) = \sum_i r_i' \psi_i(x)$
Likelihood	$L = \log \mathcal{P}[\{\phi_j\}\|\{r_i\}] \approx \sum_i r_i \log \hat{r}_i$		$L = \int_x \mathcal{P}[x\|\omega] \log \hat{\mathcal{P}}^r(x) dx$
Error	$G = \sum_i r_i \log(r_i / \hat{r}_i)$	$E = \int_x \left[\hat{\mathcal{P}}^r(x) - \mathcal{P}[x\|\omega] \right]^2 dx$	$G = \int_x \mathcal{P}[x\|\omega] \log \frac{\mathcal{P}[x\|\omega]}{\hat{\mathcal{P}}^r(x)} dx$

Table 1: A summary of the key operations with respect to the framework of the interpretation methods compared here. $h[]$ is a rounding operator to ensure integer firing rates, and $\psi_i(x) = \mathcal{N}(x_i, \sigma)$ are the kernel functions for the KDE method.

of $\hat{\phi}_j$ on successive iterations. By comparison with the linear decoding of the KDE method, Equation 4 offers a *non-linear* way of combining a set of activities $\{r_i\}$ to give a probability distribution $\hat{\mathcal{P}}^r(x)$ over the underlying variable x. The computational complexities of Equation 4 are irrelevant, since decoding is only an implicit operation that the system need never actually perform.

4 Comparing the Models

We illustrate the various models by showing the faithfulness with which they can represent two bimodal distributions. We used $\sigma = 0.3$ for the kernel functions (KDE) and the tuning functions (extended Poisson model) and used 50 units whose x_i were spaced evenly in the range $x = [-10, 10]$. Table 1 summarizes the three methods.

Figure 2a shows the decoded version of a mixture of two broad Gaussians $1/2\mathcal{N}[-2, 1] + 1/2\mathcal{N}[2, 1]$. Figure 2b shows the same for a mixture of two narrow Gaussians $\frac{1}{2}\mathcal{N}[-2, .2] + \frac{1}{2}\mathcal{N}[2, .2]$. All the models work well for representing the broad Gaussians; both forms of the KDE model have difficulty with the narrow Gaussians. The EM version of KDE puts all its weight on the nearest kernel functions, and so is too broad; the projection version 'rings' in its attempt to represent the narrow components of the distributions. The extended Poisson model reconstructs with greater fidelity.

5 Discussion

Informally, we have examined the consequences of the seemingly obvious step of saying that if a rat, for instance, is uncertain about whether it is at one of two places, then place cells representing both places could be activated. The complications

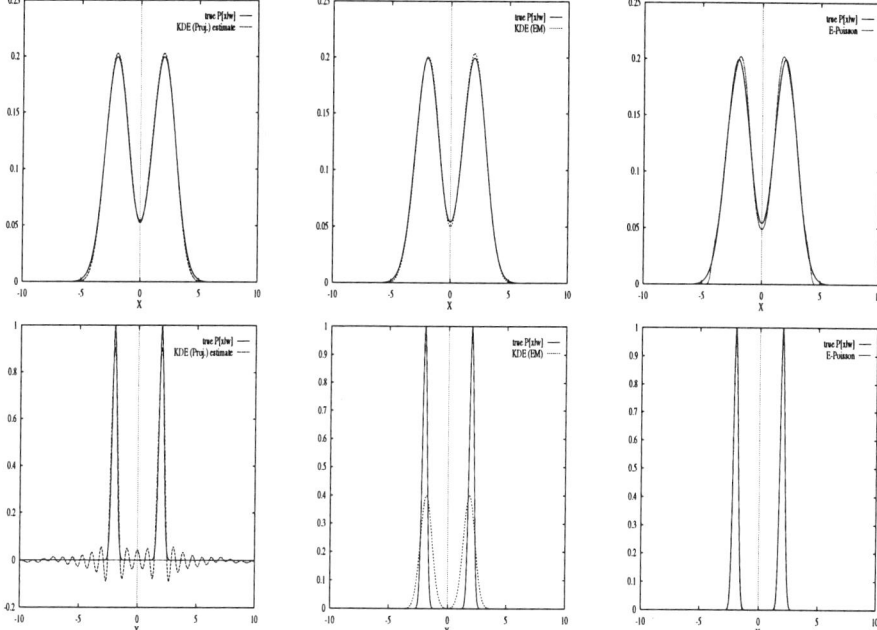

Figure 2: a) (upper) All three methods provide a good fit to the bimodal Gaussian distribution when its variance is sufficiently large ($\tau = 1.0$). b) (lower) The KDE model has difficulty when $\tau = 0.2$.

come because the structure of the interpretation changes – for instance, one can no longer think of maximum likelihood methods to extract a single value from the code directly.

One main fruit of our resulting framework is a method for encoding and decoding probability distributions that is the natural extension of the (provably inadequate) standard Poisson model for encoding and decoding single values. Cells have Poisson statistics about a mean determined by the integral of the whole probability distribution, weighted by the tuning function of the cell. We suggested a particular decoding model, based on an approximation to maximum likelihood decoding to a discretized version of the whole probability distribution, and showed that it reconstructs broad, narrow and multimodal distributions more accurately than either the standard Poisson model or the kernel density model. Stochasticity is built into our method, since the units are supposed to have Poisson statistics, and it is therefore also quite robust to noise. The decoding method is not biologically plausible, but provides a quantitative lower bound to the faithfulness with which a set of activities can code a distribution.

Stages of processing subsequent to a population code might either *extract* a single value from it to control behavior, or *integrate* it with information represented in other population codes to form a combined population code. Both operations must be performed through standard neural operations such as taking non-linear weighted sums and possibly products of the activities. We are interested in how much information is preserved by such operations, as measured against the non-biological standard of our decoding method. Modeling extraction requires modeling the loss function – there is some empirical evidence about this from a motion experiment in which electrical stimulation of MT cells was pitted against input from a moving stimulus.[10] However, much works remains to be done.

Integrating two or more population codes to generate the output in the form of another population code was stressed by Hinton,[6] who noted that it directly relates to the notion of generalized Hough transforms. We are presently studying how a system can *learn* to perform this combination, using the EM-based decoder to generate targets. One special concern for combination is how to understand noise. For instance, the visual system can be behaviorally extraordinarily sensitive – detecting just a handful of photons. However, the outputs of real cells at various stages in the system are apparently quite noisy, with Poisson statistics. If noise is added at every stage of processing and combination, then the final population code will not be very faithful to the input. There is much current research on the issue of the creation and elimination of noise in cortical synapses and neurons.

A last issue that we have not treated here is certainty or magnitude. Hinton's[6] idea of using the sum total activity of a population to code the certainty in the existence of the quantity they represent is attractive, provided that there is some independent way of knowing what the scale is for this total. We have used this scaling idea in both the KDE and the extended Poisson models. In fact, we can go one stage further, and interpret greater activity still as representing information about the existence of multiple objects or multiple motions. However, this treatment seems less appropriate for the place cell system — the rat is presumably always certain that it is somewhere. There it is plausible that the absolute level of activity could be coding something different, such as the familiarity of a location.

An entire collection of cells is a terrible thing to waste on representing just a single value of some quantity. Representing a whole probability distribution, at least with some fidelity, is not more difficult, provided that the interpretation of the encoding and decoding are clear. We suggest some steps in this direction.

References

[1] Anderson, CH (1994). *International Journal of Modern Physics C*, **5**, 135–137.

[2] Anderson, CH & Van Essen, DC (1994). In *Computational Intelligence Imitating Life*, 213–222. New York: IEEE Press.

[3] Baldi, P & Heiligenberg, W (1988). *Biological Cybernetics*, **59**, 313-318.

[4] Dempster, AP, Laird, NM & Rubin, DB (1997). *Proceedings of the Royal Statistical Society*, **B 39**, 1-38.

[5] Georgopoulos, AP, Schwartz, AB & Kettner, RE (1986). *Science*, **243**, 1416–1419.

[6] Hinton, GE (1992). *Scientific American*, **267(3)** 105-109.

[7] Newsome, WT, Britten, KH & Movshon, JA (1989). *Nature*, **341**, 52-54.

[8] O'Keefe, J & Dostrovsky, J (1971). *Brain Research*, **34**, 171-175.

[9] Salinas, E & Abbott, LF (1994). *Journal of Computational Neuroscience*, **1**, 89–107.

[10] Salzman, CD & Newsome, WT (1994). *Science*, **264**, 231-237.

[11] Seung, HS & Sompolinsky, H (1993). *Proceedings of the National Academy of Sciences, USA*, **90**, 10749–10753.

[12] Snippe, HP (1996). *Neural Computation*, **8**, 29–37.

[13] Zemel, RS & Hinton, GE (1995). *Neural Computation*, **7**, 549–564.

Part V
Implementation

VLSI Implementation of Cortical Visual Motion Detection Using an Analog Neural Computer

Ralph Etienne-Cummings
Electrical Engineering,
Southern Illinois University,
Carbondale, IL 62901

Jan Van der Spiegel
The Moore School,
University of Pennsylvania,
Philadelphia, PA 19104

Naomi Takahashi
The Moore School,
University of Pennsylvania,
Philadelphia, PA 19104

Alyssa Apsel
Electrical Engineering,
California Inst. Technology,
Pasadena, CA 91125

Paul Mueller
Corticon Inc.,
3624 Market Str,
Philadelphia, PA 19104

Abstract

Two dimensional image motion detection neural networks have been implemented using a general purpose analog neural computer. The neural circuits perform spatiotemporal feature extraction based on the cortical motion detection model of Adelson and Bergen. The neural computer provides the neurons, synapses and synaptic time-constants required to realize the model in VLSI hardware. Results show that visual motion estimation can be implemented with simple sum-and-threshold neural hardware with temporal computational capabilities. The neural circuits compute general 2D visual motion in real-time.

1 INTRODUCTION

Visual motion estimation is an area where spatiotemporal computation is of fundamental importance. Each distinct motion vector traces a unique locus in the space-time domain. Hence, the problem of visual motion estimation reduces to a feature extraction task, with each feature extractor tuned to a particular motion vector. Since neural networks are particularly efficient feature extractors, they can be used to implement these visual motion estimators. Such neural circuits have been recorded in area MT of macaque monkeys, where cells are sensitive and selective to 2D velocity (Maunsell and Van Essen, 1983).

In this paper, a hardware implementation of 2D visual motion estimation with spatiotemporal feature extractors is presented. A silicon retina with parallel, continuous time edge detection capabilities is the front-end of the system. Motion detection neural networks are implemented on a general purpose analog neural computer which is composed of programmable analog neurons, synapses, axon/dendrites and synaptic time-constants (Van der Spiegel *et al.*, 1994). The additional computational freedom introduced by the synaptic time-constants, which are unique to this neural computer, is required to realize the spatiotemporal motion estimators. The motion detection neural circuits are based on the early 1D model of Adelson and Bergen and recent 2D models of David Heeger (Adelson and Bergen, 1985; Heeger *et al.*, 1996). However, since the neurons only computed delayed weighted sum-and-threshold functions, the models must be modified. The original models require division for intensity normalization and a quadratic non-linearity to extract spatiotemporal energy. In our model, normalization is performed by the silicon retina with a large contrast sensitivity (all edges are normalized to the same output), and rectification replaces the quadratic non-linearity. Despite these modifications, we show that the model works correctly. The visual motion vector is implicitly coded as a distribution of neural activity.

Due to its computational complexity, this method of image motion estimation has not been attempted in discrete or VLSI hardware. The general purpose analog neural computer offers a unique avenue for implementing and investigating this method of visual motion estimation. The analysis, implementation and performance of spatiotemporal visual motion estimators are discussed.

2 SPATIOTEMPORAL FEATURE EXTRACTION

The technique of estimating motion with spatiotemporal feature extraction was proposed by Adelson and Bergen in 1985 (Adelson and Bergen, 1985). It emerged out of the observation that a point moving with constant velocity traces a line in the space-time domain, shown in figure 1a. The slope of the line is proportional to the velocity of the point. Hence, the velocity is represented as the orientation of the line. Spatiotemporal orientation detection units, similar to those proposed by Hubel and Wiesel for spatial orientation detection, can be used for detecting motion (Hubel and Wiesel, 1962). In the frequency domain, the motion of the point is also a line where the slope of the line is the velocity of the point. Hence orientation detection filters, shown as circles in figure 1b, can be used to measure the motion of the point relative to their tuned velocity. A population of these tuned filters, figure 1c, can be used to measure general image motion.

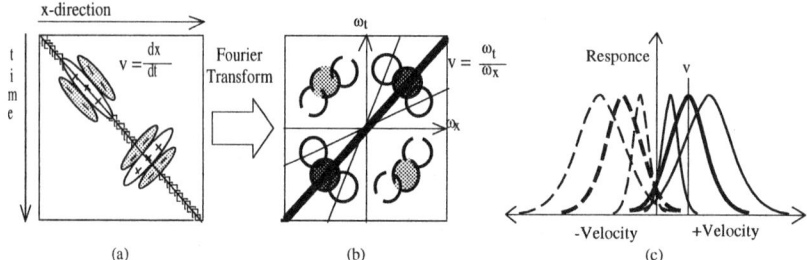

Figure 1: (a) 1D Motion as Orientation in the Space-Time Domain. (b) and (c) Motion detection with Oriented Spatiotemporal Filters.

If the point exhibits 2D motion, the problem is substantially more complicated, as observed by David Heeger (1987). A point executing 2D motion spans a plane in the frequency domain. The spatiotemporal orientation filter tuned to this motion must also span a plane (Heeger *et al.*, 1987, 1996). Figure 2a shows a filter tuned to 2D motion. Unfortunately, this torus shaped filter is difficult to realize without special mathematical tools. Furthermore, to create a general set of filters for measuring general 2D motion, the filters must cover all the spatiotemporal frequencies and all the possible velocities of the stimuli. The latter requirement is particularly difficult to obtain since there are two degrees of freedom (v_x, v_y) to cover.

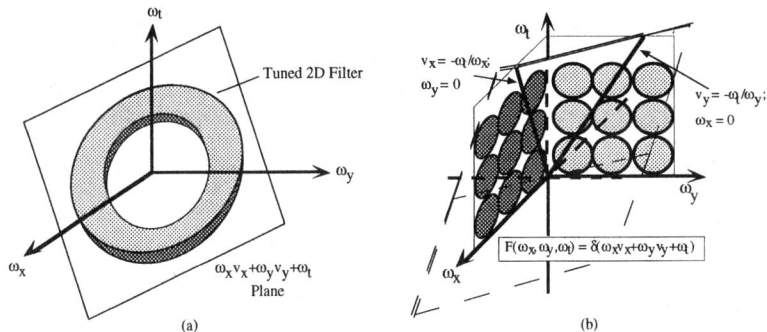

Figure 2: (a) 2D Motion Detection with 2D Oriented Spatiotemporal Filters. (b) General 2D Motion Detection with 2 Sets of 1D Filters.

To circumvent these problems, our model decomposes the image into two orthogonal images, where the perpendicular spatial variation within the receptive field of the filters are eliminated using spatial smoothing. Subsequently, 1D spatiotemporal motion detection is used on each image to measure the velocity of the stimuli. This technique places the motion detection filters, shown as the circles in figure 2b, only in the ω_x-ω_t and ω_y-ω_t planes to extract 2D motion, thereby drastically reducing the complexity of the 2D motion detection model from $O(n^2)$ to $O(2n)$.

2.1 CONSTRUCTING THE SPATIOTEMPORAL MOTION FILTERS

The filter tuned to a velocity v_{ox} (v_{0y}) is centered at ω_{ox} (ω_{oy}) and ω_{ot} where $v_{ox} = \omega_{ot}/\omega_{ox}$ ($v_{0y} = \omega_{ot}/\omega_{0y}$). To create the filters, quadrature pairs (i.e. odd and even pairs) of spatial and temporal band-pass filters centered at the appropriate spatiotemporal frequencies are summed and differenced (Adelson and Bergen, 1985). The $\pi/2$ phase relationship between the filters allows them to be combined such that they cancel in opposite quadrants, leaving the desired oriented filter, as shown in figure 3a. Equation 1 shows examples of quadrature pairs of spatial and temporal filters implemented. The coefficients of the filters balance the area under their positive and negative lobes. The spatial filters in equation 1 have a 5 x 5 receptive field, where the sampling interval is determined by the silicon retina. Figure 3b shows a contour plot of an oriented filter (α=11 rads/s, δ_2=2δ_1=40α).

$$
\begin{aligned}
S(even) &= [0.5 - 0.32Cos(\omega_x) - 0.18Cos(2\omega_x)] \quad &(a) \\
S(odd) &= [-0.66jSin(\omega_x) - 0.32jSin(2\omega_x)] \quad &(b) \\
T(even) &= \frac{-\omega_t^2 \delta_2}{(j\omega_t + \alpha)(j\omega_t + \delta_1)(j\omega_t + \delta_2)}; \alpha << \delta_1 \approx \delta_2 \quad &(c) \\
T(odd) &= \frac{j\omega_t \delta_1 \delta_2}{(j\omega_t + \alpha)(j\omega_t + \delta_1)(j\omega_t + \delta_2)}; \alpha << \delta_1 \approx \delta_2 \quad &(d) \\
\text{Left Motion} &= S(e)T(e) - S(o)T(o) \text{ or } S(e)T(o) - S(o)T(e) \quad &(e) \\
\text{Right Motion} &= S(e)T(e) + S(o)T(o) \text{ or } S(e)T(o) + S(o)T(e) \quad &(f)
\end{aligned}
\tag{1}
$$

To cover a wide range of velocity and stimuli, multiple filters are constructed with various velocity, spatial and temporal frequency selectivity. Nine filters are chosen per dimension to mosaic the ω_x-ω_t and ω_y-ω_t planes as in figure 2b. The velocity of a stimulus is given by the weighted average of the tuned velocity of the filters, where the weights are the magnitudes of each filter's response. All computations for 2D motion detection based on cortical models have been realized in hardware using a large scale general purpose analog neural computer.

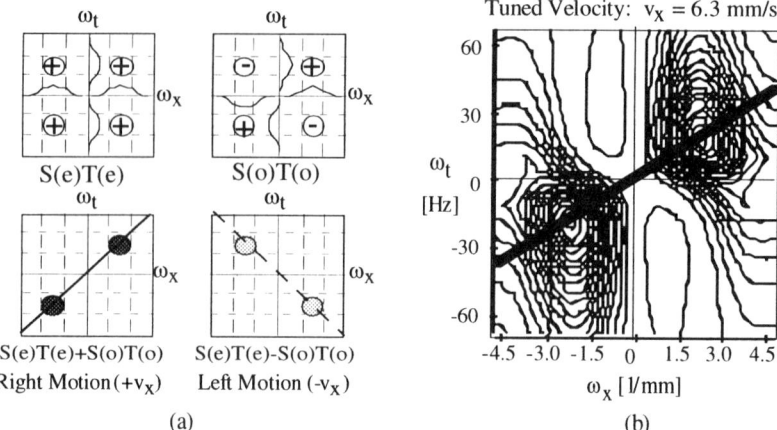

Figure 3: (a) Constructing Oriented Spatiotemporal Filters. (b) Contour Plot of One of the Filters Implemented.

3 HARDWARE IMPLEMENTATION

3.1 GENERAL PURPOSE ANALOG NEURAL COMPUTER

The computer is intended for fast prototyping of neural network based applications. It offers the flexibility of programming combined with the real-time performance of a hardware system (Mueller, 1995). It is modeled after the biological nervous system, i.e. the cerebral cortex, and consists of electronic analogs of neurons, synapses, synaptic time constants and axon/dendrites. The hardware modules capture the functional and computational aspects of the biological counterparts. The main features of the system are: configurable interconnection architecture, programmable neural elements, modular and expandable architecture, and spatiotemporal processing. These features make the network ideal to implement a wide range of network architectures and applications.

The system, shown in part in figure 4, is constructed from three types of modules (chips): (1) neurons, (2) synapses and (3) synaptic time constants and axon/dendrites. The neurons have a piece-wise linear transfer function with programmable (8bit) threshold and minimum output at threshold. The synapses are implemented as a programmable resistance whose values are variable (8 bit) over a logarithmic range between 5KOhm and 10Mohm. The time constant, realized with a load-compensated transconductance amplifier, is selectable between 0.5ms and 1s with a 5 bit resolution. The axon/dendrites are implemented with an analog cross-point switch matrix. The neural computer has a total of 1024 neurons, distributed over 64 neuron modules, with 96 synaptic inputs per neuron, a total of 98,304 synapses, 6,656 time constants and 196,608 cross point switches. Up to 3,072 parallel buffered analog inputs/outputs and a neuron output analog mulitplexer are available. A graphical interface software, which runs on the host computer, allows the user to symbolically and physically configure the network and display its behavior (Donham, 1994). Once a particular network has been loaded, the neural network runs independently of the digital host and operates in a fully analog, parallel and continuous time fashion.

3.2 NEURAL IMPLEMENTATION OF SPATIOTEMPORAL FILTERS

The output of the silicon retina, which transforms a gray scale image into a binary image of edges, is presented to the neural computer to implement the oriented spatiotemporal filters. The first and second derivatives of Gaussian functions are chosen to implement the odd and even spatial filters, respectively. They are realized by feeding the outputs of

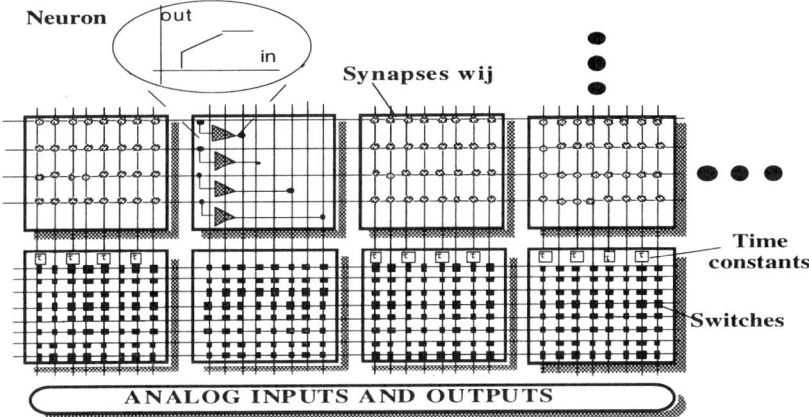

Figure 4: Block Diagram of the Overall Neural Network Architecture.

the retina, with appropriate weights, into a layer of neurons. Three parallel channels with varying spatial scales are implemented for each dimension. The output of the even (odd) spatial filter is subsequently fed to three parallel even (odd) temporal filters, which also have varying temporal tuning. Hence, three *non-oriented* pairs of spatiotemporal filters are realized for each channel. Six oriented filters are realized by summing and differencing the non-oriented pairs. The oriented filters are rectified, and lateral inhibition is used to accentuate the higher response. Figure 4 shows a schematic of the neural circuitry used to implement the orientation selective filters.

The image layer of the network in figure 5 is the direct, parallel output of the silicon retina. A 7 x 7 pixel array from the retina is decomposed into 2, 1 x 7 orthogonal linear images, and the nine motion detection filters are implemented per image. The total number of neurons used to implement this network is 152, the number of synapse is 548 and the number of time-constants is 108. The time-constant values ranges from 0.75 ms to 375 ms. After the networks have been programmed into the VLSI chips of the neural computer, the system operates in full parallel and continuous time analog mode. Consequently, this system realizes a silicon model for biological visual image motion measurement, starting from the retina to the visual cortex.

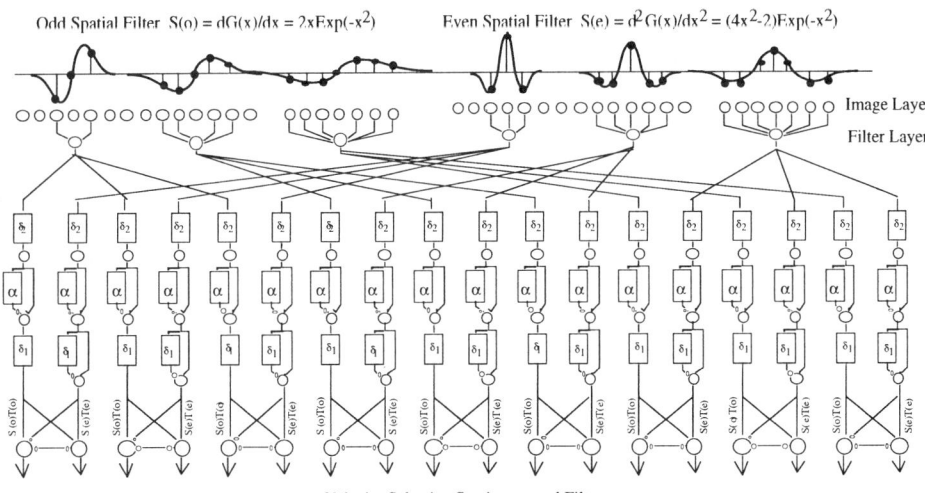

Figure 5: Neural Network Implementation of the Oriented Spatiotemporal Filters.

4 RESULTS

The response of the spatiotemporal filters implemented with the neural computer are shown in figure 6. The figure is obtained by sampling the output of the neurons at 1MHz using the on-chip analog multiplexers. In figure 6a, the impulse response of the spatial filters are shown as a point moves across their receptive field. Figure 6b shows the outputs of the even and odd temporal filters for the moving point. At the output of the filters, the even and odd signals from the spatial filters are no longer out of phase. This transformation yields to constructive or destructive interference when they are summed and differenced. When the point move in opposite direction, the odd filters changes such that the output of the temporal filters become 180° out of phase. Subsequent summing and differencing will have the opposite result. Figure 6c shows the output for all nine x-velocity selective filters as a point moves with positive velocity.

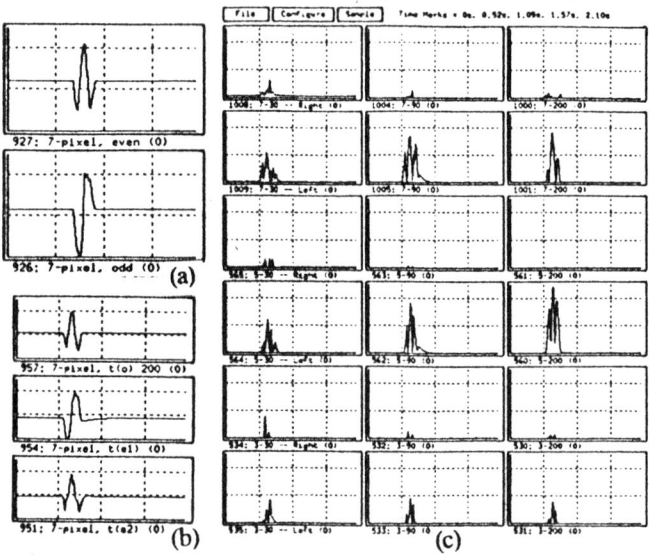

Figure 6: Output of the Neural Circuits for a Moving Point: (a) Spatial Filters, (b) Temporal Filters and (c) Motion Filters.

Figure 7 shows the tuning curves for the filters tuned to x-motion. The variations in the responses are due to variations in the analog components of the neural computer. Some aliasing is noticeable in the tuning curves when there is a minor peak in the opposite direction. This results from the discrete properties of the spatial filters, as seen in

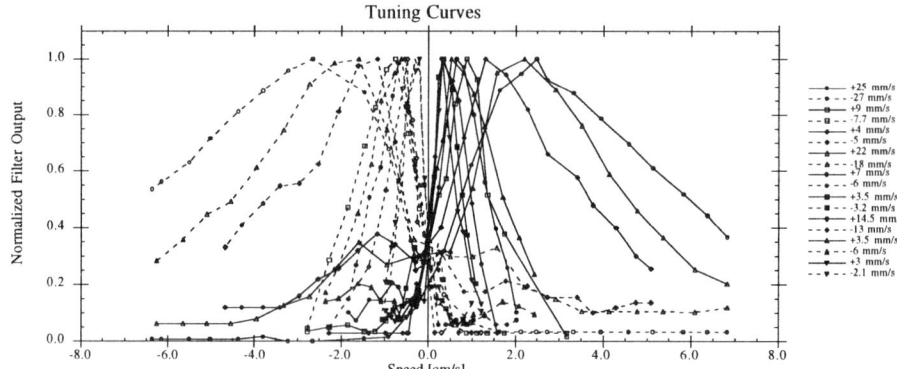

Figure 7: Tuning Curves for the Nine X-Motion Filters.

figure 3b. Due to the lateral inhibition employed, the aliasing effects are minimal. Similar curves are obtained for the y-motion tuned filters.

For a point moving with $v_x = 8.66$ mm/s and $v_y = 5$ mm/s, the output of the motion filters are shown in Table 1. Computing a weighted average using equation 2, yields $v_{xm} = 8.4$ mm/s and $v_{ym} = 5.14$ mm/s. This result agrees with the actual motion of the point.

$$v_m = \sum_i v_i^{tuned} O_i \Big/ \sum_i O_i \qquad (2)$$

Table 1: Filter Responses for a Point Moving at 10 mm/s at 30°.

	X Filters [Speed in mm/s]								Y Filters [Speed in mm/s]							
Tuned Speed	25	9	4	22	7	3.5	14.5	3.5	3	26	9.5	5	20	7.8	3.7	15	4.1	3.5
Response	0.52	0.95	0.57	0.53	0.9	0.3	0.75	0.9	0.31	0.35	0.67	0.92	0.3	0.85	0.9	0.54	0.9	0.9
Tuned Speed	-27	-7.7	-5	-18	-6	-3.2	-13	-6	-2.1	-25	-8	-4.1	-21	-7	-4	-14	-5	-2
Response	0.0	0.05	0.1	0.1	0.05	0.05	0.02	0.05	0.1	0.1	0.08	0.1	0.3	0.05	0.01	0.23	0.05	0.1

5 CONCLUSION

2D image motion estimation based on spatiotemporal feature extraction has been implemented in VLSI hardware using a general purpose analog neural computer. The neural circuits capitalize on the temporal processing capabilities of the neural computer. The spatiotemporal feature extraction approach is based on the 1D cortical motion detection model proposed by Adelson and Bergen, which was extended to 2D by Heeger *et al*. To reduce the complexity of the model and to allow realization with simple sum-and-threshold neurons, we further modify the 2D model by placing filters only in the ω_x-ω_t and ω_y-ω_t planes, and by replacing quadratic non-linearities with a rectifiers. The modifications do not affect the performance of the model. While this technique of image motion detection requires too much hardware for focal plane implementation, our results show that it is realizable when a silicon "brain," with large numbers of neurons and synaptic time constant, is available. This is very reminiscent of the biological master.

References

E. Adelson and J. Bergen, "Spatiotemporal Energy Models for the Perception of Motion," *J. Optical Society of America*, Vol. A2, pp. 284-99, 1985

C. Donham, "Real Time Speech Recognition using a General Purpose Analog Neurocomputer," *Ph.D. Thesis*, Univ. of Pennsylvania, Dept. of Electrical Engineering, Philadelphia, PA, 1995.

D. Heeger, E. Simoncelli and J. Movshon, "Computational Models of Cortical Visual Processing," *Proc. National Academy of Science*, Vol. 92, no. 2, pp. 623, 1996

D. Heeger, "Model for the Extraction of Image Flow," *J. Optical Society of America*, Vol. 4, no. 8, pp. 1455-71, 1987

D. Hubel and T. Wiesel, "Receptive Fields, Binocular Interaction and Functional Architecture in the Cat's Visual Cortex," *J. Physiology*, Vol. 160, pp. 106-154, 1962

J. Maunsell and D. Van Essen, "Functional Properties of Neurons in Middle Temporal Visual Area of the Macaque Monkey. I. Selectivity for Stimulus Direction, Speed and Orientation," *J. Neurophysiology*, Vol. 49, no. 5, pp. 1127-47, 1983

P. Mueller, J. Van der Spiegel, D. Blackman, C. Donham and R. Etienne-Cummings, "A Programmable Analog Neural Computer with Applications to Speech Recognition," *Proc. Comp. & Info. Sci. Symp.* (CISS), J. Hopkins, May 1995.

A spike based learning neuron in analog VLSI

Philipp Häfliger
Institute of Neuroinformatics
ETHZ/UNIZ
Gloriastrasse 32
CH-8006 Zürich
Switzerland
e-mail: hafliger@neuroinf.ethz.ch
tel: ++41 1 257 26 84

Misha Mahowald
Institute of Neuroinformatics
ETHZ/UNIZ
Gloriastrasse 32
CH-8006 Zürich
Switzerland
e-mail: misha@neuroinf.ethz.ch
tel: ++41 1 257 26 84

Lloyd Watts
Arithmos, Inc.
2730 San Tomas Expressway, Suite 210
Santa Clara, CA 95051-0952
USA
e-mail: lloyd@arithmos.com
tel: 408 982 4490, x219

Abstract

Many popular learning rules are formulated in terms of continuous, analog inputs and outputs. Biological systems, however, use action potentials, which are digital-amplitude events that encode analog information in the inter-event interval. Action-potential representations are now being used to advantage in neuromorphic VLSI systems as well. We report on a simple learning rule, based on the Riccati equation described by Kohonen [1], modified for action-potential neuronal outputs. We demonstrate this learning rule in an analog VLSI chip that uses volatile capacitive storage for synaptic weights. We show that our time-dependent learning rule is sufficient to achieve approximate weight normalization and can detect temporal correlations in spike trains.

1 INTRODUCTION

It is an ongoing debate how information in the nervous system is encoded and carried between neurons. In many subsystems of the brain it is now believed that it is done by the exact timing of spikes. Furthermore spike signals on VLSI chips allow the use of address-event busses to solve the problem of the large connectivity in neural networks [3, 4]. For these reasons our artificial neuron and others [2] use spike signals to communicate. Additionally the weight updates at the synapses are determined by the relative timing of presynaptic and postsynaptic spikes, a mechanism that has recently been discovered to operate in cortical synapses [5, 7, 6].

Weight normalization is a useful property of learning rules. In order to perform the normalization, some information about the whole weight vector must be available at every synapse. We use the neuron's output spikes (The neuron's output is the product of the weight and the input vector), which retrogradely propagate through the dendrites to the synapses (as has been observed in biological neurons [5]). In our model approximate normalization is an implicit property of the learning rule.

2 THE LEARNING RULE

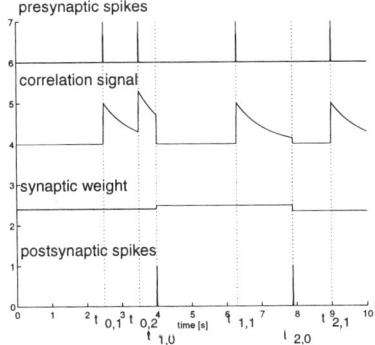

Figure 1: A snapshot of the simulation variables involved at one synapse. With $\tau = 0.83s$

The core of the learning rule is a local 'correlation signal' c at every synapse. It records the 'history' of presynaptic spikes. It is incremented by 1 with every presynaptic spike and decays in time with time constant τ:

$$c(t_{m,0}) = 0$$
$$c(t_{m,n}) = e^{-\frac{t_{m,n}-t_{m,n-1}}{\tau}} c(t_{m,n-1}) + 1 \quad , \quad n > 0 \quad , \quad t_{m,n} \leq t_{m+1,0} \quad (1)$$

$t_{m,0}$ is the time of the m'th postsynaptic spike and $t_{m,n}$ ($n > 0$) is the time of the n'th presynaptic spike after the m'th postsynaptic spike. The weight changes when the cell fires an action potential:

$$w(t_{m,0}) = w(t_{m-1,0}) + \alpha e^{-\frac{t_{m,0}-t_{m-1,s}}{\tau}} c(t_{m-1,s}) - \beta w(t_{m-1,0}) \quad (2)$$
$$s = max\{v : t_{m-1,v} \leq t_{m,0}\}$$

where w is the weight at this synapse. $t_{m-1,s}$ means the last event (presynaptic or postsynaptic spike) before the m'th postsynaptic spike. α and β are parameters influencing learning speed and weight vector normalization (see (5)).

Our learning rule is designed to react to temporal correlations between spikes in the input signals. However, to show the normalizing of the weights we analyze its behavior by making some simplifying assumptions on the input and output signals; e.g. the intervals of the presynaptic and the postsynaptic spike train are Poisson distributed and there is no correlation between single spikes. Therefore we can represent the signals by their instantaneous average frequencies O and $\vec{I}$. Now the simplified learning rule can be written as:

$$\frac{\delta}{\delta t}\vec{w} = \alpha l(O)\vec{I} - \beta \vec{w} O \quad (3)$$

$$l(O) = O\tau(1 - e^{-\frac{1}{O\tau}}) \quad (4)$$

$l(O)$ represents the average percentage to which the correlation signal is reduced between weight updates (output spikes). So when the neuron's average firing rate fulfills $O \gg \frac{1}{\tau}$, one can approximate $l(O) \approx 1$. (3) is thus reduced to the Riccati equation described by Kohonen [1]. This rule would not be Hebbian, but normalizes the weight vector (see (5)). Note that if the correlation signal does not decay, then our rule matches exactly the Riccati equation. We will further refer to it as the Modified Riccati Rule (MRR). Whereas if $O \ll \frac{1}{\tau}$ then $l(O) \approx O\tau$, which is a Hebbian learning rule also described in [1].

If we assume that the spiking mechanism preserves $O = \vec{w}^T \vec{I}$ and insert it in (3), it follows for the equilibrium state:

$$\|\vec{w}\| = \sqrt{l(O)\frac{\alpha}{\beta}} \quad (5)$$

Since $l(O) < 1$ the weight vector will never be longer than $\sqrt{\frac{\alpha}{\beta}}$. This property also holds when the simplifying assumptions are removed. The vector will always be smaller, as it is with no decay of the correlation signals, since the decay only affects the incrementing part of the rule.

Matters get much more complicated with the removal of the assumption of the pre- and postsynaptic trains being independently Poisson distributed. With an integrate-and-fire neuron for instance, or if there exist correlations between spikes of the input trains, it is no longer possible to express what happens in terms of rate coding only (with $\vec{I}$ and O). (3) is still valid as an approximation but temporal relationships between pre- and postsynaptic spikes become important. Presynaptic spikes immediately followed by an action potential will have the strongest increasing effect on the synapse's weight.

3 IMPLEMENTATION IN ANALOG VLSI

We have implemented a learning rule in a neuron circuit fabricated in a $2.0\mu m$ CMOS process. This neuron is a preliminary design that conforms only approximately to the MRR. The neuron uses an integrate-and-fire mechanism to generate action potentials (Figure 2).

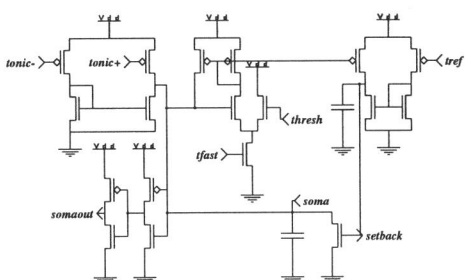

Figure 2: Integrate-and-fire neuron. The *soma* capacitor holds the somatic membrane voltage. This voltage is compared to a threshold *thresh* with a differential pair. When it crosses this threshold it gets pulled up through the mirrored current from the differential pair. This same current gets also mirrored to the right and starts to pull up a second leaky capacitor (*setback*) through a small W/L transistor, so this voltage rises slowly. This capacitor voltage finally opens a transistor that pulls *soma* back to ground where it restarts integrating the incoming current. The parameters *tonic+* and *tonic−* are used to add or subtract a constant current to the soma capacitor. *tref* allows the spike-width to be changed.

Not shown, but also part of the neuron, are two non-learning synapses: one excitatory and one inhibitory. Each of three learning synapses contains a storage capacitor for the synaptic weight and for the correlation signal (Figure 3).

The correlation signal c is simplified to a binary variable in this implementation. When an input spike occurs, the correlation signal is set to 1. It is set to 0 whenever the neuron produces an output-spike or after a fixed time-period (T in (7)) if there is no other input spike:

$$c(t_{m,0}) = 0$$
$$c(t_{m,n}) = 1 \quad , \quad n > 0 \quad , \quad t_{m,n} \le t_{m+1,0} \tag{6}$$

This approximation unfortunately tends to eliminate differences between highly active inputs and weaker inputs. Nevertheless the weight changes with every output spike:

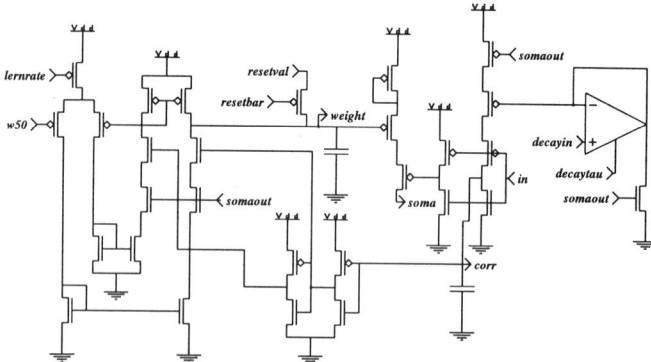

Figure 3: The CMOS learning-synapse incorporates the learning mechanism. The *weight* capacitor holds the weight, the *corr* capacitor stores the correlation signal representation. The magnitude of the weight increment and decrement are computed by a differential pair (upper left *w50*). These currents are mirrored to the synaptic weight and gated by digital switches encoding the state of the correlation signal and of the somatic action potential. The correlation signal reset is mediated by a leakage transistor, *decayin*, which has a tonic value, but is increased dramatically when the output neuron fires.

$$w(t_{m,0}) = w(t_{m-1,0}) \begin{cases} +\alpha \frac{e^{w50}}{e^{w50}+e^{w(t_{m-1,0})}} & \text{if } c(t_{m-1,s}) = 1 \text{ and } t_{m,0} - t_{m-1,s} < T \\ -\alpha \frac{e^{w(t_{m-1,0})}}{e^{w50}+e^{w(t_{m-1,0})}} & \text{otherwise} \end{cases}$$

$$s = max\{v : t_{m-1,v} \le t_{m,0}\} \tag{7}$$

w is the weight on one synapse, c is the correlation signal of that synapse, and α is a parameter that controls how fast the weight changes. (See in the previous section for a description of $t_{m,n}$.) The weight, w_{50}, is the equilibrium value of the synaptic weight when the occurrence of an input spike is fifty percent correlated with the occurrence of an output spike. This implementation differs from the Riccati rule in that either the weight increment or the weight decrement, but not both, are executed upon each output spike. Also, the weight increment is a function of the synaptic weight. The circuit was implemented this way to try and achieve an equilibrium value for the synaptic weight equal to the fraction of the time that the input neuron fired relative to the times the output neuron fired. This is the correct equilibrium value for the synaptic weight in the Riccati rule. The evolution of a synaptic weight is depicted in Figure 4.

The synaptic weight vector normalization in this implementation is accurate only when the assumptions of the design are met. These assumptions are that there is one or fewer input spikes per synapse for every output spike. This assumption is easier to meet when there are many synapses formed with the neuron, so that spikes from multiple inputs combine to drive the cell to threshold. Since we have only three synapses, this approximation is usually violated. Nevertheless, the weights compete with one another and therefore the length of the weight vector is limited. Competition between synaptic weights occurs because if one weight is stronger, it causes the output neuron to spike and this suppresses the other input that has not fired. Future revision of the chip will conform more closely to the MRR.

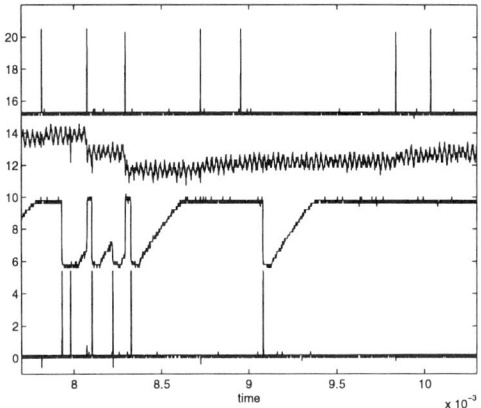

Figure 4: A snapshot of the learning behavior of a single VLSI synapse: The top trace is the neuron output (1V/division), the upper middle trace is the synaptic weight (lower voltage means a stronger synaptic weight) (25mV/division), the lower middle trace is a representation of the correlation signal (1 V/division)(it has inverted sense too) and the bottom trace is the presynaptic activity (1V/division). The weight changes only when an output spike occurs. The timeout of the correlation signal is realized with a decay and a threshold. If the correlation signal is above threshold, the weight is strengthened. If the signal has decayed below threshold at the time of an output spike, the weight is weakened. The magnitude of the change of the weight is a function of the absolute magnitude of the weight. This weight was weaker than w_{50}, so the increments are bigger than the decrements.

4 TEMPORAL CORRELATION IN INPUT SPIKE TRAINS

Figure 5 illustrates the ability of our learning rule to detect temporal correlations in spike trains. A simulated neuron strengthens those two synapses that receive 40% coincident spikes, although all four synapses get the same average spike frequencies.

5 DISCUSSION

Learning rules that make use of temporal correlations in their spike inputs/outputs provide biologically relevant mechanisms of synapse modification [5, 7, 6]. Analog VLSI implementations allow such models to operate in real time. We plan to develop such analog VLSI neurons using floating gates for weight storage and an address-event bus for interneuronal connections. These could then be used in realtime applications in adaptive 'neuromorphic' systems.

Acknowledgments

We thank the following organizations for their support: SPP Neuroinformatik des Schweizerischen Nationalfonds, Centre Swiss d'Electronique et de Microtechnique, U.S. Office of Naval Research and the Gatsby Charitable Foundation.

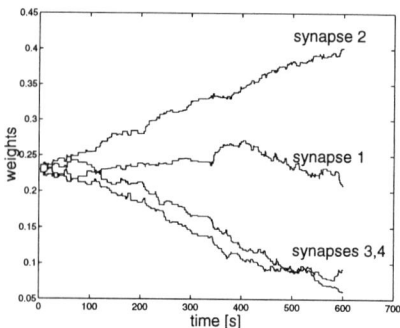

Figure 5: In this simulation we use a neuron with four synapses. All of them get input trains of the same average frequency (20Hz). Two of those input trains are the result of independent Poisson processes (synapses 3 and 4), the other two are the combination of two Poisson processes (synapses 1 and 2): One that is independent of any other (12Hz) and one that is shared by the two with slightly different time delays (8Hz): Synapse 1 gets those coincident spikes 0.01 seconds earlier than synapse 2. Synapse 2 gets stronger because when it together with synapse 1 triggered an action potential, it was the last synapse being active before the postsynaptic spike. The parameters were: $\alpha = 0.004, \beta = 0.02, \tau = 11ms$

References

[1] Tuevo Kohonen. *Self-Organization and Associative Memory*. Springer, Berlin, 1984.

[2] D.K. Ferry L.A. Akers and R.O. Grondin. Synthetic neural systems in the 1990s. *An introduction to neural and electronic networks, Academic Press (Zernetzer, Davis, Lau, McKenna)*, pages 359–387, 1995.

[3] J. Lazzaro, J. Wawrzynek, M. Mahowald, M. Sivilotti, and D. Gillespie. Silicon auditory processors as computer peripherals. *IEEE Trans. Neural Networks*, 4:523–528, 1993.

[4] A. Mortara and E. A. Vittoz. A communication architecture tailored for analog VLSI artificial neural networks: intrinsic performance and limitations. *IEEE Translation on Neural Networks*, 5:459–466, 1994.

[5] G. J. Stuart and B. Sakmann. Active propagation of somatic action potentials into neocortical pyramidal cell dendrites. *Nature*, 367:69ff, 1994.

[6] M. V. Tsodyks and H. Markram. Redistribution of synaptic efficacy between neocortical pyramidal neurons. *Nature*, 382:807–810, 1996.

[7] R. Yuste and W. Denk. Dendritic spines as basic functional units of neuronal integration. *Nature*, 375:682–684, 1995.

An Analog Implementation of the Constant Statistics Constraint For Sensor Calibration

John G. Harris and Yu-Ming Chiang
Computational Neuro-Engineering Laboratory
Department of Computer and Electrical Engineering
University of Florida
Gainesville, FL 32611

Abstract

We use the *constant statistics* constraint to calibrate an array of sensors that contains gain and offset variations. This algorithm has been mapped to analog hardware and designed and fabricated with a 2um CMOS technology. Measured results from the chip show that the system achieves invariance to gain and offset variations of the input signal.

1 Introduction

Transistor mismatches and parameter variations cause unavoidable nonuniformities from sensor to sensor. A one-time calibration procedure is normally used to counteract the effect of these fixed variations between components. Unfortunately, many of these variations fluctuate with time–either with operating point (such as data-dependent variations) or with external conditions (such as temperature). Calibrating these sensors one-time only at the "factory" is not suitable–much more frequent calibration is required. The sensor calibration problem becomes more challenging as an increasing number of different types of sensors are integrated onto VLSI chips at higher and higher integration densities. Ullman and Schechtman studied a simple gain adjustment algorithm but their method provides no mechanism for canceling additive offsets [10]. Scribner has addressed this nonuniformity correction problem in software using a neural network technique but it will be difficult to integrate this complex solution into analog hardware [9]. A number of researchers have studied sensors that output the time-derivative of the signal[9][4]. A simple time derivative cancels any additive offset in the signal but also loses all of the DC and most of the low frequency temporal information present. The offset-correction method proposed by this paper, in effect, uses a time-derivative with an extremely long time constant thereby preserving much of the low-frequency information present in the signal. However, even if an ideal time-derivative approximation is used to cancel out additive offsets, the standard deviation process described in this paper can be used to factor out gain variations.

We hope to obtain some clues for sensory adaptation from neurobiological systems which possess a tremendous ability to adapt to the surrounding environment at multiple time-scales and at multiple stages of processing. Consider the following experiments:

- After staring at a single curved line ten minutes, human subjects report that the amount of curvature perceived appears to decrease. Immediately after training, the subjects then were shown a straight line and perceived it as slightly curved in the opposite direction[5].

- After staring long enough at an object in continuous motion, the motion seems to decrease with time. Immediately after adaptation, subjects perceive motion in the opposite direction when looking at stationary objects. This experiment is called the waterfall effect[2].

- Colors tend to look less saturated over time. Color after-images are perceived containing exactly the opponent colors of the original scene[1].

Though the purpose of these biological adaptation mechanisms is not clear, some theories suggest that these methods allow for fine-tuning the visual system through long-term averaging of measured visual parameters[10]. We will apply such continuous-calibration procedures to VLSI sensor calibration.

The real-world variable $x(t)$ is transduced by a nonlinear response curve into a measured variable $y(t)$. For a single operating point, the linear approximation can be written as:

$$y(t) = ax(t) + b \qquad (1)$$

with a and b being the multiplicative gain and additive offset respectively. The gain and offset values vary from pixel to pixel and may vary slowly over time. Current infra-red focal point arrays (IRFPAs) are limited by their inability to calibrate out component variations [3]. Typically, off-board digital calibration is used to correct nonuniformities in these detector arrays; Special calibration images are used to calibrate the system at startup. One-time calibration procedures such as these do not take into account other operating points and will fail to recalibrate for any drift in the parameters.

2 Implementing Natural Constraints

A continuous calibration system must take advantage of natural constraints available during the normal operation of the sensors. One theory holds that biological systems adapt to the long-term average of the stimulus. For example, the constraints for the three psychophysical examples mentioned above (curvature, motion and color adaptation) may rely on the following constraints:

- The average line is straight.
- The average motion is zero.
- The average color is gray.

The system adapts over time in the direction of this average, where the average must be taken over a very long time: from minutes to hours. We use two additional constraints for offset/gain normalization, namely:

- The average pixel intensities are identical.
- The variances of the input for each pixel are all identical.

Each of these constraints assumes that the photoarray is periodically moving in the real-world and that the average statistics each pixels sees should be constant when averaged over a very long time. In pathological situations where humans or machines are forced to stare at a single static scene for a long time, we violate this assumption.

We estimate the time-varying mean and variance by using an exponentially shaped window into the past. The equations for mean and variance are:

$$m(t) = \frac{1}{\tau} \int_0^\infty y(t-\Delta)e^{-\Delta/\tau} d\Delta \qquad (2)$$

and

$$s(t) = \frac{1}{\tau} \int_0^\infty |y(t-\Delta) - m(t-\Delta)| e^{-\Delta/\tau} d\Delta \qquad (3)$$

The $m(t)$ and $s(t)$ in Equation 2 and 3 can be expressed as low-pass filters with inputs $y(t)$ and $|y(t) - m(t)|$ respectively. To simplify the hardware implementation further, we chose the L_1 (absolute value) definition of variance instead of the more usual L_2 definition. The L_1 definition is an equally acceptable definition of signal variation in terms of the complete calibration system. Using this definition, no squares or square roots need be calculated. An added benefit of the L_1 norm is that it provides robustness to outliers in the estimation.

A zero-mean, unity variance[1] signal can then be produced with the following shift/normalization formula:

$$x(t) = \frac{y(t) - m(t)}{s(t)} \qquad (4)$$

Equation 2, Equation 3 and Equation 4 constitute a new algorithm for continuously calibrating systems with gain and offset variations. Note that without additional apriori knowledge about the values of the gains and offsets, it is impossible to recover the true value of the signal $x(t)$ given an infinite history of $y(t)$. This is an ill-posed problem even with fixed but unknown gain and offset parameters for each sensor. All that can be done is to calibrate each sensor output to have zero offset and unity variance. After calibration, each sensor would therefore all have the same offset and variance when averaged over a long time. The fundamental assumption embedded

---

[1] For simplicity the signal $s(t)$ will be called the variance estimate throughout the rest of this paper even though technically $s(t)$ is neither the variance nor the standard deviation.

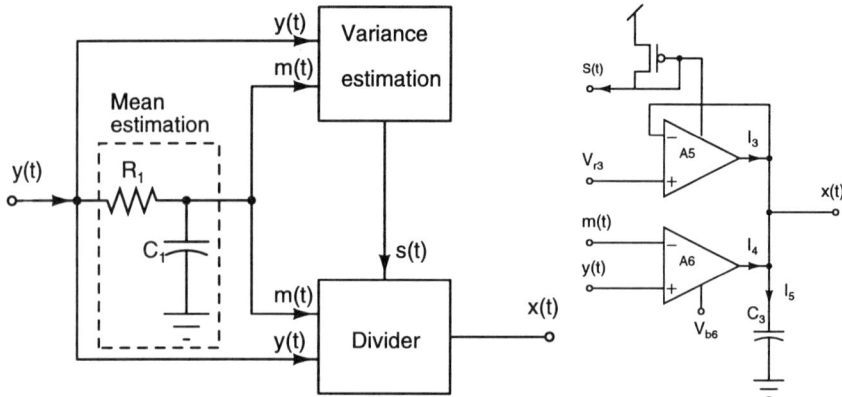

Figure 1: Left: block diagram of continuous-time calibration system, Right: schematic of the divider circuit.

in this algorithm is that each sensor measures real-world quantities with the same statistical properties (e.g., mean and variance). For example, this would mean that all pixels in a camera should eventually see the same average intensity when integrated over a long enough time. This assumption leads to other system-level constraints–in this case, the camera must be periodically moving.

We have successfully demonstrated this algorithm in software for the case of nonuniformity (gain and offset) correction of images [6]. Since there may be potentially thousands of sensors per chip, it is desirable to build calibration circuitry using subthreshold analog MOS technology to achieve ultra-low power consumption[8]. The next section describes the analog VLSI implementation of this algorithm.

3 Continuous-time calibration circuit

The block diagram of the continuous-time gain and offset calibration circuit is shown in Figure 1a. This system includes three building blocks: a mean estimation circuit, a variance estimation circuit and a divider circuit. As is shown, the mean of the signal can be easily extracted by a RC low-pass filter circuit. Since there may be potentially thousands of sensors per chip, it is desirable to build calibration circuitry using subthreshold analog MOS technology to achieve ultra-low power consumption[8].

Figure 2 shows the schematic of the variance estimation circuit. A full-wave rectifier [8] operating in the sub-threshold region is used to obtain the absolute value of the difference between the input and its mean. In the linear region, the current I_{out} is proportional to $|y(t) - m(t)|$. As indicated in Equation 3, I_{out} has to be low-pass filtered to obtain $s(t)$. In Figure 2, transconductance amplifiers A_3, A_4 and capacitor C_2 are used to form a current mode low-pass filter. For signals in the linear region, we can derive the Laplace transform of V_1 as:

$$V_1(s) = \frac{R}{RC_2 s + 1} I_{out}(s) \qquad (5)$$

which is a first-order low-pass filter for I_{out}. The value of R is a function of several

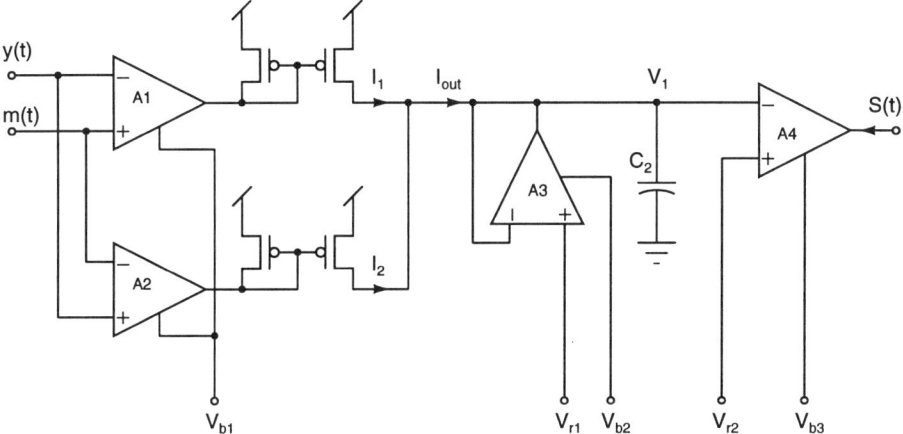

Figure 2: *Variance estimation circuit. The triangle symbols represent 5-transistor transconductance amplifiers that output a current proportional to the difference of their inputs.*

fabrication constants and an adjustable bias current. Figure 3(a) shows the expected linear relationship between the measured variance $s(t)$ and the peak-to-peak amplitude of the sine-wave input.

The third building block in the calibration system is the divider circuit shown in Figure 1b. A fed-back multiplier is used to enforce the constraint that $y(t) - m(t)$ is proportional to $x(t)s(t)$ which results in a scaled version of Equation 4. The characteristics of the divider have been measured and shown in Figure 3(b). With a fixed V_{b6} and $m(t)$, we sweep $y(t)$ from $m(t) - 0.3V$ to $m(t) + 0.3V$ and measure the the change of output. A family of input/output characteristics with $s(t) =20$, 25, 30, 40, 50, 60 and 70nA is shown in Figure 3(b). The divider circuit has been tested up to frequencies of 45kHz.

The first version of the calibration circuit has been designed and fabricated in a 2-um CMOS technology. The chip includes the major parts of this calibration circuit: the variance estimation circuit and divider circuit. In our initial design, the mean estimation circuit, which is simply a RC low-pass filter, was built off-chip. However, it can be easily integrated on-chip using a transconductance amplifier and a capacitor.

The calibration results for a signal with gain and offset variations are shown in Figure 4. The input signal is a sine wave with a severe gain and offset jump as shown at the top of Figure 4. At the middle of Figure 4, the convergence of the variance estimation is illustrated. It takes a short time for the circuit to converge after any change of the mean or variance or of the input signal. At the bottom of Figure 4, we show the calibrated signal produced by the chip. The output eventually converges to a zero-mean, constant-height sine wave independent of the values of the DC offset and amplitude of the input sine wave. Additional experiments have shown that with the input amplitude changing from 20mV to 90mV, the measured output amplitude varies by less than 3mV. Similarly, when the DC offset is varied from 1.5V to 3.5V, the amplitude of the output varies by less than 5mV. These

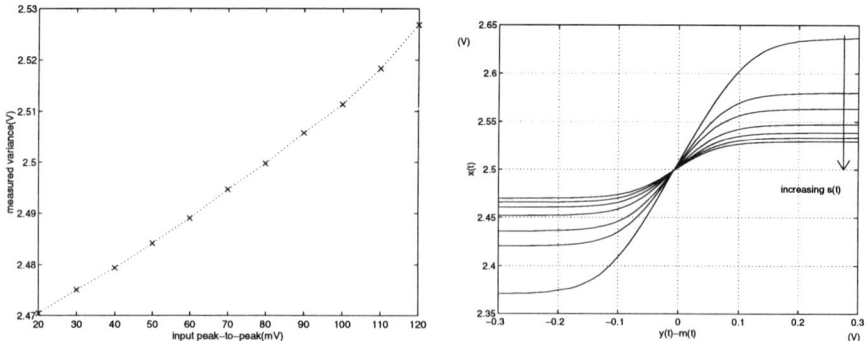

Figure 3: Left (a) shows the characteristics of measured variance $s(t)$ vs. peak-to-peak input voltage. Right (b) shows the characteristics of divider with different $s(t)$.

results demonstrate that system is invariant to gain and offset variations of the input.

4 Conclusions

The calibration circuit has been demonstrated with the time-constants on the order of 100ms. In many applications, much longer time constants will be necessarily and these cannot be reached with on-chip capacitors even with subthreshold CMOS operation. We expect to use floating-gate techniques where essentially arbitrarily long time-constants can be achieved. Mead has demonstrated a novel adaptive adaptive silicon retina that requires UV light for adaptation to occur [7]. The adaptive silicon retina implemented the constant average brightness constraint. The unoptimized layout area of one of our calibration circuits is about 250x300 um^2 in 2um CMOS technology. A future challenge will be to reduce this area and replace the large on-chip capacitors with floating gates.

Acknowledgments

The authors would like to acknowledge an NSF CAREER Award and Office of Naval Research contract #N00014-94-1-0858.

References

[1] M. Akita, C. Graham, and Y. Hsia. Maintaining an absolute hue in the presence of different background colors. *Vision Research*, 4:539–556, 1964.

[2] V.R. Carlson. Adaptation in the perception of visual velocity. *J. Exp. Psychol.*, 64(2):192–197, 1962.

[3] M.R. Kruer D.A. Scribner and J.M. Killiany. Infrared focal plane array technology. *Proc. IEEE*, 79(1):66–85, 1991.

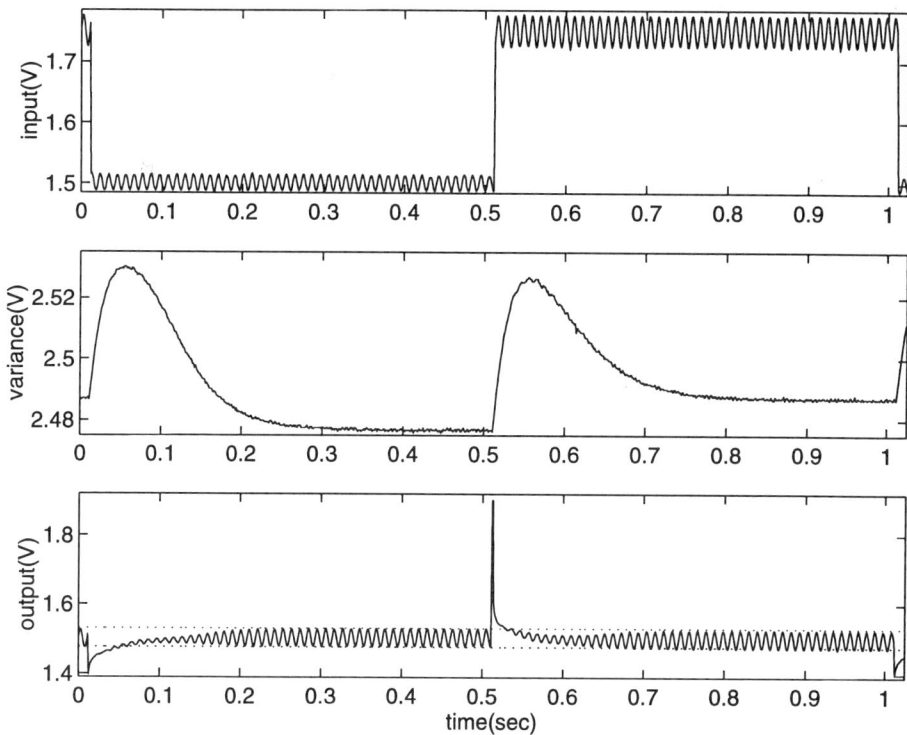

Figure 4: *Calibrating signal with offset and gain variations. Top: the input signal, $y(t)$. Middle: the computed signal variance $s(t)$. Bottom: the output signal, $x(t)$.*

[4] T. Delbrück. An electronic photoreceptor sensitive to small changes. In D. Touretzky, editor, *Advance in Neural Information Processing Systems, Volume 1*, pages 720–727. Morgan Kaufmann, Palo Alto, CA, 1989.

[5] J. Gibson. Adaptation, aftereffect and contrast in the perception of curved lines *J. Exp. Psychol.*, 16:1–16, 1933.

[6] J. G. Harris. Continuous-time calibration of VLSI sensors for gain and offset variations. In *SPIE Internatiional Symposium on Aerospace Sensing and Dual-Use Photonices:Smart Focal Plane Arrays and Focal Plane Array Testing*, pages 23–33, Orlando, FL, April 1995.

[7] C. Mead. Adaptive retina. In C. Mead and M. Ismail, editors, *Analog VLSI Implementation of Neural Systems*, pages 239–246. Kluwer Academic Publishers, 1989.

[8] C. Mead. *Analog VLSI and Neural Systems*. Addison-Wesley, 1989.

[9] D.A. Scribner, K.A. Sarkady, M.R. Kruer, J.T. Calufield, J.D. Hunt, M. Colbert, and M. Descour. Adaptive retina-like preprocessing for imaging detector arrays. In *Proc. of the IEEE International Conference on Neural Networks*, pages 1955–1960, San Francisco, CA, Feb. 1993.

[10] S. Ullman and G. Schechtman. Adaptation and gain normalization. *Proc. R. Soc. Lond. B*, 216:299–313, 1982.

Analog VLSI Circuits for Attention-Based, Visual Tracking

Timothy K. Horiuchi
Computation and Neural Systems
California Institute of Technology
Pasadena, CA 91125
timmer@klab.caltech.edu

Tonia G. Morris
Electrical and Computer Engineering
Georgia Institute of Technology
Atlanta, GA, 30332-0250
tmorris@eecom.gatech.edu

Christof Koch
Computation and Neural Systems
California Institute of Technology
Pasadena, CA 91125

Stephen P. DeWeerth
Electrical and Computer Engineering
Georgia Institute of Technology
Atlanta, GA, 30332-0250

Abstract

A one-dimensional visual tracking chip has been implemented using neuromorphic, analog VLSI techniques to model selective visual attention in the control of saccadic and smooth pursuit eye movements. The chip incorporates focal-plane processing to compute image saliency and a winner-take-all circuit to select a feature for tracking. The target position and direction of motion are reported as the target moves across the array. We demonstrate its functionality in a closed-loop system which performs saccadic and smooth pursuit tracking movements using a one-dimensional mechanical eye.

1 Introduction

Tracking a moving object on a cluttered background is a difficult task. When more than one target is in the field of view, a decision must be made to determine which target to track and what its movement characteristics are. If motion information is being computed in parallel across the visual field, as is believed to occur in the middle temporal area (MT) of primates, some mechanism must exist to preferentially extract the activity of the neurons associated with the target at the appropriate

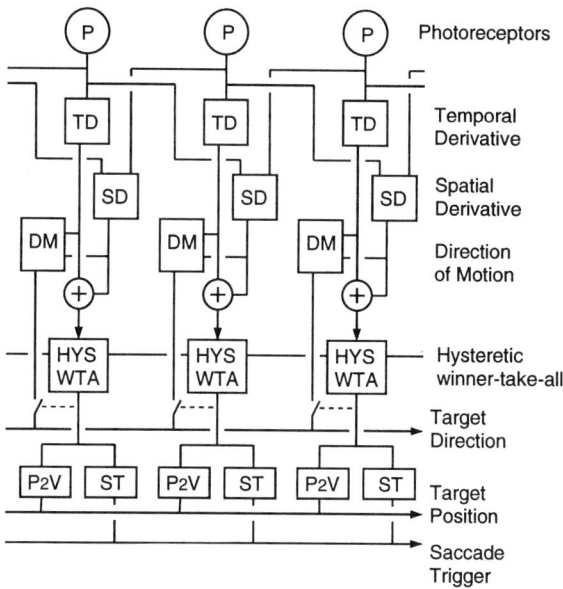

Figure 1: System Block Diagram: P = adaptive photoreceptor circuit, TD = temporal derivative circuit, SD = spatial derivative, DM = direction of motion, HYS WTA = hysteretic winner-take-all, P2V = position to voltage, ST = saccade trigger. The TD and SD are summed to form the saliency map from which the WTA finds the maximum. The output of the WTA steers the direction-of-motion information onto a common output line. Saccades are triggered when the selected pixel is outside a specified window located at the center of the array.

time. Selective visual attention is believed to be this mechanism.

In recent years, many studies have indicated that selective visual attention is involved in the generation of saccadic [10] [7] [12] [15] and smooth pursuit eye movements [9] [6] [16]. These studies have shown that attentional enhancement occurs at the target location just before a saccade as well as at the target location during smooth pursuit. In the case of saccades, attempts to dissociate attention from the target location has been shown to disrupt the accuracy or latency.

Koch and Ullman [11] have proposed a model for attentional selection based on the formation of a saliency map by combining the activity of elementary feature maps in a topographic manner. The most salient locations are where activity from many different feature maps coincide or at locations where activity from a preferentially-weighted feature map, such as temporal change, occurs. A winner-take-all (WTA) mechanism, acting as the center of the attentional "spotlight," selects the location with the highest saliency.

Previous work on analog VLSI-based, neuromorphic, hardware simulation of visual tracking include a one-dimensional, saccadic eye movement system triggered by temporal change [8] and a two-dimensional, smooth pursuit system driven by visual motion detectors [5]. Neither system has a mechanism for figure-ground discrimination of the target. In addition to this overt form of attentional shifting, covert

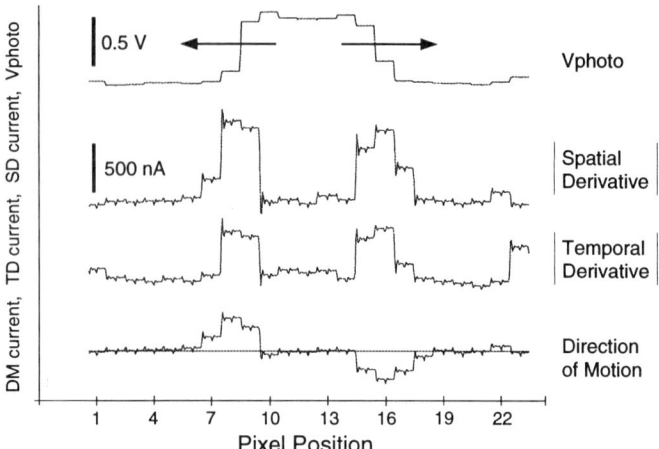

Figure 2: Example stimulus - Traces from top to bottom: Photoreceptor voltage, absolute value of the spatial derivative, absolute value of the temporal derivative, and direction-of-motion. The stimulus is a high-contrast, expanding bar, which provides two edges moving in opposite directions. The signed, temporal and spatial derivative signals are used to compute the direction-of-motion shown in the bottom trace.

attentional shifts have been modeled using analog VLSI circuits [4] [14], based on the Koch and Ullman model. These circuits demonstrate the use of delayed, transient inhibition at the selected location to model covert attentional scanning. In this paper we describe an analog VLSI implementation of an attention-based, visual tracking architecture which combines much of this previous work. Using a hardware model of the primate oculomotor system [8], we then demonstrate the use of the tracking chip for both saccadic and smooth pursuit eye movements.

2 System Description

The computational goal of this chip is the selection of a target, based on a given measure of saliency, and the extraction of its retinal position and direction of motion. Figure 1 shows a block diagram of the computation. The first few stages of processing compute simple feature maps which drive the WTA-based selection of a target to track. The circuits at the selected location signal their position and the computed direction-of-motion. This information is used by an external saccadic and smooth pursuit eye movement system to drive the eye. The saccadic system uses the position information to foveate the target and the smooth pursuit system uses the motion information to match the speed of the target.

Adaptive photoreceptors [2] (at the top of Figure 1) transduce the incoming pattern of light into an array of voltages. The temporal (TD) and spatial (SD) derivatives are computed from these voltages and are used to generate the saliency map and direction of motion. Figure 2 shows an example stimulus and the computed features. The saliency map is formed by summing the absolute-value of each derivative ($|TD| + |SD|$) and the direction-of-motion (DM) signal is a normalized product of the two

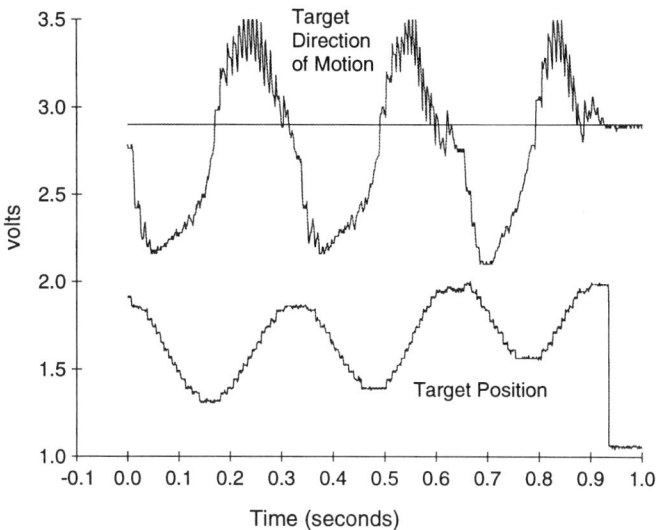

Figure 3: Extracting the target's direction of motion: The WTA output voltage is used to switch the DM current onto a common current sensing line. The output of this signal is seen in the top trace. The zero-motion level is indicated by the flat line shown at 2.9 volts. The lower trace shows the target's position from the position-to-voltage encoding circuits. The target's position and direction of motion are used to drive saccades and smooth pursuit eye movements during tracking.

derivatives. $\frac{TD \cdot SD}{|TD|+|SD|}$

In the saliency map, the temporal and spatial derivatives can be differentially weighted to emphasize moving targets over stationary targets. The saliency map provides the input to a winner-take-all (WTA) computation which finds the maximum in this map. Spatially-distributed hysteresis is incorporated in this winner-take-all computation [4] by adding a fixed current to the winner's input node and its neighbors. This distributed hysteresis is motivated by the following two ideas: 1) once a target has been selected it should continue to be tracked even if another equally interesting target comes along, and 2) targets will typically move continuously across the array. Hysteresis reduces oscillation of the winning status in the case where two or more inputs are very close to the winning input level and the local distribution of hysteresis allows the winning status to freely shift to neighboring pixels rather than to another location further away.

The WTA output signal is used to drive three different circuits: the position-to-voltage (P2V) circuit [3], the DM-current-steering circuit (see Figure 3), and the saccadic triggering (ST) circuit. The only circuits that are active are those at the winning pixel locations. The P2V circuit drives the common position output line to a voltage representing it's position in the array, the DM-steering circuit puts the local DM circuit's current onto the common motion output line, and the ST circuit drives a position-specific current onto a common line to be compared against an externally-set threshold value. By creating a "V" shaped profile of ST currents centered on the array, winning pixels away from the center will exceed the threshold

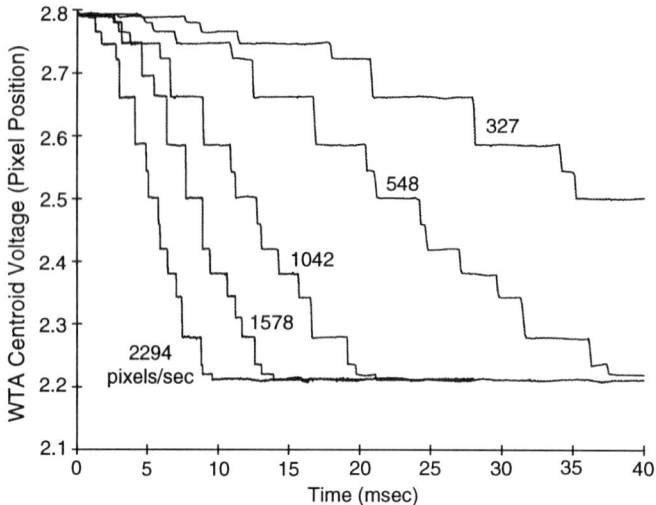

Figure 4: Position vs. time traces for the passage of a strong edge across the array at five different speeds. The speeds shown correspond to 327, 548, 1042, 1578, 2294 pixels/sec.

and send saccade requests off-chip. Figure 3 shows the DM and P2V outputs for an oscillating target.

To test the speed of the tracking circuit, a single edge was passed in front of the array at varying speeds. Figure 4 shows some of these results. The power consumption of the chip (23 pixels and support circuits, not including the pads) varies between 0.35 mW and 0.60 mW at a supply voltage of 5 volts. This measurement was taken with no clock signal driving the scanners since this is not essential to the operation of the circuit.

3 System Integration

The tracking chip has been mounted on a neuromorphic, hardware model of the primate oculomotor system [8] and is being used to track moving visual targets. The visual target is mounted to a swinging apparatus to generate an oscillating motion. Figure 5 shows the behavior of the system when the retinal target position is used to drive re-centering saccades and the target direction of motion is used drive smooth pursuit. Saccades are triggered when the selected pixel is outside a specified window centered on the array and the input to the smooth pursuit system is suppressed during saccades. The smooth pursuit system mathematically integrates retinal motion to match the eye velocity to the target velocity.

4 Acknowledgements

T. H. is supported by an Office of Naval Research AASERT grant and by the NSF Center for Neuromorphic Systems Engineering at Caltech. T. M. is supported by the Georgia Tech Research Institute.

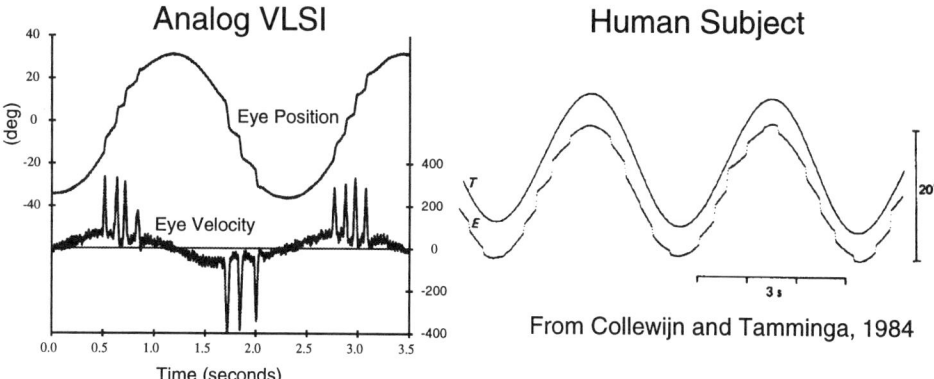

Figure 5: Saccades and Smooth Pursuit: In this example, a swinging target is tracked over a few cycles. Re-centering saccades are triggered when the target leaves a specified window centered on the array. For comparison, on the right, we show human data for the same task [1].

References

[1] H. Collewijn and E. Tamminga, "Human smooth and saccadic eye movements during voluntary pursuit of different target motions on different backgrounds" *J. Physiol.*, Vol. 351, pp. 217-250. (1984)

[2] T. Delbrück, Ph.D. Thesis, Computation and Neural Systems Program California Institute of Technology (1993)

[3] S. P. DeWeerth, "Analog VLSI Circuits for Stimulus Localization and Centroid Computation" *Intl. J. Comp. Vis.* 8(3), pp. 191-202. (1992)

[4] S. P. DeWeerth and T. G. Morris, "CMOS Current Mode Winner-Take-All with Distributed Hysteresis" *Electronics Letters*, Vol. 31, No. 13, pp. 1051-1053. (1995)

[5] R. Etienne-Cummings, J. Van der Spiegel, and P. Mueller "A Visual Smooth Pursuit Tracking Chip" *Advances in Neural Information Processing Systems 8* (1996)

[6] V. Ferrara and S. Lisberger, "Attention and Target Selection for Smooth Pursuit Eye Movements" *J. Neurosci.*, 15(11), pp. 7472-7484, (1995)

[7] J. Hoffman and B. Subramaniam, "The Role of Visual Attention in Saccadic Eye Movements" *Perception and Psychophysics*, 57(6), pp. 787-795, (1995)

[8] T. Horiuchi, B. Bishofberger, and C. Koch, "An Analog VLSI Saccadic System" *Advances in Neural Information Processing Systems 6*, Morgan Kaufmann, pp. 582-589, (1994)

[9] B. Khurana, and E. Kowler, "Shared Attentional Control of Smooth Eye Movement and Perception" *Vision Research*, 27(9), pp. 1603-1618, (1987)

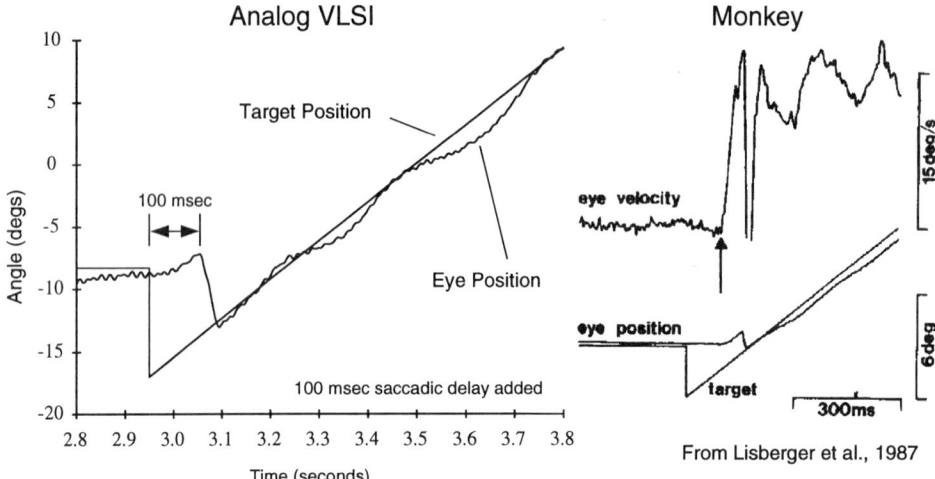

Figure 6: Step-Ramp Experiment: In this experiment, the target jumps from the fixation point to a new location and begins moving with constant velocity. On the left, the analog VLSI system tracks the target. For comparison, on the right, we show data from a monkey performing the same task [13].

[10] E. Kowler, E. Anderson, B. Dosher, E. Blaser, "The Role of Attention in the Programming of Saccades" *Vision Research*, 35(13), pp. 1897-1916, (1995)

[11] C. Koch and S. Ullman, "Shifts in selective visual attention: towards the underlying neural circuitry" *Human Neurobiology*, 4:219-227, (1985)

[12] R. Rafal, P. Calabresi, C. Brennan, and T. Scioltio, "Saccade Preparation Inhibits Reorienting to Recently Attended Locations" *J. Exp. Psych: Hum. Percep. and Perf.*, 15, pp. 673-685, (1989)

[13] S. G. Lisberger, E. J. Morris, and L. Tychsen, "Visual motion processing and sensory-motor integration for smooth pursuit eye movements." In *Ann. Rev. Neurosci.*, Cowan et al., editors. Vol. 10, pp. 97-129, (1987)

[14] T. G. Morris and S. P. DeWeerth, "Analog VLSI Circuits for Covert Attentional Shifts" *Proc. 5th Intl. Conf. on Microelectronics for Neural Networks and Fuzzy Systems* - MicroNeuro96, Feb 12-14, 1996. Lausanne, Switzerland, IEEE Computer Society Press, Los Alamitos, CA, pp. 30-37, (1996)

[15] S. Shimojo, Y. Tanaka, O. Hikosaka, and S. Miyauchi, "Vision, Attention, and Action – inhibition and facilitation in sensory motor links revealed by the reaction time and the line-motion." In *Attention and Performance XVI*, T. Inui & J. L. McClelland, editors. MIT Press, (1995)

[16] W. J. Tam and H. Ono, "Fixation Disengagement and Eye-Movement Latency" *Perception and Psychophysics*, 56(3) pp. 251-260, (1994)

Dynamically Adaptable CMOS Winner-Take-All Neural Network

Kunihiko Iizuka, Masayuki Miyamoto and Hirofumi Matsui
Information Technology Research Laboratories
Sharp
Tenri, Nara, JAPAN

Abstract

The major problem that has prevented practical application of analog neuro-LSIs has been poor accuracy due to fluctuating analog device characteristics inherent in each device as a result of manufacturing. This paper proposes a dynamic control architecture that allows analog silicon neural networks to compensate for the fluctuating device characteristics and adapt to a change in input DC level. We have applied this architecture to compensate for input offset voltages of an analog CMOS WTA (Winner-Take-All) chip that we have fabricated. Experimental data show the effectiveness of the architecture.

1 INTRODUCTION

Analog VLSI implementation of neural networks, such as silicon retinas and adaptive filters, has been the focus of much active research. Since it utilizes physical laws that electric devices obey for neural operation, circuit scale can be much smaller than that of a digital counterpart and massively parallel implementation is possible. The major problem that has prevented practical applications of these LSIs has been fluctuating analog device characteristics inherent in each device as a result of manufacturing. Historically, this has been the main reason most analog devices have been superseded by digital devices. Analog neuro VLSI is expected to conquer this problem by making use of its adaptability. This optimistic view comes from the fact that in spite of the unevenness of their components, biological neural networks show excellent competence.

This paper proposes a CMOS circuit architecture that dynamically compensates for fluctuating component characteristics and at the same time adapts device state to incoming signal levels. There are some engineering techniques available to compensate for MOS threshold fluctuation, e.g., the chopper comparator, but they need a periodical change of mode to achieve the desired effect. This is because there are two modes one for the adaptation and one for the signal processing. This is quite inconvenient because extra clock signals are needed and a break of signal processing takes place.

Incoming signals usually consist of a rapidly changing foreground component and a slowly varying background component. To process these signals incessantly, biological neural networks make use of multiple channels having different temporal/spatial scales. While a relatively slow/large channel is used to suppress background floating, a faster/smaller channel is devoted to process the foreground signal. The proposed method inspired by this biological consideration utilizes different frequency bands for adaptation and signal processing (Figure 1), where negative feedback is applied through a low pass filter so that the feedback will not affect the foreground signal processing.

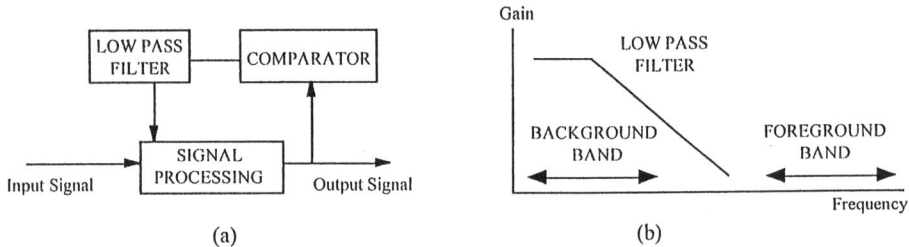

Figure 1: Dynamic adaptation by frequency divided control. (a) model diagram, (b) frequency division.

In the first part of this paper, a working analog CMOS WTA chip that we have test fabricated is introduced. Then, dynamical adaptation for this WTA chip is described and experimental results are presented.

2 ANALOG CMOS WTA CHIP

2.1 ARCHITECTURE AND SPECIFICATION

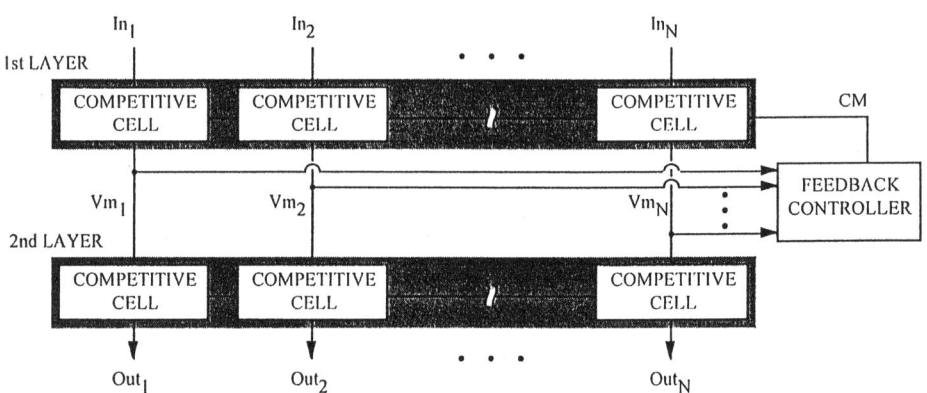

Figure 2: Analog CMOS WTA chip architecture

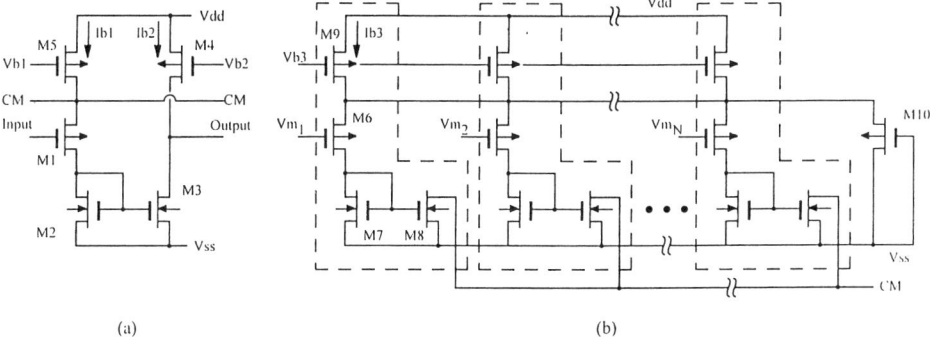

Figure 3: Circuit diagrams for (a) the competitive cell and (b) the feedback controller.

As a basic building block to construct neuro-chips, analog WTA circuits have been investigated by researchers such as [Lazzaro, 1989] and [Pedroni, 1994]. All CMOS analog WTA circuits are based on voltage follower circuits [Pedroni, 1995] to realize competition through inhibitory interaction, and they use feedback mechanisms to enhance resolution gain. The architecture of the chip that we have fabricated is shown in Figure 2 and the circuit diagram is in Figure 3. This WTA chip indicates the lowest input voltage by making the output voltage corresponds to the lowest input voltage near Vss (winner), and others nearly the power supply voltage Vdd (loser). The circuit is similar to [Sheu, 1993], but represents two advances.

1. The steering current that the feedback controller absorbs from the line CM is enlarged, allowing the winner cell can compete with others in the region where resolution gain is the largest.

2 The feedback controller originally placed after the second competitive layer is removed in order to guarantee the existence of at least one output node whose voltage is nearly zero.

Table 1 shows the specifications of the fabricated chip.

Table 1: Specifications of the fabricated WTA chip

Process	0.8 um double-metal CMOS
Number of input nodes	32
Power dissipation (measured)	< 480 µW
Power supply voltage	3V
Resolution (theoretical)	10 mV
Settling time (measured)	5 usec
Die area	1 mm × 0.5 mm

2.2 INPUT OFFSET VOLTAGE

Input offset voltages of a WTA chip may greatly deteriorate chip performance. Examples of input offset voltage distribution of the fabricated chips are shown in Figure 4. Each input offset voltage is measured relative to the first input node. The input offset voltage

ΔV_j of the j-th input node is defined as $\Delta V_j = Vin_j - Vin_1$ when the voltages of output nodes Out_j and Out_1 are equal; Vin_1 is fixed to a certain voltage and the voltage of other input nodes are fixed at a relatively high voltage.

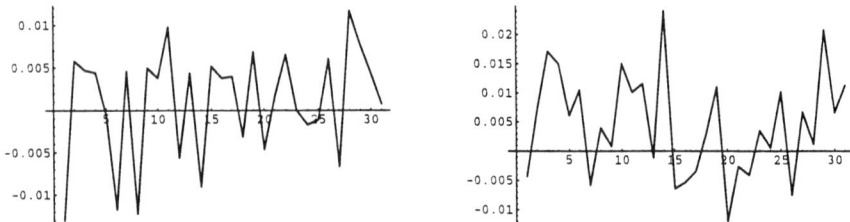

Figure 4: Examples of measured input offset voltage distribution.

The primary factor of the input offset voltage is considered to be fluctuation of MOS transistor threshold voltages in the first layer competitive cell. Then, the input offset voltage ΔV_j of this cell yielded by the small fluctuation ΔVth^i of Vth^i is calculated as follows:

$$\Delta V_j \simeq \sum_{i=1}^{4} \Delta Vth^i \frac{\partial Vin}{\partial Vth^i}$$

$$= -\Delta Vth^1 + \frac{gd_1 + gd_2 + gm_2}{gm_1}(\Delta Vth^2 - \Delta Vth^3) + \frac{gm_4(gd_1 + gd_2 + gm_2)}{gm_1 gm_3}\Delta Vth^4 ,$$

where gm_i and gd_i are the transconductance and the drain conductance of MOS Mi, respectively. Using design and process parameters, we can estimate the input offset voltage to be

$$\Delta V_j \simeq -\Delta Vth^1 + (\Delta Vth^2 - \Delta Vth^3) + 0.15\Delta Vth^4 ,$$

Based on our experiences, the maximum fluctuation of Vth^i in a chip is usually smaller than 20 mV, and it is reasonable to consider that the difference $|\Delta Vth^2 - \Delta Vth^3|$ is even smaller; perhaps less than 5 mV, because M2 and M3 compose a current mirror and are closely placed. This implies that the maximum of ΔV_j is about 28 mV, which is in rough agreement with the measured data.

3 DYNAMICAL ADAPTATION ARCHITECTURE

In Figure 5, we show circuit implementation of the dynamically adaptable WTA function. In each feedback channel, the difference between each output and the reference $Vref$ is fed back to the input node through a low pass filter consisting of R and C. The charge stored in capacitor C is controlled by this feedback signal.

Let the linear approximation of the WTA chip DC characteristic be

$$Vout_i = A (Vin_i - V0_i),$$

where Vin_i and $Vout_i$ are the voltages at the nodes In_i and Out_i respectively, and A and $V0_i$ are functions of Vin_j ($j \neq i$). The input offset voltage relative to the node In_1 is considered to be the difference between $V0_i$ and $V0_1$. On the other hand, the DC characteristic of the i-th feedback path can be approximated as

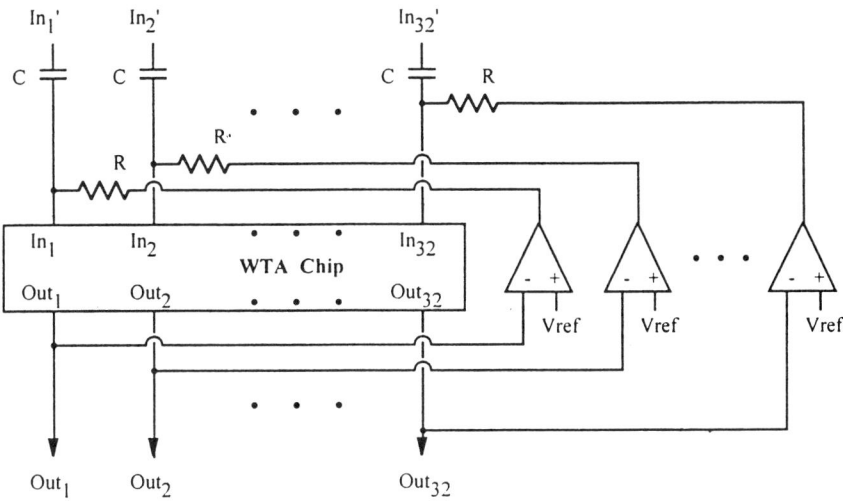

Figure 5: WTA chip equipped with adaptation circuit where R=10MΩ and C=0.33μF.

$$Vin_i = B\,(\,Vout_i - Vref).$$

It follows from the above two equations that

$$Vin_i = -\frac{AB}{1-AB}\,VO_i - \frac{B}{1-AB}\,Vref \approx VO_i\,.$$

The last term is derived using the assumptions $A \gg 1$ and $B \ll -1$. This means that the voltage difference between the DC level of the input and VO_i is clamped on the capacitor C. This in turn implies that the input offset voltage will be successfully compensated for.

The role of the low pass filters is twofold.

1. They guarantee stable dynamics of the feedback loop; we can make the cutoff frequency of the low pass filters small enough so that the gain of the feedback path is attenuated before the phase of the feedback signal is delayed by more than 180°.

2. They prevent the feed-forward WTA operation from being affected, as shown in Figure 1, the adaptive control is carried out on a different, non-overlapped frequency band than WTA operation.

4 EXPERIMENTAL RESULTS

Experiments concerning the adaptable WTA function were carried out by applying pulses of 90% duty to the input nodes In'_1 and In'_2, while other input nodes were fixed to a certain voltage. In Figures 6 (a) and 6 (b), the output waveforms of Out_1, Out_2, Out_3 and the waveform of the pulse applied to the node In'_1 are shown. Figure 6(a) shows the result when the same pulse was applied to both In'_1 and In'_2. Figure 6(b) shows the result when the amplitude of the pulse to In'_1 was greater than that of the pulse to In'_2 by 10 mV. The schematic explanation of this behavior is in Figure 7. The outputs remained at the same levels for a while after the inputs were shut off, since there was no strong inducement. As a result of adaptation, the winning frequencies of every output nodes become equal in a long time scale. This explains the unstable output during the period of quiescent inputs.

The chip used in this measurement had a relative input offset voltage of 15 mV between nodes In_1 and In_2. We can see in Figure 6 (a) that this offset voltage was completely compensated for because the output waveforms of corresponding nodes were the same.

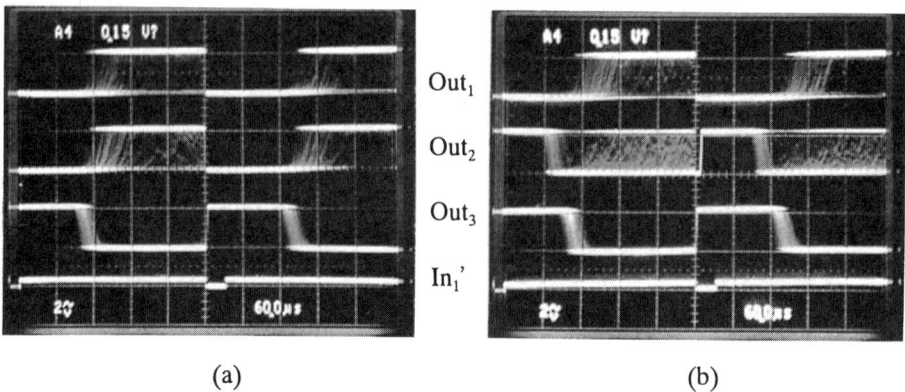

(a) (b)

Figure 6: The output waveforms of the dynamically adaptable CMOS WTA neural network. Pulse waves were applied to nodes In'_1 and In'_2; other nodes voltages were fixed. When the amplitude of each pulse was the same (a), the corresponding output waveforms were the same. When the amplitude of the pulse fed to In'_1 was greater than that to In'_2 by 10 mV (b), the output voltage at Out_1 was low (winner) and that at Out_2 was high (loser) during the period the pulse was low (on).

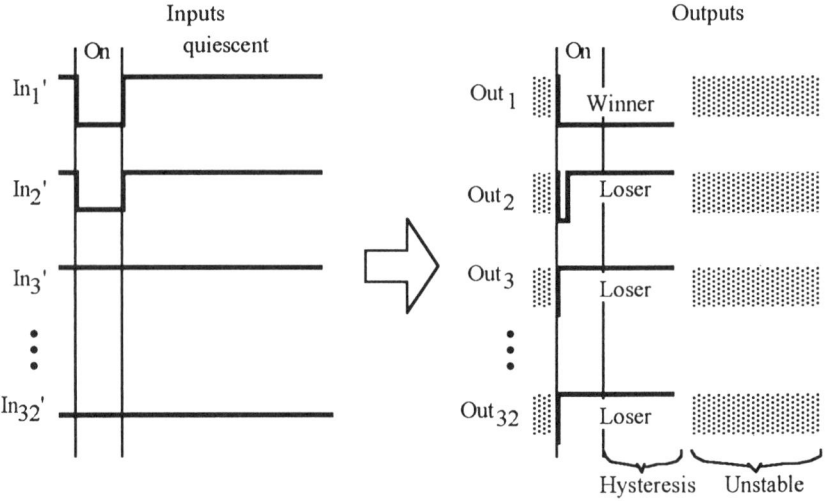

Figure 7: The schematic explanation of the dynamically adaptable WTA behavior.

5 CONCLUSION

We have proposed a dynamic adaptation architecture that uses frequency divided control and applied this to a CMOS WTA chip that we have fabricated. Experimental results show that the architecture successfully compensated for input offset voltages of the WTA chip due to inherent device characteristic fluctuations. Moreover, this architecture gives analog neuro-chips the ability to adapt to incoming signal background levels. This adaptability has a lot of applications. For example, in vision chips, the adaptation may be used to compensate for the fluctuation of photo sensor characteristics, to adapt the gain of photo sensors to background illumination level and to automatically control color balance. As another application, Figure 8 describes an analog neuron with weighted synapses, where the time constant RC is much larger than the time constant of input signals.

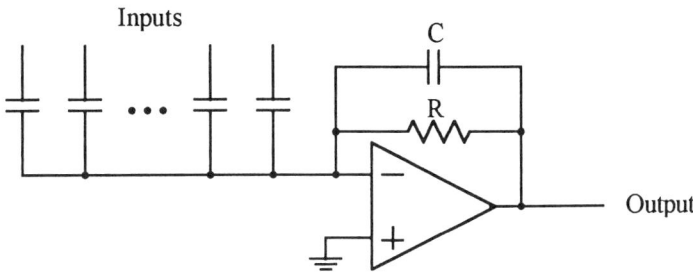

Figure 8: Analog neuron with weighted synapses where the time constant RC is much larger than that of input signals.

The key to this architecture is use of non-overlapping frequency bands for adaptation to background and foreground signal processing. For neuro-VLSIs, this requires implementing circuits with completely different time scale constants. In modern VLSI technology, however, this is not a difficult problem because processes for very high resistances, i.e., teraohms, are available.

Acknowledgment

The authors would like to thank Morio Osaka for his help in chip fabrication and Kazuo Hashiguchi for his support in experimental work.

References

Choi, J. & Sheu, B.J. (1993) A high-precision VLSI winner-take-all circuit for self-organizing neural networks. *IEEE J. Solid-State Circuits*, vol.28, no.5, pp.576-584.

Lazzaro, J., Ryckebush, S., Mahowald, M.A., & Mead, C. (1989) Winner-take-all networks of O(N) complexity. In D.S. Touretzky (eds.), *Advances in Neural Information Processing Systems* 1, pp. 703-711. Cambridge, MA: MIT Press.

Pedroni, V.A. (1994) Neural n-port voltage comparator network, Electron. Lett., vol.30, no.21, pp1774-1775.

Pedroni, V.A. (1995) Inhibitory Mechanism Analysis of Complexity O(N) MOS Winner-Take-All Networks. *IEEE Trans. Circuits Syst. I*, vol.42, no.3, pp.172-175.

An Adaptive WTA using Floating Gate Technology

W. Fritz Kruger, Paul Hasler, Bradley A. Minch, and Christof Koch
California Institute of Technology
Pasadena, CA 91125
(818) 395 - 2812
stretch@klab.caltech.edu

Abstract

We have designed, fabricated, and tested an adaptive Winner–Take–All (WTA) circuit based upon the classic WTA of Lazzaro, et al [1]. We have added a time dimension (adaptation) to this circuit to make the input derivative an important factor in winner selection. To accomplish this, we have modified the classic WTA circuit by adding floating gate transistors which slowly null their inputs over time. We present a simplified analysis and experimental data of this adaptive WTA fabricated in a standard CMOS 2μm process.

1 Winner–Take–All Circuits

In a WTA network, each cell has one input and one output. For any set of inputs, the outputs will all be at zero except for the one which is from the cell with the maximum input. One way to accomplish this is by a global nonlinear inhibition coupled with a self-excitation term [2]. Each cell inhibits all others while exciting itself; thus a cell with even a slightly greater input than the others will excite itself up to its maximal state and inhibit the others down to their minimal states. The WTA function is important for many classical neural nets that involve competitive learning, vector quantization and feature mapping. The classic WTA network characterized by Lazzaro et. al. [1] is an elegant, simple circuit that shares just one common line among all cells of the network to propagate the inhibition.

Our motivation to add adaptation comes from the idea of saliency maps. Picture a saliency map as a large number of cells each of which encodes an analog value

An Adaptive WTA using Floating Gate Technology

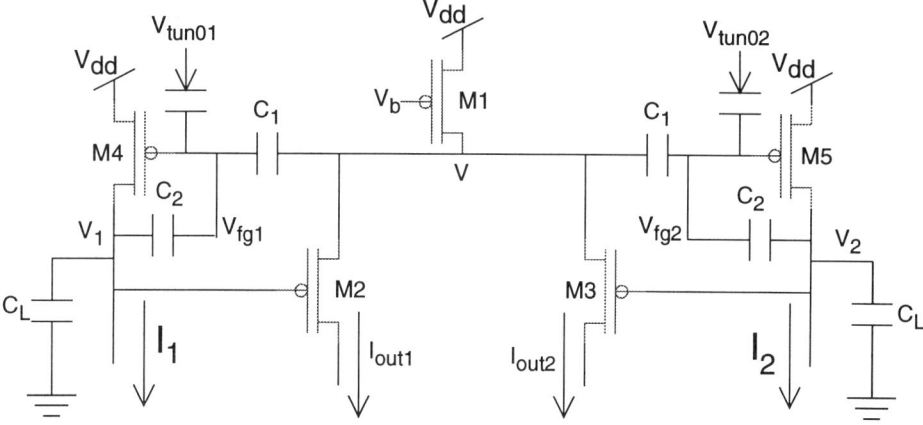

Figure 1: The circuit diagram of a two input winner-take-all circuit.

reflecting some measure of the importance (saliency) of its input. We would like to pay attention to the most salient cell, so we employ a WTA function to tell us where to look. But if the input doesn't change, we never look away from that one cell. We would like to introduce some concept of fatigue and refraction to each cell such that after winning for some time, it tires, allowing other cells to win, and then it must wait some time before it can win again. We call this circuit an adaptive WTA.

In this paper, we present an adaptive WTA based upon the classic WTA; Figure 1 shows a two-input, adaptive WTA circuit. The difference between the classic and adaptive WTA is that M_4 and M_5 are pFET single transistor synapses. A single transistor synapse [3] is either an nFET or pFET transistor with a floating gate and a tunneling junction. This enhancement results in the ability of each transistor to adapt to its input bias current. The adaptation is a result of the electron tunneling and hot-electron injection modifying the charge on the floating gate; equilibrium is established when the tunneling current equals the injection current. The circuit is devised in such a way that these are negative feedback mechanisms, consequently the output voltage will always return to the same steady state voltage determined by its bias current regardless of the DC input level. Like the autozeroing amplifier [4], the adaptive WTA is an example of a circuit where the adaptation occurs as a natural part of the circuit operation.

2 pFET hot-electron injection and electron tunneling

Before considering the behavior of the adaptive WTA, we will review the processes of electron tunneling and hot-electron injection in pFETs. In subthreshold operation, we can describe the channel current of a pFET (I_p) for a differential change in gate voltage, ΔV_g, around a fixed bias current I_{so}, as $I_p = I_{so} \exp\left(-\frac{\kappa \Delta V_g}{U_T}\right)$ where κ_p is the amount by which ΔV_g affects the surface potential of the pFET, and U_T is $\frac{kT}{q}$. We will assume for this paper that all transistors are identical.

First, we consider electron tunneling. We start with the classic model of electron

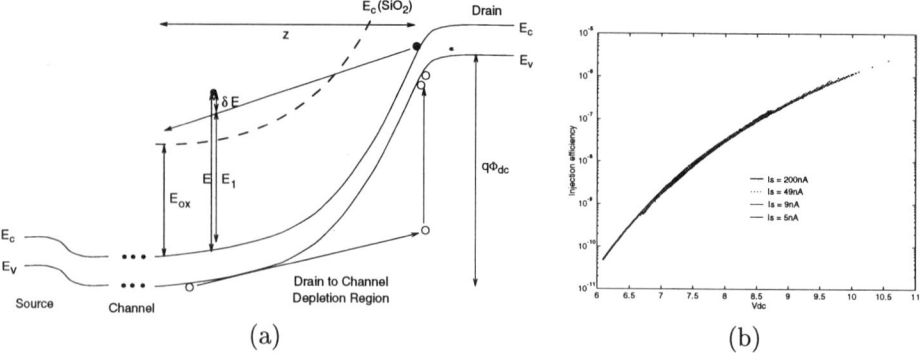

Figure 2: pFET Hot Electron Injection. (a) Band diagram of a subthreshold pFET transistor for favorable conditions for hot-electron injection. (b) Measured data of pFET injection efficiency versus the drain to channel voltage for four source currents. Injection efficiency is the ratio of injection current to source current. At Φ_{dc} equal to 8.2V, the injection efficiency increases a factor of e for an increase Φ_{dc} of 250mV.

tunneling through a silicon - SiO$_2$ system [5]. As in the autozeroing amplifier [4], the tunneling current will be only a weak function for the voltage swing on the floating gate voltage through the region of subthreshold currents; therefore we will approximate the tunneling junction as a current source supplying I_{tun0} current to the floating gate.

Second, we derive a simple model of pFET hot-electron injection. Figure 2a shows the band diagram of a pFET operating at bias conditions which are favorable for hot-electron injection. Hot-hole impact ionization creates electrons at the drain edge of the depletion region. These secondary electrons travel back into the channel region gaining energy as they go. When their energy exceeds that of the SiO$_2$ barrier, they can be injected through the oxide to the floating gate. The hole impact ionization current is proportional to the source current, and is an exponential function of the voltage drop from channel to drain (Φ_{dc}). The injection current is proportional to the hole impact ionization current and is an exponential function of the voltage drop from channel to drain. We will neglect the dependence of the floating-gate voltage for a given source current and Φ_{dc} as we did in [4]. Figure 2b shows measured injection efficiency for several source currents, where injection efficiency is the ratio of the injection current to source current. The injection efficiency is independent of source current and is approximately linear over a 1 − 2V swing in Φ_{dc}; therefore we model the injection efficiency as proportional to $\exp\left(-\frac{\Delta\Phi_{dc}}{V_{inj}}\right)$ within that 1 to 2V swing, where V_{inj} is a measured device parameter which for our process is 250mV at a bias $\Phi_{dc} = 8.2V$, and $\Delta\Phi_{dc}$ is the change in Φ_{dc} from the bias level. An increasing voltage input will increase the pFET surface potential by capacitive coupling to the floating gate. Increasing the pFET surface potential will increase the source current thereby decreasing Φ_{dc} for a fixed output voltage and lowering the injection efficiency.

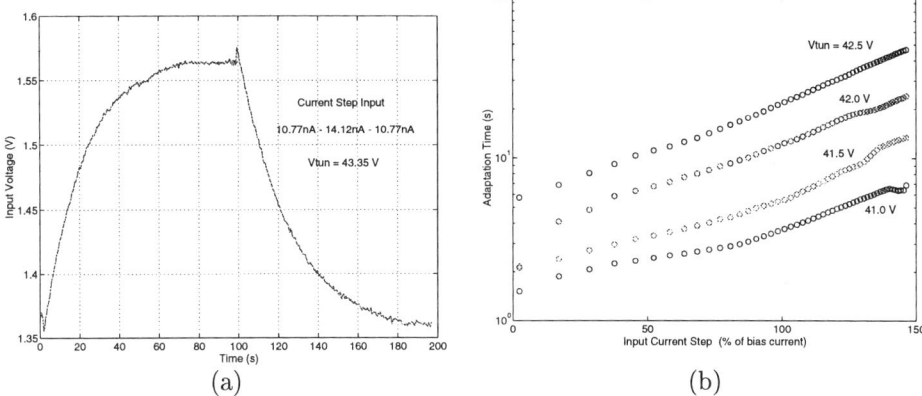

Figure 3: Illustration of the dynamics for the winning and losing input voltages. (a) Measured V_1 verses time due to an upgoing and a downgoing input current step. The initial input voltage change due to the input step is much smaller than the voltage change due to the adaptation. (b) Adaptation time of a losing input voltage for several tunneling voltages. The adaptation time is the time from the start of the input current step to the time the input voltage is within 10% of its steady state voltage. A larger tunneling current decreases the adaptation time by increasing the tunneling current supplied to the floating gate.

3 Two input Adaptive WTA

We will outline the general procedure to derive the general equations to describe the two input WTA shown in Fig. 1. We first observe that transistors M_1, M_2, and M_3 make up a differential pair. Regardless of any adaptation, the middle V node and output currents are set by the input voltages (V_1 and V_2), which are set by the input currents, as in the classic WTA [1]. The dynamics for high frequency operation are also similar to the classic WTA circuit. Next, we can write the two Kirchhoff Current Law (KCL) equations at V_1 and V_2, which relate the change in V_1 and V_2 as a function of the two input currents and the floating gate voltages. Finally, we can write the two KCL equations at the two floating gates V_{fg1} and V_{fg2}, which relates the changes in the floating gate voltages in terms of V_1 and V_2. This procedure is directly extendable to multiple inputs. A full analysis of these equations is very difficult and will be described in another paper.

For this discussion, we present a simplified analysis to develop the intuition of the circuit operation. At sufficiently high frequencies, the tunneling and injection currents do not adapt the floating gate voltages sufficiently fast to keep the input voltages at their steady state levels. At these frequencies, the adaptive WTA acts like the classic WTA circuit with one small difference. A change in the input voltages, V_1 or V_2 is linearly related to V by the capacitive coupling ($\Delta V_1 = -\frac{C_1}{C_2}\Delta V$), where this relationship is exponential in the classic WTA. There is always some capacitance C_2, even if not explicitly drawn due to the overlap capacitance from the floating gate to drain. This property gives the designer the added freedom to modify the gain. We will assume the circuit operates in its intended operating regime where the floating gate transistors settle sufficiently fast such that their channel

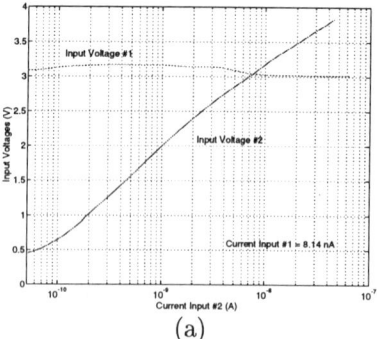
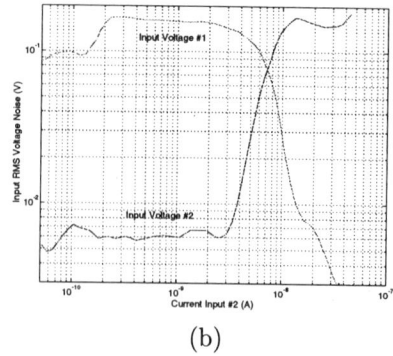

Figure 4: Measured change in steady state input voltages as a function of bias current. (a) Change in the two steady state output voltages as a function of the bias current of the second input. The bias current of the first input was held fixed at $8.14nA$. (b) Change in the RMS noise of the two output voltages as a function of the bias current of the second input. The RMS noise is much higher for the losing input than for the winning input. Note that where the two bias currents cross roughly corresponds to the location where the RMS noise on the two input voltages is equal.

current equals the input currents

$$I_i = I_{so} \exp(-\frac{\kappa \Delta V_{fgi}}{U_T}) \rightarrow \frac{dI_i}{dt} = -I_i \frac{\kappa}{U_T} \frac{dV_{fgi}}{dt} \quad (1)$$

for all inputs indexed by i, but not necessarily fast enough for the floating gates to settle to their final steady state levels.

To develop some initial intuition, we shall begin by considering one half of the two input WTA: transistors M_1, M_2 and M_4 of Figure 1. First, we notice that I_{out1} is equal to I_b (the current through transistor M_1); note that this is not true for the multiple input case. By equating these two currents we get an equation for V as $V = \kappa V_1 - \kappa V_b$, where we will assume that V_b is a fixed bias voltage. Assuming the input current equals the current through M_4, V_1 obeys the equation

$$(\kappa C_1 + C_2)\frac{dV_1}{dt} = -\frac{C_T U_T}{\kappa I_1}\frac{dI_1}{dt} + I_{tun0}\left(\frac{I_1}{I_{so}}\exp(-\frac{\Delta V_1}{V_{inj}}) - 1\right) \quad (2)$$

where C_T is the total capacitance connected to the floating gate. The steady state of (2) is

$$\Delta V_{in} = \frac{\kappa V_{inj}}{U_T} \ln\left(\frac{I_1}{I_{so}}\right) \quad (3)$$

which is exactly the same expression for each input in a multiple input WTA. We get a linear differential equation by making the substitution $X = \exp(\frac{\Delta V_1}{V_{inj}})$ [4], and we get similar solutions to the behavior of the autozeroing amplifier. Figure 3a shows measured data for an upgoing and a downgoing current step. The input current change results in an initial fast change in the input voltage, and the input voltage then adapts to its steady state voltage which is a much greater voltage change. From the voltage difference between the steady states, we get that V_{inj} is roughly $500mV$.

An Adaptive WTA using Floating Gate Technology

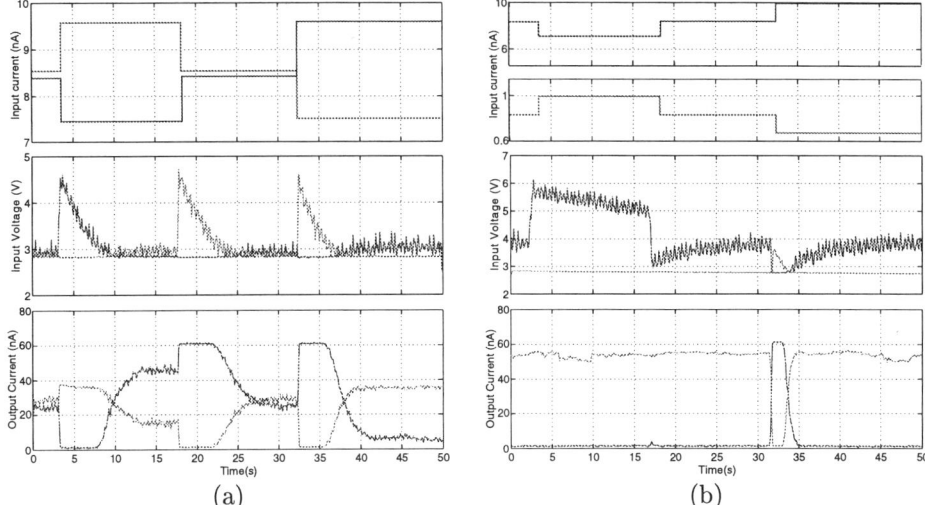

Figure 5: Experimental time traces measurements of the output current and voltage for small differential input current steps. (a) Time traces for small differential current steps around nearly identical bias currents of $8.6nA$. (b) Time traces for small differential current steps around two different bias currents of $8.7nA$ and $0.88nA$. In the classic WTA, the output currents would show no response to the input current steps.

Returning to the two input case, we get two floating gate equations by assuming that the currents through M_4 and M_5 are equal to their respective input currents and writing the KCL equations at each floating gate. If V_1 and V_2 do not cross each other in the circuit operation, then one can easily solve these KCL equations. Assume without loss of generality that V_1 is the winning voltage; which implies that $\Delta V = \kappa \Delta V_1$. The initial input voltage change before the floating gate adaptation due to a step in the two input currents of $I_1^- \to I_1^+$ and $I_2^- \to I_2^+$ is

$$\Delta V_1 = \frac{C_T}{\kappa C_1} \ln\left(\frac{I_1^+}{I_1^-}\right), \Delta V_2 \approx \frac{C_T}{C_2} \ln\left(\frac{I_1^- I_2^+}{I_1^+ I_2^-}\right) \quad (4)$$

for C_2 much less than κC_1. In this case, V_1 moves on the order of the floating gate voltage change, but V_2 moves on the order of the floating gate change amplified up by $\frac{C_T}{C_2}$. The response of ΔV_1 is governed by an identical equation to (2) of the earlier half-analysis, and therefore results in a small change in V_1. Also, any perturbation of V is only slightly amplified at V_1 due to the feedback; therefore any noise at V will only be slightly amplified into V_1. The restoration of V_2 is much quicker than the V_1 node if C_2 is much less than κC_1; therefore after the initial input step, one can safely assume that V is nearly constant. The voltage at V is amplified by $-\frac{C_1}{C_2}$ at V_2; therefore any noise at V is amplified at the losing voltage, but not at the winning voltage as the data in Fig. 4b shows. The losing dynamics are identical to the step response of an autozeroing amplifier [4]. Figure 3b shows the variation of the adaptation time verses the percent input current change for several values of tunneling voltages.

The main difficulty in exactly solving these KCL equations is the point in the dynamics where V_1 crosses V_2, since the behavior changes when the signals move through the crossover point. If we get more than a sufficient V_1 decrease to reach the starting V_2 equilibrium, then the rest of the input change is manifested by an increase in V_2. If the voltage V_2 crosses the voltage V_1, then V will be set by the new steady state, and V_1 is governed by losing dynamics until $V_1 \approx V_2$. At this point V_1 is nearly constant and V_2 is governed by losing dynamics. This analysis is directly extendible to arbitrary number of inputs.

Figure 5 shows some characteristic traces from the two-input circuit. Recall that the winning node is that with the lowest voltage, which is reflected in its corresponding high output current. In Fig. 5a, we see that as an input step is applied, the output current jumps and then begins to adapt to a steady state value. When the inputs are nearly equal, the steady state outputs are nearly equal; but when the inputs are different, the steady state output is greater for the cell with the lesser input. In general, the input current change that is the largest after reaching the previous equilibrium becomes the new equilibrium. This additional decrease in V_1 would lead to an amplified increase in the other voltage since the losing stage roughly looks like an autozeroing amplifier with the common node as the input terminal. The extent to which the inputs do not equal this largest input is manifested as a proportionally larger input voltage. The other voltage would return to equilibrium by slowly, linearly decreasing in voltage due to the tunneling current. This process will continue until V_1 equals V_2. Note in general that the inputs with lower bias currents have a slight starting advantage over the inputs with higher bias currents.

Figure 5b illustrates the advantage of the adaptive WTA over the classic WTA. In the classic WTA, the output voltage and current would not change throughout the experiment, but the adaptive WTA responds to changes in the input. The second input step does not evoke a response because there was not enough time to adapt to steady state after the previous step; but the next step immediately causes it to win. Also note in both of these traces that the noise is very large in the loosing node and small in the winner because of the gain differences (see Figure 4b).

References

[1] J. Lazzaro, S. Ryckebusch, M.A. Mahowald, and C.A. Mead "Winner–Take–All Networks of O(N) Complexity", *NIPS 1* Morgan Kaufmann Publishers, San Mateo, CA, 1989, pp 703 - 711.

[2] Grossberg S. "Adaptive Pattern Classification and Universal Recoding: I. Parallel Development and Coding of Neural Feature Detectors." *Biological Cybernetics* vol. 23, 121-134, 1988.

[3] P. Hasler, C. Diorio, B. A. Minch, and C. Mead, "Single Transistor Learning Synapses", *NIPS 7*, MIT Press, 1995, 817-824. *Also at http://www.pcmp.caltech.edu/anaprose/paul.*

[4] P. Hasler, B. A. Minch, C. Diorio, and C. Mead, "An autozeroing amplifier using pFET Hot-Electron Injection", *ISCAS*, Atlanta, 1996, III-325 - III-328. *Also at http://www.pcmp.caltech.edu/anaprose/paul.*

[5] M. Lenzlinger and E. H. Snow (1969), "Fowler-Nordheim tunneling into thermally grown SiO_2," *J. Appl. Phys.*, vol. 40, pp. 278-283, 1969.

A Micropower Analog VLSI HMM State Decoder for Wordspotting

John Lazzaro and John Wawrzynek
CS Division, UC Berkeley
Berkeley, CA 94720-1776
lazzaro@cs.berkeley.edu, johnw@cs.berkeley.edu

Richard Lippmann
MIT Lincoln Laboratory
Room S4-121, 244 Wood Street
Lexington, MA 02173-0073
rpl@sst.ll.mit.edu

Abstract

We describe the implementation of a hidden Markov model state decoding system, a component for a wordspotting speech recognition system. The key specification for this state decoder design is microwatt power dissipation; this requirement led to a continuous-time, analog circuit implementation. We characterize the operation of a 10-word (81 state) state decoder test chip.

1. INTRODUCTION

In this paper, we describe an analog implementation of a common signal processing block in pattern recognition systems: a hidden Markov model (HMM) state decoder. The design is intended for applications such as voice interfaces for portable devices that require micropower operation. In this section, we review HMM state decoding in speech recognition systems.

An HMM speech recognition system consists of a probabilistic state machine, and a method for tracing the state transitions of the machine for an input speech waveform. Figure 1 shows a state machine for a simple recognition problem: detecting the presence of keywords ("Yes," "No") in conversational speech (non-keyword speech is captured by the "Filler" state). This type of recognition where keywords are detected in unconstrained speech is called wordspotting (Lippmann et al., 1994).

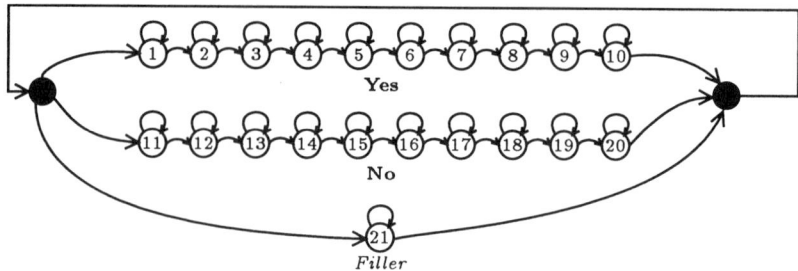

Figure 1. A two-keyword ("Yes," states 1-10, "No," states 11-20) HMM.

Our goal during speech recognition is to trace out the most likely path through this state machine that could have produced the input speech waveform. This problem can be partially solved in a local fashion, by examining short (80 ms. window) overlapping (15 ms. frame spacing) segments of the speech waveform. We estimate the probability $b_i(n)$ that the signal in frame n was produced by state i, using static pattern recognition techniques.

To improve the accuracy of these local estimates, we need to integrate information over the entire word. We do this by creating a set of state variables for the machine, called likelihoods, that are incrementally updated at every frame. Each state i has a real-valued likelihood $\phi_i(n)$ associated with it. Most states in Figure 1 have a stereotypical form: a state i that has a self-loop input, an input from state $i-1$, and an output to state $i+1$, with the self-loop and exit transitions being equally probable. For states in this topology, the update rule

$$\log(\phi_i(n)) = \log(b_i(n)) + \log(\phi_i(n-1) + \phi_{i-1}(n-1)) \tag{1}$$

lets us estimate the "log likelihood" value $\log(\phi_i(n))$ for the state i; a log encoding is used to cope with the large operating range of $\phi_i(n)$ values. Log likelihoods are negative numbers, whose magnitudes increase with each frame. We limit the range of log likelihood values by using a renormalization technique: if any log likelihood in the system falls below a minimum value, a positive constant is added to all log likelihoods in the machine.

Figure 2 shows a complete system which uses HMM state decoding to perform wordspotting. The "Feature Generation" and "Probability Generation" blocks comprise the static pattern recognition system, producing the probabilities $b_i(n)$ at each frame. The "State Decode" block updates the log likelihood variables $\log(\phi_i(n))$. The "Word Detect" block uses a simple online algorithm to flag the occurrence of a word. Keyword end-state log likelihoods are subtracted by the filler log likelihood, and when this difference exceeds a fixed threshold a keyword is detected.

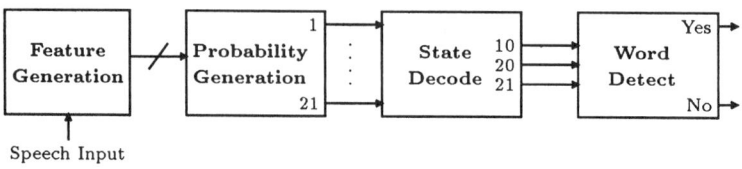

Figure 2. Block diagram for the two-keyword spotting system.

2. ANALOG CIRCUITS FOR STATE DECODING

Figure 3a shows an analog discrete-time implementation of Equation 1. The delay element (labeled Z^{-1}) acts as a edge-triggered sampled analog delay, with full-scale voltage input and output. The delay element is clocked at the frame rate of the state decoder (15 ms. clock period). The "combinatorial" analog circuits must settle within the clock period. A clock period of 15 ms. allows a relatively long settling time, which enables us to make extensive use of submicroampere currents in the circuit design. The microwatt power consumption design specification drives us to use such small currents. As a result of submicroampere circuit operation, the MOS transistors in Figure 3a are operating in the weak-inversion regime.

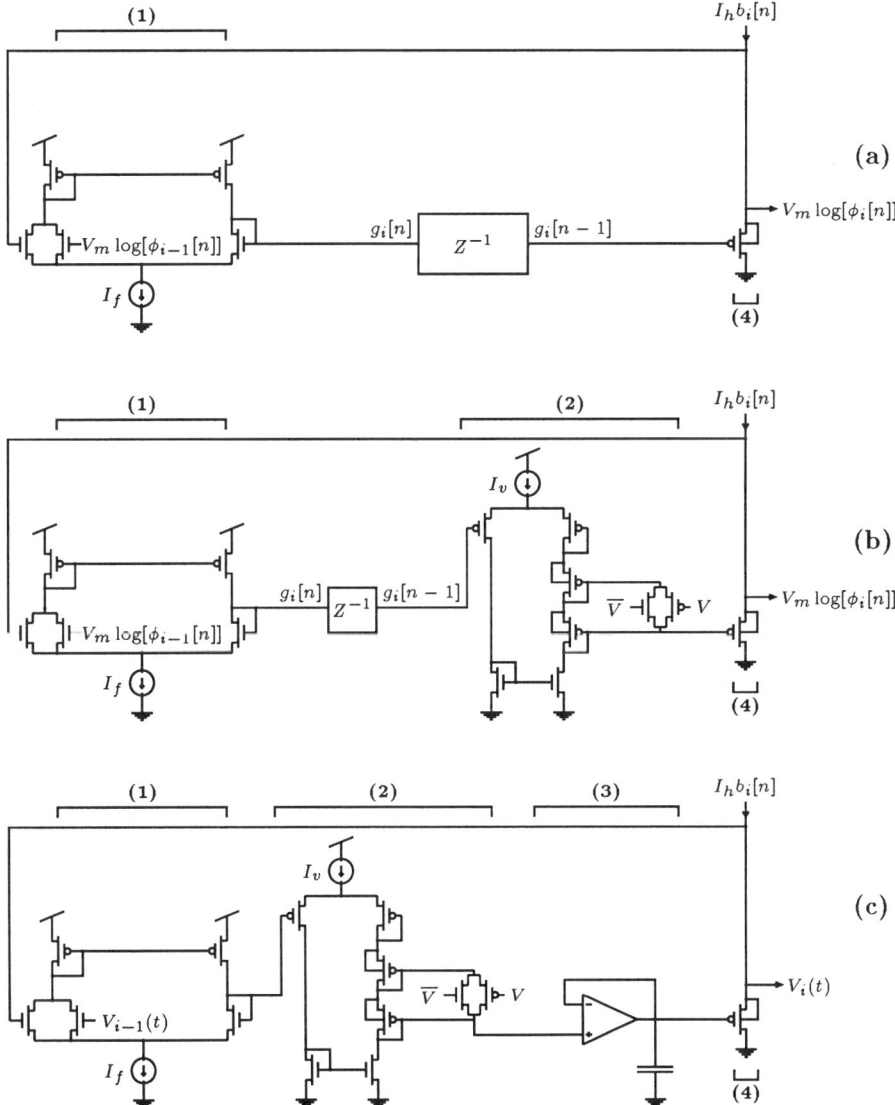

Figure 3. (a) Analog discrete-time single-state decoder. (b) Enhanced version of (a), includes the renormalization system. (c) Continuous-time extension of (b).

Equation 1 uses two types of variables: probabilities and log likelihoods. In the implementation shown in Figure 3, we choose unidirectional current as the signal type for probability, and large-signal voltage as the signal type for log likelihood. We can understand the dimensional scaling of these signal types by analyzing the floating-well transistor labeled (4) in Figure 3a. The equation

$$V_m \log(\phi_i(n)) = V_m \log(b_i(n)) + g_i(n-1) + V_m \log(\frac{I_h}{I_o}) \tag{2}$$

describes the behavior of this transistor, where $V_m = (V_o/\kappa_p)\ln(10)$, $g_i(n-1)$ is the output of the delay element, and I_o, κ and V_o are MOS parameters. Both I_o and κ in Equation 2 are functions of V_{sb}. However, the floating-well topology of the transistor ensures $V_{sb} = 0$ for this device.

The input probability $b_i(n)$ is scaled by the unidirectional current I_h, defining the current flowing through the transistor. The current I_h is the largest current that keeps the transistor in the weak-inversion regime. We define I_l to be the smallest value for $I_h b_i(n)$ that allows the circuit to settle within the clock period. The ratio I_h/I_l sets the supported range of $b_i(n)$. In the test-chip fabrication process, $I_h/I_l \approx 10,000$ is feasible, which is sufficient for accurate wordspotting. Likewise, the unitless $\log(\phi_i(n))$ is scaled by the voltage V_m to form a large-signal voltage encoding of log likelihood. A nominal value for V_m is 85mV in the test-chip process. To support a log likelihood range of 35 (the necessary range for accurate wordspotting) a large-signal voltage range of 3 volts (i.e. $35V_m$) is required.

The term $g_i(n-1)$ in Equation 2 is shown as the output of the circuit labeled (1) in Figure 3a. This circuit computes a function that approximates the desired expression $V_m \log(\phi_i(n-1) + \phi_{i-1}(n-1))$, if the transistors in the circuit operate in the weak-inversion regime.

The computed log likelihood $\log(\phi_i(n))$ in Equation 1 decreases every frame. The circuit shown in Figure 3a does not behave in this way: the voltage $V_m \log(\phi_i(n))$ *increases* every frame. This difference in behavior is attributable to the constant term $V_m \log(I_h/I_o)$ in Equation 2, which is not present in Equation 1, and is always larger than the negative contribution from $V_m \log(b_i(n))$. Figure 3b adds a new circuit (labeled (2)) to Figure 3a, that allows the constant term in Equation 2 to be altered under control of the binary input V. If V is V_{dd}, the circuit in Figure 3b is described by

$$V_m \log(\phi_i(n)) = V_m \log(b_i(n)) + g_i(n-1) + V_m \log(\frac{I_h I_o}{I_v^2}), \tag{3a}$$

where the term $V_m \log((I_h I_o)/I_v^2)$ should be less than or equal to zero. If V is grounded, the circuit is described by

$$V_m \log(\phi_i(n)) = V_m \log(b_i(n)) + g_i(n-1) + V_m \log(\frac{I_h}{I_v}), \tag{3b}$$

where the term $V_m \log(I_h/I_v)$ should have a positive value of at least several hundred millivolts. The goal of this design is to create two different operational modes for the system. One mode, described by Equation 3a, corresponds to the normal state decoder operation described in Equation 1. The other mode, described by Equation

3b, corresponds to the renormalization procedure, where a positive constant is added to all likelihoods in the system. During operation, a control system alternates between these two modes, to manage the dynamic range of the system.

Section 1 formulated HMMs as discrete-time systems. However, there are significant advantages in replacing the Z^{-1} element in Figure 3b with a continuous-time delay circuit. The switching noise of a sampled delay is eliminated. The power consumption and cell area specifications also benefit from continuous-time implementation.

Fundamentally, a change from discrete-time to continuous-time is not only an implementation change, but also an algorithmic change. Figure 3c shows a continuous-time state decoder whose observed behavior is qualitatively similar to a discrete-time decoder. The delay circuit, labeled (3), uses a linear transconductance amplifier in a follower-integrator configuration. The time constant of this delay circuit should be set to the frame rate of the corresponding discrete-time state decoder.

For correct decoder behavior over the full range of input probability values, the transconductance amplifier in the delay circuit must have a wide differential-input-voltage linear range. In the test chip presented in this paper, an amplifier with a small linear range was used. To work around the problem, we restricted the input probability currents in our experiments to a small multiple of I_l.

Figure 4 shows a state decoding system that corresponds to the grammar shown in Figure 1. Each numbered circle corresponds to the circuit shown in Figure 3c. The signal flows of this architecture support a dense layout: a rectangular array of single-state decoding circuits, with input current signal entering from the top edge of the array, and end-state log likelihood outputs exiting from the right edge of the array. States connect to their neighbors via the $V_{i-1}(t)$ and $V_i(t)$ signals shown in Figure 3c. For notational convenience, in this figure we define the unidirectional current $p_i(t)$ to be $I_h b_i(t)$.

In addition to the single-state decoder circuit, several other circuits are required. The "Recurrent Connection" block in Figure 4 implements the loopback connecting the filled circles in Figure 1. We implement this block using a 3-input version of the voltage follower circuit labeled (1) in Figure 3c. A simple arithmetic circuit implements the "Word Detect" block. To complete the system, a high fan-in/fan-out control circuit implements the renormalization algorithm. The circuit takes as input the log likelihood signals from all states in the system, and returns the binary signal V to the control input of all states. This control signal determines whether the single-state decoding circuits exhibit normal behavior (Equation 3a) or renormalization behavior (Equation 3b).

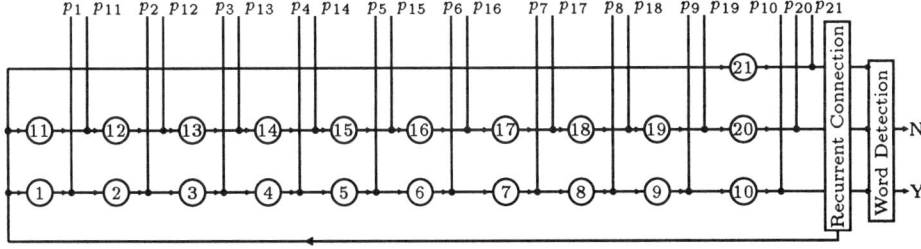

Figure 4. State decoder system for grammar shown in Figure 1.

3. STATE DECODER TEST CHIP

We fabricated a state decoder test chip in the $2\mu m$, n-well process of Orbit Semiconductor, via MOSIS. The chip has been fully tested and is functional. The chip decodes a grammar consisting of eight ten-state word models and a filler state. The state decoding and word detection sections of the chip contain 2000 transistors, and measure $586 \times 2807 \mu m$ ($586 \times 2807\lambda$, $\lambda = 1.0\mu m$). In this section, we show test results from the chip, in which we apply a temporal pattern of probability currents to the ten states of one word in the model (numbered 1 through 10) and observe the log likelihood voltage of the final state of the word (state 10).

Figure 5 contains simulated results, allowing us to show internal signals in the system. Figure 5a shows the temporal pattern of input probability currents $p_1 \ldots p_{10}$ that correspond to a simulated input word. Figure 5b shows the log likelihood voltage waveform for the end-state of the word (state 10). The waveform plateaus at L_h, the limit of the operating range of the state decoder system. During this plateau this state has the largest log likelihood in the system. Figure 5c is an expanded version of Figure 5b, showing in detail the renormalization cycles. Figure 5d shows the output computed by the "Word Detect" block in Figure 4. Note the smoothness of the waveform, unlike Figure 5c. By subtracting the filler-state log likelihood from the end-state log likelihood, the Word Detect block cancels the common-mode renormalization waveform.

Figure 6 shows a series of four experiments that confirm the qualitative behavior of the state decoder system. This figure shows experimental data recorded from the fabricated test chip. Each experiment consists of playing a particular pattern of input probability currents $p_1 \ldots p_{10}$ to the state decoder many times; for each repetition, a certain aspect of the playback is systematically varied. We measure the peak value of the end state log likelihood during each repetition, and plot this value as a function of the varied input parameter. For each experiment shown in Figure 6, the left plot describes the input pattern, while the right plot is the measured end-state log likelihood data. The experiment shown in Figure 6a involves presenting complete word patterns of varying durations to the decoder. As expected, words with unrealistically short durations have end-state responses below L_h, and would not produce successful word detection.

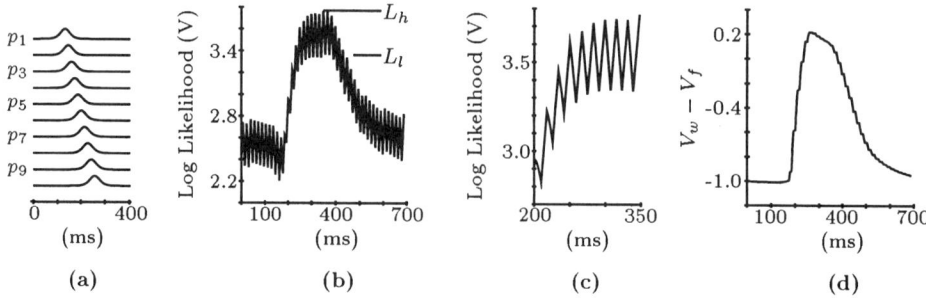

Figure 5. Simulation of state decoder: **(a)** Inputs patterns, **(b)**, **(c)** End-state response, **(d)** Word-detection response.

A Micropower Analog VLSI HMM State Decoder for Wordspotting

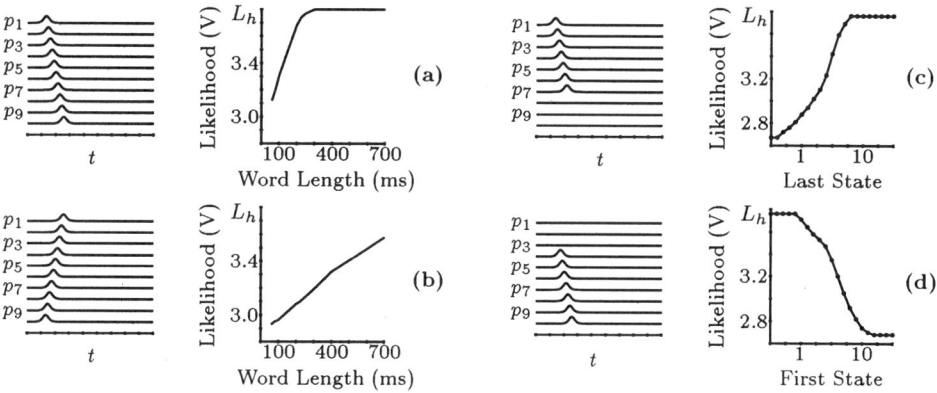

Figure 6. Measured chip data for end-state likelihoods for long, short, and incomplete pattern sequences.

The experiment shown in Figure 6b also involves presenting patterns of varying durations to the decoder, but the word patterns are presented "backwards," with input current p_{10} peaking first, and input current p_1 peaking last. The end-state response never reaches L_h, even at long word durations, and (correctly) would not trigger a word detection.

The experiments shown in Figure 6c and 6d involve presenting partially complete word patterns to the decoder. In both experiments, the duration of the complete word pattern is 250 ms. Figure 6c shows words with truncated endings, while Figure 6d shows words with truncated beginnings. In Figure 6c, end-state log likelihood is plotted as a function of the last excited state in the pattern; in Figure 6d, end-state log likelihood is plotted as a function of the first excited state in the pattern. In both plots the end-state log likelihood falls below L_h as significant information is removed from the word pattern.

While performing the experiments shown in Figure 6, the state-decoder and word-detection sections of the chip had a measured average power consumption of 141 nW ($V_{dd} = 5V$). More generally, however, the power consumption, input probability range, and the number of states are related parameters in the state decoder system.

Acknowledgments

We thank Herve Bourlard, Dan Hammerstrom, Brian Kingsbury, Alan Kramer, Nelson Morgan, Stylianos Perissakis, Su-lin Wu, and the anonymous reviewers for comments on this work. Sponsored by the Office of Naval Research (URI-N00014-92-J-1672) and the Department of Defense Advanced Research Projects Agency. Opinions, interpretations, conclusions, and recommendations are those of the authors and are not necessarily endorsed by the United States Air Force.

Reference

Lippmann, R. P., Chang, E. I., and Jankowski, C. R. (1994). "Wordspotter training using figure-of-merit back-propagation," *Proceedings International Conference on Acoustics, Speech, and Signal Processing*, Vol. 1, pp. 389-392.

Bangs, Clicks, Snaps, Thuds and Whacks: an Architecture for Acoustic Transient Processing

Fernando J. Pineda[1]
fernando.pineda@jhuapl.edu

Gert Cauwenberghs[2]
gert@jhunix.hcf.jhu.edu

R. Timothy Edwards[2]
tim@bach.ece.jhu.edu

[1]The Applied Physics Laboratory
The Johns Hopkins University
Laurel, Maryland 20723-6099

[2]Dept. of Electrical and Computer Engineering
The Johns Hopkins University
34th and Charles Streets
Baltimore Maryland 21218

ABSTRACT

We propose a neuromorphic architecture for real-time processing of acoustic transients in analog VLSI. We show how judicious normalization of a time-frequency signal allows an elegant and robust implementation of a correlation algorithm. The algorithm uses binary multiplexing instead of analog-analog multiplication. This removes the need for analog storage and analog-multiplication. Simulations show that the resulting algorithm has the same out-of-sample classification performance (~93% correct) as a baseline template-matching algorithm.

1 INTRODUCTION

We report progress towards our long-term goal of developing low-cost, low-power, low-complexity analog-VLSI processors for real-time applications. We propose a neuromorphic architecture for acoustic processing in analog VLSI. The characteristics of the architecture are explored by using simulations and real-world acoustic transients. We use acoustic transients in our experiments because information in the form of acoustic transients pervades the natural world. Insects, birds, and mammals (especially marine mammals) all employ acoustic signals with rich transient structure. Human speech, is largely composed of transients and speech recognizers based on transients can perform as well as recognizers based on phonemes (Morgan, Bourlard,Greenberg, Hermansky, and Wu, 1995). Machines also generate transients as they change state and as they wear down. Transients can be used to diagnose wear and abnormal conditions in machines.

In this paper, we consider how algorithmic choices that do not influence classification performance, make an initially difficult-to-implement algorithm, practical to implement. In particular, we present a practical architecture for performing real-time recognition of acoustic transients via a correlation-based algorithm. Correlation in analog VLSI poses two fundamental implementation challenges. First, there is the problem of template storage, second, there is the problem of accurate analog multiplication. Both problems can be solved by building sufficiently complex circuits. This solution is generally unsatisfactory because the resulting processors must have less area and consume less power than their digital counterparts in order to be competitive. Another solution to the storage problem is to employ novel floating gate devices. At present such devices can store analog values for years without significant degradation. Moreover, this approach can result in very compact, yet computationally complex devices. On the other hand, programming floating gate devices is not so straight-forward. It is relatively slow, it requires high voltage and it degrades the floating gate each time it is reprogrammed. Our "solution" is to side-step the problem completely and to develop an algorithmic solution that requires neither analog storage nor analog multiplication. Such an approach is attractive because it is both biologically plausible and electronically efficient. We demonstrate that a high level of classification performance on a real-world data set is achievable with no measurable loss of performance, compared to a baseline correlation algorithm.

The acoustic transients used in our experiments were collected by K. Ryals and D. Steigerwald and are described in (Pineda, Ryals, Steigerwald and Furth, 1995). These transients consist of isolated Bangs, Claps, Clicks, Cracks, Dinks, Pings, Pops, Slaps, Smacks, Snaps, Thuds and Whacks that were recorded on DAT tape in an office environment. The ambient noise level was uncontrolled, but typical of a single-occupant office. Approximately 221 transients comprising 10 classes were collected. Most of the energy in one of our typical transients is dissipated in the first 10 ms. The remaining energy is dissipated over the course of approximately 100 ms. The transients had durations of approximately 20-100 ms. There was considerable in-class and extra-class variability in duration. The duration of a transient was determined automatically by a segmentation algorithm described below. The segmentation algorithm was also used to align the templates in the correlation calculations.

2 THE BASELINE ALGORITHM

The baseline classification algorithm and its performance is described in Pineda, et al. (1995). Here we summarize only its most salient features. Like many biologically motivated acoustic processing algorithms, the preprocessing steps include time-frequency analysis, rectification, smoothing and compression via a nonlinearity (e.g. Yang, Wang and Shamma, 1992). Classification is performed by correlation against a template that represents a particular class. In addition, there is a "training" step which is required to create the templates. This step is described in the "correlation" section below. We turn now to a more detailed description of each processing step.

A. Time-frequency Analysis: Time-frequency analysis for the baseline algorithm and the simulations performed in this work, was performed by an ultra-low power (5.5 mW) analog VLSI filter bank intended to mimic the processing performed by the mammalian cochlea (Furth, Kumar, Andreou and Goldstein, 1994). This real-time device creates a time-frequency representation that would ordinarily require hours of computation on a high-speed workstation. More complete descriptions can be found in the references. The time-frequency representation produced by the filter bank is qualitatively similar to that produced by a wavelet transformation. The center frequencies and Q-factors of each channel are uniformly spaced in log space. The low frequency channel is tuned to a center frequency of 100 Hz and Q-factor of 1.0, while the high frequency channel is tuned to a center frequency of 6000 Hz and Q-factor 3.5. There are 31 output channels. The 31-channel cochlear output was digitized and stored on disk at a raw rate of 256K samples per second. This raw rate was distributed over 32 channels, at rates appropriate for each channel (six rates were used, 1 kHz for the lowest frequency channels up to 32 kHz for the highest-frequency channels and the unfiltered channel).

B. Segmentation: Both the template calculation and the classification algorithm rely on having a reliable segmenter. In our experiments, the transients are isolated and the noise level is low, therefore a simple segmenter is all that is needed. Figure 2. shows a segmenter that we implemented in software and which consists of a three layer neural network.

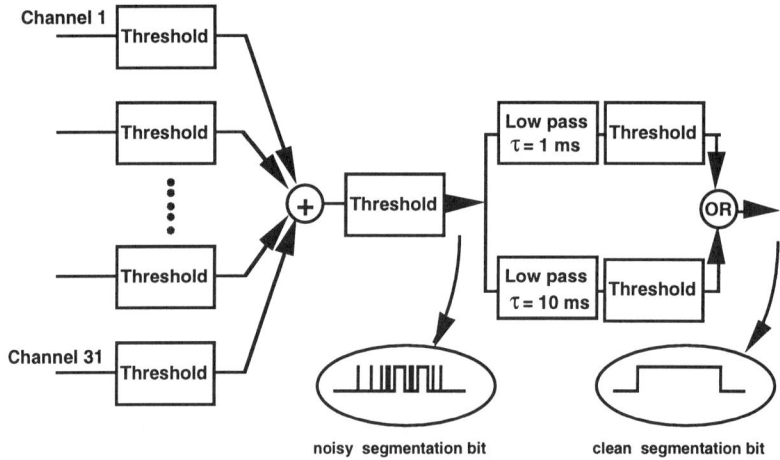

Figure 2: Schematic diagram showing the segmenter network

The input layer receives mean subtracted and rectified signals from the cochlear filters. The first layer simply thresholds these signals. The second layer consists of a single unit that accumulates and rethresholds the thresholded signals. The second layer outputs a noisy segmentation signal that is nonzero if two or more channels in the input layer exceed the input threshold. Finally, the output neuron cleans up the segmentation signal by low-pass filtering it with a time-scale of 10 ms (to fill in drop outs) and by low-pass filtering it with a time-scale of 1 ms (to catch the onset of a transient). The outputs of the two low-pass filters are OR'ed by the output neuron to produce a clean segmentation bit.

The four adjustable thresholds in the network were determined empirically so as to maximize the number of true transients that were properly segmented while minimizing the number of transients that were missed or cut in half.

C. Smoothing & Normalization: The raw output of the filter bank is rectified and smoothed with a single pole filter and subsequently normalized. Smoothing was done with a the same time-scale (1-ms) in all frequency channels. Let $\mathbf{X}(t)$ be the instantaneous vector of rectified and smoothed channel data, then the instantaneous output of the normalizer is

$\hat{\mathbf{X}}(t) = \dfrac{\mathbf{X}(t)}{\theta + \|\mathbf{X}(t)\|}$. Where θ is a positive constant whose purpose is to prevent the normalization stage from amplifying noise in the absence of a transient signal. With this normalization we have $\|\hat{\mathbf{X}}(t)\|_1 \approx 0$ if $\|\mathbf{X}(t)\|_1 << \theta$, and $\|\hat{\mathbf{X}}(t)\|_1 \approx 1$ if $\|\mathbf{X}(t)\|_1 >> \theta$. Thus θ effectively determines a soft input threshold that transients must exceed if they are to be normalized and passed on to higher level processing.

A sequence of normalized vectors over a time-window of length T is used as the feature vector for the correlation and classification stages of the algorithm. Figure 3. shows four normalized feature vectors from one class of transients (concatenated together).

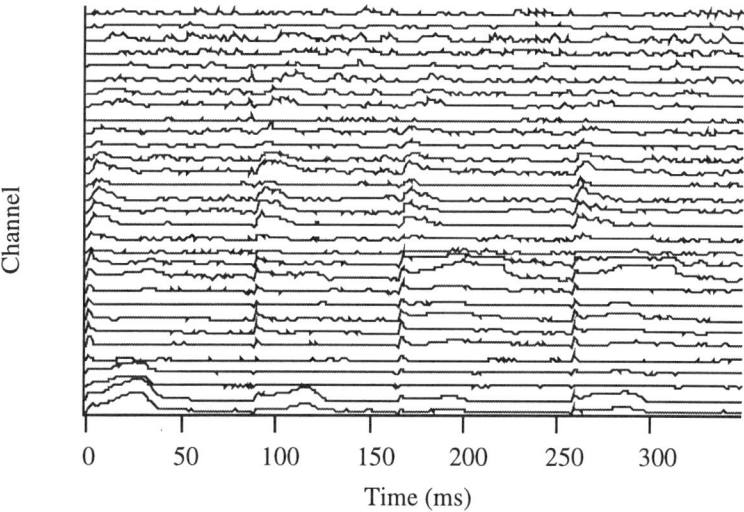

Figure 3.: Normalized representation of the first 4 exemplars from one class of transients.

D. Correlation : The feature-vectors are correlated in the time-frequency domain against a set of K time-frequency templates. The $k-th$ feature-vector-template is precalculated by averaging over a corpus of vectors from the $k-th$ class. Thus, if C_k represents the $k-th$ transient class, and if $\langle \ \rangle_k$ represents an average over the elements in a class, e.g. $\langle \hat{\mathbf{X}}(t) \rangle_k = E\{\hat{\mathbf{X}}(t)|\hat{\mathbf{X}}(t) \in C_k\}$. Then the template is of the form $b_k(t) = \langle \hat{\mathbf{X}}(t) \rangle_k$. The instantaneous output of the correlation stage is a K-dimensional vector $c(t)$ whose $k-th$ component is $c_k(t) = \sum\limits_{t'=t-T}^{t} \hat{\mathbf{X}}(t) \cdot b_k(t)$. The time-frequency window over which the correlations are performed is of length T and is advanced by one time-step between correlation calculations.

E. Classification The classification stage is a simple winner-take-all algorithm that assigns a class to the feature vector by picking the component of $c_k(t)$ that has the largest value at the appropriate time, i.e. $class = \arg\max\limits_{k}\{c_k(t_{valid})\}$.

The segmenter is used to determine the time t_{valid} when the output of the winner-take-all is to be used for classification. This corresponds to properly aligning the feature vector and the template. Leave-one-out cross-validation was used to estimate the out-of-sample classification performance of all the algorithms described in this paper. The rate of correct classification for the baseline algorithm was 92.8%. Out of a total of 221 events that were detected and segmented, 16 were misclassified.

3 A CORRELATION ALGORITHM FOR ANALOG VLSI

We now address the question of how to perform classification without performing analog-analog multiplication and without having to store analog templates. To provide a better understanding of the algorithm, we present it as a set of incremental modifications to the baseline algorithm. This will serve to make clear the role played by each modification.

Examination of the normalized representation in figure 3 suggests that the information content of any one time-frequency bin cannot be very high. Accordingly, we seek a highly compressed representation that is both easy to form and with which it is easy to compute. As a preliminary step to forming this compressed representation, consider correlating the time-derivative of the feature vector with the time-derivative of the template,

$$c_k(t) = \sum_{t'=t-T}^{t} \dot{\mathbf{X}}(t) \cdot \mathbf{b}_k(t) \quad \text{where} \quad b_k(t) = \left\langle \dot{\mathbf{X}}(t) \right\rangle_k.$$

This modification has no effect on the out-of-sample performance of the winner-take-all classification algorithm. The above representation, by itself, has very few implementation advantages. It can, in principal, mitigate the effect of any systematic offsets that might emerge from the normalization circuit. Unfortunately, the price for this small advantage would be a very complex multiplier. This is evident since the time-derivative of a positive quantity can have either sign, both the feature vector and the template are now bipolar. Accordingly the correlation hardware would now require 4-quadrant analog-analog multipliers. Moreover the storage circuits must handle bipolar quantities as well.

The next step in forming a compressed representation is to replace the time-differentiated *template* with just a sign that indicates whether the template value in a particular channel is increasing or decreasing with time. This template is $b'_k(t) = Sign\left(\left\langle \dot{\mathbf{X}}(t) \right\rangle_k\right)$. We denote this template as the [-1,+1]-representation template. The resulting classification algorithm yields *exactly* the same out-of-sample performance as the baseline algorithm. The 4-quadrant analog-analog multiply of the differentiated representation is reduced to a "4-quadrant analog-binary" multiply. The storage requirements are reduced to a single bit per time-frequency bin. To simplify the hardware yet further, we exploit the fact that the time derivative of a random unit vector $\mathbf{u}(t)$ (with respect to the 1-norm) satisfies

$$E\left\{\sum_v Sign(\langle \dot{u}_v \rangle)\dot{u}_v \right\} = 2E\left\{\sum_v \Theta(\langle \dot{u}_v \rangle)\dot{u}_v \right\}$$

where Θ is a step function. Accordingly, if we use a template whose elements are in [0,1] instead of [-1, +1], i.e. $b''_k(t) = \Theta\left(\left\langle \dot{\mathbf{X}}(t) \right\rangle_k\right)$, we expect

$$E\left\{\sum_v b'_v \dot{X}_v \right\} = 2E\left\{b''_v \dot{X}_v \right\} = \left\|\dot{\mathbf{X}}\right\|_1,$$ provided the feature vector $\dot{\mathbf{X}}(t)$ is drawn from the

same class as is used to calculate the template. Furthermore, if the feature vector and the template are statistically independent, then we expect that either representation will produce a zero correlation, $E\left\{\sum_v b'_v \dot{\hat{X}}_v\right\} = E\left\{b''_v, \dot{\hat{X}}_v\right\} = 0$. In practice, we find that the difference in correlation values between using the [0,1] and the [-1,+1] representations is simply a scale factor (approximately equal to 2 to several digits of precision). This holds even when the feature vectors and the templates do not correspond to the same class. Thus the difference between the two representations is quantitatively minor and qualitatively nonexistent, as evidenced by our classification experiments, which show that the out-of-sample performance of the [0,1] representation is *identical* to that of the [-1,+1] representation. Furthermore, changing to the [0,1] representation has no impact on the storage requirements since both representations require the storage of single bit per time-frequency bin. On the other hand, consider that by using the [0,1] representation we now have a "2-quadrant analog-binary" multiply instead of a "4-quadrant analog-binary" multiply. Finally, we observe that differentiation and correlation are commuting operations, thus rather than differentiating $\hat{X}(t)$ before correlation, we can differentiate after the correlation without changing the result. This reduces the complexity of the correlation operation still further, since the fact that both $\hat{X}(t)$ and $b'_k(t)$ are positive means that we need only implement a correlator with 1-quadrant analog-binary multiplies.

The result of the above evolution is a correlation algorithm that empirically performs as well as a baseline correlation algorithm, but only requires binary-multiplexing to perform the correlation. We find that with only 16 frequency channels and 64 time bins (1024-bits/templates), we are able to achieve the desired level of performance. We have undertaken the design and fabrication of a prototype chip. This chip has been fabricated and we will report on it's performance in the near future. Figure 4 illustrates the key architectural features of the correlator/memory implementation. The rectified and

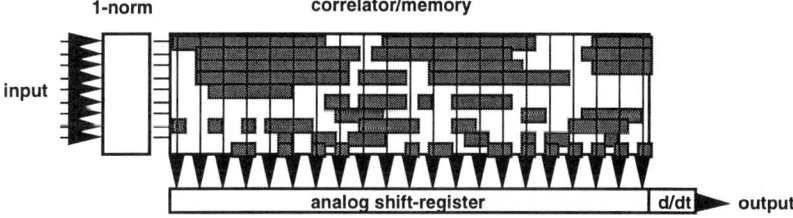

Figure 4: Schematic architecture of the k-th correlator-memory.

smoothed frequency-analyzed signals are input from the left as currents. The currents are normalized before being fed into the correlator. A binary time-frequency template is stored as a bit pattern in the correlator/memory. A single bit is stored at each time and frequency bin. If this bit is set, current is mirrored from the horizontal (frequency) lines onto vertical (aggregation) lines. Current from the aggregation lines is integrated and shifted in a bucket-brigade analog shift register. The last two stages of the shift register are differenced to estimate a time-derivative.

4   DISCUSSION AND CONCLUSIONS

The correlation algorithm described in the previous section is related to the zero-crossing representation analyzed by Yang, Wang. and Shamma (1992). This is because bit flips in the templates correspond to the zero crossings of the expected time-derivative of the normalized "energy-envelope." Note that we do not encode the incoming acoustic signal with a zero-crossing representation. Interestingly enough, if both the analog signal *and* the template are reduced to a binary representation, then the classification performance drops dramatically. It appears that maintaining some analog information in the processing path is significant.

The frequency-domain normalization approach presented above throws away absolute intensity information. Thus, low intensity resonances that remain excited after the initial burst of acoustic energy are as important in the feature vector as the initial burst of energy. These resonances can contain significant information about the nature of the transient but would have less weight in an algorithm with a different normalization scheme. Another consequence of the normalization is that even a transient whose spectrum is highly concentrated in just a few frequency channels will spread its information over the entire spectrum through the normalization denominator. The use of a normalized representation thus distributes the correlation calculation over very many frequency channels and serves to mitigate the effect of device mismatch.

We consider the proposed correlator/memory as a potential component in more sophisticated acoustic processing systems. For example, the continuously generated output of the correlators, $c(t)$, is itself a feature vector that could be used in more sophisticated segmentation and/or classification algorithms such as the time-delayed neural network approach of Unnikrishnan, Hopfield and Tank (1991).

The work reported in this report was supported by a Whiting School of Engineering/Applied Physics Laboratory Collaborative Grant. Preliminary work was supported by an APL Internal Research & Development Budget.

REFERENCES

Furth, P.M. and Kumar, N.G., Andreou, A.G. and Goldstein, M.H., "Experiments with the Hopkins Electronic EAR", 14th Speech Research Symposium, Baltimore, MD pp.183-189, (1994).

Pineda, F.J., Ryals, K., Steigerwald, D. and Furth, P., (1995). "Acoustic Transient Processing using the Hopkins Electronic Ear", World Conference on Neural Networks 1995, Washington DC.

Yang, X., Wang K. and Shamma, S.A. (1992). "Auditory Representations of Acoustic Signals", IEEE Trans. on Information Processing, 38, pp. 824-839.

Morgan, N., Bourlard, H., Greenberg, S., Hermansky, H. and Wu, S. L., (1996). "Stochastic Perceptual Models of Speech", IEEE Proc. Intl. Conference on Acoustics, Speech and Signal Processing, Detroit, MI, pp. 397-400.

Unnikrishnan, K.P., Hopfield J.J., and Tank, D.W. (1991). "Connected-Digit Speaker-Dependent Speech Recognition Using a Neural Network with Time-Delayed Connections", IEEE Transactions on Signal Processing, 39, pp. 698-713

A Silicon Model of Amplitude Modulation Detection in the Auditory Brainstem

André van Schaik, Eric Fragnière, Eric Vittoz
MANTRA Center for Neuromimetic Systems
Swiss Federal Institute of Technology
CH-1015 Lausanne
email: Andre.van_Schaik@di.epfl.ch

Abstract

Detection of the periodicity of amplitude modulation is a major step in the determination of the pitch of a sound. In this article we will present a silicon model that uses synchronicity of spiking neurons to extract the fundamental frequency of a sound. It is based on the observation that the so called 'Choppers' in the mammalian Cochlear Nucleus synchronize well for certain rates of amplitude modulation, depending on the cell's intrinsic chopping frequency. Our silicon model uses three different circuits, i.e., an artificial cochlea, an Inner Hair Cell circuit, and a spiking neuron circuit.

1. INTRODUCTION

Over the last few years, we have developed and implemented several analog VLSI building blocks that allow us to model parts of the auditory pathway [1], [2], [3]. This paper presents one experiment using these building blocks to create a model for the detection of the fundamental frequency of a harmonic complex. The estimation of this fundamental frequency by the model shows some important similarities with psycho-acoustic experiments in pitch estimation in humans [4]. A good model of pitch estimation will give us valuable insights in the way the brain processes sounds. Furthermore, a practical application to speech recognition can be expected, either by using the pitch estimate as an element in the acoustic vector fed to the recognizer, or by normalizing the acoustic vector to the pitch.

Although the model doesn't yield a complete model of pitch estimation, and explains probably only one of a few different mechanisms the brain uses for pitch estimation, it can give us a better understanding of the physiological background of psycho-acoustic results. An electronic model can be especially helpful, when the parameters of the model can be easily controlled, and when the model will operate in real time.

2. THE MODEL

The model was originally developed by Hewitt and Meddis [4], and was based on the observation that Chopper cells in the Cochlear Nucleus synchronize when the stimulus is modulated in amplitude within a particular modulation frequency range [5].

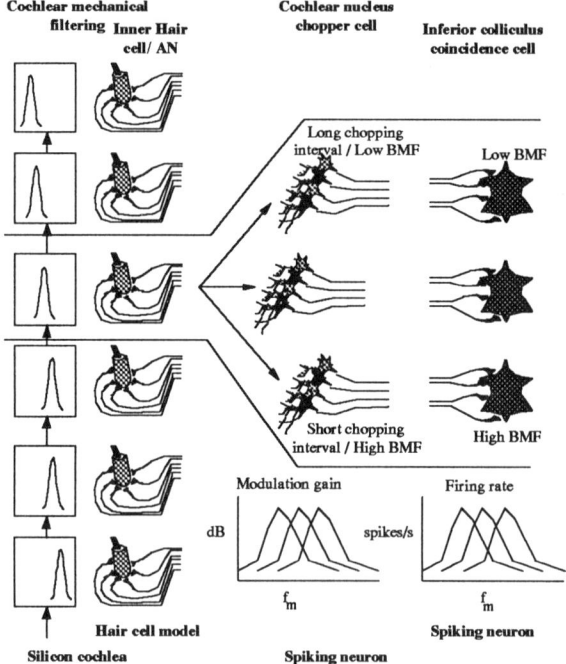

Fig. 1. Diagram of the AM detection model. BMF=Best Modulation Frequency.

The diagram shown in figure 1 shows the elements of the model. The cochlea filters the incoming sound signal. Since the width of the pass-band of a cochlear band-pass filter is proportional to its cut-off frequency, the filters will not be able to resolve the individual harmonics of a high frequency carrier (>3kHz) amplitude modulated at a low rate (<500Hz). The outputs of the cochlear filters that have their cut-off frequency slightly above the carrier frequency of the signal will therefore still be modulated in amplitude at the original modulation frequency. This modulation component will therefore synchronize a certain group of Chopper cells. The synchronization of this group of Chopper cells can be detected using a coincidence detecting neuron, and signals the presence of a particular amplitude modulation frequency. This model is biologically plausible, because it is known that the choppers synchronize to a particular amplitude modulation frequency and that they project their output towards the Inferior Colliculus (amongst others). Furthermore, neurons that can function as coincidence detectors are shown to be present in the Inferior Colliculus and the rate of firing of these neurons is a band-pass function of the amplitude modulation rate. It is not known to date however if the choppers actually project to these coincidence detector neurons.

The actual mechanism that synchronizes the chopper cells will be discussed with the measurements in section 4. In the next section, we will first present the circuits that allowed us to build the VLSI implementation of this model.

3. THE CIRCUITS

All of the circuits used in our model have already been presented in more detail elsewhere, but we will present them briefly for completeness. Our silicon cochlea has been presented in detail at NIPS'95 [1], and more details about the Inner Hair Cell circuit and the spiking neuron circuit can be found in [2].

3.1 THE SILICON COCHLEA

The silicon cochlea consists of a cascade of second order low-pass filters. Each filter section is biased using Compatible Lateral Bipolar Transistors (CLBTs) which control the cut-off frequency and the quality factor of each section. A single resistive line is used to bias all CLBTs. Because of the exponential relation between the Base-Emitter Voltage and the Collector current of the CLBTs, the linear voltage gradient introduced by the resistive line will yield a filter cascade with an exponentially decreasing cut-off frequency of the filters. The output voltage of each filter V_{out} then represents the displacement of a basilar membrane section. In order to obtain a representation of the basilar membrane velocity, we take the difference between V_{out} and the voltage on the internal node of the second order filter.

We have integrated this silicon cochlea using 104 filter stages, and the output of every second stage is connected to an output pin.

3.2 THE INNER HAIR CELL MODEL

The inner hair cell circuit is used to half-wave rectify the basilar membrane velocity signal and to perform some form of temporal adaptation, as can be seen in figure 2b. The differential pair at the input is used to convert the input voltage into a current with a compressive relation between input amplitude and the actual amplitude of the current.

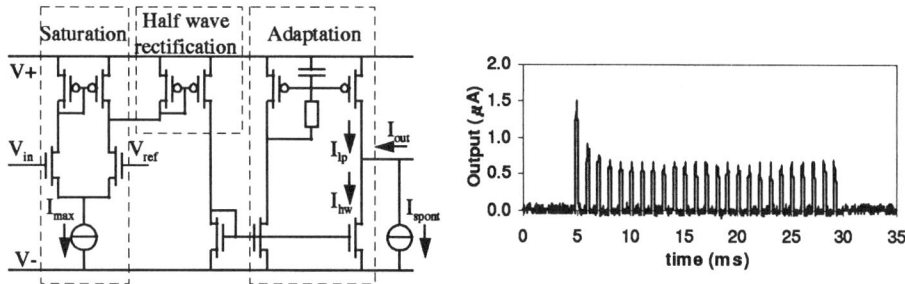

Fig. 2. a) The Inner Hair Cell circuit, b) measured output current.

We have integrated a small chip containing 4 independent inner hair cells.

3.3 THE SPIKING NEURON MODEL

The spiking neuron circuit is given in figure 3. The membrane of a biological neuron is modeled by a capacitance, C_{mem}, and the membrane leakage current is controlled by the gate voltage, V_{leak}, of an NMOS transistor. In the absence of any input ($I_{ex}=0$), the membrane voltage will be drawn to its resting potential (controlled by V_{rest}), by this leakage current. Excitatory inputs simply add charge to the membrane capacitance, whereas inhibitory inputs are simply modeled by a negative I_{ex}. If an excitatory current larger than the leakage current of the membrane is injected, the membrane potential will increase from its resting potential. This membrane potential, V_{mem}, is compared with a controllable threshold voltage V_{thres}, using a basic transconductance amplifier driving a high impedance load. If V_{mem} exceeds V_{thres}, an action potential will be generated.

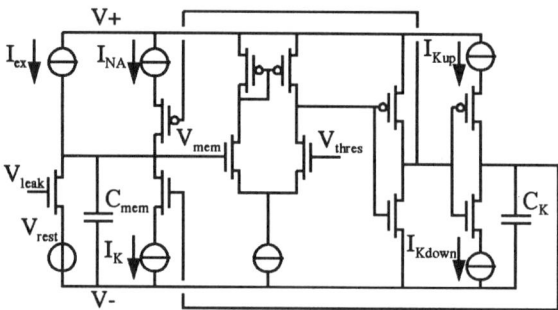

Fig. 3. The Spiking Neuron circuit

The generation of the action potential happens in a similar way as in the biological neuron, where an increased sodium conductance creates the upswing of the spike, and a delayed increase of the potassium conductance creates the downswing. In the circuit this is modeled as follows. If V_{mem} rises above V_{thres}, the output voltage of the comparator will rise to the positive power supply. The output of the following inverter will thus go low, thereby allowing the "sodium current" I_{Na} to pull up the membrane potential. At the same time however, a second inverter will allow the capacitance C_K to be charged at a speed which can be controlled by the current I_{Kup}. As soon as the voltage on C_K is high enough to allow conduction of the NMOS to which it is connected, the "potassium current" I_K will be able to discharge the membrane capacitance.

If V_{mem} now drops below V_{thres}, the output of the first inverter will become high, cutting off the current I_{Na}. Furthermore, the second inverter will then allow C_K to be discharged by the current I_{Kdown}. If I_{Kdown} is small, the voltage on C_K will decrease only slowly, and, as long as this voltage stays high enough to allow I_K to discharge the membrane, it will be impossible to stimulate the neuron if I_{ex} is smaller than I_K. Therefore I_{Kdown} can be said to control the 'refractory period' of the neuron.

We have integrated a chip, containing a group of 32 neurons, each having the same bias voltages and currents. The component mismatch and the noise ensure that we actually have 32 similar, but not completely equal neurons.

4. TEST RESULTS

Most neuro-physiological data concerning low frequency amplitude modulation of high frequency carriers exists for carriers at about 5kHz and a modulation depth of about 50%. We therefore used a 5 kHz sinusoid in our tests and a 50% modulation depth at frequencies below 550Hz.

A Silicon Model of Amplitude Modulation Detection

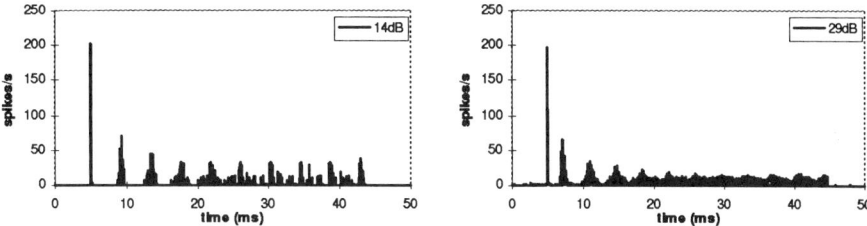

Fig. 4. PSTH of the chopper chip for 2 different sound intensities

First step in the elaboration of the model is to test if the group of spiking neurons on a single chip is capable of performing like a group of similar Choppers. Neurons in the auditory brainstem are often characterized with a Post Stimulus Time Histogram (PSTH), which is a histogram of spikes in response to repeated stimulation with a pure tone of short duration. If the choppers on the chip are really similar, the PSTH of this group of choppers will be very similar to the PSTH of a single chopper. In figure 4 the PSTH of the circuit is shown. It is the result of the summed response of the 32 neurons on chip to 20 repeated stimulations with a 5kHz tone burst. This figure shows that the response of the Choppers yields a PSTH typical of chopping neurons, and that the chopping frequency, keeping all other parameters constant, increases with increasing sound intensity. The chopping rate for an input signal of given intensity can be controlled by setting the refractory period of the spiking neurons, and can thus be used to create the different groups of choppers shown in figure 1. The chopping rate of the choppers in figure 4 is about 300Hz for a 29dB input signal.

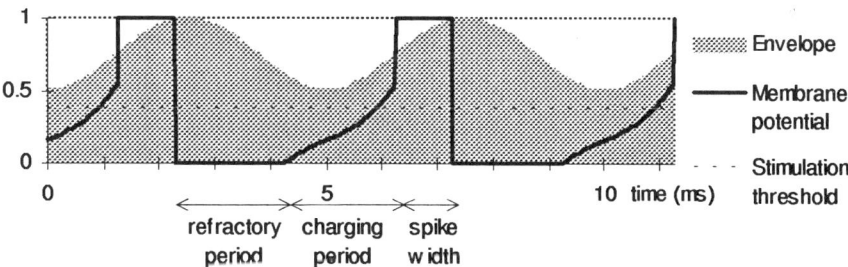

Fig. 5. Spike generation for a Chopper cell.

To understand why the Choppers will synchronize for a certain amplitude modulation frequency, one has to look at the signal envelope, which contains temporal information on a time scale that can influence the spiking neurons. The 5kHz carrier itself will not contain any temporal information that influences the spiking neuron in an important way. Consider the case when the modulation frequency is similar to the chopping frequency (figure 5). If a Chopper then spikes during the rising flank of the envelope, it will come out of its refractory period just before the next rising flank of the envelope. If the driven chopping frequency is a bit too low, the Chopper will come out of its refractory period a bit later, therefore it receives a higher average stimulation and it spikes a little higher on the rising flank of the envelope. This in turn increases the chopping frequency and thus provides a form of negative feedback on the chopping frequency. This therefore makes spiking on a certain point on the rising flank of the envelope a stable situation. With the same reasoning one can show that spiking on the falling flank is therefore an unstable situation. Furthermore, it is not possible to stabilize a cell driven above its maximum chopping rate, nor is it possible to stabilize a cell that fires more than once per modulation period. Since a group of similar choppers will stabilize at about the same point on the rising flank, their spikes will thus coincide when the modulation frequency allows them to.

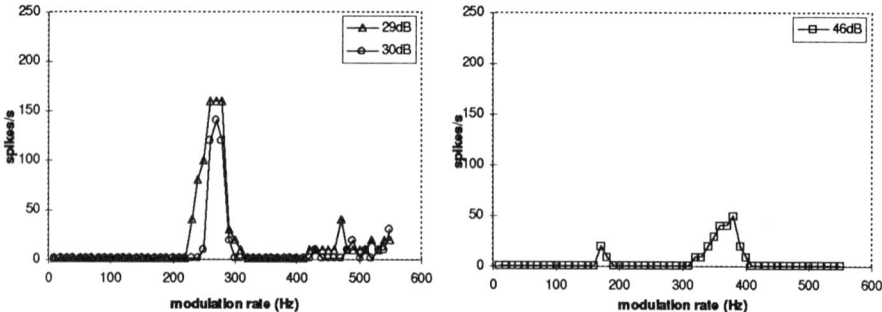

Fig. 6. AM sensitivity of the coincidence detecting neuron.

Another free parameter of the model is the threshold of the coincidence detecting neuron. If this parameter is set so that at least 60% of the choppers must spike within 1ms to be considered a coincidence, we obtain the output of figure 6. We can see that this yields the expected band-pass Modulation Transfer Function (MTF), and that the best modulation frequency for the 29dB input signal corresponds to the intrinsic chopping rate of the group of neurons. Figure 6 also shows that the best modulation frequency (BMF), just as the chopping rate, increases with increasing sound intensity, but that the maximum number of spikes per second actually decreases. This second effect is caused by the fact that the stabilizing effect of the positive flank of the signal envelope only influences the time during which the neuron is being charged, which becomes a smaller part of the total spiking period at higher intensities. The negative feedback thus has less influence on the total chopping period and therefore synchronizes the choppers less.

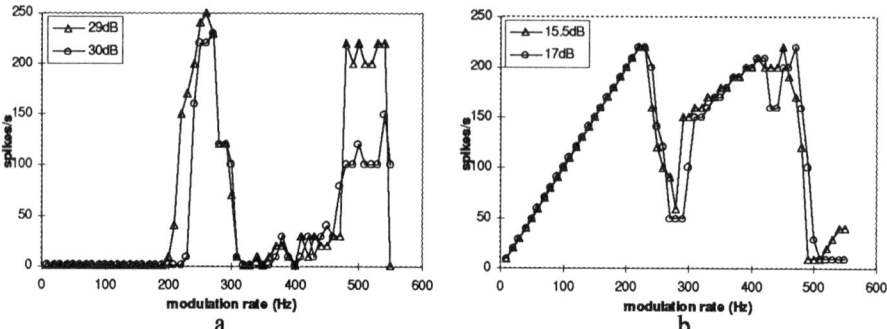

Fig. 7. AM sensitivity of the coincidence detecting neuron.

When the coincidence threshold is lowered to 50%, we can see in figure 7a that the maximum number of spikes goes up, because this threshold is more easily reached. Furthermore, a second pass-band shows up at double the BMF. This is because the choppers fire only every second amplitude modulation period, and part of the group of choppers will synchronize during the odd periods, whereas others during the even periods. The division of the group of choppers will typically be close to, but hardly ever exactly 50-50, so that either during the odd or during the even modulation period the 50% coincidence threshold is exceeded. The 60% threshold of figure 6 will only rarely be exceeded, explaining the weak second peak seen around 500Hz in this figure.

Figure 7b. shows the MTF for low intensity signals with a 50% coincidence threshold. At low intensities the effect of an additional non-linearity, the stimulation threshold, shows up. Whenever the instantaneous value of the envelope is lower than the stimulation threshold, the spiking neuron will not be stimulated because its input current will be lower than the cell's leakage current. At these low intensities the activity during the valleys of the modulation envelope will thus not be enough to stimulate the Choppers (see figure 5). For stimuli with a lower modulation frequency than the group's chopping frequency, the Choppers will come out of their refractory period in such a valley. These choppers therefore will have to wait for the envelope amplitude to increase above a certain value, before they receive anew a stimulation. This waiting period nullifies the effect of the variation of the refractory period of the Choppers, and thus synchronizes the Choppers for low modulation frequencies. A second effect of this waiting period is that in this case the firing rate of the Choppers matches the modulation frequency. When the modulation frequency becomes higher than the maximum chopping frequency, the Choppers will fire only every second period, but will still be synchronized, as can be seen between 300Hz and 500Hz in figure 7b.

5. CONCLUSIONS

In this article we have shown that it is possible to use our building blocks to build a multi-chip system that models part of the auditory pathway. Furthermore, the fact that the spiking neuron chip can be easily biased to function as a group of similar Choppers, combined with the relative simplicity of the spike generation mechanism of a single neuron on chip, allowed us to gain insight in the process by which chopping neurons in the mammalian Cochlear Nucleus synchronize to a particular range of amplitude modulation frequencies.

References

[1] A. van Schaik, E. Fragnière, & E. Vittoz, "Improved silicon cochlea using compatible lateral bipolar transistors," *Advances in Neural Information Processing Systems 8*, MIT Press, Cambridge, 1996.

[2] A. van Schaik, E. Fragnière, & E. Vittoz, "An analoge electronic model of ventral cochlear nucleus neurons," *Proc. Fifth Int. Conf. on Microelectronics for Neural Networks and Fuzzy Systems*, IEEE Computer Society Press, Los Alamitos, 1996, pp. 52-59.

[3] A. van Schaik and R. Meddis, "The electronic ear; towards a blueprint," *Neurobiology*, NATO ASI series, Plenum Press, New York, 1996.

[4] M.J. Hewitt and R. Meddis, "A computer model of amplitude-modulation sensitivity of single units in the inferior colliculus," *J. Acoust. Soc. Am.*, 95, 1994, pp. 1-15.

[5] M.J. Hewitt, R. Meddis, & T.M. Shackleton, "A computer model of a cochlear-nucleus stellate cell: responses to amplitude-modulated and pure tone stimuli," *J. Acoust. Soc. Am.*, 91, 1992, pp. 2096-2109.

PART VI
SPEECH, HANDWRITING AND SIGNAL PROCESSING

Dynamic features for visual speech-reading: A systematic comparison

Michael S. Gray[1,3], Javier R. Movellan[1], Terrence J. Sejnowski[2,3]
Departments of Cognitive Science[1] and Biology[2]
University of California, San Diego
La Jolla, CA 92093
and
Howard Hughes Medical Institute[3]
Computational Neurobiology Lab
The Salk Institute, P. O. Box 85800
San Diego, CA 92186-5800
Email: mgray, jmovellan, tsejnowski@ucsd.edu

Abstract

Humans use visual as well as auditory speech signals to recognize spoken words. A variety of systems have been investigated for performing this task. The main purpose of this research was to systematically compare the performance of a range of dynamic visual features on a speechreading task. We have found that normalization of images to eliminate variation due to translation, scale, and planar rotation yielded substantial improvements in generalization performance regardless of the visual representation used. In addition, the dynamic information in the difference between successive frames yielded better performance than optical-flow based approaches, and compression by local low-pass filtering worked surprisingly better than global principal components analysis (PCA). These results are examined and possible explanations are explored.

1 INTRODUCTION

Visual speech recognition is a challenging task in sensory integration. Psychophysical work by McGurk and MacDonald [5] first showed the powerful influence of visual information on speech perception that has led to increased interest in this area. A wide variety of techniques have been used to model speech-reading. Yuhas, Goldstein, Sejnowski, and Jenkins [8] used feedforward networks to combine gray scale images with acoustic representations of vowels. Wolff, Prasad, Stork, and Hennecke [7] explicitly computed information about the position of the lips, the shape of the mouth, and motion. This approach has the advantage of dramatically reducing the dimensionality of the input, but critical information may be lost. The visual information (mouth shape, position, and motion) was the input to a time-delay neural network (TDNN) that was trained to distinguish among consonant-vowel pairs. A separate TDNN was trained on the acoustic signal. The output probabilities for the visual and acoustic signals were then combined multiplicatively. Bregler and Konig [1] also utilized a TDNN architecture. In this work, the visual information was captured by the first 10 principal components of a contour model fit to the lips. This was enough to specify the full range of lip shapes ("eigenlips"). Bregler and Konig [1] combined the acoustic and visual information in the input representation, which gave improved performance in noisy environments, compared with acoustic information alone.

Surprisingly, the visual signal alone carries a substantial amount of information about spoken words. Garcia, Goldschen, and Petajan [2] used a variety of visual features from the mouth region of a speaker's face to recognize test sentences using hidden Markov models (HMMs). Those features that were found to give the best discrimination tended to be dynamic in nature, rather than static. Mase and Pentland [4] also explored the dynamic information present in lip images through the use of optical flow. They found that a template matching approach on the optical flow of 4 windows around the edges of the mouth yielded results similar to humans on a digit recognition task. Movellan [6] investigated the recognition of spoken digits using only visual information. The input representation for the hidden Markov model consisted of low-pass filtered pixel intensity information at each time step, as well as a delta image that showed the pixel by pixel difference between subsequent time steps.

The motivation for the current work was succinctly stated by Bregler and Konig [1]: "The real information in lipreading lies in the temporal change of lip positions, rather than the absolute lip shape." Although different kinds of dynamic visual information have been explored, there has been no careful comparison of different methods. Here we present results for four different dynamic techniques that are based on general purpose processing at the pixel level. The first approach was to combine low-pass filtered gray scale pixel values with a delta image, defined as the difference between two successive gray level images. A PCA reduction of this grayscale and delta information was investigated next. The final two approaches were motivated by the kinds of visual processing that are believed to occur in higher levels of the visual cortex. We first explored optical flow, which provides us with a representation analogous to that in primate visual area MT. Optical flow output was then combined with low-pass filtered gray-scale pixel values. Each of these four representations was tested on two different datasets: (1) the raw video images, and (2) the normalized video images.

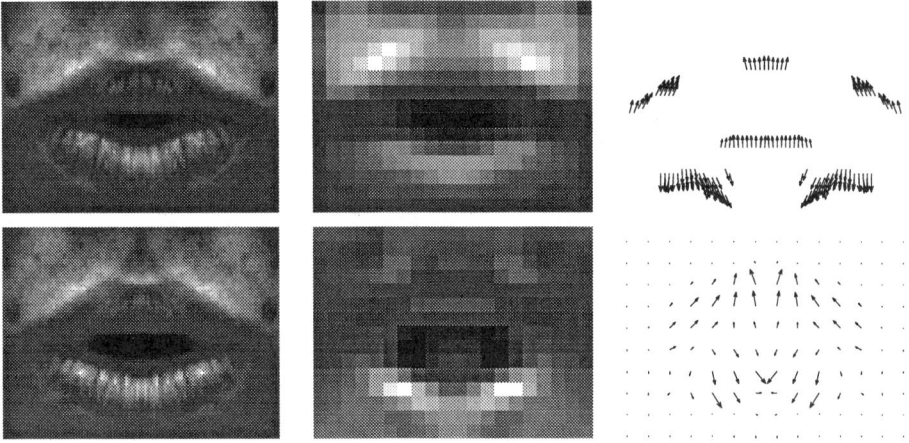

Figure 1: Image processing techniques. Left column: Two successive video frames (frames 1 and 2) from a subject saying the digit "one". These images have been made symmetric by averaging left and right pixels relative to the vertical midline. Middle column: The top panel shows gray scale pixel intensity information of frame 2 after low-pass filtering and down-sampling to a resolution of 15 x 20 pixels. The bottom panel shows the delta image (pixel-wise subtraction of frame 1 from frame 2), after low-pass filtering and downsampling. Right column: The top panel shows the optical flow for the 2 video frames in the left column. The bottom panel shows the reconstructed optical flow representation learned by a 1-state HMM. This can be considered the canonical or prototypical representation for the digit "one" across our database of 12 individuals.

2 METHODS AND MODELS

2.1 TRAINING SAMPLE

The training sample was the Tulips1 database (Movellan [6]): 96 digitized movies of 12 undergraduate students (9 males, 3 females) from the Cognitive Science Department at UC-San Diego. Video capturing was performed in a windowless room at the Center for Research in Language at UC-San Diego. Subjects were asked to talk into a video camera and to say the first four digits in English twice. Subjects could monitor the digitized images in a small display conveniently located in front of them. They were asked to position themselves so that their lips were roughly centered in the feed-back display. Gray scale video images were digitized at 30 frames per second, 100 x 75 pixels, 8 bits per pixel. The video tracks were hand segmented by selecting a few relevant frames before the beginning and after the end of activity in the acoustic track. There were an average of 9.7 frames for each movie. Two sample frames are shown in the left column of Figure 1.

2.2 IMAGE PROCESSING

We compared the performance of four different visual representations for the digit recognition task: low-pass + delta, PCA of (gray-scale + delta), flow, and low-pass

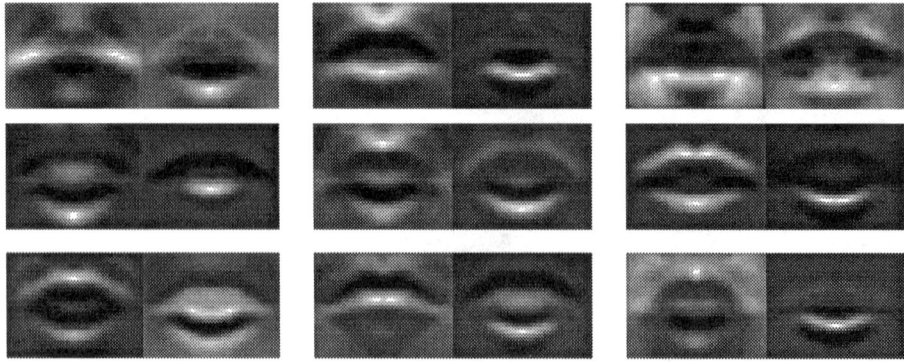

Figure 2: The first 9 principal components of the raw lip images, starting in upper left and proceeding in normal English reading order. The left half of each image contained pixel intensity information, and the right half represented the delta image.

+ flow. The video images were made symmetric by averaging pixels from the left and right side of the image (Figure 1, left column). The low-pass + delta representation (Movellan [6]) consisted of 2 parts (Figure 1, middle column). The images were low-pass filtered, and downsampled to a resolution of 15 x 20 pixels. Delta images were formed from the pixel-by-pixel difference between subsequent time frames, and then low-pass filtered and downsampled to 15 x 20 pixels. Because the images were symmetric, we used only half of the low-pass and delta images, resulting in a 300-dimensional input vector.

Our PCA of (gray-scale + delta) representation was derived from input images and delta images at the original resolution of 75 x 100 pixels. We examined the projections on to principal components (PCs) 1-300. Because the projection onto the first principal component accounted for 95% of the variance, differences between the remaining projections (2-300) were substantially reduced when the coefficients were normalized to the range [0 1] for input to the HMM. For this reason, results were also obtained for the projections on to PCs 2-301. This range of PCs gave much better performance, and it is the results on this set of PCs that are reported here. The first 9 PCs of the lip images are illustrated in Figure 2.

The delta image representation captures information about changes in the lip image over time, but does not signal the direction in which lip features are moving. To get directional information, we computed optical flow. This computation was based on the standard *brightness constraint* equation, followed by thresholding to eliminate locations without any edges or with small temporal derivatives. The resulting flow field was then low-pass filtered and downsampled to obtain our flow representation: a 140-dimensional input vector (70 for left/right motion, and 70 for up/down motion), which is illustrated in Figure 1 (right column, top panel). Finally, for the low-pass + flow inputs, low-pass filtered pixel intensities were combined with optical flow.

All four visual representations were tested on two different datasets. The first dataset contained the raw video images described above. In the second dataset, images were normalized so that variations due to translation, scale, and planar

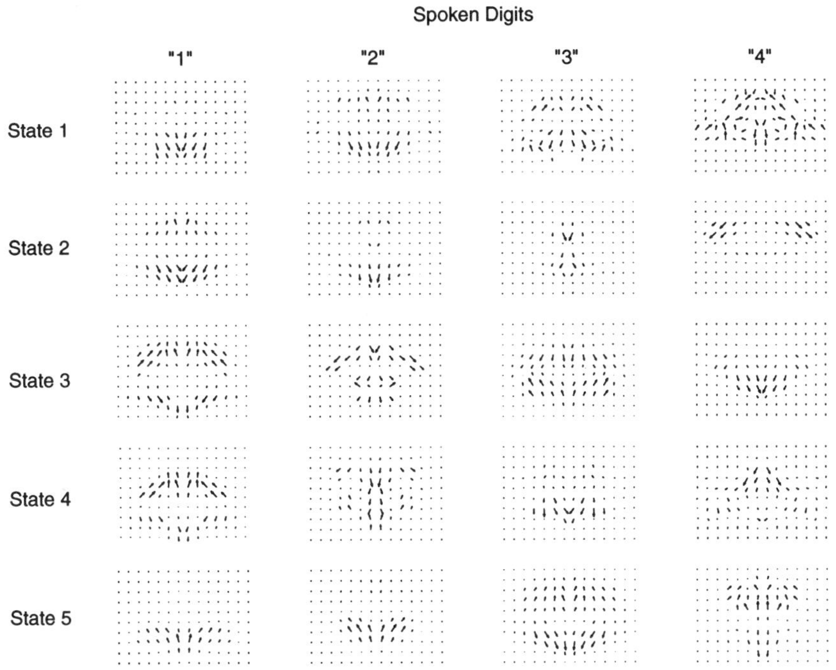

Figure 3: The optical flow representations learned by the 5-state HMMs.

rotation were eliminated. The images were normalized using parameters obtained from contour modeling of the lips by Luettin, Thacker, and Beet [3].

2.3 RECOGNITION ENGINE

The different visual representations described above formed the input to hidden Markov models which were separately trained for each word category. The images were modeled as mixtures of Gaussian distributions in pixel space. The initial state probabilities, transition probabilities, mixture coefficients, and mixture centroids were optimized using the EM algorithm. Because the probability of images rapidly approached zero when using the EM algorithm with Gaussian mixtures, we constrained the variance parameters for all the states and mixtures to be equal. In addition, the centroids of the mixtures were initialized using a linear segmentation followed by k-means clustering.

3 RESULTS

Each input representation was tested with 9 different architectures generated by combining different numbers of states (5, 7, 9) with different numbers of Gaussians (3, 5, 7) to represent each state. Each set of simulations took approximately 20 hours on a 300 MHz DEC Alpha processor. The best performance (of the 9 architectures) for each input representation is shown in Table 1. Results from the low-pass + delta representation closely matched, as expected, Movellan [6]. The small difference between Movellan [6] and the results reported here are likely due to differences in the low-pass filtering kernel, and different initializations of the parameters of the Gaussians during k-means clustering.

The flow representations (with or without low-pass pixel intensity information) gave similar results. Both of the flow representations, however, yielded better performance when the normalized images were used as input. For the PCA representation, performance was poor on the raw images, but improved markedly on the normalized dataset. The low-pass + delta representation gave excellent results for both raw and normalized images. Although the low-pass + delta representation matched the performance of normal humans (89.9%), none of these models has yet to reach the level of trained lipreaders (95.5%) on this same database (Movellan [6]).

The states learned by the HMM for these flow inputs give us information about the dynamic movement of the lips through time. These learned states (for a 5-state HMM) are shown in Figure 3, and provide an intuitive notion to the kinds of muscular activity in the face that correspond to each digit. Figure 1 (right column, bottom panel) shows the flow learned by a 1-state HMM.

Image Processing	Performance: Raw Images	Performance: Normalized Images
Low-pass + Delta	85.4	90.6
PCA of (Gray-scale + Delta)	67.7	85.4
Low-pass + Flow	61.5	68.8
Flow	63.5	66.7

Table 1: Best generalization performance (% correct) for the different visual input representations using both raw and normalized video images.

4 DISCUSSION

The purpose of this research was to compare a range of image processing techniques on a visual digit recognition task. We found that normalization of the lip images (for translation, rotation, and scale) was a crucial factor in improving the performance of the different visual representations. Normalization is important because the HMM has no mechanism to account for the wide variations in lip position and size that are present in the original dataset. It was also found that the dynamic temporal information present in the delta image contributes more to generalization performance than optical flow. Finally, compression by local low-pass filtering yielded better results than global principal components analysis.

One area of inquiry is the difference between the information provided by optical flow and the delta image. Both carry dynamic information that signals the difference between the lip images at subsequent time steps. Why should the delta image yield 15% better performance as compared to optical flow, when combined with low-pass pixel intensity information? Part of the explanation may lie in the thresholding performed in the optic flow computation, which is designed to eliminate noisy flow estimates. Unfortunately, it also leads to an optical flow output that is very sparse, as illustrated in Figure 1. The delta image, on the other hand, contains information at all points in the image. Although the significance of the delta image is not well understood, it does contain local dynamic information at all locations.

The work described here represents an exploration of the kinds of dynamic information that may be valuable for speechreading. In contrast to model-based approaches, we have sought to retain as much information as possible in the lip images by allowing the recognition engine to find relevant features of the input. This effort to combine sophisticated image processing techniques with machine learning algorithms is a valuable approach that will likely lead to new insights in a variety of applications.

Acknowledgements

We thank Dr. Juergen Luettin for the use of his parameters for normalization of the Tulips1 database. Michael S. Gray was supported by the McDonnell-Pew Center for Cognitive Neuroscience in San Diego.

References

[1] C. Bregler and Y. Konig. Eigenlips for robust speech recognition. In *Proceedings of IEEE ICASSP*, pages 669–672. Adelaide, Australia, 1991.

[2] O.N. Garcia, A.J. Goldschen, and E.D. Petajan. Feature extraction for optical automatic speech recognition or automatic lipreading. *Technical Report GWU-IIST-9232, Dept. of Electrical Engineering and Computer Science, George Washington University*, 1992.

[3] J. Luettin, N.A. Thacker, and S.W. Beet. Visual speech recognition using active shape models and hidden markov models. In *Proceedings of the IEEE International Conference on Acoustics, Speech, and Signal Processing*, volume 2, pages 817–820, Atlanta, Ga, 1996. IEEE.

[4] K. Mase and A. Pentland. Automatic lipreading by optical-flow analysis. *Systems and Computers in Japan*, 22(6):67–76, 1991.

[5] H. McGurk and J. MacDonald. Hearing lips and seeing voices. *Nature*, 264:126–130, 1976.

[6] J.R. Movellan. Visual speech recognition with stochastic networks. In G. Tesauro, D.S. Touretzky, and T. Leen, editors, *Advances in Neural Information Processing Systems*, volume 7, pages 851–858. MIT Press, Cambridge, MA, 1995.

[7] G.J. Wolff, K.V. Prasad, D.G. Stork, and M. Hennecke. Lipreading by neural networks: Visual preprocessing, learning and sensory integration. In J.D. Cowan, G. Tesauro, and J. Alspector, editors, *Advances in Neural Information Processing Systems*, volume 6, pages 1027–1034. Morgan Kaufmann, San Francisco, CA, 1994.

[8] B.P. Yuhas, Jr. Goldstein, M.H., T.J. Sejnowski, and R.E. Jenkins. Neural network models of sensory integration for improved vowel recognition. *Proceedings of the IEEE*, 78(10):1658–1668, 1990.

Blind separation of delayed and convolved sources.

Te-Won Lee
Max-Planck-Society, GERMANY,
AND Interactive Systems Group
Carnegie Mellon University
Pittsburgh, PA 15213, USA
tewon@cs.cmu.edu

Anthony J. Bell
Computational Neurobiology,
The Salk Institute
10010 N. Torrey Pines Road
La Jolla, California 92037, USA
tony@salk.edu

Russell H. Lambert
Dept of Electrical Engineering
University of South California, USA
rlambert@sipi.usc.edu

Abstract

We address the difficult problem of separating multiple speakers with multiple microphones in a real room. We combine the work of Torkkola and Amari, Cichocki and Yang, to give Natural Gradient information maximisation rules for recurrent (IIR) networks, blindly adjusting delays, separating and deconvolving mixed signals. While they work well on simulated data, these rules fail in real rooms which usually involve *non-minimum phase* transfer functions, not-invertible using stable IIR filters. An approach that sidesteps this problem is to perform infomax on a feedforward architecture in the frequency domain (Lambert 1996). We demonstrate real-room separation of two natural signals using this approach.

1 The problem.

In the linear blind signal processing problem ([3, 2] and references therein), N signals, $\mathbf{s}(t) = [s_1(t) \ldots s_N(t)]^T$, are transmitted through a medium so that an array of N sensors picks up a set of signals $\mathbf{x}(t) = [x_1(t) \ldots x_N(t)]^T$, each of which has been mixed, delayed and filtered as follows:

$$x_i(t) = \sum_{j=1}^{N} \sum_{k=0}^{M-1} a_{ijk} s_j(t - D_{ij} - k) \quad (1)$$

(Here D_{ij} are entries in a matrix of delays and there is an M-point filter, $\mathbf{a}_{ij}$, between the the jth source and the ith sensor.) The problem is to invert this mixing without knowledge of it, thus recovering the original signals, $\mathbf{s}(t)$.

2 Architectures.

The obvious architecture for inverting eq.1 is the *feedforward* one:

$$u_i(t) = \sum_{j=1}^{N} \sum_{k=0}^{M-1} w_{ijk} x_j(t - d_{ij} - k). \quad (2)$$

which has filters, $\mathbf{w}_{ij}$, and delays, d_{ij}, which supposedly reproduce, at the u_i, the original uncorrupted source signals, s_i. This was the architecture implicitly assumed in [2]. However, it cannot solve the delay-compensation problem, since in eq.1 each delay, D_{ij}, delays a single source, while in eq.2 each delay, d_{ij} is associated with a mixture, x_j.

Torkkola [8], has addressed the problem of solving the delay-compensation problem with a *feedback* architecture. Such an architecture can, in principle, solve this problem, as shown earlier by Platt & Faggin [7]. Torkkola [9] also generalised the feedback architecture to remove dependencies across time, to achieve the deconvolution of mixtures which have been filtered, as in eq.1.

Here we propose a slightly different architecture than Torkkola's ([9], eq.15). His architecture could fail since it is missing feedback cross-weights for $t = 0$, ie: w_{ij0}. A full feedback system looks like:

$$u_i(t) = x_i - \sum_{j=1}^{N} \sum_{k=0}^{M-1} w_{ijk} u_j(t - d_{ij} - k). \quad (3)$$

and is illustrated in Fig.1. Because terms in $u_i(t)$ appear on both sides, we rewrite this in vector terms: $\mathbf{u}(t) = \mathbf{x}(t) - \mathbf{W}_0 \mathbf{u}(t) - \sum_{k=1}^{M-1} \mathbf{W}_k \mathbf{u}(t-k)$, in order to solve it as follows:

$$\mathbf{u}(t) = (\mathbf{I} + \mathbf{W}_0)^{-1}(\mathbf{x}(t) - \sum_{k=1}^{M-1} \mathbf{W}_k \mathbf{u}(t-k)) \quad (4)$$

In these equations, there is a feedback unmixing matrix, $\mathbf{W}_k$, for each time point of the filter, but the 'leading matrix', $\mathbf{W}_0$ has a special status in solving for $\mathbf{u}(t)$. The delay terms are useful since one metre of distance in air at an 8kHz sampling rate, corresponds to a whole 25 zero-taps of a filter. Reintroducing them gives us:

$$\mathbf{u}(t) = (\mathbf{I} + \mathbf{W}_0)^{-1}(\mathbf{x}(t) - \mathbf{net}(t)), \quad net_i(t) = \sum_{j=1}^{N} \sum_{k=1}^{M-1} w_{ijk} u(t - d_{ij} - k)) \quad (5)$$

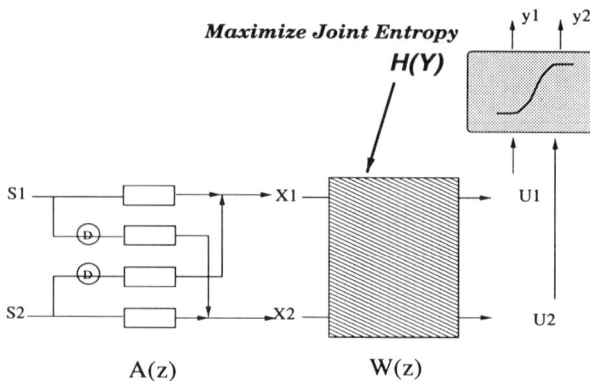

Figure 1: The feedback neural architecture of eq.9, which is used to separate and deconvolve signals. Each box represents a causal filter and each circle denotes a time delay.

3 Algorithms.

Learning in this architecture is performed by maximising the joint entropy, $H(\mathbf{y}(t))$, of the random vector $\mathbf{y}(t) = g(\mathbf{u}(t))$, where g is a bounded monotonic nonlinear function (a sigmoid function). The success of this for separating sources depends on four assumptions: (1) that the sources are statistically independent, (2) that each source is white, ie: there are no dependencies between time points, (3) that the non-linearity, g, has a derivative which has higher kurtosis than the probability density functions (pdf's) of the sources, and (4) that a stable IIR (feedback) inverse of the mixing exists; ie: that a is *minimum phase* (see section 5).

Assumption (1) is reasonable and Assumption (3) allows some tailoring of our algorithm to fit data of different types. Assumption (2), on the other hand, is not true for natural signals. Our algorithm will whiten: it will remove dependencies across time which already existed in the original source signals, s_i. However, it is possible to restore the characteristic autocorrelations (amplitude spectra) of the sources by post-processing. For the reasoning behind Assumption (3) see [2]. We will discuss Assumption 4 in section 5.

In the static feedback case of eq.5, when $M = 1$, the learning rule for the feedback weights $\mathbf{W}_0$ is just a co-ordinate transform of the rule for feedforward weights, $\hat{\mathbf{W}}_0$, in the equivalent architecture of $\mathbf{u}(t) = \hat{\mathbf{W}}_0 \mathbf{x}(t)$. Since $\hat{\mathbf{W}}_0 \equiv (\mathbf{I} + \mathbf{W}_0)^{-1}$, we have $\mathbf{W}_0 = \hat{\mathbf{W}}_0^{-1} - \mathbf{I}$, which, due to the quotient rule for matrix differentiation, differentiates as:

$$\Delta \mathbf{W}_0 = -(\hat{\mathbf{W}}^{-1}) \Delta \hat{\mathbf{W}} (\hat{\mathbf{W}}^{-1}) \qquad (6)$$

The best way to maximise entropy in the feedforward system is not to follow the entropy gradient, as in [2], but to follow its 'natural' gradient, as reported by Amari et al [1]:

$$\Delta \hat{\mathbf{W}} \propto \frac{\partial H(\mathbf{y})}{\partial \hat{\mathbf{W}}} \hat{\mathbf{W}}^T \hat{\mathbf{W}} \qquad (7)$$

This is an optimal rescaling of the entropy gradient [1, 3]. It simplifies the learning rule and speeds convergence considerably. Evaluated, it gives [2]:

$$\Delta \hat{\mathbf{W}}_0 \propto (\mathbf{I} + \hat{\mathbf{y}} \mathbf{u}^T) \hat{\mathbf{W}}_0, \qquad \hat{y}_i = \frac{\partial}{\partial y_i} \frac{\partial y_i}{\partial u_i} \tag{8}$$

Substituting into eq.7 gives the natural gradient rule for static feedback weights:

$$\Delta \mathbf{W}_0 \propto -(\mathbf{I} + \mathbf{W}_0)(\mathbf{I} + \hat{\mathbf{y}} \mathbf{u}^T), \tag{9}$$

This reasoning may be extended to networks involving filters. For the feedforward filter architecture $\mathbf{u}(t) = \sum_{k=0}^{M-1} \hat{\mathbf{W}}_k \mathbf{x}(t-k)$, we derive a natural gradient rule (for $k > 0$) of:

$$\Delta \hat{\mathbf{W}}_k \propto \hat{\mathbf{y}} \mathbf{u}_{t-k}^T \hat{\mathbf{W}}_k \tag{10}$$

where, for convenience, time has become subscripted. Performing the same coordinate transforms as for $\mathbf{W}_0$ above, gives the rule:

$$\Delta \mathbf{W}_k \propto -(\mathbf{I} + \mathbf{W}_k) \hat{\mathbf{y}} \mathbf{u}_{t-k}^T \tag{11}$$

(We note that learning rules similar to these have been independently derived by Cichocki et al [4]). Finally, for the delays in eq.5, we derive [2, 8]:

$$\Delta d_{ij} \propto \frac{\partial H(\mathbf{y})}{\partial d_{ij}} = -\hat{y}_i \sum_{k=1}^{M-1} \frac{\partial}{\partial t} w_{ijk} u(t - d_{ij} - k) \tag{12}$$

This rule is different from that in [8] because it uses the collected temporal gradient information from all the taps. The algorithms of eq.9, eq.11 and eq.12 are the ones we use in our experiments on the architecture of eq.5.

4 Simulation results for the feedback architecture

To test the learning rules in eq.9, eq.11 and eq.12 we used an IIR filter system to recover two sources which had been mixed and delayed as follows (in Z-transform notation):

$$\begin{aligned}
A_{11}(z) &= 0.9 + 0.5 z^{-1} + 0.3 z^{-2} \\
A_{21}(z) &= -0.7 z^{-5} - 0.3 z^{-6} - 0.2 z^{-7} \\
A_{12}(z) &= 0.5 z^{-5} + 0.3 z^{-6} + 0.2 z^{-7} \\
A_{22}(z) &= 0.8 - 0.1 z^{-1}
\end{aligned} \tag{13}$$

The mixing system, $\mathbf{A}(z)$, is a minimum-phase system with all its zeros inside the unit circle. Hence, $\mathbf{A}(z)$ can be inverted using a stable causal IIR system since all poles of the inverting systems are also inside the unit circle. For this experiment, we chose an artificially-generated source: a white process with a Laplacian distribution $[f_x(x) = \exp(-|x|)]$. In the frequency domain the deconvolving system looks as follows:

$$\begin{bmatrix} U_1(z) \\ U_2(z) \end{bmatrix} = \frac{1}{D(z)} \begin{bmatrix} W_{11}(z) & W_{21}(z) \\ W_{12}(z) & W_{22}(z) \end{bmatrix} \begin{bmatrix} X_1(z) \\ X_2(z) \end{bmatrix} \tag{14}$$

where $D(z) = W_{11}(z) W_{22}(z) - W_{12}(z) W_{21}(z))$. This leads to the following solution for the weight filters:

$$\begin{aligned}
W_{11}(z) &= A_{22}(z) & W_{22}(z) &= A_{11}(z) \\
W_{21}(z) &= -A_{21}(z) & W_{12}(z) &= -A_{12}(z)
\end{aligned} \tag{15}$$

The learning rule we used was that of eq.9 and eq.11 with the logistic non-linearity, $y_i = 1/\exp(-u_i)$. Fig.2A shows the four filters learnt by our IIR algorithm. The bottom row shows the inverting system convolved with the mixing system, proving that $\mathbf{W} * \mathbf{A}$ is approximately the identity mapping. Delay learning is not demonstrated here, though for periodic signals like speech we observed that it is subject to local minima problems [8, 9].

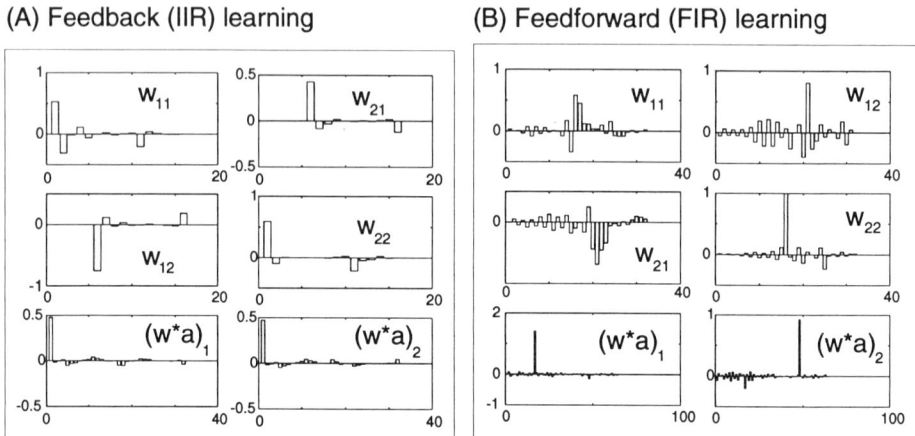

Figure 2: Top two rows: learned unmixing filters for (A) IIR learning on minimum-phase mixing, and (B) FIR freq.-domain learning on non-minimum phase mixing. Bottom row: the convolved mixing and unmixing systems. The delta-like response indicates successful blind unmixing. In (B) this occurs acausally with a time-shift.

5 Back to the feedforward architecture.

The feedback architecture is elegant but limited. It can only invert minimum-phase mixing (all zeros are inside the unit circle meaning that all poles of the inverting system are as well). Unfortunately, real room acoustics usually involves non-minimum phase mixing.

There does exist, however, a stable *non-causal* feedforward (FIR) inverse for non-minimum phase mixing systems. The learning rules for such a system can be formulated using the FIR polynomial matrix algebra as described by Lambert [5]. This may be performed in the time or frequency domain, the only requirements being that the inverting filters are long enough and their main energy occurs more-or-less in their centre. This allows for the non-causal expansion of the non-minimum phase roots, causing the roughly symmetrical "flanged" appearance of the filters in Fig.2B.

For convenience, we formulate the infomax and natural gradient infomax rules [2, 1] in the frequency domain:

$$\Delta \underline{\mathbf{W}} \propto \underline{\mathbf{W}}^{-H} + \text{fft}(\hat{\mathbf{y}})\underline{\mathbf{X}}^H \tag{16}$$

$$\Delta \underline{\mathbf{W}} \propto (\mathbf{I} + \text{fft}(\hat{\mathbf{y}})\underline{\mathbf{U}}^H)\underline{\mathbf{W}} \tag{17}$$

where the H superscript denotes the Hermitian transpose (complex conjugate). In these rules, as in eq.14, $\underline{\mathbf{W}}$ is a matrix of filters and $\underline{\mathbf{U}}$ and $\underline{\mathbf{X}}$ are blocks of multi-sensor signal in the frequency domain. Note that the nonlinearity $\hat{y}_i = \frac{\partial}{\partial y_i} \frac{\partial y_i}{\partial u_i}$ still operates in the time domain and the fft is applied at the output.

6 Simulation results for the feedforward architecture

To show the learning rule in eq.17 working, we altered the transfer function in eq.13 as follows:
$$A_{11}(z) = 1 + 1.0z^{-1} - 0.75z^{-2}. \tag{18}$$
This system is now non-minimum phase, having zeros outside the unit circle. The inverse system can be approximated by stable non-causal FIR filters. These were learnt using the learning rule of eq.17 (again, with the logistic non-linearity). The resulting learnt filters are shown in Fig.2B where the leading weights were chosen to be at half the filter size ($M/2$). Non-causality of the filters can be clearly observed for $\mathbf{w}_{12}$ and $\mathbf{w}_{21}$, where there are non-zero coefficients before the maximum amplitude weights. The bottom row of Fig.2B shows the successful separation by plotting the complete unmixing/mixing transfer function: $\mathbf{W} * \mathbf{A}$.

7 Experiments with real recordings

To demonstrate separation in a real room, we set up two microphones and recorded firstly two people speaking and then one person speaking with music in the background. The microphones and the sources were both 60cm apart and 60cm from each other (arranged in a square), and the sampling was 16kHz. Fig.3A shows the two recordings of a person saying the digits "one" to "ten" while loud music plays in the background. The IIR system of eq.5, eq.9 and eq.11 was unable to separate these signals, presumably due to the non-minimum-phase nature of the room transfer functions. However, the algorithm of eq.17, converged after 30 passes through the 10 second recordings. The filter lengths were 256 (corresponding to 16ms). The separated signals are shown in Fig.3B. Listening to them conveys a sense of almost-clean separation, though interference is audible. The results on the two people speaking were similar.

An important application is in spontaneous speech recognition tasks where the best recognizer may fail completely in the presence of background music or competing speakers (as in the teleconferencing problem). To test this application, we fed into a speech recognizer, ten sentences recorded with loud music in the background and ten sentences recorded with a simultaneous speaker interference. After separation, the recognition rate increased considerably for both cases. These results are reported in detail in [6].

8 Conclusions

Starting with 'Natural gradient infomax' IIR learning rules for blind time delay adjustment, separation and deconvolution, we showed how these worked well on minimum-phase mixing, but not on non-minimum-phase mixing, as usually occurs in rooms. This led us to an FIR frequency domain infomax approach suggested by Lambert [5]. The latter approach shows much better separation of speech and music mixed in a real-room. Based on these techniques, it should now be possible to develop real-world applications.

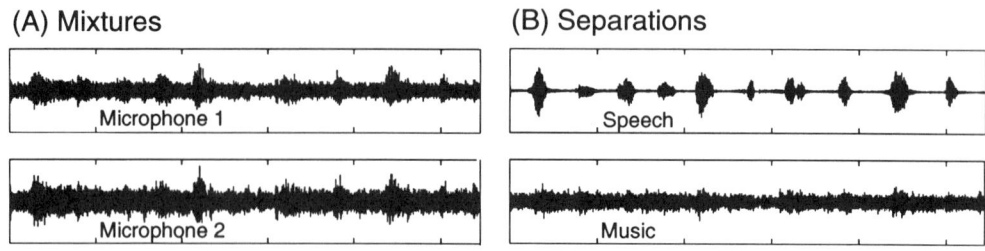

Figure 3: Real-room separation/deconvolution. (A) recorded mixtures (B) separated speech (spoken digits 1-10) and music.

Acknowledgments

T.W.L. is supported by the Daimler-Benz-Fellowship, and A.J.B. by a grant from the Office of Naval Research. We are grateful to Kari Torkkola for sharing his results with us, and to Jürgen Fritsch, Terry Sejnowski and Alex Waibel for discussions and comments.

References

[1] Amari S-I. Cichocki A. & Yang H.H. 1996. A new learning algorithm for blind signal separation, *Advances in Neural Information Processing Systems 8*, MIT press.

[2] Bell A.J. & Sejnowski T.J. 1995. An information maximisation approach to blind separation and blind deconvolution, *Neural Computation*, 7, 1129-1159

[3] Cardoso J-F. & Laheld B. 1996. Equivariant adaptive source separation, *IEEE Trans. on Signal Proc.*, Dec. 1996

[4] Cichocki A., Amari S-I & Cao J. 1996. Blind separation of delayed and convolved signals with self-adaptive learning rate, in *Proc. Intern. Symp. on Nonlinear Theory and Applications (NOLTA*96)*, Kochi, Japan.

[5] Lambert R. 1996.Multichannel blind deconvolution: FIR matrix algebra and separation of multipath mixtures, *PhD Thesis*, University of Southern California, Department of Electrical Engineering, May 1996.

[6] Lee T-W. & Orglmeister R. Blind source separation of real-world signals. submitted to *Proc. ICNN*, Houston, USA, 1997.

[7] Platt J.C. & Faggin F. 1992. Networks for the separation of sources that are superimposed and delayed, in Moody J.E et al (eds) *Advances in Neural Information Processing Systems 4*, Morgan-Kaufmann

[8] Torkkola K. 1996. Blind separation of delayed sources based on information maximisation, *Proc IEEE ICASSP*, Atlanta, May 1996.

[9] Torkkola K. 1996. Blind separation of convolved sources based on information maximisation, *Proc. IEEE Workshop on Neural Networks and Signal Processing*, Kyota, Japan, Sept. 1996

A Constructive RBF Network for Writer Adaptation

John C. Platt and Nada P. Matić
Synaptics, Inc.
2698 Orchard Parkway
San Jose, CA 95134
platt@synaptics.com, nada@synaptics.com

Abstract

This paper discusses a fairly general adaptation algorithm which augments a standard neural network to increase its recognition accuracy for a specific user. The basis for the algorithm is that the output of a neural network is characteristic of the input, even when the output is incorrect. We exploit this characteristic output by using an *Output Adaptation Module* (OAM) which maps this output into the correct user-dependent confidence vector. The OAM is a simplified Resource Allocating Network which constructs radial basis functions on-line. We applied the OAM to construct a writer-adaptive character recognition system for on-line hand-printed characters. The OAM decreases the word error rate on a test set by an average of 45%, while creating only 3 to 25 basis functions for each writer in the test set.

1 Introduction

One of the major difficulties in creating any statistical pattern recognition system is that the statistics of the training set is often different from the statistics in actual use. The creation of a statistical pattern recognizer is often considered as a regression problem, where class probabilities are estimated from a fixed training set. Statistical pattern recognizers tend to work well for typical data that is similar to the training set data, but do not work well for atypical data that is not well represented in the training set. Poor performance on atypical data is a problem for human interfaces, because people tend to provide drastically non-typical data (for example, see figure 1).

The solution to this difficulty is to create an adaptive recognizer, instead of treating recognition as a static regression problem. The recognizer must adapt to new statistics during use. As applied to on-line handwriting recognition, an adaptive

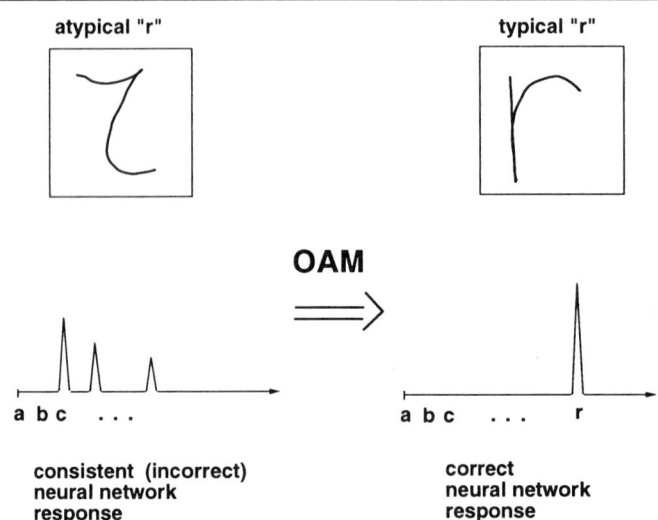

Figure 1: When given atypical input data, the neural network produces a consistent incorrect output pattern. The OAM recognizes the consistent pattern and produces a corrected user-adaptive output.

recognizer improves the accuracy for a particular user by adapting the recognizer to that user.

This paper proposes a novel method for creating an adaptive recognizer, which we call the *Output Adaptation Module* or OAM. The OAM was inspired by the development of a writer-independent neural network handwriting recognizer. We noticed that the output of this neural network was characteristic of the input: if a specific style of character was shown to the network, the network's output was almost always consistent for that specific style, even when the output was incorrect.

To exploit the consistency of the incorrect outputs, we decided to add an OAM on top of the network. The OAM learns to recognize these consistent incorrect output vectors, and produces a more correct output vector (see figure 1). The units of the OAM are radial basis functions (RBF) [5]. Adaptation of these RBF units is performed using a simplified version of the Resource Allocating Network (RAN) algorithm of Platt [4][2]. The number of units that RAN allocates scales sub-linearly with the number of presented learning examples, in contrast to other algorithms which allocate a new unit for every learned example.

The OAM has the following properties, which are useful for a user-adaptive recognizer:

- The adaptation is very fast: the user need only provide a few additional examples of his own data.
- There is very little recognition speed degradation.
- A modest amount of additional memory per user is required.
- The OAM is not limited to neural network recognizers.
- The output of the OAM is a corrected vector of confidences, which is more useful for contextual post-processing than a single label.

1.1 Relationship to Previous Work

The OAM is related to previous work in user adaptation of neural recognizers for both speech and handwriting.

A previous example of user adaptation of a neural handwriting recognizer employed a Time Delay Neural Network (TDNN), where the last layer of a TDNN was replaced with a tunable classifier that is more appropriate for adaptation [1][3]. In Guyon, et al. [1], the last layer of a TDNN was replaced by a k-nearest neighbor classifier. This work was further extended in Matić, et al. [3], where the last layer of the TDNN was replaced with an optimal hyperplane classifier which is retrained for adaptation purposes. The optimal hyperplane classifier retained the same accuracy as the k-nearest neighbor classifier, while reducing the amount of computation and memory required for adaptation.

The present work improves upon these previous user-adaptive handwriting systems in three ways. First, the OAM does not require the retraining and storage of the entire last layer of the network. The OAM thus further reduces both CPU and memory requirements. Second, the OAM produces an output vector of confidences, instead of simply an output label. This vector of confidences can be used effectively by a contextual post-processing step, while a label cannot. Third, our adaptation experiments are performed on a neural network which recognizes a full character set. These previous papers only experimented with neural networks that recognized character subsets, which is a less difficult adaptation problem.

The OAM is related to stacking [6]. In stacking, outputs of multiple recognizers are combined via training on partitions of the training set. With the OAM, the multiple outputs of a recognizer are combined using memory-based learning. The OAM is trained on the idiosyncratic statistics of actual use, not on a pre-defined training set partition.

2 The Output Adaptation Module (OAM)

Section 2 of this paper describes the OAM in detail, while section 3 describes its application to create a user-adaptive handwriting recognizer.

The OAM maps the output of a neural network V_i into a user-adapted output O_i, by adding an adaptation vector A_i:

$$O_i = V_i + A_i. \qquad (1)$$

Depending on the neural network training algorithm used, both the output of the neural network V_i and the user-adapted output O_i can estimate *a posteriori* class probabilities, suitable for further post-processing.

The goal of the OAM is to bring the output O_i closer to an ideal response T_i. In our experiments, the target T_i is 0.9 for the neuron corresponding to the correct character and 0.1 for all other neurons.

The adaptation vector A_i is computed by a radial basis function network that takes V_i as an input:

$$O_i = V_i + A_i = V_i + \sum_j C_{ij} \Phi_j(\vec{V}), \qquad (2)$$

$$\Phi_j(\vec{V}) = f\left(\frac{d(\vec{V}, \vec{M_j})}{R_j}\right). \qquad (3)$$

where $\vec{M_j}$ is the center of the jth radial basis function, d is a distance metric between $\vec{V}$ and $\vec{M_j}$, R_j is a parameter that controls the width of the jth basis function, f is

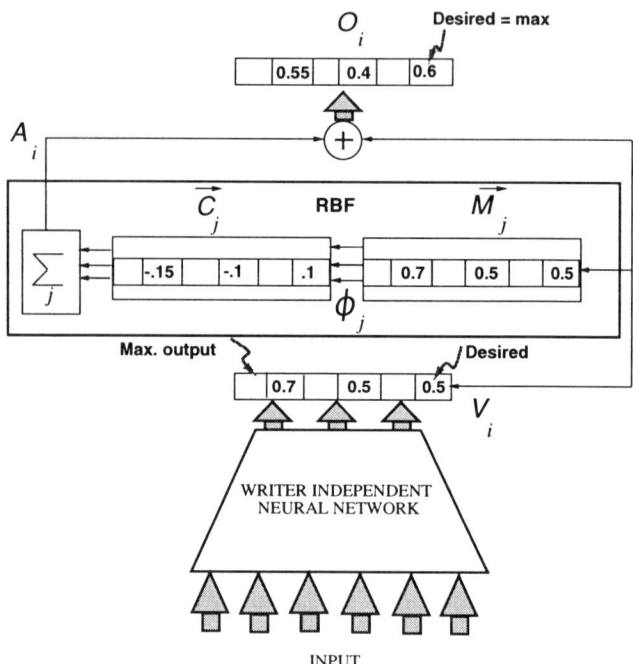

Figure 2: The architecture of the OAM.

a decreasing function that controls the shape of the basis functions, and C_{ij} is the amount of correction that the jth basis function adds to the output. We call $\vec{M}_j$ the memories in the adaptation module, and we call $\vec{C}_j$ the correction vectors (see figure 2).

The function f is a decreasing polynomial function:

$$f(x) = \begin{cases} \left(1 - x^2\right)^2, & \text{if } x < 1; \\ 0, & \text{otherwise.} \end{cases} \quad (4)$$

The distance function d is a Euclidean distance metric that first clips both of its input vectors to the range $[0.1, 0.9]$ in order to reduce spurious noise.

The algorithm for constructing the radial basis functions is a simplification of the RAN algorithm [4][2]. The OAM starts with no memories or corrections. When the user corrects a recognition error, the OAM finds the distance $d_{\min}$ from the nearest memory to the vector V_i. If the distance $d_{\min}$ is greater than a threshold δ, then a new RBF unit is allocated, with a new memory that is set to the vector V_i, and a corresponding correction vector that is set to correct the error with a step size a:

$$C_{ik} = a(T_i - O_i). \quad (5)$$

If the distance $d_{\min}$ is less than δ, no new unit is allocated: the correction vector of the nearest memory to V_i is updated to correct the error by a step size b.

$$\Delta C_{ik} = b(T_i - O_i)\Phi_k(\vec{V}). \quad (6)$$

For our experiments, we set $\delta = 0.1$, $a = 0.25$, and $b = 0.2$. The values a and b are chosen to be less than 1 to sacrifice learning speed to gain learning stability.

The number of radial basis functions grows sub-linearly with the number of errors, because units are only allocated for novel errors that the OAM has not seen before.

For errors similar to those the OAM has seen before, the algorithm updates one of the correction vectors using a simplified LMS rule (eq. 6).

In the computation of the nearest memory, we always consider an additional phantom memory: the target $\vec{Q}$ that corresponds to the highest output in $\vec{V}$. This phantom memory is considered in order to prevent the OAM from allocating memories when the neural network output is unambiguous. The phantom memory prevents the OAM from affecting the output for neatly written characters.

The adaptation algorithm used is described as pseudo-code, below:

```
For every character shown to the network {
    If the user indicates an error {
        T⃗ = target vector of the correct character
        Q⃗ = target vector of the highest element in V⃗
        d_min = min(min_j d(V⃗, M⃗_j), d(V⃗, Q⃗))
        If d_min > δ {  // allocate a new memory
            k = index of the new memory
            C_ik = a(T_i − O_i)
            M⃗_k = V⃗
            R_j = d_min
        }
        else if memories exist and min_j d(V⃗, M⃗_j) < d(V⃗, Q⃗) {
            k = arg min_j d(V⃗, M⃗_j)
            C_ik = C_ik + b(T_i − O_i)Φ_k(V⃗)
        }
    }
}
```

3   Experiments and Results

To test the effectiveness of the OAM, we used it to create a writer-adaptive handwriting recognition system. The OAM was connected to the outputs of a writer-independent neural network trained to recognize characters hand-printed in boxes. This neural network was a carefully tuned multilayer feed-forward network, trained with the back-propagation algorithm. The network has 510 inputs, 200 hidden units, and 72 outputs.

The input to the OAM was a vector of 72 confidences, one per class. These confidences were in the range $[0, 1]$. There is one input for every upper case character, lower case character, and digit. There is also one input for each member of a subset of punctuation characters (!$&',-:;=?).

The OAM was tested interactively. Tests of the OAM were performed by five writers disjoint from the training writers for the writer-independent neural network. These writers had atypical writing styles which were difficult for the network to recognize. Test characters were entered word-by-word on a tablet. The writers were instructed to write more examples of characters that reflected their atypical writing style. The words that these writers used were not taken from a word list, and could consist of any combination of the 72 available characters. Users were shown the results of the OAM, combined into words and further processed by a dictionary. Whenever the system failed to recognize a word correctly, all misclassified characters and their corresponding desired labels were used by the OAM to adapt the system to the

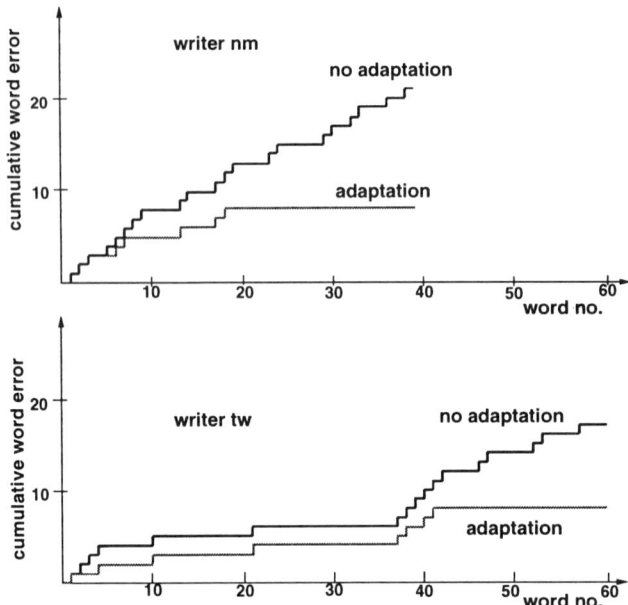

Figure 3: The cumulative number of word errors for the writer "nm" and the writer "tw", with and without adaptation

Writer	% word error no OAM	% word error OAM	Memories stored during test	Words written during test
rag	25%	17%	6	93
mfe	62%	36%	12	53
qm	42%	31%	25	80
nm	54%	21%	4	39
tw	28%	10%	3	60

Table 1: Quantitative test results for the OAM.

particular user.

Figure 3 shows the performance of the OAM for the writer "nm" and for the writer "tw". The total number of word errors since adaptation started is plotted against the number of words shown to the OAM. The baseline cumulative error without the OAM is also given. The slope of each curve gives the estimate of the instantaneous error rate. The OAM causes the slope for both writers to decrease dramatically as the adaptation progresses. Over the last third of the test set, the word error rate for writer "nm" was 0%, while the word error rate for writer "tw" was 5%. These examples show the the OAM can substantially improve the accuracy of a writer-independent neural network.

Quantitative results are shown in table 1, where the word error rates obtained with the OAM are compared to the baseline word error rates without the OAM. The right two columns contain the number of stored basis functions and the number of words tested by the OAM.

The OAM corrects an average of 45% of the errors in the test set. The accuracy rates with the OAM were taken for the entire test run, and therefore count the errors that were made while adaptation was taking place. By the end of the test, the true error rates for these writers would be even lower than those shown in table 1, as can be seen in figure 3.

These experiments showed that the OAM adapts very quickly and requires a small amount of additional memory and computation. For most writers, only 2-3 presentations of a writer-dependent variant of a character were sufficient for the OAM to adapt. The maximum number of stored basis functions were 25 in these experiments. The OAM did not substantially affect the recognition speed of the system.

4 Conclusions

We have designed a widely applicable *Output Adaptation Module* (OAM) to place on top of standard neural networks. The OAM takes the output of the network as input, and determines an additional adaptation vector to add to the output. The adaptation vector is computed via a radial basis function network, which is learned with a simplification of the RAN algorithm. The OAM has many nice properties: only a few examples are needed to learn atypical inputs, the number of stored memories grows sub-linearly with the number of errors, the recognition rate of the writer-independent neural network is unaffected by adaptation and the output of the module is a confidence vector suitable for further post-processing.

The OAM addresses the difficult problem of creating a high-perplexity adaptive recognizer. We applied the OAM to create a writer-adaptive handwriting recognition system. On a test set of five difficult writers, the adaptation module decreased the error rate by 45%, and only stored between 3 and 25 basis functions per writer.

5 Acknowledgements

We wish to thank Steve Nowlan for helpful suggestions during the development of the OAM algorithm and for his work on the writer-independent neural network. We would also like to thank Joe Decker for his work on the writer-independent neural network.

References

[1] I. Guyon, D. Henderson, P. Albrecht, Y. Le Cun, and J. Denker. Writer independent and writer adaptive neural network for on-line character recognition. In S. Impedovo, editor, *From Pixels to Features III*, Amsterdam, 1992. Elsevier.

[2] V. Kadirkamanathan and M. Niranjan. A function estimation approach to sequential learning with neural networks. *Neural Computation*, 5(6):954–976, 1993.

[3] N. Matić, I. Guyon, J. Denker, and V. Vapnik. Writer adaptation for on-line handwritten character recognition. In *ICDAR93*, Tokyo, 1993. IEEE Computer Society Press.

[4] J. Platt. A resource-allocating network for function interpolation. *Neural Computation*, 3(2):213–225, 1991.

[5] M. Powell. Radial basis functions for multivariate interpolation: A review. In J. C. Mason and M. G. Cox, editors, *Algorithms for Approximation*, Oxford, 1987. Clarendon Press.

[6] D. Wolpert. Stacked generalization. *Neural Networks*, 5(2):241–260, 1992.

A New Approach to Hybrid HMM/ANN Speech Recognition Using Mutual Information Neural Networks

G. Rigoll, C. Neukirchen
Gerhard-Mercator-University Duisburg
Faculty of Electrical Engineering
Department of Computer Science
Bismarckstr. 90, Duisburg, Germany

ABSTRACT

This paper presents a new approach to speech recognition with hybrid HMM/ANN technology. While the standard approach to hybrid HMM/ANN systems is based on the use of neural networks as posterior probability estimators, the new approach is based on the use of mutual information neural networks trained with a special learning algorithm in order to maximize the mutual information between the input classes of the network and its resulting sequence of firing output neurons during training. It is shown in this paper that such a neural network is an optimal neural vector quantizer for a discrete hidden Markov model system trained on Maximum Likelihood principles. One of the main advantages of this approach is the fact, that such neural networks can be easily combined with HMM's of any complexity with context-dependent capabilities. It is shown that the resulting hybrid system achieves very high recognition rates, which are now already on the same level as the best conventional HMM systems with continuous parameters, and the capabilities of the mutual information neural networks are not yet entirely exploited.

1 INTRODUCTION

Hybrid HMM/ANN systems deal with the optimal combination of artificial neural networks (ANN) and hidden Markov models (HMM). Especially in the area of automatic speech recognition, it has been shown that hybrid approaches can lead to very powerful and efficient systems, combining the discriminative capabilities of neural networks and the superior dynamic time warping abilities of HMM's. The most popular hybrid approach is described in (Hochberg, 1995) and replaces the component modeling the emission probabilities of the HMM by a neural net. This is possible, because it is shown in (Bourlard, 1994) that neural networks can be trained so that the output of the m-th neuron approximates the posterior probability $p(\Omega_m|\underline{x})$. In this paper, an alternative method for constructing a hybrid system is presented. It is based on the use of discrete HMM's which are combined with a neural vector quantizer (VQ) in order to form a hybrid system. Each speech feature vector is presented to the neural network, which generates a firing neuron in its output layer. This neuron is processed as VQ label by the HMM's. There are the following arguments for this alternative hybrid approach:

- The neural vector quantizer has to be trained on a special information theory criterion, based on the mutual information between network input and resulting neuron firing sequence. It will be shown that such a network is the optimal acoustic processor for a discrete HMM system, resulting in a profound mathematical theory for this approach.
- Resulting from this theory, a formula can be derived which jointly describes the behavior of the HMM and the neural acoustic processor. In that way, both systems can be described in a unified manner and both major components of the hybrid system can be trained using a unified learning criterion.
- The above mentioned theoretical background leads to the development of new neural network paradigms using novel training algorithms that have not been used before in other areas of neurocomputing, and therefore represent major challenges and issues in learning and training for neural systems.
- The neural networks can be easily combined with any HMM system of arbitrary complexity. This leads to the combination of optimally trained neural networks with very powerful HMM's, having all features useful for speech recognition, e.g. triphones, function words, crossword triphones, etc.. Context-dependency, which is very desirable but relatively difficult to realize with a pure neural approach, can be left to the HMM's.
- The resulting hybrid system has still the basic structure of a discrete system, and therefore has all the effective features associated with discrete systems, e.g. quick and easy training as well as recognition procedures, real-time capabilities, etc..
- The work presented in this paper has been also successfully implemented for a demanding speech recognition problem, the 1000 word speaker-independent continuous Resource Management speech recognition task. For this task, the hybrid system produces one of the best recognition results obtained by any speech recognition system.

In the following section, the theoretical foundations of the hybrid approach are briefly explained. A unified probabilistic model for the combined HMM/ANN system is derived, describing the interaction of the neural and the HMM component. Furthermore, it is shown that the optimal neural acoustic processor can be obtained from a special information theoretic network training algorithm.

2 INFORMATION THEORY PRINCIPLES FOR NEURAL NETWORK TRAINING

We are considering now a neural network of arbitrary topology used as neural vector quantizer for a discrete HMM system. If K patterns are presented to the hybrid system during training, the feature vectors resulting from these patterns using any feature extraction method can be denoted as $\underline{x}(k)$, k=1...K. If these feature vectors are presented to the input layer of a neural network, the network will generate one firing neuron for each presentation. Hence, all K presentations will generate a stream of firing neurons with length K resulting from the output layer of the neural net. This label stream is denoted as Y=y(1)...y(K). The label stream Y will be presented to the HMM's, which calculate the probability that this stream has been observed while a pattern of a certain class has been presented to the system. It is assumed, that M different classes Ω_m are active in the system, e.g. the words or phonemes in speech recognition. Each feature vector $\underline{x}(k)$ will belong to one of these classes. The class Ω_m, to which feature vector $\underline{x}(k)$ belongs is denoted as $\Omega(k)$. The major training issue for the neural network can be now formulated as follows: How should the weights of the network be trained, so that the network produces a stream of firing neurons that can be used by the discrete HMM's in an optimal way? It is known that HMM's are usually trained with information theory methods which mostly rely on the Maximum Likelihood (ML) principle. If the parameters of the hybrid system (i.e. transition and emission probabilities and network weights) are summarized in the vector $\underline{\theta}$, the probability $p_{\underline{\theta}}(\underline{x}(k)|\Omega(k))$ denotes the probability of the pattern $\underline{x}$ at discrete time k, under the assumption that it has been generated by the model representing class $\Omega(k)$, with parameter set $\underline{\theta}$. The ML principle will then try to maximize the joint probability of all presented training patterns $\underline{x}(k)$, according to the following Maximum Likelihood function:

$$\underline{\theta}^* = \arg\max_{\underline{\theta}} \left\{ \frac{1}{K} \sum_{k=1}^{K} \log p_{\underline{\theta}}(\underline{x}(k)|\Omega(k)) \right\} \quad (1)$$

where $\underline{\theta}^*$ is the optimal parameter vector maximizing this equation. Our goal is to feed the feature vector $\underline{x}$ into a neural network and to present the neural network output to the Markov model. Therefore, one has to introduce the neural network output in a suitable manner into the above formula. If the vector $\underline{x}$ is presented to the network input layer, and we assume that there is a chance that any neuron y_n, n=1...N (with network output layer size N) can fire with a certain probability, then the output probability $p(\underline{x}|\Omega)$ in (1) can be written as:

$$p(\underline{x}|\Omega) = \sum_{n=1}^{N} p(\underline{x},y_n|\Omega) = \sum_{n=1}^{N} p(y_n|\Omega) \cdot p(\underline{x}|y_n,\Omega) \quad (2)$$

Now, the combination of the neural component with the HMM can be made more obvious: In (2), typically the probability $p(y_n|\Omega)$ will be described by the Markov model, in terms of the emission probabilities of the HMM. For instance, in continuous parameter HMM's, these probabilities are interpreted as weights for Gaussian mixtures. In the case of semi-continuous systems or discrete HMM's, these probabilities will serve as discrete emission probabilities of the codebook labels. The probability $p(\underline{x}|y_n,\Omega)$ describes the acoustic processor of the system and is characterizing the relation between the vector $\underline{x}$ as input to the acoustic processor and the label y_n, which can be considered as the n-th output component of the acoustic processor. This n-th output component may characterize e.g. the n-th Gaussian mixture component in continuous parameter HMM's, or the generation of the n-th label of a vector quantizer in a discrete system. This probability is often considered as independent of the class Ω and can then be expressed as $p(\underline{x}|y_n)$. It is exactly this probability, that can be modeled efficiently by our neural network. In this case, the vector $\underline{x}$ serves as input to the neural network and y_n characterizes the n-th neuron in the output layer of the network. Using Bayes law, this probability can be written as:

$$p(\underline{x}|y_n) = \frac{p(y_n|\underline{x}) \cdot p(\underline{x})}{p(y_n)} \quad (3)$$

yielding for (2):

$$p(\underline{x}|\Omega) = p(\underline{x}) \cdot \sum_{n=1}^{N} p(y_n|\Omega) \cdot \frac{p(y_n|\underline{x})}{p(y_n)} \quad (4)$$

Using again Bayes law to express

one obtains from (4):

$$p(y_n|\Omega) = \frac{p(\Omega|y_n) \cdot p(y_n)}{p(\Omega)} \qquad (5)$$

$$p(\underline{x}|\Omega) = \frac{p(\underline{x})}{p(\Omega)} \cdot \sum_{n=1}^{N} p(\Omega|y_n) \cdot p(y_n|\underline{x}) \qquad (6)$$

We have now modified the class-dependent probability of the feature vector $\underline{x}$ in a way that allows the incorporation of the probability $p(y_n|\underline{x})$. This probability allows a better characterization of the behavior of the neural network, because it describes the probability of the various neurons y_n, if the vector $\underline{x}$ is presented to the network input. Therefore, these probabilities give a good description of the input/output behavior of the neural network. Eq. (6) can therefore be considered as probabilistic model for the hybrid system, where the neural acoustic processor is characterized by its input/output behavior. Two cases can be now distinguished: In the first case, the neural network is assumed to be a probabilistic paradigm, where each neuron fires with a certain probability, if an input vector is presented. In this case all neurons contribute to the information forwarded to the HMM's. As already mentioned, in this paper, the second possible case is considered, namely that only one neuron in the output layer fires and will be fed as observed label to the HMM. In this case, we have a deterministic decision, and the probability $p(y_n|\underline{x})$ describes what neuron y_{n*} fires if vector $\underline{x}$ is presented to the input layer. Therefore, this probability reduces to

$$p(y_n|\underline{x}) = \begin{cases} 1 & \text{if } y_n = y_{n*} \\ 0 & \text{else} \end{cases} \qquad (7)$$

Then, (6) yields:

$$p(\underline{x}|\Omega) = \frac{p(\underline{x})}{p(\Omega)} \cdot p(\Omega|y_{n*}) \qquad (8)$$

Now, the class-dependent probability $p(\underline{x}|\Omega)$ is expressed through the probability $p(\Omega|y_{n*})$, involving directly the firing neuron y_{n*}, when feature vector $\underline{x}$ is presented. One has now to turn back to (1), recalling the fact, that this equation describes the fact that the Markov models are trained with the ML criterion. It should also be recalled, that the entire sequence of feature vectors, $\underline{x}(k)$, k=1...K, results in a label stream of firing neurons $y_{n*}(k)$, k=1...K, where $y_{n*}(k)$ is the firing neuron if the k-th vector $\underline{x}(k)$ is presented to the neural network. Now, (8) can be substituted into (1) for each presentation k, yielding the modified ML criterion:

$$\underline{\theta}^* = \arg\max_{\underline{\theta}} \left\{ \sum_{k=1}^{K} \log \frac{p(\underline{x}(k))}{p(\Omega(k))} \cdot p(\Omega(k)|y_{n*}(k)) \right\}$$

$$= \arg\max_{\underline{\theta}} \left\{ \sum_{k=1}^{K} \log p(\underline{x}(k)) - \sum_{k=1}^{K} \log p(\Omega(k)) + \sum_{k=1}^{K} \log p(\Omega(k)|y_{n*}(k)) \right\} \qquad (9)$$

Usually, in a continuous parameter system, the probability $p(\underline{x})$ can be expressed as:

$$p(\underline{x}) = \sum_{n=1}^{N} p(\underline{x}|y_n) \cdot p(y_n) \qquad (10)$$

and is therefore dependent of the parameter vector $\underline{\theta}$, because in this case, $p(\underline{x}|y_n)$ can be interpreted as the probability provided by the Gaussian distributions, and the parameters of the Gaussians will depend on $\underline{\theta}$. As just mentioned before, in a discrete system, only one firing neuron y_{n*} survives, resulting in the fact that only the n*-th member remains in the sum in (10). This would correspond to only one "firing Gaussian" in the continuous case, leading to the following expression for $p(\underline{x})$:

$$p(\underline{x}) = p(\underline{x} | y_{n*}) \cdot p(y_{n*}) = p(\underline{x}, y_{n*}) = p(y_{n*} | \underline{x}) \cdot p(\underline{x}) \qquad (11)$$

Considering now the fact, that the acoustic processor is not represented by a Gaussian but instead by a vector quantizer, where the probability $p(y_{n*}|\underline{x})$ of the firing neuron is equal to 1, then (11) reduces to $p(\underline{x}) = p(\underline{x})$ and it becomes obvious that this probability is not affected by any distribution that depends on the parameter vector $\underline{\theta}$. This would be different, if $p(y_{n*}|\underline{x})$ in (11) would not have binary characteristics as in (7), but would be computed by a continuous function which in this case would depend on the parameter vector $\underline{\theta}$. Thus, without consideration of $p(\underline{x})$, the remaining expression to be maximized in (9) reduces to:

$$\underline{\theta}^* = \arg\max_{\underline{\theta}} \left[-\sum_{k=1}^{K} \log p(\Omega(k)) + \sum_{k=1}^{K} \log p(\Omega(k) | y_{n*}(k)) \right] \qquad (12)$$

$$= \arg\max_{\underline{\theta}} \left[-E\{\log p(\Omega)\} + E\{\log p(\Omega | y_{n*})\} \right]$$

These expectations of logarithmic probabilities are also defined as entropies. Therefore, (9) can be also written as

$$\underline{\theta}^* = \arg\max_{\underline{\theta}} \{H(\Omega) - H(\Omega | Y)\} \qquad (13)$$

This equation can be interpreted as follows: The term on the right side of (13) is also known as the mutual information $I(\Omega, Y)$ between the probabilistic variables Ω and Y, i.e.:

$$I(\Omega, Y) = H(\Omega) - H(\Omega | Y) = H(Y) - H(Y | \Omega) \qquad (14)$$

Therefore, the final information theory-based training criterion for the neural network can be formulated as follows: The synaptic weights of the neural network should be chosen as to maximize the mutual information between the string representing the classes of the vectors presented to the network input layer during training and the string representing the resulting sequence of firing neurons in the output layer of the neural network. This can be also expressed as the Maximum Mutual Information (MMI) criterion for neural network training. This concludes the proof that MMI neural networks are indeed optimal acoustic processors for HMM's trained with maximum likelihood principles.

3 REALIZATION OF MMI TRAINING ALGORITHMS FOR NEURAL NETWORKS

Training the synaptic weights of a neural network in order to achieve mutual information maximization is not easy. Two different algorithms have been developed for this task and can only be briefly outlined in this paper. A detailed description can be found in (Rigoll, 1994) and (Neukirchen, 1996). The first experiments used a single-layer neural network with Euclidean distance as propagation function. The first implementation of the MMI training paradigm has been realized in (Rigoll, 1994) and is based on a self-organizing procedure, starting with initial weights derived from k-means clustering of the training vectors, followed by an iterative procedure to modify the weights. The mutual information increases in a self-organizing way from a low value at the start to a much higher value after several iteration cycles. The second implementation has been realized recently and is described in detail in (Neukirchen, 1996). It is based on the idea of using gradient methods for finding the MMI value. This technique has not been used before, because the maximum search for finding the firing neuron in the output layer has prevented the calculation of derivatives. This maximum search can be approximated using the softmax function, denoted as s_n for the n-th neuron. It can be computed from the activations z_l of all neurons as:

$$s_n = e^{z_n/T} / \sum_{l=1}^{N} e^{z_l/T} \qquad (15)$$

where a small value for parameter T approximates a crisp maximum selection. Since the string Ω in (14) is always fixed during training and independent of the parameters in $\underline{\theta}$, only the function $H(\Omega|Y)$ has to be minimized. This function can also be expressed as

$$H(\Omega|Y) = -\sum_{m=1}^{M} \sum_{n=1}^{N} p(y_n, \Omega_m) \cdot \log p(\Omega_m | y_n)$$

$$= -\sum_{m=1}^{M} \sum_{n=1}^{N} p(y_n, \Omega_m) \cdot \log \frac{p(y_n, \Omega_m)}{\sum_{l=1}^{M} p(y_n, \Omega_l)} = -\sum_{m=1}^{M} \sum_{n=1}^{N} p^*[p(y_n, \Omega_m)] \qquad (16)$$

A derivative with respect to a weight w_{lj} of the neural network yields:

$$\frac{\partial H(\Omega|Y)}{\partial w_{lj}} = -\sum_{m=1}^{M} \sum_{n=1}^{N} \left\{ \frac{\partial p^*[p(y_n, \Omega_m)]}{\partial p(y_n, \Omega_m)} \cdot \frac{\partial p(y_n, \Omega_m)}{\partial s_n} \cdot \frac{\partial s_n}{\partial z_n} \cdot \frac{\partial z_n}{\partial w_{lj}} \right\} \qquad (17)$$

As shown in (Neukirchen, 1996), all the required terms in (17) can be computed effectively and it is possible to realize a gradient descend method in order to maximize the mutual information of the training data. The great advantage of this method is the fact that it is now possible to generalize this algorithm for use in all popular neural network architectures, including multilayer and recurrent neural networks.

4 RESULTS FOR THE HYBRID SYSTEM

The new hybrid system has been developed and extensively tested using the Resource Management 1000 word speaker-independent continuous speech recognition task. First, a baseline discrete HMM system has been built up with all well-known features of a context-dependent HMM system. The performance of that baseline system is shown in column 2 of Table 1. The 1st column shows the performance of the hybrid system with the neural vector quantizer. This network has some special features not mentioned in the previous sections, e.g. it uses multiple frame input and has been trained on context-dependent classes. That means that the mutual information between the stream of firing neurons and the corresponding input stream of triphones has been maximized. In this way, the firing behavior of the network becomes sensitive to context-dependent units. Therefore, this network may be the only existing context-dependent acoustic processor, carrying the principle of triphone modeling from the HMM structure to the acoustic front end. It can be seen, that a substantially higher recognition performance is obtained with the hybrid system, that compares well with the leading continuous system (HTK, in column 3). It is expected, that the system will be further improved in the near future through various additional features, including full exploitation of multilayer neural VQ's and several conventional HMM improvements, e.g. the use of crossword triphones. Recent results on the larger Wall Street Journal (WSJ) database have shown a 10.5% error rate for the hybrid system compared to a 13.4% error rate for a standard discrete system, using the 5k vocabulary test with bigram language model of perplexity 110. This error rate can be further reduced to 8.9% using crossword triphones and 6.6% with a trigram language model. This rate compares already quite favorably with the best continuous systems for the same task. It should be noted that this hybrid WSJ system is still in its initial stage and the neural component is not yet as sophisticated as in the RM system.

5 CONCLUSION

A new neural network paradigm and the resulting hybrid HMM/ANN speech recognition system have been presented in this paper. The new approach performs already very well and is still perfectible. It gains its good performance from the following facts: (1) The use of information theory-based training algorithms for the neural vector quantizer, which can be shown to be optimal for the hybrid approach. (2) The possibility of introducing context-dependency not only to the HMM's, but also to the neural quantizer. (3) The fact that this hybrid approach allows the combination of an optimal neural acoustic processor with the most advanced context-dependent HMM system. We will continue to further implement various possible improvements for our hybrid speech recognition system.

REFERENCES

Rigoll, G. (1994) Maximum Mutual Information Neural Networks for Hybrid Connectionist-HMM Speech Recognition Systems, *IEEE Transactions on Speech and Audio Processing*, Vol. 2, No. 1, Special Issue on Neural Networks for Speech Processing, pp. 175-184

Neukirchen, C. & Rigoll, G. (1996) Training of MMI Neural Networks as Vector Quantizers, *Internal Report, Gerhard-Mercator-University Duisburg, Faculty of Electrical Engineering,* available via http://www.fb9-ti.uni-duisburg.de/veroeffentl.html

Bourlard, H. & Morgan, N. (1994) *Connectionist Speech Recognition: A Hybrid Approach*, Kluwer Academic Publishers

Hochberg, M., Renals, S., Robinson, A., Cook, G. (1995) Recent Improvements to the ABBOT Large Vocabulary CSR System, *in Proc. IEEE-ICASSP*, Detroit, pp. 69-72

Rigoll, G., Neukirchen, C., Rottland, J. (1996) A New Hybrid System Based on MMI-Neural Networks for the RM Speech Recognition Task, *in Proc. IEEE-ICASSP*, Atlanta

Table 1: Comparison of recognition rates for different speech recognition systems

test set	RM SI word recognition rate with word pair grammar: correctness (accuracy)		
	hybrid MMI-NN system	baseline k-means VQ system	continuous pdf system (HTK)
Feb.'89	**96,3 %** (**95,6 %**)	94,3 % (93,6 %)	96,0 % (95,5 %)
Oct.'89	**95,4 %** (**94,5 %**)	93,5 % (92,0 %)	95,4 % (94,9 %)
Feb.'91	**96,7 %** (**95,9 %**)	94,4 % (93,5 %)	96,6 % (96,0 %)
Sep.'92	**93,9 %** (**92,5 %**)	90,7 % (88,9 %)	93,6 % (92,6 %)
average	**95,6 %** (**94,6 %**)	93,2 % (92,0 %)	95,4 % (94,7 %)

Neural Network Modeling of Speech and Music Signals

Axel Röbel
Technical University Berlin, Einsteinufer 17, Sekr. EN-8, 10587 Berlin, Germany
Tel: +49-30-314 25699, FAX: +49-30-314 21143, email: roebel@kgw.tu-berlin.de

Abstract

Time series prediction is one of the major applications of neural networks. After a short introduction into the basic theoretical foundations we argue that the iterated prediction of a dynamical system may be interpreted as a model of the system dynamics. By means of RBF neural networks we describe a modeling approach and extend it to be able to model instationary systems. As a practical test for the capabilities of the method we investigate the modeling of musical and speech signals and demonstrate that the model may be used for synthesis of musical and speech signals.

1 Introduction

Since the formulation of the reconstruction theorem by Takens [10] it has been clear that a nonlinear predictor of a dynamical system may be directly derived from a systems time series. The method has been investigated extensively and with good success for the prediction of time series of nonlinear systems. Especially the combination of reconstruction techniques and neural networks has shown good results [12].

In our work we extend the ideas of predicting nonlinear systems by the more demanding task of building system models, which are able to resynthesize the systems time series. In the case of chaotic or strange attractors the resynthesis of identical time series is known to be impossible. However, the modeling of the underlying attractor leads to the possibility to resynthesis time series which are consistent with the system dynamics. Moreover, the models may be used for the analysis of the system dynamics, for example the estimation of the Lyapunov exponents [6]. In the following we investigate the modeling of music and speech signals, where the system dynamics are known to be instationary. Therefore, we develop an extension of the modeling approach, such that we are able to handle instationary systems.

In the following, we first give a short review concerning the state space reconstruction from time series by delay coordinate vectors, a method that has been introduced by Takens [10] and later extended by Sauer et al. [9]. Then we explain the structure of the neural networks we used in the experiments and the enhancements necessary to be able to model instationary dynamics. As an example we apply the neural models to a saxophone tone and a speech signal and demonstrate that the signals may be resynthesized using the neural models. Furthermore, we discuss some of the problems and outline further developments of the application.

2 Reconstructing attractors

Assume an n-dimensional dynamical system $f(\cdot)$ evolving on an attractor A. A has fractal dimension d, which often is considerably smaller then n. The system state $\vec{z}$ is observed through a sequence of measurements $h(\vec{z})$, resulting in a time series of measurements $y_t = h(\vec{z}(t))$. Under weak assumptions concerning $h(\cdot)$ and $f(\cdot)$ the fractal embedding theorem[9] ensures that, for $D > 2d$, the set of all *delayed coordinate vectors*

$$Y_{D,T} = \{t > t_0 : (y_t, y_{t-T}, \ldots, y_{t-(D-1)T})\}, \qquad (1)$$

with an arbitrary delay time T, forms an embedding of A in the D-dimensional *reconstruction* space. We call the minimal D, which yields an embedding of A, the *embedding dimension* D_e. Because an embedding preserves characteristic features of A, especially it is one to one, it may be employed for building a system model. For this purpose the reconstruction of the attractor is used to uniquely identify the systems state thereby establishing the possibility of uniquely predicting the systems evolution. The prediction function may be represented by a hyperplane over the attractor in an $(D+1)$ dimensional space. By iterating this prediction function we obtain a vector valued system model which, however, is valid only at the respective attractor.

For the reconstruction of instationary systems dynamics we confine ourselves to the case of slowly varying parameters and model the instationary system using a sequence of attractors.

3 RBF neural networks

There are different topologies of neural networks that may be employed for time series modeling. In our investigation we used radial basis function networks which have shown considerably better scaling properties, when increasing the number of hidden units, than networks with sigmoid activation function [8]. As proposed by Verleysen et. al [11] we initialize the network using a vector quantization procedure and then apply backpropagation training to finally tune the network parameters. The tuning of the parameters yields an improvement factor of about ten in prediction error compared to the standard RBF network approach [8, 3]. Compared to earlier results [7] the normalization of the hidden layer activations yields a small improvement in the stability of the models.

The resulting network function for m-dimensional vector valued output is of the form

$$\vec{N}(\vec{x}) = \sum_j \vec{w}_j \frac{\exp\left(-(\frac{\vec{c}_j - \vec{x}}{\sigma_j})^2\right)}{\sum_i \exp(-(\frac{\vec{c}_i - \vec{x}}{\sigma_i})^2)} + \vec{b}, \qquad (2)$$

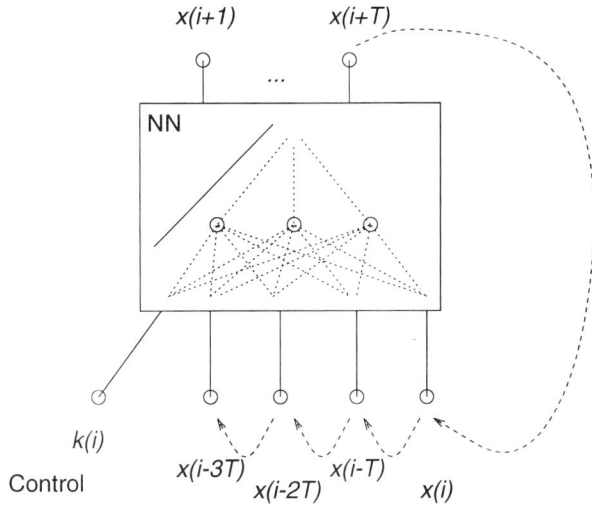

Fig. 1: Input/Output structure of the neural model.

where σ_j represents the standard deviation of the Gaussian, the input $\vec{x}$ and the centers $\vec{c}$ are n-dimensional vectors and $\vec{b}$ and $\vec{w}_j$ are m-dimensional parameters of the network. Networks of the form eq. (2) with a finite number of hidden units are able to approximate arbitrary closely all continuous mappings $R^n \to R^m$ [4]. This universal approximation property is the foundation of using neural networks for time series modeling, where we denote them as *neural models*. In the context of the previous section the neural models are approximating the systems prediction function.

To be able to represent instationary dynamics, we extend the network according to figure 1 to have an additional input, that enables the control of the actual mapping

$$\vec{N}(\vec{x}, k) = \sum_j \vec{w}_j \frac{\exp\left(-(\frac{\vec{c}_j - \vec{x}}{\sigma_j})^2 - (\frac{t_j - k}{\sigma_{tj}})^2\right)}{\sum_i \exp\left(-(\frac{\vec{c}_i - \vec{x}}{\sigma_i})^2 - (\frac{t_i - k}{\sigma_{ti}})^2\right)} + \vec{b}. \qquad (3)$$

This model is close to the Hidden Control Neural Network described in [2]. From the universal approximation properties of the RBF-networks stated above it follows, that eq. (3) with appropriate control sequence $k(i)$ is able to approximate any sequence of functions. In the context of time series prediction the value i represents the actual sample time. The control sequence may be optimized during training, as described in [2], The optimization of $k(i)$ requires prohibitively large computational power if the number of different control values, the domain of k is large. However, as long as the systems instationarity is described by a smooth function of time, we argue that it is possible to select $k(i)$ to be a fixed linear function of i. With the preselected $k(i)$ the training of the network adapts the parameters t_j and σ_{tj} such that the model evolution closely follows the systems instationarity.

4 Neural models

As is shown in figure 1 we use the delayed coordinate vectors and a selected control sequence to train the network to predict the sequence of the following T time samples. The vector valued prediction avoids the need for a further interpolation of the predicted samples. Otherwise, an interpolation would be necessary to obtain the original sample frequency, but, because the Nyquist frequency is not regarded in choosing T, is not straightforward to achieve.

After training we initialize the network input with the first input vector $(\vec{x}_0, k(0))$ of the time series and iterate the network function shifting the network input and using the latest output unit to complete the new input. The control input may be copied from the training phase to resynthesize the training signal or may be varied to emulate another sequence of system dynamics.

The question that has to be posed in this context is concerned with the stability of the model. Due to the prediction error of the model the iteration will soon leave the reconstructed attractor. Because there exists no training data from the neighborhood of the attractor the minimization of the prediction error of the network does not guaranty the stability of the model [5]. Nevertheless, as we will see in the examples, the neural models are stable for at least some parameters D and T.

Due to the high density of training data the method for stabilizing dynamical models presented in [5] is difficult to apply in our situation. Another approach to increase the model stability is to lower the gradient of the prediction function for the directions normal to the attractor. This may be obtained by disturbing the network input during training with a small noise level. While conceptually straightforward, we found that this method is only partly successful. While the resulting prediction function is smoother in the neighborhood of the attractor, the prediction error for training with noise is considerably higher as expected from the noise free results, such that the overall effect often is negative. To circumvent the problems of training with noise further investigations will consider a optimization function with regularization that directly penalizes high derivatives of the network with respect to the input units [1]. The stability of the models is a major subject of further research.

5 Practical results

We have applied our method to two acoustic time series, a single saxophone tone, consisting of 16000 samples sampled at 32kHz and a speech signal of the word *manna*[1]. The latter time series consists of 23000 samples with a sampling rate of 44.1kHz. Both time series have been normalized to stay within the interval $[-1, 1]$. The estimation of the dimension of the underlying attractors yields a dimension of about 2-3 in both cases.

We chose the control input $k(i)$ to be linear increasing from -0.8 to 0.8. Stable models we found for both time series using $D > 5$. Namely for the parameter T we observed considerable impact on the model quality. While smaller T results in better one step ahead prediction, the iterated model often becomes unstable. This might be explained by the decrease in variation within the prediction hyperplane, that has to be learned. For small T the model tends to become linear and does not capture the nonlinear characteristics of the system. Therefore the iteration of those models failed.

To large values of T results in an insufficient one step ahead prediction error, which pushes the model far away from the attractor also producing unstable behavior.

---

[1]The name of our parallel computer

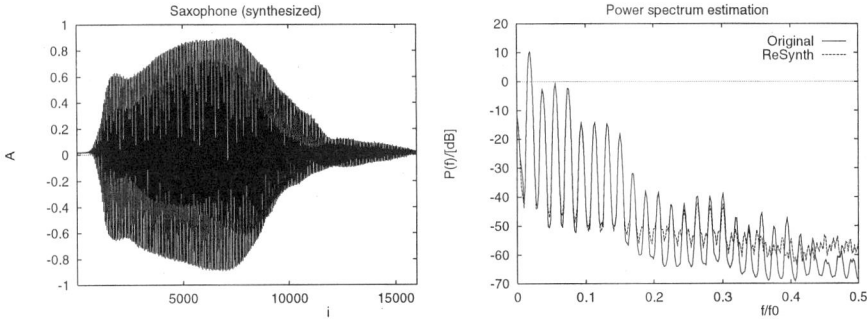

Fig. 2: Synthesized saxophone signal and power spectrum estimation for the original (solid) and synthesized (dashed) signal.

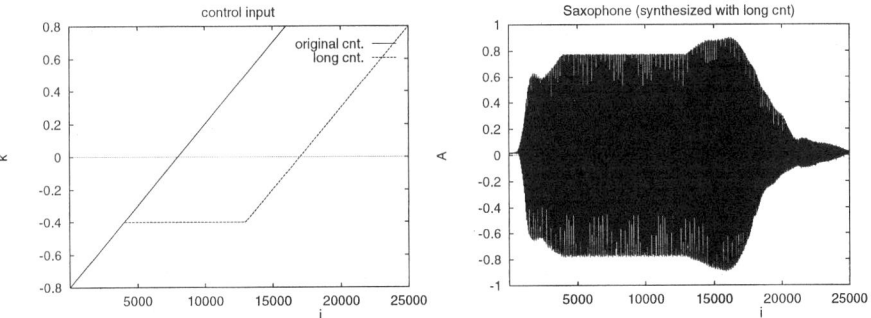

Fig. 3: Varying the synthesized tone by varying the control input sequence.

5.1 Modeling a saxophone

In the following we consider the results for the saxophone model. The model we present consists of 10 input units, 200 hidden units and 5 output units and was trained with additional Gaussian noise at the input. The standard deviation of the noise is 0.0005 and the RMS training error obtained is 0.005. The resulting saxophone model is able to resynthesize a signal which is nearly indistinguishable from the original one. The resynthesized time series is shown in figure 2. The time series follows the original one with a small phase shift, which stems from a small difference in the onset of the model. Also in figure 2 the power spectrum of the saxophone signal and the neural model is shown. From the spectrum we see the close resemblance of the sound.

One major demand for the practical application of the proposed musical instrument models is the possibility to control the synthesized sound. At the present state there exists only one control input to the model. Nevertheless, it is interesting to investigate the effect of varying the control input of the model. We tried different control input sequences to synthesize saxophone tones. It turns out that the model remains stable such that we are able to control the envelope of the sound. An example of a tone with increased duration is shown in figure 3. In this example the control input first follows the trained version, then remains constant to produce a longer duration of the tone and then increases to reproduce the decay of the tone from the trained time series.

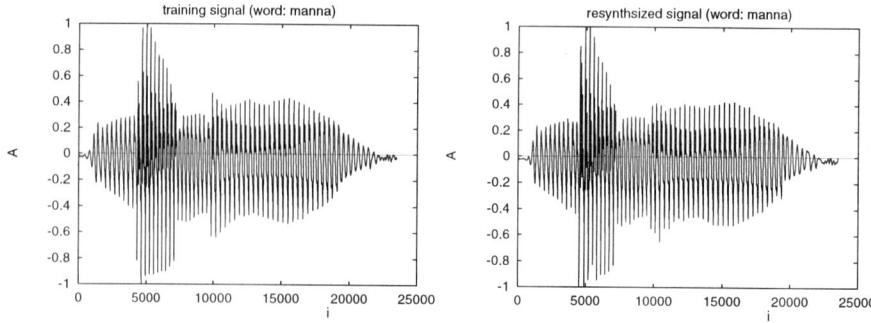

Fig. 4: Original and synthesized signal of the word *manna*.

5.2 Modeling a speech signal

For modeling the time series of the spoken word *manna* we used a similar network compared to the saxophone model. Due to the increased instationarity in the signal we needed an increased number of RBF units in the network. The best results up to now has been obtained with a network of 400 hidden units, delay time $T = 8$, output dimension 8 and input dimension 11.

In figure 4 we show the original and the resynthesized signal. The quality of the model is not as high as in the case of the saxophone. Nevertheless, the word is quite understandable. From the figure we see, that the main problems stem from the transitions between consecutive phonemes. These transitions are rather quick in time and, therefore, there exists only a small amount of data describing the dynamics of the transitions. We assume that more training examples of the same word will cure the problem. However, it will probably require a well trained speaker to reproduce the dynamics in speaking the same word twice.

6 Further developments

There are two practical applications that directly follow from the presented results. The first one is to synthesize music signals. To consider musicians demands, we need to enhance the control of the synthesized signals. Therefore, in the future we will try to enlarge the models, incorporating different flavors of sound into the same model and adding additional control inputs. Especially we plan to build models for different volume and pitch.
As a second application we will further investigate the possibilities for using the neural models as a speech synthesizer. An interesting topic of further research would be the extension of the model with an intonation control input that incorporates the possibility to synthesize different intonations of the same word from one model.

7 Summary

The article describes a methodology to build instationary models from time series of dynamical systems. We give theoretical arguments for the universality of the models and discuss some of the restrictions and actual problems. As practical test for the method we apply the models to the demanding task of the synthesis of musical and speech signals. It is demonstrated that the models are capable to resynthesize the trained signals. At the present state the envelope and duration of the synthesized signals may be controlled. Intended further developments have been shortly described.

References

[1] C. M. Bishop. Training with noise is equivalent to tikhonov regularization. *Neural Computation*, 7(1):108–116, 1995.

[2] E. Levin. Hidden control neural architecture modelling of nonlinear time varying systems and its applications. *IEEE Transactions on Neural Networks*, 4(2):109–116, 1993.

[3] J. Moody and C. Darken. Fast learning in networks of locally-tuned processing units. *Neural Computation*, 1:281–294, 1989.

[4] J. Park and I. Sandberg. Universal approximation using radial-basis-function networks. *Neural Computation*, 3(2):246–257, 1991.

[5] J. C. Principe and J.-M. Kuo. Dynamic modelling of chaotic time series with neural networks. In G. Tesauro, D. S. Touretzky, and T. Leen, editors, *Neural Information Processing Systems 7 (NIPS 94)*, 1995.

[6] A. Röbel. Neural models for estimating lyapunov exponents and embedding dimension from time series of nonlinear dynamical systems. In *Proceedings of the Intern. Conference on Artificial Neural Networks, ICANN'95, Vol. II*, pages 533–538, Paris, 1995.

[7] A. Röbel. Rbf networks for synthesis of speech and music signals. In *3. Workshop Fuzzy-Neuro-Systeme'95*, Darmstadt, 1995. Deutsche Gesellschaft für Informatik e.V.

[8] A. Röbel. Scaling properties of neural networks for the prediction of time series. In *Proceedings of the 1996 IEEE Workshop on Neural Networks for Signal Processing VI*, 1996.

[9] T. Sauer, J. A. Yorke, and M. Casdagli. Embedology. *Journal of Statistical Physics*, 65(3/4):579–616, 1991.

[10] F. Takens. *Detecting Strange Attractors in Turbulence*, volume 898 of *Lecture Notes in Mathematics (Dynamical Systems and Turbulence, Warwick 1980)*, pages 366–381. D.A. Rand and L.S. Young, Eds. Berlin: Springer, 1981.

[11] M. Verleysen and K. Hlavackova. An optimized RBF network for approximation of functions. In *Proceedings of the European Symposium on Artificial Neural Networks, ESANN'94*, 1994.

[12] A. S. Weigend and N. A. Gershenfeld. *Time Series Prediction: Forecasting the Future and Understanding the Past*. Addison-Wesley Pub. Comp., 1993.

A Constructive Learning Algorithm for Discriminant Tangent Models

Diego Sona   Alessandro Sperduti   Antonina Starita

Dipartimento di Informatica, Università di Pisa
Corso Italia, 40, 56125 Pisa, Italy
email: {sona,perso,starita}di.unipi.it

Abstract

To reduce the computational complexity of classification systems using tangent distance, Hastie et al. (HSS) developed an algorithm to devise rich models for representing large subsets of the data which computes automatically the "best" associated tangent subspace. Schwenk & Milgram proposed a discriminant modular classification system (*Diabolo*) based on several autoassociative multilayer perceptrons which use tangent distance as error reconstruction measure.

We propose a gradient based constructive learning algorithm for building a tangent subspace model with discriminant capabilities which combines several of the the advantages of both HSS and Diabolo: devised tangent models hold discriminant capabilities, space requirements are improved with respect to HSS since our algorithm is discriminant and thus it needs fewer prototype models, dimension of the tangent subspace is determined automatically by the constructive algorithm, and our algorithm is able to learn new transformations.

1 Introduction

Tangent distance is a well known technique used for transformation invariant pattern recognition. State-of-the-art accuracy can be achieved on an isolated handwritten character task using tangent distance as the classification metric within a nearest neighbor algorithm [SCD93]. However, this approach has a quite high computational complexity, owing to the inefficient search and large number of Euclidean and tangent distances that need to be calculated. Different researchers have shown how such time complexity can be reduced [Sim94, SS95] at the cost of increased space complexity.

A different approach to the problem was used by Hastie et al. [HSS95] and Schwenk & Milgram [SM95b, SM95a]. Both of them used learning algorithms for reducing the classification time and space requirements, while trying to preserve the same accuracy. Hastie et al. [HSS95] developed rich models for representing large subsets of the prototypes. These models are learned from a training set through a Singular Value Decomposition based algorithm which minimizes the average 2-sided tangent distance from a subset of the training images. A nice feature of this algorithm is that it computes automatically the "best" tangent subspace associated with the prototypes. Schwenk & Milgram [SM95b] proposed a modular classification system (*Diabolo*) based on several autoassociative multilayer perceptrons which use tangent distance as the error reconstruction measure. This original model was then improved by adding discriminant capabilities to the system [SM95a].

Comparing Hastie et al. algorithm (HSS) versus the discriminant version of Diabolo, we observe that: Diabolo seems to require less memory than HSS, however, learning is faster in HSS; Diabolo is discriminant while HSS is not; the number of hidden units to be used in Diabolo's autoassociators must be decided heuristically through a trial and error procedure, while the dimension of the tangent subspaces in HSS can be controlled more easily; Diabolo uses predefined transformations, while HSS is able to learn new transformations (like style transformations).

In this paper, we introduce the *tangent distance neuron* (TD-neuron), which implements the 1-sided version of the tangent distance, and we devise a gradient based constructive learning algorithm for building a tangent subspace model with discriminant capabilities. In this way, we are able to combine the advantages of both HSS and Diabolo: the model holds discriminant capabilities, learning is just a bit slower than HSS, space requirements are improved with respect to HSS since the TD-neuron is discriminant and thus it needs fewer prototype models, the dimension of the tangent subspace is determined automatically by the constructive algorithm, and TD-neuron is able to learn new transformations.

2 Tangent Distance

In several pattern recognition problems Euclidean distance fails to give a satisfactory solution since it is unable to account for invariant transformations of the patterns. Simard et al. [SCD93] suggested dealing with this problem by generating a parameterized 7-dimensional manifold for each image, where each parameter accounts for one such invariance. The underlying idea consists in approximating the considered transformations locally through a linear model.

For the sake of exposition, consider rotation. Given a digitalized image X_i of a pattern i, the rotation operation can be approximated by $\tilde{X}_i(\theta) = X_i + T_{X_i}\theta$, where θ is the rotation angle, and T_{X_i} is the tangent vector to the rotation curve generated by the rotation operator for X_i. The tangent vector T_{X_i} can easily be computed by finite difference. Now, instead of measuring the distance between two images as $D(X_i, X_j) = \|X_i - X_j\|$ for any norm $\|\cdot\|$, Simard et al. proposed using the *tangent distance* $D_T(X_i, X_j) = \min_{\theta_i, \theta_j} \|\tilde{X}_i(\theta_i) - \tilde{X}_j(\theta_j)\|$.

If k types of transformations are considered, there will be k different tangent vectors per pattern. If $\|\cdot\|$ is the Euclidean norm, computing the tangent distance is a simple least-squares problem. A solution for this problem[1] can be found in Simard et al. [SCD93], where the authors used D_T to drive a 1-NN classification rule.

---

[1] A special case of tangent distance, i.e., the one sided tangent distance $D_T^{1-sided}(X_i, X_j) = \min_{\theta_i} \|\tilde{X}_i(\theta_i) - X_j\|$, can be computed more efficiently [SS95].

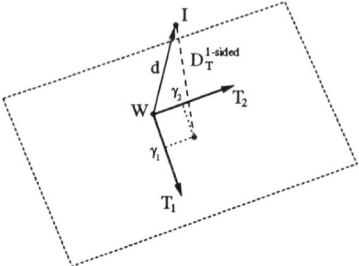

Figure 1: Geometric interpretation of equation 1. Note that $net = (D_T^{1-sided})^2$.

Unfortunately, 1-NN is expensive. To reduce the complexity of the above approach, Hastie et al. [HSS95] proposed an algorithm for the generation of rich models representing large subsets of patterns. This algorithm computes for each class a prototype (the *centroid*), and an associated subspace (described by the tangent vectors), such that the total tangent distance of the centroid with respect to the prototypes in the training set is minimised. Note that the associated subspace is not predefined as in the case of standard tangent distance, but is computed on the basis of the training set.

3 Tangent Distance Neuron

In this section we define the Tangent Distance neuron (TD-neuron), which is the computational model studied in this paper. A TD-neuron is characterized by a set of $n+1$ vectors, of the same dimension as the input vectors (in our case, images). One of these vectors, W is used as reference vector (*centroid*), while the remaining vectors, T_i ($i = 1, \ldots, n$), are used as *tangent* vectors. Moreover, the set of *tangent* vectors constitutes an *ortho-normal basis*.

Given an input vector I the input net of the TD-neuron is computed as the square of the 1-sided tangent distance between I and the tangent model $\{W, T_1, \ldots, T_n\}$ (see Figure 1)

$$net = \|\underbrace{I - W}_{d}\|^2 - \sum_{i=1}^{n}[(I-W)^t T_i]^2 = d^t d - \sum_{i=1}^{n}[\underbrace{d^t T_i}_{\gamma_i}]^2 \qquad (1)$$

where we have used the fact that the *tangent* vectors constitute an ortho-normal basis. For the sake of notation, d denotes the difference between the input pattern and the centroid, and the projection of d over the i-th tangent vector is denoted by γ_i. Note that, by definition, net is non-negative.

The output o of the TD-neuron is then computed by transforming the net through a nonlinear monotone function f. In our experiments, we have used the following function

$$o = f(\alpha, net) = \frac{1}{1 + \alpha\, net} \qquad (2)$$

where α controls the steepness of the function. Note that o is positive since net is always positive and within the range $(0, 1]$.

4 Learning

The TD-neuron can be trained to discriminate between patterns belonging to two different classes through a gradient descent technique. Thus, given a training set $\{(I_1, t_1), \ldots, (I_N, t_N)\}$, where $t_i \in \{0, 1\}$ is the i-th desired output, and N is the total number of patterns in the training set, we can define the error function as

$$E = \frac{1}{2} \sum_{k=1}^{N} (t_k - o_k)^2 \qquad (3)$$

where o_k is the output of the TD-neuron for the k-th input pattern.

Using equations (1-2), it is trivial to compute the changes for the tangent vectors, the centroid and α:

$$\Delta T_i = -\eta \left(\frac{\delta E}{\delta T_i} \right) = 2\alpha\eta \sum_{k=1}^{N} (t_k - o_k) o_k^2 \gamma_{ik} d_k \qquad (4)$$

$$\Delta W = -\eta \left(\frac{\delta E}{\delta W} \right) = 2\alpha\eta \sum_{k=1}^{N} (t_k - o_k) o_k^2 (d_k - \sum_{i=1}^{n} \gamma_{ik} T_i) \qquad (5)$$

$$\Delta \alpha = -\eta_\alpha \left(\frac{\delta E}{\delta \alpha} \right) = -\sum_{k=1}^{N} net_k \, \eta_\alpha (t_k - o_k) o_k^2 \qquad (6)$$

where η and η_α are learning parameters.

The learning algorithm initializes the centroid W to the average of the patterns with target 1, i.e., $W = \frac{1}{N_1} \sum_{k=1}^{N_1} I_k$, where N_1 is the number of patterns with target equal to 1, and the tangent vectors to random vectors with small modulus. Then α, the centroid W and the tangent vectors T_i are changed according to equations (4-6). Moreover, since the tangent vectors must constitute an ortho-normal basis, after each epoch of training the vectors T_i are ortho-normalized.

5 The Constructive Algorithm

Before training the TD-neuron using equations (4-6), we have to set the tangent subspace dimension. The same problem is present in HSS and Diabolo (i.e., number of hidden units). To solve this problem we have developed a constructive algorithm which adds tangent vectors one by one according to the computational needs.

The key idea is based on the observation that a typical run of the learning algorithm described in Section 4 leads to the sequential convergence of the vectors according to their relative importance. This means that the tangent vectors all remain random vectors while the centroid converges first.

Then one of the tangent vectors converges to the most relevant transformation (while the remaining tangent vectors are still immature), and so on till all the tangent vectors converge, one by one, to less and less relevant transformations.

This behavior suggests starting the training using only the centroid (i.e., without tangent vectors) and allow it to converge. Then, as in other constructive algorithms, the centroid is frozen and one random tangent vector T_1 is added. Learning is resumed till changes in T_1 become irrelevant. During learning, however, T_1 is normalized after each epoch. At convergence, T_1 is frozen, a new random tangent vector T_2 is added, and learning is resumed. New tangent vectors are iteratively added till changes in the classification accuracy becomes irrelevant.

	HSS		TD-neuron		
# Tang.	% Cor	% Err	% Cor	% Rej	% Err
0	—	—	73.78	7.24	18.98
1	78.74	21.26	72.06	10.48	17.46
2	79.10	20.90	77.99	8.05	13.96
3	79.94	20.06	81.14	7.17	11.69
4	81.47	18.53	82.68	6.84	10.48
5	76.87	23.13	84.25	5.63	10.12
6	71.29	28.71	85.21	5.14	9.65
7	—	—	86.16	4.76	9.08
8	—	—	86.37	4.89	8.74

Table 1: The results obtained by the HSS algorithm and the TD-neuron.

6 Results

We have tested our constructive algorithm versus the HSS algorithm (which uses the 2-sided tangent distance) on 10587 binary digits from the NIST-3 dataset. The binary 128x128 digits were transformed into a 64-grey level 16x16 format by a simple local counting procedure. **No other pre-processing transformation was performed.** The training set consisted of 3000 randomly chosen digits, while the remaining digits where used in the test set. A single tangent model for each class of digit was computed using both algorithms. The classification of the test digits was performed using the label of the closest model for HSS and the output of the TD-neurons for our system. The TD-neurons used a rejection criterion with parameters adapted during training.

In Table 1 we have reported the performances on the test set of both HSS and our system. Different numbers of tangent vectors were tested for both of them. From the results it is clear that the models generated by HSS reach a peak in performance with 4 tangent vectors and then a sharp degradation of the generalization is observed by adding more tangent vectors. On the contrary, the TD-neurons are able to steadily increase the performance with an increasing number of tangent vectors. The improvement in the performance, however, seems to saturate when using many tangent vectors. Table 2 presents the confusion matrix obtained by the TD-neurons with 8 tangent vectors.

For comparison, we display some of the tangent models computed by HSS and by our algorithm in Figure 2. Note how tangent models developed by the HSS algorithm tend to be more blurred than the ones developed by our algorithm. This is due to the lake of discriminant capabilities by the HSS algorithm and it is the main cause of the degradation in performance observed when using more than 4 tangent vectors.

It must be pointed out that, for a fixed number of tangent vectors, the HSS algorithm is faster than ours, because it needs only a fraction of the training examples (only one class). However, our algorithm is remarkably more efficient when a family of tangent models with an increasing number of tangent vectors must be generated[2]. Moreover, since a TD-neuron uses the one sided tangent distance, it is faster in computing the output.

7 Conclusion

We introduced the *tangent distance neuron* (TD-neuron), which implements the 1-sided version of the tangent distance and gave a constructive learning algorithm for building a tangent subspace with discriminant capabilities. As stated in the in-

---
[2]The tangent model computed by HSS depends on the number of tangent vectors.

A Constructive Learning Algorithm for Discriminant Tangent Models

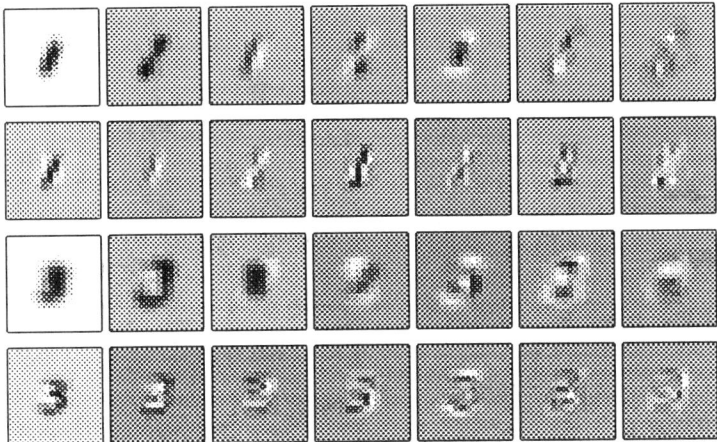

Figure 2: The tangent models obtained for digits '1' and '3' by the HSS algorithm (row 1 and 3, respectively) and our TD-neuron (row 2 and 4, respectively). The centroids are shown in the first column.

troduction, there are many advantages of using the proposed computational model versus other techniques like HSS and Diabolo. Specifically, we believe that the proposed approach is particularly useful in those applications where it is very important to have a classification system which is both discriminant and semantically transparent, in the sense that it is very easy to understand how it works. One among these applications is the classification of ancient book scripts. In fact, the description, the comparison, and the classification of forms are the main tasks of paleographers. Until now, however, these tasks have been generally performed without the aid of a universally accepted and quantitatively based method or technique. Consequently, very often it is impossible to reach a definitive date attribution of a document to within 50 years. In this field, it is very important to have a system which is both discriminant and explanatory, so that paleographers can learn from it which are the relevant features of the script of a given epoch. These requirements rule out systems like Diabolo, which is not easily interpretable, and also tangent models developed by HSS, which are not discriminant. In Figure 3 we have reported some preliminary results we obtained within this field.

Perhaps most importantly, our work suggests a number of research avenues. We used just a single TD-neuron; presumably having several neurons arranged as an adaptive pre-processing layer within a standard feed-forward neural network can yield a remarkable increase in the transformation invariant features of the network.

	o_0	o_1	o_2	o_3	o_4	o_5	o_6	o_7	o_8	o_9	Rej	% Cor	% Rej	% Err
C_0	661	4	2	5	27	8	2	1	9	0	42	86.86	5.52	7.62
C_1	4	842	0	1	1	1	1	11	8	0	9	95.90	1.03	3.08
C_2	4	1	650	2	13	2	10	6	9	0	69	84.86	9.01	6.14
C_3	1	3	22	656	0	26	1	11	18	4	28	85.19	3.64	11.17
C_4	0	0	2	0	633	3	4	5	7	48	32	86.24	4.36	9.40
C_5	1	1	3	39	2	535	7	1	7	3	44	83.20	6.84	9.95
C_6	0	4	1	2	6	11	680	0	4	0	33	91.77	4.45	3.78
C_7	1	1	3	0	4	3	0	727	12	24	27	90.65	3.37	5.99
C_8	1	4	7	18	14	12	0	7	607	11	62	81.70	8.34	9.96
C_9	0	0	0	12	43	1	0	70	36	562	25	75.03	3.34	21.63
Total			Correct:	86.37%			Rejected	4.89%				Errors	8.74%	

Table 2: The confusion matrix for the TD-neurons with 8 tangent vectors.

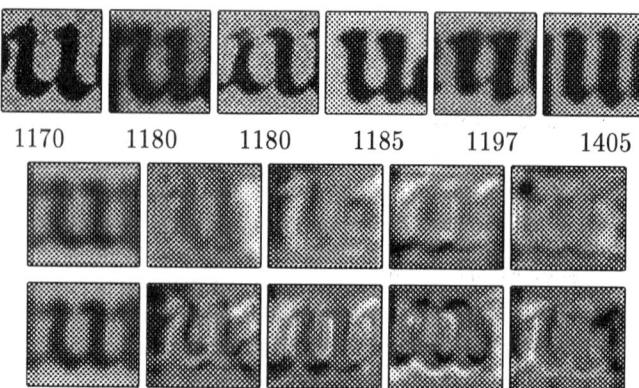

Figure 3: **Top:** samples of "u" from documents of different ages. **Bottom:** the tangent model for the 1180 devised by HSS (first row) and by our algorithm (second row). Note how the model obtained by our algorithm is more clearly understandable.

Clustering algorithms can also be used to devise computationally efficient discriminant classifiers.

References

[HSS95] T. Hastie, P.Y. Simard, and E. Säckinger. Learning prototype models for tangent distance. In G. Tesauro, D. Touretzky, and T. Leen, editors, *Advances in Neural Information Processing Systems 7*, pages 999–1006. San Mateo, CA: Morgan Kaufmann, 1995.

[SCD93] P.Y. Simard, Y. Le Cun, and J. Denker. Efficient pattern recognition using a new transformation distance. In S.J. Hanson, J.D. Cowan, and C.L. Giles, editors, *Advances in Neural Information Processing Systems 5*, pages 50–58. San Mateo, CA: Morgan Kaufmann, 1993.

[Sim94] P.Y. Simard. Efficient computation of complex distance metrics using hierarchical filtering. In J.D. Cowan, G. Tesauro, and J. Alspector, editors, *Advances in Neural Information Processing Systems 6*, pages 168–175. San Mateo, CA: Morgan Kaufmann, 1994.

[SM95a] H. Schwenk and M. Milgram. Learning discriminant tangent models for handwritten character recognition. In *International Conference on Artificial Neural Networks*, pages 585–590. Springer-Verlag, 1995.

[SM95b] H. Schwenk and M. Milgram. Transformation invariant autoassociation with application to handwritten character recognition. In G. Tesauro, D. Touretzky, and T. Leen, editors, *Advances in Neural Information Processing Systems 7*, pages 991–998. San Mateo, CA: Morgan Kaufmann, 1995.

[SS95] A. Sperduti and D.G. Stork. A rapid graph-based method for arbitrary transformation-invariant pattern classification. In G. Tesauro, D.S. Touretzky, and T. Leen, editors, *Advances in Neural Information Processing Systems 7*, pages 665–672. Boston, MA: MIT Press, 1995.

Dual Kalman Filtering Methods for Nonlinear Prediction, Smoothing, and Estimation

Eric A. Wan
ericwan@ee.ogi.edu

Alex T. Nelson
atnelson@ee.ogi.edu

Department of Electrical Engineering
Oregon Graduate Institute
P.O. Box 91000 Portland, OR 97291

Abstract

Prediction, estimation, and smoothing are fundamental to signal processing. To perform these interrelated tasks given noisy data, we form a time series model of the process that generates the data. Taking noise in the system explicitly into account, maximum-likelihood and Kalman frameworks are discussed which involve the dual process of estimating both the model parameters and the underlying state of the system. We review several established methods in the linear case, and propose several extensions utilizing dual Kalman filters (DKF) and forward-backward (FB) filters that are applicable to neural networks. Methods are compared on several simulations of noisy time series. We also include an example of nonlinear noise reduction in speech.

1 INTRODUCTION

Consider the general autoregressive model of a noisy time series with both process and additive observation noise:

$$x(k) = f(x(k-1), ...x(k-M), \mathbf{w}) + v(k-1) \quad (1)$$
$$y(k) = x(k) + r(k), \quad (2)$$

where $x(k)$ corresponds to the true underlying time series driven by process noise $v(k)$, and $f(\cdot)$ is a nonlinear function of past values of $x(k)$ parameterized by $\mathbf{w}$.

The only available observation is $y(k)$ which contains additional additive noise $r(k)$. *Prediction* refers to estimating an $\hat{x}(k)$ given past observations. (For purposes of this paper we will restrict ourselves to univariate time series.) In *estimation*, $\hat{x}(k)$ is determined given observations up to and including time k. Finally, *smoothing* refers to estimating $\hat{x}(k)$ given all observations, past and future.

The minimum mean square nonlinear prediction of $x(k)$ (or of $y(k)$) can be written as the conditional expectation $E[x(k)|\mathbf{x}(k-1)]$, where $\mathbf{x}(k) = [x(k), x(k-1), \cdots x(0)]$. If the time series $x(k)$ were directly available, we could use this data to generate an approximation of the optimal predictor. However, when $x(k)$ is not available (as is generally the case), the common approach is to use the noisy data directly, leading to an approximation of $E[y(k)|\mathbf{y}(k-1)]$. However, this results in a biased predictor: $E[y(k)|\mathbf{y}(k-1)] = E[x(k)|\mathbf{x}(k-1) + R(k-1)] \neq E[x(k)|\mathbf{x}(k-1)]$.

We may reduce the above bias in the predictor by exploiting the knowledge that the observations $y(k)$ are measurements arising from a time series. Estimates $\hat{x}(k)$ are found (either through *estimation* or *smoothing*) such that $||x(k) - \hat{x}(k)|| < ||x(k) - y(k)||$. These estimates are then used to form a predictor that approximates $E[x(k)|\hat{\mathbf{x}}(k-1)]$.[1]

In the remainder of this paper, we will develop methods for the dual estimation of both states $\hat{x}$ and weights $\hat{\mathbf{w}}$. We show how a maximum-likelihood framework can be used to relate several existing algorithms and how established linear methods can be extended to a nonlinear framework. New methods involving the use of dual Kalman filters are also proposed and experiments are provided to compare results.

2 DUAL ESTIMATION

Given only noisy observations $y(k)$, the dual estimation problem requires consideration of both the standard prediction (or output) errors $e_p(k) = y(k) - f(\hat{\mathbf{x}}(k-1), \mathbf{w})$ as well as the observation (or input) errors $e_o(k) = y(k) - \hat{x}(k)$. The minimum observation error variance equals the noise variance σ_r^2. The prediction error, however, is correlated with the observation error since $y(k) - f(\mathbf{x}(k-1)) = r(k-1) + v(k)$, and thus has a minimum variance of $\sigma_r^2 + \sigma_v^2$. Assuming the errors are Gaussian, we may construct a log-likelihood function which is proportional to $\mathbf{e}^T \Sigma^{-1} \mathbf{e}$, where $\mathbf{e}^T = [e_o(0), e_o(1)....e_o(N), e_p(M), e_p(M+1), ...e_p(N)]$, a vector of all errors up to time N, and

$$\Sigma \triangleq E[\mathbf{e}\mathbf{e}^T] = \begin{bmatrix} \sigma_r^2 I_N & 0 & 0 \\ & \sigma_r^2 I_{N-M} & 0 \\ \hline 0 & \sigma_r^2 I_{N-M} & (\sigma_r^2 + \sigma_v^2) I_{N-M} \\ 0 & 0 & \end{bmatrix} \quad (3)$$

Minimization of the log-likelihood function leads to the maximum-likelihood estimates for both $\hat{x}(k)$ and $\mathbf{w}$. (Although we may also estimate the noise variances σ_r^2 and σ_v^2, we will assume in this paper that they are known.) Two general frameworks for optimization are available:

---

[1]Because models are trained on estimated data $\hat{x}(k)$, it is important that estimated data still be used for prediction of out-of training set (on-line) data. In other words, if our model was formed as an approximation of $E[x(k)|\hat{\mathbf{x}}(k-1)]$, then we should not provide it with $y(k-1)$ as an input in order to avoid a model mismatch.

2.1 Errors-In-Variables (EIV) Methods

This method comes from the statistics literature for nonlinear regression (see Seber and Wild, 1989), and involves batch optimization of the cost function in Equation 3. Only minor modifications are made to account for the time series model. These methods, however, are memory intensive (Σ is approx. $2N \times 2N$) and also do not accommodate new data in an efficient manner. Retraining is necessary on all the data in order to produce estimates for the new data points.

If we ignore the cross correlation between the prediction and observation error, then Σ becomes a diagonal matrix and the cost function may be expressed as simply $\sum_{k=1}^{N} \gamma e_p^2(k) + e_o^2(k)$, with $\gamma = \sigma_r^2/(\sigma_r^2 + \sigma_v^2)$. This is equivalent to the *Clearning* (CLRN) cost function (Weigend, 1995), developed as a heuristic method for cleaning the inputs in neural network modelling problems. While this allows for stochastic optimization, the assumption in the time series formulation may lead to severely biased results. Note also that no estimate is provided for the last point $\hat{x}(N)$.

When the model $f = \mathbf{w}^T \mathbf{x}$ is known and linear, EIV reduces to a standard (batch) weighted least squares procedure which can be solved in closed form to generate a maximum-likelihood estimate of the noise free time series. However, when the linear model is unknown, the problem is far more complicated. The inner product of the parameter vector $\mathbf{w}$ with the vector $\mathbf{x}(k-1)$ indicates a bilinear relationship between these unknown quantities. Solving for $x(k)$ requires knowledge of $\mathbf{w}$, while solving for $\mathbf{w}$ requires $x(k)$. Iterative methods are necessary to solve the nonlinear optimization, and a Newton's-type batch method is typically employed. An EIV method for nonlinear models is also readily developed, but the computational expense makes it less practical in the context of neural networks.

2.2 Kalman Methods

Kalman methods involve reformulation of the problem into a state-space framework in order to efficiently optimize the cost function in a recursive manner. At each time point, an optimal estimation is achieved by combining both a prior prediction and new observation. Connor (1994), proposed using an Extended Kalman filter with a neural network to perform state estimation alone. Puskorious and Feldkamp (1994) and others have posed the weight estimation in a state-space framework to allow Kalman training of a neural network. Here we extend these ideas to include the dual Kalman estimation of both states and weights for efficient maximum-likelihood optimization. We also introduce the use of forward-backward *information* filters and further explicate relationships to the EIV methods.

A state-space formulation of Equations 1 and 2 is as follows:

$$\mathbf{x}(k) = F[\mathbf{x}(k-1)] + Bv(k-1) \qquad (4)$$
$$y(k) = C\mathbf{x}(k) + r(k) \qquad (5)$$

where

$$\mathbf{x}(k) = \begin{bmatrix} x(k) \\ x(k-1) \\ \vdots \\ x(k-M+1) \end{bmatrix} \quad F[\mathbf{x}(k)] = \begin{bmatrix} f(x(k), \ldots, x(k-M+1), \mathbf{w}) \\ x(k) \\ \vdots \\ x(k-M+2) \end{bmatrix} \quad B = \begin{bmatrix} 1 \\ 0 \\ \vdots \\ 0 \end{bmatrix}, \qquad (6)$$

and $C = B^T$. If the model is linear, then $f(\mathbf{x}(k))$ takes the form $\mathbf{w}^T\mathbf{x}(k)$, and $F[\mathbf{x}(k)]$ can be written as $A\mathbf{x}(k)$, where A is in controllable canonical form.

If the model is linear, and the parameters $\mathbf{w}$ are known, the Kalman filter (KF) algorithm can be readily used to estimate the states (see Lewis, 1986). At each time step, the filter computes the linear least squares estimate $\hat{x}(k)$ and prediction $\hat{x}^-(k)$, as well as their error covariances, $P_\mathbf{x}(k)$ and $P_\mathbf{x}^-(k)$. In the linear case with Gaussian statistics, the estimates are the minimum mean square estimates. With no prior information on x, they reduce to the maximum-likelihood estimates.

Note, however, that while the Kalman filter provides the maximum-likelihood estimate at each instant in time given all *past* data, the EIV approach is a batch method that gives a *smoothed* estimate given *all* data. Hence, only the estimates $\hat{x}(N)$ at the final time step will match. An exact equivalence for all time is achieved by combining the Kalman filter with a backwards *information filter* to produce a forward-backward (FB) smoothing filter (Lewis, 1986).[2] Effectively, an inverse covariance is propagated backwards in time to form backwards state estimates that are combined with the forward estimates. When the data set is large, the FB filter offers significant computational advantages over the batch form.

When the model is nonlinear, the Kalman filter cannot be applied directly, but requires a linearization of the nonlinear model at the each time step. The resulting algorithm is known as the extended Kalman filter (EKF) and effectively approximates the nonlinear function with a time-varying linear one.

2.2.1 Batch Iteration for Unknown Models

Again, when the linear model is unknown, the bilinear relationship between the time series estimates, $\hat{x}$, and the weight estimates, $\hat{\mathbf{w}}$ requires an iterative optimization. One approach (referred to as LS-KF) is to use a Kalman filter to estimate $\hat{x}(k)$ with $\hat{\mathbf{w}}$ fixed, followed by least-squares optimization to find $\hat{\mathbf{w}}$ using the current $\hat{x}(k)$. Specifically, the parameters are estimated as $\hat{\mathbf{w}} = (\mathbf{X}_{KF}^T \mathbf{X}_{KF})^{-1} \mathbf{X}_{KF} \mathbf{y}$, where $\mathbf{X}_{KF}$ is a matrix of KF state estimates, and $\mathbf{y}$ is a $1 \times N$ vector of observations.

For nonlinear models, we use a feedforward neural network to approximate $f(\cdot)$, and replace the LS and KF procedures by backpropagation and extended Kalman filtering, respectively (referred to here as BP-EKF, see Connor 1994). A disadvantage of this approach is slow convergence, due to keeping a set of *inaccurate* estimates fixed at each batch optimization stage.

2.2.2 Dual Kalman Filter

Another approach for unknown models is to concatenate both $\mathbf{w}$ and $\mathbf{x}$ into a joint state vector. The model and time series are then estimated simultaneously by applying an EKF to the nonlinear joint state equations (see Goodwin and Sin, 1994 for the linear case). This algorithm, however, has been known to have convergence problems.

An alternative is to construct a separate state-space formulation for the underlying weights as follows:
$$\mathbf{w}(k) = \mathbf{w}(k-1) \tag{7}$$
$$y(k) = f(\hat{\mathbf{x}}(k-1), \mathbf{w}(k)) + n(k), \tag{8}$$

---
[2] A slight modification of the cost in Equation 3 is necessary to account for initial conditions in the Kalman form.

where the state transition is simply an identity matrix, and $f(\hat{\mathbf{x}}(k-1), \mathbf{w}(k))$ plays the role of a time-varying nonlinear observation on $\mathbf{w}$.

When the unknown model is linear, the observation takes the form $\hat{\mathbf{x}}(k-1)^T \mathbf{w}(k)$. Then a pair of dual Kalman filters (DKF) can be run in parallel, one for state estimation, and one for weight estimation (see Nelson, 1976). At each time step, all current estimates are used. The dual approach essentially allows us to separate the non-linear optimization into two linear ones. Assumptions are that $\hat{\mathbf{x}}$ and $\hat{\mathbf{w}}$ remain uncorrelated and that statistics remain Gaussian. Note, however, that the error in each filter should be accounted for by the other. We have developed several approaches to address this coupling, but only present one here for the sake of brevity. In short, we write the variance of the noise $n(k)$ as $CP_{\mathbf{x}}^-(k)C^T + \sigma_r^2$. in Equation 8, and replace $v(k-1)$ by $v(k-1) + (\mathbf{w}(k)^T - \hat{\mathbf{w}}^T(k))\mathbf{x}(k-1)$ in Equation 4 for estimation of $\hat{\mathbf{x}}(k)$. Note that the ability to couple statistics in this manner is not possible in the batch approaches.

We further extend the DKF method to nonlinear neural network models by introducing a dual extended Kalman filtering method (DEKF). This simply requires that Jacobians of the neural network be computed for both filters at each time step. Note, by feeding $\hat{\mathbf{x}}(k)$ into the network, we are implicitly using a recurrent network.

2.2.3 Forward-Backward Methods

All of the Kalman methods can be reformulated by using forward-backward (FB) Kalman filtering to further improve state smoothing. However, the dual Kalman methods require an interleaving of the forward and backward state estimates in order to generate a smooth update at each time step. In addition, using the FB estimates requires caution because their noncausal nature can lead to a biased $\hat{\mathbf{w}}$ if they are used improperly. Specifically, for LS-FB the weights are computed as: $\hat{\mathbf{w}} = (\mathbf{X}_{KF}^T \mathbf{X}_{FB})^{-1} \mathbf{X}_{KF} \mathbf{y}$, where $\mathbf{X}_{FB}$ is a matrix of FB (smooth) state estimates. Equivalent adjustments are made to the dual Kalman methods. Furthermore, a model of the time-reversed system is required for the nonlinear case. The explication and results of these algorithms will be appear in a future publication.

3 EXPERIMENTS

Table 1 compares the different approaches on two linear time series, both when the linear model is known and when it is unknown. The least square (LS) estimation for the weights in the bottom row represents a baseline performance wherein no noise model is used. In-sample training set predictions must be interpreted carefully as all training set data is being used to optimize for the weights. We see that the Kalman-based methods perform better out of training set (recall the model-mismatch issue[1]). Further, only the Kalman methods allow for on-line estimations (on the test set, the state-estimation Kalman filters continue to operate with the weight estimates fixed). The forward-backward method further improves performance over KF methods. Meanwhile, the clearning-equivalent cost function sacrifices both state and weight estimation MSE for improved in-sample prediction; the resulting test set performance is significantly worse.

Several time series were used to compare the nonlinear methods, with the results summarized in Table 2. Conclusions parallel those for the linear case. Note, the DEKF method performed better than the baseline provided by standard backprop-

Table 1: Comparison of methods for two linear models
Model Known

	Train 1		Test 1			Train 2		Test 2		
	Est.	Pred.	Est.	Pred.	w	Est.	Pred.	Est.	Pred.	w
MLE	.094	.322	-	1.09	-	.165	.558	-	1.32	-
CLRN	.203	.134	-	1.08	-	.343	.342	-	1.32	-
KF	.134	.559	.132	0.59	-	.197	.778	.221	0.85	-
FB	.094	.559	.132	0.59	-	.165	.778	.221	0.85	-

Model Unknown

	Est.	Pred.	Est.	Pred.	w	Est.	Pred.	Est.	Pred.	w
EIV						.172	.545	-	1.81	.122
CLRN						.278	.049	-	14.1	11.28
LS-KF	.138	.563	.139	.605	.134	.197	.778	.226	0.85	.325
LS-FB	.099	.347	.136	.603	.281	.169	.612	.229	0.89	.369
DKF	.135	.557	.133	.595	.212	.198	.779	.221	.863	.149
DFB	.096	.329	.134	.596	.187	.165	.587	.221	.859	.065
LS	-	.886	-	1.09	.612	-	1.08	-	1.32	0.590

MSE values for estimation (Est.), prediction (Pred.) and weights (w) (normalized to signal var.). 1 - AR(11) model, $\sigma_r^2 = 4$, $\sigma_v^2 = 1$, 2000 training samples, 1000 testing samples. EIV and CLRN were not computed for the unknown model due to memory constraints. 2 - AR(5) model, $\sigma_r^2 = .7.$, $\sigma_v^2 = .5.$, 375 training, 125 testing.

Table 2: Comparison of methods on nonlinear time series

	NNet 1				NNet 2				NNet 3			
	Train		Test		Train		Test		Train		Test	
	Es.	Pr.	Es.	Pr.	Es.	Pr.	Es.	Pr.	Es.	Pr.	Es.	Pr.
BP-EKF	.17	.58	.15	.63	.08	.31	.08	.33	.16	.59	.17	.59
DEKF	.14	.57	.13	.59	.07	.30	.06	.32	.14	.56	.14	.55
BP	.35	.57	.35	.69	.22	.30	.23	.36	.32	.68	.32	.68

The series Nnet 1,2,3 are generated by autoregressive neural networks which exhibit limit cycle and chaotic behavior. $\sigma_v^2 = .16$, $\sigma_r^2 = .81$, 2700 training samples, 1300 testing samples. All network models fit using 10 inputs and 5 hidden units. Cross-validation was not used in any of the methods.

agation (wherein no model of the noise is used). The DEKF method exhibited fast convergence, requiring only 10-20 epochs for training. A DEFB method is under development.

The DEKF was tested on a speech signal corrupted with simulated bursting white noise (Figure 1). The method was applied to successive 64ms (512 point) windows of the signal, with a new window starting every 8ms (64 points). The results in the figure were computed assuming both σ_v^2 and σ_r^2 were known. The average SNR is improved by 9.94 dB. We also ran the experiment when σ_r^2 and σ_v^2 were estimated using only the noisy signal (Nelson and Wan, 1997), and acheived an SNR improvement of 8.50 dB. In comparison, available "state-of-the-art" techniques of *spectral subtraction* (Boll, 1979) and *RASTA* processing (Hermansky et al., 1995), achieve SNR improvements of only .65 and 1.26 dB, respectively. We extend the algorithms to the colored noise case in a second paper (Nelson and Wan, 1997).

4 CONCLUSIONS

We have described various methods under a Kalman framework for the dual estimation of both states and weights of a noisy time series. These methods utilize both

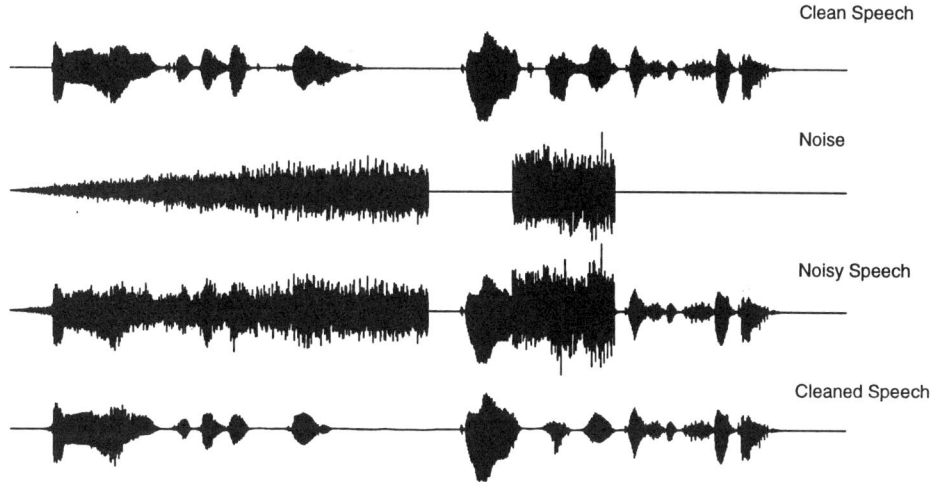

Figure 1: Cleaning Noisy Speech With The DEKF. 33,000 pts (5 sec.) shown.

process and observation noise models to improve estimation performance. Work in progress includes extensions for colored noise, blind signal separation, forward-backward filtering, and noise estimation. While further study is needed, the dual extended Kalman filter methods for neural network prediction, estimation, and smoothing offer potentially powerful new tools for signal processing applications.

Acknowledgements

This work was sponsored in part by NSF under grant ECS-9410823 and by ARPA/AASERT Grant DAAH04-95-1-0485.

References

S.F. Boll. Suppression of acoustic noise in speech using spectral subtraction. *IEEE ASSP-27*, pp. 113-120. April 1979.

J. Connor, R. Martin, L. Atlas. Recurrent neural networks and robust time series prediction. *IEEE Tr. on Neural Networks*. March 1994.

F. Lewis. *Optimal Estimation* John Wiley & Sons, Inc. New York. 1986.

G. Goodwin, K.S. Sin. *Adaptive Filtering Prediction and Control.* Prentice-Hall, Inc., Englewood Cliffs, NJ. 1994.

H. Hermansky, E. Wan, C. Avendano. Speech enhancement based on temporal processing. *ICASSP Proceedings*. 1995.

A. Nelson, E. Wan. Neural speech enhancement using dual extended Kalman filtering. Submitted to *ICNN'97*.

L. Nelson, E. Stear. The simultaneous on-line estimation of parameters and states in linear systems. *IEEE Tr. on Automatic Control*. February, 1976.

G. Puskorious, L. Feldkamp. Neural control of nonlinear dynamic systems with kalman filter trained recurrent networks. *IEEE Trn. on NN*, vol. 5, no. 2. 1994.

G. Seber, C. Wild. *Nonlinear Regression.* John Wiley & Sons. 1989.

A. Weigend, H.G. Zimmerman. Clearning. University of Colorado Computer Science Technical Report CU-CS-772-95. May, 1995.

Ensemble Methods for Phoneme Classification

Steve Waterhouse **Gary Cook**
Cambridge University Engineering Department
Cambridge CB2 1PZ, England, Tel: [+44] 1223 332754
Email: srw1001@eng.cam.ac.uk, gdc@eng.cam.ac.uk

Abstract

This paper investigates a number of ensemble methods for improving the performance of phoneme classification for use in a speech recognition system. Two ensemble methods are described; boosting and mixtures of experts, both in isolation and in combination. Results are presented on two speech recognition databases: an isolated word database and a large vocabulary continuous speech database. These results show that principled ensemble methods such as boosting and mixtures provide superior performance to more naive ensemble methods such as averaging.

INTRODUCTION

There is now considerable interest in using ensembles or committees of learning machines to improve the performance of the system over that of a single learning machine. In most neural network ensembles, the ensemble members are trained on either the same data (Hansen & Salamon 1990) or different subsets of the data (Perrone & Cooper 1993). The ensemble members typically have different initial conditions and/or different architectures. The subsets of the data may be chosen at random, with prior knowledge or by some principled approach e.g. clustering. Additionally, the outputs of the networks may be combined by any function which results in an output that is consistent with the form of the problem. The expectation of ensemble methods is that the member networks pick out different properties present in the data, thus improving the performance when their outputs are combined.

The two techniques described here, boosting (Drucker, Schapire & Simard 1993) and mixtures of experts (Jacobs, Jordan, Nowlan & Hinton 1991), differ from simple ensemble methods.

In boosting, each member of the ensemble is trained on patterns that have been filtered by previously trained members of the ensemble. In mixtures, the members of the ensemble, or "experts", are trained on data that is stochastically selected by a gate which additionally learns how to best combine the outputs of the experts.

The aim of the work presented here is twofold and inspired from two differing but complimentary directions. Firstly, how does one select which data to train the ensemble members on and secondly, given these members how does one combine them to achieve the optimal result? The rest of the paper describes how a combination of boosting and mixtures may be used to improve phoneme error rates.

PHONEME CLASSIFICATION

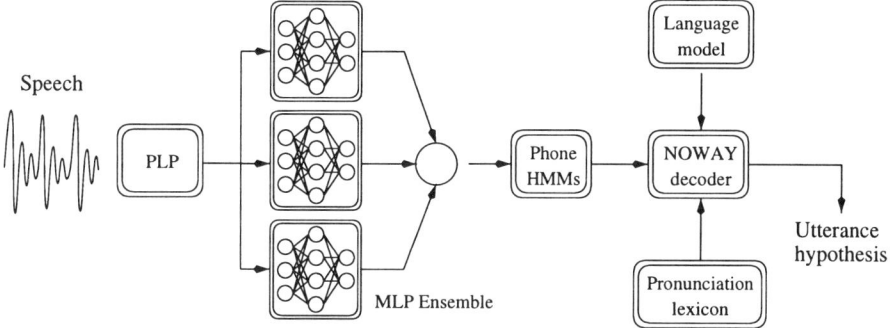

Figure 1: The ABBOT hybrid connectionist-HMM speech recognition system with an MLP ensemble acoustic model

The Cambridge University Engineering Department connectionist speech recognition system (ABBOT) uses a hybrid connectionist - hidden Markov model (HMM) approach. This is shown in figure 1. A connectionist acoustic model is used to map each frame of acoustic data to posterior phone probabilities. These estimated phone probabilities are then used as estimates of the observation probabilities in an HMM framework. Given new acoustic data and the connectionist-HMM framework, the maximum a posteriori word sequence is then extracted using a single pass, start synchronous decoder. A more complete description of the system can be found in (Hochberg, Renals & Robinson 1994).

Previous work has shown how a novel boosting procedure based on utterance selection can be used to increase the performance of the recurrent network acoustic model (Cook & Robinson 1996). In this work a combined boosting and mixtures-of-experts approach is used to improve the performance of MLP acoustic models. Results are presented for two speech recognition tasks. The first is phonetic classification on a small isolated digit database. The second is a large vocabulary continuous speech recognition task from the Wall Street Journal corpus.

ENSEMBLE METHODS

Most ensemble methods can be divided into two separate methods; network selection and network combination. Network selection addresses the question of how to choose the data each network is trained on. Network combination addresses the question of what is the best way to combine the outputs of these trained networks. The simplest method for network selection is to train separate networks on separate regions of the data, chosen either randomly, with prior knowledge or according to some other criteria, e.g. clustering.

The simplest method of combining the outputs of several networks is to form an average, or simple additive merge: $y(t) = \frac{1}{K}\sum_{k=1}^{K} y_k(t)$, where $y_k(t)$ is the output of the kth network at time t.

Boosting

Boosting is a procedure which results in an ensemble of networks. The networks in a boosting ensemble are trained sequentially on data that has been filtered by the previously trained networks in the ensemble. This has the advantage that only data that is likely to result in improved generalization performance is used for training. The first practical application of a boosting procedure was for the optical character recognition task (Drucker et al. 1993). An ensemble of feedforward neural networks was trained using supervised learning. Using boosting the authors reported a reduction in error rate on ZIP codes from the United States Postal Service of 28% compared to a single network. The boosting procedure is as follows: train a network on a randomly chosen subset of the available training data. This network is then used to filter the remaining training data to produce a training set for a second network with an even distribution of cases which the first network classifies correctly and incorrectly. After training the second network the first and second networks are used to produce a training set for a third network. This training set is produced from cases in the remaining training data that the first two networks disagree on.

The boosted networks are combined using either a voting scheme or a simple add as described in the previous section. The voting scheme works as follows: if the first two networks agree, take their answer as the output, if they disagree, use the third network's answer as the output.

Mixtures of Experts

The mixture of experts (Jacobs et al. 1991) is a different type of ensemble to the two considered so far. The ensemble members or *experts* are trained with data which is stochastically selected by a *gate*. The gate in turn learns how to best combine the experts given the data. The training of the experts, which are typically single or multi-layer networks, proceeds as for standard networks, with an additional weighting of the output error terms by the posterior probabilty $h_i(t)$ of selecting expert i given the current data point at time (t): $h_i(t) = g_i(t).P_i(t) \Big/ \sum_j g_j(t).P_j(t)$, where $g_i(t)$ is the output of the gate for expert i, and $P_i(t)$ is the probability of obtaining the correct output given expert i. In the case of classification, considered here, the experts use softmax output units. The gate, which is typically a single or multi-layered network with softmax output units is trained using the posterior probabilities as targets. The overall output $y(t)$ of the mixture of experts is given by the weighted combination of the gate and expert outputs: $y(t) = \sum_{k=1}^{K} g_k(t).y_k(t)$, where $y_k(t)$ is the output of the kth expert, and $g_k(t)$ is the output of the gate for expert k at time t.

The mixture of experts is based on the principle of divide and conquer, in which a relatively hard problem is broken up into a series of smaller easier to solve problems. By using the posterior probabilities to weight the experts and provide targets for the gate, the effective data sets used to train each expert may overlap.

SPEECH RECOGNITION RESULTS

This section describes the results of experiments on two speech databases: the Bellcore isolated digits database and the Wall Street Journal Corpus (Paul & Baker 1992). The inputs to the networks consist of 9 frames of acoustic feature vectors; the frame on which the network is currently performing classification, plus 4 frames of left context and 4 frames of right context. The context frames allow the network to take account of the dynamical nature of speech. Each acoustic feature vector consists of 8th order PLP plus log energy coefficients along with the dynamic delta coeficients of these coefficients, computed with an analysis window of 25ms, every 12.5 ms at a sampling rate of 8kHz. The speech is labelled with 54 phonemes according to the standard ABBOT phone set.

Bellcore Digits

The Bellcore digits database consists of 150 speakers saying the words "zero" through "nine", "oh", "no" and "yes". The database was divided into a training set of 122 speakers, a cross validation set of 13 speakers and a test set of 15 speakers. Each method was evaluated over 10 partitions of the data into different training, cross validation and test sets. In all the experiments on the Bellcore digits multi-layer perceptrons with 200 hidden units were used as the basic network members in the ensembles. The gates in the mixtures were also multi-layer perceptrons with 20 hidden units.

Ensemble	Combination Method	Phone Error Rate Average	σ
Simple ensemble	cheat	14.7 %	0.9
Simple ensemble	vote	20.3 %	1.2
Simple ensemble	average	19.3 %	1.2
Simple ensemble	soft gated	20.9 %	1.2
Simple ensemble	hard gated	19.3 %	1.0
Simple ensemble	mixed	17.1 %	1.3
Boosted ensemble	cheat	11.9 %	1.0
Boosted ensemble	vote	17.8 %	1.1
Boosted ensemble	average	17.4 %	1.1
Boosted ensemble	soft gated	17.8 %	1.0
Boosted ensemble	hard gated	17.4 %	1.2
Boosted ensemble	mixed	16.4 %	1.0

Table 1: Comparison of phone error rates using different ensemble methods on the Bellcore isolated digits task.

Table 1 summarises the results obtained on the Bellcore digits database. The meaning of the entries are as follows. Two types of ensemble were trained:

Simple Ensemble: consisting of 3 networks each trained on 1/3 of the training data each (corresponding to 40 speakers used for training and 5 for cross validation for each network),

Boosted Ensemble: consisting of 3 networks trained according to the boosting algorithm of the previous section. Due to the relatively small size of the data set, it was necessary to ensure that the distributions of the randomly chosen data were consistent with the overall training data distribution.

Given each set of ensemble networks, 6 combination methods were evaluated:

cheat: The cheat scheme uses the best ensemble member for each example in the data set. The best ensemble member is determined by looking at the correct label in the labelled test set (hence *cheating*). This method is included as a lower bound on the error. Since the tests are performed on unseen data, this bound can only be approached by learning an appropriate combination function of the ensemble member outputs.

average: The ensemble members' outputs are combined using a simple average.

vote: The voting scheme outlined in the previous section.

gated: In the gated combination method, the ensemble networks were kept fixed whilst the gate was trained. Two types of gating were evaluated, standard or *soft* gating, and *hard* or winner take all (WTA) training. In WTA training the targets for the gate are binary, with a target of 1.0 for the output corresponding to the expert whose probability of generating the current data point correctly is greatest, and 0.0 for the other outputs.

mixed: In contrast to the *gated* method, the *mixed* combination method both trains a gate and retrains the ensemble members using the mixture of experts framework.

From these results it can be concluded that boosting provides a significant improvement in performance over a simple ensemble. In addition, by training a gate to combine the boosted networks performance can be further enhanced. As might be expected, re-training both the boosted networks and the gate provides the biggest improvement, as shown by the result for the mixed boosted networks.

Wall Street Journal Corpus

The training data used in these experiments is the short term speakers from the Wall Street Journal corpus. This consists of approximately 36,400 sentences from 284 different speakers (SI284). The first network is trained on 1.5 million frames randomly selected from the available training data (15 million frames). This is then used to filter the unseen training data to select frames for training the second network. The first and second networks are then used to select data for the third network as described previously. The performance of the boosted MLP ensemble

Test Set	Language Model	Lexicon	Word Error Rate			
			Single MLP	Boosted	Gated	Mixed
et_h2_93	trigram	20k	16.0%	12.9%	12.9%	11.2 %
dt_s5_93	bigram	5k	20.4%	16.5%	16.5%	15.1%

Table 2: Evaluation of the performance of boosting MLP acoustic models

was evaluated on a number of ARPA benchmark tests. The results are summarised in Table 2.

Initial experiments use the November 1993 Hub 2 evaluation test set (et_h2_93). This is a 5,000 word closed vocabulary, non-verbalised punctuation test. It consists of 200 utterances, 20 from each of 10 different speakers, and is recorded using a Sennheiser HMD 410 microphone. The prompting texts are from the Wall Street Journal. Results are reported for a system using the standard ARPA 5k bigram language model.

The Spoke 5 test (dt_s5_93) is designed for evaluation of unsupervised channel adaptation algorithms. It consists of a total of 216 utterances from 10 different speakers. Each speaker's data was recorded with a different microphone. In all cases simultaneous recordings were made using a Sennheiser microphone. The task is a 5,000 word, closed vocabulary, non-verbalised punctuation test. Results are only reported for the data recorded using the Sennheiser microphone. This is a matched test since the same microphone is used to record the training data. The standard ARPA 5k bigram language model was used for the tests. Further details of the November 1993 spoke 5 and hub 2 tests, can be found in (Pallett, Fiscus, Fisher, Garofolo, Lund & Pryzbocki 1994).

Four techniques were evaluated on the WSJ corpus; a single network with 500 hidden units, a boosted ensemble with 3 networks with 500 hidden units each, a gated ensemble of the boosted networks and a mixture trained from boosted ensembles. As can be seen from the table, boosting has resulted in significant improvements in performance for both the test sets over a single model. In addition, in common with the results on the Bellcore digits, whilst the gating combination method does not give an improvement over simple averaging, the retraining of the whole ensemble using the mixed combination method gives an average improvement of a further 8% over the averaging method.

CONCLUSION

This paper has described a number of ensemble methods for use with neural network acoustic models. It has been shown that through the use of principled methods such as boosting and mixtures the performance of these models may be improved over standard ensemble techniques. In addition, by combining the techniques via boot-strapping mixtures using the boosted networks the performance of the models can be improved further. Previous work, which focused on boosting at the word level showed improvements for a recurrent network:HMM hybrid at the word level over the baseline system (Cook & Robinson 1996). This paper has shown how the performance of a static MLP system can also be improved by boosting at the frame level.

Acknowledgements

Many thanks to Bellcore for providing the digits data set to our partners, ICSI; Nikki Mirghafori for help with datasets; David Johnson for providing the starting point for our code development; and Dan Kershaw for his invaluable advice.

References

Cook, G. & Robinson, A. (1996), Boosting the performance of connectionist large-vocabulary speech recognition, *in* 'International Conference on Spoken Language Processing'.

Drucker, H., Schapire, R. & Simard, P. (1993), Improving Performance in Neural Networks Using a Boosting Algorithm, *in* S. Hanson, J. Cowan & C. Giles, eds, 'Advances in Neural Information Processing Systems 5', Morgan Kauffmann, pp. 42–49.

Hansen, L. & Salamon, P. (1990), 'Neural Network Ensembles', *IEEE Transactions on Pattern Analysis and Machine Intelligence* **12**, 993–1001.

Hochberg, M., Renals, S. & Robinson, A. (1994), 'ABBOT: The CUED hybrid connectionist-HMM large-vocabulary recognition system', *Proc. of Spoken Language Systems Technology Worshop, ARPA*.

Jacobs, R. A., Jordan, M. I., Nowlan, S. J. & Hinton, G. E. (1991), 'Adaptive mixtures of local experts', *Neural Computation* **3**(1), 79–87.

Pallett, D., Fiscus, J., Fisher, W., Garofolo, J., Lund, B. & Pryzbocki, M. (1994), '1993 Benchmark Tests for the ARPA Spoken Language Program', *ARPA Workshop on Human Language Technology* pp. 51–73. Merrill Lynch Conference Center, Plainsboro, NJ.

Paul, D. & Baker, J. (1992), The Design for the Wall Street Journal-based CSR Corpus, *in* 'DARPA Speech and Natural Language Workshop', Morgan Kaufman Publishers, Inc., pp. 357–62.

Perrone, M. P. & Cooper, L. N. (1993), When networks disagree: Ensemble methods for hybird neural networks, *in* 'Neural Networks for Speech and Image Processing', Chapman-Hall.

Effective Training of a Neural Network Character Classifier for Word Recognition

Larry Yaeger	**Richard Lyon**	**Brandyn Webb**
Apple Computer	Apple Computer	The Future
5540 Bittersweet Rd.	1 Infinite Loop, MS301-3M	4578 Fieldgate Rd.
Morgantown, IN 46160	Cupertino, CA 95014	Oceanside, CA 92056
larryy@apple.com	lyon@apple.com	brandyn@brainstorm.com

Abstract

We have combined an artificial neural network (ANN) character classifier with context-driven search over character segmentation, word segmentation, and word recognition hypotheses to provide robust recognition of hand-printed English text in new models of Apple Computer's Newton MessagePad. We present some innovations in the training and use of ANNs as character classifiers for word recognition, including normalized output error, frequency balancing, error emphasis, negative training, and stroke warping. A recurring theme of reducing *a priori* biases emerges and is discussed.

1 INTRODUCTION

We have been conducting research on bottom-up classification techniques based on trainable artificial neural networks (ANNs), in combination with comprehensive but weakly-applied language models. To focus our work on a subproblem that is tractable enough to lead to usable products in a reasonable time, we have restricted the domain to hand-printing, so that strokes are clearly delineated by pen lifts. In the process of optimizing overall performance of the recognizer, we have discovered some useful techniques for architecting and training ANNs that must participate in a larger recognition process. Some of these techniques—especially the normalization of output error, frequency balancing, and error emphasis—suggest a common theme of significant value derived by reducing the effect of *a priori* biases in training data to better represent low frequency, low probability samples, including second and third choice probabilities.

There is ample prior work in combining low-level classifiers with various search strategies to provide integrated segmentation and recognition for writing (Tappert *et al* 1990) and speech (Renals *et al* 1992). And there is a rich background in the use of ANNs as classifiers, including their use as a low-level, character classifier in a higher-level word recognition system (Bengio *et al* 1995). But many questions remain regarding optimal strategies for deploying and combining these methods to achieve acceptable (to a real user) levels of performance. In this paper, we survey some of our experiences in exploring refinements and improvements to these techniques.

2 SYSTEM OVERVIEW

Our recognition system, the Apple-Newton Print Recognizer (ANPR), consists of three conceptual stages: Tentative Segmentation, Classification, and Context-Driven Search. The primary data upon which we operate are simple sequences of (x,y) coordinate pairs, plus pen-up/down information, thus defining stroke primitives. The Segmentation stage decides which strokes will be combined to produce *segments*—the tentative groupings of strokes that will be treated as possible characters—and produces a sequence of these segments together with legal transitions between them. This process builds an implicit graph which is then scored in the Classification stage and examined for a maximum likelihood interpretation in the Search stage.

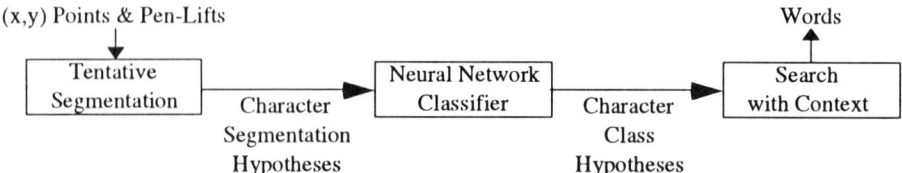

Figure 1: A Simplified Block Diagram of Our Hand-Print Recognizer.

3 TRAINING THE NEURAL NETWORK CLASSIFIER

Except for an *integrated multiple-representations* architecture (Yaeger *et al* 1996) and the training specifics detailed here, a fairly standard multi-layer perceptron trained with BP provides the ANN character classifier at the heart of ANPR. Training an ANN character classifier for use in a word recognition system, however, has different constraints than would training such a system for stand-alone character recognition. All of the techniques below, except for the annealing schedule, at least modestly *reduce* individual character recognition accuracy, yet dramatically *increase* word recognition accuracy.

A large body of prior work exists to indicate the general applicability of ANN technology as classifiers providing good estimates of *a posteriori* probabilities of each class given the input (Gish 1990, Richard and Lippmann 1991, Renals and Morgan 1992, Lippmann 1994, Morgan and Bourlard 1995, and others cited herein).

3.1 NORMALIZING OUTPUT ERROR

Despite their ability to provide good first choice *a posteriori* probabilities, we have found that ANN classifiers do a poor job of representing second and third choice probabilities when trained in the classic way—minimizing mean squared error for target vectors that are all 0's, except for a single 1 corresponding to the target class. This results in erratic word recognition failures as the net fails to accurately represent the legitimate ambiguity between characters. We speculated that reducing the "pressure towards 0" relative to the "pressure towards 1" as seen at the output units, and thus reducing the large bias towards 0 in target vectors, might permit the net to better model these inherent ambiguities.

We implemented a technique for "normalizing output error" (*NormOutErr*) by reducing the BP error for non-target classes relative to the target class by a factor that normalizes the total non-target error seen at a given output unit relative to the total target error seen at that unit. Assuming a training set with equal representation of classes, this normalization should then be based on the number of non-target versus target classes in a typical training vector, or, simply, the number of output units (minus one). Hence for *non-target* output units, we scale the error at each unit by a constant:

$$e' = Ae$$

where e is the error at an output unit, and A is defined to be:

$$A = 1 / \left[d(N_{outputs} - 1) \right]$$

where $N_{outputs}$ is the number of output units, and d is a user-adjusted tuning parameter, typically ranging from 0.1 to 0.2. Error at the *target* output unit is unchanged. Overall, this raises the activation values at the output units, due to the reduced pressure towards zero, particularly for low-probability samples. Thus the learning algorithm no longer converges to a minimum mean-squared error (MMSE) estimate of $P(class|input)$, but to an MMSE estimate of a nonlinear function $f(P(class|input), A)$ depending on the factor A by which we reduced the error pressure toward zero.

Using a simple version of the technique of Bourlard and Wellekens (1990), we worked out what that resulting nonlinear function is. The net will attempt to converge to minimize the modified quadratic error function

$$\langle \hat{E}^2 \rangle = p(1-y)^2 + A(1-p)y^2$$

by setting its output y for a particular class to

$$y = p/(A - Ap + p)$$

where $p = P(class|input)$, and A is as defined above. The inverse function is

$$p = yA/(yA + 1 - y)$$

We verified the fit of this function by looking at histograms of character-level empirical percentage-correct versus y, as in Figure 2.

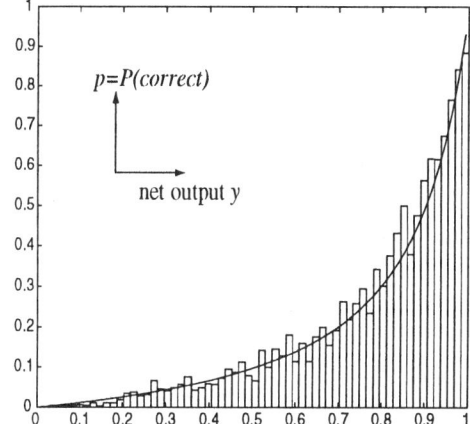

Figure 2: Empirical p vs. y Histogram for a Net Trained with $A=0.11$ ($d=.1$), with the Corresponding Theoretical Curve.

Note that the lower-probability samples have their output activations raised significantly, relative to the 45° line that $A = 1$ yields.

The primary benefit derived from this technique is that the net does a much better job of representing second and third choice probabilities, and low probabilities in general. Despite a small drop in top choice character accuracy when using NormOutErr, we obtain a very significant increase in word accuracy by this technique. Figure 3 shows an exaggerated example of this effect, for an atypically large value of d (0.8), which overly penalizes character accuracy; however, the 30% decrease in word error rate is normal for this technique. (Note: These data are from a multi-year-old experiment, and are not necessarily representative of current levels of performance on any absolute scale.)

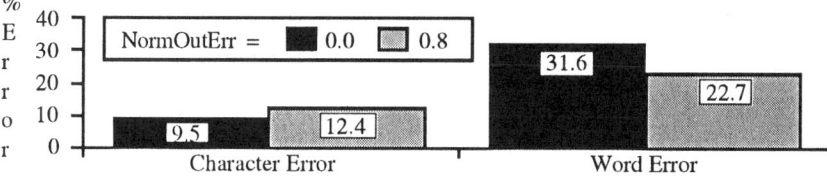

Figure 3: Character and Word Error Rates for Two Different Values of NormOutErr (d). A Value of 0.0 Disables NormOutErr, Yielding Normal BP. The Unusually High Value of 0.8 ($A=0.013$) Produces Nearly Equal Pressures Towards 0 and 1.

3.2 FREQUENCY BALANCING

Training data from natural English words and phrases exhibit very non-uniform priors for the various character classes, and ANNs readily model these priors. However, as with NormOutErr, we find that reducing the effect of these priors on the net, in a controlled way, and thus forcing the net to allocate more of its resources to low-frequency, low-probability classes is of significant benefit to the overall word recognition process. To this end, we explicitly (partially) balance the frequencies of the classes during training. We do this by probabilistically skipping and repeating patterns, based on a precomputed *repetition factor*. Each presentation of a repeated pattern is "warped" uniquely, as discussed later.

To compute the repetition factor for a class i, we first compute a normalized frequency of that class:

$$F_i = S_i / \overline{S}$$

where S_i is the number of samples in class i, and $\overline{S}$ is the average number of samples over all classes, computed in the obvious way:

$$\overline{S} = (\frac{1}{C}\sum_{i=1}^{C} S_i)$$

with C being the number of classes. Our repetition factor is then defined to be:

$$R_i = (a/F_i)^b$$

with a and b being user controls over the amount of skipping vs. repeating and the degree of prior normalization, respectively. Typical values of a range from 0.2 to 0.8, while b ranges from 0.5 to 0.9. The factor $a < 1$ lets us do more skipping than repeating; e.g. for $a = 0.5$, classes with relative frequency equal to half the average will neither skip nor repeat; more frequent classes will skip, and less frequent classes will repeat. A value of 0.0 for b would do nothing, giving $R_i = 1.0$ for all classes, while a value of 1.0 would provide "full" normalization. A value of b somewhat less than one seems to be the best choice, letting the net keep some bias in favor of classes with higher prior probabilities.

This explicit prior-bias reduction is related to Lippmann's (1994) and Morgan and Bourlard's (1995) recommended method for converting from the net's estimate of posterior probability, *p(class|input)*, to the value needed in an HMM or Viterbi search, *p(input|class)*, which is to divide by *p(class)* priors. Besides eliminating potentially noisy estimates of low probability classes and a possible need for renormalization, our approach forces the net to actually learn a better model of these lower frequency classes.

3.3 ERROR EMPHASIS

While frequency balancing corrects for under-represented classes, it cannot account for under-represented writing styles. We utilize a conceptually related probabilistic skipping of patterns, but this time for just those patterns that the net correctly classifies in its forward/recognition pass, as a form of "error emphasis", to address this problem. We define a *correct-train probability* (0.1 to 1.0) that is used as a biased coin to determine whether a particular pattern, having been correctly classified, will also be used for the backward/training pass or not. This only applies to correctly segmented, or "positive" patterns, and misclassified patterns are never skipped.

Especially during early stages of training, we set this parameter fairly low (around 0.1), thus concentrating most of the training time and the net's learning capability on patterns that are more difficult to correctly classify. This is the only way we were able to get the net to learn to correctly classify unusual character variants, such as a 3-stroke "5" as written by only one training writer.

Variants of this scheme are possible in which misclassified patterns would be repeated, or different learning rates would apply to correctly and incorrectly classified patterns. It is also related to techniques that use a training subset, from which easily-classified patterns are replaced by randomly selected patterns from the full training set (Guyon *et al* 1992).

3.4 NEGATIVE TRAINING

Our recognizer's tentative segmentation stage necessarily produces a large number of invalid segments, due to inherent ambiguities in the character segmentation process. During recognition, the network must classify these invalid segments just as it would any valid segment, with no knowledge of which are valid or invalid. A significant increase in word-level recognition accuracy was obtained by performing *negative training* with these invalid segments. This consists of presenting invalid segments to the net during training, with all-zero target vectors. We retain control over the degree of negative training in two ways. First is a *negative-training factor* (0.2 to 0.5) that modulates the learning rate (equivalently by modulating the error at the output layer) for these negative patterns. This reduces the impact of negative training on positive training, and modulates the impact on characters that specifically look like elements of multi-stroke characters (e.g., I, 1, 1, o, O, 0). Secondly, we control a *negative-training probability* (0.05 to 0.3), which determines the probability that a particular negative sample will actually be trained on (for a given presentation). This both reduces the overall impact of negative training, and significantly reduces training time, since invalid segments are more numerous than valid segments. As with NormOutErr, this modification hurts character-level accuracy a little bit, but helps word-level accuracy a lot.

3.5 STROKE WARPING

During training (but not during recognition), we produce random variations in stroke data, consisting of small changes in skew, rotation, and x and y linear and quadratic scalings. This produces alternate character forms that are consistent with stylistic variations within and between writers, and induces an explicit aspect ratio and rotation invariance within the framework of standard back-propagation. The amounts of each distortion to apply were chosen through cross-validation experiments, as just the amount needed to yield optimum generalization. We also examined a number of such samples by eye to verify that they represent a natural range of variation. A small set of such variations is shown in Figure 4.

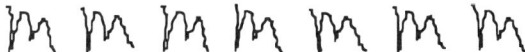

Figure 4: A Few Random Stroke Warpings of the Same Original "m" Data.

Our stroke warping scheme is somewhat related to the ideas of Tangent Dist and Tangent Prop (Simard *et al* 1992, 1993), in terms of the use of predetermined families of transformations, but we believe it is much easier to implement. It is also somewhat distinct in applying transformations on the original coordinate data, as opposed to using distortions of images. The voice transformation scheme of Chang and Lippmann (1995) is also related, but they use a static replication of the training set through a small number of transformations, rather than dynamic random transformations of infinite variety.

3.6 ANNEALING & SCHEDULING

Many discussions of back-propagation seem to assume the use of a single fixed learning rate. We view the stochastic back-propagation process as more of a simulated annealing, with a learning rate starting very high and decreasing only slowly to a very low value. We typically start with a rate near 1.0 and reduce the rate by a *decay factor* of 0.9 until it gets down to about 0.001. The rate decay factor is applied following any epoch for which the total squared error increased on the training set. Repeated tests indicate that this approach yields better results than low (or even moderate) initial learning rates, which we speculate to be related to a better ability to escape local minima.

In addition, we find that we obtain best overall results when we also allow some of our many training parameters to change over the course of a training run. In particular, the correct train probability needs to start out very low to give the net a chance to learn unusual character styles, but it should finish up at 1.0 in order to not introduce a general posterior probability bias in favor of classes with lots of ambiguous examples. We typically train a net in four "phases" according to parameters such as in Figure 5.

Phase	Epochs	Learning Rate	Correct Train Prob	Negative Train Prob
1	25	1.0 - 0.5	0.1	0.05
2	25	0.5 - 0.1	0.25	0.1
3	50	0.1 - 0.01	0.5	0.18
4	30	0.01 - 0.001	1.0	0.3

Figure 5: A Typical Multi-Phase Schedule of Learning Rates and Other Parameters for Training a Character-Classifier Net.

4 DISCUSSION AND FUTURE DIRECTIONS

The normalization of output error, frequency balancing, and error emphasis network-training methods discussed previously share a unifying theme: Reducing the effect of *a priori* biases in the training data on network learning significantly improves the network's performance in an integrated recognition system, despite a modest reduction in the network's accuracy for individual characters. Normalization of output error prevents over-represented non-target classes from biasing the net against under-represented target classes. Frequency balancing prevents over-represented target classes from biasing the net against under-represented target classes. And error emphasis prevents over-represented writing styles from biasing the net against under-represented writing styles. One could even argue that negative training eliminates an absolute bias towards properly segmented characters, and that stroke warping reduces the bias towards those writing styles found in the training data, although these techniques provide wholly new information to the system as well.

Though we've offered arguments for why each of these techniques, individually, helps the overall recognition process, it is unclear why prior-bias reduction, in general, should be so consistently valuable. The general effect may be related to the technique of dividing out priors, as is sometimes done to convert from $p(class|input)$ to $p(input|class)$. But we also believe that forcing the net, during learning, to allocate resources to represent less frequent sample types may be directly beneficial. In any event, it is clear that paying attention to such biases and taking steps to modulate them is a vital component of effective training of a neural network serving as a classifier in a maximum likelihood recognition system.

We speculate that a method of modulating the learning rate at each output unit—based on a measure of its accuracy relative to the other output units—may be possible, and that such a method might yield the combined benefits of several of these techniques, with fewer user-controllable parameters.

Acknowledgements

This work was done in collaboration with Bill Stafford, Apple Computer, and Les Vogel, Angel Island Technologies. We are also indebted to our many colleagues in the connectionist community and at Apple Computer.

Some techniques in this paper have pending U.S. and foreign patent applications.

References

Y. Bengio, Y. LeCun, C. Nohl, and C. Burges, "LeRec: A NN/HMM Hybrid for On-Line Handwriting Recognition," Neural Computation, Vol. 7, pp. 1289-1303, 1995.

H. Bourlard and C. J. Wellekens, "Links between Markov Models and Multilayer Perceptrons," *IEEE Trans. PAMI*, Vol. 12, pp. 1167-1178, 1990.

E. I. Chang and R. P. Lippmann, "Using Voice Transformations to Create Additional Training Talkers for Word Spotting," in *Advances in Neural Information Processing Systems 7*, Tesauro et al. (eds.), pp. 875-882, MIT Press, 1995.

H. Gish, "A Probabilistic Approach to Understanding and Training of Neural Network Classifiers," *Proc. IEEE Intl. Conf. on Acoustics, Speech, and Signal Processing* (Albuquerque, NM), pp. 1361-1364, 1990.

I. Guyon, D. Henderson, P. Albrecht, Y. LeCun, and P. Denker, "Writer independent and writer adaptive neural network for on-line character recognition," in *From pixels to features III*, S. Impedovo (ed.), pp. 493-506, Elsevier, Amsterdam, 1992.

R. A. Jacobs, M. I. Jordan, S. J. Nowlan, and G. E. Hinton, "Adaptive Mixtures of Local Experts," *Neural Computation*, Vol. 3, pp. 79-87, 1991.

R. P. Lippmann, "Neural Networks, Bayesian *a posteriori* Probabilities, and Pattern Classification," pp. 83-104 in: *From Statistics to Neural Networks—Theory and Pattern Recognition Applications*, V. Cherkassky, J. H. Friedman, and H. Wechsler (eds.), Springer-Verlag, Berlin, 1994.

N. Morgan and H. Bourlard, "Continuous Speech Recognition—An introduction to the hybrid HMM/connectionist approach," IEEE Signal Processing Mag., Vol. 13, no. 3, pp. 24-42, May 1995.

S. Renals and N. Morgan, "Connectionist Probability Estimation in HMM Speech Recognition," TR-92-081, International Computer Science Institute, 1992.

S. Renals and N. Morgan, M. Cohen, and H. Franco "Connectionist Probability Estimation in the Decipher Speech Recognition System," *Proc. IEEE Intl. Conf. on Acoustics, Speech, and Signal Processing* (San Francisco), pp. I-601-I-604, 1992.

M. D. Richard and R. P. Lippmann, "Neural Network Classifiers Estimate Bayesian *a Posteriori* Probabilities," *Neural Computation*, Vol. 3, pp. 461-483, 1991.

P. Simard, B. Victorri, Y. LeCun and J. Denker, "Tangent Prop—A Formalism for Specifying Selected Invariances in an Adaptive Network," in *Advances in Neural Information Processing Systems 4*, Moody et al. (eds.), pp. 895-903, Morgan Kaufmann, 1992.

P. Simard, Y. LeCun and J. Denker, "Efficient Pattern Recognition Using a New Transformation Distance," in *Advances in Neural Information Processing Systems 5*, Hanson et al. (eds.), pp. 50-58, Morgan Kaufmann, 1993.

C. C. Tappert, C. Y. Suen, and T. Wakahara, "The State of the Art in On-Line Handwriting Recognition," *IEEE Trans. PAMI*, Vol. 12, pp. 787-808, 1990.

L. Yaeger, B. Webb, and R. Lyon, "Combining Neural Networks and Context-Driven Search for On-Line, Printed Handwriting Recognition", (unpublished).

PART VII
VISUAL PROCESSING

Viewpoint invariant face recognition using independent component analysis and attractor networks

Marian Stewart Bartlett
University of California San Diego
The Salk Institute
La Jolla, CA 92037
marni@salk.edu

Terrence J. Sejnowski
University of California San Diego
Howard Hughes Medical Institute
The Salk Institute, La Jolla, CA 92037
terry@salk.edu

Abstract

We have explored two approaches to recognizing faces across changes in pose. First, we developed a representation of face images based on independent component analysis (ICA) and compared it to a principal component analysis (PCA) representation for face recognition. The ICA basis vectors for this data set were more spatially local than the PCA basis vectors and the ICA representation had greater invariance to changes in pose. Second, we present a model for the development of viewpoint invariant responses to faces from visual experience in a biological system. The temporal continuity of natural visual experience was incorporated into an attractor network model by Hebbian learning following a lowpass temporal filter on unit activities. When combined with the temporal filter, a basic Hebbian update rule became a generalization of Griniasty et al. (1993), which associates temporally proximal input patterns into basins of attraction. The system acquired representations of faces that were largely independent of pose.

1 Independent component representations of faces

Important advances in face recognition have employed forms of principal component analysis, which considers only second-order moments of the input (Cottrell & Metcalfe, 1991; Turk & Pentland 1991). Independent component analysis (ICA) is a generalization of principal component analysis (PCA), which decorrelates the higher-order moments of the input (Comon, 1994). In a task such as face recognition, much of the important information is contained in the high-order statistics of the images. A representational basis in which the high-order statistics are decorrelated may be more powerful for face recognition than one in which only the second order statistics are decorrelated, as in PCA representations. We compared an ICA-based representation to a PCA-based representation for recognizing faces across changes in pose.

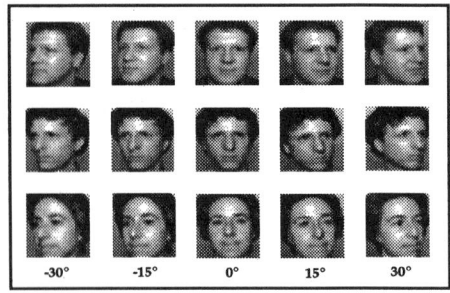

Figure 1: Examples from image set (Beymer, 1994).

The image set contained 200 images of faces, consisting of 40 subjects at each of five poses (Figure 1). The images were converted to vectors and comprised the rows of a 200 x 3600 data matrix, X. We consider the face images in X to be a linear mixture of an unknown set of statistically independent source images S, where A is an unknown mixing matrix (Figure 2). The sources are recovered by a matrix of learned filters, W, which produce statistically independent outputs, U.

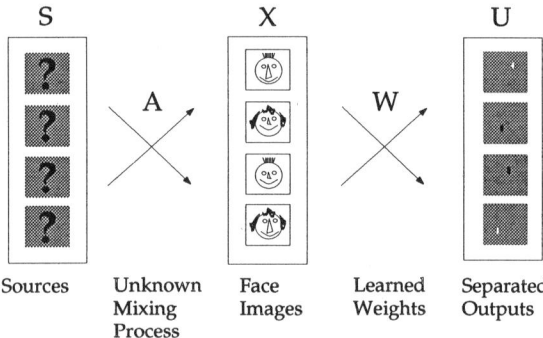

Figure 2: Image synthesis model.

The weight matrix, W, was found through an unsupervised learning algorithm that maximizes the mutual information between the input and the output of a nonlinear transformation (Bell & Sejnowski, 1995). This algorithm has proven successful for separating randomly mixed auditory signals (the cocktail party problem), and has recently been applied to EEG signals (Makeig et al., 1996) and natural scenes (see Bell & Sejnowski, this volume). The independent component images contained in the rows of U are shown in Figure 3. In contrast to the principal components, all 200 independent components were spatially local. We took as our face representation the rows of the matrix $A = W^{-1}$ which provide the linear combination of source images in U that comprise each face image in X.

1.1 Face Recognition Performance: ICA vs. Eigenfaces

We compared the performance of the ICA representation to that of the PCA representation for recognizing faces across changes in pose. The PCA representation of a face consisted of its component coefficients, which was equivalent to the "Eigenface"

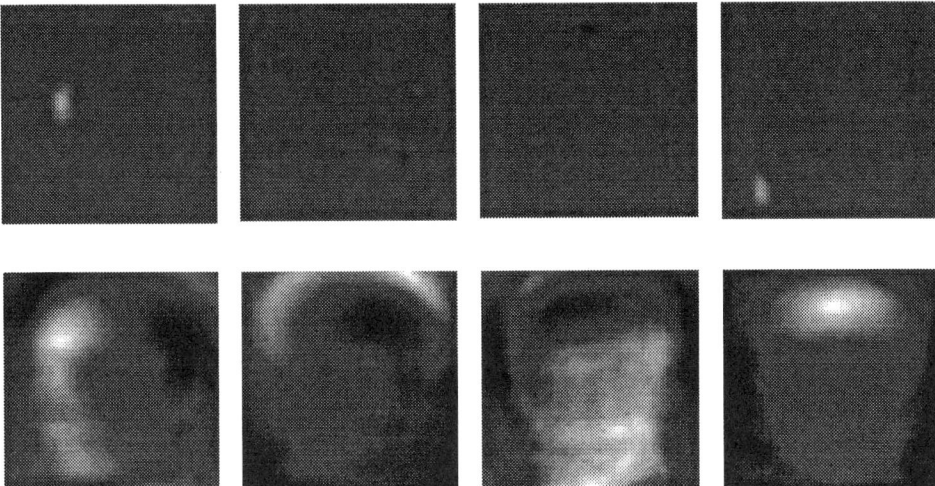

Figure 3: Top: Four independent components of the image set. Bottom: First four principal components.

representation (Turk & Pentland, 1991). A test image was recognized by assigning it the label of the nearest of the other 199 images in Euclidean distance.

Classification error rates for the ICA and PCA representations and for the original graylevel images are presented in Table 1. For the PCA representation, the best performance was obtained with the 120 principal components corresponding to the highest eigenvalues. Dropping the first three principal components, or selecting ranges of intermediate components did not improve performance. The independent component sources were ordered by the magnitude of the weight vector, row of W, used to extract the source from the image.[1] Best performance was obtained with the 130 independent components with the largest weight vectors. Performance with the ICA representation was significantly superior to Eigenfaces by a paired t-test ($\alpha < 0.05$).

	Mutual Information	Percent Correct Recognition
Graylevel Images	.89	.83
PCA	.10	.84
ICA	.007	.87

Table 1: Mean mutual information between all pairs of 10 basis images, and between the original graylevel images. Face recognition performance is across all 200 images.

For the task of recognizing faces across pose, a statistically independent basis set provided a more powerful representation for face images than a principal component representation in which only the second order statistics are decorrelated.

---

[1] The magnitude of the weight vector for optimally projecting the source onto the sloping part of the nonlinearity provides a measure of the variance of the original source (Tony Bell, personal communication).

2 Unsupervised Learning of Viewpoint Invariant Representations of Faces in an Attractor Network

Cells in the primate inferior temporal lobe have been reported that respond selectively to faces despite substantial changes in viewpoint (Hasselmo, Rolls, Baylis, & Nalwa, 1989). Some cells responded independently of viewing angle, whereas other cells gave intermediate responses between a viewer-centered and an object centered representation. This section addresses how a system can acquire such invariance to viewpoint from visual experience.

During natural visual experience, different views of an object or face tend to appear in close temporal proximity as an animal manipulates the object or navigates around it, or as a face changes pose. Capturing such temporal relationships in the input is a way to automatically associate different views of an object without requiring three dimensional descriptions.

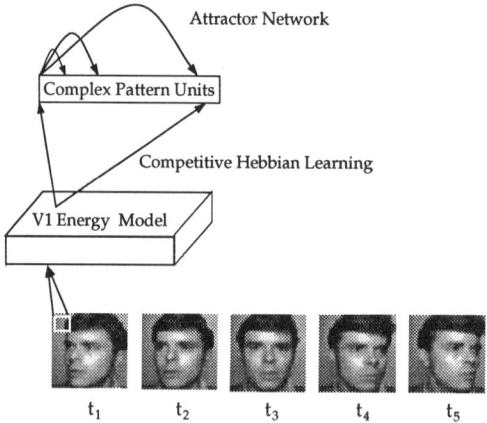

Figure 4: Model architecture.

Hebbian learning can capture these temporal relationships in a feedforward system when the output unit activities are passed through a lowpass temporal filter (Foldiak, 1991; Wallis & Rolls, 1996). Such lowpass temporal filters have been related to the time course of the modifiable state of a neuron based on the open time of the NMDA channel for calcium influx (Rhodes, 1992). We show that 1) this lowpass temporal filter increases viewpoint invariance of face representations in a feedforward system trained with competitive Hebbian learning, and 2) when the input patterns to an attractor network are passed through a lowpass temporal filter, then a basic Hebbian weight update rule associates sequentially proximal input patterns into the same basin of attraction.

This simulation used a subset of 100 images from Section 1, consisting of twenty faces at five poses each. Images were presented to the model in sequential order as the subject changed pose from left to right (Figure 4). The first layer is an energy model related to the output of V1 complex cells (Heeger, 1991). The images were filtered by a set of sine and cosine Gabor filters at 4 spatial scales and 4 orientations at 255 spatial locations. Sine and cosine outputs were squared and summed. The set of V1 model outputs projected to a second layer of 70 units, grouped into two inhibitory pools. The third stage of the model was an attractor network produced by lateral interconnections among all of the complex pattern units. The feedforward and lateral connections were trained successively.

2.1 Competitive Hebbian learning of temporal relationships

The Competitive Learning Algorithm (Rumelhart & Zipser, 1985) was extended to include a temporal lowpass filter on output unit activities (Bartlett & Sejnowski, 1996). This manipulation gives the winner in the previous time steps a competitive advantage for winning, and therefore learning, in the current time step.

$$\Delta w_{ij} = \begin{cases} \alpha(\frac{x_{iu}}{s_u} - w_{ij}) & \text{if winner} = j \\ 0.1\alpha(\frac{x_{iu}}{s_u} - w_{ij}) & \text{if winner} \neq j \end{cases}$$

$$winner = max_j[\overline{y_j}^{(t)}]$$
$$\overline{y_j}^{(t)} = \lambda y_j^t + (1-\lambda)\overline{y_j}^{(t-1)} \qquad (1)$$

The output activity of unit j at time t, $\overline{y_j}^{(t)}$, is determined by the trace, or running average, of its activation, where y_j^t is the weighted sum of the feedforward inputs, α is the learning rate, x_{iu} is the value of input unit i for pattern u, and s_u is the total amount of input activation for pattern u. The weight to each unit was constrained to sum to one. This algorithm was used to train the feedforward connections. There was one face pattern per time step and λ was set to 1 between individuals.

2.2 Lateral connections in the output layer form an attractor network

Hebbian learning of lateral interconnections, in combination with a lowpass temporal filter on the unit activities in (1), produces a learning rule that associates temporally proximal inputs into basins of attraction. We begin with a simple Hebbian learning rule

$$W_{ij} = \frac{1}{N}\sum_{t=1}^{P}(y_i^t - y^0)(y_j^t - y^0) \qquad (2)$$

where N is the number of units, P is the number of patterns, and y^0 is the mean activity over all of the units. Replacing y_i^t with the activity trace $\overline{y_i}^{(t)}$ defined in (1), substituting $y^0 = \lambda y^0 + (1-\lambda)y^0$ and multiplying out the terms leads to the following learning rule:

$$W_{ij} = \frac{1}{N}\sum_{t=1}^{P}(y_i^t - y^0)(y_j^t - y^0) + k_1\left[(y_i^t - y^0)(\overline{y_j}^{(t-1)} - y^0) + (\overline{y_i}^{(t-1)} - y^0)(y_j^t - y^0)\right]$$
$$+ k_2\left[(\overline{y_i}^{(t-1)} - y^0)(\overline{y_j}^{(t-1)} - y^0)\right] \qquad (3)$$

where $k_1 = \frac{\lambda(1-\lambda)}{\lambda^2}$ and $k_2 = \frac{(1-\lambda)^2}{\lambda^2}$

The first term in this equation is basic Hebbian learning, the second term associates pattern t with pattern $t-1$, and the third term is Hebbian association of the trace activity for pattern $t-1$. This learning rule is a generalization of an attractor network learning rule that has been shown to associate random input patterns into basins of attraction based on serial position in the input sequence (Griniasty, Tsodyks & Amit, 1993). The following update rule was used for the activation V of unit i at time t from the lateral inputs (Griniasty, Tsodyks, & Amit, 1993):

$$V_i(t + \delta t) = \phi \left[\sum W_{ij} V_j(t) - \theta \right]$$

Where θ is a neural threshold and $\phi(x) = 1$ for $x > 0$, and 0 otherwise. In these simulations, $\theta = 0.007$, $N = 70$, $P = 100$, $y^0 = 0.03$, and $\lambda = 0.5$ gave $k_1 = k_2 = 1$.

2.3 Results

Temporal association in the feedforward connections broadened the pose tuning of the output units (Figure 5 Left). When the lateral connections in the output layer were added, the attractor network acquired responses that were largely invariant to pose (Figure 5 Right).

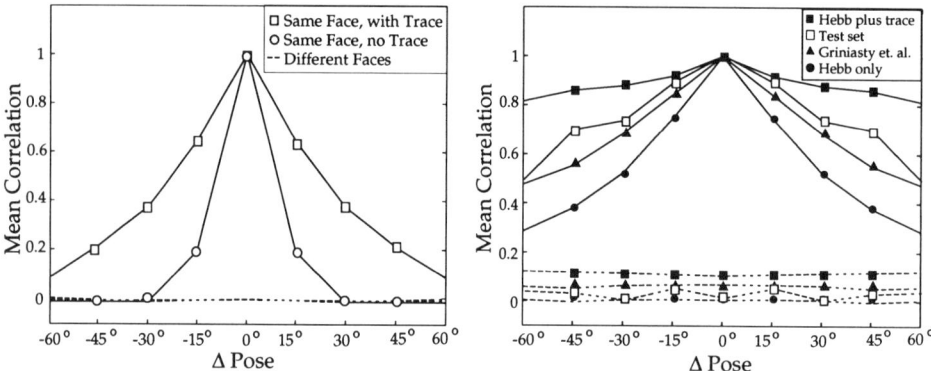

Figure 5: Left: Correlation of the outputs of the feedforward system as a function of change in pose. Correlations across different views of the same face (-) are compared to correlations across different faces (--) with the temporal trace parameter $\lambda = 0.5$ and $\lambda = 0$. Right: Correlations in sustained activity patterns in the attractor network as a function of change in pose. Results obtained with Equation 3 (Hebb plus trace) are compared to Hebb only, and to the learning rule in Griniasty et al. (1993). Test set results for Equation 3 (open squares) were obtained by alternately training on four poses and testing on the fifth, and then averaging across all test cases.

		Attractor Network		ICA
F	N	F/N	% Correct	% Correct
5	70	.07	1.00	.96
10	70	.14	.90	.86
20	70	.29	.61	.89
20	160	.13	.73	.89

Table 2: Face classification performance of the attractor network for four ratios of the number of desired memories, F, to the number of units, N. Results are compared to ICA for the same subset of faces.

Classification accuracy of the attractor network was calculated by nearest neighbor on the activity states (Table 2). Performance of the attractor network depends both on the performance of the feedforward system, which comprises its input, and on the ratio of the number of patterns to be encoded in memory, F, to the number of units, N, where each individual in the face set comprises one memory pattern. The attractor network performed well when this ratio was sufficiently high. The ICA representation also performed well, especially for N=20.

The goal of this simulation was to begin with structured inputs similar to the responses of V1 complex cells, and to explore the performance of unsupervised learning mechanisms that can transform these inputs into pose invariant responses. We showed that a lowpass temporal filter on unit activities, which has been related to the time course of the modifiable state of a neuron (Rhodes, 1992), cooperates with Hebbian learning to (1) increase the viewpoint invariance of responses to faces in a feedforward system, and (2) create basins of attraction in an attractor network which associate temporally proximal inputs. These simulations demonstrated that viewpoint invariant representations of complex objects such as faces can be developed from visual experience by accessing the temporal structure of the input.

Acknowledgments

This project was supported by Lawrence Livermore National Laboratory ISCR Agreement B291528, and by the McDonnell-Pew Center for Cognitive Neuroscience at San Diego.

References

Bartlett, M. Stewart, & Sejnowski, T., 1996. Unsupervised learning of invariant representations of faces through temporal association. *Computational Neuroscience: Int. Rev. Neurobio. Suppl. 1* J.M Bower, Ed., Academic Press, San Diego, CA:317-322.

Beymer, D. 1994. Face recognition under varying pose. In *Proceedings of the 1994 IEEE Computer Society Conference on Computer Vision and Pattern Recognition.* Los Alamitos, CA: IEEE Comput. Soc. Press: 756-61.

Bell, A. & Sejnowski, T., (1997). The independent components of natural scenes are edge filters. *Advances in Neural Information Processing Systems 9.*

Bell, A., & Sejnowski, T., 1995. An information Maximization approach to blind separation and blind deconvolution. *Neural Comp.* 7: 1129-1159.

Comon, P. 1994. Independent component analysis - a new concept? *Signal Processing* 36:287-314.

Cottrell & Metcalfe, 1991. Face, gender and emotion recognition using Holons. In *Advances in Neural Information Processing Systems 3*, D. Tourctzky, (Ed.), Morgan Kaufman, San Mateo, CA: 564 - 571.

Foldiak, P. 1991. Learning invariance from transformation sequences. *Neural Comp.* 3:194-200.

Griniasty, M., Tsodyks, M., & Amit, D. 1993. Conversion of temporal correlations between stimuli to spatial correlations between attractors. *Neural Comp.* 5:1-17.

Hasselmo M. Rolls E. Baylis G. & Nalwa V. 1989. Object-centered encoding by face-selective neurons in the cortex in the superior temporal sulcus of the monkey. *Experimental Brain Research* 75(2):417-29.

Heeger, D. (1991). Nonlinear model of neural responses in cat visual cortex. *Computational Models of Visual Processing,* M. Landy & J. Movshon, Eds. MIT Press, Cambridge, MA.

Makeig, S, Bell, AJ, Jung, T-P, and Sejnowski, TJ 1996. Independent component analysis of Electroencephalographic data, In: *Advances in Neural Information Processing Systems* 8, 145-151.

Rhodes, P. 1992. The long open time of the NMDA channel facilitates the self-organization of invariant object responses in cortex. *Soc. Neurosci. Abst.* 18:740.

Rumelhart, D. & Zipser, D. 1985. Feature discovery by competitive learning. *Cognitive Science* 9: 75-112.

Turk, M., & Pentland, A. 1991. Eigenfaces for Recognition. *J. Cog. Neurosci.* 3(1):71-86.

Wallis, G. & Rolls, E. 1996. A model of invariant object recognition in the visual system. Technical Report, Oxford University Department of Experimental Psychology.

Learning temporally persistent hierarchical representations

Suzanna Becker
Department of Psychology
McMaster University
Hamilton, Ont. L8S 4K1
becker@mcmaster.ca

Abstract

A biologically motivated model of cortical self-organization is proposed. Context is combined with bottom-up information via a maximum likelihood cost function. Clusters of one or more units are modulated by a common contextual gating signal; they thereby organize themselves into mutually supportive predictors of abstract contextual features. The model was tested in its ability to discover viewpoint-invariant classes on a set of real image sequences of centered, gradually rotating faces. It performed considerably better than supervised back-propagation at generalizing to novel views from a small number of training examples.

1 THE ROLE OF CONTEXT

The importance of context effects[1] in perception has been demonstrated in many domains. For example, letters are recognized more quickly and accurately in the context of words (see e.g. McClelland & Rumelhart, 1981), words are recognized more efficiently when preceded by related words (see e.g. Neely, 1991), individual speech utterances are more intelligible in the context of continuous speech, etc. Further, there is mounting evidence that neuronal responses are modulated by context. For example, even at the level of the LGN in the thalamus, the primary source of visual input to the cortex, Murphy & Sillito (1987) have reported cells with "end-stopped" or length-tuned receptive fields which depend on top-down inputs from the cortex. The end-stopped behavior disappears when the top-down connections are removed, suggesting that the cortico-thalamic connections are providing contextual modulation to the LGN. Moving a bit higher up the visual hierarchy, von der Heydt et al. (1984) found cells which respond to "illusory contours", in the absence of a contoured stimulus within the cells' classical receptive fields. These examples demonstrate that neuronal responses can be modulated by secondary sources of information in complex ways, provided the information is consistent with their expected or preferred input.

---

[1] We use the term context rather loosely here to mean any secondary source of input. It could be from a different sensory modality, a different input channel within the same modality, a temporal history of the input, or top-down information.

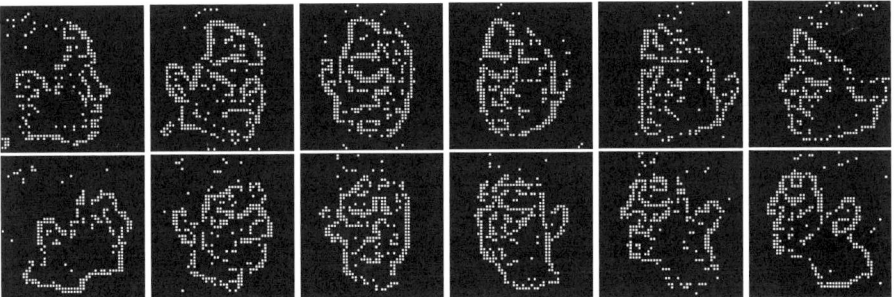

Figure 1: *Two sequences of 48 by 48 pixel images digitized with an IndyCam and preprocessed with a Sobel edge filter. Eleven views of each of four to ten faces were used in the simulations reported here. The alternate (odd) views of two of the faces are shown above.*

Why would contextual modulation be such a pervasive phenomenon? One obvious reason is that if context can influence *processing*, it can help in disambiguating or cleaning up a noisy stimulus. A less obvious reason may be that if context can influence *learning*, it may lead to more compact representations, and hence a more powerful processing system. To illustrate, consider the benefits of incorporating temporal history into an unsupervised classifier. Given a continuous sensory signal as input, the classifier must try to discover important partitions in its training data. If it can discover features that are *temporally persistent*, and thus insensitive to transformations in the input, it should be able to represent the signal compactly with a small set of features. Further, these features are more likely to be associated with the identity of objects rather than lower-level attributes.

However, most classifiers group patterns together on the basis of spatial overlap. This may be reasonable if there is very little shift or other form of distortion between one time step and the next, but is not a reasonable assumption about the sensory input to the cortex. Pre-cortical stages of sensory processing, certainly in the visual system (and probably in other modalities), tend to remove low-order correlations in space and time, e.g. with centre-surround filters. Consider the image sequences of gradually rotating faces in Figure 1. They have been preprocessed by a simple edge-filter, so that successive views of the same face have relatively little pixel overlap. In contrast, identical views of different faces may have considerable overlap. Thus, a classifier such as k-means, which groups patterns based on their Euclidean distance, would not be expected to do well at classifying these patterns. So how are people (and in fact very young children) able to learn to classify a virtually infinite number of objects based on relatively brief exposures? It is argued here that the assumption of *temporal persistence* is a powerful constraining factor for achieving this, and is one which may be used to advantage in artificial neural networks as well. Not only does it lead to the development of higher-order feature analyzers, but it can result in more compact codes which are important for applications like image compression. Further, as the simulations reported here show, improved generalization may be achieved by allowing high-level expectations (e.g. of class labels) to influence the development of lower-level feature detectors.

2 THE MODEL

Competitive learning (for a review, see Becker & Plumbley, 1996) is considered by many to be a reasonably strong candidate model of cortical learning. It can be implemented, in its simplest form, by a Hebbian learning rule in a network with lateral inhibition. However, a major limitation of competitive learning, and the majority of unsupervised learning procedures (but see the Discussion section), is that they treat the input as a set of independent identically distributed (iid) samples. They fail to take into account context. So they are unable to take advantage of the temporal continuity in signals. In contrast, real sensory signals may be better viewed as discretely sampled, continuously varying time-series rather than iid samples.

The model described here extends maximum likelihood competitive learning (MLCL) (Nowlan, 1990) in two important ways: (i) modulation by context, and (ii) the incorporation of several "canonical features" of neocortical circuitry. The result is a powerful framework for modelling cortical self-organization.

MLCL retains the benefits of competitive learning mentioned above. Additionally, it is more easily extensible because it maximizes a global cost function:

$$L = \sum_{\alpha=1}^{n} \log \left[\sum_{i=1}^{m} \pi_i y_i^{(\alpha)} \right] \qquad (1)$$

where the π_i's are positive weighting coefficients which sum to one, and the y_i's are the clustering unit activations:

$$y_i^{(\alpha)} = N(\vec{I}^{(\alpha)}, \vec{w}_i, \Sigma_i) \qquad (2)$$

where $\vec{I}^{(\alpha)}$ is the input vector for pattern α, and $N()$ is the probability of $\vec{I}^{(\alpha)}$ under a Gaussian centred on the ith unit's weight vector, $\vec{w}_i$, with covariance matrix Σ_i. For simplicity, Nowlan used a single global variance parameter for all input dimensions, and allowed it to shrink during learning. MLCL actually maximizes the log likelihood (L) of the data under a mixture of Gaussians model, with mixing proportions equal to the π's. L can be maximized by online gradient ascent[2] with learning rate ε:

$$\Delta w_{ij} = \varepsilon \frac{\partial L}{\partial w_{ij}} = \varepsilon \sum_{\alpha} \frac{\pi_i\, y_i^{(\alpha)}}{\sum_k \pi_k\, y_k^{(\alpha)}} \left(I_j^{(\alpha)} - w_{ij} \right) \qquad (3)$$

Thus, we have a Hebbian update rule with normalization of post-synaptic unit activations (which could be accomplished by shunting inhibition) and weight decay.

2.1 Contextual modulation

To integrate a contextual information source into MLCL, our first extension is to replace the mixing proportions (π_i's) by the outputs of *contextual gating units* (see Figure 2). Now the π_i's are computed by separate processing units receiving their own separate stream of input, the "context". The role of the gating signals here is analagous to that of the gating network in the (supervised) "competing experts" model (Jacobs et al., 1991).[3] For the network shown in Figure 2, the context is simply a time-delayed version of the outputs of a *module* (explained in the next subsection). However, more general forms of context are possible (see Discussion). In the simulations reported here, the context units computed their outputs according to a *softmax* function of their weighted summed inputs x_i:

$$\pi_i^{(\alpha)} = \frac{e^{x_i(\alpha)}}{\sum_j e^{x_j(\alpha)}} \qquad (4)$$

We refer to the action of the gating units (the π_i's) as *modulatory* because of the

---

[2]Nowlan (1990) used a slightly different online weight update rule that more closely approximates the batch update rule of the EM algorithm (Dempster et al., 1977)

[3]However, in the competing experts architecture, both the experts and gating network receive a common source of input. The competing experts model could be thought of as fitting a mixture model of the training signal.

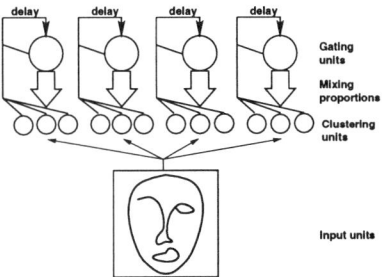

Figure 2: *The architecture used in the simulations reported here. Except where indicated, the gating units received all their inputs across unit delay lines with fixed weights of 1.0.*

multiplicative effect they have on the activities of the clustering units (the y_i's). This multiplicative interaction is built into the cost function (Equation 1), and consequently, arises in the learning rule (Equation 3). Thus, clustering units are encouraged to discover features that agree with the current context signal they receive. If their context signal is weak or if they fail to capture enough of the activation relative to the other clustering units, they will do very little learning. Only if a unit's weight vector is sufficiently close to the current input vector *and* it's corresponding gating unit is strongly active will it do substantial learning.

2.2 Modular, hierarchical architecture

Our second modification to MLCL is required to apply it to the architecture shown in Figure 2, which is motivated by several ubiquitous features of the neocortex: a laminar structure, and a functional organization into "cortical clusters" of spatially nearby columns with similar receptive field properties (see e.g. Calvin, 1995). The cortex, when flattened out, is like a large six-layered sheet. As Calvin (1995, pp. 269) succinctly puts it, "... the bottom layers are like a subcortical 'out' box, the middle layer like an 'in' box, and the superficial layers somewhat like an 'interoffice' box connecting the columns and different cortical areas". The middle and superficial layer cells are analagous to the first-layer clustering units and gating units respectively. Thus, we propose that the superficial cells may be providing the contextual modulation. (The bottom layers are mainly involved in motor output and are not included in the present model.) To induce a functional modularity in our model analogous to cortical clusters, clustering units within the same module receive a *shared gating signal*. The cost function and learning rule are now:

$$L = \sum_{\alpha=1}^{n} \log \left[\sum_{i=1}^{m} \pi_i^{(\alpha)} \frac{1}{l} \sum_{j=1}^{l} y_{ij}^{(\alpha)} \right] \quad (5)$$

$$\Delta w_{ijk} = \varepsilon \sum_{\alpha} \frac{\pi_i^{(\alpha)} \, y_{ij}^{(\alpha)}}{\sum_q \pi_q^{(\alpha)} \sum_r y_{qr}^{(\alpha)}} \left(I_k^{(\alpha)} - w_{ijk} \right) \quad (6)$$

Thus, units in the same module form predictions $y_{ij}^{(\alpha)}$ of the same contextual feature $\pi_i^{(\alpha)}$. Fortunately, there is a disincentive to all of them discovering identical weights: they would then do poorly at modelling the input.

3 EXPERIMENTS

As a simple test of this model, it was first applied to a set of image sequences of four centered, gradually rotating faces (see Figure 1), divided into training and test

		Training Set	Test Set
no context, 4 faces:	Layer 1	59.2 (2.4)	65 (3.5)
context, 4 faces:	Layer 1	88.4 (3.9)	74.5 (4.2)
	Layer 2	88.8 (4.0)	72.7 (4.8)
context, 10 faces:	Layer 1	96.3 (1.2)	71.0 (3.0)
	Layer 2	91.8 (2.4)	70.2 (4.3)

Table 1: *Mean percent (and standard error) correctly classified faces, across 10 runs, for unsupervised clustering networks trained for 2000 iterations with a learning rate of 0.5, with and without temporal context. Layer 1: clustering units. Layer 2: gating units. Performance was assessed as follows: Each unit was assigned to predict the face class for which it most frequently won (was the most active). Then for each pattern, the layer's activity vector was counted as correct if the winner correctly predicted the face identity.*

sets by taking alternating views. It was predicted that the clustering units should discover "features" such as individual views of specific faces. Further, different views of the same face should be clustered together within a module because they will be observed in the same temporal context, while the gating units should discover the identity of faces, independent of viewpoint.

First, the baseline effect of the temporal context on clustering performance was assessed by comparing the network shown in Figure 2 to the same network with the input connections to the gating layer removed. The latter is equivalent to MLCL with fixed, equal π_i's. The results are summarized in Table 1. As predicted, the temporal context provides incentive for the clustering units to group successive instances of the same face together, and the gating layer can therefore do very well at classifying the faces with a much smaller number of units - i.e., independently of viewpoint. In contrast, the clustering units without the contextual signal are more likely to group together similar views of different people's faces.

Next, to explore the scaling properties of the model, a network like the one shown in Figure 2 but with 10 modules was presented with a set of 10 faces, 11 views each. As before, the odd-numbered views were trained on and the even-numbered views were tested on. To achieve comparable performance to the smaller network, the weights on the self-pointing connections on the gating units were increased from 1.0 to 3.0, which increased the time constant of temporal agveraging. The model then had no difficulty scaling up to the larger training set size, as shown in Table 1.

Based on the unexpected success of this model, it's classification performance was then compared against supervised back-propagation networks on the four face sequences. The first supervised network we tried was a simple recurrent network with essentially the same architecture: one layer of Gaussian units followed by one layer of recurrent softmax units with fixed delay lines. Over ten runs of each model, although the unsupervised classifier did worse on the training set (it averaged 88% while the supervised model always scored 100% correct), it outperformed the supervised model in its generalization ability by a considerable margin (it averaged 73% while the supervised model averaged 45% correct).

Finally, a feedforward back-propagation network with sigmoid units was trained. The following constraint on the hidden layer activations, $h_j(t)$: [4]

$$\text{hidden state cost} = \lambda \sum_j (h_j(t) - h_j(t-1))^2$$

---

[4] As Geoff Hinton pointed out, the above constraint, if normalized by the variance, maximizes the mutual information between hidden unit states at adjacent time steps.

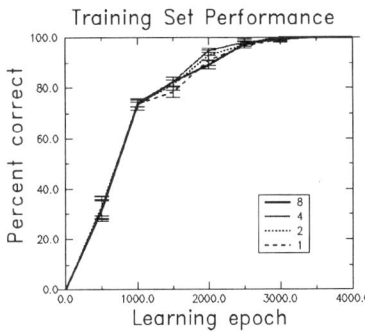 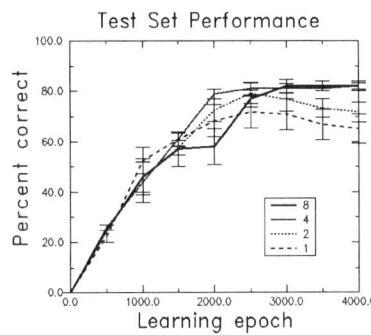

Figure 3: *Learning curves, averaged over five runs, for feedforward supervised net with a temporal smoothness constraint, for each of four levels of the parameter λ.*

was added to the cost function to encourage temporal smoothness. As the results in Figure 3 show, a feedforward network with no contextual input was thereby able to perform as well as our unsupervised model when it was constrained to develop hidden layer representations that clustered temporally adjacent patterns together.

4 DISCUSSION

The unsupervised model's markedly better ability to generalize stems from it's cost function; it favors hidden layer features which contribute to temporally coherent predictions at the output (gating) layer. Multiple views of a given object are therefore more likely to be detected by a given clustering unit in the unsupervised model, leading to considerably improved interpolation of novel views. The poor generalization performance of back-propagation is not just due to overtraining, as the learning curves in Figure 3 show. Even with early stopping, the network with the lowest value of λ would not have done as well as the unsupervised network. There is simply no reason why supervised back-propagation should cluster temporally adjacent views together unless it is explicitly forced to do so.

A "contextual input" stream was implemented in the simplest possible way in the simulations reported here, using fixed delay lines. However, the model we have proposed provides for a completely general way of incorporating arbitrary contextual information, and could equally well integrate other sources of input. The incoming weights to the gating units could also be learned. In fact, the gating unit activities actually represent the probabilities of each clustering unit's Gaussian model fitting the data, conditioned on the temporal history; hence, the entire model could be viewed as a Hidden Markov Model (Geoff Hinton, personal communication). However, current techniques for fitting HMMs are intractable if state dependencies span arbitrarily long time intervals.

The model in its present implementation is not meant to be a realistic account of the way humans learn to recognize faces. Viewpoint-invariant recognition is achieved, if at all, in a hierarchical, multi-stage system. One could easily extend our model to achieve this, by connecting together a sequence of networks like the one shown in Figure 2, each having progressively larger receptive fields.

A number of other unsupervised learning rules have been proposed based on the assumption of temporally coherent inputs (Földiák, 1991; Becker, 1993; Stone, 1996). Phillips et al. (1995) have proposed an alternative model of cortical self-organization they call *coherent Infomax* which incorporates contextual modulation. In their model, the outputs from one processing stream modulate the activity in another stream, while the mutual information between the two streams is maximized.

A wide range of perceptual and cognitive abilities could be modelled by a network that can learn features of its primary input in particular contexts. These include multi-sensor fusion, feature segregation in object recognition using top-down cues, and semantic disambiguation in natural language understanding. Finally, it is widely believed that memories are stored rapidly in the hippocampus and related brain structures, and gradually incorporated into the slower-learning cortex for long-term storage. The model proposed here may be able to explain how such interactions between disparate information sources are learned.

Acknowledgements

This work evolved out of discussions with Ron Racine and Larry Roberts. Thanks to Geoff Hinton for contributing several valuable insights, as mentioned in the paper, and to Ken Seergobin for the face images. Software was developed using the Xerion neural network simulation package from Hinton's lab, with programming assistance from Lianxiang Wang. This work was supported by a McDonnell-Pew Cognitive Neuroscience research grant and a research grant from the Natural Sciences and Engineering Research Council of Canada.

References

Becker, S. (1993). Learning to categorize objects using temporal coherence. In S. J. Hanson, J. D. Cowan, & C. L. Giles (Eds.), *Advances in Neural Information Processing Systems 5* (pp. 361–368). San Mateo, CA: Morgan Kaufmann.

Becker, S. & Plumbley, M. (1996). Unsupervised neural network learning procedures for feature extraction and classification. *International Journal of Applied Intelligence*, 6(3).

Calvin, W. H. (1995). Cortical columns, modules, and Hebbian cell assemblies. In M. Arbib (Ed.), *The handbook of brain theory and neural networks*. Cambridge, MA: MIT Press.

Dempster, A. P., Laird, N. M., & Rubin, D. B. (1977). Maximum likelihood from incomplete data via the EM algorithm. *Proceedings of the Royal Statistical Society, B-39*:1–38.

Földiák, P. (1991). Learning invariance from transformation sequences. *Neural Computation*, 3(2):194–200.

Jacobs, R. A., Jordan, M. I., Nowlan, S. J., & Hinton, G. E. (1991). Adaptive mixtures of local experts. *Neural Computation*, 3(1):79–87.

McClelland, J. L. & Rumelhart, D. E. (1981). An interactive activation model of context effects in letter perception, part I: An account of basic findings. *Psychological Review*, 88:375–407.

Murphy, C. & Sillito, A. M. (1987). Corticofugal feedback influences the generation of length tuning in the visual pathway. *Nature*, 329:727–729.

Neely, J. (1991). Semantic priming effects in visual word recognition: A selective review of current findings and theories. In D. Besner & G. W. Humphreys (Eds.), *Basic processes in reading: Visual Word Recognition* (pp. 264–336). Hillsdale, NJ: Lawrence Erlbaum Associates.

Nowlan, S. J. (1990). Maximum likelihood competitive learning. In D. S. Touretzky (Ed.), *Neural Information Processing Systems, Vol. 2* (pp. 574–582). San Mateo, CA: Morgan Kaufmann.

Phillips, W. A., Kay, J., & Smyth, D. (1995). The discovery of structure by multi-stream networks of local processors with contextual guidance. *Network*, 6:225–246.

Stone, J. (1996). Learning perceptually salient visual parameters using spatiotemporal smoothness constraints. *Neural Computation*, 8:1463–1492.

von der Heydt, R., Peterhans, E., & Baumgartner, G. (1984). Illusory contours and cortical neural responses. *Science*, 224:1260–1262.

Edges are the 'Independent Components' of Natural Scenes.

Anthony J. Bell and Terrence J. Sejnowski
Computational Neurobiology Laboratory
The Salk Institute
10010 N. Torrey Pines Road
La Jolla, California 92037
tony@salk.edu, terry@salk.edu

Abstract

Field (1994) has suggested that neurons with line and edge selectivities found in primary visual cortex of cats and monkeys form a sparse, distributed representation of natural scenes, and Barlow (1989) has reasoned that such responses should emerge from an unsupervised learning algorithm that attempts to find a factorial code of independent visual features. We show here that non-linear 'infomax', when applied to an ensemble of natural scenes, produces sets of visual filters that are localised and oriented. Some of these filters are Gabor-like and resemble those produced by the sparseness-maximisation network of Olshausen & Field (1996). In addition, the outputs of these filters are as independent as possible, since the infomax network is able to perform Independent Components Analysis (ICA). We compare the resulting ICA filters and their associated basis functions, with other decorrelating filters produced by Principal Components Analysis (PCA) and zero-phase whitening filters (ZCA). The ICA filters have more sparsely distributed (kurtotic) outputs on natural scenes. They also resemble the receptive fields of simple cells in visual cortex, which suggests that these neurons form an information-theoretic co-ordinate system for images.

1 Introduction.

Both the classic experiments of Hubel & Wiesel [8] on neurons in visual cortex, and several decades of theorising about feature detection in vision, have left open the question most succinctly phrased by Barlow "Why do we have edge detectors?" That is: are there any coding principles which would predict the formation of localised, oriented receptive fields? Barlow's answer is that edges are suspicious coincidences in an image. Formalised information-theoretically, this means that our visual cortical feature detectors might be the end result of a *redundancy reduction* process [4, 2], in which the activation of each feature detector is supposed to be as *statistically independent* from the others as possible. Such a 'factorial code' potentially involves dependencies of all orders, but most studies [9, 10, 2] (and many others) have used only the second-order statistics required for *decorrelating* the outputs of a set of feature detectors. Yet there are multiple decorrelating solutions, including the 'global' unphysiological Fourier filters produced by PCA, so further constraints are required.

Field [7] has argued for the importance of sparse, or 'Minimum Entropy', coding [4], in which each feature detector is activated as rarely as possible. Olshausen & Field demonstrated [12] that such a sparseness criterion could be used to self-organise localised, oriented receptive fields.

Here we present similar results using a direct information-theoretic criterion which maximises the joint entropy of a non-linearly transformed output feature vector [5]. Under certain conditions, this process will perform Independent Component Analysis (or ICA) which is equivalent to Barlow's redundancy reduction problem. Since our ICA algorithm, applied to natural scenes, does produce local edge filters, Barlow's reasoning is vindicated. Our ICA filters are more sparsely distributed than those of other decorrelating filters, thus supporting some of the arguments of Field (1994) and helping to explain the results of Olshausen's network from an information-theoretic point of view.

2   Blind separation of natural images.

A perceptual system is exposed to a series of small image patches, drawn from an ensemble of larger images. In the *linear image synthesis* model [12], each image patch, represented by the vector $\mathbf{x}$, has been formed by the linear combination of N basis functions. The basis functions form the columns of a fixed matrix, $\mathbf{A}$. The weighting of this linear combination (which varies with each image) is given by a vector, $\mathbf{s}$. Each component of this vector has its own associated basis function, and represents an underlying 'cause' of the image. Thus: $\mathbf{x}=\mathbf{As}$. The goal of a perceptual system, in this simplified framework, is to linearly transform the images, $\mathbf{x}$, with a matrix of filters, $\mathbf{W}$, so that the resulting vector: $\mathbf{u}=\mathbf{Wx}$, recovers the underlying causes, $\mathbf{s}$, possibly in a different order, and rescaled. For the sake of argument, we will define the ordering and scaling of the causes so that $\mathbf{W}=\mathbf{A}^{-1}$. But what should determine their form? If we choose decorrelation, so that $\langle\mathbf{uu}^T\rangle=\mathbf{I}$, then the solution for $\mathbf{W}$ must satisfy:

$$\mathbf{W}^T\mathbf{W} = \langle\mathbf{xx}^T\rangle^{-1} \tag{1}$$

There are several ways to constrain the solution to this:

(1) Principal Components Analysis $\mathbf{W}_P$ (PCA), is the Orthogonal (global) solution [$\mathbf{WW}^T=\mathbf{I}$]. The PCA solution to Eq.(1) is $\mathbf{W}_P = \mathbf{D}^{-\frac{1}{2}}\mathbf{E}^T$, where $\mathbf{D}$ is the diagonal matrix of eigenvalues, and $\mathbf{E}$ is the matrix who's columns are the eigenvectors. The filters (rows of $\mathbf{W}_P$) are orthogonal, are thus the same as the PCA basis functions, and are typically *global* Fourier filters, ordered according to the amplitude spectrum of the image. Example PCA filters are shown in Fig.1a.

(2) Zero-phase Components Analysis $\mathbf{W}_Z$ (ZCA), is the Symmetrical (local) solution [$\mathbf{WW}^T=\mathbf{W}^2$]. The ZCA solution to Eq.(1) is $\mathbf{W}_Z=\langle\mathbf{xx}^T\rangle^{-1/2}$ (matrix square root). ZCA is the polar opposite of PCA. It produces *local* (centre-surround type) whitening fil-

ters, which are ordered according to the phase spectrum of the image. That is, each filter whitens a given pixel in the image, preserving the spatial arrangement of the image and flattening its frequency (amplitude) spectrum. $\mathbf{W}_Z$ is related to the transforms described by Atick & Redlich [3]. Example ZCA filters and basis functions are shown in Fig.1b.

(3) Independent Components Analysis $\mathbf{W}_I$ (ICA), is the Factorised (semi-local) solution $[f_{\mathbf{u}}(\mathbf{u}) = \prod_i f_{u_i}(u_i)]$. Please see [5] for full references. The 'infomax' solution we describe here is related to the approaches in [5, 1, 6].

As we will show, in Section 5, ICA on natural images produces decorrelating filters which are sensitive to both phase (locality) and spatial frequency information, just as in transforms involving oriented Gabor functions or wavelets. Example ICA filters are shown in Fig.1d and their corresponding basis functions are shown in Fig.1e.

3 An ICA algorithm.

It is important to recognise two differences between finding an ICA solution, $\mathbf{W}_I$, and other decorrelation methods. (1) there may be no ICA solution, and (2) a given ICA algorithm may not find the solution even if it exists, since there are approximations involved. In these senses, ICA is different from PCA and ZCA, and cannot be calculated analytically, for example, from second order statistics (the covariance matrix), except in the gaussian case.

The approach which we developed in [5] (see there for further references to ICA) was to maximise by stochastic gradient ascent the joint entropy, $H[g(\mathbf{u})]$, of the linear transform squashed by a sigmoidal function, g. When the non-linear function is the same (up to scaling and shifting) as the cumulative density functions (c.d.f.s) of the underlying independent components, it can be shown (Nadal & Parga 1995) that such a non-linear 'infomax' procedure also minimises the mutual information between the u_i, exactly what is required for ICA. In most cases, however, we must pick a non-linearity, g, without any detailed knowledge of the probability density functions (p.d.f.s) of the underlying independent components. In cases where the p.d.f.s are super-gaussian (meaning they are peakier and longer-tailed than a gaussian, having kurtosis greater than 0), we have repeatedly observed, using the logistic or tanh nonlinearities, that maximisation of $H[g(\mathbf{u})]$ still leads to ICA solutions, when they exist, as with our experiments on speech signal separation [5]. Although the infomax algorithm is described here as an ICA algorithm, a fuller understanding needs to be developed of under exactly what conditions it may fail to converge to an ICA solution.

The basic infomax algorithm changes weights according to the entropy gradient. Defining $y_i = g(u_i)$ to be the sigmoidally transformed output variables, the stochastic gradient learning rule is:

$$\Delta \mathbf{W} \propto \frac{\partial H(\mathbf{y})}{\partial \mathbf{W}} = E\left[\frac{\partial \ln |J|}{\partial \mathbf{W}}\right] = E[\mathbf{W}^{-T} + \hat{\mathbf{y}}\mathbf{x}^T] \qquad (2)$$

In this, E denotes expected value, $\mathbf{y} = [g(u_1)\ldots g(u_N)]^T$, and $|J|$ is the absolute value of the determinant of the Jacobian matrix: $J = \det [\partial y_i/\partial x_j]_{ij}$, and $\hat{\mathbf{y}} = [\hat{y}_1 \ldots \hat{y}_N]^T$, the elements of which depend on the nonlinearity according to: $\hat{y}_i = \partial/\partial y_i(\partial y_i/\partial u_i)$.

Amari, Cichocki & Yang [1] have proposed a modification of this rule which utilises the *natural* gradient rather than the *absolute* gradient of $H(\mathbf{y})$. The natural gradient exists for objective functions which are functions of matrices, as in this case, and is the same as the *relative* gradient concept developed by Cardoso & Laheld (1996). It amounts to multiplying the absolute gradient by $\mathbf{W}^T\mathbf{W}$, giving, in our case, the following altered version of Eq.(2):

$$\Delta \mathbf{W} \propto \frac{\partial H(\mathbf{y})}{\partial \mathbf{W}} \mathbf{W}^T \mathbf{W} = (\mathbf{I} + \hat{\mathbf{y}} \mathbf{u}^T) \mathbf{W} \qquad (3)$$

This rule has the twin advantages over Eq.(2) of avoiding the matrix inverse, and of converging several orders of magnitude more quickly, for data, $\mathbf{x}$, that is not prewhitened. The speedup is explained by the fact that convergence is no longer dependent on the conditioning of the underlying basis function matrix, $\mathbf{A}$. Writing Eq.(3) for one weight gives $\Delta w_{ij} \propto w_{ij} + \hat{y}_i \sum_k w_{kj} u_k$. This rule is 'almost local' requiring a backwards pass.

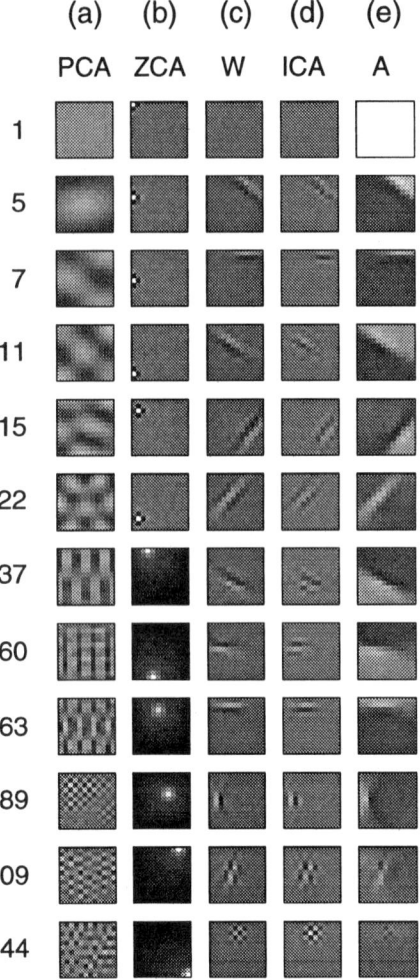

Figure 1: Selected decorrelating filters and their basis functions extracted from the natural scene data. Each type of decorrelating filter yielded 144 12x12 filters, of which we only display a subset here. Each column contains filters or basis functions of a particular type, and each of the rows has a number relating to which row of the filter or basis function matrix is displayed. (a) PCA ($\mathbf{W}_P$): The 1st, 5th, 7th etc Principal Components, showing increasing spatial frequency. There is no need to show basis functions and filters separately here since for PCA, they are the same thing. (b) ZCA ($\mathbf{W}_Z$): The first 6 entries in this column show the one-pixel wide centre-surround filter which whitens while preserving the phase spectrum. All are identical, but shifted. The lower 6 entries (37, 60 show the basis functions instead, which are the columns of the inverse of the $\mathbf{W}_Z$ matrix. (c) $\mathbf{W}$: the weights learnt by the ICA network trained on $\mathbf{W}_Z$-whitened data, showing (in descending order) the DC filter, localised oriented filters, and localised checkerboard filters. (d) $\mathbf{W}_I$: The corresponding ICA filters, calculated according to $\mathbf{W}_I = \mathbf{W}\mathbf{W}_Z$, looking like whitened versions of the $\mathbf{W}$-filters. (e) $\mathbf{A}$: the corresponding basis functions, or columns of $\mathbf{W}_I^{-1}$. These are the patterns which optimally stimulate their corresponding ICA filters, while not stimulating any other ICA filter, so that $\mathbf{W}_I \mathbf{A} = \mathbf{I}$.

4 Methods.

We took four natural scenes involving trees, leafs etc., and converted them to greyscale values between 0 and 255. A training set, $\{\mathbf{x}\}$, was then generated of 17,595 12x12 samples from the images. This was 'sphered' by subtracting the mean and multiplying by twice the local symmetrical (zero-phase) whitening filter: $\{\mathbf{x}\} \leftarrow 2\mathbf{W}_Z(\{\mathbf{x}\} - \langle\mathbf{x}\rangle)$. This removes both first and second order statistics from the data, and makes the covariance matrix of $\mathbf{x}$ equal to $4\mathbf{I}$. This is an appropriately scaled starting point for further training since infomax (Eq.(3)) on raw data, with the logistic function, $y_i = (1 + e^{-u_i})^{-1}$, produces a $\mathbf{u}$-vector which approximately satisfies $\langle\mathbf{u}\mathbf{u}^T\rangle = 4\mathbf{I}$. Therefore, by prewhitening $\mathbf{x}$ in this way, we can ensure that the subsequent transformation, $\mathbf{u} = \mathbf{W}\mathbf{x}$, to be learnt should approximate an orthonormal matrix (rotation without scaling), roughly satisfying the relation $\mathbf{W}^T\mathbf{W} = \mathbf{I}$. The matrix, $\mathbf{W}$, is then initialised to the identity matrix, and trained using the logistic function version of Eq.(3), in which $\hat{y}_i = 1 - 2y_i$. Thirty sweeps through the data were performed, at the end of each of which, the order of the data vectors was permuted to avoid cyclical behaviour in the learning. In each sweep, the weights were updated in batches of 50 presentations. The learning rate (proportionality constant in Eq.(3)) followed 21 sweeps at 0.001, and 3 sweeps at each of 0.0005, 0.0002 and 0.0001, taking 2 hours running MATLAB on a Sparc-20 machine, though a reasonable result for 12x12 filters can be achieved in 30 minutes. To verify that the result was not affected by the starting condition of $\mathbf{W} = \mathbf{I}$, the training was repeated with several randomly initialised weight matrices, and also on data that was not prewhitened. The results were qualitatively similar, though convergence was much slower.

The full ICA transform from the raw image was calculated as the product of the sphering (ZCA) matrix and the learnt matrix: $\mathbf{W}_I = \mathbf{W}\mathbf{W}_Z$. The basis function matrix, $\mathbf{A}$, was calculated as $\mathbf{W}_I^{-1}$. A PCA matrix, $\mathbf{W}_P$, was calculated. The original (unsphered) data was then transformed by all three decorrelating transforms, and for each the kurtosis of each of the 144 filters was calculated. Then the mean kurtosis for each filter type (ICA, PCA, ZCA) was calculated, averaging over all filters and input data.

5 Results.

The filters and basis functions resulting from training on natural scenes are displayed in Fig.1 and Fig.2. Fig.1 displays example filters and basis functions of each type. The PCA filters, Fig.1a, are spatially global and ordered in frequency. The ZCA filters and basis functions are spatially local and ordered in phase. The ICA filters, whether trained on the ZCA-whitened images, Fig.1c, or the original images, Fig.1d, are semi-local filters, most with a specific orientation preference. The basis functions, Fig.1e, calculated from the Fig.1d ICA filters, are not local, and naturally have the spatial frequency characteristics of the original images. Basis functions calculated from Fig.1d (as with PCA filters) are the same as the corresponding filters since the matrix $\mathbf{W}$ (as with $\mathbf{W}_P$) is orthogonal.

In order to show the full variety of ICA filters, Fig.2 shows, with lower resolution, all 144 filters in the matrix $\mathbf{W}$, in reverse order of the vector-lengths of the filters, so that the filters corresponding to higher-variance independent components appear at the top. The general result is that ICA filters are localised and mostly oriented. Unlike the basis functions displayed in Olshausen & Field (1996), they do not cover a broad range of spatial frequencies. However, the appropriate comparison to make is between the ICA basis functions, and the basis functions in Olshausen & Field's Figure 4. The ICA basis functions in our Fig.1e are oriented, but not localised and therefore it is difficult to observe any multiscale properties. However, when we ran the ICA algorithm on Olshausen's images, which were preprocessed with a whitening/lowpass filter, our algorithm yielded basis functions which were localised multiscale Gabor patches qualitatively similar to those in Olshausen's Figure 4. Part of the difference in our results is therefore attributable to different preprocessing techniques.

The distributions (image histograms) produced by PCA, ZCA and ICA are generally double-exponential ($e^{-|u_i|}$), or 'sparse', meaning peaky with a long tail, when compared to a gaussian, as predicted by Field [7]. The log histograms are seen to be roughly linear across 5 orders of magnitude. The histogram for the ICA filters, however, departs slightly from linearity, being more peaked, and having a longer tail than the ZCA and PCA histograms. This spreading of the tail signals the greater sparseness of the outputs of the ICA filters, and this is reflected in a calculated kurtosis measure of 10.04 for ICA, compared to 3.74 for PCA, and 4.5 for ZCA.

In conclusion, these simulations show that the filters found by the ICA algorithm of Eq.(3) with a logistic non-linearity are localised, oriented, and produce outputs distributions of very high sparseness. It is notable that this is achieved through an information theoretic learning rule which (1) has no noise model, (2) is sensitive to higher-order statistics (spatial coincidences), (3) is non-Hebbian (it is closer to anti-Hebbian) and (4) is simple enough to be almost locally implementable. Many other levels of higher-order invariance (translation, rotation, scaling, lighting) exist in natural scenes. It will be interesting to see if information-theoretic techniques can be extended to address these invariances.

Acknowledgements

This work emerged through many extremely useful discussions with Bruno Olshausen and David Field. We are very grateful to them, and also to Paul Viola and Barak Pearlmutter. The work was supported by the Howard Hughes Medical Institute.

References

[1] Amari S. Cichocki A. & Yang H.H. 1996. A new learning algorithm for blind signal separation, *Advances in Neural Information Processing Systems 8*, MIT press.

[2] Atick J.J. 1992. Could information theory provide an ecological theory of sensory processing? *Network* 3, 213-251

[3] Atick J.J. & Redlich A.N. 1993. Convergent algorithm for sensory receptive field development, *Neural Computation* 5, 45-60

[4] Barlow H.B. 1989. Unsupervised learning, *Neural Computation* 1, 295-311

[5] Bell A.J. & Sejnowski T.J. 1995. An information maximization approach to blind separation and blind deconvolution, *Neural Computation*, 7, 1129-1159

[6] Cardoso J-F. & Laheld B. 1996. Equivariant adaptive source separation, *IEEE Trans. on Signal Proc.*, Dec.1996.

[7] Field D.J. 1994. What is the goal of sensory coding? *Neural Computation* 6, 559-601

[8] Hubel D.H. & Wiesel T.N. 1968. Receptive fields and functional architecture of monkey striate cortex, *J. Physiol.*, 195: 215-244

[9] Linsker R. 1988. Self-organization in a perceptual network. *Computer*, 21, 105-117

[10] Miller K.D. 1988. Correlation-based models of neural development, in *Neuroscience and Connectionist Theory*, M. Gluck & D. Rumelhart, eds., 267-353, L.Erlbaum, NJ

[11] Nadal J-P. & Parga N. 1994. Non-linear neurons in the low noise limit: a factorial code maximises information transfer. *Network*, 5, 565-581.

[12] Olshausen B.A. & Field D.J. 1996. Natural image statistics and efficient coding, *Network: Computation in Neural Systems*, 7, 2.

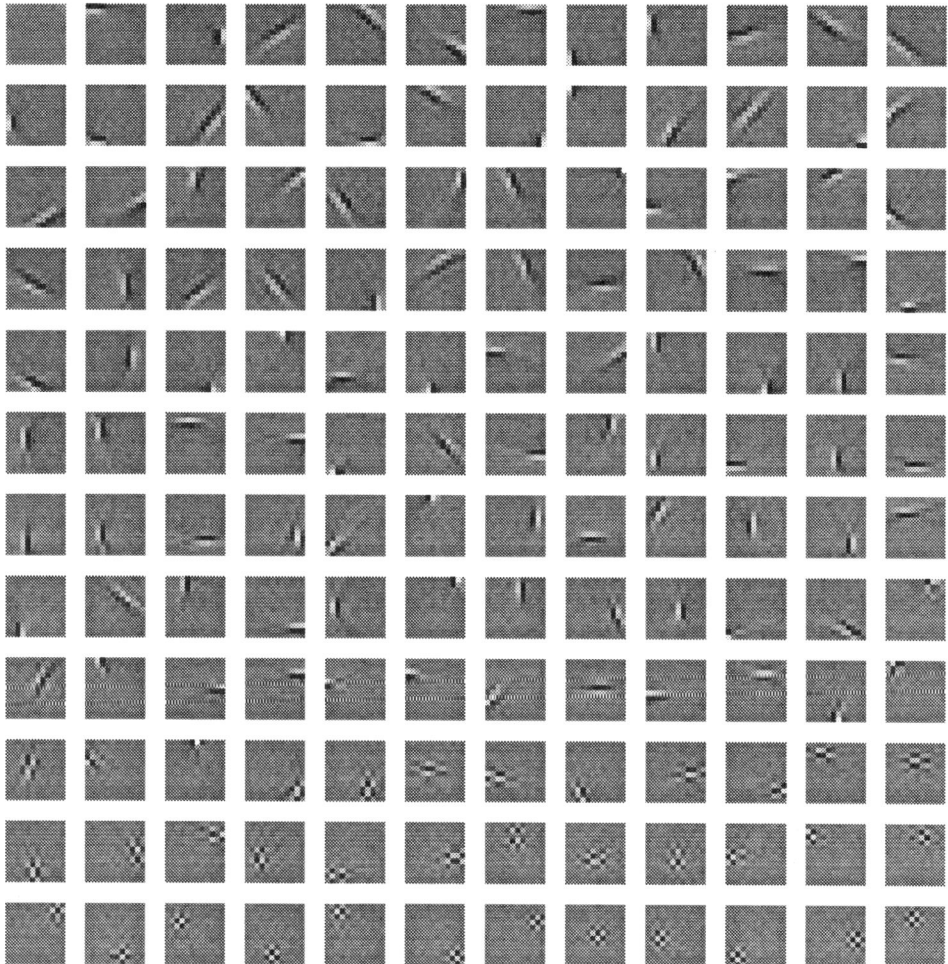

Figure 2: The matrix of 144 filters obtained by training on ZCA-whitened natural images. Each filter is a row of the matrix **W**, and they are ordered left-to-right, top-to-bottom in reverse order of the length of the filter vectors. In a rough characterisation, and more-or-less in order of appearance, the filters consist of one DC filter (top left), 106 oriented filters (of which 35 were diagonal, 37 were vertical and 34 horizontal), and 37 localised checkerboard patterns. The diagonal filters are longer than the vertical and horizontal due to the bias induced by having square, rather than circular, receptive fields.

Compositionality, MDL Priors, and Object Recognition

Elie Bienenstock (elie@dam.brown.edu)
Stuart Geman (geman@dam.brown.edu)
Daniel Potter (dfp@dam.brown.edu)
Division of Applied Mathematics,
Brown University, Providence, RI 02912 USA

Abstract

Images are ambiguous at each of many levels of a contextual hierarchy. Nevertheless, the high-level interpretation of most scenes is unambiguous, as evidenced by the superior performance of humans. This observation argues for global vision models, such as deformable templates. Unfortunately, such models are computationally intractable for unconstrained problems. We propose a compositional model in which primitives are recursively composed, subject to syntactic restrictions, to form tree-structured objects and object groupings. Ambiguity is propagated up the hierarchy in the form of multiple interpretations, which are later resolved by a Bayesian, equivalently minimum-description-length, cost functional.

1 Bayesian decision theory and compositionality

In his Essay on Probability, Laplace (1812) devotes a short chapter—his "Sixth Principle"—to what we call today the Bayesian decision rule. Laplace observes that we interpret a "regular combination," e.g., an arrangement of objects that displays some particular symmetry, as having resulted from a "regular cause" rather than arisen by chance. It is not, he argues, that a symmetric configuration is less likely to happen by chance than another arrangement. Rather, it is that among all possible combinations, which are equally favored by chance, there are very few of the regular type: *"On a table we see letters arranged in this order,* Constantinople, *and we judge that this arrangement is not the result of chance, not because it is less possible than the others, for if this word were not employed in any language we should not suspect it came from any particular cause, but this word being in use amongst us, it is incomparably more probable that some person has thus arranged the aforesaid letters than that this arrangement is due to chance."* In this example, regularity is not a mathematical symmetry. Rather, it is a convention shared among language users, whereby *Constantinople* is a word, whereas *Ipctneolnosant*, a string containing the same letters but arranged in a random order, is not.

Central in Laplace's argument is the observation that the number of words in the language is smaller, indeed "incomparably" smaller, than the number of possible arrangements of letters. Indeed, if the collection of 14-letter words in a language made up, say, half of all 14-letter strings—a rich language indeed—we would, upon seeing the string *Constantinople* on the table, be far less inclined to deem it a word, and far more inclined to accept it as a possible coincidence. The sparseness of allowed combinations can be observed at all linguistic articulations (phonetic-syllabic, syllabic-lexical, lexical-syntactic, syntactic-pragmatic, to use broadly defined levels), and may be viewed as a form of *redundancy*—by analogy to error-correcting codes. This redundancy was likely devised by evolution to ensure efficient communication in spite of the ambiguity of elementary speech signals. The hierarchical compositional structure of natural visual scenes can also be thought of as redundant: the rules that govern the composition of edge elements into object boundaries, of intensities into surfaces etc., all the way to the assembly of 2-D projections of named objects, amount to a collection of drastic combinatorial restrictions. Arguably, this is why in all but a few—generally hand-crafted—cases, natural images have a unique high-level interpretation in spite of pervasive low-level ambiguity—this being amply demonstrated by the performances of our brains.

In sum, compositionality appears to be a fundamental aspect of cognition (see also von der Malsburg 1981, 1987; Fodor and Pylyshyn 1988; Bienenstock, 1991, 1994, 1996; Bienenstock and Geman 1995). We propose here to account for mental computation in general and scene interpretation in particular in terms of *elementary composition operations*, and describe a mathematical framework that we have developed to this effect. The present description is a cursory one, and some notions are illustrated on two simple examples rather than formally defined—for a detailed account, see Geman et al. (1996), Potter (1997). The *binary-image* example refers to an $N \times N$ array of binary-valued pixels, while the *Laplace-Table* example refers to a one-dimensional array of length N, where each position can be filled with one of the 26 letters of the alphabet or remain blank.

2 Labels and composition rules

The *objects* operated upon are denoted $\omega_i, i = 1, 2, \ldots, k$. Each *composite* object ω carries a *label*, $l = L(\omega)$, and the list of its constituents, $(\omega_1, \omega_2, \cdots)$. These uniquely determine ω, so we write $\omega = l(\omega_1, \omega_2, \cdots)$. A *scene* S is a collection of *primitive* objects. In the binary-image case, a scene S consists of a collection of black pixels in the $N \times N$ array. All these primitives carry the same label, $L(\omega) = p$ (for "Point"), and a parameter $\pi(\omega)$ which is the position in the image. In Laplace's Table, a scene S consists of an arrangement of characters on the table. There are 26 primitive labels, "A","B",...,"Z", and the parameter of a primitive ω is its position $1 \leq \pi(\omega) \leq N$ (all primitives in such a scene must have different positions).

An example of a composite ω in the binary-image case is an arrangement composed of a black pixel at any position except on the rightmost column and another black pixel to the immediate right of the first one. The label is "Horizontal Linelet," denoted $L(\omega) = hl$, and there are $N(N-1)$ possible horizontal linelets. Another non-primitive label, "Vertical Linelet," or vl, is defined analogously. An example of a composite ω for Laplace's Table is an arrangement of 14 neighboring primitives carrying the labels "C", "O", "N", "S", ..., "E" in that order, wherever that arrangement will fit. We then have $L(\omega) = Constantinople$, and there are $N-13$ possible Constantinople objects.

The *composition rule* for label type l consists of a *binding function*, B_l, and a set of allowed binding-function values, or *binding support*, S_l: denoting by Ω the set of *all* objects in the model, we have, for any $\omega_1, \cdots, \omega_k \in \Omega$, $B_l(\omega_1, \cdots, \omega_k) \in S_l \Leftrightarrow l(\omega_1, \cdots, \omega_k) \in \Omega$. In the binary-image example, $B_{hl}(\omega_1, \omega_2) = B_{vl}(\omega_1, \omega_2) = (L(\omega_1), L(\omega_2), \pi(\omega_2) - \pi(\omega_1))$, $S_{hl} = \{(p, p, (1, 0))\}$ and $S_{vl} = \{(p, p, (0, 1))\}$ define the hl- and vl-composition rules, $p + p \to hl$ and $p + p \to vl$. In Laplace's Table, $C + O + \cdots + E \to Constantinpole$ is an example of a 14-ary composition rule, where we must check the label and position of each constituent. One way to define the binding function and support for this rule is: $B(\omega_1, \cdots, \omega_{14}) = (L(\omega_1), \cdots, L(\omega_{14}), \pi(\omega_2) - \pi(\omega_1), \pi(\omega_3) - \pi(\omega_1), \cdots, \pi(\omega_{14}) - \pi(\omega_1))$ and $S = (C, \cdots, E, 1, 2, \cdots, 13)$.

We now introduce *recursive* labels and composition rules: the label of the composite object is identical to the label of one or more of its constituents, and the rule may be applied an arbitrary number of times, to yield objects of arbitrary complexity. In the binary-image case, we use a recursive label c, for *Curve*, and an associated binding function which creates objects of the form $hl + p \to c$, $vl + p \to c$, $c + p \to c$, $p + hl \to c$, $p + vl \to c$, $p + c \to c$, and $c + c \to c$. The reader may easily fill in the details, i.e., define a binding function and binding support which result in "c"-objects being precisely curves in the image, where a curve is of length at least 3 and may be self-intersecting. In the previous examples, primitives were composed into compositions; here compositions are further composed into more complex compositions. In general, an object ω is a *labeled tree*, where each vertex carries the name of an object, and each leaf is associated with a primitive (the association is not necessarily one-to-one, as in the case of a self-intersecting curve).

Let $\mathcal{M}$ be a *model*—i.e., a collection of labels with their binding functions and binding supports—and Ω the set of all objects in $\mathcal{M}$. We say that object $\omega \in \Omega$ covers S if S is precisely the set of primitives that make up ω's leaves. An *interpretation* I of S is any finite collection of objects in Ω such that the union of the sets of primitives they cover is S. We use the convention that, for all $\mathcal{M}$ and S, I_0 denotes the *trivial* interpretation, defined as the collection of (unbound) primitives in S. In most cases of interest, a model $\mathcal{M}$ will allow many interpretations for a scene S. For instance, given a long curve in the binary-image model, there will be many ways to recursively construct a "c"-labeled tree that covers exactly that curve.

3 The MDL formulation

In Laplace's Table, a scene consisting of the string *Constantinople* admits, in addition to I_0, the interpretation $I_1 = \{\omega_1\}$, where ω_1 is a "*Constantinople*"-object. We wish to define a probability distribution D on interpretations such that $D(I_1) \gg D(I_0)$, in order to realize Laplace's "incomparably more probable". Our definition of D will be motivated by the following use of the Minimum Description Length (MDL) principle (Rissanen 1989). Consider a scene S and pretend we want to transmit S as quickly as possible through a noiseless channel, hence we seek to *encode* it as efficiently as possible, i.e., with the shortest possible binary code c. We can always use the trivial interpretation I_0: the codeword $c(I_0)$ is a mere list of n locations in S. We need not specify labels, since there is only one primitive label in this example. The length, or *cost*, of this code for S is $|c(I_0)| = n \log_2(N^2)$.

Now however we want to take advantage of regularities, in the sense of Laplace, that we *expect* to be present in S. We are specifically interested in compositional regularities, where some arrangements that occur more frequently than by chance can be interpreted *advantageously* using an appropriate compositional model $\mathcal{M}$. Interpretation I is advantageous if $|c(I)| < |c(I_0)|$. An example in the binary-image case is a linelet scene S. The trivial encoding of this scene costs us $|c(I_0)| = 2[\log_2 3 + \log_2(N^2)]$ bits, whereas the cost of the compositional interpretation $I_1 = \{\omega_1\}$ is $|c(I_1)| = \log_2 3 + \log_2(N(N-1))$, where ω_1 is an hl or vl object, as the case may be. The first $\log_2 3$ bits encode the label $L(\omega_1) \in \{p, hl, vl\}$, and the rest encodes the position in the image. The compositional $\{p, hl, vl\}$ model is therefore advantageous for a linelet scene, since I_1 affords us a gain in encoding cost of about $2 \log_2 N$ bits.

In general, the gain realized by encoding $\{\omega\} = \{l(\omega_1, \omega_2)\}$ instead of $\{\omega_1, \omega_2\}$ may be viewed as a *binding energy*, measuring the affinity that ω_1 and ω_2 exhibit for each other as they assemble into ω. This binding energy is $\mathcal{E}_l = |c(\omega_1)| + |c(\omega_2)| - |c(l(\omega_1, \omega_2))|$, and an efficient $\mathcal{M}$ is one that contains *judiciously chosen* cost-saving composition rules. In effect, if, say, linelets were very rare, we would be better off with the trivial model. The inclusion of non-primitive labels would force us to add at least one bit to the code of every object—to specify its label—and this would increase the *average* encoding cost, since the infrequent use of non-primitive labels would not balance the extra small cost incurred on primitives. In practical applications, the construction of a sound $\mathcal{M}$ is no trivial issue. Note however the simple rationale for including a rule such as $p + p \to hl$. Giving ourselves the label hl renders redundant the independent encoding of the positions of horizontally adjacent pixels. In general, a good model should allow one to hierarchically compose with each other *frequently occurring* arrangements of objects.

This use of MDL leads in a straightforward way to an equivalent Bayesian formulation. Setting $P'(\omega) = 2^{-|c(\omega)|} / \sum_{\omega' \in \Omega} 2^{-|c(\omega')|}$ yields a probability distribution P' on Ω for which c is approximately a Shannon code (Cover and Thomas 1991). With this definition, the decision to include the label hl—or the label *Constantinople*— would be viewed, in principle, as a statement about the prior probability of finding horizontal linelets—or *Constantinople* strings—in the scene to be interpreted.

4 The observable-measure formulation

The MDL formulation however has a number of shortcomings; in particular, computing the binding energy for composite objects can be problematic. We outline now an alternative approach (Geman et al. 1996, Potter 1997), where a probability distribution $P(\omega)$ on Ω is defined through a family of *observable measures* Q_l. These measures assign probabilities to each possible binding-function value, $s \in S_l$, and also to the primitives. We require $\sum_{l \in \mathcal{M}} \sum_{s \in S_l} Q_l(s) = 1$, where the notion of binding function has been extended to primitives via $B_{prim}(\omega) = \pi(\omega)$ for primitive

ω. The probabilities induced on Ω by Q_l are given by $P(\omega) = Q_{prim}(B_{prim}(\omega))$ for a primitive ω, and $P(\omega) = Q_l(B_l(\omega_1, \omega_2)) P^2(\omega_1, \omega_2 | B_l(\omega_1, \omega_2))$ for a composite object $\omega = l(\omega_1, \omega_2)$.[1] Here $P^2 = P \times P$ is the product probability, i.e., the *free*, or *not-bound*, distribution for the pair $(\omega_1, \omega_2) \in \Omega^2$. For instance, with $C + \cdots + E \to Constantinople$, $P^{14}(\omega_1, \omega_2, \ldots, \omega_{14} | B_{Cons\ldots}(\omega_1, \ldots, \omega_{14}) = (C, O, \cdots, 13))$ is the conditional probability of observing a *particular* string *Constantinople*, under the free distribution, given that $(\omega_1, \ldots, \omega_{14})$ constitutes such a string. With the reasonable assumption that, under Q, primitives are uniformly distributed over the table, this conditional probability is simply the inverse of the number of possible *Constantinople* strings, i.e., $1/(N-13)$.

The binding energy, defined, by analogy to the MDL approach, as $\mathcal{E}_l = \log_2(P(\omega)/(P(\omega_1)P(\omega_2)))$, now becomes $\mathcal{E}_l = \log_2(Q_l(B_l(\omega_1, \omega_2))) - \log_2(P \times P(B_l(\omega_1, \omega_2)))$. Finally, if $\mathcal{I}$ is the collection of all finite interpretations $I \subset \Omega$, we define the probability of $I \in \mathcal{I}$ as $D(I) = \Pi_{\omega \in I} P(\omega)/Z$, with $Z = \sum_{I' \in \mathcal{I}} \Pi_{\omega \in I'} P(\omega)$. Thus, the probability of an interpretation containing several free objects is obtained by assuming that these objects occurred in the scene independently of each other. Given a scene $\mathcal{S}$, recognition is formulated as the task of maximizing D over all the I's in $\mathcal{I}$ that are interpretations of $\mathcal{S}$.

We now illustrate the use of D on our two examples. In the binary-image example with model $\mathcal{M} = \{p, hl, vl\}$, we use a parameter $q, 0 \le q \le 1$, to adjust the prior probability of linelets. Thus, $Q_{prim}(B_{prim}(\omega)) = (1-q)/N^2$ for primitives, and $Q_{hl}((p,p,0,1)) = Q_{vl}((p,p,1,0)) = q/2$ for linelets. It is easily seen that regardless of the normalizing constant Z, the binding energy of two adjacent pixels into a linelet is $\mathcal{E}_{hl} = \mathcal{E}_{vl} = \log_2(q/2) - \log_2[\frac{(1-q)^2}{N^4} N(N-1)]$. Interestingly, as long as $q \ne 0$ and $q \ne 1$, the binding energy, for large N, is approximately $2 \log_2 N$, which is independent of q. Thus, the linelet interpretation is "incomparably" more likely than the independent occurrence of two primitives at neighboring positions. We leave it to the reader to construct a prior P for the model $\{p, hl, vl, c\}$, e.g. by distributing the Q-mass evenly between all composition rules. Finally, in Laplace's Table, if there are M equally likely non-primitive labels—say city names—and q is their total mass, the binding energy for *Constantinople* is $\mathcal{E}_{Cons\ldots} = \log_2 \frac{q}{M(N-13)} - \log_2[\frac{1-q}{26N}]^{14}$, and the "regular" cause is again "incomparably" more likely.

There are several advantages to this reformulation from codewords into probabilities using the Q-parameters. First, the Q-parameters can in principle be adjusted to better account for a particular world of images. Second, we get an explicit formula for the binding energy, (namely $\log_2(Q/P \times P)$). Of course, we need to evaluate the product probability $P \times P$, and this can be highly non-trivial—one approach is through sampling, as demonstrated in Potter (1997). Finally, this formulation is well-suited for parameter estimation: the Q's, which are the parameters of the distribution P, are indeed observables, i.e., directly available empirically.

5 Concluding remarks

The approach described here was applied by X. Xing to the recognition of "on-line" handwritten characters, using a binary-image-type model as above, enriched

---

[1] This is actually an implicit definition. Under reasonable conditions, it is well defined—see Geman et al. (1996).

with higher-level labels including curved lines, straight lines, angles, crossings, T-junctions, L-junctions (right angles), and the 26 letters of the alphabet. In such a model, the search for an optimal solution cannot be done exhaustively. We experimented with a number of strategies, including a two-step algorithm which first generates *all* possible objects in the scene, and then selects the "best" objects, i.e., the objects with highest *total* binding energy, using a greedy method, to yield a final scene interpretation. (The total binding energy of ω is the sum of the binding energies $\mathcal{E}_l$ over all the composition rules l used in the composition of ω. Equivalently, the total binding energy is the log-likelihood ratio $\log_2(P(\omega)/\Pi_i P(\omega_i))$, where the product is taken over all the primitives ω_i covered by ω.)

The first step of the algorithm typically results in high-level objects partly overlapping on the set of primitives they cover, i.e., competing for the interpretation of shared primitives. Ambiguity is thus propagated in a "bottom-up" fashion. The ambiguity is resolved in the second "top-down" pass, when high-level composition rules are used to select the best compositions, at all levels including the lower ones. A detailed account of our experiments will be given elsewhere. We found the results quite encouraging, particularly in view of the potential scope of the approach. In effect, we believe that this approach is in principle capable of addressing unrestricted vision problems, where images are typically very ambiguous at lower levels for a variety of reasons—including occlusion and mutual overlap of objects—hence purely bottom-up segmentation is impractical.

Turning now to biological implications, note that dynamic binding in the nervous system has been a subject of intensive research and debate in the last decade. Most interesting in the present context is the suggestion, first clearly articulated by von der Malsburg (1981), that composition may be performed thanks to a dual mechanism of accurate synchronization of spiking activity—not necessarily relying on periodic firing—and fast reversible synaptic plasticity. If there is some neurobiological truth to the model described in the present paper, the binding mechanism proposed by von der Malsburg would appear to be an attractive implementation. In effect, the use of fine temporal structure of neural activity opens up a large realm of possible high order codes in networks of neurons.

In the present model, constituents always bind *in the service* of a new object, an operation one may refer to as *triangular binding*. Composite objects can engage in further composition, thus giving rise to arbitrarily deep tree-structured constructs. Physiological evidence of triangular binding in the visual system can be found in Sillito et al. (1994); Damasio (1989) describes an approach derived from neuroanatomical data and lesion studies that is largely consistent with the formalism described here.

An important requirement for the neural representation of the tree-structured objects used in our model is that the doing and undoing of links operating on some constituents, say ω_1 and ω_2, while affecting in some *useful* way the high-order patterns that represent these objects, leaves these patterns, as representations of ω_1 and ω_2, intact. A family of biologically plausible patterns that would appear to satisfy this requirement is provided by *synfire* patterns (Abeles 1991). We hypothesized elsewhere (Bienenstock 1991, 1994, 1996) that synfire chains could be dynamically bound via weak synaptic couplings; such couplings would synchronize the wave-like activities of two synfire chains, in much the same way as coupled oscillators lock their phases. Recursiveness of compositionality could, in principle, arise from the further binding of these composite structures.

Acknowledgements

Supported by the Army Research Office (DAAL03-92-G-0115), the National Science Foundation (DMS-9217655), and the Office of Naval Research (N00014-96-1-0647).

References

Abeles, M. (1991) *Corticonics: Neuronal circuits of the cerebral cortex*, Cambridge University Press.

Bienenstock, E. (1991) Notes on the growth of a composition machine, in *Proceedings of the Royaumont Interdisciplinary Workshop on Compositionality in Cognition and Neural Networks—I*, D. Andler, E. Bienenstock, and B. Laks, Eds., pp. 25–43. (1994) A Model of Neocortex. *Network: Computation in Neural Systems*, 6:179–224. (1996) Composition, In *Brain Theory: Biological Basis and Computational Principles*, A. Aertsen and V. Braitenberg eds., Elsevier, pp 269–300.

Bienenstock, E., and Geman, S. (1995) Compositionality in Neural Systems, In *The Handbook of Brain Theory and Neural Networks*, M.A. Arbib ed., M.I.T./Bradford Press, pp 223–226.

Cover, T.M., and Thomas, J.A. (1991) *Elements of Information Theory*, Wiley and Sons, New York.

Damasio, A. R. (1989) Time-locked multiregional retroactivation: a systems-level proposal for the neural substrates of recall and recognition, *Cognition*, 33:25–62.

Fodor, J.A., and Pylyshyn, Z.W. (1988) Connectionism and cognitive architecture: a critical analysis, *Cognition*, 28:3–71.

Geman, S., Potter, D., and Chi, Z. (1996) *Compositional Systems*, Technical Report, Division of Applied Mathematics, Brown University.

Laplace, P.S. (1812) *Esssai philosophique sur les probabilités*. Translation of Truscott and Emory, New York, 1902.

Potter, D. (1997) *Compositional Pattern Recognition*, PhD Thesis, Division of Applied Mathematics, Brown University, In preparation.

Rissanen, J. (1989) *Stochastic Complexity in Statistical Inquiry* World Scientific Co, Singapore.

Sillito, A.M., Jones, H.E, Gerstein, G.L., and West, D.C. (1994) Feature-linked synchronization of thalamic relay cell firing induced by feedback from the visual cortex, *Nature*, 369: 479-482

von der Malsburg, C. (1981) *The correlation theory of brain function*. Internal report 81-2, Max-Planck Institute for Biophysical Chemistry, Dept. of Neurobiology, Göttingen, Germany. (1987) Synaptic plasticity as a basis of brain organization, in *The Neural and Molecular Bases of Learning* (J.P. Changeux and M. Konishi, Eds.), John Wiley and Sons, pp. 411–432.

Learning Appearance Based Models: Mixtures of Second Moment Experts

Christoph Bregler and Jitendra Malik

Computer Science Division
University of California at Berkeley
Berkeley, CA 94720
email: bregler@cs.berkeley.edu, malik@cs.berkeley.edu

Abstract

This paper describes a new technique for object recognition based on learning appearance models. The image is decomposed into local regions which are described by a new texture representation called "Generalized Second Moments" that are derived from the output of multiscale, multiorientation filter banks. Class-characteristic local texture features and their global composition is learned by a hierarchical mixture of experts architecture (Jordan & Jacobs). The technique is applied to a vehicle database consisting of 5 general car categories (Sedan, Van with back-doors, Van without back-doors, old Sedan, and Volkswagen Bug). This is a difficult problem with considerable in-class variation. The new technique has a 6.5% misclassification rate, compared to eigen-images which give 17.4% misclassification rate, and nearest neighbors which give 15.7% misclassification rate.

1 Introduction

Until a few years ago neural network and other statistical learning techniques were not very popular in computer vision domains. Usually such techniques were only applied to artificial visual data or non-mainstream problems such as handwritten digit recognition.

A significant shift has occurred recently with the successful application of appearance-based or viewer-centered techniques for object recognition, supplementing the use of 3D models. Appearance-based schemes rely on collections of images of the object. A principal advantage is that they implicitly capture both shape and photometric information(e.g. surface reflectance variation). They have been most sucessfully applied in the domain of human faces [15, 11, 1, 14] though other 3d objects under fixed lighting have also been considered [13]. View-based representations lend themselves very naturally to learning from examples– principal component analysis[15, 13] and radial basis functions[1] have been used.

Approaches such as principal component analysis (or "eigen-images") use global representations at the image level. The objective of our research was to develop a representation which would be more 'localist', where representations of different 'parts' of the object would be composed together to form the representation of the object as a whole. This appears to be essential in order to obtain robustness to occlusion and ease of generalization when different objects in a class may have variations in particular parts but not others. A part based view is also more consistent with what is known about human object recognition (Tanaka and collaborators).

In this paper, we propose a domain independent part decomposition using a 2D grid representation of overlapping local image regions. The image features of each local patch are represented using a new texture descriptor that we call "Generalized Second Moments". Related representations have already been successfully applied to other early-vision tasks like stereopsis, motion, and texture discrimination. Class-based local texture features and their global relationships are induced using the "Hierarchical Mixtures of Experts" Architecture (HME) [8].

We apply this technique to the domain of vehicle classification. The vehicles are seen from behind by a camera mounted above a freeway(Figure 1). We urge the reader to examine Figure 3 to see examples of the in class variations in the 5 different categories. Our technique could classify five broader categories with an error of as low as 6.5% misclassification, while the best results using eigen-images and nearest neighbor techniques were 17.4% and 15.7% mis-classification error.

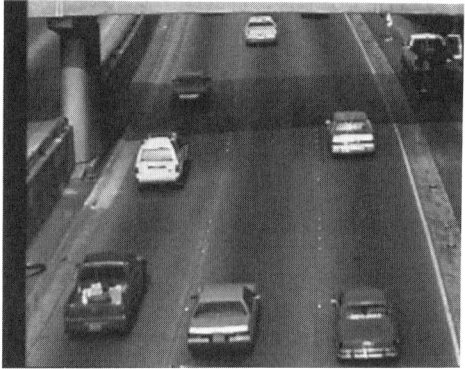

Figure 1: Typical shot of the freeway segment

2 Representation

An appearance based representation should be able to capture features that discriminate the different object categories. It should capture both local textural and global structural information. This corresponds roughly to the notion in 3D object models of (i) parts (ii) relationship between parts.

2.1 Structural Description

Objects usually can be decomposed into parts. A face consists of eyes, nose, and mouth. Cars are made out of window screens, tail lights, license plates etc. The question is what granularity is appropriate and how much domain knowledge should be exploited. A car could be a single part in a scene, a license plate could be a part, or the letters in the license plate could be the decomposed parts. Eyes, nose, and mouth could be the most important parts of a face for recognition, but maybe other parts are important as well.

It would be advantageous if each part could be described in a decoupled way using a representation that was most appropriate for it. Object classification should be based on these local part descriptions and the relationship between the parts. The partitioning reduces the complexity greatly and invariance to the precise relation between the parts could be achieved.

For our domain of vehicle classification we don't believe it is appropriate to explicitly code any part decomposition. The kind and number of useful parts might vary across different car makes. The resolution of the images (100x100 pixel) restricts us to a certain degree of granularity. We decided to decompose the image using a 2D grid of overlapping tiles or Gaussian windows but only local classification for each tile region is done. The content of each local tile is represented by a feature vector (next section). The generic grid representation allows the mixture of experts architecture to induce class-based part decomposition, and extract local texture and global shape features. For example the outline of a face could be represented by certain orientation dominances in the local tiles at positions of the face boundary. The eyes are other characteristic features in the tiles.

2.2 Local Features

We wanted to extract characteristic features from each local tile. The traditional computer vision approach would be to find edges and junctions. The weakness of these representations is that they do not capture the richness of textured regions, and the hard decision thresholds make the measurement process non–robust.

An alternative view is motivated by our understanding of processing in biological vision systems. We start by convolving image regions with a large number of spatial filters, at various orientations, phases, and scales. The response values of such filters contain much more general information about the local neighborhood, a fact that has now been recognized and exploited in a number of early vision tasks like stereopsis, motion and texture analysis [16, 9, 6, 12, 7].

Although this approach is loosely inspired by the current understanding of processing in the early stages of the primate visual system, the use of spatial filters has many advantages from a pure analytical viewpoint[9, 7]. We use as filter kernels, orientation selective elongated Gaussian derivatives. This enables one to gain the power of orientation specific features, such as edges, without the disadvantage of non-robustness due to hard thresholds. If multiple orientations are present at a single point (e.g. junctions), they are represented in a natural way. Since multiple scales are used for the filters, no *ad hoc* choices have to be made for the scale parameters of the feature detectors. Interestingly the choices of these filter kernels can also be motivated in a learning paradigm as they provide very useful intermediate layer units in convolutional neural networks [3].

The straightforward approach would then be to characterize each image pixel by such a vector of feature responses. However note that there is considerable redundancy in the filter responses– particularly at coarse scales, the responses of filters at neighboring pixels are strongly correlated. We would like to compress the representation in some way. One approach might be to subsample at coarse scales, another might be to choose feature locations with local magnitude maxima or high responses across several directions. However there might be many such interesting points in an image region. It is unclear how to pick the right number of points and how to order them.

Leaving this issue of compressing the filter response representation aside for the moment, let us study other possible representations of low level image data. One way of representing the texture in a local region is to calculate a windowed second moment matrix [5]. Instead of finding maxima of filter responses, the second moments of brightness gradients in the local neighborhood are weighted and averaged with a circular Gaussian window. The gradient is a special case of Gaussian oriented filter banks. The windowed second moment matrix takes into account the response of all filters in this neighborhood. The disadvantage is that gradients are not very orientation selective and a certain scale has to be selected beforehand. Averaging the gradients "washes" out the detailed orientation information in complex texture regions.

Orientation histograms would avoid this effect and have been applied successfully for classification [4]. Elongated families of oriented and scaled kernels could be used to estimate the orientation at each point. But as pointed out already, there might be more than one orientation at each point, and significant information is lost.

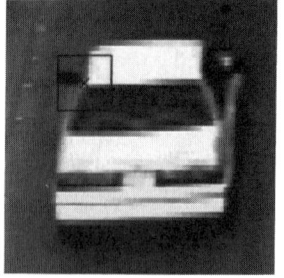 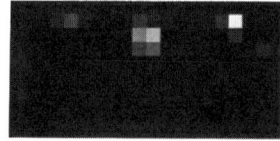

Figure 2: Left image: The black rectangle outlines the selected area of interest. Right image: The reconstructed scale and rotation distribution of the Generalized Second Moments. The horizontal axis are angles between 0 and 180 degrees and the vertical axis are different scales.

3 Generalized Second Moments

We propose a new way to represent the texture in a local image patch by combining the filter bank approach with the idea of second moment matrices.

The goal is to compute a feature vector for a local image patch that contains information about the orientation and scale distribution. We compute for each pixel in the image patch the R basis kernel responses (using X-Y separable steerable scalable approximations of a rich filter family). Given a spatial weighting function of the patch (e.g. Gaussian), we compute the covariance matrix of the weighted set of R dimensional vectors. In [2] we show that this covariance matrix can be used to reconstruct for any desired oriented and scaled version of the filter family the weighted sum of all filter response energies:

$$E(\theta, \sigma) = \sum_{x,y} W(x, y)[F_{\theta,\sigma}(x, y)]^2 \qquad (1)$$

Using elongated kernels produces orientation/scale peaks, therefore the sum of all orientation/scale responses doesn't "wash" out high peaks. The height of each individual peak corresponds to the intensity in the image. Little noisy orientations have no high energy responses in the sum. $E(\theta, \sigma)$ is somehow a "soft" orientation/scale histogram of the local image patch. Figure 2 shows an example of such a scale/orientation reconstruction based on the covariance matrix (see [2] for details). Three peaks are seen, representing the edge lines along three directions and scales in the local image patch.

This representation greatly reduces the dimensionality without being domain specific or applying any hard decisions. It is shift invariant in the local neighborhood and decouples scale in a nice way. Dividing the $R \times R$ covariance matrix by its trace makes this representation also illumination invariant.

Using a 10x10 grid and a kernel basis of 5 first Gaussian derivatives and 5 second Gaussian derivatives represents each input image as an $10 \cdot 10 \cdot (5+1) \cdot 5 = 3000$ dimensional vector (a 5×5 covariance matrix has $(5+1) \cdot 5$ independent parameters). Potentially we could represent the full image with one generalized second moment matrix of dimension 20 if we don't care about capturing the part decomposition.

4 Mixtures of Experts

Even if we only deal with the restricted domain of man-made object categories (e.g. cars), the extracted features still have a considerable in-class variation. Different car shapes and poses produce nonlinear class subspaces. Hierarchical Mixtures of Experts (HME by Jordan & Jacobs) are able to model such nonlinear decision surfaces with a soft hierarchical decomposition of the

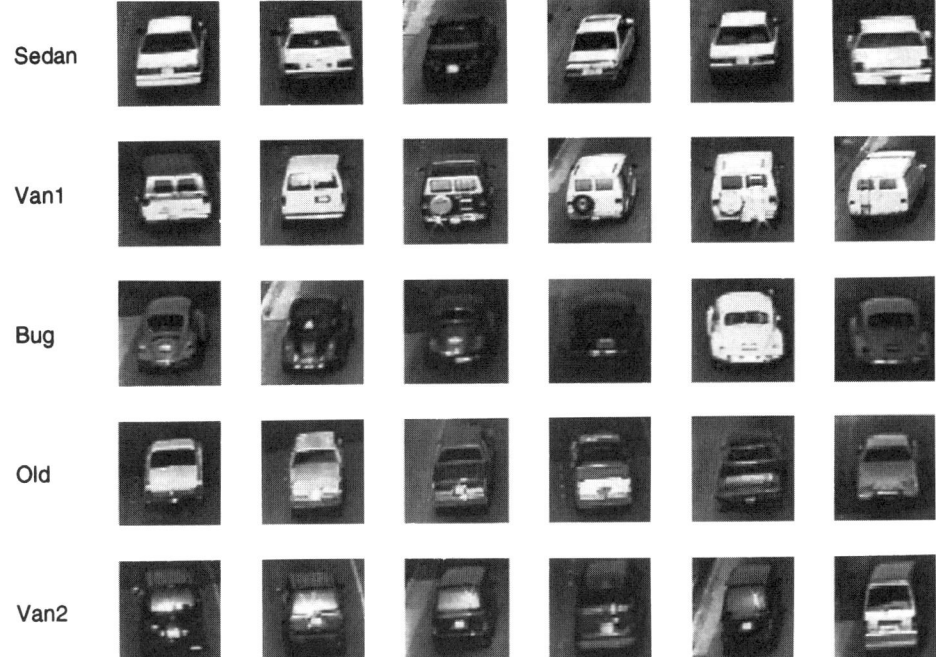

Figure 3: Example images of the five vehicle classes.

feature space and local linear classification experts. Potentially different experts are "responsible" for different object poses or sub-categories.

The gating functions decompose the feature space into a nested set of regions using a hierarchical structure of soft decision boundaries. Each region is the domain for a specific expert that classifies the feature vectors into object categories. We used generalized linear models (GLIM). Given the training data and output labels, the gating functions and expert functions can be estimated using an iterative version of the EM-algorithm. For more detail see [8].

In order to reduce training time and storage requirements, we trained such nonlinear decision surfaces embedded in one global linear subspace. We choose the dimension of this linear subspace to be large enough, so that it captures most of the lower-dimensional nonlinearity (3000 dimensional feature space projected into an 64 dimensional subspace estimated by principal components analysis).

5 Experiments

We experimented with a database consisting of images taken from a surveillance camera on a bridge covering normal daylight traffic on a freeway segment (Figure 1). The goal is to classify different types of vehicles. We are able to segment each moving object based on motion cues [10]. We chose the following 5 vehicle classes: Modern Sedan, Old Sedan, Van with back-doors, Van without back-door, and Volkswagen Bug. The images show the rear of the car across a small set of poses (Figure 3). All images are normalized to 100x100 pixel using bilinear interpolation. For this reason the size or aspect ratio can not be used as a feature.

We ran our experiments using two different image representations:

- Generalized Second Moments: A 10×10 grid was used. Generalized second moments

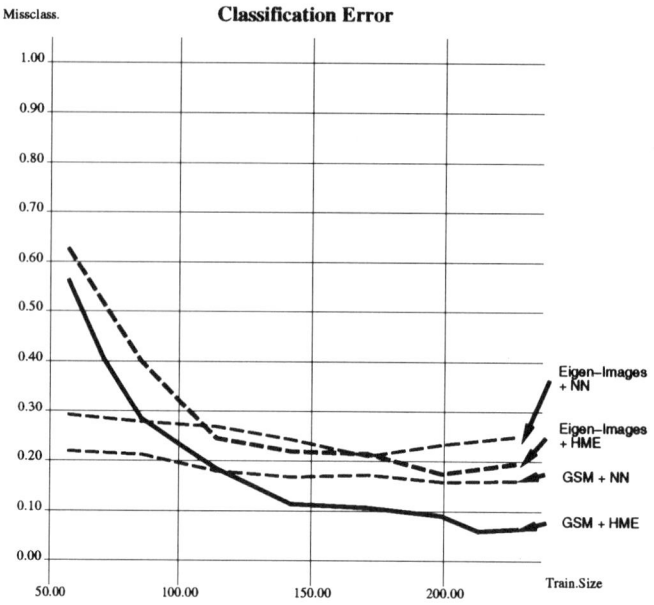

Figure 4: The classification errors of four different techniques. The X-axis shows the size of the training set, and the Y-axis shows the percentage of misclassified test images. HME stands for Hierarchical Mixtures of Experts, GSM stands for Generalized Second Moments, and 1-NN stands for Nearest Neighbors.

were computed [1] using a window of $\sigma = 6$ pixel, and 5 filter bases of 3:1 elongated first and second Gaussian derivatives on a scale range between 0.25 and 1.0.

- Principal Components Analysis ("Eigen-Images"): We used no grid decomposition and projected the global graylevel vector into a 64 dimensional linear space.

Two different classifiers were used:

- HME architecture with 8 local experts.
- A simple 1-Nearest-Neighbor Classifier (1-NN).

Figure 4 shows the classification error rate for all 4 combinations as a function of the size of the training set. Each experiment is run 5 times with different sampling of training and test images[2]. The database consists of 285 example images. Therefore the number of test images are (285− number of training images).

Across all experiments the HME architecture based on Generalized Moments was superior to all other techniques. The best performance with a misclassification of 6.5% was achieved using 228 training images. When fewer than 120 training images are used, the HME architecture performed worse than nearest neighbors.

The most common confusion was between sedans and "old" sedans. The second most confusion was between vans with back-doors, vans without back-doors, and old sedans.

---

[1] We experimented also with grid sizes between 6x6 to 16x16, and with 8 filter bases and a rectangle window for the second moment statistics without getting significant improvement.

[2] For a given training size n we trained 5 classifiers on 5 different training and test sets and computed the average error rate. The training and test set for each classifier was generated by the same database. The n training examples were randomly sampled from the database, and the remaining examples were used for the test set.

6   Conclusion

We have demonstrated a new technique for appearance-based object recognition based on a 2D grid representation, generalized second moments, and hierarchical mixtures of experts. Experiments have shown that this technique has significant better performance than other representation techniques like eigen-images and other classification techniques like nearest neighbors.

We believe that learning such appearance-based representations offers a very attractive methodology. Hand-coding features that could discriminant object categories like the different car types in our database seems to be a nearly impossible task. The only choice in such domains is to estimate discriminating features from a set of example images automatically.

The proposed technique can be applied to other domains as well. We are planning to experiment with face databases, as well as larger car databases and categories to further investigate the utility of hierarchical mixtures of experts and generalized second moments.

Acknowledgments   We would like to thank Leo Breiman, Jerry Feldman, Thomas Leung, Stuart Russell, and Jianbo Shi for helpful discussions and Michael Jordan, Lawrence Saul, and Doug Shy for providing code.

References

[1] D. Beymer, A. Shashua, and T. Poggio. Example based image analysis and synthesis. *M.I.T. A.I. Memo No. 1431*, Nov 1993.

[2] C. Bregler and J. Malik. Learning Appearance Based Models: Hierarchical Mixtures of Experts Approach based on Generalized Second Moments. Technical Report UCB//CSD-96-897, Comp. Sci. Dep., U.C. Berkeley, http://www.cs/ bregler/soft.html, 1996.

[3] Y. Le Cun, B. Boser, J.S. Denker, S. Solla, R. Howard, and L. Jackel. Back-propagation applied to handwritten zipcode recognition. *Neural Computation*, 1(4), 1990.

[4] W. Freeman and M. Roth. Orientation histograms for hand gesture recognition. In *International Workshop on Automatic Face- and Gesture-Recognition*, 1995.

[5] J. Garding and T. Lindeberg. Direct computation of shape cues using scale-adapted spatial derivative operators. *Int. J. of Computer Vision*, 17, February 1996.

[6] D.J. Heeger. Optical flow using spatiotemporal filters. *Int. J. of Computer Vision*, 1, 1988.

[7] D. Jones and J. Malik. Computational framework for determining stereo correspondence from a set of linear spatial filters. *Image and Vision Computing*, 10(10), 1992.

[8] M.I. Jordan and R. A. Jacobs. Hierarchical mixtures of experts and the em algorithm. *Neural Computation*, 6(2), March 1994.

[9] J.J. Koenderink. Operational significance of receptive field assemblies. *Biol. Cybern.*, 58:163–171, 1988.

[10] D. Koller, J. Weber, and J. Malik. Robust multiple car tracking with occlusion reasoning. In *Proc. Third European Conference on Computer Vision*, pages 189–196, May 1994.

[11] M. Lades, J.C. Vorbrueggen, J. Buhmann, J. Lange, C. von der Malsburg, and R.P. Wuertz. Distortion invariant object recognition in the dynamic link architecure. In *IEEE Transactions on Computers*, volume 42, 1993.

[12] J. Malik and P. Perona. Preattentive texture discrimination with early vision mechanisms. *J. Opt. Soc. Am. A*, 7(5):923–932, 1990.

[13] H. Murase and S.K. Nayar. Visual learning and recognition of 3-d objects from appearance. *Int. J. Computer Vision*, 14(1):5–24, January 1995.

[14] H.A. Rowley, S. Baluja, and T. Kanade. Human face detection in visual scenes. In *NIPS*, volume 8, 1996.

[15] M. Turk and A. Pentland. Eigenfaces for recognition. *Journal of Cognitive Neuroscience*, 3(1):71–86, 1991.

[16] R.A. Young. The gaussian derivative theory of spatial vision: Analysis of cortical cell receptive field line-weighting profiles. Technical Report GMR-4920, General Motors Research, 1985.

Spatial Decorrelation in Orientation Tuned Cortical Cells

Alexander Dimitrov
Department of Mathematics
University of Chicago
Chicago, IL 60637
a-dimitrov@uchicago.edu

Jack D. Cowan
Department of Mathematics
University of Chicago
Chicago, IL 60637
cowan@math.uchicago.edu

Abstract

In this paper we propose a model for the lateral connectivity of orientation-selective cells in the visual cortex based on information-theoretic considerations. We study the properties of the input signal to the visual cortex and find new statistical structures which have not been processed in the retino-geniculate pathway. Applying the idea that the system optimizes the representation of incoming signals, we derive the lateral connectivity that will achieve this for a set of local orientation-selective patches, as well as the complete spatial structure of a layer of such patches. We compare the results with various physiological measurements.

1 Introduction

In recent years much work has been done on how the structure of the visual system reflects properties of the visual environment (Atick and Redlich 1992; Attneave 1954; Barlow 1989). Based on the statistics of natural scenes compiled and studied by Field (1987) and Ruderman and Bialek (1993), work was done by Atick and Redlich (1992) on the assumption that one of the tasks of early vision is to reduce the redundancy of input signals, the results of which agree qualitatively with numerous physiological and psychophysical experiments. Their ideas were further strengthened by research suggesting the possibility that such structures develop via simple correlation-based learning mechanisms (Atick and Redlich 1993; Dong 1994).

As suggested by Atick and Li (1994), further higher-order redundancy reduction of the luminosity field in the visual processing system is unlikely, since it gives little benefit in information compression. In this paper we apply similar ideas to a different input signal which is readily available to the system and whose statistical properties are lost in the analysis of the luminosity signal. We note that after the application of the retinal "mexican hat" filter the most obvious salient features that are left in images are sharp changes in luminosity, for which the filter is not optimal, i.e. local edges. Such edges have correlations which are very different from the luminosity autocorrelation of natural images (Field 1987), and have zero probability measure in visual scenes, so they are lost in the ensemble averages used to compute the autocorrelation function of natural images. We know that this signal is projected to a set of direction-sensitive units in V1 for each distinct retinal position, thereby introducing new redundancy in the signal. Thus the necessity for compression and use of factorial codes arises once again.

Since local edges are defined by sharp changes in the luminosity field, we can use a derivative operation to pick up the pertinent structure. Indeed, if we look at the gradient of the luminosity as a vector field, its magnitude at a point is proportional to the change of luminosity, so that a large magnitude signals the possible presence of a discontinuity in the luminosity profile. Moreover, in two dimensions, the direction of the gradient vector is perpendicular to the direction of the possible local edge, whose presence is given by the magnitude. These properties define a one-to-one correspondence between large gradients and local edges.

The structure of the network we use reflects what is known about the structure of V1. We select as our system a layer of direction sensitive cells which are laterally connected to one another, each receiving input from the previous layer. We assume that each unit receives as input the directional derivative of the luminosity signal along the preferred visuotopic axis of the cell. This implies that locally the input to a cell is proportional to the cosine of the angle between the unit's preferred direction and the local gradient (edge). Thus each unit receives a broadly tuned signal, with HW-HH approximately $60°$. With this feed-forward structure, the idea that the system is trying to decorrelate its inputs suggests a way to calculate the lateral connections that will perform this task. This calculation, and a further study of the statistical properties of the input is the topic of the paper.

2 Mathematical Model

Let $G(x) = (G_1(x), G_2(x))$ be the gradient of luminosity at x. Assume that there is a set of N detectors with activity O_i at x, each with a preferred direction n_i. Let the input from the previous layer to each detector be the directional derivative along its preferred direction.

$$V_i(x) = |Grad(L(x)).n_i| = |\frac{d}{dn_i}L(x)| \qquad (1)$$

There are long range correlations in the inputs to the network due both to the statistical structure of the natural images and the structure of the input. The simplest of them are captured in the two-point correlation matrix $R_{ij}(x_1, x_2) = < V_i(x_1)V_j(x_2) >$, where the averaging is done across images. Then R is a block matrix, with an $N \times N$ matrix at each spatial position (x_1, x_2).

We formulate the problem in terms of a recurrent kernel W, so that

$$O = V + W * O \qquad (2)$$

The biological interpretation of this is that V is the effective input to V1 from the LGN and W specifies the lateral connectivity in V1. This equation describes the steady state of the linear dynamical system $\dot{O} = -O + W * O + V$. The above recurrent system has a solution for O not an eigenfunction of W in the form $O = (\delta - W)^{-1} * V = K * V$. This suggests that there is an equivalent feed-forward system with a transfer function $K = (\delta - W)^{-1}$ and we can consider only such systems.

The corresponding feed-forward system is a linear system that acts on the input $V(x)$ to produce an output $O(x) = (K \cdot V)(x) \equiv \int K(x,y) \cdot V(y) dy$. If we use Barlow's redundancy reduction hypothesis (Barlow 1989), this filter should decorrelate the output signal. This is achieved by requiring that

$$\begin{aligned} \delta(x_1 - x_2) &\sim\; <O(x_1) \circ O(x_2)> = <(K \cdot V)(x_1) \circ (K \cdot V)(x_2)> \Leftrightarrow \\ \delta(x_1 - x_2) &\sim\; K \cdot R \cdot K^T \end{aligned} \quad (3)$$

The aim then is to solve (3) for K. Obviously, this is equivalent to $K^T \cdot K \sim R^{-1}$ (assuming K and R are non-singular), which has a solution $K \sim R^{-\frac{1}{2}}$, unique up to a unitary transformation. The corresponding recurrent filter is then

$$W = \delta - K^{-1} = \delta - \rho\; R^{\frac{1}{2}} \quad (4)$$

This expression suggests an immediate benefit in the use of lateral kernels by the system. As (4) shows, the filter does not now require inverting the correlation matrix and thus is more stable than a feed-forward filter. This also helps preserve the local structure of the autocorrelator in the optimal filter, while, because of the inversion process, a feed-forward system will in general produce non-local, non-topographic solutions.

To obtain a realistic connectivity structure, we need to explicitly include the effects of noise on the system. The system is then described by $O_1 = V + N_1 + M * W * (O_1 + N_2)$, where N_1 is the input noise and N_2 is the noise, generated by individual units in the recurrently connected layer. Similarly to a feed-forward system (Atick and Redlich 1992), we can modify the decorrelation kernel W derived from (2) to $M * W$. The form of the correction M, which minimizes the effects of noise on the system, is obtained by minimizing the distance between the states of the two systems. If we define $\chi^2(M) = <|O - O_1|^2>$ as the distance function, the solution to $\frac{\partial \chi^2(M)}{\partial M} = 0$ will give us the appropriate kernel. A solution to this problem is

$$M * W = \delta - (R + N_1^2 + N_2^2) * (\rho\; R^{1/2} + N_2^2)^{-1} \quad (5)$$

We see that it has the correct asymptotics as N_1, N_2 approach zero. The filter behaves well for large N_2, turning mostly into a low-pass filter with large attenuation. It cannot handle well large N_1 and reaches $-\infty$ proportionally to N_1^2.

3 Results

3.1 Local Optimal Linear Filter

As a first calculation with this model, consider its implications for the connectivity between units in a single hypercolumn. This allows for a very simple application of the theory and does not require any knowledge of the input signal under very general assumptions.

We assume that direction selective cells receive as input from the previous layer the projection of the gradient onto their preferred direction. Thus they act as directional derivatives, so that their response to a signal with the luminosity profile $L(x)$ and no input from other lateral units is $V_i(x) = |Grad(L(x)).n_i| = |d/dn_i(L(x))|$

With this assumption the outputs of the edge detectors are correlated. Define a (local) correlation matrix $R_{ij} = <V_i V_j>$. By assumption (1), $V_k = |a \, Cos(\alpha - \alpha_k)|$, where a and α are random, independent variables, denoting the magnitude and direction of the local gradient and α_k is the preferred angle of the detector. Assuming spatially isotropic local structure for natural scenes, we can calculate the average of R by integrating over a uniform probability measure in α. Then

$$R_{ij} = A \int_0^\pi |Cos(\alpha - \alpha_i) Cos(\alpha - \alpha_j)| \, d\alpha \qquad (6)$$

where $A = <a^2>$ can be factored because of the assumption of statistical independence. By the homogeneity assumption, R_{ij} is a function of the relative angle $|\alpha_i - \alpha_j|$ only. This allows us to easily calculate the integral in (6) from its Fourier series. Indeed, in Fourier space $\hat{R}$ is just the square of the power spectrum of the underlying signal, i.e., $\cos(\alpha)$ on $[0, \pi]$. Thus we obtain the form of R analytically.

Knowing the local correlations, we can find a recurrent linear filter which decorrelates the outputs after it is applied. This filter is $W = \delta - \rho \, R^{-\frac{1}{2}}$ (Sec.2), unique up to a unitary transformation.

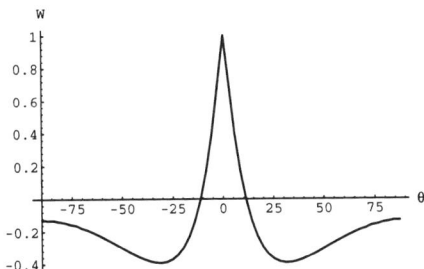

Figure 1: Local recurrent filter in the presence of noise. The connection strength W depends only on the relative angle θ between units.

If we include noise in the calculation according to (5), we obtain a filter which depends on the signal to noise ratio of the input level. We model the noise process here as a set of independent noise processes for each unit, with $(N_1)_i$ being the input noise and $(N_2)_i$ the output noise for unit i. All noise processes are assumed statistically independent. The result for $S/N_2 \sim 3$ is shown on Fig.1. We observe the broadening of the central connections, caused by the need to average local results in order to overcome the noise. It was calculated at very low N_1 level, since, as mentioned in Section 2, the filter is unstable with respect to input noise.

With this filter we can directly compare calculations obtained from applying it to a specific input signal, with physiological measurements of the orientation selectivity of cells in the cortex. The results of such comparisons are presented in Fig.2, in which we plot the activity of orientation selective cells in arbitrary units vs stimulus angle in degrees. We see very good matches with experimental results of Celebrini, Thorpe, Trotter, and Imbert (1993), Schiller, Finlay, and Volman (1976) and Orban (1984). We expect some discrepancies, such as in Figures 2.D and 2.F, which can be attributed to the threshold nature of real neural units. We see that we can use the model to classify physiologically distinct cells by the value of the N_2 parameter that describes them. Indeed, since this parameter models the intrinsic noise of a neural unit, we expect it to differ across populations.

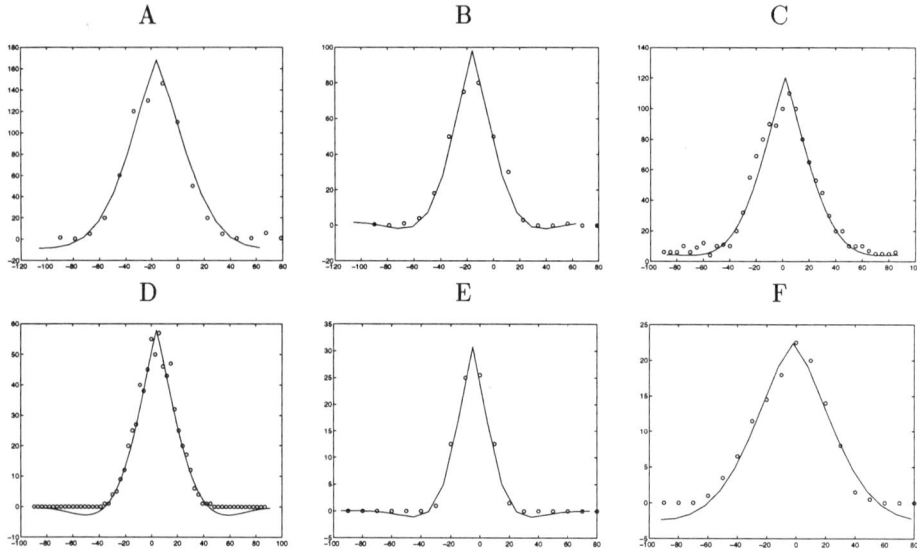

Figure 2: Comparison with experimental data. The activity of orientation selective cells in arbitrary units is plotted against stimulus angle in degrees. Experimental points are denoted with circles, calculated result with a solid line. The variation in the forms of the tuning curves could be accounted for by selecting different noise levels in our noise model. A - data from cell CAJ4 in Celebrini et.al. and fit for $N_1 = 0.1, N_2 = 0.2$. B - data from cell CAK2 in Celebrini et.al. and fit for $N_1 = 0.35, N_2 = 0.1$. C - data from a complex cell from Orban and fit for $N_1 = 0.3, N_2 = 0.45$. D - data from a simple cell from Orban and fit for $N_1 = 1.0, N_2 = 0.45$. E - data from a simple cells in Schiller et.al. and fit for $N_1 = 0.06, N_2 = 0.001$. F - data from a simple cells in Schiller et.al. and fit for $N_1 = 15.0, N_2 = 0.01$.

3.2 Non-Local Optimal Filter

We can perform a similar analysis of the non-local structure of natural images to design a non-local optimal filter. This time we have a set of detectors $V_k(x) = |a(x) \ Cos(\alpha(x) - k \ \pi/N)|$ and a correlation function $R_{ij}(x,y) =< V_i(x) \ V_j(y) >$, averaged over natural scenes. We assume that the function is spatially translation invariant and can be represented as $R_{ij}(x,y) = R_{ij}(x-y)$. The averaging was done over a set of about 100 different pictures, with 10-20 256^2 samples taken from each picture.

The structure of the correlation matrix depends both on the autocorrelator of the gradient field and the structure of the detectors, which are correlated. Obviously the fact that the output units compute $|a(x) \ Cos(\alpha(x) - k\pi/N)|$ creates many local correlations between neighboring units. Any non-local structure in the detector set is due to a similar structure, present in the gradient field autocorrelator.

The structure of the translation-invariant correlation matrix $R(x)$ is shown in Fig.3A. This can be interpreted as the correlation between the input to the center hypercolumn with the input to rest of the hypercolumns. The result of the complete model (5) can be seen in Fig.3B. Since the filter is also assumed to be translation invariant, the pictures can be interpreted as the connectivity of the center hypercolumn with the rest of the network. This is seen to be concentrated near the diagonal,

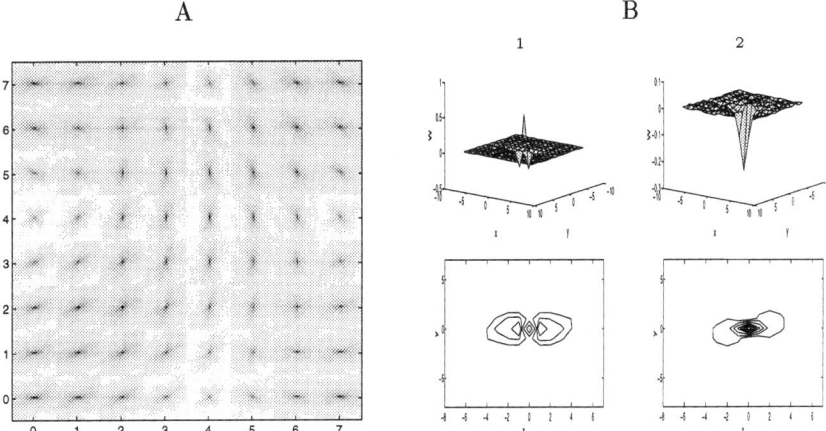

Figure 3: **A.** The autocorrelation function of a set with 8 detectors. Dark represents high correlation, light - low correlation. The sets are indexed by the preferred angles θ_i, θ_j in units of $\frac{\pi}{8}$ and each R_{ij} has spatial structure, which is represented as a 32×32 square. **B.** The lateral connectivity for the central horizontal selective unit with neighboring horizontal (1) and $\pi/4$ (2) selective units. Note the anisotropic connectivity and the rotation of the connectivity axis on the second picture.

and weak in the two adjacent bands, which represent connections to edge detectors with a perpendicular preferred direction. The noise minimizing filter is a low pass filter, as expected, and thus decreases the high frequency component of the power spectrum of the respective decorrelating filter.

4 Conclusions and Discussion

We have shown that properties of orientation selective cells in the visual cortex can be partially described by some very simple linear systems analysis. Using this we obtain results which are in very good agreement with physiological and anatomical data of single-cell recordings and imaging. We can use the parameters of the model to classify functionally and structurally differing cells in the visual cortex.

We achieved this by using a recurrent network as the underlying model. This was chosen for several reasons. One is that we tried to give the model biological plausibility and recurrency is well established on the cortical level. Another related heuristic argument is that although there exists a feed-forward network with equivalent properties, as shown in Section 2, such a network will require an additional layer of cells, while the recurrent model allows both for feed-forward processing (the input to our model) as well as manipulation of the output of that (the decorrelation procedure in our model). Finally, while a feed-forward network needs large weights to amplify the signal, a recurrent network is able to achieve very high gains on the input signal with relatively small weights by utilizing special architecture. As can be seen from our equivalence model, $K = (\delta - W)^{-1}$, so if W is so constructed as to have an eigenvalues close to 1, it will produce enormous amplification.

Our work is based on previous suggestions relating the structure of the visual environment to the structure of the visual pathway. It was thought before (Atick and Li 1994) that this particular relation can describe only early visual pathways, but is insufficient to account for the structure of the striate cortex. We show here that redundancy reduction is still sufficient to describe many of the complexities of the visual cortex, thus strengthening the possibility that this is a basic building principle for the visual system and one should anticipate its appearance in later regions of the latter.

What is even more intriguing is the possibility that this method can account for the structure of other sensory pathways and cortices. We know e.g. that the somatosensory pathway and cortex are similar to the visual ones, because of the similar environments that they encounter (luminosity, edges and textures have analogies in somesthesia). Similar analogies may be expected for the auditory pathway.

We expect even better results if we consider a more realistic non-linear model for the neural units. In fact this improves tremendously the information-processing abilities of a bounded system, since it captures higher order correlations in the signal and allows for true minimization of the mutual information in the system, rather than just decorrelating. Very promising results in this direction have been recently described by Bell and Sejnowski (1996) and Lin and Cowan (1997) and we intend to consider the implications for our model.

Acknowledgements

Supported in part by Grant # 96-24 from the James S. McDonnell Foundation.

References

Atick, J. J. and Z. Li (1994). Towards a theory of the striate cortex. *Neural Computation 6*, 127–146.

Atick, J. J. and N. N. Redlich (1992). What does the retina know about natural scenes? *Neural Computation 4*, 196–210.

Atick, J. J. and N. N. Redlich (1993). Convergent algorithm for sensory receptive field developement. *Neural Computation 5*, 45–60.

Attneave, F. (1954). Some informational aspects of visual perception. *Psychological Review 61*, 183–193.

Barlow, H. B. (1989). Unsupervised learning. *Neural Computation 1*, 295–311.

Bell, A. T. and T. J. Sejnowski (1996). The "independent components" of natural scences are edge filters. *Vision Research* (submitted).

Celebrini, S., S. Thorpe, Y. Trotter, and M. Imbert (1993). Dynamics of orientation coding in area V1 of the awake primate. *Visual Neuroscience 10*, 811–825.

Dong, D. (1994). Associative decorrelation dynamics: a theory of self-organization and optimization in feedback networks. Volume 7 of *Advances in Neural Information Processing Systems*, pp. 925–932. The MIT Press.

Field, D. J. (1987). Relations between the statistics of natural images and the response properties of cortical cells. *J. Opt. Soc. Am. 4*, 2379–2394.

Lin, J. K. and J. D. Cowan (1997). Faithful representation of separable input distributions. *Neural Computation*, (to appear).

Orban, G. A. (1984). *Neuronal Operations in the Visual Cortex*. Springer-Verlag, Berlin.

Ruderman, D. L. and W. Bialek (1993). Statistics of natural images: Scaling in the woods. In J. D. Cowan, G. Tesauro, and J. Alspector (Eds.), *Advances in Neural Information Processing Systems*, Volume 6. Morgan Kaufman, San Mateo, CA.

Schiller, P., B. Finlay, and S. Volman (1976). Quantitative studies of single-cell properties in monkey striate cortex. II. Orientation specificity and ocular dominance. *J. Neuroph. 39*(6), 1320–1333.

Spatiotemporal Coupling and Scaling of Natural Images and Human Visual Sensitivities

Dawei W. Dong

California Institute of Technology
Mail Code 139-74
Pasadena, CA 91125

dawei@hope.caltech.edu

Abstract

We study the spatiotemporal correlation in natural time-varying images and explore the hypothesis that the visual system is concerned with the optimal coding of visual representation through spatiotemporal decorrelation of the input signal. Based on the measured spatiotemporal power spectrum, the transform needed to decorrelate input signal is derived analytically and then compared with the actual processing observed in psychophysical experiments.

1 Introduction

The visual system is concerned with the perception of objects in a dynamic world. A significant fact about natural time-varying images is that they do not change randomly over space-time; instead image intensities at different times and/or spatial positions are highly correlated. We measured the spatiotemporal correlation function – equivalently the power spectrum – of natural images and we find that it is non-separable, i.e., coupled in space and time, and exhibits a very interesting scaling behaviour. When expressed as a function of an appropriately scaled frequency variable, the spatiotemporal power spectrum is given by a simple power-law. We point out that the same kind of spatiotemporal coupling and scaling exists in human visual sensitivity measured in psychophysical experiments. This poses the intriguing question of whether there is a quantitative relationship between the power spectrum of natural images and visual sensitivity. We answer this question by showing that the latter can be predicted from measurements of the power spectrum.

2 Spatiotemporal Coupling and Scaling

Interest in properties of time-varying images dates back to the early days of development of the television [1]. But systematic studies have not been possible previously primarily due to technical obstacles, and our knowledge of the regularities of time-varying images has so far been very limited.

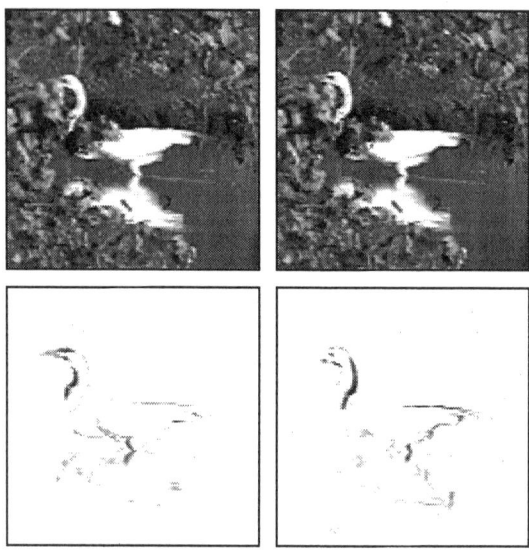

Figure 1: Natural time-varying images are highly correlated in space and time. Shown on the top are two frames of a motion scene separated by thirty three milliseconds. These two frames are highly repetitive, in fact the light intensities of most corresponding pixels are similar. Shown on the bottom are light increase (on the left) and light decrease (on the right) between the above two snapshots indicated by greyscale of pixels (white means no change). One can immediately see that only a small portion of the image changes significantly over this time scale. Our methods have been described previously [3]. To summarize, more than one thousand segments of videos on 8mm video tape (NTSC format RGB) are digitized to 8 bits greyscale using a Silicon Graphics Video board with default factory settings. Two types of segments are analyzed. The first are segments from movies on video tapes (e.g. "Raiders of the Lost Ark", "Uncommon Valor"). The second type of segments that we analyzed are videos made by the authors. The scene of the moving egret shown here is taken at Central Park in New York City.

We have systematically measured the two point correlation matrix or covariance matrix of $10°\times10°\times2s$ (horizontal×vertical×temporal digitized to $64\times64\times64$) segments of natural time-varying images by averaging over 1049 movie segments. An example of two consecutive frames from a typical segment is given in Figure 1. The Fourier transform of the correlation matrix, or the power spectrum, turns out to be a non-separable function of spatial and temporal frequencies and exhibits an interesting scaling behaviour. From our measurements (see Figure 2) we find

$$R(f, w) = R(f_w)$$

where f_w is a scaled frequency which is simply the spatial frequency f scaled by $G(w/f)$, a function of the ratio of temporal and spatial frequencies, i.e., $f_w = G(w/f)f$. This behaviour is revealed most clearly by plotting the power spectrum as a function of f for fixed w/f ratio: the curves for different w/f ratios are just a horizontal shift from each other.

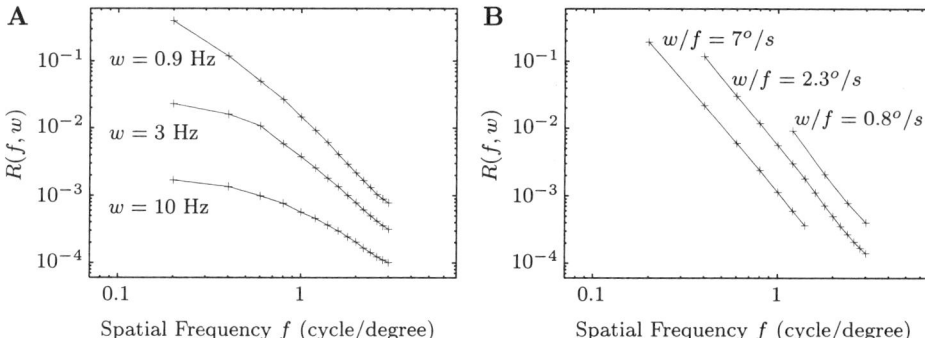

Figure 2: Spatiotemporal power spectra of natural time-varying images. (**A**) plotted as a function of spatial frequency for three temporal frequencies (0.9, 3, 10) Hz; (**B**) plotted for three velocities — ratios of temporal and spatial frequencies — (0.8, 2.3, 7) degree/second. There are some important conclusions that can be drawn from this measurement. First, it is obvious that the power spectrum cannot be separated into pure spatial and pure temporal parts; space and time are coupled in a non-trivial way. The power spectrum at low temporal frequency decreases more rapidly with increasing spatial frequency. Second, underlying this data is an interesting scaling behaviour which can be easily seen from the curves for constant w/f ratios: each curve is simply shifted horizontally from each other in the log-log plot. Thus curves for constant w/f ratio overlap with each other when shifted by an amount of $G(w/f)$, i.e., when plotted against a scaled frequency $f_w = G(w/f)f$. The similar spatio-temporal coupling and scaling for hunam visual sensitivity is shown in Figure 3.

Interestingly, the human visual system seems to be designed to take advantage of such regularity in natural images. The spatiotemporal contrast sensitivity of human $K(f, w)$, i.e., the visual responses to a sinewave grating of spatial frequency f modulated at temporal frequency w, exhibits the same kind of spatiotemporal coupling and scaling (see Figure 3),

$$K(f, w) = K(f_w).$$

Again, when the contrast sensitivity curves are plotted as a function of f for fixed w/f ratios, the curves have the same shape and are only shifted from each other [2].

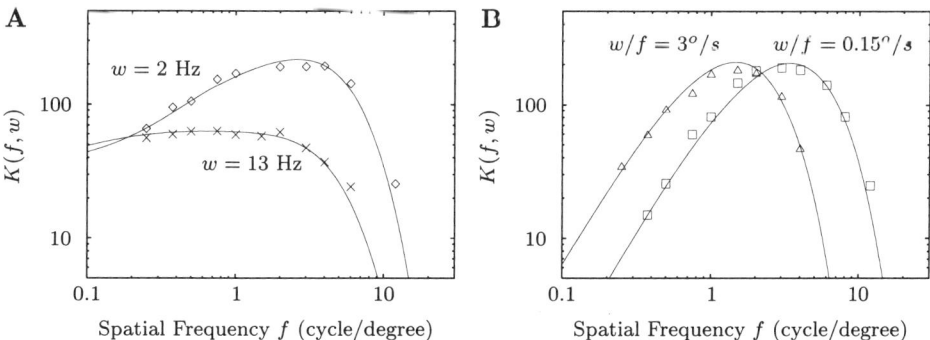

Figure 3: Spatiotemporal contrast sensitivities of human vision. (**A**) plotted as a function of spatial frequency for two temporal frequencies (2, 13) Hz; (**B**) plotted for two w/f ratios (0.15, 3) degree/second. The solid lines in both A and B are the empirical fits. The experimental data points and empirical fitting curves are from reference [2]. First, it can be seen that the human visual sensitivity curve is band-pass filter at low temporal frequency and approaches low-pass filter for higher temporal frequency. The space and time are coupled. Second, it is clear that the curves for different w/f ratios have the same shape and are only shifted horizontally from each other in the log-log plot. Again, curves for constant w/f ratio overlap with each other when shifted by an amount of $G(w/f)$, i.e., when plotted against a scaled frequency $f_w = G(w/f)f$. The similar behaviour of spatiotemporal coupling and scaling for the power spectra of natural images is shown in Figure 2.

3 Relative Motion of Visual Scene

Why does the human visual sensitivity have the same spatiotemporal coupling and scaling as natural images?

The intuition underlying the spatiotemporal coupling and scaling of natural images is that when viewing a real visual scene the natural eye and/or body movements translate the entire scene across the retina and every spatial Fourier component of the scene moves at the same velocity. Thus it is reasonable to assume that for constant velocity, i.e., w/f ratio, the power spectrum show the same universal behaviour. This assumption is tested quantitatively in the following.

Our measurements reveal that the spatiotemporal power spectrum has a simple form
$$R(f_w) \sim f_w^{-3}$$
which is shown in Figure 6A. This behaviour can be accounted for if the dominant component in the temporal signal comes from motion of objects with static power spectra of $R_s(f) \sim f^{-2}$. The static power spectra for the same collection of images is measured by treating frames as snapshots (Figure 4A); the measurement confirmed the above assumption and is in agreement with earlier works on the statistical properties of static natural images [5, 6, 7].

It is easy to derive that for a rotationally symmetric static spectrum $R_s(f) = K/f^2$ (K is a constant), the spatiotemporal power spectrum of moving images is

$$R(f, w) = \frac{K}{f^3} P(\frac{w}{f}), \tag{1}$$

where $P(\frac{w}{f})$ is the function of velocity distribution, which is shown as the solid curve in Figure 4B (measured independently from the optical flows between frames).

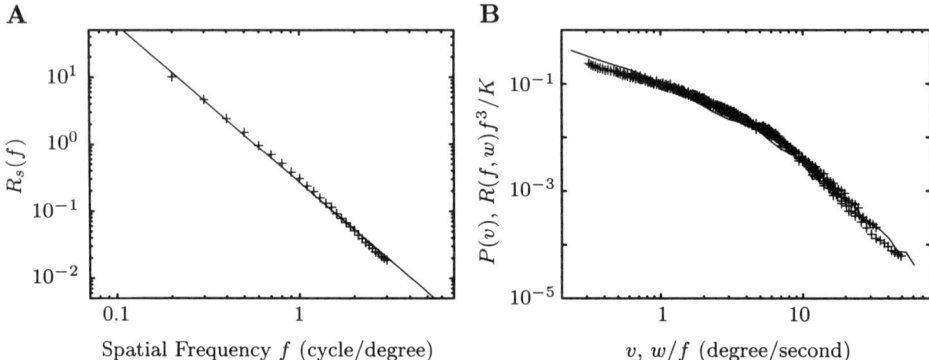

Figure 4: Spatial power spectrum and velocity distribution. (**A**) the measured spatial power spectrum of snap shot images, which shows that $R_s(f) \sim K/f^2$ is a good approximation to the spectrum; (**B**) the measured velocity distribution $P(v)$ (solid curve), in which the data of Figure 2 for the power spectrum were replotted as a function of w/f after multiplication by f^3 — all the data points fall on the $P(v)$ curve.

In summary, the measured spatiotemporal power spectrum is dominated by images of spatial power spectrum $\sim 1/f^2$ moving with a velocity distribution $P(v) \sim 1/(v + v_0)^2$ (similar velocity distribution has been proposed earlier [8, 3] . Thus $R(f, w) = K/f^3(w/f + v_0)^2$ and $G(w/f) \sim (w/f + v_0)^{2/3}$.

Based on the assumption that the visual system is optimized to transmit information from natural scenes, we have derived and pointed out in references [3, 4] that the spatiotemporal contrast sensitivity K is a function of the power spectrum R, and thus the spatiotemporal coupling and scaling of R of natural images translates directly to the spatiotemporal coupling and scaling of K of visual sensitivity i.e., R is a function of f_w only, so is K.

4 Spatiotemporal Decorrelation

The theory of spatiotemporal decorrelation is based on ideas of optimal coding from information theory: decorrelation of inputs to make statistically independent representations when signal is strong and smoothing where noise is significant. The end result is that by chosing the correct degree of decorrelation the signal is compressed by elimination of what is irrelevant without significant loss of information.

The following relationship can be derived for the visual sensitivity K and the power spectrum R in the presence of noise power N:

$$K = R^{-1/2}(1 + N/R)^{-3/2}$$

The figure below illustrates the predicted filter for the case of white noise (constant N).

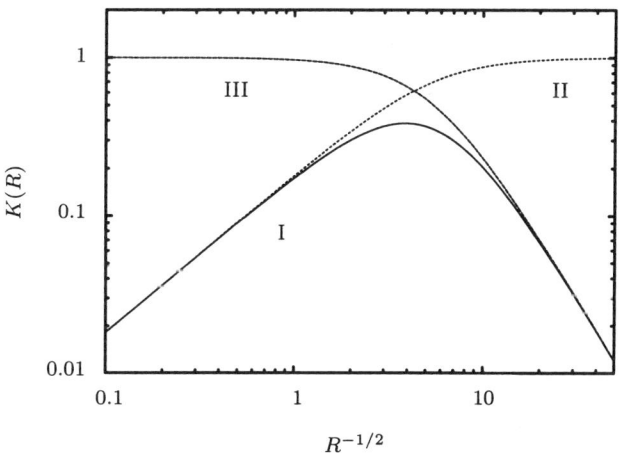

Figure 5: Predicted optimal filter (curve I): in the low noise regime, it is given by whitening filter $R^{-1/2}$ (curve II), which achieves spatiotemporal decorrelation; while at high noise regime it asymptotes the low-pass filter (curve III) which suppresses noise.

As shown in Figure 6, the relation between the contrast sensitivity and the power spectrum predicts

$$K(f_w) \sim \left(\frac{f_w}{1 + Nf_w^3}\right)^{\frac{3}{2}}$$

in which N is the power of the white noise. This prediction is compared with psychophysical data in Figure 6B where we have used the scaling function $G(w/f) = (w/f + v_0)^{2/3}$ which has the same asymptotic behaviour as we have shown for the natural time-varying images [3]. We find that for $v_0 = 1$ degree/second, the human contrast sensitivity curves for w/f from 0.1 to 4 degree/second, measured in reference [2], overlap very well with the theoretical prediction from the power spectrum of our measurements.

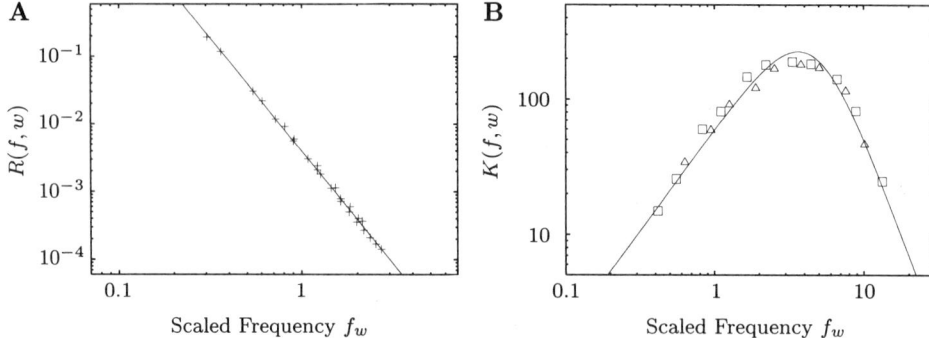

Figure 6: Relation between the power spectrum of natural images and the human visual sensitivities. (**A**) the measured spatiotemporal power spectrum (Figure 2B) replotted as a function of the scaled frequency can be fit very well by $R \sim f_w^{-3}$ (solid line); (**B**) the spatiotemporal contrast sensitivities of human vision (Figure 3B) replotted as a function of the scaled frequency can be fit very well by our theoretical prediction (solid line). Our theory on the relation between the visual sensitivity K and the power spectrum of natural time-varying images R in the presence of noise power N has been described in detail in reference [4]. To summarize, the visual sensitivity in Fourier space is simply $K = R^{-1/2}(1 + N/R)^{-3/2}$. In a linear system, this is proportional to the visual response to a sinewave of spatial frequency f modulated at temporal frequency w, i.e., the contrast sensitivity curves shown in Figure 3. In the case of white noise, i.e., N is independent of f and w, K depends on f and w through the power spectrum R. Since R is a function of the scaled frequency f_w only, so is K. From our measurement $R \sim f_w^3$, thus $K \sim f_w^{3/2}(1 + Nf_w^3)^{-3/2}$. This curve is plotted in the figure as the solid line with $N = 0.01$. The agreement is very good.

5 Conclusions and Discussions

A simple relationship is revealed between the statistical structure of natural time-varying images and the spatiotemporal sensitivity of human vision. The existence of this relationship supports the hypothesis that visual processing is optimized to compress as much information as possible about the outside world into the limited dynamic range of the visual channels.

We should point out that this scaling behaviour is expected to break down for very high temporal and spatial frequency where the effect of the temporal and spatial modulation function of the eye [9, 10] cannot be ignored.

Finally while our predictions show that, in general, the human visual sensitivity is strongly space-time coupled, we do predict a regime where decoupling is a good approximation. This is based on the fact that in the regime of relatively high temporal frequency and relatively low spatial frequency we find that the power spectrum of natural images is separable into spatial and temporal parts [3]. In a previous work we have used this decoupling to model response properties of cat LGN cells where we have shown that these can be accounted for by the theoretical prediction based on the power spectrum in that regime [4].

Acknowledgements

The author gratefully acknowledges the discussions with Dr. Joseph Atick.

References

[1] Kretzmer ER, 1952. Statistics of television signals. The bell system technical journal. 751-763.

[2] Kelly DH, 1979 Motion and vision. II. Stabilized spatio-temporal threshold surface. J. Opt. Soc. Am. 69, 1340-1349.

[3] Dong DW, Atick JJ, 1995 Statistics of natural time-varying images. Network: Computation in Neural Systems, 6, 345-358.

[4] Dong DW, Atick JJ, 1995 Temporal decorrelation: a theory of lagged and nonlagged responses in the lateral geniculate nucleus. Network: Computation in Neural Systems, 6, 159-178.

[5] Burton GJ, Moorhead IR, 1987. Color and spatial structure in natural scenes. Applied Optics. 26(1): 157-170.

[6] Field DJ, 1987. Relations between the statistics of natural images and the response properties of cortical cells.. J. Opt. Soc. Am. A 4: 2379-2394.

[7] Ruderman DL, Bialek W, 1994. Statistics of natural images: scaling in the woods. Phy. Rev. Let. 73(6): 814-817.

[8] Van Hateren JH, 1993. Spatiotemporal Contrast sensitivity of early vision. Vision Res. 33(2): 257-267.

[9] Campbell FW, Gubisch RW, 1966. Optical quality of the human eye. J. Physiol. 186: 558-578.

[10] Schnapf JL, Baylor DA, 1987. How photoreceptor cells respond to light. Scientific American 256(4): 40-47.

Selective Integration: A Model for Disparity Estimation

Michael S. Gray, Alexandre Pouget, Richard S. Zemel,
Steven J. Nowlan, Terrence J. Sejnowski
Departments of Biology and Cognitive Science
University of California, San Diego
La Jolla, CA 92093
and
Howard Hughes Medical Institute
Computational Neurobiology Lab
The Salk Institute, P. O. Box 85800
San Diego, CA 92186-5800
Email: michael, alex, zemel, nowlan, terry@salk.edu

Abstract

Local disparity information is often sparse and noisy, which creates two conflicting demands when estimating disparity in an image region: the need to spatially average to get an accurate estimate, and the problem of not averaging over discontinuities. We have developed a network model of disparity estimation based on disparity-selective neurons, such as those found in the early stages of processing in visual cortex. The model can accurately estimate multiple disparities in a region, which may be caused by transparency or occlusion, in real images and random-dot stereograms. The use of a selection mechanism to selectively integrate reliable local disparity estimates results in superior performance compared to standard back-propagation and cross-correlation approaches. In addition, the representations learned with this selection mechanism are consistent with recent neurophysiological results of von der Heydt, Zhou, Friedman, and Poggio [8] for cells in cortical visual area V2. Combining multi-scale biologically-plausible image processing with the power of the mixture-of-experts learning algorithm represents a promising approach that yields both high performance and new insights into visual system function.

1 INTRODUCTION

In many stereo algorithms, the local correlation between images from the two eyes is used to estimate relative depth (Jain, Kasturi, & Schunk [5]). Local correlation measures, however, convey no information about the reliability of a particular disparity measurement. In the model presented here, we introduce a separate *selection* mechanism to determine which locations of the visual input have consistent disparity information. The focus was on several challenging viewing situations in which disparity estimation is not straightforward. For example, can the model estimate the disparity of more than one object in a scene? Does occlusion lead to poorer disparity estimation? Can the model determine the disparities of two transparent surfaces? Does the model estimate accurately the disparities present in real world images? Datasets corresponding to these different conditions were generated and used to test the model.

Our goal is to develop a neurobiologically plausible model of stereopsis that accurately estimates disparity. Compared to traditional cross-correlation approaches that try to compute a depth map for all locations in space, the mixture-of-experts model used here searches for sparse, reliable patterns or configurations of disparity stimuli that provide evidence for objects at different depths. This allows partial segmentation of the image to obtain a more compact representation of disparities. Local disparity estimates are sufficient in this case, as long as we selectively segment those regions of the image with reliable disparity information.

The rest of the paper is organized as follows. First, we describe the architecture of the mixture-of-experts model. Second, we provide a brief qualitative description of the model's performance followed by quantitative results on a variety of datasets. In the third section, we compare the activity of units in the model to recent neurophysiological data. Finally, we discuss these findings, and consider remaining open questions.

2 MIXTURE-OF-EXPERTS MODEL

The model of stereopsis that we have explored is based on the filter model for motion detection devised by Nowlan and Sejnowski [6]. The motion problem was readily adapted to stereopsis by changing the time domain of motion to the left/right image domain for stereopsis. Our model (Figure 1) consisted of several stages and computed its output using only feed-forward processing, as described below (see also Gray, Pouget, Zemel, Nowlan, and Sejnowski [2] for more detail). The output of the first stage (disparity energy filters) became the input to two different primary pathways: (1) the local disparity networks, and (2) the selection networks. The activation of each of the four disparity-tuned output units in the model was the product of the outputs of the two primary pathways (summed across space). An objective function based on the mixture-of-experts framework (Jacobs, Jordan, Nowlan, & Hinton [4]) was used to optimize the weights from the disparity energy units to the local disparity networks and to the selection networks. The weights to the output units from the local disparity and selection pathways were fixed at 1.0. Once the model was trained, we obtained a scalar disparity estimate from the model by computing a nonlinear least squares Gaussian fit to the four output values. The mean of the Gaussian was our disparity estimate. When two objects were present

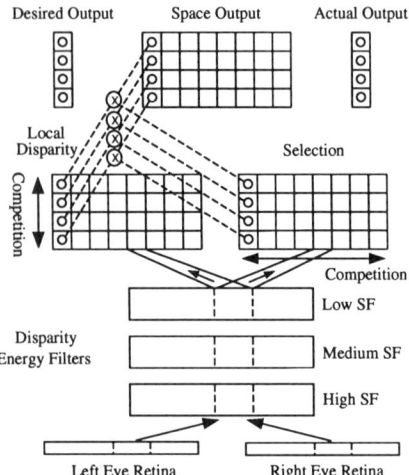

Figure 1: The mixture-of-experts architecture.

in the input, we fit the sum of two Gaussians to the four output values.

2.1 DISPARITY ENERGY FILTERS

The retinal layer in the model consisted of one-dimensional right eye and left eye images, each 82 pixels in length. These images were the input to disparity energy filters, as developed by Ohzawa, DeAngelis, and Freeman [7]. At the energy filter layer, there were 51 receptive field (RF) locations which received input from partially overlapping regions of the retinae. At each of these RF locations, there were 30 energy units corresponding to 10 phase differences at 3 spatial frequencies. These phase differences were proportional to disparity. An energy unit consisted of 4 energy filter pairs, each of which was a Gabor filter. The outputs of the disparity energy units were normalized at each RF location and within each spatial frequency using a soft-max nonlinearity.

2.2 LOCAL DISPARITY NETWORKS

In the local disparity pathway, there were 8 RF locations, and each received a weighted input from 9 disparity energy locations. Each RF location corresponded to a local disparity network and contained a pool of 4 disparity-tuned units. Neighboring locations received input from overlapping sets of disparity energy units. Weights were shared across all RF locations for each disparity. Soft-max competition occurred *within* each local disparity network (across disparity), and insured that only one disparity was strongly activated at each RF location.

2.3 SELECTION NETWORKS

Like the local disparity networks, the selection networks were organized into a grid of 8 RF locations with a pool of 4 disparity-tuned units at each location. These 4 units represented the local support for each of the different disparity hypotheses. It is more useful to think of the selection networks, however, as 4 separate layers each of which responded to a specific disparity across all regions of the image. Like the local disparity pathway, neighboring RF locations received input from overlapping disparity energy units, and weights were shared across space for each disparity. In addition, the outputs of the selection network were normalized with the softmax operation. This competition, however, occurred separately for each of the 4 disparities in a global fashion *across space*.

3 RESULTS

Figure 2 shows the pattern of activations in the model when presented with a single object at a disparity of 2.1 pixels. The visual layout of the model in this figure is identical to the layout in Figure 1. The stimulus appears at bottom, with the 3 disparity energy filter banks directly above it. On the left above the disparity energy filters are the local disparity networks. The selection networks are on the right. The summed output (across space) appears in the upper right corner of the figure. Note that the selection network for a 2 pixel disparity (2nd row from the bottom in the selection pathway) is active for the spatial location at far left. The corresponding location is also highly active in the local disparity pathway, and this combination leads to strong activation for a 2 pixel disparity in the output of the model.

The mixture-of-experts model was optimized individually on a variety of different datasets and then tested on novel stimuli from the same datasets. The model's ability to discriminate among different disparities was quantified as the disparity threshold — the disparity difference at which one can correctly see a difference in depth 75% of the time. Disparity thresholds for the test stimuli were computed using signal-detection theory (Green & Swets [3]). Sample stimuli and their disparity thresholds are shown in Table 1. The model performed best on single object stimuli (top row). This disparity threshold (0.23 pixels) was substantially less than the input resolution of the model (1 pixel) and was thus exhibiting stereo hyperacuity. The model also performed well when there were multiple, occluding objects (2nd row). When both the stimulus and the background were generated from a uniform random distribution, the disparity threshold rose to 0.55 pixels. The model estimated disparity accurately in random-dot stereograms and real world images. Binary stereograms containing two transparent surfaces, however, were a challenging stimulus, and the threshold rose to 0.83 pixels. Part of the difficulty with this stimulus (containing two objects) was fitting the sum of 2 Gaussians to 4 data points.

We have compared our mixture-of-experts model (containing both a selection pathway and a local disparity pathway) with standard backpropagation and cross-correlation techniques (Gray et al [2]). The primary difference is that the back-propagation and cross-correlation models have no separate selection mechanism. In essence, one mechanism must compute both the segmentation and the disparity estimation. In our tests with the back-propagation model, we found that disparity thresholds for single object stimuli had risen by a factor of 3 (to 0.74 pixels) compared to the mixture-of-experts model. Disparity estimation of the cross-correlation model was similarly poor. Thresholds rose by a factor of 2 (compared to the mixture-of-experts model) for both single object stimuli and the noise stimuli (threshold = 0.46, 1.28 pixels, respectively).

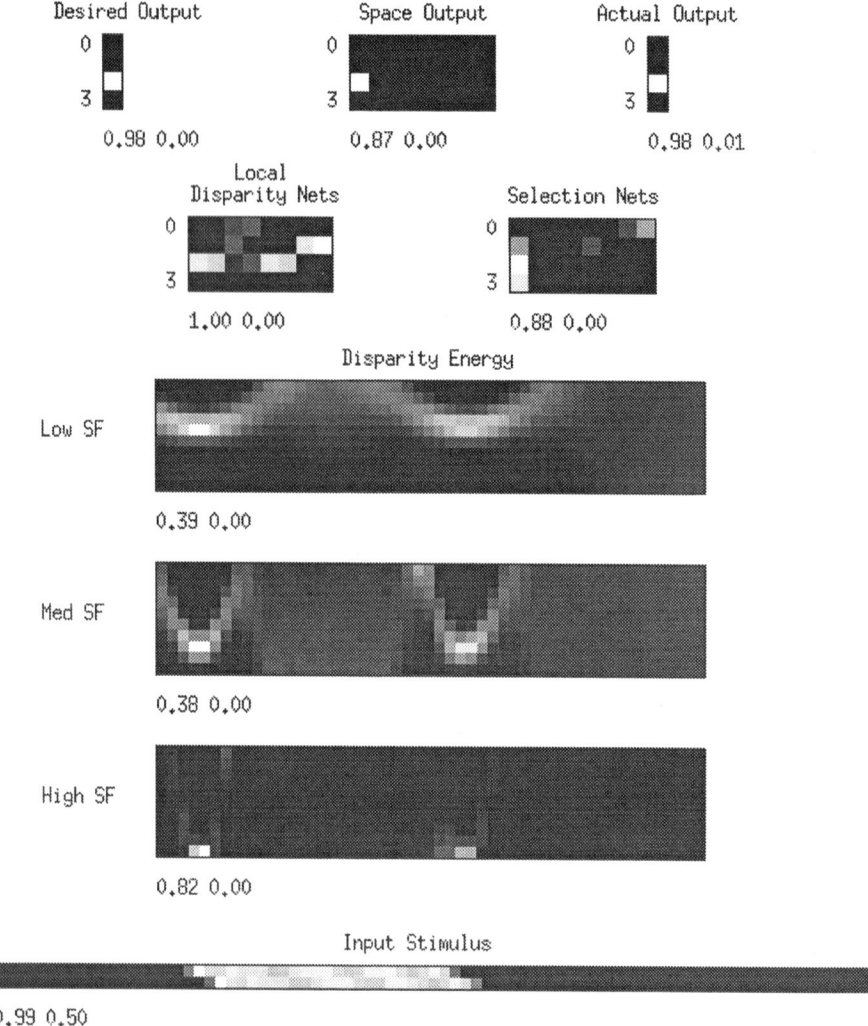

Figure 2: The activity in the mixture-of-experts model in response to an input stimulus containing a single object at a disparity of 2.10 pixels. At bottom is the input stimulus. The 3 regions in the middle represent the output of the disparity energy filters. Above the disparity energy output are the two pathways of the model. The local disparity networks appear to the left and the selection networks are to the right. Both the local disparity networks and the selection networks receive topographically organized input from the disparity energy filters. The selection and local disparity networks are displayed so that the top row represents a disparity of 0 pixels, the next row a 1 pixel disparity, then 2 and 3 pixel disparities in the remaining rows. At the top left part of the figure is the desired output for the given input stimulus. In the top middle is the output for each local region of space. On the top right is the actual output of the model collapsed across space. The numbers at the bottom left of each part of the network indicate the maximum and minimum activation values within that part. White indicates maximum activation level, black is minimum.

Stimulus Type	Sample Stimulus	Threshold
Single		0.23
Double		0.41
Noise		0.55
Random-Dot		0.36
Transparent		0.83
Real		0.30

Table 1: Sample stimuli for each of the datasets, and corresponding disparity thresholds (in pixels) for the mixture-of-experts model.

4 COMPARISON WITH NEUROPHYSIOLOGICAL DATA

To gain insight into the response properties of the selection units in our model, we mapped their activations as a function of space and disparity. Specifically, we measured the activation of a unit as a single high-contrast edge was moved across the spatial extent of the receptive field. At each spatial location, we tested all possible disparities. An example of this mapping is shown in Figure 3. This selection unit is sensitive to changes in disparity as we move across space. We refer to this property as *disparity contrast*. In other words, the selection unit learned that a reliable indicator for a given disparity is a change in disparity across space. This type of detector can be behaviorally significant, because disparity contrast may play a role in signaling object boundaries. These selection units could thus provide valuable information in the construction of a 3D model of the world. Recent neurophysiological studies by von der Heydt, Zhou, Friedman, and Poggio [8] is consistent with this interpretation. They found that neurons of awake, behaving monkeys in area V2 responded to edges of 4° by 4° random-dot stereograms. Because random-dot stereograms have no monocular form cues, these neurons must be responding to edges in depth. This sensitivity to edges in a depth map corresponds directly to the response profile of the selection units.

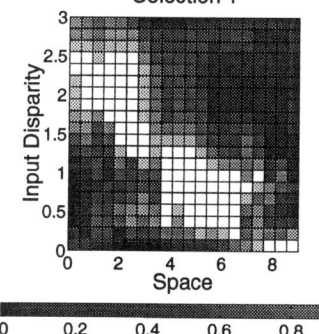

Figure 3: Selection unit activity

5 DISCUSSION

A major difficulty in estimating the disparities of objects in a visual scene in realistic circumstances (i.e., with clutter, transparency, occlusion, noise) is knowing which cues are most reliable and should be integrated, and which regions have ambiguous or unreliable information. Nowlan and Sejnowski [6] found that selection units learned to respond strongly to image regions that contained motion energy in several different directions. The role of those selection units is similar to layered analysis techniques for computing support maps in the motion domain (Darrell & Pentland [1]). The operation of the dual pathways in our model bears some similarities to the pathways developed in the motion model of Nowlan and Sejnowski [6]. In the stereo domain, we have found that our selection units develop into edge detectors on a disparity map. They thus responded to regions rich in disparity information, analogous to the salient motion information captured in the motion [6] selection units.

We have also found that the model matches psychophysical data recorded by Westheimer and McKee [9] on the effects of spatial frequency filtering on disparity thresholds (Gray et al [2]). They found, in human psychophysical experiments, that disparity thresholds increased for any kind of spatial frequency filtering of line targets. In particular, disparity sensitivity was more adversely affected by high-pass filtering than by low-pass filtering.

In summary, we propose that the functional division into *local response* and *selection* represents a general principle for image interpretation and analysis that may be applicable to many different visual cues, and also to other sensory domains. In our approach to this problem, we utilized a multi-scale neurophysiologically-realistic implementation of binocular cells for the input, and then combined it with a neural network model to learn reliable cues for disparity estimation.

References

[1] T. Darrell and A.P. Pentland. Cooperative robust estimation using layers of support. *IEEE Transactions on Pattern Analysis and Machine Intelligence*, 17(5):474–87, 1995.

[2] M.S. Gray, A. Pouget, R.S. Zemel, S.J. Nowlan, and T.J. Sejnowski. Reliable disparity estimation through selective integration. *INC Technical Report 9602, Institute for Neural Computation, University of California, San Diego*, 1996.

[3] D.M. Green and J.A. Swets. *Signal Detection Theory and Psychophysics*. John Wiley and Sons, New York, 1966.

[4] R.A. Jacobs, M.I. Jordan, S.J. Nowlan, and G.E. Hinton. Adaptive mixtures of local experts. *Neural Computation*, 3:79–87, 1991.

[5] R. Jain, R. Kasturi, and B.G. Schunck. *Machine Vision*. McGraw-Hill, New York, 1995.

[6] S.J. Nowlan and T.J. Sejnowski. Filter selection model for motion segmentation and velocity integration. *Journal of the Optical Society of America A*, 11(12):3177–3200, 1994.

[7] I. Ohzawa, G.C. DeAngelis, and R.D. Freeman. Stereoscopic depth discrimination in the visual cortex: Neurons ideally suited as disparity detectors. *Science*, 249:1037–1041, 1990.

[8] R. von der Heydt, H. Zhou, H. Friedman, and G.F. Poggio. Neurons of area V2 of visual cortex detect edges in random-dot stereograms. *Soc. Neurosci. Abs.*, 21:18, 1995.

[9] G. Westheimer and S.P. McKee. Stereoscopic acuity with defocus and spatially filtered retinal images. *Journal of the Optical Society of America*, 70:772–777, 1980.

ARTEX: A Self-Organizing Architecture for Classifying Image Regions

Stephen Grossberg and James R. Williamson
{steve, jrw}@cns.bu.edu
Center for Adaptive Systems and
Department of Cognitive and Neural Systems
Boston University
677 Beacon Street,
Boston, MA 02215

Abstract

A self-organizing architecture is developed for image region classification. The system consists of a preprocessor that utilizes multi-scale filtering, competition, cooperation, and diffusion to compute a vector of image boundary and surface properties, notably texture and brightness properties. This vector inputs to a system that incrementally learns noisy multidimensional mappings and their probabilities. The architecture is applied to difficult real-world image classification problems, including classification of synthetic aperture radar and natural texture images, and outperforms a recent state-of-the-art system at classifying natural textures.

1 INTRODUCTION

Automatic processing of visual scenes often begins by detecting regions of an image with common values of simple local features, such as texture, and mapping the pattern of feature activation into a predicted region label. We develop a self-organizing neural architecture, called the ARTEX algorithm, for automatically extracting a novel and effective array of such features and mapping them to output region labels. ARTEX is made up of biologically motivated networks, the Boundary Contour System and Feature Contour System (BCS/FCS) networks for visual feature extraction (Cohen & Grossberg, 1984; Grossberg & Mingolla, 1985a, 1985b; Grossberg & Todorović, 1988; Grossberg, Mingolla, & Williamson, 1995), and the Gaussian ARTMAP (GAM) network for classification (Williamson, 1996).

ARTEX is first evaluated on a difficult real-world task, classifying regions of synthetic aperture radar (SAR) images, where it reliably achieves high resolution (single pixel) classification results, and creates accurate probability maps for its class predictions. ARTEX is then evaluated on classification of natural textures, where it outperforms the texture classification system in Greenspan, Goodman, Chellappa, & Anderson (1994) using comparable preprocessing and training conditions.

2 FEATURE EXTRACTION NETWORKS

Filled-in surface brightness. Regions of interest in an image can often be segmented based on first-order differences in pixel intensity. An improvement over raw pixel intensities can be obtained by compensating for variable illumination of the image to yield a local brightness feature. A further improvement over local brightness features can be obtained with a surface brightness feature, which is obtained by smoothing local brightness values when they belong to the same region, while maintaining differences when they belong to different regions. Such a procedure tends to maximize the separability of different regions in brightness space by minimizing within-region variance while maximizing between-region variance.

In Grossberg et al. (1995) a multiple-scale BCS/FCS network was used to process noisy SAR images for use by human operators by normalizing and segmenting the SAR intensity distributions and using these transformed data to fill-in surface representations that smooth over noise while maintaining informative structures. The single-scale BCS/FCS used here employs the middle-scale BCS/FCS used in that study. The BCS/FCS equations and parameters are fully described in Grossberg et al. (1995). The BCS/FCS is herein applied to SAR images that are spatially consolidated to half the size (in each dimension) of the images used in that study, and so is comparable to the large-scale BCS/FCS used there.

Multiple-scale oriented contrast. In addition to surface brightness, another image property that is useful for region segmentation is texture. One popular approach for analyzing texture, for which there is a great deal of supporting biological and computational evidence, decomposes an image, at each image location, into a set of energy measures at different oriented spatial frequencies. This may be done by applying a bank of orientation-selective bandpass filters followed by simple non-linearities and spatial pooling, to extract multiple-scale oriented contrast features. The early stages of the BCS, which define a Static Oriented Contrast (or SOC) filtering network, carry out these operations, and variants of them have been used in many texture segregation algorithms (Bergen, 1991; Greenspan et al., 1994).

Here, the SOC network produces $K=4$ oriented contrast features at each of four spatial scales. The first stage of the SOC network is a shunting on-center off-surround network that compensates for variable illumination, normalizes, and computes ratio contrasts in the image. Given an input image, I, the output at pixel (i,j) and scale g in the first stage of the SOC network is

$$a_{ij}^g = \frac{I_{ij} - (G^g * I)_{ij} - DE}{D + I_{ij} + (G^g * I)_{ij}}, \tag{1}$$

where $E=0.5$, and G^g is a Gaussian kernel defined by

$$G_{ij}^g(p,q) = \frac{1}{2\pi\sigma_g^2} \exp[-((i-p)^2 + (j-q)^2)/2\sigma_g^2], \tag{2}$$

with $\sigma_g = 2^g$, for the spatial scales $g=0,1,2,3$. The value of D is determined by the range of pixel intensities in the input image. We use $D=2000$ for SAR images and $D=255$ for natural texture images. The next stage obtains a local measure of orientational contrast by convolving the output of (1) with Gabor filters, H_k^g, which are defined at four orientations, and then full-wave rectifying the result:

$$b^g_{ijk} = |(H^g_k * a^g)_{ij}|. \qquad (3)$$

The horizontal Gabor filter ($k=0$) is defined by:

$$H^g_{ij0}(p,q) = G^g_{ij}(p,q) \cdot \sin[0.75\pi(j-q)/\sigma_g]. \qquad (4)$$

Orientational contrast responses may exhibit high spatial variability. A smooth, reliable measure of orientational contrast is obtained by spatially pooling the responses within the same orientation:

$$c^g_{ijk} = (G^g * b^g_k)_{ij}. \qquad (5)$$

Equation (5) yields an *orientationally variant*, or OV, representation of oriented contrast. A further optional stage yields an *orientationally invariant*, or OI, representation by shifting the oriented responses at each scale into a canonical ordering, to yield a common representation for rotated versions of the same texture:

$$d^g_{ijk} = c^g_{ijk'}, \text{ where } k' = [k + \arg\max_{k''}(c^g_{ijk''})] \bmod K. \qquad (6)$$

3 CLASSIFICATION NETWORK

GAM is a constructive, incremental-learning network which self-organizes internal category nodes that learn a Gaussian mixture model of the M-dimensional input space, as well as mappings to output class labels. Here, mappings are learned from 17-dimensional input vectors (composed of a filled-in brightness feature and 16 oriented contrast features) to a class label representing a shadow, road, grass, or tree region. The jth category's receptive field is parametrized by two M-dimensional vectors: its mean, $\vec{\mu}_j$, and standard deviation, $\vec{\sigma}_j$. A scalar, n_j, also represents the node's cumulative credit. Category j is activated only if its *match*, G_j, satisfies the match criterion, which is determined by a vigilance parameter, ρ. Match is a measure, obtained from the category's unit-height Gaussian distribution, of how close an input, $\vec{x}$, is to the category's mean, relative to its standard deviation:

$$G_j = \exp\left(-\frac{1}{2}\sum_{i=1}^M \left(\frac{x_i - \mu_{ji}}{\sigma_{ji}}\right)^2\right). \qquad (7)$$

The match criterion is a threshold: the category is activated only if $G_j > \rho$; otherwise, the category is *reset*. The input strength, g_j, is determined by

$$g_j = \frac{n_j}{\prod_{i=1}^M \sigma_{ji}} G_j \text{ if } G_j > \rho; \quad g_j = 0 \text{ otherwise}. \qquad (8)$$

The category's activation, y_j, which represents $P(j|\vec{x})$, is obtained by

$$y_j = \frac{g_j}{D + \sum_{l=1}^N g_l}, \qquad (9)$$

where N is the number of categories and D is a shunting decay term that maintains sensitivity to the input magnitude in the activation level ($D = 0.01$ here).

When category j is first chosen, it learns a permanent mapping to the output class, k, associated with the current training sample. All categories that map to the same class prediction belong to the same *ensemble*: $j \in E(k)$. Each time an input is presented, the categories in each ensemble sum their activations to generate a net probability estimate, z_k, of the class prediction k that they share:

$$z_k = \sum_{j \in E(k)} y_j. \qquad (10)$$

The system prediction, K, is determined by the maximum probability estimate,
$$K = \arg\max_k(z_k), \tag{11}$$
which determines the chosen ensemble. Once the class prediction K is chosen, we obtain the category's "chosen-ensemble" activation, y_j^*, which represents $P(j|\vec{x}, K)$:
$$y_j^* = \frac{y_j}{\sum_{l \in E(K)} y_l} \text{ if } j \in E(K); \quad y_j^* = 0 \text{ otherwise.} \tag{12}$$

If K is the correct prediction, then the network resonates and learns; otherwise, match tracking is invoked: ρ is raised to the average match of the chosen ensemble.
$$\rho = \exp\left(-\frac{1}{2} \sum_{j \in E(K)} y_j^* \sum_{i=1}^{M} \left(\frac{x_i - \mu_{ji}}{\sigma_{ji}}\right)^2\right). \tag{13}$$

In addition, all categories in the chosen ensemble are reset. Equations (8)–(11) are then re-evaluated. Based on the remaining non-reset categories, a new prediction K in (11), and its corresponding ensemble, are chosen. This automatic search cycle continues until the correct prediction is made, or until all committed categories are reset and an uncommitted category is chosen. Upon presentation of the next training sample, ρ is reassigned its baseline value: $\rho = \bar{\rho}$. Here, $\bar{\rho} \approx 0$.

When category j learns, n_j is updated to represent the amount of training data the node has been assigned credit for:
$$n_j := n_j + y_j^*. \tag{14}$$
The vectors $\vec{\mu}_j$ and $\vec{\sigma}_j$ are then updated to learn the input statistics:
$$\mu_{ji} := (1 - y_j^* n_j^{-1})\mu_{ji} + y_j^* n_j^{-1} x_i, \tag{15}$$
$$\sigma_{ji} := \sqrt{(1 - y_j^* n_j^{-1})\sigma_{ji}^2 + y_j^* n_j^{-1}(x_i - \mu_{ji})^2}, \tag{16}$$

GAM is initialized with $N=0$. When a category is first chosen, N is incremented, and the new category, indexed by $J=N$, is initialized with $n_J = 1$, $\vec{\mu} = \vec{x}$, $\sigma_{ji} = \gamma$, and with a permanent mapping to the correct output class. Initializing $\sigma_{ji} = \gamma$ is necessary to make (7) and (8) well-defined. Varying γ has a marked effect on learning: as γ is raised, learning becomes slower, but fewer categories are created. The input vectors are normalized to have the same standard deviation in each dimension so that γ has the same meaning in each dimension.

4 SIMULATION RESULTS

Classifying SAR image regions. Figure 1 illustrates the classification results obtained on one SAR image after training on the other eight images in the data set. The final classification result (bottom, right) closely resembles the hand-labeled regions (middle, left). The caption summarizes the average results obtained on all nine images. ARTEX learns this problem very quickly, using a small number of self-organized categories, as shown in Figure 2 (left). The best classification result of 84.2% correct is obtained by filling-in the probability estimates from equation (10) within the BCS boundaries, using an FCS diffusion equation as described in Grossberg et al. (1995). These filled-in probability estimates predict the actual classification rates with remarkable accuracy (Figure 2, right).

Classifying natural textures. ARTEX performance is now compared to that of a texture analysis system described in Greenspan et al. (1994), which we refer to as the "hybrid system" because it is a hybrid architecture made up of a

ARTEX: A Self-organizing Architecture for Classifying Image Regions

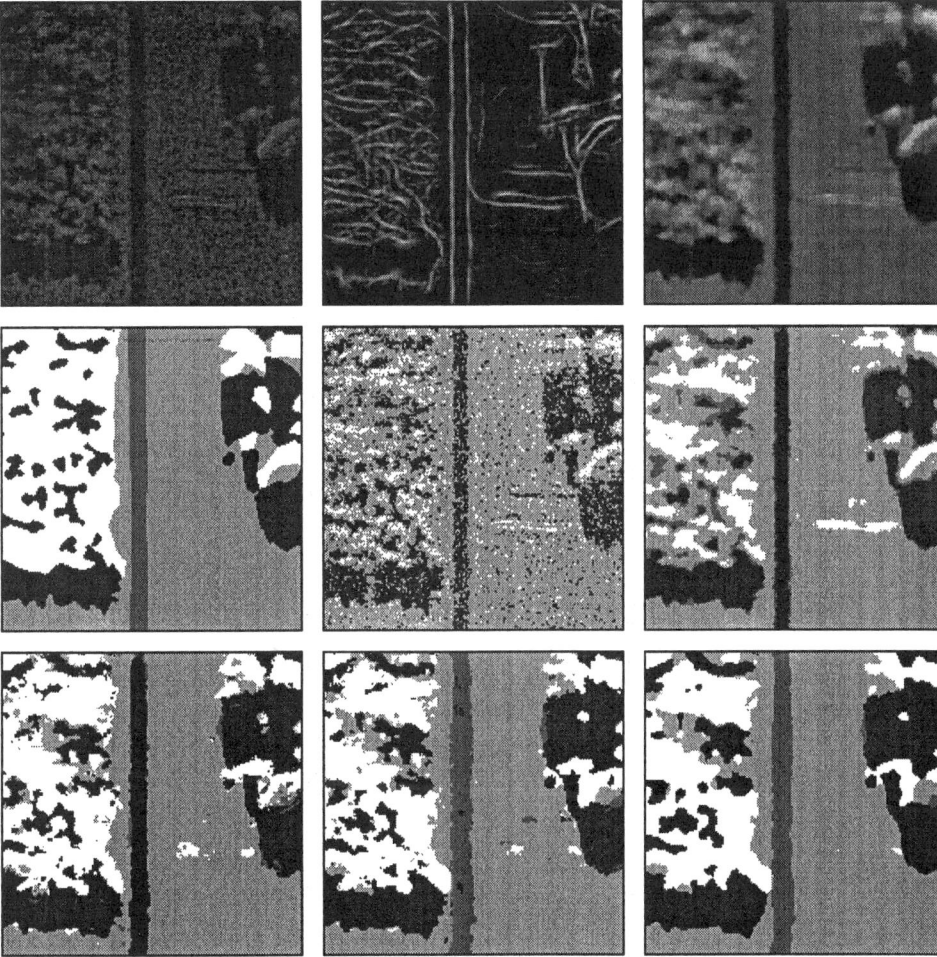

Figure 1: Results are shown on a 180x180 pixel SAR image, which is one of nine images in data set. Top row: Center/surround, first stage output (left); BCS boundaries to FCS filling-in (middle); final BCS/FCS filled-in output (right). Note that BCS accurately localizes region boundaries, and that FCS improves appearance by smoothing intensities within regions while maintaining sharp differences between regions. Middle row: Hand-labeled regions corresponding to shadow, road, grass, trees (left); Gaussian classifier results based on center/surround feature (middle, 59.6% correct), and based on filled-in feature (right, 70.7%). Note that filling-in greatly improves classification by reducing brightness variability within regions. However, the lack of textural information results in errors, such as the misclassification of the vertical road as a shadow region. Bottom row: GAM results ($\gamma = 4$) based on 16 SOC features in addition to the filled-in brightness feature: using the OV representation (left, 81.9%), using the OI representation (middle, 83.2%), and using filled-in OI prediction probabilities (right, 84.2%). With the OV representation (bottom, left), the thin vertical road is misclassified as shadows because there are no thin vertical roads in the training set. With the OI representation, however (bottom, middle), the road is classified correctly because the training set includes thin roads at other orientations. Finally, the classification results are improved by filling-in the prediction probabilities from equation (10) within the BCS boundaries, thereby taking advantage of spatial and structural context (bottom, right).

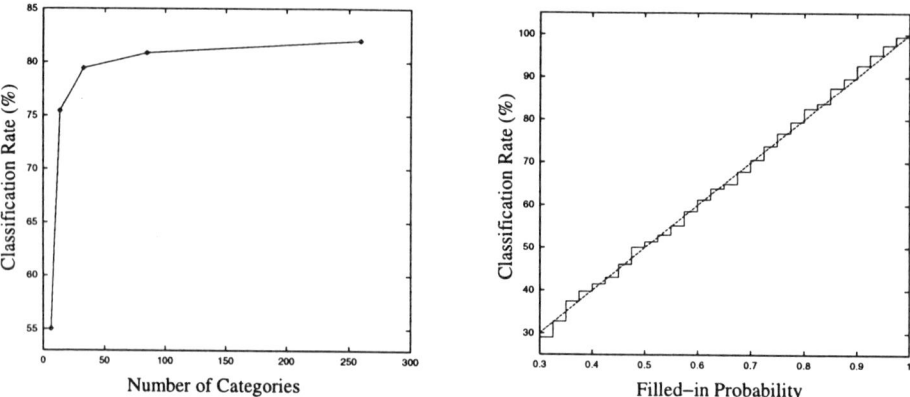

Figure 2: Left: classification rate is plotted as a function of the number of categories after training on different sized subsets of the SAR training data: (left-to-right) 0.01%, 0.1%, 1%, 10%, and 100% of the training set. Right: classification rate is plotted as a function of filled-in probability estimates.

log-Gabor pyramid representation, followed by unsupervised k-means clustering in the feature space, followed by batch learning of mappings from clusters to output classes using a rule-based classifier. The hybrid system uses three pyramid levels and four orientations at each level. Each level of the pyramid is produced via three blurring/decimation steps, resulting in an 8x8 pixel resolution. For a fair comparison, sufficient blurring/decimation was added as a postprocessing step to ARTEX features to yield the same net amount of blurring. Both ARTEX and the hybrid system use an OV representation for these problems because the textures are not rotated. The first task is classification of a library of ten separate structured and unstructured textures after training on different example images. ARTEX obtains better performance, achieving 96.3% correct after 40 training epochs (with $\gamma = 1$, 34 categories) versus 94.3% for the hybrid system. Even after only one training epoch, ARTEX achieves better results (94.9%, 23 categories). The second task (Figure 3) is classification of a five-texture mosaic, which requires discriminating texture boundaries, after training on examples of the five textures, plus an additional texture (sand). ARTEX achieves 93.6% correct after 40 training epochs (33 categories), and produces results which appear to be better than those produced by the hybrid system on a similar problem (see Greenspan et al., 1994, Figure 5).

In summary, the ARTEX system demonstrates the utility of combining BCS texture and FCS brightness measures for image preprocessing. These features may be effectively classified by the GAM network, whose self-calibrating matching and search operations enable it to carry out fast, incremental, distributed learning of recognition categories and their probabilities. BCS boundaries may be further used to constrain the diffusion of these probabilities according to FCS rules to improve prediction probability.

Acknowledgements

Stephen Grossberg was supported by the Office of Naval Research (ONR N00014-95-1-0409 and ONR N00014-95-1-0657). James Williamson was supported by the Advanced Research Projects Agency (ONR N00014-92-J-4015), the Air Force Office of Scientific Research (AFOSR F49620-92-J-0225 and AFOSR F49620-92-J-0334), the National Science Foundation (NSF IRI-90-00530 and NSF IRI-90-24877), and

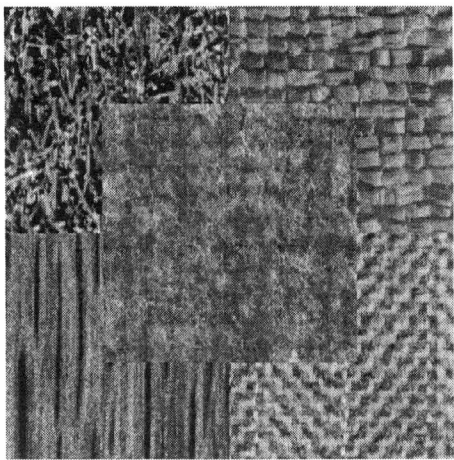 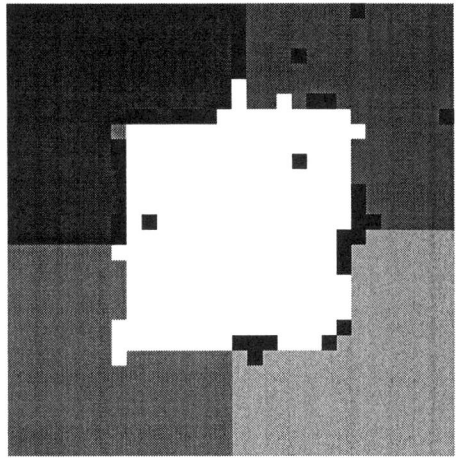

Figure 3: Left: mosaic of five natural textures. Right: ARTEX classification (93.6% correct) after training on examples of five textures and an additional texture (sand).

the Office of Naval Research (ONR N00014-91-J-4100 and ONR N00014-95-1-0409).

References

Bergen, J.R. "Theories of visual texture perception," in *Spatial Vision*, D. M. Regan Ed. New York: Macmillan, 1991, pp. 114-134.

Cohen, M. & Grossberg, S., (1984). Neural dynamics of brightness perception: Features, boundaries, diffusion, and resonance. *Perception & Psychophysics*, **36**, 428-456.

Greenspan, H., Goodman, R., Chellappa, R., & Anderson, C.H. (1994). Learning texture discrimination rules in a multiresolution system. *IEEE Trans. PAMI*, **16**, 894-901.

Grossberg, S. & Mingolla, E. (1985a). Neural dynamics of form perception: Boundary completion, illusory figures, and neon color spreading. *Psychological Review*, **92**, 173-211.

Grossberg, S. & Mingolla, E. (1985b). Neural dynamics of perceptual grouping: Textures, boundaries, and emergent segmentations. *Perception & Psychophysics*, **38**, 141-171.

Grossberg, S., Mingolla, E., & Williamson, J. (1995). Synthetic aperture radar processing by a multiple scale neural system for boundary and surface representation. *Neural Networks*, **8**, 1005-1028.

Grossberg, S. & Todorović, D. (1988). Neural dynamics of 1-D and 2-D brightness perception: A unified model of classical and recent phenomena. *Perception & Psychophysics*, **43**, 241-277.

Grossberg, S., & Williamson, J.R. (1996). A self-organizing system for classifying complex images: Natural textures and synthetic aperture radar. Technical Report CAS/CNS TR-96-002, Boston, MA: Boston University.

Williamson, J.R. (1996). Gaussian ARTMAP: A neural network for fast incremental learning of noisy multidimensional maps. *Neural Networks*, **9**, 881-897.

Contour Organisation with the EM Algorithm

J. A. F. Leite and E. R. Hancock
Department of Computer Science
University of York, York, Y01 5DD, UK.

Abstract

This paper describes how the early visual process of contour organisation can be realised using the EM algorithm. The underlying computational representation is based on fine spline coverings. According to our EM approach the adjustment of spline parameters draws on an iterative weighted least-squares fitting process. The expectation step of our EM procedure computes the likelihood of the data using a mixture model defined over the set of spline coverings. These splines are limited in their spatial extent using Gaussian windowing functions. The maximisation of the likelihood leads to a set of linear equations in the spline parameters which solve the weighted least squares problem. We evaluate the technique on the localisation of road structures in aerial infra-red images.

1 Introduction

Dempster, Laird and Rubin's EM (expectation and maximisation) [1] algorithm was originally introduced as a means of finding maximum likelihood solutions to problems posed in terms of incomplete data. The basic idea underlying the algorithm is to iterate between the expectation and maximisation modes until convergence is reached. Expectation involves computing *a posteriori* model probabilities using a mixture density specified in terms of a series of model parameters. In the maximisation phase, the model parameters are recomputed to maximise the expected value of the incomplete data likelihood. In fact, when viewed from this perspective, the updating of *a posteriori* probabilities in the expectation phase would appear to have much in common with the probabilistic relaxation process extensively exploited in low and intermediate level vision [9, 2]. Maximisation of the incomplete data likelihood is reminiscent of robust estimation where outlier reject is employed in the iterative re-computation of model parameters [7].

It is these observations that motivate the study reported in this paper. We are interested in the organisation of the output of local feature enhancement operators into meaningful global contour structures [13, 2]. Despite providing one of the classical applications of relaxation labelling in low-level vision [9], successful solutions to the iterative curve reinforcement problem have proved to be surprisingly elusive [8, 12, 2]. Recently, two contrasting ideas have offered practical relaxation operators. Zucker *et al* [13] have sought biologically plausible operators which draw on the idea of computing a global curve organisation potential and locating consistent structure using a form of local snake dynamics [11]. In essence this biologically inspired model delivers a fine arrangement of local splines that minimise the curve organisation potential. Hancock and Kittler [2], on the other hand, appealed to a more information theoretic motivation [4]. In an attempt to overcome some of the well documented limitations of the original Rosenfeld, Hummel and Zucker relaxation operator [9] they have developed a Bayesian framework for relaxation labelling [4]. Of particular significance for the low-level curve enhancement problem is the underlying statistical framework which makes a clear-cut distinction between the roles of uncertain image data and prior knowledge of contour structure. This framework has allowed the output of local image operators to be represented in terms of Gaussian measurement densities, while curve structure is represented by a dictionary of consistent contour structures [2].

While both the fine-spline coverings of Zucker [13] and the dictionary-based relaxation operator of Hancock and Kittler [2] have delivered practical solutions to the curve reinforcement problem, they each suffer a number of shortcomings. For instance, although the fine spline operator can achieve quasi-global curve organisation, it is based on an essentially *ad hoc* local compatibility model. While being more information theoretic, the dictionary-based relaxation operator is limited by virtue of the fact that in most practical applications the dictionary can only realistically be evaluated over at most a 3x3 pixel neighbourhood. Our aim in this paper is to bridge the methodological divide between the biologically inspired fine-spline operator and the statistical framework of dictionary based relaxation. We develop an iterative spline fitting process using the EM algorithm of Dempster *et al* [1]. In doing this we retain the statistical framework for representing filter responses that has been used to great effect in the initialisation of dictionary-based relaxation. However, we overcome the limited contour representation of the dictionary by drawing on local cubic splines.

2 Prerequisites

The practical goal in this paper is the detection of line-features which manifest themselves as intensity ridges of variable width in raw image data. Each pixel is characterised by a vector of measurements, z_i where i is the pixel-index. This measurement vector is computed by applying a battery of line-detection filters of various widths and orientations to the raw image. Suppose that the image data is indexed by the pixel-set I. Associated with each image pixel is a cubic spline parameterisation which represents the best-fit contour that couples it to adjacent feature pixels. The spline is represented by a vector of parameters denoted by

$\underline{q}_i = (q_i^0, q_i^1, q_i^2, q_i^3)^T$. Let (x_i, y_i) represent the position co-ordinates of the pixel indexed i. The spline variable, $s_{i,j} = x_i - x_j$ associated with the contour connecting the pixel indexed j is the horizontal displacement between the pixels indexed i and j. We can write the cubic spline as an inner product $F(s_{i,j}, \underline{q}_i) = \underline{q}_i^T \cdot \underline{S}_{i,j}$ where $\underline{S}_{i,j} = (1, s_{i,j}, s_{i,j}^2, s_{i,j}^3)^T$. Central to our EM algorithm will be the comparison of the predicted vertical spline displacement with its measured value $r_{i,j} = y_i - y_j$.

In order to initialise the EM algorithm, we require a set of initial spline probabilities which we denote by $\pi(\underline{q}_i^{(0)})$. Here we use the multi-channel combination model recently reported by Leite and Hancock [5] to compute an initial multi-scale line-feature probability. Accordingly, if Σ is the variance-covariance matrix for the components of the filter bank, then

$$\pi(\underline{q}_i^{(0)}) = 1 - \exp\left[-\frac{1}{2}\underline{z}_i^T \Sigma^{-1} \underline{z}_i\right] \quad (1)$$

The remainder of this paper outlines how these initial probabilities are iteratively refined using the EM algorithm. Because space is limited we only provide an algorithm sketch. Essential algorithm details such as the estimation of spline orientation and the local receptive gating of the spline probabilities are omitted for clarity. Full details can be found in a forthcoming journal article [6].

3 Expectation

Our basic model of the spline organisation process is as follows. Associated with each image pixel is a spline parameterisation. Key to our philosophy of exploiting a mixture model to describe the global contour structure of the image is the idea that the pixel indexed i can associate to each of the putative splines residing in a local Gaussian window N_i. We commence by developing a mixture model for the conditional probability density for the filter response $\underline{z}_i$ given the current global spline description. If $\Phi^{(n)} = \{\underline{q}_i^{(n)}, \forall i \in I\}$ is the global spline description at iteration n of the EM process, then we can expand the mixture distribution over a set of putative splines that may associate with the image pixel indexed i

$$p(\underline{z}_i | \Phi^{(n)}) = \sum_{j \in N_i} p(\underline{z}_i | \underline{q}_j^{(n)}) \pi(\underline{q}_j^{(n)}) \quad (2)$$

The components of the above mixture density are the conditional measurement densities $p(\underline{z}_i | \underline{q}_j^{(n)})$ and the spline mixing proportions $\pi(\underline{q}_j^{(n)})$. The conditional measurement densities represent the likelihood that the datum $\underline{z}_i$ originates from the spline centred on pixel j. The mixing proportions, on the other hand, represent the fractional contribution to the data arising from the jth parameter vector i.e. $\underline{q}_j^{(n)}$. Since we are interested in the maximum likelihood estimation of spline parameters, we turn our attention to the likelihood of the raw data, i.e.

$$p(\underline{z}_i, \forall i \in I | \Phi^{(n)}) = \prod_{i \in I} p(\underline{z}_i | \Phi^{(n)}) \quad (3)$$

The expectation step of the EM algorithm is aimed at estimating the log-likelihood using the parameters of the mixture distribution. In other words, we need to average the likelihood over the space of potential pixel-spline assignments. In fact, it was Dempster, Laird and Rubin [1] who observed that maximising the weighted log-likelihood was equivalent to maximising the conditional expectation of the likelihood for a new parameter set given an old parameter set. For our spline fitting problem, maximisation of the expectation of the conditional likelihood is equivalent to maximising the weighted log-likelihood function

$$Q(\Phi^{(n+1)}|\Phi^{(n)}) = \sum_{i \in I} \sum_{j \in N_i} P(\underline{q}_j^{(n)}|\underline{z}_i) \ln p(\underline{z}_i|\underline{q}_j^{(n+1)}) \qquad (4)$$

The *a posteriori* probabilities $P(\underline{q}_j^{(n)}|\underline{z}_i)$ may be computed from the corresponding components of the mixture density $p(\underline{z}_i|\underline{q}_j^{(n)})$ using the Bayes formula

$$P(\underline{q}_j^{(n)}|\underline{z}_i) = \frac{p(\underline{z}_i|\underline{q}_j^{(n)})\pi(\underline{q}_j^{(n)})}{\sum_{k \in N_i} p(\underline{z}_i|\underline{q}_k^{(n)})\pi(\underline{q}_k^{(n)})} \qquad (5)$$

For notational convenience, and to make the weighting role of the *a posteriori* probabilities explicit we use the shorthand $w_{i,j}^{(n)} = P(\underline{q}_j^{(n)}|\underline{z}_i)$. Once updated parameter estimates $\underline{q}_i^{(n)}$ become available through the maximisation of this criterion, improved estimates of the mixture components may be obtained by substitution into equation (6). The updated mixing proportions, $\pi(\underline{q}_i^{(n+1)})$, required to determine the new weights $w_{i,j}^{(n)}$ are computed from the newly available density components using the following estimator

$$\pi(\underline{q}_i^{(n+1)}) = \sum_{j \in N_i} \frac{p(\underline{z}_j|\underline{q}_i^{(n)})\pi(\underline{q}_i^{(n)})}{\sum_{k \in I} p(\underline{z}_j|\underline{q}_k^{(n)})\pi(\underline{q}_k^{(n)})} \qquad (6)$$

In order to proceed with the development of a spline fitting process we require a model for the mixture components, i.e. $p(\underline{z}_i|\underline{q}_j^{(n)})$. Here we assume that the required model can be specified in terms of Gaussian distribution functions. In other words, we confine our attention to Gaussian mixtures. The physical variable of these distributions is the squared error residual for the position prediction of the ith datum delivered by the jth spline. Accordingly we write

$$p(\underline{z}_i|\underline{q}_j^{(n)}) = \sqrt{\frac{\beta}{2\pi}} \exp\left[-\beta\left(r_{i,j} - F(s_{i,j}, \underline{q}_j^{(n)})\right)^2\right] \qquad (7)$$

where β is the inverse variance of the fit residuals. Rather than estimating β, we use it in the spirit of a control variable to regulate the effect of fit residuals.

Equations (5), (6) and (11) therefore specify a recursive procedure that iterates the weighted residuals to compute a new mixing proportions based on the quality of the spline fit.

4 Maximisation

The maximisation step aims to optimize the quantity $Q(\Phi^{(n+1)}|\Phi^{(n)})$ with respect to the spline parameters. Formally this corresponds to finding the set of spline parameters which satisfy the condition

$$\Phi^{(n+1)} = \arg\max_{\Phi} Q(\Phi|\Phi^{(n)}) \qquad (8)$$

We find a local approximation to this condition by solving the following set of linear equations

$$\frac{\partial Q(\Phi^{(n+1)}|\Phi^{(n)})}{\partial (q_i^k)^{(n+1)}} = 0 \qquad (9)$$

for each spline parameter $(q_i^k)^{(n+1)}$ in turn, i.e. for k=0,1,2,3. Recovery of the splines is most conveniently expressed in terms of the following matrix equation for the components of the parameter-vector $\underline{q}_i^{(n)}$

$$\underline{q}_i^{(n+1)} = (A_i^{(n)})^{-1} \underline{X}_i^{(n)} \qquad (10)$$

The elements of the vector $X^{(n)}$ are weighted cross-moments between the parallel and perpendicular spline distances in the Gaussian window, i.e.

$$\underline{X}_i^{(n)} = \begin{pmatrix} \sum_{j \in N_i} w_{i,j}^{(n)} r_{i,j} \\ \sum_{j \in N_i} w_{i,j}^{(n)} r_{i,j} s_{i,j} \\ \sum_{j \in N_i} w_{i,j}^{(n)} r_{i,j} s_{i,j}^2 \\ \sum_{j \in N_i} w_{i,j}^{(n)} r_{i,j} s_{i,j}^3 \end{pmatrix} \qquad (11)$$

The elements of the matrix $A_i^{(n)}$, on the other hand, are weighted moments computed purely in terms of the parallel distance $s_{i,j}$. If k and l are the row and column indices, then the (k,l)th element of the matrix $A_i^{(n)}$ is

$$[A_i^{(n)}]_{k,l} = \sum_{j \in N_i} w_{i,j}^{(n)} s_{i,j}^{k+l-2} \qquad (12)$$

5 Experiments

We have evaluated our iterative spline fitting algorithm on the detection of line-features in aerial infra-red images. Figure 1a shows the original picture. The initial feature probabilities (i.e. $\pi(q_i^{(0)})$) assigned according to equation (1) are shown in Figure 1b. Figure 1c shows the final contour-map after the EM algorithm has converged. Notice that the line contours exhibit good connectivity and that the junctions are well reconstructed. We have highlighted a subregion of the original image. There are two features in this subregion to which we would like to draw attention. The first of these is centred on the junction structure. The second feature is a neighbouring point on the descending branch of the road.

Figure 2 shows the iterative evolution of the cubic splines at these two locations. The spline shown in Figure 2a adjusts to fit the upper pair of road segments. Notice also that although initially displaced, the final spline passes directly through the junction. In the case of the descending road-branch the spline shown in Figure 2b recovers from an initially poor orientation estimate to align itself with the underlying road structure. Figure 2c shows how the spline probabilities (i.e. $\pi(q_i^{(n)})$) evolve with iteration number. Initially, the neighbourhood is highly ambiguous. Many neighbouring splines compete to account for the local image structure. As a result the detected junction is several pixels wide. However, as the fitting process iterates, the splines move from the inconsistent initial estimate to give a good local estimate which is less ambiguous. In other words the two splines illustrated in Figure 2 have successfully arranged themselfs to account for the junction structure.

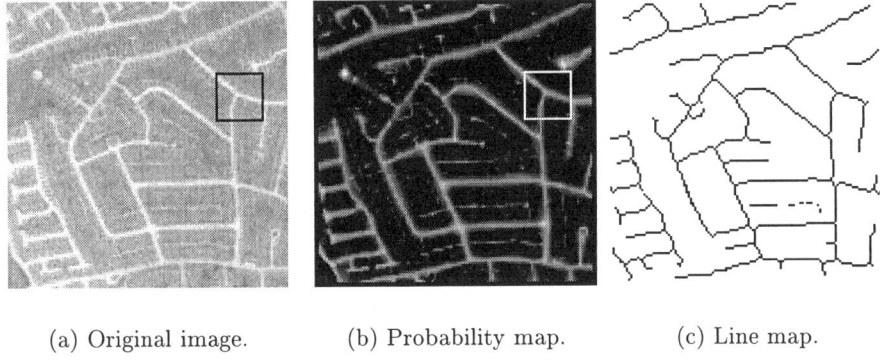

(a) Original image.　　　(b) Probability map.　　　(c) Line map.

Figure 1: Infra-red aerial picture with corresponding probability map showing region containing pixel under study and correspondent line map.

6 Conclusions

We have demonstrated how the process of parallel iterative contour refinement can be realised using the classical EM algorithm of Dempster, Laird and Rubin [1]. The refinement of curves by relaxation operations has been a preoccupation in the literature since the seminal work of Rosenfeld, Hummel and Zucker [9]. However, it is only recently that successful algorithms have been developed by appealing to more sophisticated modelling methodologies [13, 2]. Our EM approach not only delivers comparable performance, it does so using a very simple underlying model. Moreover, it allows the contour re-enforcement process to be understood in a weighted least-squares optimisation framework which has many features in common with snake dynamics [11] without being sensitive on the initial positioning of control points. Viewed from the perspective of classical relaxation labelling [9, 4], the EM framework provides a natural way of evaluating support beyond the immediate object neighbourhood. Moreover, the framework for spline fitting in 2D is readily extendible to the reconstruction of surface patches in 3D [10].

References

[1] Dempster A., Laird N. and Rubin D., "Maximum-likelihood from incomplete data via the EM algorithm", J. Royal Statistical Soc. Ser. B (methodological), **39**, pp 1-38, 1977.

[2] Hancock E.R. and Kittler J., "Edge Labelling using Dictionary-based Probabilistic Relaxation", IEEE PAMI, **12**, pp. 161-185, 1990.

[3] Jordan M.I. and Jacobs R.A, "Hierarchical Mixtures of Experts and the EM Algorithm", *Neural Computation*, **6**, pp. 181-214, 1994.

[4] Kittler J. and Hancock, E.R., "Combining Evidence in Probabilistic relaxation", International Journal of Pattern Recognition and Artificial Intelligence, **3**, N1, pp 29-51, 1989.

[5] Leite J.A.F. and Hancock, E.R., " Statistically Combining and Refining Multichannel Information", *Progress in Image Analysis and Processing III: Edited by S Impedovo, World Scientific*, pp. 193-200, 1994.

[6] Leite J.A.F. and Hancock, E.R., "Iterative curve organisation with the EM algorithm", *to appear in Pattern Recognition Letters*, 1997.

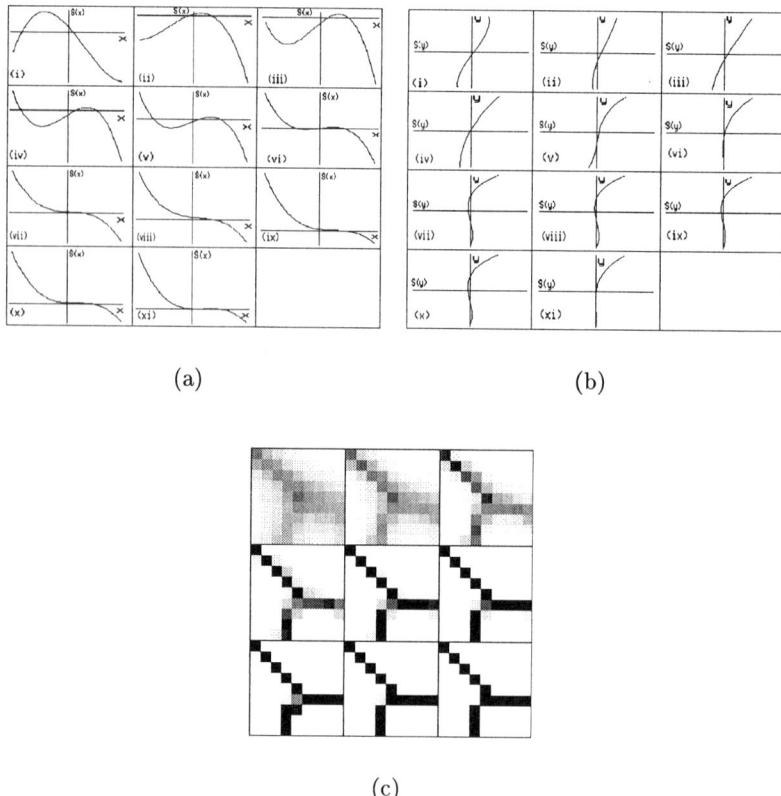

Figure 2: Evolution of the spline in the fitting process. The image in (a) is the junction spline while the image in (b) is the branch spline. The first spline is shown in (i), and the subsequent ones from (ii) to (xi). The evolution of the corresponding spline probabilities is shown in (c).

[7] Meer P., Mintz D., Rosenfeld A. and Kim D.Y., "Robust Regression Methods for Computer Vision - A Review", *International Journal of Computer vision*, **6**, pp. 59–70, 1991.

[8] Peleg S. and Rosenfeld A., "Determining Compatibility Coefficients for curve enhancement relaxation processes", *IEEE SMC*, **8**, pp. 548–555, 1978.

[9] Rosenfeld A., Hummel R.A. and Zucker S.W., "Scene labelling by relaxation operations", IEEE Transactions SMC, SMC-6, pp400-433, 1976.

[10] Sander P.T. and Zucker S.W., "Inferring surface structure and differential structure from 3D images", IEEE PAMI, **12**, pp 833-854, 1990.

[11] Terzopoulos D., "Regularisation of inverse problems involving discontinuities", IEEE PAMI, **8**, pp 129-139, 1986.

[12] Zucker, S.W., Hummel R.A., and Rosenfeld A., "An application of relaxation labelling to line and curve enhancement", *IEEE TC*, **C-26**, pp. 394–403, 1977.

[13] Zucker S., David C., Dobbins A. and Iverson L., "The organisation of curve detection: coarse tangent fields and fine spline coverings", *Proceedings of the Second International Conference on Computer Vision*, pp. 577–586, 1988.

Visual Cortex Circuitry and Orientation Tuning

Trevor Mundel
Department of Neurology
University of Chicago
Chicago, IL 60637
mundel@math.uchicago.edu

Alexander Dimitrov
Department of Mathematics
University of Chicago
Chicago, IL 60637
a-dimitrov@uchicago.edu

Jack D. Cowan
Departments of Mathematics and Neurology
University of Chicago
Chicago, IL 60637
cowan@math.uchicago.edu

Abstract

A simple mathematical model for the large–scale circuitry of primary visual cortex is introduced. It is shown that a basic cortical architecture of recurrent local excitation and lateral inhibition can account quantitatively for such properties as orientation tuning. The model can also account for such local effects as cross–orientation suppression. It is also shown that non–local state–dependent coupling between similar orientation patches, when added to the model, can satisfactorily reproduce such effects as non–local iso–orientation suppression, and non–local cross–orientation enhancement. Following this an account is given of perceptual phenomena involving object segmentation, such as "pop–out", and the direct and indirect tilt illusions.

1 INTRODUCTION

The edge detection mechanism in the primate visual cortex (V1) involves at least two fairly well characterized circuits. There is a local circuit operating at sub–hypercolumn dimensions comprising strong orientation specific recurrent excitation and weakly orientation specific inhibition. The other circuit operates between hypercolumns, connecting cells with similar orientation preferences separated by several millimetres of cortical tissue. The horizontal connections which mediate this circuit have been extensively studied. These connections are ideally structured to provide local cortical processes with information about the global nature of stimuli. Thus they have been invoked to explain a wide variety of context dependent visual processing. A good example of this is the tilt illusion (TI), where surround stimulation causes a misperception of the angle of tilt of a grating.

The interaction between such local and long–range circuits has also been investigated. Typically these experiments involve the separate stimulation of a cells receptive field (the *classical* receptive field or "center") and the immediate region outside the receptive field (the *non–classical* receptive field or "surround"). In the first part of this work we present a simple model of cortical center–surround interaction. Despite the simplicity of the model we are able to quantitatively reproduce many experimental findings. We then apply the model to the TI. We are able to reproduce the principle features of both the direct and indirect TI with the model.

2 PRINCIPLES OF CORTICAL OPERATION

Recent work with voltage–sensitive dyes (Blasdel, 1992) augments the early work of Hubel & Wiesel (1962) which indicated that clusters of cortical neurons corresponding to cortical columns have similar orientation preferences. An examination of local field potentials (Victor et al., 1994) which represent potentials averaged over cortical volumes containing many hundreds of cells show orientation preferences. These considerations suggest that the appropriate units for an analysis of orientation selectivity are the localized clusters of neurons preferring the same orientation. This choice of a population model immediately simplifies both analysis and computation with the model. For brevity we will refer to elements or edge detectors, however these are to be understood as referring to localized populations of neurons with a common orientation preference. We view the cortex as a lattice of hypercolumns, in which each hypercolumn comprises a continuum of iso–orientation patches distinguished by their preferred orientation ϕ. All space coordinates refer to distances between hypercolumn centers. The population model we adopt throughout this work is a simplified form of the Wilson–Cowan equations.

2.1 LOCAL MODEL

Our local model is a ring ($\phi = -90° to + 90°$) of coupled iso–orientation patches and inhibitors with the following characteristics

- Weakly tuned orientation biased inputs to V1. These may arise either from slight orientation biases of lateral geniculate nucleus (LGN) neurons or from converging thalamocortical afferents
- Sharply tuned (space constant $\pm 7.5°$) recurrent excitation between iso–orientation populations
- Broadly tuned inhibition to all iso–orientation populations with a cut-off of inhibition interactions at between $45°$ and $60°$ separation

The principle constraint is that of a critical balance between excitatory and inhibitory currents. Recent theoretical studies (Tsodyks & Sejnowski 1995; Vreeswijk & Sompolinsky 1996) have focused on this condition as an explanation for certain features of the dynamics of natural neuronal assemblies. These features include the irregular temporal firing patterns of cortical neurons, the sensitivity of neuronal assemblies in vivo to small fluctuations in total synaptic input and the distribution of firing rates in cortical networks which is markedly skewed towards low mean rates. Vreeswijk & Sompolinsky demonstrate that such a balance emerges naturally in certain large networks of excitatory and inhibitory populations. We implement this critical balance by explicitly tuning the strength of connection weights between excitatory and inhibitory populations so that the system state is subcritical to a bifurcation point with respect to the relative strength of excitation/inhibition.

2.2 HORIZONTAL CONNECTIONS

We distinguish three potential patterns of horizontal connectivity

- connections between edge detectors along an axis parallel to the detectors preferred orientation (visuotopic connection)
- connections along an axis orthogonal to the detectors preferred orientation, with or without visuotopic connections
- radially symmetric connection to all detectors of the same orientation in surrounding hypercolumns

Recent experimental work in the tree shrew (Fitzpatrick et al., 1996) and preliminary work in the macaque (Blasdel, personal communication) indicate that visuotopic connection is the predominant pattern of long–range connectivity. This connectivity pattern allows for the following reduction in dimension of the problem for certain experimental conditions.

Consider the following experiment. A particular hypercolumn designated the "center" is stimulated with a grating at orientation ϕ resulting in a response from the ϕ–edge detector. The region outside the receptive area of this hypercolumn (in the "surround") is also stimulated with a grating at some uniform orientation ϕ' resulting in responses from ϕ'–edge detectors at each hypercolumn in the surround. In order to study the interactions between center and surround, then to first order approximation only the center hypercolumn and interaction with the surround along the ϕ visuotopic axis (defined by the center) and the ϕ' visuotopic axis (once again defined by the center) need be considered. In fact, except when $\phi = \phi'$ the effect of the center on the surround will be negligible in view of the modulatory nature of the horizontal connections detailed above. Thus we can reduce the problem (a priori three dimensional – one angle and two space dimensions) to two dimensions (one angle and one space dimension) with respect to a fixed center. This reduction is the key to providing a simple analysis of complex neurophysiological and psychophysical data.

3 RESULTS

3.1 CENTER–SURROUND INTERACTIONS

Although, we have modeled the state–dependence of the horizontal connections, many of the center–surround experiments we wish to model have not taken this dependence explicitly into account. In general the surround has been found to be suppressive on the center, which accords with the fact that the center is usually stimulated with high contrast stimuli. A typical example of the surround suppressive effect is shown in figure 1.

The basic finding is that stimulation in the surround of a visual cortical cell's receptive field generally results in a suppression of the cell's tuning response that is maximal for surround stimulation at the orientation of the cell's peak tuning

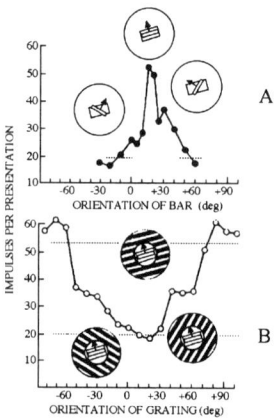

Figure 1: Non-local effects on orientation tuning - experimental data. Response to constant center stimulation at 15° and surround stimulation at angles $[-90°, 90°]$ (open circles), Local tuning curve (filled circles). Redrawn from Blakemore and Tobin (1972)

response and falls off with stimulation at other orientations in a characteristic manner. Further examples of surround suppression can be found in the paper of Sillito et al. (1995). Figure 2 depicts simulations in which long–range connections to local inhibitory populations are strong compared to connections to local excitatory populations.

These experiments and simulations appear to conflict with the consistent experimental finding that stimulating a hypercolumn with an orthogonal stimulus suppresses the response to the original stimulus.

The relevant results can be summarised as follows: cross–orientation suppression (with orthogonal gratings) originates within the receptive field of most cells examined and is a consistent finding in both complex and simple cells. The degree of suppression depends linearly on the size of the orthogonal grating up to a critical dimension which is smaller than the classical receptive field dimension. It is possible to suppress a response to the baseline firing rate by either increasing the size or the contrast of the orthogonal grating.

The model outlined earlier can account for all these observations, and similar measurements recently described by Sillitto et. al. (1995), in a strikingly simple fashion in the setting of single mode bifurcations. Orthogonal inputs are of the form $a/2[1 + \cos 2s(\phi - \phi_0)] + b/2[1 + \cos 2s(\phi - \phi_0 + 90°)]$, where a and b are amplitudes with $a > b$ and $\phi \in [-90°, 90°]$. By simple trigonometry this simplifies to $(a+b)/2 + (a-b)/2 \cos 2s(\phi - \phi_0)$ Thus the input of amplitude b reduces the amplitude of the orthogonal input and hence gives rise to a smaller response. This is then the mechanism by which local double orthogonal stimulation leads to suppression.

The center–surround case is different in that the orthogonal input originates from the horizontal connections and (in the suppressive setting) is input primarily to the orthogonal inhibitory population. It can be shown rigorously that for small amplitude stimuli this is equivalent to an orthogonal input to the excitatory population with opposite sign. Thus we have a total input $(a+b)/2[1 + \cos(2s(\phi - \phi_0)]$ where b arises from the horizontal input and hence increases the amplitude of the fundamental component of the input.

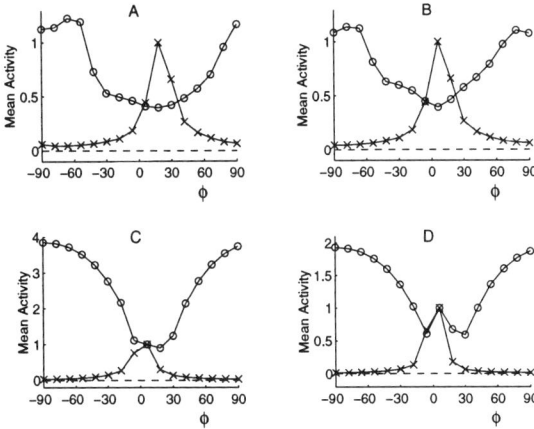

Figure 2: Non-local effects on orientation tuning. (o-o-o) = Center response to preferred orientation at different surround orientations, (x-x-x) = Center orientation tuning without surround stimulation, (—) = Center response to surround stimulation alone. A - response of population with 20° orientation preference. B, C and D - response of populations with 5° orientation preference.

More realistically, multiple modes may bifurcate simultaneously, though in the small amplitude linear regime where orientation preference is determined these can all be treated separately in the manner detailed above and lead to the same result.

3.2 POPOUT AND GAIN CONTROL

"Stimulus" dependent horizontal connections have recently been used to model a possible physiological correlate for the psychophysical phenomena of " pop–out " and enhancement (Stemmler, Usher & Niebur, 1995). In this model the horizontal input to excitatory neurons is via sodium channels which are dependent in the conventional manner on the differential between the membrane voltage and the sodium equilibrium potential. For such sodium channels the synaptic currents are attenuated as the membrane depolarizes towards the sodium equilibrium potential. This effect is opposite to that observed for the sodium channels mediating the horizontal input (Hirsch & Gilbert, 1991) which show increased synaptic currents as the membrane is depolarized. Thus although this model reproduces the phenomena described above it does not do so on the basis of the known physiology. We have confirmed with our model that weak stimulus enhancement and strong stimulus pop–out can be modelled with a variety of formulations for the excitatory neuron horizontal input, including a formulation which attenuates with increasing activity as in the model of Stemmler et. al.

It is interesting to note that one overall effect of the horizontal connections is to act as a type of gain control uniformizing the local response over a range of stimulus strengths. This gain control function has been discussed by Somers, Nelson & Sur (1994).

3.3 THE TILT ILLUSION

The tilt illusion (TI) is one of the basic orientation–based visual illusion. A TI occurs when viewing a test line against an inducing grating of uniformly oriented lines with an angle of θ between the orientation of the test line and the inducing grating. Two components of the TI have been described (Wenderoth & Johnstone, 1988), the *direct* TI where the test line appears to be repelled by the grating–the orientation differential appears increased, and the *indirect* TI where the test line appears attracted to the orientation of the grating–the orientation differential appears decreased. Figure 3 depicts a typical plot of magnitude of the tilt effect versus the angle differential between inducing grating and test line reproduced from Wenderoth & Beh (1977). The TI thus provides compelling evidence that local

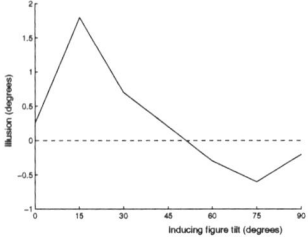

Figure 3: Direct (positive) and indirect (negative) tilt effects

detection of edges is dependent on information from more distant points in the visual field. It is generally believed, that the direct TI is due to lateral inhibition between cortical neurones (Wenderoth & Johnstone, 1988: Carpenter & Blakemore, 1973). It has been postulated that the indirect TI occurs at a higher level of visual processing. We show here that both the direct and indirect TI are a consequence of the lateral and local connections in our model.

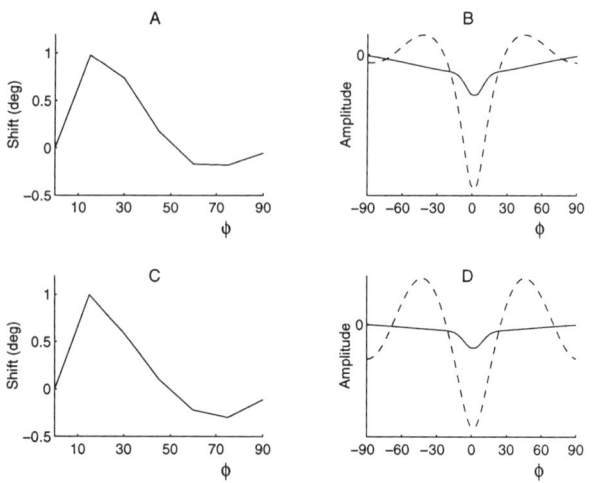

Figure 4: Model simulations of the tilt effect (A and C). B and D show the corresponding kernels mediating long–range interactions. Solid lines indicate the absolute kernel and dashed lines indicate the effective kernel

In figure 4 we give examples of the TI obtained from the model system. The effective kernels for long–range interactions are obtained by filtering the absolute kernels with the local filter which has a band–pass characteristic. It is this effective kernel which determines the tilt effect in keeping with our simulations and analysis which show that orientation preference is determined at the small amplitude linear stage of system development.

4 SUMMARY AND DISCUSSION

We have shown that a very simple center–surround organization, operating in the orientation domain can successfully account for a wide range of neurophysiological and psychophysical phenomena, all involving the effects of visual context on the responses of assemblies of spiking neurons. We expect to be able to show that such an organization can be seen in many parts of the cortex, and that it plays an important role in many forms of information processing in the brain.

Acknowledgements

Supported in part by Grant # 96-24 from the James S. McDonnell Foundation.

References

C. Blakemore and E.A. Tobin, Lateral Inhibition Between Orientation Detectors in the Cat's Visual Cortex, Exp. Brain Res., **15**, 439–440, (1972)

G.G. Blasdel, Orientation selectivity, preference, and continuity in monkey striate cortex, J. Neurosci. **12** No 8, 3139–3161 (1992)

R.H.S. Carpenter and C. Blakemore, Interactions between orientations in human vision, Expl. Brain. Res., **18**, 287–303, (1973)

G.C. DeAngelis, J.G. Robson, I. Ohzawa and R.D. Freeman, Organization of Suppression in Receptive Fields of Neurons in Cat Visual Cortex, J. Neurophysiol., **68** No 1, 144–163, (1992)

D. Fitzpatrick, The Functional Organization of Local Circuits in Visual Cortex: Insights from the Study of Tree Shrew Striate Cortex, Cerebral Cortex **6**, 329–341, (1996)

J.D. Hirsch and C.D. Gilbert, Synaptic physiology of horizontal connections in the cat's visual cortex, J. Neurosci., **11**, 1800–1809, (1991)

A.M. Sillito, K.L. Grieve, H.E. Jones, J. Cudeiro & J. Davis, Visual cortical mechanisms detecting focal orientation discontinuities, Nature, 378, 492–496, (1995)

D.C. Somers, S. Nelson and M. Sur, Effects of long range connections on gain control in an emergent model of visual cortical orientation selectivity, Soc. Neurosci.,**20**, 646.7, (1994)

M. Stemmler, M. Usher and E. Niebur, Lateral Interactions in Primary Visual Cortex: A Model Bridging Physiology and Psychophysics, Science, **269**, 1877–1880, (1995)

M.V. Tsodyks and T. Sejnowski, Rapid state switching in balanced cortical network models, Network, **6** No 2, 111–124, (1995)

J.D. Victor, K. Purpura, E. Katz and B. Mao, Population encoding of spatial frequency, orientation and color in macaque V1, J. Neurophysiol., **72** No 5, (1994)

C. Vreeswijk and H. Sompolinsky, Chaos in neuronal networks with balanced excitatory and inhibitory activity. Science **274**, 1724–1726, (1996)

P. Wenderoth and H. Beh, Component analysis of orientation illusions, Perception, **6** 57–75, (1977)

P. Wenderoth and S. Johnstone, The different mechanisms of the direct and indirect tilt illusions, Vision Res., **28** No 2, 301–312, (1988)

Representing Face Images for Emotion Classification

Curtis Padgett
Department of Computer Science
University of California, San Diego
La Jolla, CA 92034

Garrison Cottrell
Department of Computer Science
University of California, San Diego
La Jolla, CA 92034

Abstract

We compare the generalization performance of three distinct representation schemes for facial emotions using a single classification strategy (neural network). The face images presented to the classifiers are represented as: full face projections of the dataset onto their eigenvectors (eigenfaces); a similar projection constrained to eye and mouth areas (eigenfeatures); and finally a projection of the eye and mouth areas onto the eigenvectors obtained from 32x32 random image patches from the dataset. The latter system achieves 86% generalization on novel face images (individuals the networks were not trained on) drawn from a database in which human subjects consistently identify a single emotion for the face.

1 Introduction

Some of the most successful research in machine perception of complex natural image objects (like faces), has relied heavily on reduction strategies that encode an object as a set of values that span the principal component sub-space of the object's images [Cottrell and Metcalfe, 1991, Pentland et al., 1994]. This approach has gained wide acceptance for its success in classification, for the efficiency in which the eigenvectors can be calculated, and because the technique permits an implementation that is biologically plausible. The procedure followed in generating these face representations requires normalizing a large set of face views ("mug-shots") and from these, identifying a statistically relevant sub-space. Typically the sub-space is located by finding either the eigenvectors of the faces [Pentland et al., 1994] or the weights of the connections in a neural network [Cottrell and Metcalfe, 1991].

In this work, we classify face images based on their emotional content and examine how various representational strategies impact the generalization results of a classifier. Previous work using whole face representations for emotion classification by

Cottrell and Metcalfe [Cottrell and Metcalfe, 1991] was less encouraging than results obtained for face recognition. We seek to determine if the problem in Cottrell and Metcalfe's work stems from bad data (i.e., the inability of the undergraduates to demonstrate emotion), or an inadequate representation (i.e. eigenfaces).

Three distinct representations of faces are considered in this work– a whole face representation similar to that used in previous work on recognition, sex, and emotion [Cottrell and Metcalfe, 1991]; a more localized representation based on the eyes (eigeneyes and eigenmouths) and mouth [Pentland et al., 1994]; and a representation of the eyes and mouth that makes use of basis vectors obtained by principal components of random image blocks. By examining the generalization rate of the classifiers for these different face representations, we attempt to ascertain the sensitivity of the representation and its potential for broader use in other vision classification problems.

2 Face Data

The dataset used in Cottrell and Metcalfe's work on emotions consisted of the faces of undergraduates who were asked to pose for particular expressions. However, feigned emotions by untrained individuals exhibit significant differences from the prototypical face expression [Ekman and Friesen, 1977]. These differences often result in disagreement between the observed emotion and the expression the actor is attempting to feign. A feigned smile for instance, differs around the eyes when compared with a "natural" smile. The quality of the displayed emotion is one of the reasons cited by Cottrell and Metcalfe for the poor recognition rates achieved by their classifier.

To reduce this possibility, we made use of a validated facial emotion database (Pictures of Facial Affect) assembled by Ekman and Friesen [Ekman and Friesen, 1976]. Each of the face images in this set exhibits a substantial agreement between the labeled emotion and the observed response of human subjects. The actors used in this database were trained to reliably produce emotions using Facial Action Coding System [Ekman and Friesen, 1977] and their images were presented to undergraduates for testing. The agreement between the emotion the actor was required to express and the students' observations was at least 70% on all the images incorporated in the database. We digitized a total of 97 images from 12 individuals (6 male, 6 female). Each portrays one of 7 emotions– happy, sad, fear, anger, surprise, disgust or neutral. With the exception of the neutral faces, each image in the set is labeled with a response vector of the remaining six emotions indicating the fraction of total respondents classifying the image with a particular emotion.

Each of the images was linearly stretched over the 8 bit greyscale range to reduce lighting variations. Although care was taken in collecting the original images, natural variations in head size and the mouth's expression resulted in significant variation in the distance between the eyes (2.7 pixels) and in the vertical distance from the eyes to the mouth (5.0 pixels). To achieve scale invariance, each image was scaled so that prominent facial features were located in the same image region. Eye and mouth templates were constructed from a number of images, and the most correlated template was used to localize the respective feature. Similar techniques have been employed in previous work on faces [Brunelli and Poggio, 1993]. Examples of the normalized images and typical facial expressions can be found in Figure 1.

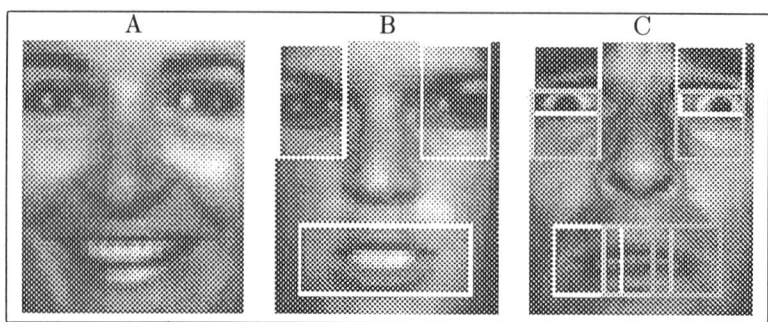

Figure 1: The image regions from which the representations are derived. Image A is a typical normalized and cropped image used to generate the full face eigenvectors. Image B depicts the feature regions from which the feature eigenvectors are calculated. Image C indicates each of the block areas projected onto the random block eigenvectors.

3 Representation

From the normalized database, we develop three distinct representations that form independent pattern sets for a single classification scheme. The selected representations differ in their scope (features or whole face) and in the nature of the sub-space (eigen- faces/features or eigenvectors of random image patches). The more familiar representational schemes (eigenfaces, eigenfeatures) are based on PCA of aligned features or faces. They have been shown to provide a reasonably compact representation for recognition purposes but little is known about their suitability for other classification tasks.

Random image patches are used to identify an alternative sub-space from which a set of localized face feature patterns are generated. This space is different in that the sub-space is more general, the variance captured by the leading eigenvectors is derived from patches drawn randomly over the set of face images. As we seek to develop generalizations across the rather small portion of image space containing faces or features, perturbations in this space will hopefully reflect more about class characteristics than individual distinctions.

For each of the pattern sets, we normalized the resultant set of values obtained from their projections on the eigenvectors by their standard deviation to produce Z scores. The Z score obtained from each image constitutes a single input to the neural network classifier. The highest valued eigenvectors typically contain more average features so that presumably they would be more suitable for object classification. All the representations will make use of the top k principal components.

The full-faced pattern has proved to be quite useful in identification and the same techniques using face features have also been valuable [Pentland et al., 1994, Cottrell and Metcalfe, 1991]. However representations useful for identification of individuals may not be suitable for emotion recognition. In determining the appropriate emotion, structural differences in faces need to be suppressed. One way to accomplish this is to eliminate portions of the face image where variation provides little information with respect to emotion. Local changes in facial muscles around the eyes and mouth are generally associated with our perception of emotions [Ekman and Friesen, 1977]. The full face images presumably contain much information that is simply irrelevant to the task at hand which could impact the ability of the classifier to uncover the signal.

The feature based representations are derived from local windows around the eyes and mouth of the normalized whole face images (see Fig. 1B). The eigenvectors of the feature sub-space are determined independently for each feature (left/right eye and mouth). A face pattern is generated by projecting the particular facial features on their respective eigenvectors.

The random block pattern set is formed from image blocks extracted around the feature locations (see Fig. 1C). The areas around each eye are divided into two vertically overlapping blocks of size 32x32 and the mouth is sectioned into three. However, instead of performing PCA on each individual block or all of them together, a more general PCA of random 32x32 blocks taken over the entire image was used to generate the eigenvectors. We used random blocks to reduce the uniqueness of a projection for a single individual and provide a more reasonable model of the early visual system. The final input pattern consists of the normalized projection of the seven extracted blocks for the image on the top n principal components.

4 Classifier design and training

The principal goal of classification for this study is to examine how the different representational spaces facilitate a classifiers ability to generalize to novel individuals. Comparing expected recognition rate error using the same classification technique with different representations should provide an indication of how well the signal of interest is preserved by the respective representation. A neural network with a hidden layer employing a non-linear activation function (sigmoid) is trained to learn the input-output mapping between the representation of the face image and the associated response vector given by human subjects.

A simple, fully connected, feed-forward neural network containing a single hidden layer with 10 nodes, when trained using back propagation, is capable of correctly classifying the input of training sets from each of the three representations (tested for pattern sizes up to 140 dimensions). The architecture of the network is fixed for a particular input size (based on the number of projections on the respective sub-space) and the generalization of the network is found on a set of images from a novel individual. An overview of the network design is shown in Fig. 2.

To minimize the impact of choosing a poor hold out set from the training set, each of the 11 individuals in the training set was in turn used as a hold out. The results of the 11 networks were then combined to evaluate the classification error on the test set. A number of different techniques are possible: winner take all, weighted average output, voting, etc. The method that we found to consistently give the highest generalization rate involved combining Z scores from the 11 networks. The average output for each possible emotion across all the networks was calculated along with its deviation over the entire training set. These values were used to normalize each output of the 11 networks and the highest weighted sum for a particular input was the associated emotion.

Due to the limited amount of data available for testing and training, a cross-validation technique using each set of an individual's images for testing was employed to increase the confidence of the generalization measurement. Thus, for each individual, 11 networks were combined to evaluate the generalization on the single test individual, and this procedure is repeated for all 12 individuals to give an average generalization error. This results in a total of 132 networks to evaluate the entire database. A single trial consisted of the generalization rate obtained over the whole database for a particular size of input pattern. By varying the initial weights of the network, we can determine the expected generalization performance of this type

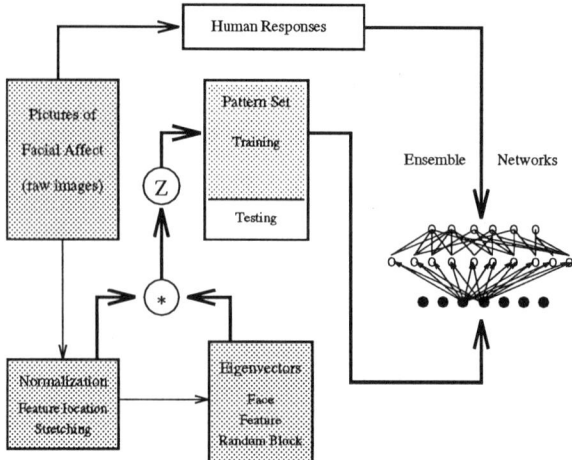

Figure 2: The processing path used to evaluate the pattern set of each representation scheme. The original image data (after normalization) is used to generate the eigenvectors and construct the pattern sets. Human responses are used in training the classifiers and determining generalization percentages on the test data.

classifier on each representation. The number of projections on the relevant space is also varied to determine a generalization curve for each representation. Constructing, training, and evaluating the 132 networks takes approximately 2 minutes on a SparcStation 10 for input pattern size of 15 and 4 minutes for an input pattern size of 80.

5 Results

Fig. 3 provides the expected generalization achieved by the neural network architecture initially seeded with small random weights for an increasing number of projections in the respective representational spaces. Each data point represents the average of 20 trials, 1 σ error bars show the amount of error with respect to the mean. The curve (generalization rate vs. input pattern size) was evaluated at 6 points for the whole face and at 8 points for each feature based approach. The eigenfeature representation made use of up to 40 eigenvectors for the three regions while the random block representation made use of up to 17 eigenvectors for each of its seven regions.

For the most part, all the representations show improvement as the number of projections increase. Variations as input size increases are most likely due to a combination of two factors: lower signal to noise ratios (SNR) for higher order projections; and the increasing number of parameters with a fixed number of patterns, making generalization difficult. The highest average recognition rate achieved by the neural network ensembles is 86%, found using the random block representation with 15 projections per block. The results indicate that the generalization rate for emotion classification varies significantly depending on the representational strategy. Both local feature-based approaches (eigenfeatures and random block) did significantly better over their shared range than the eigenface representation. Over most of the range, the random block representation is clearly superior to the eigenfeature representation even though both are derived from the same image area.

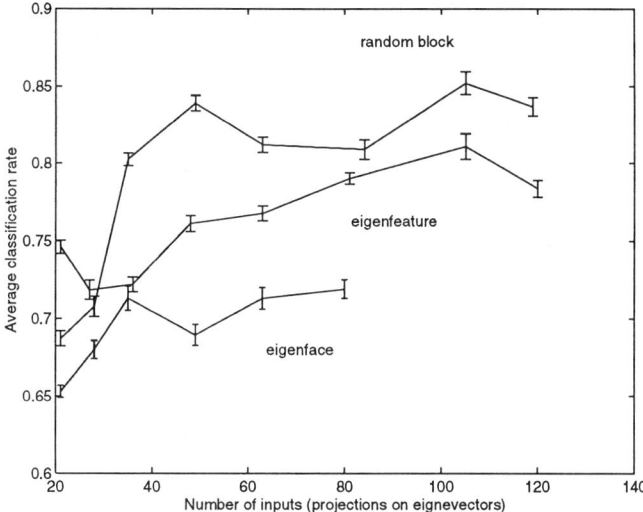

Figure 3: Generalization curves for feature-based representation and full-face representation.

6 Discussion

Fig. 3 clearly demonstrates that reasonable recognition rates can be obtained for novel individuals using representational techniques that were found useful for identity. The 86% generalization rate achieved by the neural network ensemble using random block patterns with 105 projections compares favorably with the results obtained from techniques that use an expression sequence (neutral to expression) [Mase, 1991, Yacoob and Davis, 1996, Bartlett et al., 1996]. Such schemes make use of a neutral mask which enhances the sequence's expression by simple subtraction, a technique that is not possible on novel, static face images. That our technique works as well or better indicates the possibility that the human visual system need not rely on difference image strategies over sequences of images in classifying emotions. As many psychological studies are performed on static images of individuals, models that can accommodate this aspect of emotion recognition can make predictions that directly guide research [Padgett et al., 1996].

As for the suitability of the various representations for fine grained discrimination over different individual objects (as required by emotion classification), Fig. 3 clearly demonstrates the benefits accrued by concentrating on facial features important to emotion. The generalization of the trained networks making use of the two local feature-based representations averages 6-15% higher than do the networks trained using projections on the eigenfaces. The increased performance can be attributed to a better signal to noise ratio for the feature regions. As much of the face is rigid (e.g. the chin and forehead), these regions provide little in the way of information useful in classifying emotions. However, there are substantial differences in these areas between individuals, which will be expressed by the principal component analysis of the images and thus reflected in the projected values. These variations are essentially noise with respect to emotion recognition making it more difficult for the classifier to extract useful generalizations during learning.

The final point is the superiority of the random block representation over the range examined. One possible explanation for its significant performance edge is that major feature variations (e.g. open mouth, open eyes, etc.) are more effectively preserved by this representation than the eigenfeature approach, which covers the same image area. Due to individual differences in mouth/eye structure, one would expect that many of the eigenvectors of the feature space would be devoted to this variance. Facial expressions could be substantially orthogonal to this variance, so that information pertinent to emotion discrimination is effectively hidden. This of course would imply that the eigenfeature representation should be better than the random block representation for face recognition purposes. However, this is not the case. Nearest neighbor classification of individuals using the same pattern sets shows that the random block representation does better for this task as well (results not shown). We are currently developing a noise model that looks promising as an explanation for this phenomenon.

7 Conclusion

We have demonstrated that average generalization rates of 86% can be obtained for emotion recognition on novel individuals using techniques similar to work done in face recognition. Previous work on emotion recognition has relied on image sequences and obtained recognition rates of nearly the same generalization. The model we developed here is potentially of more interest to researchers in emotion that make use of static images of novel individuals in conducting their tests. Future work will compare aspects of the network model with human performance.

References

[Bartlett et al., 1996] Bartlett, M., Viola, P., Sejnowski, T., Larsen, J., Hager, J., and Ekman, P. (1996). Classifying facial action. In Touretzky, D., Mozer, M., and Hasselmo, M., editors, *Advances in Neural Information Processing Systems 8*, Cambridge, MA. MIT Press.

[Brunelli and Poggio, 1993] Brunelli, R. and Poggio, T. (1993). Face recognition: Feature versus templates. *IEEE Trans. Patt. Anal. Machine Intell.*, 15(10).

[Cottrell and Metcalfe, 1991] Cottrell, G. W. and Metcalfe, J. (1991). Empath: Face, gender and emotion recognition using holons. In Lippman, R., Moody, J., and Touretzky, D., editors, *Advances in Neural Information Processing Systems 3*, pages 564–571, San Mateo. Morgan Kaufmann.

[Ekman and Friesen, 1976] Ekman, P. and Friesen, W. (1976). Pictures of facial affect.

[Ekman and Friesen, 1977] Ekman, P. and Friesen, W. (1977). *Facial Action Coding System*. Consulting Psychologists, Palo Alto, CA.

[Mase, 1991] Mase, K. (1991). Recognition of facial expression from optical flow. *IEICE Transactions*, 74(10):3474–3483.

[Padgett et al., 1996] Padgett, C., Cottrell, G., and Adolphs, R. (1996). Categorical perception in facial emotion classification. In Cottrell, G., editor, *Proceedings of the 18th Annual Cognitive Science Conference, San Diego CA*.

[Pentland et al., 1994] Pentland, A. P., Moghaddam, B., and Starner, T. (1994). View-based and modular eigenspaces for face recognition. In *IEEE Conference on Computer Vision & Pattern Recognition*.

[Yacoob and Davis, 1996] Yacoob, Y. and Davis, L. (1996). Recognizing human facial expressions from long image sequences using optical flow. *IEEE Transactions on Pattern Analysis and Machine Intelligence*, 18:636–642.

Rapid Visual Processing using Spike Asynchrony

Simon J. Thorpe & Jacques Gautrais
Centre de Recherche Cerveau & Cognition
F-31062 Toulouse
France
email thorpe@cerco.ups-tlse.fr

Abstract

We have investigated the possibility that rapid processing in the visual system could be achieved by using the order of firing in different neurones as a code, rather than more conventional firing rate schemes. Using SPIKENET, a neural net simulator based on integrate-and-fire neurones and in which neurones in the input layer function as analog-to-delay converters, we have modeled the initial stages of visual processing. Initial results are extremely promising. Even with activity in retinal output cells limited to one spike per neuron per image (effectively ruling out any form of rate coding), sophisticated processing based on asynchronous activation was nonetheless possible.

1. INTRODUCTION

We recently demonstrated that the human visual system can process previously unseen natural images in under 150 ms (Thorpe et al, 1996). Such data, together with previous studies on processing speeds in the primate visual system (see Thorpe & Imbert, 1989) put severe constraints on models of visual processing. For example, temporal lobe neurones respond selectively to faces only 80-100 ms after stimulus onset (Oram & Perrett, 1992; Rolls & Tovee, 1994). To reach the temporal lobe in this time, information from the retina has to pass through roughly ten processing stages (see Fig. 1). If one takes into account the surprisingly slow conduction velocities of intracortical axons (< 1 ms-1, see Nowak & Bullier, 1997) it appears that the computation time within any cortical stage will be as little as 5-10 ms. Given that most cortical neurones will be firing below 100 spikes.s^{-1}, it is difficult to escape the conclusion that processing can be achieved with only one spike per neuron.

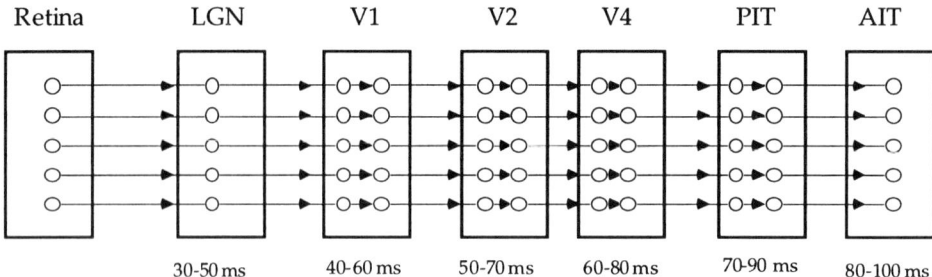

Figure 1 : Approximate latencies for neurones in different stages of the visual primate visual system (see Thorpe & Imbert, 1989; Nowak & Bullier, 1997).

Such constraints pose major problems for conventional firing rate codes since at least two spikes are needed to estimate a neuron's instantaneous firing rate. While it is possible to use the number of spikes generated by a population of cells to code analog values, this turns out to be expensive, since to code n analog values, one needs $n-1$ neurones. Furthermore, the roughly Poisson nature of spike generation would also seriously limit the amount of information that can be transmitted. Even at 100 spikes.s^{-1}, there is a roughly 35% chance that the neuron will generate no spike at all within a particular 10 ms window, again forcing the system to use large numbers of redundant cells.

An alternative is to use information encoded in the temporal pattern of firing produced in response to transient stimuli (Mainen & Sejnowski, 1995). In particular, one can treat neurones not as *analog to frequency converters* (as is normally the case) but rather as *analog to delay converters*(Thorpe, 1990, 1994). The idea is very simple and uses the fact that the time taken for an integrate-and-fire neuron to reach threshold depends on input strength. Thus, in response to an intensity profile, the 6 neurones in figure 2 will tend to fire in a particular order - the most strongly activated cells firing first. Since each neuron fires one and only one spike, the firing rates of the cells contain no information, but there *is* information in the *order* in which the cells fire (see also Hopfield, 1995).

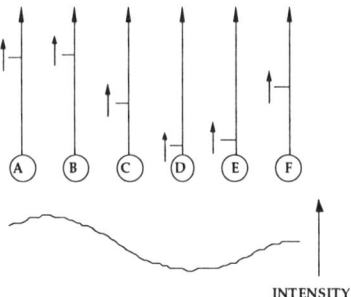

Figure 2 : An example of spike order coding. Because of the intrinsic properties of neurones the most strongly activated neurones will fire first. The sequence B>A>F>C>E>D is one ot the 720 (i.e. 6!) possible orders in which the 6 neurones can fire, each of which reflects a different intensity profile. Note that such a code can be used to send information very quickly.

To test the plausibility of using spike order rather than firing rate as a code, we have developed a neural network simulator "SPIKENET" and used it to model the initial stages of visual processing. Initial results are very encouraging and demonstrate that sophisticated visual processing can indeed be achieved in a visual system in which only one spike per neuron is available.

2. SPIKENET SIMULATIONS

SPIKENET has been developed in order to simulate the activity of large numbers of integrate-and-fire neurones. The basic neuronal elements are simple, and involve only a limited number of parameters, namely, an activation level, a threshold and a membrane time constant. The basic propagation mechanism involves processing the list of neurones that fired during the previous time step. For each spiking neuron, we add a synaptic weight value to each of its targets, and, if the target neuron's activation level exceeds its threshold, we add it to the list of spiking neurones for the next time step and reset its activation level by subtracting the threshold value. When a target neuron is affected for the first time on any particular time step, its activation level is recalculated to simulate an exponential decay over time. One of the great advantages of this kind of "event-driven" simulator is its computational efficiency - even very large networks of neurones can be simulated because no processor time is wasted on inactive neurones.

2.1 ARCHITECTURE

As an initial test of the possibility of single spike processing, we simulated the propagation of activity in a visual system architecture with three levels (see Figure 3). Starting from a gray-scale image (180 x 214 pixels) we calculate the levels of activation in two retinal maps, one corresponding to ON-center retinal ganglion cells, the other to OFF-center cells. This essentially corresponds to convolving the image with two Mexican-hat type operators. However, unlike more classic neural net models, these activation levels are not used to determine a continuous output value for each neuron, nor to calculate a firing rate. Instead, we treat the cells as analog-to-delay converters and calculate at which time step each retinal unit will fire. Because of their receptive field organization, cells which fire at the shortest latencies will correspond to regions in the image where the local contrast is high. Note, however, that each retinal ganglion cell will fire once and once only. While this is clearly not physiologically realistic (normally, cells firing at a short latencies go on to fire further spikes at short intervals) our aim was to see what sort of processing can be achieved in the absence of rate coding.

The ON- and OFF-center cells each make excitatory connections to a large number of cortical maps in the second level of the network. Each map contains neurones with a different pattern of afferent connections which results in orientation and spatial frequency selectivity similar to that described for simple-type neurones in striate cortex. In these simulations we used 32 different filters corresponding to 8 different orientations (each separated by 45°) and four different scales or spatial frequencies. This is functionally equivalent to having one single cortical map (equivalent to area V1) in which each point in visual space corresponds to a hypercolumn containing a complete set of orientation and spatial frequency tuned filters.

Units in the third layer receive weighted inputs from all the simple units corresponding to a particular region of space with the same orientation preference and thus roughly correspond to complex cells in area V1.

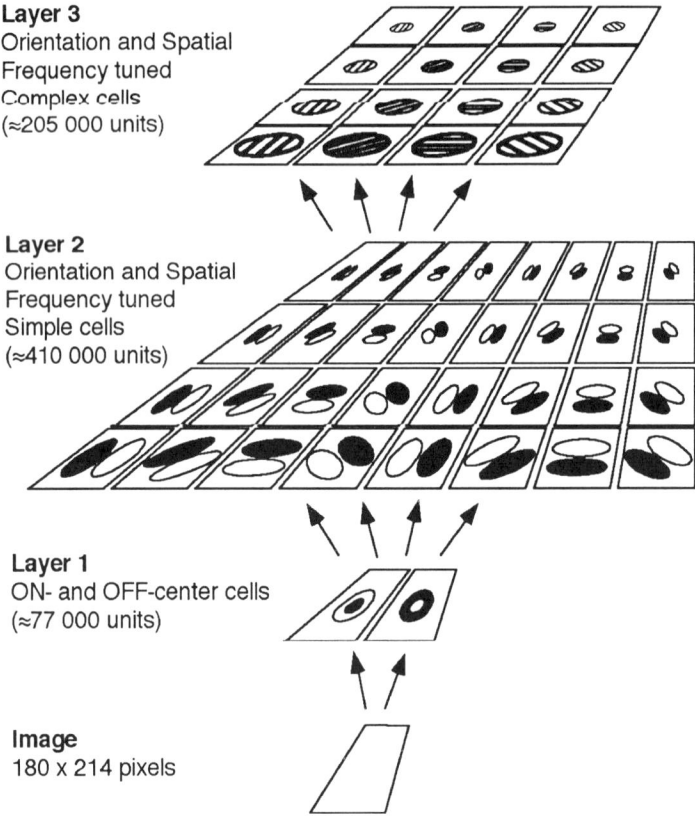

Figure 3 : Architecture used in the present simulations

One unusual feature of the propagation process used in SPIKENET is that the post-synaptic effect of activating a synapse is not fixed, but depends on how many inputs have already been activated. Thus, the earliest firing cells produce a maximal post-synaptic effect (100%), but those which fire later produce less and less response. Specifically, the sensitivity of the post-synaptic neuron decreases by a fixed percentage each time one of its inputs fires. The phenomenon is somewhat similar to the sorts of activity-dependent synaptic depression described recently by Markram & Tsodyks (1996) and others, but differs in that the depression affects all the inputs to a particular neuron. The net result is to make the post-synaptic cell sensitive to the *order* in which its inputs are activated.

2.2 SIMULATION RESULTS

When a new image is presented to the network, spikes are generated asynchronously in the ON- and OFF-center cells of the retina in such a way that information about regions of the image with high local contrast (i.e. where there are contours present) are sent to the cortex first. Progressively, neurons in the second layer become more and more excited, and, after a variable number of time steps, the first cells in the second layer will start to reach threshold and fire. Note that, as in the first layer, the earliest firing units will be those for whom the pattern of input activation best matches their receptive field structure.

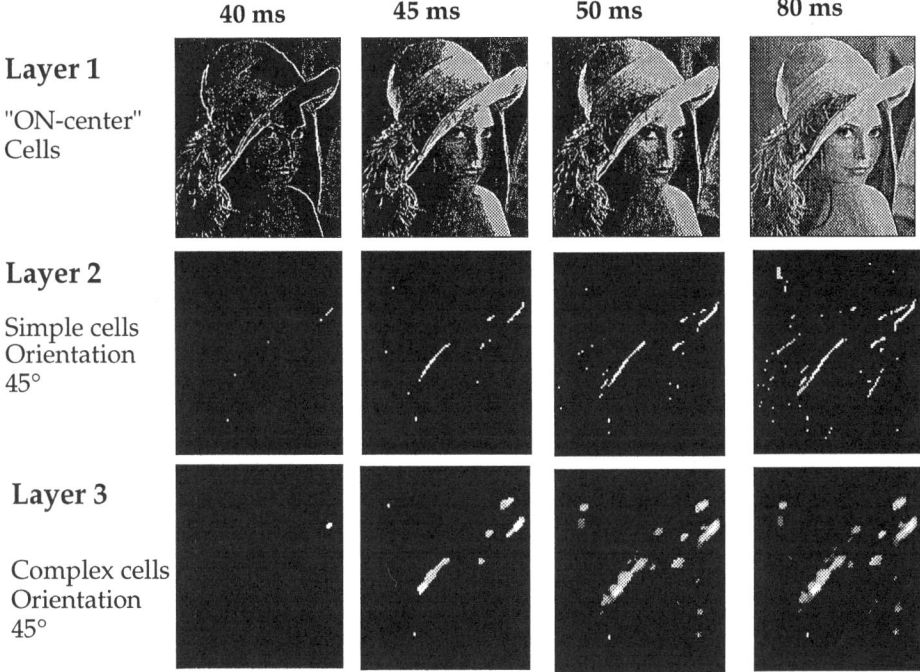

Figure 4 : Development of activity in 3 of the maps

Figure 4 illustrates this process for just three maps. The top row shows the location of units in the ON-center retinal map that have fired after various delays. After 40 msec, the main outlines of the figure can be seen but progressively more details are seen after 45 and then 50 ms. Note that the representation used here uses pixel intensity to code the order in which the cells have fired - bright white spots correspond to places in the image where the cells fired earliest. In the final frame (taken at 80 ms) the vast majority of ON-center cells have already fired and the resulting image is quite similar to a high spatial frequency filtered version of the original image.

The middle row of images shows activity in one of the second level maps - the one corresponding to medium spatial frequency components oriented at 45°. Note that in the first timeslice (40 ms) very few cells have fired, but that the proportion increases progressively over the next 10 or so milliseconds. However, even at the end of the propagation process, the proportion of cells that have actually fired remains low. Finally, the lowest row shows activity in the corresponding third layer map - again corresponding to contours oriented at 45°, but this time with less precise position specificity as a result of the grouping process.

Figure 5 plots the total number of spikes occurring per millisecond in each of the three layers during the first 100 ms following the onset of processing. It is perhaps not surprising that the onset of firing occurs later for layers 2 and 3. However, there is a huge amount of overlap in the onset latencies of cells in the three layers, and indeed, it is doubtful whether there would be any systematic differences in mean onset latency between the three layers.

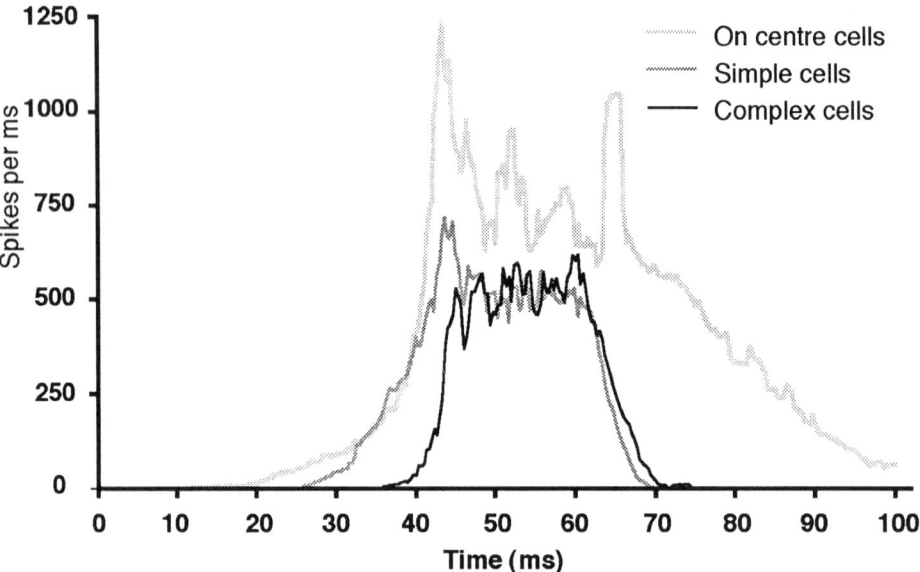

Figure 5 : Amount of activity measured in spikes/ms for the three layers of neurones as a function of time

But perhaps one of the most striking features of these simulations is the way in which the onset latency of cells can be seen to vary with the stimulus. The small number of cells in each layer which fire early are in fact very special because only the most optimally activated cells will fire at such short latencies. The implications of this effect for visual processing are far reaching because it means that the earliest information arriving at later processing stages will be particularly informative because the cells involved are very unambiguous. Interestingly, such changes in onset latency have been observed experimentally in neurones in area V1 of the awake primate in response to changes in orientation. In these experiments it was shown that shifting the orientation of a grating away from a neuron's preferred orientation could result in changes in not only the firing rate of the cell, but also increases in onset latency of as much as 20-30 ms (Celebrini, Thorpe, Trotter & Imbert, 1993).

3. CONCLUSIONS

A number of points can be made on the basis of these results. Perhaps the most important is that visual processing can indeed be performed under conditions in which spike frequency coding is effectively ruled out. Clearly, under normal conditions, neurones in the visual system that respond to a visual input will almost invariably generate more than one spike. However, as we have argued previously, processing in the visual system is so fast that most cells will not have time to generate more than one spike before processing in later stages has to be initiated. The present results indicate that the use of temporal order coding may provide a key to understanding this remarkable efficiency.

The simulations presented here are clearly very limited, but we are currently looking at spike propagation in more complex architectures that include extensive horizontal connections between neurones in a particular layer as well as additional layers of processing. As an example, we have recently developed an application capable of digit recognition. SPIKENET is well suited for such large scale simulations because of the event-driven nature of the propagation process. For instance, the propagation presented here, which involved roughly 700 000 neurones and over 35 million connections, took roughly 15 seconds on a 150 MHz PowerMac, and even faster simulations are possible using parallel processing. With this is view we have developed a version of SPIKENET that uses PVM (Parallel Virtual Machine) to run on a cluster of workstations.

References

Celebrini S., Thorpe S., Trotter Y. & Imbert M. (1993). Dynamics of orientation coding in area V1 of the awake primate *Visual Neuroscience* **10**, 811-25.

Hopfield J. J. (1995). Pattern recognition computation using action potential timing for stimulus representation. *Nature*, **376**, 33-36.

Mainen Z. F. & Sejnowski T. J. (1995). Reliability of spike timing in neocortical neurons *Science*, **268**, 1503-6.

Markram H. & Tsodyks M. (1996) Redistribution of synaptic efficacy between neocortical pyramidal neurons. *Nature,* **382,** 807-810

Nowak L.G. & Bullier J (1997) The timing of information transfer in the visual system. In Kaas J., Rocklund K. & Peters A. (eds). Extrastriate Cortex in Primates (in press). Plenum Press.

Oram M. W. & Perrett D. I. (1992). Time course of neural responses discriminating different views of the face and head *Journal of Neurophysiology*, **68**, 70-84.

Rolls E. T. & Tovee M. J. (1994). Processing speed in the cerebral cortex and the neurophysiology of visual masking *Proc R Soc Lond B Biol Sci*, **257**, 9-15.

Thorpe S., Fize D. & Marlot C. (1996). Speed of processing in the human visual system *Nature*, **381,** 520-522.

Thorpe S. J. (1990). Spike arrival times: A highly efficient coding scheme for neural networks. In R. Eckmiller, G. Hartman & G. Hauske (Eds.), *Parallel processing in neural systems* (pp. 91-94). North-Holland: Elsevier. Reprinted in H. Gutfreund & G. Toulouse (1994), *Biology and computation : A physicist's choice.* Singapour: World Scientific.

Thorpe S. J. & Imbert M. (1989). Biological constraints on connectionist models. In R. Pfeifer, Z. Schreter, F. Fogelman-Soulié & L. Steels (Eds.), *Connectionism in Perspective.* (pp. 63-92). Amsterdam: Elsevier.

Interpreting images by propagating Bayesian beliefs

Yair Weiss
Dept. of Brain and Cognitive Sciences
Massachusetts Institute of Technology
E10-120, Cambridge, MA 02139, USA
yweiss@psyche.mit.edu

Abstract

A central theme of computational vision research has been the realization that reliable estimation of local scene properties requires propagating measurements across the image. Many authors have therefore suggested solving vision problems using architectures of locally connected units updating their activity in parallel. Unfortunately, the convergence of traditional relaxation methods on such architectures has proven to be excruciatingly slow and in general they do not guarantee that the stable point will be a global minimum.

In this paper we show that an architecture in which *Bayesian Beliefs* about image properties are propagated between neighboring units yields convergence times which are several orders of magnitude faster than traditional methods and avoids local minima. In particular our architecture is non-iterative in the sense of Marr [5]: at every time step, the local estimates at a given location are optimal given the information which has already been propagated to that location. We illustrate the algorithm's performance on real images and compare it to several existing methods.

1 Theory

The essence of our approach is shown in figure 1. Figure 1a shows the prototypical ill-posed problem: interpolation of a function from sparse data. Figure 1b shows a traditional relaxation approach to the problem: a dense array of units represents the value of the interpolated function at discretely sampled points. The activity of a unit is updated based on the local data (in those points where data is available) and the activity of the neighboring points. As discussed below, the local update rule can

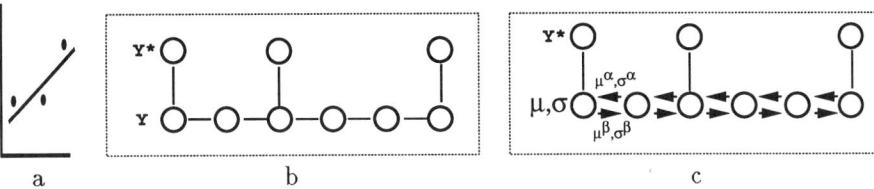

Figure 1: a. a prototypical ill-posed problem b. Traditional relaxation approach: dense array of units represent the value of the interpolated function. Units update their activity based on local information and the activity of neighboring units. c. The Bayesian Belief Propagation (BBP) approach. Units transmit probabilities and combine them according to probability calculus in two non-interacting streams.

be defined such that the network converges to a state in which the activity of each unit corresponds to the value of the globally optimal interpolating function. Figure 1c shows the Bayesian Belief Propagation (BBP) approach to the problem. As in the traditional approach the function is represented by the activity of a dense array of units. However the units transmit probabilities rather than single estimates to their neighbors and combine the probabilities according to the probability calculus.

To formalize the above discussion, let y_k represent the activity of a unit at location k, and let y_k^* be noisy samples from the true function. A typical interpolation problem would be to minimize:

$$J(Y) = \sum_k w_k (y_k - y_k^*)^2 + \lambda \sum_i (y_i - y_{i+1})^2 \qquad (1)$$

Where we have defined $w_k = 0$ for grid points with no data, and $w_k = 1$ for points with data. Since J is quadratic, any local update in the direction of the gradient will converge to the optimal estimate. This yields updates of the sort:

$$y_k \leftarrow y_k + \eta_k (\lambda (\frac{y_{k-1} + y_{k+1}}{2} - y_k) + w_k (y_k^* - y_k)) \qquad (2)$$

Relaxation algorithms differ in their choice of η: $\eta = 1/(\lambda + w_k)$ corresponds to Gauss-Seidel relaxation and $\eta = 1.9/(\lambda + w_k)$ corresponds to successive over relaxation (SOR) which is the method of choice for such problems [10].

To derive a BBP update rule for this problem, note that that minimizing $J(Y)$ is equivalent to maximizing the posterior probability of Y given Y^* assuming the following generative model:

$$y_{i+1} = y_i + \nu \qquad (3)$$
$$y_i^* = w_i y_i + \eta \qquad (4)$$

Where $\nu \sim N(0, \sigma_R)$, $\eta \sim N(0, \sigma_D)$. The ratio of σ_D to σ_R plays a role similar to that of λ in the original cost functional.

The advantage of considering the cost functional as a posterior is that it enables us to use the methods of Hidden Markov Models, Bayesian Belief Nets and Optimal Estimation to derive local update rules (cf. [6, 7, 1]). Denote the posterior by $P_i(u) = P(Y_i = u | Y^*)$, the Markovian property allows us to factor $P_i(u)$ into three terms: one depending on the local data, another depending on data to the left of i and a third depending on data to the right of i. Thus:

$$P_i(u) = c \alpha_i(u) L_i(u) \beta_i(u) \qquad (5)$$

where $\alpha_i(u) = P(Y_i = u | Y_{1,i-1}^*), \beta_i(u) = P(Y_i = u | Y_{i+1,N}^*), L_i(u) = P(Y_i^* | Y_i = u)$ and c denotes a normalizing constant. Now, denoting the conditional $C_i(u, v) =$

$P(Y_i = u | Y_{i-1} = v)$, $\alpha_i(u)$ can be written in terms of $\alpha_{i-1}(v)$:

$$\alpha_i(u) = c \int_v \alpha_{i-1}(v) C_i(u,v) L_{i-1}(v) \tag{6}$$

where c denotes another normalizing constant. A symmetric equation can be written for $\beta_i(u)$.

This suggests a propagation scheme where units represent the probabilities given in the left hand side of equations 5–6 and updates are based on the right hand side, i.e. on the activities of neighboring units. Specifically, for a Gaussian generating process the probabilities can be represented by their mean and variance. Thus denote $P_i \sim N(\mu_i, \sigma_i)$, and similarly $\alpha_i \sim N(\mu_i^\alpha, \sigma_i^\alpha)$ and $\beta_i \sim N(\mu_i^\beta, \sigma_i^\beta)$. Performing the integration in 6 gives a Kalman-Filter like update for the parameters:

$$\mu_i \leftarrow \frac{\frac{w_i}{\sigma_D} Y_i^* + \frac{1}{\sigma_i^\alpha} \mu_i^\alpha + \frac{1}{\sigma_i^\beta} \mu_i^\beta}{\frac{w_i}{\sigma_D} + \frac{1}{\sigma_i^\alpha} + \frac{1}{\sigma_i^\beta}} \tag{7}$$

$$\mu_i^\alpha \leftarrow \frac{\frac{1}{\sigma_{i-1}^\alpha} \mu_{i-1}^\alpha + \frac{w_{i-1}}{\sigma_D} Y_{i-1}^*}{\frac{1}{\sigma_{i-1}^\alpha} + \frac{w_{i-1}}{\sigma_D}} \tag{8}$$

$$\sigma_i^\alpha \leftarrow \sigma_R + (\frac{1}{\sigma_{i-1}^\alpha} + \frac{w_{i-1}}{\sigma_D})^{-1} \tag{9}$$

(the update rules for the parameters of β are analogous)

So far we have considered continuous estimation problems but identical issues arise in labeling problems, where the task is to estimate a label L_k which can take on M discrete values. We will denote $L_k(m) = 1$ if the label takes on value m and zero otherwise. Typically one minimizes functionals of the form:

$$J(L) = \sum_m \sum_k V_k(m) L_k(m) - \lambda \sum_m \sum_k L_k(m) L_{k+1}(m) \tag{10}$$

Traditional relaxation labeling algorithms minimize this cost functional with updates of the form:

$$L_k \leftarrow f(V_k, L_{k-1}, L_k, L_{k+1}) \tag{11}$$

Again different relaxation labeling algorithms differ in their choice of f. A linear sum followed by a threshold gives the discrete Hopfield network updates, a linear sum followed by a "soft" threshold gives the continuous or mean-field Hopfield updates and yet another form gives the relaxation labeling algorithm of Rosenfeld et al. (see [3] for a review of relaxation labeling methods).

To derive a BBP algorithm for this case one can again rewrite J as the posterior of a Markov generating process, and calculate $P(L_k(m) = 1)$ for this process.[1]. This gives the same expressions as in equations 5–6 with the integral replaced by a linear sum. Since the probabilities here are not Gaussian, the α_i, β_i, P_i will not be represented by their mean and variances, but rather by a vector of length M. Thus the update rule for α_i will be:

$$\alpha_i(k) \leftarrow c \sum_l \alpha_{i-1}(l) C_i(k,l) L_{i-1}(l) \tag{12}$$

(and similarly for β.)

---

[1] For certain special cases, knowing $P(L_k(m) = 1)$ is not sufficient for choosing the sequence of labels that minimizes J. In those cases one should do belief revision rather than propagation [6]

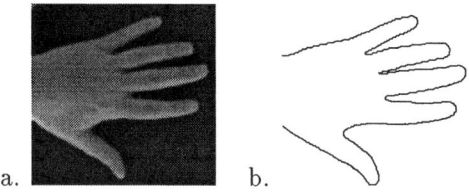

Figure 2: **a.** the first frame of a sequence. The hand is translated to the left. **b.** contour extracted using standard methods

1.1 Convergence

Equations 5–6 are mathematical identities. Hence, it is possible to show [6] that after N iterations the activity of units P_i will converge to the correct posteriors, where N is the maximal distance between any two units in the architecture, and an iteration refers to one update of all units. Furthermore, we have been able to show that after $n < N$ iterations, the activity of unit P_i is guaranteed to represent the probability of the hidden state at location i given all data within distance n.

This guarantee is significant in the light of a distinction made by Marr (1982) regarding local propagation rules. In a scheme where units only communicate with their neighbors, there is an obvious limit on how fast the information can reach a given unit: i.e. after n iterations the unit can only know about information within distance n. Thus there is a minimal number of iterations required for all data to reach all units. Marr distinguished between two types of iterations – those that are needed to allow the information to reach the units, versus those that are used to refine an estimate based on information that has already arrived. The significance of the guarantee on P_i is that it shows that BBP only uses the first type of iteration – iterations are used only to allow more information to reach the units. Once the information has arrived, P_i represents the correct posterior given that information and no further iterations are needed to refine the estimate. Moreover, we have been able to show that propagations schemes that do not propagate probabilities (such as those in equations 2) will in general *not* represent the optimal estimate given information that has already arrived.

To summarize, both traditional relaxation updates as in equation 2 and BBP updates as in equations 7–9 give simple rules for updating a unit's activity based on local data and activities of neighboring units. However, the fact that BBP updates are based on the probability calculus guarantees that a unit's activity will be optimal given information that has already arrived and gives rise to a qualitative difference between the convergence of these two types of schemes. In the next section, we will demonstrate this difference in image interpretation problems.

2 Results

Figure 2a shows the first frame of a sequence in which the hand is translated to the left. Figure 2b shows the bounding contour of the hand extracted using standard techniques.

2.1 Motion propagation along contours

Local measurements along the contour are insufficient to determine the motion. Hildreth [2] suggested to overcome the local ambiguity by minimizing the following

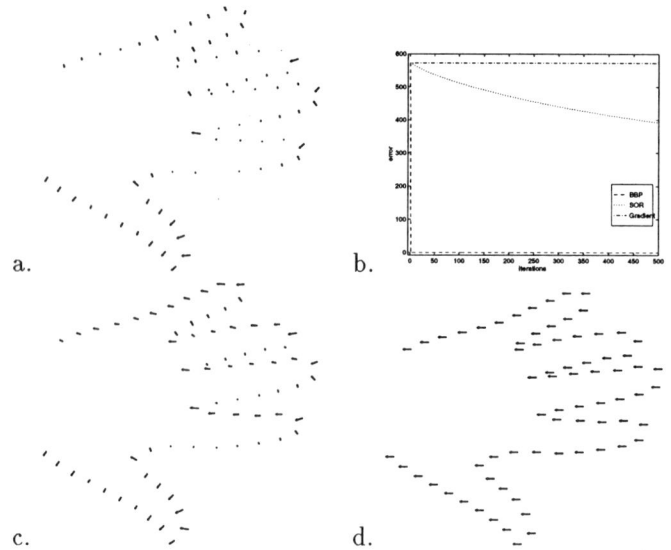

Figure 3: **a.** Local estimate of velocity along the contour. **b.** Performance of SOR, gradient descent and BBP as a function of time. BBP converges orders of magnitude faster than SOR. **c.** Motion estimate of SOR after 500 iterations. **d.** Motion estimate of BBP after 3 iterations.

cost functional:

$$J(V) = \sum_k (dx_k^t v_k + dt_k)^2 + \lambda \sum_k ||v_{k+1} - v_k||^2 \qquad (13)$$

where dx, dt denote the spatial and temporal image derivatives and v_k denotes the velocity at point k along the contour. This functional is analogous to the interpolation functional (eq. 1) and the derivation of the relaxation and BBP updates are also analogous.

Figure 3a shows the estimate of motion based solely on local information. The estimates are wrong due to the aperture problem. Figure 3b shows the performance of three propagation schemes: gradient descent, SOR and BBP. Gradient descent converges so slowly that the improvement in its estimate can not be discerned in the plot. SOR converges much faster than gradient descent but still has significant error after 500 iterations. BBP gets the correct estimate after 3 iterations ! (Here and in all subsequent plots an iteration refers to one update of all units in the network). This is due to the fact that after 3 iterations, the estimate at location k is the optimal one given data in the interval $[k-3, k+3]$. In this case, there is enough data in every such interval along the contour to correctly estimate the motion. Figure 3c shows the estimate produced by SOR after 500 iterations. Even with simple visual inspection it is evident that the estimate is quite wrong. Figure 3d shows the (correct) estimate produced by BBP after 3 iterations.

2.2 Direction of figure propagation

The extracted contour in figure 2 bounds a dark and a light region. *Direction of figure* (DOF) (e.g. [9]) refers to which of these two regions is figure and which is ground. A local cue for DOF is convexity - given three neighboring points along the contour we prefer the DOF that makes the angle defined by those points acute

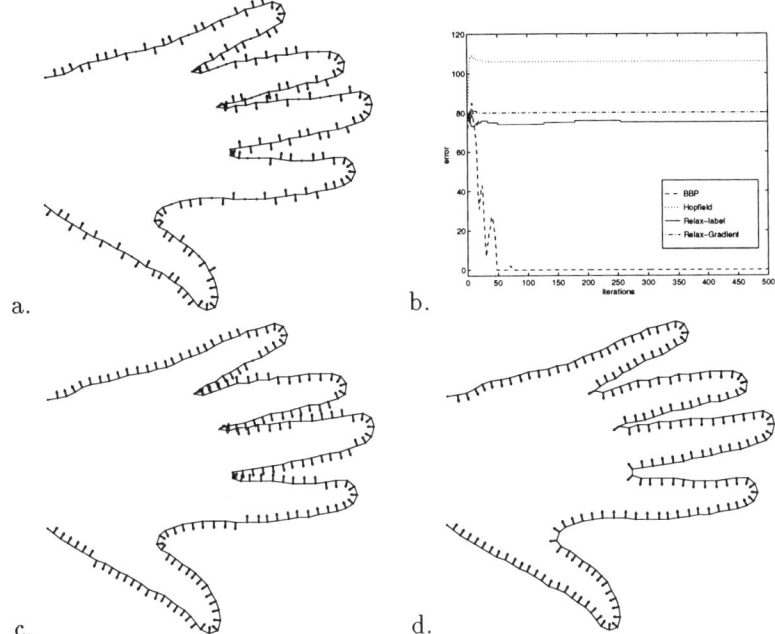

Figure 4: **a.** Local estimate of DOF along the contour. **b.** Performance of Hopfield, gradient descent, relaxation labeling and BBP as a function of time. BBP is the only method that converges to the global minimum. **c.** DOF estimate of Hopfield net after convergence. **d.** DOF estimate of BBP after convergence.

rather than obtuse. Figure 4a shows the results of using this local cue on the hand contour. The local cue is not sufficient.

We can overcome the local ambiguity by minimizing a cost functional that takes into account the DOF at neighboring points in addition to the local convexity. Denote by $L_k(m)$ the DOF at point k along the contour and define

$$J(L) = \sum_m \sum_k V_k(m) L_k(m) - \lambda \sum_m \sum_k L_k(m) L_{k+1}(m) \qquad (14)$$

with $V_k(m)$ determined by the acuteness of the angle at location k.

Figure 4b shows the performance of four propagation algorithms on this task: three traditional relaxation labeling algorithms (MF Hopfield, Rosenfeld et al, constrained gradient descent) and BBP. All three traditional algorithms converge to a local minimum, while the BBP converges to the global minimum. Figure 4c shows the local minimum reached by the Hopfield network and figure 4d shows the correct solution reached by the BBP algorithm. Recall (section 1.1) that BBP is guaranteed to converge to the correct posterior given all the data.

2.3 Extensions to 2D

In the previous two examples ambiguity was reduced by combining information from other points on the same contour. There exist, however, cases when information should be propagated to all points in the image. Unfortunately, such propagation problems correspond to Markov Random Field (MRF) generative models, for which calculation of the posterior cannot be done efficiently. However, Willsky and his colleagues [4] have recently shown that MRFs can be approximated with hierarchical or multi-resolution models. In current work, we have been using the multi-resolution generative model to derive local BBP rules. In this case, the Bayesian beliefs are propagated between neighboring units in a pyramidal representation of the image. Although this work is still in preliminary stages, we find encouraging results in comparison with traditional 2D relaxation schemes.

3 Discussion

The update rules in equations 5–6 differ slightly from those derived by Pearl [6] in that the quantities α, β are conditional probabilities and hence are constantly normalized to sum to unity. Using Pearl's original algorithm for sequences as long as the ones we are considering will lead to messages that become vanishingly small. Likewise our update rules differ slightly from the forward-backward algorithm for HMMs [7] in that ours are based on the assumption that all states are equally likely apriore and hence the updates are symmetric in α and β. Finally, equation 9 can be seen as a variant of a Riccati equation [1].

In addition to these minor notational differences, the context in which we use the update rules is different. While in HMMs and Kalman Filters, the updates are seen as interim calculations toward calculating the posterior, we use these updates in a parallel network of local units and are interested in how the estimates of units in this network improve as a function of iteration. We have shown that an architecture that propagates Bayesian beliefs according to the probability calculus yields orders of magnitude improvements in convergence over traditional schemes that do not propagate probabilities. Thus image interpretation provides an important example of a task where it pays to be a Bayesian.

Acknowledgments

I thank E. Adelson, P. Dayan, J. Tenenbaum and G. Galperin for comments on versions of this manuscript; M.I. Jordan for stimulating discussions and for introducing me to Bayesian nets. Supported by a training grant from NIGMS.

References

[1] Arthur Gelb, editor. *Applied Optimal Estimation*. MIT Press, 1974.

[2] E. C. Hildreth. *The Measurement of Visual Motion*. MIT Press, 1983.

[3] S.Z. Li. *Markov Random Field Modeling in Computer Vision*. Springer-Verlag, 1995.

[4] Mark R. Luettgen, W. Clem Karl, and Allan S. Willsky. Efficient multiscale regularization with application to the computation of optical flow. *IEEE Transactions on image processing*, 3(1):41–64, 1994.

[5] D. Marr. *Vision*. H. Freeman and Co., 1982.

[6] Judea Pearl. *Probabilistic Reasoning in Intelligent Systems: Networks of Plausible Inference*. Morgan Kaufmann, 1988.

[7] Lawrence Rabiner and Biing-Hwang Juang. *Fundamentals of Speech recognition*. PTR Prentice Hall, 1993.

[8] A. Rosenfeld, R. Hummel, and S. Zucker. Scene labeling by relaxation operations. *IEEE Transactions on Systems, Man and Cybernetics*, 6:420–433, 1976.

[9] P. Sajda and L. H. Finkel. Intermediate-level visual representations and the construction of surface perception. *Journal of Cognitive Neuroscience*, 1994.

[10] Gilbert Strang. *Introduction to Applied Mathematics*. Wellesley-Cambridge, 1986.

Salient Contour Extraction by Temporal Binding in a Cortically-Based Network

Shih-Cheng Yen and **Leif H. Finkel**
Department of Bioengineering and
Institute of Neurological Sciences
University of Pennsylvania
Philadelphia, PA 19104, U. S. A.
syen@jupiter.seas.upenn.edu
leif@jupiter.seas.upenn.edu

Abstract

It has been suggested that long-range intrinsic connections in striate cortex may play a role in contour extraction (Gilbert *et al.*, 1996). A number of recent physiological and psychophysical studies have examined the possible role of long range connections in the modulation of contrast detection thresholds (Polat and Sagi, 1993,1994; Kapadia *et al.*, 1995; Kovács and Julesz, 1994) and various pre-attentive detection tasks (Kovács and Julesz, 1993; Field *et al.*, 1993). We have developed a network architecture based on the anatomical connectivity of striate cortex, as well as the temporal dynamics of neuronal processing, that is able to reproduce the observed experimental results. The network has been tested on real images and has applications in terms of identifying salient contours in automatic image processing systems.

1   INTRODUCTION

Vision is an active process, and one of the earliest, preattentive actions in visual processing is the identification of the salient contours in a scene. We propose that this process depends upon two properties of striate cortex: the pattern of horizontal connections between orientation columns, and temporal synchronization of cell responses. In particular, we propose that perceptual salience is directly related to the degree of cell synchronization.

We present results of network simulations that account for recent physiological and psychophysical "pop-out" experiments, and which successfully extract salient contours from real images.

2   MODEL ARCHITECTURE

Linear quadrature steerable filter pyramids (Freeman and Adelson, 1991) are used to model the response characteristics of cells in primary visual cortex. Steerable filters are computationally efficient as they allow the energy at any orientation and spatial frequency to be calculated from the responses of a set of basis filters. The fourth derivative of a Gaussian and its Hilbert transform were used as the filter kernels to approximate the shape of the receptive fields of simple cells.

The model cells are interconnected by long-range horizontal connections in a pattern similar to the co-circular connectivity pattern of Parent and Zucker (1989), as well as the "association field" proposed by Field *et al.* (1993). For each cell with preferred orientation, θ, the orientations, ϕ, of the pre-synaptic cell at position (i,j) relative to the post-synaptic cell, are specified by:

$$\phi(\theta, i, j) = 2 \tan^{-1}\left(\frac{j}{i}\right) - \theta$$

(see Figure 1a). These excitatory connections are confined to two regions, one flaring out along the axis of orientation of the cell (co-axial), and another confined to a narrow zone extending orthogonally to the axis of orientation (trans-axial). The fan-out of the co-axial connections is limited to low curvature deviations from the orientation axis while the trans-axial connections are limited to a narrow region orthogonal to the cell's orientation axis. These constraints are expressed as:

$$\Gamma(\theta, i, j, \psi) = \begin{cases} 1, & \textit{if } \tan^{-1}\left(\frac{j}{i}\right) - \theta < \kappa, \\ 1, & \textit{if } \tan^{-1}\left(\frac{j}{i}\right) - \theta = \frac{\pi}{2} \pm \varepsilon, \\ 0, & \textit{otherwise.} \end{cases}$$

where κ represents the maximum angular deviation from the orientation axis of the post-synaptic cell and ε represents the maximum angular deviation from the orthogonal axis of the post-synaptic cell. Connection weights decrease for positions with increasing angular deviation from the orientation axis of the cell, as well as positions with increasing distance, in agreement with the physiological and psychophysical findings. Figure 1b illustrates the connectivity pattern. There is physiological, anatomical and psychophysical evidence consistent with the existence of both sets of connections (Nelson and Frost, 1985; Kapadia *et al.*, 1995; Rockland and Lund, 1983; Lund *et al.*, 1985; Fitzpatrick, 1996; Polat and Sagi, 1993, 1994).

Cells that are facilitated by the connections inhibit neighboring cells that lie outside the facilitatory zones. The magnitude of the inhibition is such that only cells receiving strong support are able to remain active. This is consistent with the physiological findings of Nelson and Frost (1985) and Kapadia *et al.* (1995) as well as the intra-cellular recordings of Weliky et al. (1995) which show EPSPs followed by IPSPs when the long-distance connections were stimulated. This inhibition is thought to occur through di-synaptic pathways.

In the model, cells are assumed to enter a "bursting mode" in which they synchronize with other bursting cells. In cortex, bursting has been associated with supragranular "chattering cells" (Gray and McCormick (1996). In the model, cells that enter the bursting

Salient Contour Extraction by Temporal Binding in a Cortically-based Network

mode are modeled as homogeneous coupled neural oscillators with a common fundamental frequency but different phases (Kopell and Ermentrout, 1986; Baldi and Meir, 1990). The phase of each oscillator is modulated by the phase of the oscillators to which it is coupled. Oscillators are coupled only to other oscillators with which they have strong, reciprocal, connections. The oscillators synchronize using a simple phase averaging rule:

$$\Theta_i(t) = \frac{\sum w_{ij} \Theta_j(t-1)}{\sum w_{ij}}, \quad w_{ii} = 1$$

where Θ represents the phase of the oscillator and w_{ij} represents the weight of the connection between oscillator i and j. The oscillators synchronize iteratively with synchronization defined as the following condition:

$$|\Theta_i(t) - \Theta_j(t)| < \delta, \quad i, j \in C, \quad t < t_{max}$$

where C represents all the coupled oscillators on the same contour, δ represents the maximum phase difference between oscillators, and t_{max} represents the maximum number of time steps the oscillators are allowed to synchronize. The salience of the chain is then represented by the sum of the activities of all the synchronized elements in the group, C. The chain with the highest salience is chosen as the output of the network. This allows us to compare the output of the model to psychophysical results on contour extraction.

It has been postulated that the 40 Hz oscillations observed in the cortex may be responsible for perceptual binding across different cortical regions (Singer and Gray, 1995). Recent studies have questioned the functional significance and even the existence of these oscillations (Ghose and Freeman, 1992; Bair et al., 1994). We use neural oscillators only as a simple functional means of computing synchronization and make no assumption regarding their possible role in cortex.

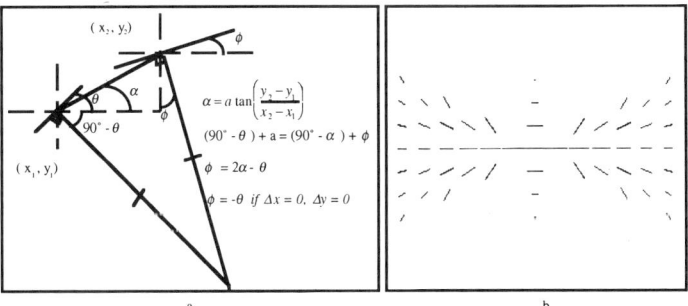

Figure 1: a) Co-circularity constraint. b) Connectivity pattern of a horizontally oriented cell. Length of line indicates connection strength.

3 RESULTS

This model was tested by simulating a number of psychophysical experiments. A number of model parameters remain to be defined through further physiological and psychophysical experiments, thus we only attempt a qualitative fit to the data. All simulations were conducted with the same parameter set.

3.1 EXTRACTION OF SALIENT CONTOURS

Using the same methods as Field et al. (1993), we tested the model's ability to extract contours embedded in noise (see Figure 2). Pairs of stimulus arrays were presented to the network, one array contains a contour, the other contains only randomly oriented elements. The network determines the stimulus containing the contour with the highest salience. Network performance was measured by computing the percentage of correct detection. The network was tested on a range of stimulus variables governing the target contour: 1) the angle, β, between elements on a contour, 2) the angle between elements on a contour but with the elements aligned orthogonal to the contour passing through them, 3) the angle between elements with a random offset angle, $\pm\alpha$, with respect to the contour passing through them, and 4) average separation of the elements. 500 simulations were run at each data point. The results are shown in Figure 2. The model shows good qualitative agreement with the psychophysical data. When the elements are aligned, the performance of the network is mostly modulated by the co-axial connections, whereas when the elements are oriented orthogonal to the contour, the trans-axial connections mediate performance. Both the model and human subjects are adversely affected as the weights between consecutive elements decrease in strength. This reduces the length of the contour and thus the saliency of the stimulus.

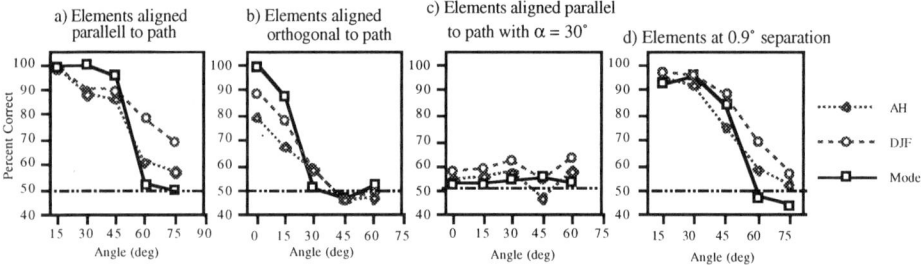

Figure 2: Simulation results are compared to the data from 2 subjects (AH, DJF) in Field *et al.* (1993). Stimuli consisted of 256 randomly oriented Gabor patches with 12 elements aligned to form a contour. Each data point represents results for 500 simulations.

3.2 EFFECTS OF CONTOUR CLOSURE

In a series of experiments using similar stimuli to Field *et al.* (1993), Kovács and Julesz (1993) found that closed contours are much more salient than open contours. They reported that when the inter-element spacing between all elements was gradually increased, the maximum inter-element separation for detecting closed contours, Δ_c (defined at 75% performance), is higher than that for open contours, Δ_o. In addition, they showed that when elements spaced at Δ_o are added to a "jagged" (open) contour, the saliency of the contour increases monotonically but when elements spaced at Δ_c are added to a circular contour, the saliency does not change until the last element is added and the contour becomes closed. In fact, at Δ_c, the contour is not salient until it is closed, at which point it suddenly "pops-out" (see Figure 3c). This finding places a strong constraint on the computation of saliency in visual perception.

Interestingly, it has been shown that synchronization in a chain of coupled neural oscillators is enhanced when the chain is closed (Kopell and Ermentrout, 1986; Ermentrout, 1985; Somers and Kopell, 1993). This property seems to be related to the differences in boundary effects on synchronization between open and closed chains and appears to hold across different families of coupled oscillators. It has also been shown that synchronization is dependent on the coupling between oscillators -- the stronger the coupling, the better the synchronization, both in terms of speed and coherence (Somers and Kopell, 1993; Wang, 1995). We believe these findings may apply to the psychophysical results.

As in Kovács and Julesz (1993), the network is presented with two stimuli, one containing a contour and the other made up of all randomly oriented elements. The network picks the stimulus containing the synchronized contour with the higher salience. In separate trials, the threshold for maximum separation between elements was determined for open and closed contours. The ratio of the separation of the background elements to the that of elements on a closed curve, φ_c, was found to be 0.6 (which is similar to the threshold of 0.65 recently reported by Kovács et al., 1996), whereas the ratio for open contours, φ_o, was found to be 0.9. (Δ is the threshold separation of contour elements, φ, at a particular background separation). We then examined the changes in salience for open and closed contours. The performance of the network was measured as additional elements were added to an initial short contour of elements. The results are shown in Figure 3b. At φ_o, both open and closed contours are synchronized but at φ_c, elements are synchronized only when the chains are closed. If salience can only be computed for synchronized contours, then as additional elements are added to an open chain at φ_o, the salience would increase since the whole chain is synchronized. On the other hand, at φ_c, as long as the last element is missing, the chain is really an open chain, and since φ_c is smaller than φ_o, the elements on the chain will not be able to synchronize and adding elements has no effect on salience. Once the last element is added, the chain is immediately able to synchronize and the salience of the contour increases dramatically and causes the contour to "pop-out".

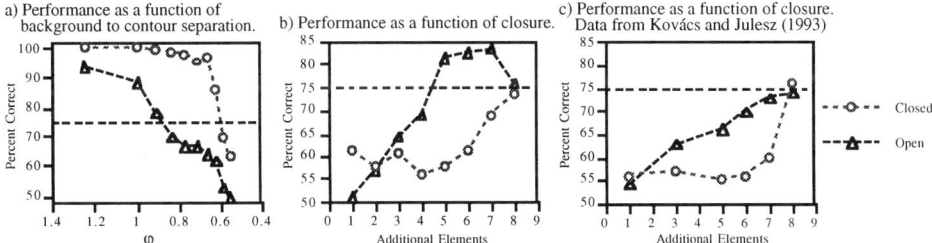

Figure 3. Simulation of the experiments of Kovács and Julesz (1993). Stimuli consisted of 2025 randomly oriented Gabor patches, with 24 elements aligned to form a contour. Each data point represents results from 500 trials. a) Plot of the performance of the model with respect to the ratio of the separation of the background elements to the contour elements. Results show closed contours are salient to a more salient than open contours. b) Changes in salience as additional elements are added to open and closed contours. Results show that the salience of open contours increase monotonically while the salience of closed contours only change with the addition of the last element. Open contours were initially made up of 7 elements while closed contours were made up of 17 elements. c) The data from Kovács and Julesz (1993) are re-plotted for comparison.

3.3 REAL IMAGES

A stringent test of the model's capabilities is the ability to extract perceptually salient contours in real images. Figure 4 and 5 show results for a typical image. The original grayscale image, the output of the steerable filters, and the output of the model are shown in Figure 4a,b,c and Figure 5a,b,c respectively. The network is able to extract some of the more salient contours and ignore other high contrast edges detected by the steerable filters. Both simulations used filters at only one spatial scale and could be improved through interactions across multiple spatial frequencies. Nevertheless, the model shows promise for automated image processing applications

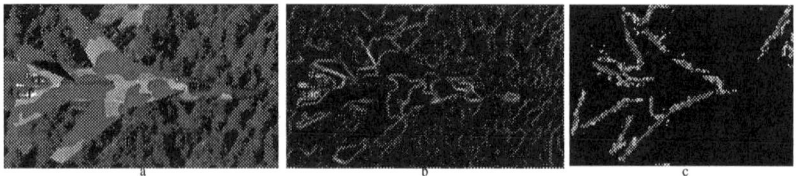

Figure 4: a) Plane image. b) Steerable filter response. c) Result of model showing the most salient contours.

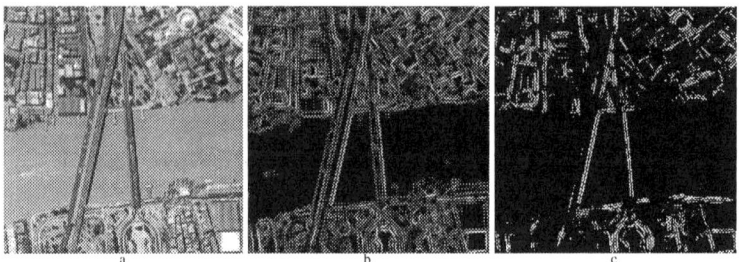

Figure 5: a) Satellite image of Bangkok. b) Steerable filter response. c) Salient contours extracted from the image. The model included filters at only one spatial frequency.

4 CONCLUSION

We have presented a cortically-based model that is able to identify perceptually salient contours in images containing high levels of noise. The model is based on the use of long distance intracortical connections that facilitate the responses of cells lying along smooth contours. Salience is defined as the combined activity of the synchronized population of cells responding to a particular contour. The model qualitatively accounts for a range of physiological and psychophysical results and can be used in extracting salient contours in real images.

Acknowledgements

Supported by the Office of Naval Research (N00014-93-1-0681), The Whitaker Foundation, and the McDonnell-Pew Program in Cognitive Neuroscience.

References

Bair, W., Koch, C., Newsome, W. & Britten, K. (1994). Power spectrum analysis of bursting cells in area MT in the behaving monkey. *Journal of Neuroscience, 14*, 2870-2892.

Baldi, P. & Meir, R. (1990). Computing with arrays of coupled oscillators: An application to preattentive texture discrimination. *Neural Computation, 2,* 458-471.

Ermentrout, G. B. (1985). The behavior of rings of coupled oscillators. *Journal of Mathematical Biology, 23,* 55-74.

Field, D. J., Hayes, A. & Hess, R. F. (1993). Contour integration by the human visual system: Evidence for a local "Association Field". *Vision Research, 33*, 173-193.

Fitzpatrick, D. (1996). The functional-organization of local circuits in visual-cortex – insights from the study of tree shrew striate cortex. *Cerebral Cortex, 6,* 329-341.

Freeman, W. T. & Adelson, E. H. (1991). The design and use of steerable filters. *IEEE Transactions on Pattern Analysis and Machine Intelligence, 13,* 891-906.

Gilbert, C. D., Das, A., Ito, M., Kapadia, M. & Westheimer, G. (1996). Spatial integration and cortical dynamics. *Proceedings of the National Academy of Sciences USA, 93*, 615-622.

Ghose, G. M. & Freeman, R. D. (1992). Oscillatory discharge in the visual system: Does it have a functional role? *Journal of Neurophysiology, 68*, 1558-1574.

Gray, C. M. & McCormick, D. A. (1996). Chattering cells -- superficial pyramidal neurons contributing to the generation of synchronous oscillations in the visual-cortex. *Science, 274*, 109-113.

Kapadia, M. K., Ito, M., Gilbert, C. D. & Westheimer. G. (1995). Improvement in visual sensitivity by changes in local context: Parallel studies in human observers and in V1 of alert monkeys. *Neuron,15*, 843-856.

Kopell, N. & Ermentrout, G. B. (1986). Symmetry and phaselocking in chains of weakly coupled oscillators. *Communications on Pure and Applied Mathematics, 39*, 623-660.

Kovács, I. & Julesz, B. (1993). A closed curve is much more than an incomplete one: Effect of closure in figure-ground segmentation. *Proceedings of National Academy of Sciences, USA, 90*, 7495-7497.

Kovács, I. & Julesz, B. (1994). Perceptual sensitivity maps within globally defined visual shapes. *Nature, 370*, 644-646.

Kovács, I., Polat, U. & Norcia, A. M. (1996). Breakdown of binding mechanisms in amblyopia. *Investigative Ophthalmology & Visual Science, 37*, 3078.

Lund, J., Fitzpatrick, D. & Humphrey, A. L. (1985). The striate visual cortex of the tree shrew. In Jones, E. G. & Peters, A. (Eds), *Cerebral Cortex* (pp. 157-205). New York: Plenum.

Nelson, J. I. & Frost, B. J. (1985). Intracortical facilitation among co-oriented, co-axially aligned simple cells in cat striate cortex. *Experimental Brain Research, 61*, 54-61.

Parent, P. & Zucker, S. W. (1989). Trace inference, curvature consistency, and curve detection. *IEEE Transactions on Pattern Analysis and Machine Intelligence, 11*, 823-839.

Polat, U. & Sagi, D. (1993). Lateral interactions between spatial channels: Suppression and facilitation revealed by lateral masking experiments. *Vision Research, 33*, 993-999.

Polat, U. & Sagi, D. (1994). The architecture of perceptual spatial interactions. *Vision Research, 34*, 73-78.

Rockland, K. S. & Lund, J. S. (1983). Intrinsic laminar lattice connections in primate visual cortex. *Journal of Comparative Neurology, 216*, 303-318.

Singer, W. & Gray, C. M. (1995). Visual feature integration and the temporal correlation hypothesis. *Annual Review of Neuroscience, 18*, 555-586.

Somers, D. & Kopell, N. (1993). Rapid synchronization through fast threshold modulation. *Biological Cybernetics, 68*, 393-407.

Wang, D. (1995). Emergent synchrony in locally coupled neural oscillators. *IEEE Transactions on Neural Networks, 6*, 941-948.

Weliky M., Kandler, K., Fitzpatrick, D. & Katz, L. C. (1995). Patterns of excitation and inhibition evoked by horizontal connections in visual cortex share a common relationship to orientation columns. *Neuron, 15*, 541-552.

Part VIII
Applications

An Orientation Selective Neural Network for Pattern Identification in Particle Detectors

Halina Abramowicz, David Horn, Ury Naftaly, Carmit Sahar–Pikielny
School of Physics and Astronomy, Tel Aviv University
Tel Aviv 69978, Israel
halina@post.tau.ac.il, horn@neuron.tau.ac.il
ury@post.tau.ac.il, carmit@post.tau.ac.il

Abstract

We present an algorithm for identifying linear patterns on a two-dimensional lattice based on the concept of an orientation selective cell, a concept borrowed from neurobiology of vision. Constructing a multi-layered neural network with fixed architecture which implements orientation selectivity, we define output elements corresponding to different orientations, which allow us to make a selection decision. The algorithm takes into account the granularity of the lattice as well as the presence of noise and inefficiencies. The method is applied to a sample of data collected with the ZEUS detector at HERA in order to identify cosmic muons that leave a linear pattern of signals in the segmented calorimeter. A two dimensional representation of the relevant part of the detector is used. The algorithm performs very well. Given its architecture, this system becomes a good candidate for fast pattern recognition in parallel processing devices.

I Introduction

A typical problem in experiments performed at high energy accelerators aimed at studying novel effects in the field of Elementary Particle Physics is that of preselecting interesting interactions at as early a stage as possible, in order to keep the data volume manageable. One class of events that have to be eliminated is due to cosmic muons that pass all trigger conditions.

The most characteristic feature of cosmic muons is that they leave in the detector a path of signals aligned along a straight line. The efficiency of pattern recognition algorithms depends strongly on the granularity with which such a line is probed, on the level of noise and the response efficiency of a given detector. Yet the efficiency of a visual scan is fairly independent of those features [1] . This lead us to look for a new approach through application of ideas from the field of vision.

The main tool that we borrow from the neuronal circuitry of the visual cortex is the orientation selective simple cell [2]. It is incorporated in the hidden layers of a feed forward neural network, possessing a predefined receptive field with excitatory and inhibitory connections. Using these elements we have developed [3] a method for identifying straight lines of varying slopes and lengths on a grid with limited resolution. This method is then applied to the problem of identifying cosmic muons in accelerator data, and compared with other tools.

By using a network with a fixed architecture we deviate from conventional approaches of neural networks in particle physics [4]. One advantage of this approach is that the number of free parameters is small, and it can, therefore, be determined using a small data set. The second advantage is the fact that it opens up the possibility of a relatively simple implementation in hardware. This is an important feature for particle detectors, since high energy physics experiments are expected to produce in the next decade a flux of data that is higher than present analysis methods can cope with.

II Description of the Task

In a two-dimensional representation, the granularity of the rear part of the ZEUS calorimeter [6] can be emulated roughly by a 23×23 lattice of 20×20 cm^2 squares. While such a representation does not use the full information available in the detector, it is sufficient for our study. In our language each cell of this lattice will be denoted as a pixel. A pixel is activated if the corresponding calorimeter cell is above a threshold level predetermined by the properties of the detector.

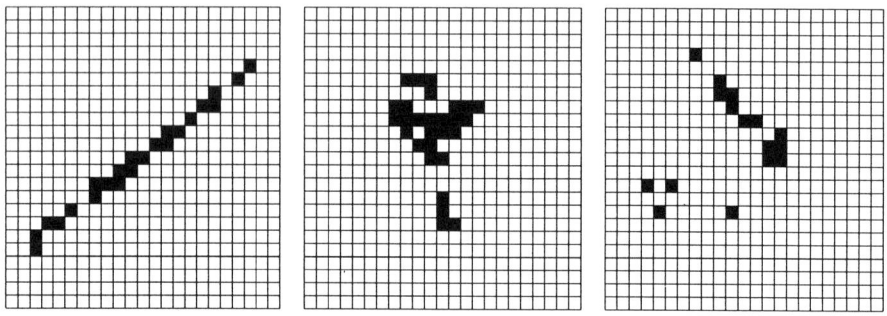

Figure 1: Example of patterns corresponding to a cosmic muon (left), a typical accelerator event (middle), and an accelerator event that looks like a muon (right), as seen in a two dimensional projection.

A cosmic muon, depending on its angle of incidence, activates along its linear path typically from 3 to 25 neighboring pixels anywhere on the 23×23 grid. The pattern of signals generated by accelerator events consists on average of 3 to 8 clusters, of typically 4 adjacent activated pixels, separated by empty pixels. The clusters

Orientation Selective Neural Network

tend to populate the center of the 23 × 23 lattice. Due to inherent dynamics of the interactions under study, the distribution of clusters is not isotropic. Examples of events, as seen in the two-dimensional projection in the rear part of the ZEUS calorimeter, are shown in figure 1.

The lattice discretizes the data and distorts it. Adding conventional noise levels, the decision of classification of the data into accelerator events and cosmic muon events is difficult to obtain through automatic means. Yet, it is the feeling of experimentalists dealing with these problems, that any expert can distinguish between the two cases with high efficiency (identifying a muon as such) and purity (not misidentifying an accelerator event). We define our task as developing automatic means of doing the same.

III The Orientation Selective Neural Network

Our analysis is based on a network of orientation selective neurons (OSNN) that will be described in this chapter. We start out with an input layer of pixels on a two dimensional grid with discrete labeling $i = (x, y)$ of the neuron (pixel) that can get the values $S_i = 1$ or 0, depending on whether the pixel is activated or not.

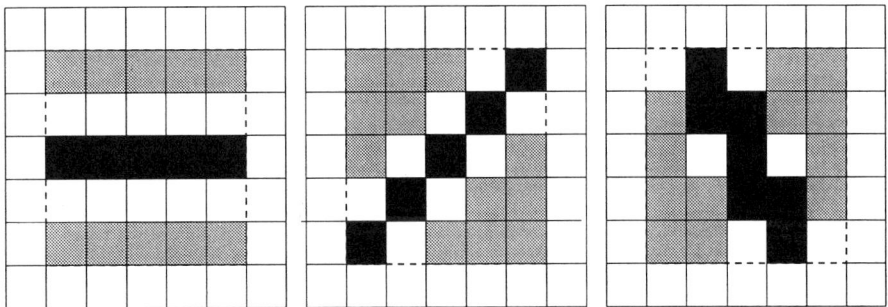

Figure 2: Connectivity patterns for orientation selective cells on the second layer of the OSNN. From left to right are examples of orientations of 0, $\pi/4$ and $5\pi/8$. Non-zero weights are defined only within a 5 × 5 grid. The dark pixels have weights of +1, and the grey ones have weights of -1. White pixels have zero weights.

The input is being fed into a second layer that is composed of orientation selective neurons $V_2^{i,\alpha}$ at location i with orientation θ_α where α belongs to a discrete set of 16 labels, i.e. $\theta_\alpha = \alpha\pi/16$. The neuron $V_2^{i,\alpha}$ is the analog of a simple cell in the visual cortex. Its receptive field consists of an array of dimension 5 × 5 centered at pixel i. Examples of the connectivity, for three different choices of α, are shown in Fig. 2. The weights take the values of 1,0 and -1.

The second layer consists then of $23 \times 23 \times 16$ neurons, each of which may be thought of as one of 16 orientation elements at some (x, y) location of the input layer. Next we employ a modified Winner Take All (WTA) algorithm, selecting the leading orientation $\alpha_{max}(i)$ for which the largest $V_2^{i,\alpha}$ is obtained at the given location i. If we find that several $V_2^{i,\alpha}$ at the same location i are close in value to the maximal one, we allow up to five different $V_2^{i,\alpha}$ neurons to remain active at this stage of the processing, provided they all lie within a sector of $\alpha_{max} \pm 2$, or $\theta_{max} \pm \pi/8$. All other $V_2^{i,\alpha}$ are reset to zero. If, however, at a given location i we obtain several large values of $V_2^{i,\alpha}$ that correspond to non-neighboring orientations, all are being discarded.

The third layer also consists of orientation selective cells. They are constructed with a receptive field of size 7×7, and receive inputs from neurons with the same orientation on the second layer. The weights on this layer are defined in a similar fashion to the previous ones, but here negative weights are assigned the value of -3, not -1. For linear patterns, the purpose of this layer is to fill in the holes due to fluctuations in the pixel activation, i.e. complete the lines of same orientation of the second layer. As before, we keep also here up to five highest values at each location, following the same WTA procedure as on the second layer.

The fourth layer of the OSNN consists of only 16 components, D^α, each corresponding to one of the discrete orientations α. For each orientation we calculate the convolution of the first and third layers, $D^\alpha = \sum_i V_3^{i,\alpha} S_i$. The elements D^α carry the information about the number of the input pixels that contribute to a given orientation θ_α. Cosmic muons are characterized by high values of D^α whereas accelerator events possess low values, as shown in figure 3 below.

The computational complexity of this algorithm is $\mathcal{O}(n)$ where n is the number of pixels, since a constant number of operations is performed on each pixel. There are basically four free parameters in the algorithm. These are the sizes of the receptive fields on the second and third layer and the corresponding activation thresholds. Their values can be tuned for the best performance, however they are well constrained by the spatial resolution, the noise level in the system and the activation properties of the input pixels. The size of the receptive field determines to a large extent the number of orientations allowed to survive in the modified WTA algorithm.

IV OSNN and a Selection Criterion on the Training Set

The details of the design of the OSNN and the tuning of its parameters were fixed while training it on a sample of 250 cosmic muons and a similar amount of accelerator events. The sample was obtained by preselection with existing algorithms and a visual scan as a cross-check.

For cosmic muon events the highest value of D^α, $D_{\max}$, determines the orientation of the straight line. In figure 3 we present the correlation between $D_{\max}$ and the number n_p of activated input pixels for cosmic muon and accelerator events. As expected one observes a linear correlation between $D_{\max}$ and n_p for the muons while almost no correlation is observed for accelerator events. This allows us to set a selection criterion defined by the separator in this figure. We quantify the quality of our selection by quoting the efficiency of properly identifying a cosmic muon for 100% purity, corresponding to no accelerator event misidentified as a muon. In OSNN-D, which we define according to the separator shown in Fig 3, we obtain 93.0% efficiency on the training set.

On the right hand side of Fig 3 we present results of a conventional method for detecting lines on a grid, the Hough transform [7, 8, 9]. This is based on the analysis of a parameter space describing locations and slopes of straight lines. The cells of this space with the largest occupation number, $N_{\max}$, are the analogs of our $D_{\max}$. In the figure we show the correlation of $N_{\max}$ with n_p which allows us to draw a separator between cosmic muons and accelerator events, leading to an efficiency of 88% for 100% purity. Although this number is not much lower than the

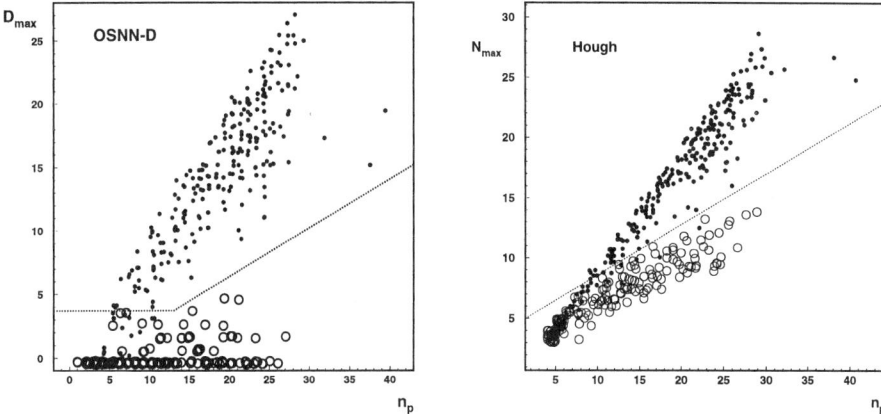

Figure 3: Left: Correlation between the maximum value of D^α, $D_{\max}$, and the number n_p of input pixels for cosmic muon (dots) and accelerator events (open circles). The dashed line defines a separator such that all events above it correspond to cosmic muons (100% purity). This selection criterion has 93% efficiency. Right: Using the Hough Transform method, we compare the values of the largest accumulation cell $N_{\max}$ with n_p and find that the two types of events have different slopes, thus allowing also the definition of a separator. In this case, the efficiency is 88%.

efficiency of OSNN-D, we note that the difference between the two types of event distributions is not as significant as in OSNN-D. In the test set, to be discussed in the next chapter, we will consider 40,000 accelerator events contaminated by less than 100 cosmic muons. Clearly the expected generalization quality of OSNN-D will be higher than that of the Hough transform. It should of course be noted that the OSNN is a multi-layer network, whereas the Hough transform method that we have described is a single-layer operation, i.e. it calculates global characteristics. If one wishes to employ some quasi-local Hough transform one is naturally led back to a network that has to resemble our OSNN.

V Training and Testing of OSNN-S

If instead of applying a simple cut we employ an auxiliary neural network to search for the best classification of events using the OSNN outputs, we obtain still better results. The auxiliary network has 6 inputs, one hidden layer with 5 nodes and one output unit. The input consists of a set of five consecutive D^α centered around $D_{\max}$ and the total number of activated input pixels, n_p. The cosmic muons are assigned an output value $s = 1$ and the accelerator events $s = 0$. The net is trained on our sample with error back-propagation. This results in an improved separation of cosmic muon events from the rest. Whereas in OSNN-D we find a continuum of cosmic muons throughout the range of $D_{\max}$, here we obtain a clear bimodal distribution, as seen in Figure 4. For $s \geq 0.1$ no accelerator events are found and the muons are selected with an efficiency of 94.7%. This selection procedure will be denoted as OSNN-S.

As a test of our method we apply OSNN-S to a sample of 38,606 data events that passed the standard physics cuts [5]. The distribution of the neural network output s is presented in Figure 4. It looks very different from the one obtained with the training sample. Whereas the former consisted of approximately 500 events distributed equally among accelerator events and cosmic muons, this one contains mostly accelerator events, with a fraction of a percent of muons. This proportion is characteristic of physics samples. The vast majority of accelerator events are found in the first bin, but a long tail extends throughout s. The last bin in s is indeed dominated by cosmic muons.

We performed a visual scan of all 181 events with $s \geq 0.1$ using the full information from the detector. This allowed us to identify the cosmic-muon events represented by shaded areas in figure 4. For $s \geq 0.1$ we find 55 cosmic-muon events and 123 accelerator events, 55 of which resemble muons on the rear segment of the calorimeter. The latter, together with the genuine cosmic muons, populate mainly the region of large s values.

We conclude that our method picked out the cosmic muons from the very large sample of data, in spite of the fact that it relied just on two-dimensional information from the rear part of the detector. This fact is, however, responsible for the contamination of the high s region by accelerator events that resemble cosmic muons. Even with all its limitations, our method reduces the problem of rejecting cosmic-muon events down to scanning less than one percent of all the events. We conclude that we have achieved the goal that we set for ourselves, that of replacing a laborious visual scan by a computer algorithm with similar reliability.

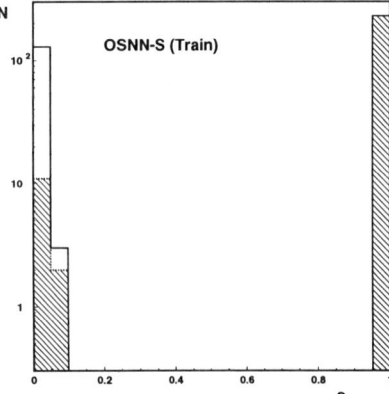 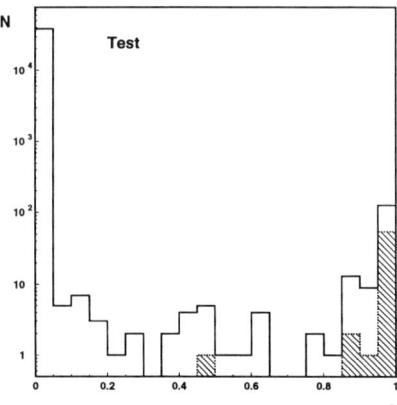

Figure 4: Left: Number of events as a function of the output s of an auxiliary neural net. Choosing the separator to be $s = 0.1$ we obtain an efficiency of 94.7% on our training set. This bimodal distribution holds the promise of better generalization than the OSNN-D method depicted in Figure 3. Muons are represented by shaded areas. Right: Distribution of the auxiliary neural network output s obtained with the OSNN-S selector for the test sample of 38,606 events. The tail of the distribution of accelerator events leads to 123 accelerator events with $s > 0.1$, including 55 that resemble straight lines on the input layer. 55 genuine cosmic muons were identified in the high s region.

VI Summary

We have presented an algorithm for identifying linear patterns on a two-dimensional lattice based on the concept of an orientation selective cell, a concept borrowed from neurobiology of vision. Constructing a multi-layered neural network with fixed architecture that implements orientation selectivity, we define output elements corresponding to different orientations, that allow us to make a selection decision. The algorithm takes into account the granularity of the lattice as well as the presence of noise and inefficiencies.

Our feed-forward network has a fixed set of synaptic weights. Hence, although the number of neurons is very high, the complexity of the system, as determined by the number of free parameters, is low. This allows us to train our system on a small data set. We are gratified to see that, nontheless, it generalizes well and performs excellently on a test sample that is larger by two orders of magnitude.

One may regard our method as a refinement of the Hough transform, since each of our orientation selective cells acts as a filter of straight lines on a limited grid. The major difference from conventional Hough transforms is that we perform semi-local calculations, and proceed in several stages, reflected by the different layers of our network, before evaluating global parameters.

The task that we have set to ourselves in the application described here is only one example of problems of pattern recognition that are encountered in the analysis of particle detectors. Given the large flux of data in these experiments, one is faced by two requirements: correct identification and fast performance. Using a structure like our OSNN for data classification, one can naturally meet the speed requirement through its realization in hardware, taking advantage of the basic features of distributed parallel computation.

Acknowledgements

We are indebted to the ZEUS Collaboration for allowing us to use the sample of data for this analysis. This work was partly supported by a grant from the Israel Science Foundation.

References

[1] ZEUS Collab., The ZEUS Detector, Status Report 1993, DESY 1993; M. Derrick et al., Phys. Lett. B 293 (1992) 465.

[2] D. H. Hubel and T. N. Wiesel, J. Physiol. 195 (1968) 215.

[3] H. Abramowicz, D. Horn, U. Naftaly and C. Sahar-Pikielny, Nuclear Instrum. and Methods in Phys. Res. A378 (1996) 305.

[4] B. Denby, Neural Computation, 5 (1993) 505.

[5] ZEUS Calorimeter Group, A. Andresen et al., Nucl. Inst. Meth. A 309 (1991) 101.

[6] P. V. Hough, "Methods and means to recognize complex patterns", U.S. patent 3.069.654.

[7] D. H. Ballard, Pattern Recognition 3 (1981) 11.

[8] R. O. Duda and P. E. Hart, Commun. ACM. 15 (1972) 1.

[9] ZEUS collab., M. Derrick et al., Phys. Lett. B 316 (1993) 412; ZEUS collab., M. Derrick et al., Zeitschrift f. Physik C 69 (1996) 607-620

Adaptive Access Control Applied to Ethernet Data

Timothy X Brown
Dept. of Electrical and Computer Engineering
University of Colorado, Boulder, CO 80309-0530
timxb@colorado.edu

Abstract

This paper presents a method that decides which combinations of traffic can be accepted on a packet data link, so that quality of service (QoS) constraints can be met. The method uses samples of QoS results at different load conditions to build a neural network decision function. Previous similar approaches to the problem have a significant bias. This bias is likely to occur in any real system and results in accepting loads that miss QoS targets by orders of magnitude. Preprocessing the data to either remove the bias or provide a confidence level, the method was applied to sources based on difficult-to-analyze ethernet data traces. With this data, the method produces an accurate access control function that dramatically outperforms analytic alternatives. Interestingly, the results depend on throwing away more than 99% of the data.

1 INTRODUCTION

In a communication network in which traffic sources can be dynamically added or removed, an access controller must decide when to accept or reject a new traffic source based on whether, if added, acceptable service would be given to all carried sources. Unlike *best-effort* services such as the internet, we consider the case where traffic sources are given *quality of service* (QoS) guarantees such as maximum delay, delay variation, or loss rate. The goal of the controller is to accept the maximal number of users while guaranteeing QoS. To accommodate diverse sources such as constant bit rate voice, variable-rate video, and bursty computer data, packet-based protocols are used. We consider QOS in terms of lost packets (i.e. packets discarded due to resource overloads). This is broadly applicable (e.g. packets which violate delay guarantees can be considered lost) although some QoS measures can not fit this model.

The access control task requires a classification function—analytically or empirically derived—that specifies what conditions will result in QoS not being met. Analytic functions have been successful only on simple traffic models [Gue91], or they are so conservative that they grossly under utilize the network. This paper describes a neural network method that adapts an access control function based on historical data on what conditions packets have and have not been successfully carried. Neural based solutions have been previously applied to the access control problem [Hir90][Tra92][Est94], but these approaches have a distinct bias that under real-world conditions leads to accepting combinations of calls that miss QoS targets by orders of magnitude. Incorporating preprocessing methods to eliminate this bias is critical and two methods from earlier work will be described. The combined data preprocessing and neural methods are applied to difficult-to-model ethernet traffic.

2 THE PROBLEM

Since the decision to accept a multilink connection can be decomposed into decisions on the individual links, we consider only a single link. A link can accept loads from different source types. The loads consist of packets modeled as discrete events. Arriving packets are placed in a buffer and serviced in turn. If the buffer is full, excess packets are discarded and treated as lost. The precise event timing is not critical as the concern is with the number of lost packets relative to the total number of packets received in a large sample of events, the so-called *loss rate*. The goal is to only accept load combinations which have a loss rate below the QoS target denoted by $p*$.

Load combinations are described by a feature vector, $\bar{\phi}$, consisting of load types and possibly other information such as time of day. Each feature vector, $\bar{\phi}$, has an associated loss rate, $p(\bar{\phi})$, which can not be measured directly. Therefore, the goal is to have a classifier function, $C(\bar{\phi})$, such that $C(\bar{\phi}) >, <, = 0$ if $p(\bar{\phi}) <, >, = p*$.

Since analytic $C(\bar{\phi})$ are not in general available, we look to statistical classification methods. This requires training samples, a desired output for each sample, and a significance or weight for each sample. Loads can be dynamically added or removed. Training samples are generated at load transitions, with information since the last transition containing the number of packet arrivals, T, the number of lost packets, s, and the feature vector, $\bar{\phi}$.

A sample $(\bar{\phi}_i, s_i, T_i)$, requires a desired classification, $d(\bar{\phi}_i, s_i, T_i) \in \{+1, -1\}$, and a weight, $w(\bar{\phi}_i, s_i, T_i) \in (0, \infty)$. Given a data set $\{(\bar{\phi}_i, s_i, T_i)\}$, a classifier, C, is then chosen that minimizes the weighted sum squared error $E = \sum_i [w(\bar{\phi}_i, s_i, T_i)(C(\bar{\phi}_i) - d(\bar{\phi}_i, s_i, T_i))^2]$.

A classifier, with enough degrees of freedom will set $C(\bar{\phi}_i) = d(\bar{\phi}_i, s_i, T_i)$ if all the $\bar{\phi}_i$ are different. With multiple samples at the same $\bar{\phi}$ then we see that the error is minimized when

$$C(\bar{\phi}) = \left(\sum_{\{i | \bar{\phi}_i = \bar{\phi}\}} [w(\bar{\phi}_i, s_i, T_i) d(\bar{\phi}_i, s_i, T_i)] \right) / \left(\sum_{\{i | \bar{\phi}_i = \bar{\phi}\}} w(\bar{\phi}_i, s_i, T_i) \right). \quad (1)$$

Thus, the optimal $C(\bar{\phi})$ is the weighted average of the $d(\bar{\phi}_i, s_i, T_i)$ at $\bar{\phi}$. If the classifier has fewer degrees of freedom (e.g. a low dimension linear classifier), $C(\bar{\phi})$ will be the average of the $d(\bar{\phi}_i, s_i, T_i)$ in the neighborhood of $\bar{\phi}$, where the neighborhood is, in general, an unspecified function of the classifier.

A more direct form of averaging would be to choose a specific neighborhood around $\bar{\phi}$ and average over samples in this neighborhood. This suffers from having to store all the samples in the decision mechanism, and incurs a significant computational burden. More significant is how to decide the size of the neighborhood. If it is fixed, in sparse regions no samples may be in the neighborhood. In dense regions near decision boundaries, it may average over too wide a range for accurate estimates. Dynamically setting the neighborhood so that it always contains the k nearest neighbors solves this problem, but does not account for the size of the samples. We will return to this in Section 4.

3 THE SMALL SAMPLE PROBLEM

Neural networks have previously been applied to the access control problem [Hir91] [Tra92][Est94]. In [Hir90] and [Tra92], $d(\bar{\phi}_i, s_i, T_i) = +1$ when $s_i/T_i < p*$, $d(\bar{\phi}_i, s_i, T_i) = -1$ otherwise, and the weighting is a uniform $w(\bar{\phi}_i, s_i, T_i) = 1$ for all i. This desired out and uniform weighting we call the *normal* method. For a given load combination, $\bar{\phi}$, assume an idealized system where packets enter and with probability $p(\bar{\phi})$ independent of earlier or later packets, the packet is labeled as lost. In a sample of T such Bernoulli trials with s the number packets lost, let $P_B = P\{s/T > p*\}$. Since with the normal method $d(\bar{\phi}, s, T) = -1$ if $s/T > p*$, $P_B = P\{d(\bar{\phi}, s, T) = -1\}$. From (1), with uniform weighting the decision boundary is where $P_B = 0.5$. If the samples are small (i.e. $T < (\ln 2)/p* < 1/p*$), $d(\bar{\phi}, s, T) = -1$ for all $s > 0$. In this case $P_B = 1 - (1 - p(\bar{\phi}))^T$. Solving for $p(\bar{\phi})$ at $P_B = 0.5$ using $\ln(1 - x) \approx -x$, the decision boundary is at $p(\bar{\phi}) \approx (\ln 2)/T > p*$. So, for small sample sizes, the normal method boundary is biased to greater than $p*$ and can be made orders of magnitude larger as T becomes smaller. For larger T, e.g. $Tp* > 10$, this bias will be seen to be negligible.

One obvious solution is to have large samples. This is complicated by three effects. The first is that desired loss rates in data systems are often small; typically in the range 10^{-6}–10^{-12}. This implies that to be large, samples must be at least 10^7–10^{13} packets. For the latter, even at Gbps rates, short packets, and full loading this translates into samples of several hours of traffic. Even for the first at typical rates, this can translate into minutes of traffic. The second, related problem is that in dynamic data networks, while individual connections may last for significant periods, on the aggregate a given combination of loads may not exist for the requisite period. The third more subtle problem is that in any queueing system even with uncorrelated arrival traffic the buffering introduces memory in the system. A typical sample with losses may contain 100 losses, but a loss trace would show that all of the losses occurred in a single short overload interval. Thus the number of independent trials can be several orders of magnitude smaller than indicated by the raw sample size indicating that the loads must be stable for hours, days, or even years to get samples that lead to unbiased classification.

An alternative approach used in [Hir95] sets $d(\bar{\phi}, s, T) = s/T$ and models $p(\bar{\phi})$ directly. The probabilities can vary over orders of magnitude making accurate estimates difficult. Estimating the less variable $\log(p(\bar{\phi}))$ with $d = \log(s/T)$ is complicated by the logarithm being undefined for small samples where most samples have no losses so that $s = 0$.

4 METHODS FOR TREATING BIAS AND VARIANCE

We present without proof two preprocessing methods derived and analyzed in [Bro96]. The first eliminates the sample bias by choosing an appropriate d and w that directly solves (1) s.t. $C(\bar{\phi}) >, <, = 0$ if and only if $p(\bar{\phi}) <, >, = p*$ i.e. it is an unbiased estimate as to whether the loss rate is above and below $p*$. This is the *weighting* method shown in Table 1. The relative weighting of samples with loss rates above and below the critical loss rate is plotted in Figure 1. For large T, as expected, it reduces to the normal method.

The second preprocessing method assigns uniform weighting, but classifies $d(\bar{\phi}, s, T) = 1$ only if a certain confidence level, L, is met that the sample represents a combination where $p(\bar{\phi}) < p*$. Such a confidence was derived in [Bro96]:

Table 1: Summary of Methods.

Method	Sample Class $d(\bar{\phi}_i, s_i, T_i) = +1$ if	Weighting, $w(\bar{\phi}_i, s_i, T_i)$, when	
		$d(\bar{\phi}_i, s_i, T_i) = +1$ (i.e. w^+)	$d(\bar{\phi}_i, s_i, T_i) = -1$ (i.e. w^-)
Normal	$s_i \leq \lfloor p*T \rfloor$	1	1
Weighting	$s_i \leq \lfloor p*T \rfloor$	$T \sum_{i > \lfloor p*T \rfloor} \binom{T}{i} p*^i (1-p*)^{T-i}$	$T \sum_{i \leq \lfloor p*T \rfloor} \binom{T}{i} p*^i (1-p*)^{T-i}$
Aggregate	Table 2	1	1

$$P\{p(\bar{\phi}) > p^* | s, T\} \cong e^{-Tp^*} \sum_{i=0}^{s} \frac{(Tp^*)^i}{i!} \qquad (2)$$

For small T (e.g. $T < 1/p^*$ and $L > 1 - 1/e$), even if $s = 0$ (no losses), this level is not met. But, a neighborhood of samples with similar load combinations may all have no losses indicating that this sample can be classified as having $p(\bar{\phi}) < p^*$. Choosing a neighborhood requires a metric, m, between feature vectors, $\bar{\phi}$. In this paper we simply use Euclidean distance. Using the above and solving for T when $s = 0$, the smallest meaningful neighborhood size is the smallest k such that the aggregate sample is greater than a critical size, $T^* = -\ln(1-L)/p^*$. From (2), this guarantees that if no packets in the aggregate sample are lost we can classify it as having $p(\bar{\phi}) < p^*$ within our confidence level. For larger samples, or where samples are more plentiful and k can afford to be large, (2) can be used directly. Table 2 summarizes this *aggregate* method.

The above preprocessing methods assume that the training samples consist of independent samples of Bernoulli trials. Because of memory introduced by the buffer and possible correlations in the arrivals, this is decidedly not true. The methods can still be applied, if samples can be subsampled at every Ith trial where I is large enough so that the samples are pseudo-independent, i.e. the dependency is not significant for our application.

A simple graphical method for determining I is as follows. Observing Figure 1, if the number of trials is artificially increased, for small samples the weighting method will tend to under weight the trials with errors, so that its decision boundary will be at erroneously high loss rates. This is the case with correlated samples. The sample size, T, overstates the number of independent trials. As the subsample factor is increased, the subsample size becomes smaller, the trials become increasingly independent, the weighting becomes more appropriate, and the decision boundary moves closer to the true decision boundary. At some point, the samples are sufficiently independent so that sparser subsampling does not change the decision boundary. By plotting the decision boundary of the classifier as a function of I, the point where the boundary is independent of the subsample factor indicates a suitable choice for I.

In summary, the procedure consists of collecting traffic samples at different combinations of traffic loads that do and do not meet quality of service. These are then subsampled with a factor I determined as above. Then one of the sample preprocessing methods, summarized in Table 1, are applied to the data. These preprocessed samples are then used in any neural network or classification scheme. Analysis in [Bro96] derives the expected bias (shown in Figure 2) of the methods when used with an ideal classifier. The normal method can be arbitrarily biased, the weighting method is unbiased, and the aggregate method chooses a conservative boundary. Simulation experiments in [Bro96] applying it to a well characterized M/M/1 queueing system to determine acceptable loads showed that the weighting method was able to produce unbiased threshold estimates over a range of val-

Table 2: Aggregate Classification Algorithm

1. Given Sample $(\bar{\phi}_i, s_i, T_i) \in \{(\bar{\phi}_i, s_i, T_i)\}$, metric, m, and confidence level, L.
2. Calculate $T^* = -\ln(1-L)/p^*$.
3. Find nearest neighbors $n_0, n_1, \ldots$ where $n_0 = i$ and $m(\bar{\phi}_{n_j}, \bar{\phi}_i) \leq m(\bar{\phi}_{n_{j+1}}, \bar{\phi}_i)$ for $j \geq 0$.
4. Choose smallest k s.t. $T' = \sum_{j=0}^{k} T_{n_j} \geq T^*$. Let $s' = \sum_{j=0}^{k} s_{n_j}$.
5. Using (2), $d(\bar{\phi}_i, s_i, T_i) = \begin{cases} +1 & \text{if } P\{p(\bar{\phi}) > p^* \| s', T'\} < (1-L) \\ -1 & \text{o.w.} \end{cases}$

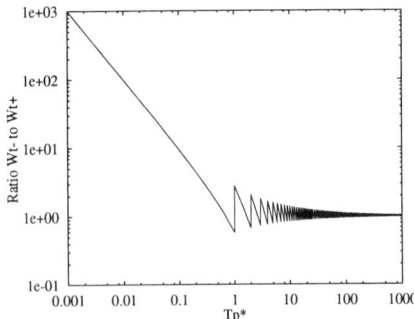
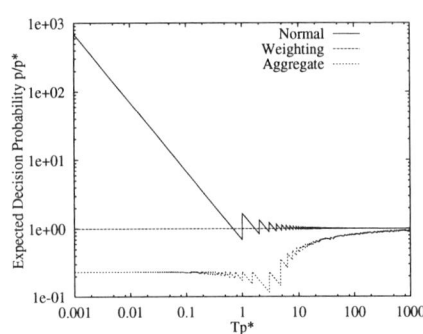

Figure 1: Plot of Relative Weighting of Samples with Losses Below (w^-) and Above (w^+) the Critical Loss Rate.

Figure 2: Expected Decision Normalized by $p*$. The nominal boundary is $p/p* = 1$. The aggregate method uses $L = 0.95$.

ues; and the aggregate method produced conservative estimates that were always below the desired threshold, although in terms of traffic load were only 5% smaller. Even in this simple system where the input traffic is uncorrelated (but the losses become correlated due the memory in the queue), the subsample factor was 12, meaning that good results required more than 90% of the data be thrown out.

5 EXPERIMENTS WITH ETHERNET TRAFFIC DATA

This paper set out to solve the problem of access control for real world data. We consider a system where the call combinations consist of individual computer data users trunked onto a single output link. This is modeled as a discrete-time single-server queueing model where in each time slot one packet can be processed and zero or more packets can arrive from the different users. The server has a buffer of fixed length 1000. To generate a realistic arrival process, we use ethernet data traces. The bandwidth of the link was chosen at from 10–100Mbps. With 48 byte packets, the queue packet service rate was the bandwidth divided by 384. All arrival rates are normalized by the service rate.

5.1 THE DATA

We used ethernet data described in [Lel93] as the August 89 busy hour containing traffic ranging from busy file-servers/routers to users with just a handful of packets. The detailed data set records every packet's arrival time (to the nearest 100μsec), size, plus source and destination tags. From this, 108 "data traffic" sources were generated, one for each computer that generated traffic on the ethernet link. To produce uniform size packets, each ethernet packet (which ranged from 64 to 1518 bytes) was split into 2 to 32 48-byte packets (partial packets were padded to 48 bytes). Each ethernet packet arrival time was mapped into a particular time slot in the queueing model. All the packets arriving in a timeslot are immediately added to the buffer, any buffer overflows would be discarded (counted as lost), and if the buffer was non-empty at the start of the timeslot, one packet sent. Ethernet contains a collision protocol so that only one of the sources is sending packets at any one time onto a 10Mbps connection. Decorrelating the sources via random starting offsets, produced independent data sources with the potential for overloads. Multiple copies at different offsets produced sufficient loads even for bandwidths greater than 10Mbps.

The peak data rate with this data is fixed, while the load (the average rate over the one hour trace normalized by the peak rate) ranges over five orders of magnitude. Also troubling, analysis of this data [Lel93] shows that the aggregate traffic exhibits chaotic self-similar properties and suggests that it may be due to the sources' distribution of packet inter-arrival times following an extremely heavy tailed distribution with infinite higher order moments. No tractable closed form solution exists for such data to predict whether a particular load will result in an overload. Thus, we apply adaptive access control.

5.2 EXPERIMENT AND RESULTS

We divided the data into two roughly similar groups of 54 sources each; one for training and one for testing. To create sample combinations we assign a distribution over the different training sources, choose a source combination from this distribution, and choose a random, uniform (over the period of the trace) starting time for each source. Simulations that reach the end of a trace wrap around to the beginning of the trace. The sources are described by a single feature corresponding to the average load of the source over the one hour data trace. A group of sources is described by the sum of the average loads. The source distribution was a uniformly chosen 0–M copies of each of the 54 training samples. M was dynamically chosen so that the link would be sufficiently loaded to cause losses. Each sample combination was processed for 3×10^7 time slots, recording the load combination, the number of packets serviced correctly, and the number blocked. The experiment was repeated for a range of bandwidths. The bandwidths and number of samples at each bandwidth are shown in Table 3

We applied the three methods of Table 1 based on $p* = 10^{-6}$ ($L = 95\%$ for the aggregate method) and used the resulting data in a linear classifier. Since the feature is the load and larger loads will always cause more blocking, $p(\phi)$ is a one variable monotonic function. A linear classifier is sufficient for this case and its output is simply a threshold on the load.

To create pseudo-independent trials necessary for the aggregate and weighting methods, we subsampled every Ith packet. Using the graphical method of Section 4, the resulting I are shown in column 4 of Table 3. A typical subsample factor is 200. The sample sizes ranged from 10^5 to 10^7 trials, But, after subsampling by a factor of 200, even for the largest samples, $p*T < 0.05 \ll 1$.

The thresholds found by each method are shown in Table 3. To get loss rate estimates at these thresholds, the average loss rate of the 20% of source combinations below each method's threshold is computed. Since accepted loads would be below the threshold this is a typical loss rate. The normal scheme is clearly flawed with losses 10 times higher than $p*$, the weighting scheme's loss rate is apparently unbiased with results around $p*$, while the aggregate scheme develops a conservative boundary below $p*$. To test the boundaries, we repeated the experiment generating source combination samples using the 54 sources not used in the training. Table 3 also shows the losses on this test set and indicates that the training set boundaries produce similar results on the test data.

The boundaries are compared with those of more conventional, model-based techniques. One proposed technique for detecting overloads appears in [Gue91]. This paper assumes the sources are based on a Markov On/Off model. Applying the method to this ethernet data (treating each packet arrival as an On period and calculating necessary parameters from there), all but the very highest loads in the training sets are classified as acceptable indicating that the loss rate would be orders of magnitude higher than $p*$. A conservative technique is to accept calls only as long as the sum of the peak source transmission rates is less than the link bandwidth. For the 10Mbps link, since this equals the original ethernet

Table 3: Results from Experiments at Different Link Bandwidth.

Band-width (Mbps)	Number of Samples		Sub-sample Factor	Threshold Found & Loss Rate at Threshold on (train/test) Set		
	Train	Test		Normal	Weighting	Aggregate
10	1569	1080	230	0.232 (1e–5/4e–6)	0.139 (8e–7/1e–6)	0.105 (1e–7/8e–8)
17.5	2447	3724	180	0.415 (2e–5/3e–5)	0.268 (5e–7/9e–7)	0.215 (3e–9/4e–7)
30	6696	4219	230	0.508 (7e–6/4e–5)	0.333 (4e–6/5e–8)	0.286 (3e–7/2e–8)
100	1862	N.A.	180	0.688 (1e–5/N.A.)	0.566 (5e–7/N.A.)	0.494 (0e–0/N.A.)

data rate, this peak rate method will accept exactly one source. Averaging over all sources, the average load would be 0.0014 and would not increase with increasing bandwidth. The neural method takes advantage of better trunking at increasing bandwidths, and carries two orders of magnitude more traffic.

6 CONCLUSION

Access control depends on a classification function that decides if a given set of load conditions will violate quality of service constraints. In this paper quality of service was in terms of a maximum packet loss rate, $p*$. Given that analytic methods are inadequate when given realistic traffic sources, a neural network classification method based on samples of traffic results at different load conditions is a practical alternative. With previous neural network approaches, the synthetic nature of the experiments obscured a significant bias that exists with more realistic data. This bias, due to the small sample sizes relative to $1/p*$, is likely to occur in any real system and results in accepting loads with losses that are orders of magnitude greater than $p*$.

Preprocessing the data to either remove the bias or provide a confidence level, the neural network was applied to sources based on difficult-to-analyze ethernet data traces. A group of sources was characterized by its total load so that the goal was to simply choose a threshold on how much load the link would accept. The neural network was shown to produce accurate estimates of the correct threshold. Interestingly these good results depend on creating traffic samples representing independent packet transmissions. This requires more than 99% of the data to be thrown away indicating that for good performance an easy-to-implement sparse sampling of the packet fates is sufficient. It also indicates that unless the total number of packets that is observed is orders of magnitude larger than $1/p*$, the samples are actually small and preprocessing methods such as in this paper must be applied for accurate loss rate classification.

In comparison to analytic techniques, all of the methods, are more accurate at identifying overloads. In comparison to the best safe alternative that works even on this ethernet data, the neural network method was able to carry two orders of magnitude more traffic. The techniques in this paper apply to a range of network problems from routing, to bandwidth allocation, network design, as well as access control.

References

[Bro96] Brown, T.X, "Classifying Loss Rates with Small Samples," Submitted to *IEEE Tran. on Comm.*, April 1996.

[Est94] Estrella, A.D., Jurado, A., Sandoval, F., "New Training Pattern Selection Method for ATM Call Admission Neural Control," *Elec. Let.*, Vol. 30, No. 7, pp. 577–579, Mar. 1994.

[Gue91] Guerin, R., Ahmadi, H., Naghshineh, M., "Equivalent Capacity and its Application to Bandwidth Allocation in High-Speed Networks," *IEEE JSAC*, vol. 9, no. 7, pp. 968–981, 1991.

[Hir90] Hiramatsu, A., "ATM Communications Network Control by Neural Networks," *IEEE Trans. on Neural Networks*, vol. 1, no. 1, pp. 122–130, 1990.

[Hir95] Hiramatsu, A., "Training Techniques for Neural Network Applications in ATM," *IEEE Comm. Mag.*, October, pp. 58–67, 1995.

[Lel93] Leland, W.E., Taqqu, M.S., Willinger, W., Wilson, D.V., "On the Self-Similar Nature of Ethernet Traffic," in *Proc. of ACM SIGCOMM* 1993. pp. 183–193.

[Tra92] Tran-Gia, P., Gropp, O., "Performance of a Neural Net used as Admission Controller in ATM Systems," *Proc. Globecom 92*, Orlando, FL, pp. 1303–1309.

Predicting Lifetimes in Dynamically Allocated Memory

David A. Cohn
Adaptive Systems Group
Harlequin, Inc.
Menlo Park, CA 94025
cohn@harlequin.com

Satinder Singh
Department of Computer Science
University of Colorado
Boulder, CO 80309
baveja@cs.colorado.edu

Abstract

Predictions of lifetimes of dynamically allocated objects can be used to improve time and space efficiency of dynamic memory management in computer programs. Barrett and Zorn [1993] used a simple lifetime predictor and demonstrated this improvement on a variety of computer programs. In this paper, we use decision trees to do lifetime prediction on the same programs and show significantly better prediction. Our method also has the advantage that during training we can use a large number of features and let the decision tree automatically choose the relevant subset.

1 INTELLIGENT MEMORY ALLOCATION

Dynamic memory allocation is used in many computer applications. The application requests blocks of memory from the operating system or from a memory manager when needed and explicitly frees them up after use. Typically, all of these requests are handled in the same way, without any regard for how or for how long the requested block will be used. Sometimes programmers use runtime profiles to analyze the typical behavior of their program and write special purpose memory management routines specifically tuned to dominant classes of allocation events. Machine learning methods offer the opportunity to automate the process of tuning memory management systems.

In a recent study, Barrett and Zorn [1993] used two allocators: a special allocator for objects that are short-lived, and a default allocator for everything else. They tried a simple prediction method on a number of public-domain, allocation-intensive programs and got mixed results on the lifetime prediction problem. Nevertheless, they showed that for all the cases where they were able to predict well, their strategy of assigning objects predicted to be short-lived to the special allocator led to savings in program running times. Their results imply that if we could predict well in all cases we could get similar savings for all programs. We concentrate on the lifetime prediction task in this paper and show that using axis-parallel decision trees does indeed lead to significantly better prediction on all the programs studied by Zorn and Grunwald and some others that we included. Another advantage of our approach is that we can use a large number of features about the allocation requests and let the decision tree decide on their relevance.

There are a number of advantages of using lifetime predictions for intelligent memory management. It can improve CPU usage, by using special-purpose allocators, e.g., short-lived objects can be allocated in small spaces by incrementing a pointer and deallocated together when they are all dead. It can decrease memory fragmentation, because the short-lived objects do not pollute the address space of long lived objects. Finally, it can improve program locality, and thus program speed, because the short-lived objects are all allocated in a small part of the heap.

The advantages of prediction must be weighed against the time required to examine each request and make that prediction about its intended use. It is frequently argued that, as computers and memory become faster and cheaper, we need to be less concerned about the speed and efficiency of machine learning algorithms. When the purpose of the algorithm is to save space and computation, however, these concerns are paramount.

1.1 RELATED WORK

Traditionally, memory management has been relegated to a single, general-purpose allocator. When performance is critical, software developers will frequently build a custom memory manager which they believe is tuned to optimize the performance of the program. Not only is this hand construction inefficient in terms of the programming time required, this "optimization" may seriously degrade the program's performance if it does not accurately reflect the program's use [Wilson et al., 1995].

Customalloc [Grunwald and Zorn, 1992] monitors program runs on benchmark inputs to determine the most commonly requested block sizes. It then produces a set of memory allocation routines which are customized to efficiently allocate those block sizes. Other memory requests are still handled by a general purpose allocator.

Barrett and Zorn [1993] studied lifetime prediction based on benchmark inputs. At each allocation request, the call graph (the list of nested procedure/function calls in effect at the time) and the object size was used to identify an *allocation site*. If all allocations from a particular site were short-lived on the benchmark inputs, their algorithm predicted that future allocations would also be short-lived. Their method produced mixed results at lifetime prediction, but demonstrated the savings that such predictions could bring.

In this paper, we discuss an approach to lifetime prediction which uses learned decision trees. In the next section, we first discuss the identification of relevant state features by a decision tree. Section 3 discusses in greater detail the problem of lifetime prediction. Section 4 describes the empirical results of applying this approach to several benchmark programs, and Section 5 discusses the implications of these results and directions for future work.

2 FEATURE SELECTION WITH A DECISION TREE

Barrett and Zorn's approach captures state information in the form of the program's call graph at the time of an allocation request, which is recorded to a fixed predetermined depth. This graph, plus the request size, specifies an allocation "site"; statistics are gathered separately for each site. A drawback of this approach is that it forces a division for each distinct call graph, preventing generalization across irrelevant features. Computationally, it requires maintaining an explicit call graph (information that the program would not normally provide), as well as storing a potentially large table of call sites from which to make predictions. It also ignores other potentially useful information, such as the *parameters* of the functions on the call stack, and the contents of heap memory and the program registers at the time of the request.

Ideally, we would like to examine as much of the program state as possible at the time of each allocation request, and automatically extract those pieces of information that best allow predicting how the requested block will be used. Decision tree algorithms are useful for this sort of task. A decision tree divides inputs on basis of how each input feature improves "purity" of the tree's leaves. Inputs that are statistically irrelevant for prediction are not used in any splits; the tree's final set of decisions examine only input features that improve its predictive performance.

Regardless of the parsimony of the final tree however, training a tree with the entire program state as a feature vector is computationally infeasible. In our experiments, detailed below, we arbitrarily used the top 20 words on the stack, along with the request size, as an approximate indicator of program state. On the target machine (a Sparcstation), we found that including program registers in the feature set made no significant difference, and so dropped them from consideration for efficiency.

3 LIFETIME PREDICTION

The characteristic of memory requests that we would like to predict is the lifetime of the block – how long it will be before the requested memory is returned to the central pool. Accurate lifetime prediction lets one segregate memory into short-term, long-term and permanent storage. To this end, we have used a decision tree learning algorithm to derive rules that distinguish "short-lived" and "permanent" allocations from the general pool of allocation requests.

For short-lived blocks, one can create a very simple and efficient allocation scheme [Barrett and Zorn, 1993]. For "permanent" blocks, allocation is also simple and cheap, because the allocator does not need to compute and store any of the information that would normally be required to keep track of the block and return it to the pool when freed.

One complication is that of unequal loss for different types of incorrect predictions. An appropriately routed memory request may save dozens of instruction cycles, but an inappropriately routed one may cost hundreds. The cost in terms of memory may also be unequal: a short-lived block that is incorrectly predicted to be "permanent" will permanently tie up the space occupied by the block (if it is allocated via a method that can not be freed). A "permanent" block, however, that is incorrectly predicted to be short-lived may pollute the allocator's short-term space by preventing a large segment of otherwise free memory from being reclaimed (see Barrett and Zorn for examples).

These risks translate into a time-space tradeoff that depends on the properties of the specific allocators used and the space limitations of the target machine. For our experiments, we arbitrarily defined false positives and false negatives to have equal loss, except where noted otherwise. Other cases may be handled by reweighting the splitting criterion, or by rebalancing the training inputs (as described in the following section).

4 EXPERIMENTS

We conducted two types of experiments. The first measured the ability of learned decision trees to predict allocation lifetimes. The second incorporated these learned trees into the target applications and measured the change in runtime performance.

4.1 PREDICTIVE ACCURACY

We used the OC1 decision tree software (designed by Murthy et al. [1994]) and considered only axis-parallel splits, in effect, conditioning each decision on a single stack feature. We chose the sum minority criterion for splits, which minimizes the number of training examples misclassified after the split. For tree pruning, we used the cost complexity heuristic, which holds back a fraction (in our case 10%) of the data set for testing, and selects the smallest pruning of the original tree that is within one standard error squared of the best tree [Breiman et al. 1984]. The details of these and other criteria may be found in Murthy et al. [1994] and Breiman et al. [1984]. In addition to the automatically-pruned trees, we also examined trees that had been truncated to four leaves, in effect examining no more than two features before making a decision.

OC1 includes no provisions for explicitly specifying a loss function for false positive and false negative classifications. It would be straightforward to incorporate this into the sum minority splitting criterion; we chose instead to incorporate the loss function into the training set itself, by duplicating training examples to match the target ratios (in our case, forcing an equal number of positive and negative examples).

In our experiments, we used the set of benchmark applications reported on by Barrett and Zorn: *Ghostscript*, a PostScript interpreter, *Espresso*, a PLA logic optimizer, and *Cfrac*, a program for factoring large numbers, *Gawk*, an AWK programming language interpreter and *Perl*, a report extraction language. We also examined *Gcc*, a public-domain C compiler, based on our company's specific interest in compiler technology.

The experimental procedure was as follows: We linked the application program with a modified *malloc* routine which, in addition to allocating the requested memory, wrote to a trace file the size of the requested block, and the top 20 machine words on the program stack. Calls to *free* allowed tagging the existing allocations, which, following Barrett and Zorn, were labeled according to how many bytes had been allocated during their lifetime.[1]

It is worth noting that these experiments were run on a Sparcstation, which frequently optimizes away the traditional stack frame. While it would have been possible to force the system to maintain a traditional stack, we wished to work from whatever information was available from the program "in the wild", without overriding system optimizations.

---

[1]We have also examined, with comparable success, predicting lifetimes in terms of the number of intervening calls to malloc, which may be argued as an equally useful measure. We focus on number of bytes for the purposes of comparison with the existing literature.

Input files were taken from the public ftp archive made available by Zorn and Grunwald [1993]. Our procedure was to take traces of three of the files (typically the largest three for which we could store an entire program trace). Two of the traces were combined to form a training set for the decision tree, and the third was used to test the learned tree.

Ghostscript training files: manual.ps and large.ps; test file: ud-doc.ps
Espresso training files: cps and mlp4; test file: Z5xp1
Cfrac training inputs: 41757646344123832613190542166099121 and 32790560067400421458831903; test input: 41757646344124860145938030302877
Gawk training file: adj.awk/words-small.awk; test file: adj.awk/words-large.awk[2]
Perl training files: endsort.perl (endsort.perl as input), hosts.perl (hosts-data.perl as input); test file: adj.perl(words-small.awk as input)
Gcc training files: cse.c and combine.c; test file: expr.c

4.1.1 SHORT-LIVED ALLOCATIONS

First, we attempted to distinguish short-lived allocations from the general pool. For comparison with Barrett and Zorn [1993], we defined "short-lived" allocations as those that were freed before 32k subsequent bytes had been allocated. The experimental results of this section are summarized in Table 1.

application	Barrett & Zorn		OC1	
	false pos %	false neg %	false pos %	false neg %
ghostscript	0	25.2	0.13 (0.72)	1.7 (13.5)
espresso	0.006	72	0.38 (1.39)	6.58 (14.9)
cfrac	3.65	52.7	2.5 (0.49)	16.9 (19.4)
gawk	0	_[3]	0.092 (0.092)	0.34 (0.34)
perl	1.11	78.6	5.32 (10.8)	33.8 (34.3)
gcc	-	-	0.85 (2.54)	31.1 (31.0)

Table 1: Prediction errors for "short-lived" allocations, in percentages of misallocated bytes. Values in parentheses are for trees that have been truncated to two levels. Barrett and Zorn's results included for comparison where available.

4.1.2 "PERMANENT" ALLOCATIONS

We then attempted to distinguish "permanent" allocations from the general pool (Barrett and Zorn only consider the short-lived allocations discussed in the previous section). "Permanent" allocations were those that were not freed until the program terminated. Note that there is some ambiguity in these definitions — a "permanent" block that is allocated near the end of the program's lifetime may also be "short-lived". Table 2 summarizes the results of these experiments.

We have not had the opportunity to examine the function of each of the "relevant features" in the program stacks; this is a subject for future work.

---

[2] For *Gawk*, we varied the training to match that used by Barrett and Zorn. They used as training input a single gawk program file run with one data set, and tested on the same gawk program run with another.

[3] We were unable to compute Barrett and Zorn's exact results here, although it appears that their false negative rate was less than 1%.

application	false pos %	false neg %
ghostscript	0	0.067
espresso	0	1.27
cfrac	0.019	3.3
gcc	0.35	19.5

Table 2: Prediction errors for "permanent" allocations (% misallocated bytes).

4.2 RUNTIME PERFORMANCE

The raw error rates we have presented above indicate that it is possible to make accurate predictions about the lifetime of allocation requests, but not whether those predictions are good enough to improve program performance. To address that question, we have incorporated predictive trees into three of the above applications and measured the effect on their runtimes.

We used a hybrid implementation, replacing the single monolithic decision tree with a number of simpler, site-specific trees. A "site" in this case was a lexical instance of a call to malloc or its equivalent. When allocations from a site were exclusively short-lived or permanent, we could directly insert a call to one of the specialized allocators (in the manner of Barrett and Zorn). When allocations from a site were mixed, a site-specific tree was put in place to predict the allocation lifetime.

Requests predicted to be short-lived were routed to a "quick malloc" routine similar to the one described by Barrett and Zorn; those predicted to be permanent were routed to another routine specialized for the purpose. On tests with random data these specialized routines were approximately four times faster than "malloc".

Our experiments targeted three applications with varying degrees of predictive accuracy: ghostscript, gcc, and cfrac. The results are encouraging (see Table 3). For ghostscript and gcc, which have the best predictive accuracies on the benchmark data (from Section 4.1), we had a clear improvement in performance. For cfrac, with much lower accuracy, we had mixed results: for shorter runs, the runtime performance was improved, but on longer runs there were enough missed predictions to pollute the short-lived memory area and degrade performance.

5 DISCUSSION

The application of machine learning to computer software and operating systems is a largely untapped field with promises of great benefit. In this paper we have described one such application, producing efficient and accurate predictions of the lifetimes of memory allocations.

Our data suggest that, even with a feature set as large as a runtime program stack, it is possible to characterize and predict the memory usage of a program after only a few benchmark runs. The exceptions appear to be programs like Perl and gawk which take both a script and a data file. Their memory usage depends not only upon characterizing typical scripts, but the typical data sets those scripts act upon.[4]

Our ongoing research in memory management is pursuing a number of other con-

---

[4] Perl's generalization performance is significantly better when tested on the same script with different data. We have reported the results using different scripts for comparison with Barrett and Zorn.

application	benchmark test error			run time	
(training set)	short	long	permanent	normal	predictive
ghostscript, trained on ud-doc.ps; 7 sites, 1 tree					
manual.ps	16/256432	0/3431	0/0	96.29	95.43
large.ps				17.22	16.75
thesis.ps				40.27	37.57
gcc, trained on combine, cse, c-decl; 17 sites, 4 trees					
expr.c	0/11988	2786/11998	301/536875	12.59	12.40
loop.c				5.16	5.16
reload1.c				7.02	6.81
cfrac, trained on 100···057; 8 sites, 4 trees					
327···903	24/7970099	13172/22332	106/271	7.75	7.23
417···771				67.93	74.57
417···121				225.31	245.64

Table 3: Running times in seconds for applications with site-specific trees. Times shown are averages over 24-40 runs, and with the exception of loop.c, are statistically significant with probability greater than 99%.

tinuations of the results described here, including lifetime clustering and intelligent garbage collection.

REFERENCES

D. Barrett and B. Zorn (1993) Using lifetime predictors to improve memory allocation performance. SIGPLAN'93 – Conference on Programming Language Design and Implementation, June 1993, Albuquerque, New Mexico, pp. 187-196.

L. Breiman, J. Friedman, R. Olshen and C. Stone (1984) *Classification and Regression Trees*, Wadsworth International Group, Belmont, CA.

D. Grunwald and B. Zorn (1992) CUSTOMALLOC: Efficient synthesized memory allocators. Technical Report CU-CS-602-92, Dept. of Computer Science, University of Colorado.

S. Murthy, S. Kasif and S. Salzberg (1994) A system for induction of oblique decision trees. *Journal of Artificial Intelligence Research* **2**:1-32.

P. Wilson, M. Johnstone, M. Neely and D. Boles (1995) Dynamic storage allocation: a survey and critical review. Proc. 1995 Intn'l Workshop on Memory Management, Kinross, Scotland, Sept. 27-29, Springer Verlag.

B. Zorn and D. Grunwald (1993) A set of benchmark inputs made publicly available, in ftp archive `ftp.cs.colorado.edu:/pub/misc/malloc-benchmarks/`.

Multi-Task Learning for Stock Selection

Joumana Ghosn
Dept. Informatique et
Recherche Opérationnelle
Université de Montréal
Montreal, Qc H3C-3J7
ghosn@iro.umontreal.ca

Yoshua Bengio [*]
Dept. Informatique et
Recherche Opérationnelle
Université de Montréal
Montreal, Qc H3C-3J7
bengioy@iro.umontreal.ca

Abstract

Artificial Neural Networks can be used to predict future returns of stocks in order to take financial decisions. Should one build a separate network for each stock or share the same network for all the stocks? In this paper we also explore other alternatives, in which some layers are shared and others are not shared. When the prediction of future returns for different stocks are viewed as different tasks, sharing some parameters across stocks is a form of multi-task learning. In a series of experiments with Canadian stocks, we obtain yearly returns that are **more than 14% above various benchmarks**.

1 Introduction

Previous applications of ANNs to financial time-series suggest that several of these prediction and decision-taking tasks present sufficient non-linearities to justify the use of ANNs (Refenes, 1994; Moody, Levin and Rehfuss, 1993). These models can incorporate various types of explanatory variables: so-called technical variables (depending on the past price sequence), micro-economic stock-specific variables (such as measures of company profitability), and macro-economic variables (which give information about the business cycle).

One question addressed in this paper is whether the way to treat these different variables should be different for different stocks, i.e., should one use the same network for all the stocks or a different network for each stock? To explore this question

---
[*]also, AT&T Labs, Holmdel, NJ 07733

we performed a series of experiments in which different subsets of parameters are shared across the different stock models. When the prediction of future returns for different stocks are viewed as **different tasks** (which may nonetheless have something in common), sharing some parameters across stocks is a form of **multi-task learning**.

These experiments were performed on 9 years of data concerning 35 large capitalization companies of the Toronto Stock Exchange (TSE). Following the results of previous experiments (Bengio, 1996), the networks were not trained to predict the future return of stocks, but instead to directly optimize a financial criterion. This has been found to yield returns that are significantly superior to training the ANNs to minimize the mean squared prediction error.

In section 2, we review previous work on multi-task. In section 3, we describe the financial task that we have considered, and the experimental setup. In section 4, we present the results of these experiments. In section 5, we propose an extension of this work in which the models are re-parameterized so as to automatically learn what must be shared and what need not be shared.

2   Parameter Sharing and Multi-Task Learning

Most research on ANNs has been concerned with *tabula rasa* learning. The learner is given a set of examples $(x_1, y_1), (x_2, y_2), ..., (x_N, y_N)$ chosen according to some unknown probability distribution. Each pair (x, y) represents an input x, and a desired value y. One defines a training criterion C to be minimized in function of the desired outputs and of the outputs of the learner $f(x)$. The function f is parameterized by the parameters of the network and belongs to a set of hypotheses H, that is the set of all functions that can be realized for different values of the parameters. The part of generalization error due to variance (due to the specific choice of training examples) can be controlled by making strong assumptions on the model, i.e., by choosing a small hypotheses space H. But using an incorrect model also worsens performance.

Over the last few years, methods for automatically choosing H based on similar tasks have been studied. They consider that a learner is embedded in a world where it faces **many related tasks** and that the knowledge acquired when learning a task can be used to learn better and/or faster a new task. Some methods consider that the related tasks are not always all available at the same time (Pratt, 1993; Silver and Mercer, 1995): knowledge acquired when learning a previous task is transferred to a new task. Instead, all tasks may be learned in parallel (Baxter, 1995; Caruana, 1995), and this is the approach followed here. Our objective is not to use multi-task learning to improve the speed of learning the training data (Pratt, 1993; Silver and Mercer, 1995), but instead to improve generalization performance. For example, in (Baxter, 1995), several neural networks (one for each task) are trained simultaneouly. The networks share their first hidden layers, while all the remaining layers are specific to each network. The shared layers use the knowledge provided from the training examples of all the tasks to build an internal representation suitable for all these tasks. The remaining layers of each network use the internal representation to learn a specific task.

In the multitask learning method used by Caruana (Caruana, 1995), all the hidden layers are shared. They serve as mutual sources of inductive bias. It was also suggested that besides the relevant tasks that are used for learning, it may be possible to use other related tasks that we do not want to learn but that may help to further bias the learner (Caruana, Baluja and Mitchell, 1996; Intrator and Edelman, 1996).

In the family discovery method (Omohundro, 1996), a parameterized family of models is built. Several learners are trained separately on different but related tasks and their parameters are used to construct a manifold of parameters. When a new task has to be learned, the parameters are chosen so as to maximize the data likelihood on the one hand, and to maximize a "family prior" on the other hand which restricts the chosen parameters to lie on the manifold.

In all these methods, the values of some or all the parameters are constrained. Such models restrict the size of the hypotheses space sufficiently to ensure good generalization performance from a small number of examples.

3 Application to Stock Selection

We apply the ideas of multi-task learning to a problem of stock selection and portfolio management. We consider a universe of 36 assets, including 35 risky assets and one risk-free asset. The risky assets are 35 Canadian large-capitalization stocks from the Toronto Stock Exchange. The risk-free asset is represented by 90-days Canadian treasury bills. The data is monthly and spans 8 years, from February 1986 to January 1994 (96 months). Each month, one can buy or sell some of these assets in such a way as to distribute the current worth between these assets. We do not allow borrowing or short selling, so the weights of the resulting portfolio are all non-negative (and they sum to 1).

We have selected 5 explanatory variables, 2 of which represent macro-economic variables which are known to influence the business cycle, and 3 of which are micro-economic variables representing the profitability of the company and previous price changes of the stock. The macro-economic variables were derived from yields of long-term bonds and from the Consumer Price Index. The micro-economic variables were derived from the series of dividend yields and from the series of ratios of stock price to book value of the company. Spline **extrapolation** (not interpolation) was used to obtain monthly data from the quarterly or annual company statements or macro-economic variables. For these variables, we used the dates at which their value was made public, not the dates to which they theoretically refer.

To take into account the non-stationarity of the financial and economic time-series, and estimate performance over a variety of economic situations, multiple training experiments were performed on different training windows, each time testing on the following 12 months. For each architecture, 5 such trainings took place, with training sets of size 3, 4, 5, 6, and 7 years respectively. Furthermore, multiple such experiments with different initial weights were performed to verify that we did not obtain "lucky" results due to particular initial weights. The 5 concatenated test periods make an overall 5-year test period from February 1989 to January 1994.

The training algorithm is described in (Bengio, 1996) and is based on the optimization of the neural network parameters with respect to a financial criterion (here maximizing the overall profit). The outputs of the neural network feed a trading module. The trading module has as input at each time step the output of the network, as well as, the weights giving the current distribution of worth between the assets. These weights depend on the previous portfolio weights and on the relative change in value of each asset (due to different price changes). The outputs of the trading module are the current portfolio weights for each of the assets. Based on the difference between these desired weights and the current distribution of worth, transactions are performed. Transaction costs of 1% (of the absolute value of each buy or sell transaction) are taken into account. Because of transaction costs, the actions of the trading module at time t influence the profitability of its future actions. The financial criterion depends in a non-additive way on the performance of the network over the whole sequence. To obtain gradients of this criterion with respect to the network output we have to backpropagate gradients backward through time, through the trading module, which computes a differentiable function of its inputs. Therefore, a gradient step is performed only after presenting the whole training sequence (in order, of course). In (Bengio, 1996), we have found this procedure to yield significantly larger profits (around 4% better annual return), at comparable risks, in comparison to training the neural network to predict expected future returns with the mean squared error criterion. In the experiments, the ANN was trained for 120 epochs.

4 Experimental Results

Four sets of experiments with different types of parameter sharing were performed, with two different architectures for the neural network: 5-3-1 (5 inputs, a hidden layer of 3 units, and 1 output), 5-3-2-1 (5 inputs, 3 units in the first hidden layer, 2 units in the second hidden layer, and 1 output). The output represents the belief that the value of the stock is going to increase (or the expected future return over three months when training with the MSE criterion).

Four types of parameter sharing between the different models for each stock are compared in these experiments: sharing everything (the same parameters for all the stocks), sharing only the parameters (weights and biases) of the first hidden layers, sharing only the output layer parameters, and not sharing anything (independent models for each stock).

The main results for the test period, using the 5-3-1 architecture, are summarized in Table 1, and graphically depicted in Figure 1 with the worth curves for the four types of sharing. The results for the test period, using the 5-3-2-1 architecture are summarized in Table 2. The ANNs were compared to two benchmarks: a buy-and-hold benchmark (with uniform initial weights over all 35 stocks), and the TSE300 Index. Since the buy-and-hold benchmark performed better (8.3% yearly return) than the TSE300 Index (4.4% yearly return) during the 02/89-01/94 test period, Tables 1, and 2 give comparisons with the buy-and-hold benchmark. Variations of average yearly return on the test period due to different initial weights were computed by performing each of the experiments 18 times with different random seeds. The resulting standard deviations are less than 3.7 when no parameters or all the parameters are shared, less than 2.7 when the parameters of the first hidden layers are shared, and less than 4.2 when the output layer is shared.

The values of **beta** and **alpha** are computed by fitting the monthly return of the portfolio r_p to the return of the benchmark r_M, both adjusted for the risk-free return

Table 1: Comparative results for the 5-3-1 architecture: four types of sharing are compared with the buy-and-hold benchmark (see text).

	buy & hold	share all	share hidden	share output	no sharing
Average yearly return	8.3%	13%	23.4%	24.8%	22.8%
Standard deviation (monthly)	3.5%	4.3%	5.3%	5.3%	5.2%
Beta	1	1.07	1.30	1.26	1.26
Alpha (yearly)	0	9%	20.6%	21.8%	19.9%
t-statistic for alpha = 0	NA	11	14.9	15	14
Reward to variability	0.9%	9.6%	22.9%	24.7%	22.3%
Excess return above benchmark	0	4.7%	15.1%	16.4%	14.5%
Maximum drawdown	15.7%	13.3%	13.4%	13.3%	13.3%

Table 2: Comparative results for the 5-3-2-1 architecture: three types of sharing are compared with the buy-and-hold benchmark (see text).

	buy & hold	share all	share first hidden	share all hidden	no sharing
Average yearly return	8.3%	12.5%	22.7%	23%	9.1%
Standard deviation (monthly)	3.5%	4.%	5.2%	5.2%	3.1%
Beta	1	1.02	1.25	1.28	0.87
Alpha (yearly)	0	8.2%	19.7%	20.1%	4.%
t-statistic for alpha = 0	NA	12.1	14.1	14.8	21.2
Reward to variability	0.9%	9.3%	22.2%	22.5%	2.5%
Excess return above benchmark	0	4.2%	14.4%	14.7%	0.8%
Maximum drawdown	15.7%	13%	12.6%	13.4%	10%

r_i (interest rates), according to the linear regression $E(r_p - r_i) = \text{alpha} + \text{beta}(r_M - r_i)$. Beta is simply the ratio of the covariance between the portfolio return and the market return with the variance of the market. According to the Capital Asset Pricing Model (Sharpe, 1964), beta gives a measure of "systematic" risk, i.e., as it relates to the risk of the market, whereas the variance of the return gives a measure of total risk. The value of alpha in the tables is annualized (as a compound return): it represents a measure of excess return (over the market benchmark) adjusted for market risk (beta). The hypothesis that alpha = 0 is clearly rejected in all cases (with t-statistics above 9, and corresponding p-values very close to 0). The **reward to variability** (or "Sharpe ratio") as defined in (Sharpe, 1966), is another risk-adjusted measure of performance: $\frac{(r_p - r_i)}{\sigma_p}$, where σ_p is the standard deviation of the portfolio return (monthly returns were used here). The excess return above benchmark is the simple difference (not risk-adjusted) between the return of the portfolio and that of the benchmark. The maximum drawdown is another measure of risk, and it can be defined in terms of the worth curve: worth[t] is the ratio between the value of the portfolio at time t and its value at time 0. The maximum drawdown is then defined as $\max_t \frac{((\max_{s \leq t} \text{worth}[s]) - \text{worth}[t])}{(\max_{s \leq t} \text{worth}[s])}$.

Three conclusions clearly come out of the tables and figure: (1) The main improvement is obtained by allowing some parameters to be not shared (for the 5-3-1 architecture, although the best results are obtained with a shared hidden and a free output layer, there are no significant differences between the different types of partial sharing, or no sharing at all). (2) Sharing some parameters yielded more consistent results (across architectures) than when not sharing at all. (3) The performance obtained in this way is very much better than that obtained by the benchmarks (buy-and-hold or TSE300), i.e., the yearly return is more than 14% above the best benchmark, while the risks are comparable (as measured by standard deviation of

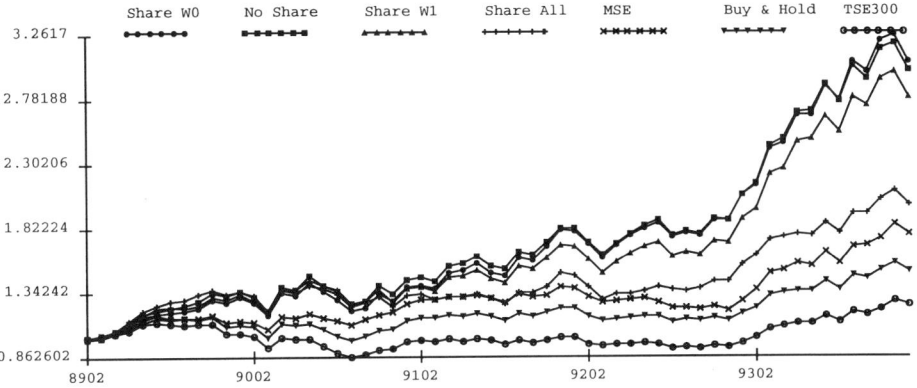

Figure 1: Evolution of total worth in the 5-year test period 02/89-01/94, for the 5-3-1 architecture, and different types of sharing. From top to bottom: sharing the hidden layer, no sharing across stocks, sharing the output layer, sharing everything, sharing everything with MSE training, Buy and Hold benchmark, TSE300 benchmark.

return or by maximum drawdown).

5 Future Work

We will extend the results presented here in two directions. Firstly, given the impressive results obtained with the described approach, we would like to repeat the experiment on different data sets, for different markets. Secondly, we would like to generalize the type of multi-task learning by allowing for more freedom in the way the different tasks influence each other.

Following (Omohundro, 1996), the basic idea is to re-parameterize the parameters $\theta_i \in R^{n_1}$ of the ith model, for all n models in the following way: $\theta_i = f(p_i, \omega)$ where $p_i \in R^{n_2}$, $\omega \in R^{n_3}$, and $n \times n_1 < n \times n_2 + n_3$. For example, if $f()$ is an affine function, this forces the parameters of each the n different networks to lie on the same linear manifold. The position of a point on the manifold is given by a n_2-dimensional vector p_i, and the manifold itself is specified by the n_3 parameters of ω. The expected advantage of this approach with respect to the one used in this paper is that different models (e.g., corresponding to different stocks) may "share" more or less depending on how far their p_i is from the p_j's for other models. One does not have to specify which parameters are free and which are shared, but one has to specify how many are really free (n_2) per model, and the shape of the manifold.

6 Conclusion

The results presented of this paper show an interesting application of the ideas of multi-task learning to stock selection. In this paper we have addressed the question of whether ANNs trained for stock selection or portfolio management should be different for each stock or shared across all the stocks. We have found significantly better results when some or (sometimes) all of the parameters of the stock models are free (not shared). Since a parcimonuous model is always preferable, we conclude that partially sharing the parameters is even preferable, since it does not yield a deterioration in performance, and it yields more consistent results. Another interesting conclusion of this paper is that very large returns can be obtained at risks comparable to the market using a combination of partial parameter sharing and training with respect to a financial training criterion, with a small number of explanatory input features that include technical, micro-economic and macro-economic information.

References

Baxter, J. (1995). Learning internal representations. In *Proceedings of the Eighth International Conference on Computational Learning Theory*, pages 311–320, Santa Cruz, California. ACM Press.

Bengio, Y. (1996). Using a financial training criterion rather than a prediction criterion. Technical Report #1019, Dept. Informatique et Recherche Operationnelle, Universite de Montreal.

Caruana, R. (1995). Learning many related tasks at the same time with backpropagation. In Tesauro, G., Touretzky, D. S., and Leen, T. K., editors, *Advances in Neural Information Processing Systems*, volume 7, pages 657–664, Cambridge, MA. MIT Press.

Caruana, R., Baluja, S., and Mitchell, T. (1996). Using the future to "sort out" the present: Rankprop and multitask learning for medical risk evaluation. In *Advances in Neural Information Processing Systems*, volume 8.

Intrator, N. and Edelman, S. (1996). How to make a low-dimensional representation suitable for diverse tasks. *Connection Science, Special issue on Transfer in Neural Networks*. to appear.

Moody, J., Levin, U., and Rehfuss, S. (1993). Predicting the U.S. index of industrial production. *Neural Network World*, 3(6):791–794.

Omohundro, S. (1996). Family discovery. In Mozer, M., Touretzky, D., and Perrone, M., editors, *Advances in Neural Information Processing Systems 8*. MIT Press, Cambridge, MA.

Pratt, L. Y. (1993). Discriminability-based transfer between neural networks. In Giles, C. L., Hanson, S. J., and Cowan, J., editors, *Advances in Neural Information Processing Systems 5*, pages 204–211, San Mateo, CA. Morgan Kaufmann.

Refenes, A. (1994). Stock performance modeling using neural networks: a comparative study with regression models. *Neural Networks*, 7(2):375–388.

Sharpe, W. (1964). Capital asset prices: A theory of market equilibrium under conditions of risk. *Journal of Finance*, 19:425–442.

Sharpe, W. (1966). Mutual fund performance. *Journal of Business*, 39(1):119–138.

Silver, D. L. and Mercer, R. E. (1995). Toward a model of consolidation: The retention and transfer of neural net task knowledge. In *Proceedings of the INNS World Congress on Neural Networks*, volume 3, pages 164–169, Washington, DC.

The Neurothermostat: Predictive Optimal Control of Residential Heating Systems

Michael C. Mozer[†], Lucky Vidmar[†], Robert H. Dodier[‡]
[†]Department of Computer Science
[‡]Department of Civil, Environmental, and Architectural Engineering
University of Colorado, Boulder, CO 80309–0430

Abstract

The *Neurothermostat* is an adaptive controller that regulates indoor air temperature in a residence by switching a furnace on or off. The task is framed as an optimal control problem in which both comfort and energy costs are considered as part of the control objective. Because the consequences of control decisions are delayed in time, the Neurothermostat must anticipate heating demands with predictive models of occupancy patterns and the thermal response of the house and furnace. Occupancy pattern prediction is achieved by a hybrid neural net / look-up table. The Neurothermostat searches, at each discrete time step, for a decision sequence that minimizes the expected cost over a fixed planning horizon. The first decision in this sequence is taken, and this process repeats. Simulations of the Neurothermostat were conducted using artificial occupancy data in which regularity was systematically varied, as well as occupancy data from an actual residence. The Neurothermostat is compared against three conventional policies, and achieves reliably lower costs. This result is robust to the relative weighting of comfort and energy costs and the degree of variability in the occupancy patterns.

For over a quarter century, the home automation industry has promised to revolutionize our lifestyle with the so-called Smart House® in which appliances, lighting, stereo, video, and security systems are integrated under computer control. However, home automation has yet to make significant inroads, at least in part because software must be tailored to the home occupants.

Instead of expecting the occupants to program their homes or to hire someone to do so, one would ideally like the home to essentially *program itself* by observing the lifestyle of the occupants. This is the goal of the Neural Network House (Mozer et al., 1995), an actual residence that has been outfitted with over 75 sensors—including temperature, light, sound, motion—and actuators to control air heating, water heating, lighting, and ventilation. In this paper, we describe one research project within the house, the *Neurothermostat*, that learns to regulate the indoor air temperature automatically by observing and detecting patterns in the occupants' schedules and comfort preferences. We focus on the problem of air heating with a whole-house furnace, but the same approach can be taken with alternative or multiple heating devices, and to the problems of cooling and ventilation.

1 TEMPERATURE REGULATION AS AN OPTIMAL CONTROL PROBLEM

Traditionally, the control objective of air temperature regulation has been to minimize energy consumption while maintaining temperature within an acceptable comfort margin during certain times of the day and days of the week. This is sensible in commercial settings, where occupancy patterns follow simple rules and where energy considerations dominate individual preferences. In a residence, however, the desires and schedules of occupants need to be weighted equally with energy considerations. Consequently, we frame the task of air temperature regulation as a problem of maximizing occupant comfort *and* minimizing energy costs.

These two objectives clearly conflict, but they can be integrated into a unified framework via an optimal control aproach in which the goal is to heat the house according to a policy that minimizes the cost

$$J = \lim_{\kappa \to \infty} \frac{1}{\kappa} \sum_{t=t_0+1}^{t_0+\kappa} [e(u_t) + m(\mathbf{x}_t)],$$

where time, t, is quantized into nonoverlapping intervals during which we assume all environmental variables remain constant, t_0 is the interval ending at the current time, u_t is the control decision for interval t (e.g., turn the furnace on), $e(u)$ is the energy cost associated with decision u, $\mathbf{x}_t$ is the environmental state during interval t, which includes the indoor temperature and the occupancy status of the home, and $m(\mathbf{x})$ is the *misery* of the occupant given state $\mathbf{x}$. To add misery and energy costs, a common currency is required. Energy costs are readily expressed in dollars. We also determine misery in dollars, as we describe later.

While we have been unable to locate any earlier work that combined energy and comfort costs in an optimal control framework, optimal control has been used in a variety of building energy system control applications (e.g., Henze & Dodier, 1996; Khalid & Omatu, 1995).

2 THE NEUROTHERMOSTAT

Figure 1 shows the system architecture of the Neurothermostat and its interaction with the environment. The heart of the Neurothermostat is a controller that, at time intervals of δ minutes, can switch the house furnace on or off. Because the consequences of control decisions are delayed in time, the controller must be *predictive* to anticipate heating demands. The three boxes in the Figure depict components that predict or model various aspects of the environment. We explain their purpose via a formal description of the controller operation.

The controller considers sequences of κ decisions, denoted $\mathbf{u}$, and searches for the sequence that minimizes the expected total cost, $\bar{J}_\mathbf{u}$, over the planning horizon of $\kappa\delta$ minutes:

$$\bar{J}_\mathbf{u} = \sum_{t=t_0+1}^{t_0+\kappa} E_{\mathbf{x}|\mathbf{u}}[e(u_t) + m(\mathbf{x}_t)] = \sum_{t=t_0+1}^{t_0+\kappa} e(u_t) + \bar{m}_\mathbf{u}(\mathbf{x}_t),$$

where the expectation is computed over future states of the environment conditional on the decision sequence $\mathbf{u}$. The energy cost in an interval depends only on the control decision during that interval. The misery cost depends on two components

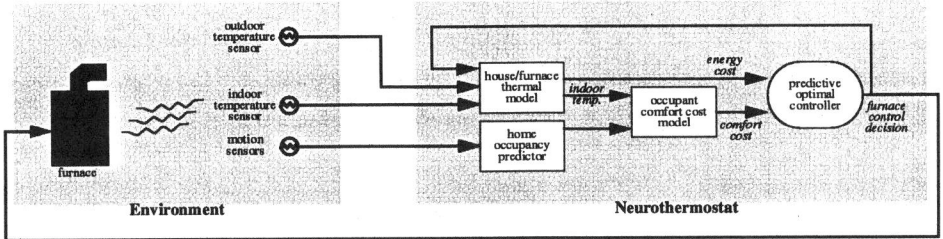

Figure 1: The Neurothermostat and its interaction with the environment

of the state—the house occupancy status, $o(t)$ (0 for empty, 1 for occupied), and the indoor air temperature, $h_{\mathbf{u}}(t)$:

$$\bar{m}_{\mathbf{u}}(o(t), h_{\mathbf{u}}(t)) = p[o(t) = 1]\, m(1, h_{\mathbf{u}}(t)) + p[o(t) = 0]\, m(0, h_{\mathbf{u}}(t))$$

Because the true quantities e, $h_{\mathbf{u}}$, m, and p are unknown, they must be estimated. The house thermal model of Figure 1 provides $\hat{e}$ and $\hat{h}_{\mathbf{u}}$, the occupant comfort cost model provides $\hat{m}$, and the home occupancy predictor provides $\hat{p}$.

We follow a tradition of using neural networks for prediction in the context of building energy system control (e.g., Curtiss, Kreider, & Brandemuehl, 1993; Ferrano & Wong, 1990; Miller & Seem, 1991), although in our initial experiments we require a network only for the occupancy prediction.

2.1 PREDICTIVE OPTIMAL CONTROLLER

We propose a closed-loop controller that combines prediction with fixed-horizon planning, of the sort proposed by Clarke, Mohtadi, and Tuffs (1987). At each time step, the controller considers all possible decision sequences over the planning horizon and selects the sequence that minimizes the expected total cost, $\bar{J}$. The first decision in this sequence is then performed. After δ minutes, the planning and execution process is repeated. This approach assumes that beyond the planning horizon, all costs are independent of the first decision in the sequence.

While dynamic programming is an efficient search algorithm, it requires a discrete state space. Wishing to avoid quantizing the continuous variable of indoor temperature, and the errors that might be introduced, we performed performed exhaustive search through the possible decision sequences, which was tractable due to relatively short horizons and two additional domain constraints. First, because the house occupancy status can reasonably be assumed to be independent of the indoor temperature, $\hat{p}$ need not be recalculated for every possible decision sequence. Second, the current occupancy status depends on the recent occupancy history. Consequently, one needs to predict occupancy *patterns* over the planning horizon, $\mathbf{o} \in \{0, 1\}^\kappa$ to compute $\hat{p}$. However, because most occupancy sequences are highly improbable, we find that considering only the most likely sequences—those containing at most two occupancy state transitions—produces the same decisions as doing the search over the entire distribution, reducing the cost from $O(2^\kappa)$ to $O(\kappa^2)$.

2.2 OCCUPANCY PREDICTOR

The basic task of the occupancy predictor is to estimate the probability that the occupant will be home δ minutes in the future. The occupancy predictor can be run iteratively to estimate the probability of an occupancy pattern.

If occupants follow a deterministic daily schedule, a look up table indexed by time of day and current occupancy state should capture occupancy patterns. We thus use a look up table to encode whatever structure possible, and a neural network to encode residual structure. The look up table divides time into fixed δ minute bins. The neural network consisted of the following inputs: current time of day; day of the week; average proportion of time home was occupied in the 10, 20, and 30 minutes from the present time of day on the previous three days and on the same day of the week during the past four weeks; and the proportion of time the home was occupied during the past 60, 180, and 360 minutes. The network, a standard three-layer architecture, was trained by back propagation. The number of hidden units was chosen by cross validation.

2.3 THERMAL MODEL OF HOUSE AND FURNACE

A thermal model of the house and furnace predicts future indoor temperature(s) as a function of the outdoor temperature and the furnace operation. While one could perform system identification using neural networks, a simple parameterized resistance-capacitance (RC) model provides a reasonable first-order approximation. The RC model assumes that: the inside of the house is at a uniform temperature, and likewise the outside; a homogeneous flat wall separates the inside and outside, and this wall has a thermal resistance R and thermal capacitance C; the entire wall mass is at the inside temperature; and the heat input to the inside is Q when the furnace is running or zero otherwise. Assuming that the outdoor temperature, denoted g, is constant, the the indoor temperature at time t, $\hat{h}_\mathbf{u}(t)$, is:

$$\hat{h}_\mathbf{u}(t) = \hat{h}_\mathbf{u}(t-1)\exp(-60\delta/RC) + (RQu(t) + g)(1 - \exp(-60\delta/RC)),$$

where $\hat{h}_\mathbf{u}(t_0)$ is the actual indoor temperature at the current time. R and C were determined by architectural properties of the Neural Network House to be 1.33 Kelvins/kilowatt and 16 megajoules/Kelvin, respectively. The House furnace is rated at 133,000 Btu/hour and has 92.5% fuel use efficiency, resulting in an output of $Q = 36.1$ kilowatts. With natural gas at \$.485 per CCF, the cost of operating the furnace, $\hat{e}$, is \$.7135 per hour.

2.4 OCCUPANT COMFORT COST MODEL

In the Neural Network House, the occupant expresses discomfort by adjusting a setpoint temperature on a control panel. However, for simplicity, we assume in this work the setpoint is a constant, λ. When the home is occupied, the misery cost is a monotonic function of the deviation of the actual indoor temperature from the setpoint. When the home is empty, the misery cost is zero regardless of the temperature.

There is a rich literature directed at measuring thermal comfort in a given environment (i.e., dry-bulb temperature, relative humidity, air velocity, clothing insulation, etc.) for the average building occupant (e.g., Fanger, 1972; Gagge, Stolwijk, & Nishi, 1971). Although the measurements indicate the fraction of the population which is uncomfortable in a particular environment, one might also interpret them as a measure of an individual's level of discomfort. As a function of dry-bulb temperature, this curve is roughly parabolic. We approximate it with a measure of misery in a δ-minute period as follows:

$$\hat{m}(o, h) = o\alpha \frac{\delta}{24 \times 60} \frac{\max(0, |\lambda - h| - \epsilon)^2}{25}.$$

The first term, o, is a binary variable indicating the home occupancy state. The second term is a conversion factor from arbitrary "misery" units to dollars. The third term scales the misery cost from a full day to the basic update interval. The fourth term produces the parabolic relative misery function, scaled so that a temperature difference of 5° C produces one unit of misery, with a *deadband* region from $\lambda - \epsilon$ to $\lambda + \epsilon$.

We have chosen the conversion factor α using an economic perspective. Consider the lost productivity that results from trying to work in a home that is 5° C colder than desired for a 24 hour period. Denote this loss ρ, measured in hours. The cost in dollars of this loss is then $\alpha = \gamma\rho$, where γ is the individual's hourly salary. With this approch, α can be set in a natural, intuitive manner.

3 SIMULATION METHODOLOGY

In all experiments we report below, $\delta = 10$ minutes, $\kappa = 12$ steps (120 minute planning horizon), $\lambda = 22.5°$ C, $\epsilon = 1$, and $\gamma = 28$ dollars per hour. The productivity loss, ρ, was varied from 1 to 3 hours.

We report here results from the Neurothermostat operating in a simulated environment, rather than in the actual Neural Network House. The simulated environment incorporates the house/furnace thermal model described earlier and occupants whose preferences follow the comfort cost model. The outdoor temperature is assumed to remain a constant 0° C. Thus, the Neurothermostat has an accurate model of its environment, except for the occupancy patterns, which it must predict based on training data. This allows us to evaluate the performance of the Neurothermostat and the occupancy model as occupancy patterns are varied, uncontaminated by the effect of inaccuracy in the other internal models.

We have evaluated the Neurothermostat with both real and artificial occupancy data. The real data was collected from the Neural Network House with a single resident over an eight month period, using a simple algorithm based on motion detector output and the opening and closing of outside doors. The artificial data was generated by a simulation of a single occupant. The occupant would go to work each day, later on the weekends, would sometimes come home for lunch, sometimes go out on weekend nights, and sometimes go out of town for several days. To examine performance of the Neurothermostat as a function of the variability in the occupant's schedule, the simulation model included a parameter, the *variability index*. An index of 0 means that the schedule is entirely deterministic; an index of 1 means that the schedule was very noisy, but still contained statistical regularities. The index determined factors such as the likelihood and duration of out-of-town trips and the variability in departure and return times.

3.1 ALTERNATIVE HEATING POLICIES

In addition to the Neurothermostat, we examined three nonadaptive control policies. These policies produce a *setpoint* at each time step, and the furnace is switched on if the temperature drops below the setpoint and off if the temperature rises above the setpoint. (We need not be concerned about damage to the furnace by cycling because control decisions are made ten minutes apart.) The *constant-temperature* policy produces a fixed setpoint of 22.5° C. The *occupancy-triggered* policy produces a setpoint of 18° C when the house is empty, 22.5° C when the house is occupied. The *setback-thermostat* policy lowers the setpoint from 22.5° C to 18° C half an hour before the mean work departure time for that day of the week, and raises it back to 22.5° C half an hour before the mean work return time for that day of the week. The setback temperature for the occupancy-triggered and setback-thermostat policies was determined empirically to minimize the total cost.

4 RESULTS

4.1 OCCUPANCY PREDICTOR

Performance of three different predictors was evaluated using artificial data across a range of values for the variability index. For each condition, we generated eight training/test sets of artificial data, each training and test set consisting of 150 days of data. Table 1 shows the normalized mean squared error (MSE) on the test set, averaged over the eight replications. The normalization involved dividing the MSE for each replication by the error obtained by predicting the future occupancy state

Table 1: Normalized MSE on Test Set for Occupancy Prediction—Artificial Data

	variability index				
	0	.25	.50	.75	1
lookup table	.49	.81	.94	.92	.94
neural net	.02	.63	.83	.86	.91
lookup table + neural net	.02	.60	.78	.77	.74

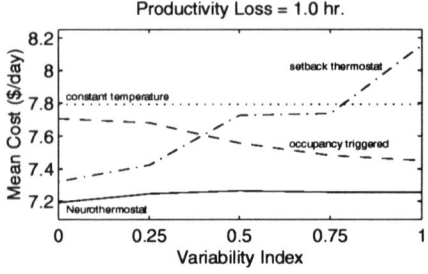
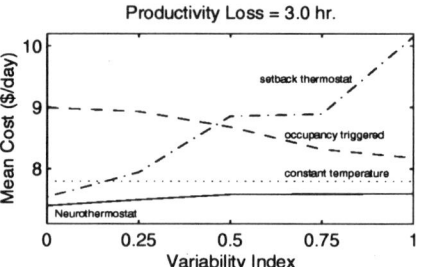

Figure 2: Mean cost per day incurred by four control policies on (artificial) test data as a function of the data's variability index for $\rho = 1$ (comfort lightly weighted, left panel) and $\rho = 3$ (comfort heavily weighted, right panel).

is the same as the present state. The main result here is that the combination of neural network and look up table perform better than either component in isolation (ANOVA: $F(1,7) = 1121, p < .001$ for combination vs. table; $F(1,7) = 64, p < .001$ for combination vs. network), indicating that the two components are capturing different structure in the data.

4.2 CONTROLLER WITH ARTIFICIAL OCCUPANCY DATA

Having trained eight occupancy predictors with different (artificial data) training sets, we computed misery and energy costs for the Neurothermostat on the corresponding test sets. Figure 2 shows the mean total cost per day as a function of variability index, control policy, and relative comfort cost. The robust result is that the Neurothermostat outperforms the three nonadaptive control policies for all levels of the variability index and for both a wide range of values of ρ.

Other patterns in the data are noteworthy. Costs for the Neurothermostat tend to rise with the variability index, as one would expect because the occupant's schedule becomes less predictable. The constant-temperature policy is worst if occupant comfort is weighted lightly, and begins to approach the Neurothermostat in performance as comfort costs are increased. If comfort costs overwhelm energy costs, then the constant-temperature policy and the Neurothermostat converge.

4.3 CONTROLLER WITH REAL OCCUPANCY DATA

Eight months of real occupancy data collected in the Neural Network House beginning in September 1994 was also used to generate occupancy models and test controllers. Three training/test splits were formed by training on five consecutive months and testing on the next month. Table 2 shows the mean daily cost for the four controllers. The Neurothermostat significantly outperforms the three nonadaptive controllers, as it did with the artificial data.

5 DISCUSSION

The simulation studies reported here strongly suggest that adaptive control of residential heating and cooling systems is worthy of further investigation. One is

Table 2: Mean Daily Cost Based on Real Occupancy Data

	productivity loss	
	$\rho = 1$	$\rho = 3$
Neurothermostat	$6.77	$7.05
constant temperature	$7.85	$7.85
occupancy triggered	$7.49	$8.66
setback thermostat	$8.12	$9.74

tempted to trumpet the conclusion that adaptive control lowers heating costs, but before doing so, one must be clear that the cost being lowered is a combination of comfort and energy costs. If one is merely interested in lowering energy costs, then simply shut off the furnace. A central contribution of this work is thus the framing of the task of air temperature regulation as an optimal control problem in which both comfort and energy costs are considered as part of the control objective.

A common reaction to this research project is, "My life is far too irregular to be predicted. I don't return home from work at the same time every day." An important finding of this work is that even a highly nondeterministic schedule contains sufficient statistical regularity to be exploited by a predictive controller. We found this for both artificial data with a high variability index and real occupancy data.

A final contribution of our work is to show that for periodic data such as occupancy patterns that follow a weekly schedule, the combination of a look up table to encode the periodic structure and a neural network to encode the residual structure can outperform either method in isolation.

Acknowledgements

Support for this research has come from Lifestyle Technologies, NSF award IRI-9058450, and a CRCW grant-in-aid from the University of Colorado. This project owes its existence to the dedication of many students, particularly Marc Anderson, Josh Anderson, Paul Kooros, and Charles Myers. Our thanks to Reid Hastie and Gary McClelland for their suggestions on assessing occupant misery.

References

Clarke, D. W., Mohtadi, C., & Tuffs, P. S. (1987). Generalized predictive control-Part I. The basic algorithm. *Automatica, 23*, 137-148

Curtiss, P., Kreider, J. F., & Brandemuehl, M. J. (1993). Local and global control of commercial building HVAC systems using artificial neural networks. *Proceedings of the American Control Conference, 3*, 3029-3044.

Fanger, P. O. (1972). *Thermal comfort.* New York: McGraw-Hill.

Ferrano, F. J., & Wong, K. V. (1990). Prediction of thermal storage loads using a neural network. *ASHRAE Transactions, 96*, 723-726.

Gagge, A. P., Stolwijk, J. A. J., & Nishi, Y. (1971). An effective temperature scale based on a simple model of human physiological regulatory response. *ASHRAE Transactions, 77*, 247-262.

Henze, G. P., & Dodier, R. H. (1996). Development of a predictive optimal controller for thermal energy storage systems. Submitted for publication.

Khalid, M., & Omatu, S. (1995). Temperature regulation with neural networks and alternative control schemes. *IEEE Transactions on Neural Networks, 6*, 572-582.

Miller, R. C., & Seem, J. E. (1991). Comparison of artificial neural networks with traditional methods of predicting return time from night or weekend setback. *ASHRAE Transactions, 97*, 500-508.

Mozer, M. C., Dodier, R. H., Anderson, M., Vidmar, L., Cruickshank III, R. F., & Miller, D. (1995). The neural network house: An overview. In L. Niklasson & M. Boden (Eds.), *Current trends in connectionism* (pp. 371-380). Hillsdale, NJ: Erlbaum.

Sequential Tracking in Pricing Financial Options using Model Based and Neural Network Approaches

Mahesan Niranjan
Cambridge University Engineering Department
Cambridge CB2 1PZ, England
niranjan@eng.cam.ac.uk

Abstract

This paper shows how the prices of option contracts traded in financial markets can be tracked sequentially by means of the Extended Kalman Filter algorithm. I consider call and put option pairs with identical strike price and time of maturity as a two output nonlinear system. The Black-Scholes approach popular in Finance literature and the Radial Basis Functions neural network are used in modelling the nonlinear system generating these observations. I show how both these systems may be identified recursively using the EKF algorithm. I present results of simulations on some FTSE 100 Index options data and discuss the implications of viewing the pricing problem in this sequential manner.

1 INTRODUCTION

Data from the financial markets has recently been of much interest to the neural computing community. The complexity of the underlying macro-economic system and how traders react to the flow of information leads to highly nonlinear relationships between observations. Further, the underlying system is essentially time varying, making any analysis both difficult and interesting. A number of problems, including forecasting a univariate time series from past observations, rating credit risk, optimal selection of portfolio components and pricing options have been thrown at neural networks recently.

The problem addressed in this paper is that of sequential estimation, applied to pricing of options contracts. In a nonstationary environment, such as financial markets, sequential estimation is the natural approach to modelling. This is because data arrives at the modeller sequentially, and there is the need to build and apply the best possible model with available data. At the next point in time, some additional data is available and the task becomes one of optimally updating the model to account for the new data. This can either be done by reestimating the model with a moving window of data or by sequentially propagating the estimates of model parameters and some associated information (such as the error covariance matrices in the Kalman filtering framework discussed in this paper).

2 SEQUENTIAL ESTIMATION

Sequential estimation of nonlinear models via the Extended Kalman Filter algorithm is well known (e.g. Candy, 1986; Bar-Shalom & Li, 1993). This approach has also been widely applied to the training of Neural Network architectures (e.g. Kadirkamanathan & Niranjan, 1993; Puskorius & Feldkamp, 1994). In this section, I give the necessary equations for a second order EKF, i.e. Taylor series expansion of the nonlinear output equations, truncated at order two, for the state space model simplified to the system identification framework considered here.

The parameter vector or state vector, θ, is assumed to have the following simple random walk dynamics.

$$\underline{\theta}(n+1) = \underline{\theta}(n) + \underline{u}(n),$$

where $\underline{u}(n)$ is a noise term, known as process noise. $\underline{u}(n)$ is of the same dimensionality as the number of states used to represent the system. The process noise gives a random walk freedom to the state dynamics facilitating the tracking behaviour desired in nonstationary environments. In using the Kalman filtering framework, we assume the covariance matrix of this noise process, denoted Q, is known. In practice, we set Q to some small diagonal matrix.

The observations from the system are given by the equation

$$\underline{z}(n) = \underline{f}(\underline{\theta}, \underline{U}) + \underline{w}(n),$$

where, the vector $\underline{z}(n)$ is the output of the system consisting of the call and put option prices at time n. $\underline{U}$ denotes the input information. In the problem considered here, $\underline{U}$ consists of the price of the underlying asset and the time to maturity if the option. $\underline{w}$ is known as the measurement noise, covariance matrix of which, denoted R, is also assumed to be known. Setting the parameters R and Q is done by trial and error and knowledge about the noise processes. In the estimation framework considered here, Q and R determine the tracking behaviour of the system. For the experiments reported in this paper, I have set these by trial and error, but more systematic approaches involving multiple models is possible (Niranjan et al, 1994).

The prior estimates at time $(n+1)$, using all the data upto time (n) and the model of the dynamical system, or the prediction phase of the Kalman algorithm is given by the equations:

$$\hat{\underline{\theta}}(n+1|n) = \hat{\underline{\theta}}(n|n)$$
$$\hat{P}(n+1|n) = \hat{P}(n|n) + Q(n)$$
$$\hat{\underline{z}}(n+1|n) = \underline{J}_\theta(\underline{\theta}(n+1|n)) + \frac{1}{2} \sum_{i=1}^{n_\theta} \underline{e}_i \, \text{tr}\left(\underline{H}^i_{\theta\theta}(n+1) \hat{P}(n+1|n)\right)$$

where $\underline{J}_\theta$ and $\underline{H}^i_{\theta\theta}$ are the Jacobian and Hessians of the output $\underline{z}$; also $n_\theta = 2$. $\underline{e}_i$ are unit vectors in direction i. tr(.) denotes trace of a matrix. The posterior estimates or the correction phase of the Kalman algorithm are given by the equations:

$$S(n+1) = \underline{J}_\theta(n+1)\hat{P}(n+1|n)\underline{J}'_\theta(n+1)$$
$$+ \frac{1}{2}\sum_{i=1}^{n_\theta}\sum_{j=1}^{n_\theta} \underline{e}_i\underline{e}_j \left(\underline{H}^i_{\theta\theta}(n+1)\,\hat{P}(n+1|n)\underline{H}^j_{\theta\theta}(n+1)\,\hat{P}(n+1|n)\right)$$
$$+ R$$
$$K(n+1) = \hat{P}(n+1|n)\underline{J}_\theta(n+1)S^{-1}(n+1)$$
$$\underline{v}(n+1) = \underline{z}(n+1) - \underline{J}_\theta(n+1)\hat{\underline{\theta}}(n+1|n)$$
$$\hat{\underline{\theta}}(n+1|n+1) = \hat{\underline{\theta}}(n+1|n) + K(n+1)\underline{v}(n+1)$$
$$\hat{P}(n+1|n+1) = (I - K(n+1)\underline{J}_\theta(n+1))\,\hat{P}(n+1|n)\,(I - K(n+1)\underline{J}_\theta(n+1))'$$
$$+ K(n+1)\,R\,K(n+1)'$$

Here, $K(n+1)$ is the Kalman Gain matrix and $\underline{v}(n+1)$ is the innovation signal.

3 BLACK-SCHOLES MODEL

The Black-Scholes equation for calculating the price of an European style call option (Hull, 1993) is

$$C = S\,\mathcal{N}(d_1) - X\,e^{-r\,t_m}\,\mathcal{N}(d_2),$$

where,

$$d_1 = \frac{\ln(S/X) + (r + \frac{\sigma^2}{2})\sqrt{t_m}}{\sigma\sqrt{t_m}}$$
$$d_2 = d_1 - \sigma\sqrt{t_m}$$

Here, C is the price of the call option, S the underlying asset price, X the strike price of the option at maturity, t_m the time to maturity and r is the risk free interest rate. σ is a term known as volatility and may be seen as an instantaneous variance of the time variation of the asset price. $\mathcal{N}(.)$ is the cumulative normal function. For a derivation of the formula and the assumptions upon which it is based see Hull, 1993. Readers unfamiliar with financial terms only need to know that all the quantities in the above equation, except σ, can be directly observed. σ is usually estimated from a small moving window of data of about 50 trading days.

The equivalent formula for the price of a put option is given by

$$P = -S\,\mathcal{N}(-d_1) + X\,e^{-r\,t_m}\,\mathcal{N}(-d_2),$$

For recursive estimation of the option prices with this model, I assume that the instantaneous picture given by the Black Scholes model is correct. The state vector is two dimensional and consists of the volatility σ and the interest rate r. The Jacobian and Hessian required for applying EKF algorithm are

$$\underline{J}_\theta = \begin{pmatrix} \frac{\partial C}{\partial \sigma} & \frac{\partial C}{\partial r} \\ \frac{\partial P}{\partial \sigma} & \frac{\partial P}{\partial r} \end{pmatrix} ;\ \underline{H}^1_{\theta\theta} = \begin{pmatrix} \frac{\partial^2 C}{\partial \sigma^2} & \frac{\partial^2 C}{\partial \sigma \partial r} \\ \frac{\partial^2 C}{\partial \sigma \partial r} & \frac{\partial^2 C}{\partial r^2} \end{pmatrix} ;\ \underline{H}^2_{\theta\theta} = \begin{pmatrix} \frac{\partial^2 P}{\partial \sigma^2} & \frac{\partial^2 P}{\partial \sigma \partial r} \\ \frac{\partial^2 P}{\partial \sigma \partial r} & \frac{\partial^2 P}{\partial r^2} \end{pmatrix}$$

Expressions for the terms in these matrices are given in table 1.

Table 1: First and Second Derivatives of the Black Scholes Model

$\frac{\partial C}{\partial \sigma} = \frac{\partial P}{\partial \sigma}$		$S\sqrt{t_m}\,\mathcal{N}'(d_1)$
$\frac{\partial C}{\partial r}$		$Xt_m\exp(-rt_m)\mathcal{N}(d_2)$
$\frac{\partial P}{\partial r}$		$-Xt_m\exp(-rt_m)\mathcal{N}(-d_2)$
$\frac{\partial^2 C}{\partial \sigma^2} = \frac{\partial^2 P}{\partial \sigma^2}$		$\frac{S\sqrt{t_m}\,d_1 d_2}{\sigma}\mathcal{N}'(d_1)$
$\frac{\partial^2 C}{\partial r^2}$		$-Xt_m\exp(-rt_m)\left(t_m\mathcal{N}(d_2) - \frac{d_2\sqrt{t_m}}{\sigma}\mathcal{N}'(d_2)\right)$
$\frac{\partial^2 P}{\partial r^2}$		$Xt_m\exp(-rt_m)\left(t_m\mathcal{N}(-d_2) - \frac{d_2\sqrt{t_m}}{\sigma}\mathcal{N}'(-d_2)\right)$
$\frac{\partial^2 C}{\partial \sigma \partial r} = \frac{\partial^2 P}{\partial \sigma \partial r}$		$\frac{-Sd_1 t_m}{\sigma}\mathcal{N}'(d_1)$

4 NEURAL NETWORK MODELS

The data driven neural network model considered here is the Radial Basis Functions Network (RBF). Following Hutchinson et al, I use the following architecture:

$$\hat{C}/X = \sum_{j=1}^{m} \lambda_j \, \phi\left(\left(\underline{U} - \underline{\mu}_j\right)^t \Sigma^{-1} \left(\underline{U} - \underline{\mu}_j\right)\right) + \underline{W}^t \underline{Y} + w_0$$

where $\underline{U}$ is the two dimensional input data vector consisting of the asset price and time to maturity. The asset price S is normalised by the strike price of the option X. The time to maturity, t_m, is also normalised such that the full lifetime of the option gets a value 1.0. These normalisations is the reason for considering options in pairs with the same strike price and time of maturity in this study. The nonlinear function $\phi(.)$ is set to $\phi(\alpha) = \sqrt{\alpha}$ and $m = 4$. With the nonlinear part of the network fixed, Kalman filter training of the RBF model is straightforward (see Kadirkamanathan & Niranjan, 1993). In the simulations studied in this paper, I used two approaches to fix the nonlinear functions. The first was to use the $\underline{\mu}_j$s and the Σ published in Hutchinson et al. The second was to select the $\underline{\mu}_j$ terms as random subsets of the training data and set Σ to I. The estimation problem is now linear and hence the Kalman filter equations become much simpler than the EKF equations used in the training of the Black-Scholes model.

In addition to training by EKF, I also implemented a batch training of the RBF model in which a moving window of data was used, training on data from $(n - 50)$ to n days and testing on day $(n+1)$. Since it is natural to assume that data closer to the test day is more appropriate than data far back in time, I incorporated a weighting function to weight the errors linearly, in the minimisation process. The least squares solution, with a weighting function, is given by the modified pseudo

Table 2: Comparison of the Approximation Errors for Different Methods

Strike Price	Trivial	RBF Batch	RBF Kalman	BS Historic	BS Kalman
2925	0.0790	0.0632	0.0173	0.0845	0.0180
3025	0.0999	0.1109	0.0519	0.1628	0.0440
3125	0.0764	0.0455	0.0193	0.0343	0.0112
3225	0.1116	0.0819	0.0595	0.0885	0.0349

inverse

$$\underline{l} = (Y' W Y)^{-1} Y' W \underline{t}$$

Matrix W is a diagonal matrix, consisting of the weighting function in its diagonal elements, $\underline{t}$ is the target values of options prices, and $\underline{l}$ is the vector containing the unknown coefficients $\lambda_1, ..., \lambda_m$. The elements of Y are given by $y_{ij} = \phi_j(\underline{U}_i)$, with $j = 1, ..., m$ and $i = n - 50, ..., n$.

5 SIMULATIONS

The data set for teh experiments consisted of call and put option contracts on the FTSE-100 Index, during the period February 1994 to December 1994. The date of maturity of all contracts was December 1994. Five pairs (Call and Put) of contracts at strike prices of 2925, 3025, 3125, 3225, and 3325.

The tracking behaviour of the EKF for one of the pairs is shown in Fig. 1 for a call/put pair with strike price 3125. Fig. 2 shows the trajectories of the underlying state vector for four different call/put option pairs. Table 2 shows the squared errors in the approximation errors computed over the last 100 days of data (allowing for an initial period of convergence of the recursive algorithms).

6 DISCUSSION

This paper presents a sequential approach to tracking the price of options contracts. The sequential approach is based on the Extended Kalman Filter algorithm, and I show how it may be used to identify a parametric model of the underlying nonlinear system. The model based approach of the finance community and the data driven approach of neural computing community lead to good estimates of the observed price of the options contracts when estimated in this manner.

In the state space formulation of the Black-Scholes model, the volatility and interest rate are estimated from the data. I trust the instantaneous picture presented by the model based approach, but reestimate the underlying parameters. This is different from conventional wisdom, where the risk free interest rate is set to some figure observed in the bond markets. The value of volatility that gives the correct options price through Black Scholes equation is called option implied volatility, and is usually different for different options. Option traders often use the differences in implied volatility to take trading positions. In the formulation presented here, there is an extra freedom coming in the form what one might call *implied interest rates*. It's difference from the interest rates observed in the markets might explain trader speculation about risk associated with a particular currency.

The derivatives of the RBF model output with respect to its inputs is easy to compute. Hutchinson *et al* use this to define a highly relevant performance measure

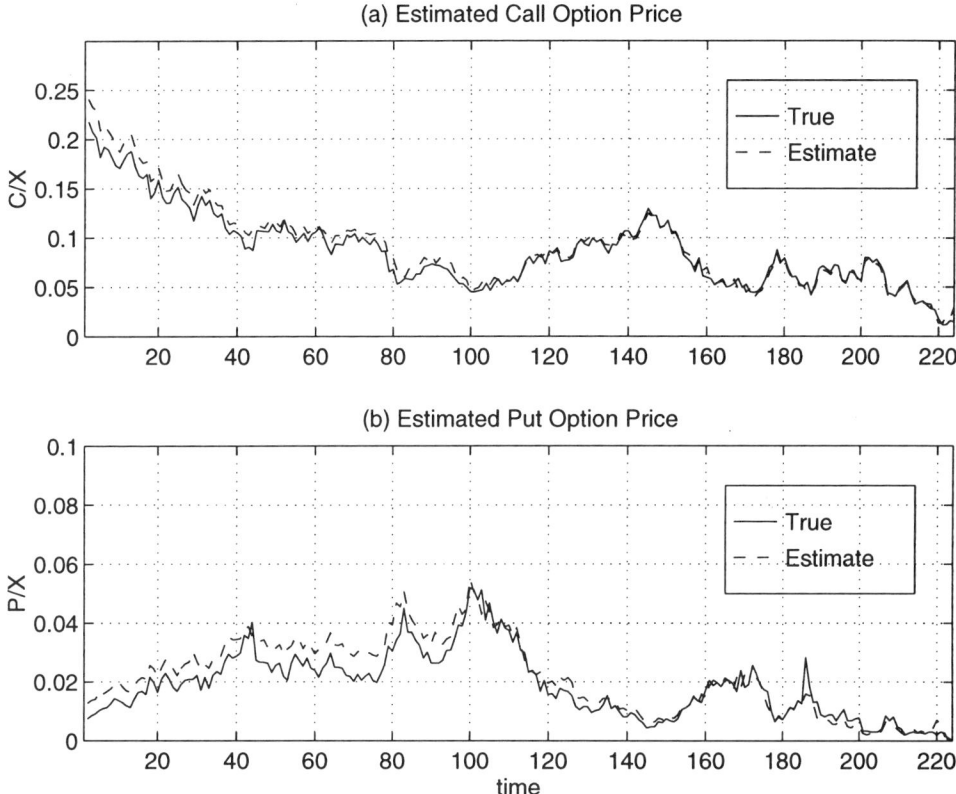

Figure 1: Tracking Black-Scholes Model with EKF; Estimates of Call and Put Prices

suitable to this particular application, namely the tracking error of a delta neutral portfolio. This is an evaluation that is somewhat unfair to the RBF model since at the time of training, the network is not shown the derivatives. An interesting combination of the work presented in this paper and Hutchinson et al's performance measure is to train the neural network to approximate the observed option prices and simultaneously force the derivative network to approximate the delta observed in the markets.

References

Bar-Shalom, Y. & Li, X-R. (1993), 'Estimation and Tracking: Principles, Techniques and Software', Artech House, London.

Candy, J. V. (1986), 'Signal Processing: The Model Based Aproach', McGraw-Hill, New York.

Hull, J. (1993), 'Options, Futures and Other Derivative Securities', Prentice Hall, NJ.

Hutchinson, J. M., Lo, A. W. & Poggio, T. (1994), 'A Nonparametric Approach to Pricing and Hedging Derivative Securities Via Learning Networks', The Journal of Finance, Vol XLIX, No. 3., 851-889.

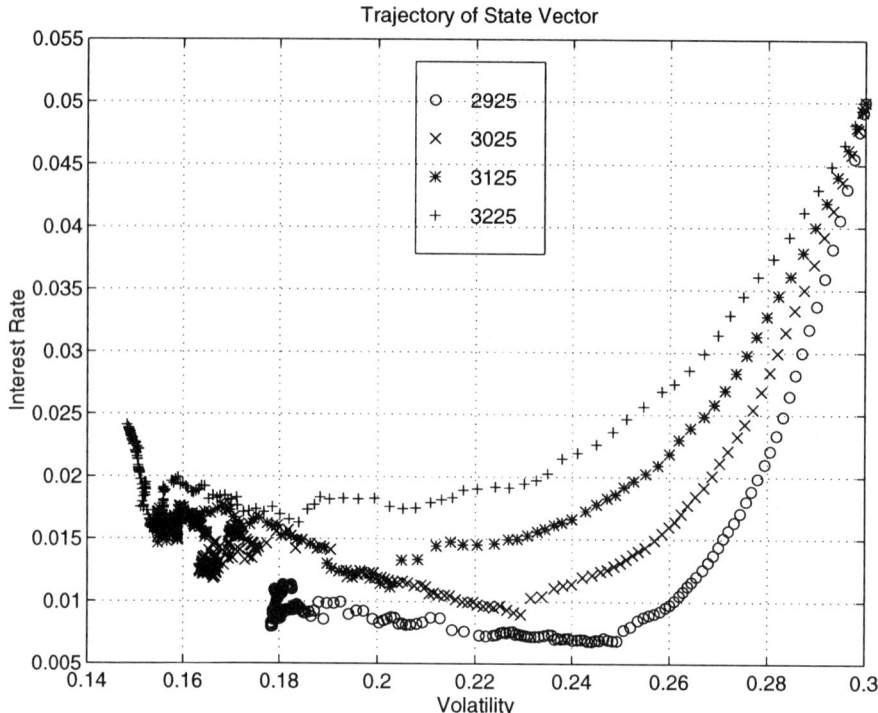

Figure 2: Tracking Black-Scholes Model with EKF; Estimates of Call and Put Prices and the Trajectory of the State Vector

Kadirkamanathan, V. & Niranjan, M (1993), 'A Function Estimation Approach to Sequential Learning with Neural Networks', *Neural Computation* **5**, pp. 954-975.

Lowe, D. (1995), 'On the use of Nonlocal and Non Positive Definite Basis Functions in Radial Basis Function Networks', Proceedings of the IEE Conference on Artificial Neural Networks, IEE Conference Publication No. 409, pp 206-211.

Niranjan, M., Cox, I. J., Hingorani, S. (1994), 'Recursive Estimation of Formants in Speech', Proceedings of the International Conference on Acoustics, Speech and Signal Processing, ICASSP '94, Adelaide.

Puskorius, G.V. & Feldkamp, L.A. (1994), 'Neurocontrol of Nonlinear Dynamical Systems with Kalman Filter-Trained Recurrent Networks', IEEE Transactions on Neural Networks, 5 (2), pp 279-297.

A comparison between neural networks and other statistical techniques for modeling the relationship between tobacco and alcohol and cancer

Tony Plate
BC Cancer Agency
601 West 10th Ave, Epidemiology
Vancouver BC Canada V5Z 1L3
tap@comp.vuw.ac.nz

Pierre Band
BC Cancer Agency
601 West 10th Ave, Epidemiology
Vancouver BC Canada V5Z 1L3

Joel Bert
Dept of Chemical Engineering
University of British Columbia
2216 Main Mall
Vancouver BC Canada V6T 1Z4

John Grace
Dept of Chemical Engineering
University of British Columbia
2216 Main Mall
Vancouver BC Canada V6T 1Z4

Abstract

Epidemiological data is traditionally analyzed with very simple techniques. Flexible models, such as neural networks, have the potential to discover unanticipated features in the data. However, to be useful, flexible models must have effective control on overfitting. This paper reports on a comparative study of the predictive quality of neural networks and other flexible models applied to real and artificial epidemiological data. The results suggest that there are no major unanticipated complex features in the real data, and also demonstrate that MacKay's [1995] Bayesian neural network methodology provides effective control on overfitting while retaining the ability to discover complex features in the artificial data.

1 Introduction

Traditionally, very simple statistical techniques are used in the analysis of epidemiological studies. The predominant technique is logistic regression, in which the effects of predictors are linear (or categorical) and additive on the log-odds scale. An important virtue of logistic regression is that the relationships identified in the data can be interpreted and explained in simple terms, such as "the odds of developing lung cancer for males who smoke between 20 and 29 cigarettes per day are increased by a factor of 11.5 over males who do not smoke". However, because of their simplicity, it is difficult to use these models to discover unanticipated complex relationships, i.e., non-linearities in the effect of a predictor or interactions between predictors. Interactions and non-linearities can of course be introduced into logistic regressions, but must be pre-specified, which tends to be impractical unless there are only a few variables or there are a priori reasons to test for particular effects.

Neural networks have the potential to automatically discover complex relationships. There has been much interest in using neural networks in biomedical applications; witness the recent series of articles in *The Lancet*, e.g., Wyatt [1995] and Baxt [1995]. However, there are not yet sufficient comparisons or theory to come to firm conclusions about the utility of neural networks in biomedical data analysis. To date, comparison studies, e.g, those by Michie, Spiegelhalter, and Taylor [1994], Burke, Rosen, and Goodman [1995], and Lippmann, Lee, and Shahian [1995], have had mixed results, and Jefferson et al's [1995] complaint that many "successful" applications of neural networks are not compared against standard techniques appears to be justified. The intent of this paper is to contribute to the body of useful comparisons by reporting a study of various neural-network and statistical modeling techniques applied to an epidemiological data analysis problem.

2 The data

The original data set consisted of information on 15,463 subjects from a study conducted by the Division of Epidemiology and Cancer Prevention at the BC Cancer Agency. In this study, detailed questionnaire reported personal information, lifetime tobacco and alcohol use, and lifetime employment history for each subject. The subjects were cancer patients in BC with diagnosis dates between 1983 and 1989, as ascertained by the population-based registry at the BC Cancer Agency. Six different tobacco and alcohol habits were included: cigarette (C), cigar (G), and pipe (P) smoking, and beer (B), wine (W), and spirit drinking (S). The models reported in this paper used up to 27 predictor variables: age at first diagnosis (AGE), and 26 variables related to alcohol and tobacco consumption. These included four variables for each habit: total years of consumption (CYR etc), consumption per day or week (CDAY, BWK etc), years since quitting (CYQUIT etc), and a binary variable indicating any indulgence (CSMOKE, BDRINK etc). The remaining two binary variables indicated whether the subject ever smoked tobacco or drank alcohol. All the binary variables were non-linear (threshold) transforms of the other variables. Variables not applicable to a particular subject were zero, e.g., number of years of smoking for a non-smoker, or years since quitting for a smoker who did not quit.

Of the 15,463 records, 5901 had missing information in some of the fields related to tobacco or alcohol use. These were not used, as there are no simple methods for dealing with missing data in neural networks. Of the 9,562 complete records, a randomly selected 3,195 were set aside for testing, leaving 6,367 complete records to be used in the modeling experiments.

There were 28 binary outcomes: the 28 sites at which a subject could have cancer (subjects had cancers at up to 3 different sites). The number of cases for each site varied, e.g., for LUNGSQ (Lung Squamous) there were 694 cases among the complete records, for ORAL (Oral Cavity and Pharynx) 306, and for MEL (Melanoma) 464.

All sites were modeled individually using carefully selected subjects as controls. This is common practice in cancer epidemiology studies, due to the difficulty of collecting an unbiased sample of non-cancer subjects for controls. Subjects with cancers at a site suspected of being related to tobacco usage were not used as controls. This eliminated subjects with any sites other than COLON, RECTUM, MEL (Melanoma), NMSK (Non-melanoma skin), PROS (Prostate), NHL (Non-Hodgkin's lymphoma), and MMY (Multiple-Myeloma), and resulted in between 2959 and 3694 controls for each site. For example, the model for LUNGSQ (lung squamous cell) cancer was fitted using subjects with LUNGSQ as the positive outcomes (694 cases), and subjects all of whose sites were among COLON, RECTUM, MEL, NMSK, PROS, NHL, or MMY as negative outcomes (3694 controls).

3 Statistical methods

A number of different types of statistical methods were used to model the data. These ranged from the non-flexible (logistic regression) through partially flexible (Generalized Additive Models or GAMs) to completely flexible (classification trees and neural networks). Each site was modeled independently, using the log likelihood of the data under the binomial distribution as the fitting criterion. All of the modeling, except for the neural networks and ridge regression, was done using the the S-plus statistical software package [StatSci 1995].

For several methods, we used Breiman's [1996] *bagging* technique to control overfitting. To "bag" a model, one fits a set of models independently on bootstrap samples. The bagged prediction is then the average of the predictions of the models in the set. Breiman suggests that bagging will give superior predictions for unstable models (such as stepwise selection, pruned trees, and neural networks).

Preliminary analysis revealed that the predictive power of non-flexible models could be improved by including non-linear transforms of some variables, namely AGESQ and the binary indicator variables SMOKE, DRINK, CSMOKE, etc. Flexible models should be able to discover useful non-linear transforms for themselves and so these derived variables were not included in the flexible models. In order to allow comparisons to test this, one of non-flexible models (ONLYLIN-STEP) also did not use any of these derived variables.

Null model: (NULL) The predictions of the null model are just the frequency of the outcome in the training set.

Logistic regression: The FULL model used the full set of predictor variables, including a quadratic term for age: AGESQ.

Stepwise logistic regression: A number of stepwise regressions were fitted, differing in the set of variables considered. Outcome-balanced 10-fold cross validation was used to select the model size giving best generalization. The models were as follows: AGE-STEP (AGE and AGESQ); CYR-AGE-STEP (CYR, AGE and AGESQ); ALC-CYR-AGE-STEP (all alcohol variables, CYR, AGE and AGESQ); FULL-STEP (all variables including AGESQ); and ONLYLIN-STEP (all variables except for the derived binary indicator variables SMOKE, CSMOKE, etc, and only a linear AGE term).

Ridge regression: (RIDGE) Ridge regression penalizes a logistic regression model by the sum of the squared parameter values in order to control overfitting. The evidence framework [MacKay 1995] was used to select seven shrinkage parameters: one for each of the six habits, and one for SMOKE, DRINK, AGE and AGESQ.

Generalized Additive Models: GAMs [Hastie and Tibshirani 1990] fit a smoothing spline to each parameter. GAMs can model non-linearities, but not interactions. A stepwise procedure was used to select the degree (0,1,2, or 4) of the smoothing spline for each parameter. The procedure started with a model having a smoothing spline of degree 2 for each parameter, and stopped when the AIC statistic could not reduced any further. Two stepwise GAM models were fitted: GAM-FULL used the full set of variables, while GAM-CIG used the cigarette variables and AGE.

Classification trees: [Breiman et al. 1984] The same cross-validation procedure as used with stepwise regression was used to select the best size for TREE, using the implementation in S-plus, and the function shrink.tree() for pruning. A bagged version with 50 replications, TREE-BAGGED, was also used. After constructing a tree for the data in a replication, it was pruned to perform optimally on the training data not included in that replication.

Ordinary neural networks: The neural network models had a single hidden layer of tanh functions and a small weight penalty (0.01) to prevent parameters going to infinity. A conjugate-gradient procedure was used to optimize weights. For the NN-ORD-H2 model, which had no control on complexity, a network with two hidden units was trained three times from different small random starting weights. Of these three, the one with best performance on the training data was selected as "the model". The NN-ORD-HCV used common method for controlling overfitting in neural networks: 10-fold CV for selecting the optimal number of hidden units. Three random starting points for each partition were used calculate the average generalization error for networks with one, two and three hidden units Three networks with the best number of hidden units were trained on the entire set of training data, and the network having the lowest training error was chosen.

Bagged neural networks with early stopping: Bagging and early stopping (terminating training before reaching a minimum on training set error in order to prevent overfitting) work naturally together. The training examples omitted from each bootstrap replication provide a validation set to decide when to stop, and with early stopping, training is fast enough to make bagging practical. 100 networks with two hidden units were trained on separate bootstrap replications, and the best 50 (by their performance on the omitted examples) were included in the final bagged model, NN-ESTOP-BAGGED. For comparison purposes, the mean individual performance of these early-stopped networks is reported as NN-ESTOP-AVG.

Neural networks with Bayesian regularization: MacKay's [1995] Bayesian evidence framework was used to control overfitting in neural networks. Three random starts for networks with 1, 2, 3 or 4 hidden units and three different sets of regularization (penalty) parameters were used, giving a total of 36 networks for each site. The three possibilities for regularization parameters were: (a) three penalty parameters – one for each of input to hidden, bias to hidden, and hidden to output; (b) partial Automatic Relevance Determination (ARD) [MacKay 1995] with seven penalty parameters controlling the input to hidden weights – one for each habit and one for AGE; and (c) full ARD, with one penalty parameter for each of the 19 inputs. The "evidence" for each network was evaluated and the best 18 networks were selected for the equally-weighted committee model NN-BAYES-CMTT. NN-BAYES-BEST was the single network with the maximum evidence.

4 Results and Discussion

Models were compared based on their performance on the held-out test data, so as to avoid overfitting bias in evaluation. While there are several ways to measure performance, e.g., 0-1 classification error, or area under the ROC curve (as in Burke, Rosen and Goodman [1995]), we used the test-set deviance as it seems appropriate to compare models using the same criterion as was used for fitting. Reporting performance is complicated by the fact that there were 28 different modeling tasks (i.e., sites), and some models did better on some sites and worse on others. We report some overall performance figures and some pairwise comparisons of models.

Neural Networks in Cancer Epidemiology

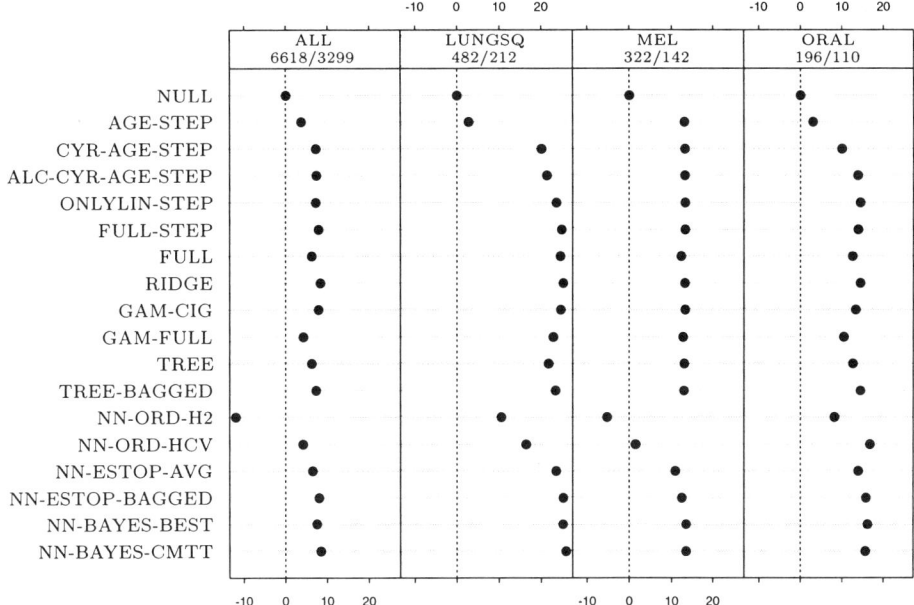

Figure 1: Percent improvement in deviance on test data over the null model.

Figure 1 shows aggregate deviances across sites (i.e., the sum of the test deviance for one model over the 28 sites) and deviances for selected sites. The horizontal scale in each column indicates the percentage reduction in deviance over the null model. Zero percent (the dotted line) is the same performance as the null model, and 100% would be perfect predictions. Numbers below the column labels are the number of positive outcomes in the training and test sets, respectively. The best predictions for LUNGSQ can reduce the null deviance by just over 25%. It is interesting to note that much of the information is contained in AGE and CYR: The CYR-AGE-STEP model achieved a 7.1% reduction in overall deviance, while the maximum reduction (achieved by NN-BAYES-CMTT) was only 8.3%.

There is no single threshold at which differences in test-set deviance are "significant", because of strong correlations between predictions of different models. However, the general patterns of superiority apparent in Figure 1 were repeated across the other sites, and various other tests indicate they are reliable indicators of general performance. For example, the best five models, both in terms of aggregate deviance across all sites and median rank of performance on individual sites, were, in order NN-BAYES-CMTT, RIDGE, NN-ESTOP-BAGGED, GAM-CIG, and FULL-STEP. The ONLYLIN-STEP model ranked sixth in median rank, and tenth in aggregate deviance.

Although the differences between the best flexible models and the logistic models were slight, they were consistent. For example, NN-BAYES-CMTT did better than FULL-STEP on 21 sites, and better than ONLYLIN-STEP on 23 sites, while FULL-STEP drew with ONLYLIN-STEP on 14 sites and did better on 9. If the models had no effective difference, there was only a 1.25%. chance of one model doing better than the other 21 or more times out of 28. Individual measures of performance were also consistent with these findings. For example, for LUNGSQ a bootstrap test of test-set deviance revealed that the predictions of NN-BAYES-CMTT were on average better than those of ONLYLIN-STEP in 99.82% of resampled test sets (out of 10,000), while the predictions of NN-BAYES-CMTT beat FULL-STEP in 93.75% of replications and FULL-STEP beat ONLYLIN-STEP in 98.48% of replications.

These results demonstrate that good control on overfitting is essential for this task. Ordinary neural networks with no control on overfitting do worse than guessing (i.e., the null model). Even when the number of hidden units is chosen by cross-validation, the performance is still worse than a simple two-variable stepwise logistic regression (CYR-AGE-STEP). The inadequacy of the simple AIC-based stepwise procedure for choosing the complexity of GAMs is illustrated by the poor performance of the GAM-FULL model (the more restricted GAM-CIG model does quite well).

The effective methods for controlling overfitting were bagging and Bayesian regularization. Bagging improved the performance of trees and early-stopped neural networks to good levels. Bayesian regularization worked very well with neural networks and with ridge regression. Furthermore, examination of the performance of individual networks indicates that networks with fine-grained ARD were frequently superior to those with coarser control on regularization.

5 Artificial sites with complex relationships

The very minor improvement achieved by neural networks and trees over logistic models provokes the following question: are complex relationships are really relatively unimportant in this data, or is the strong control on overfitting preventing identification of complex relationships? In order to answer this question, we created six artificial "sites" for the subjects. These were designed to have very similar properties to the real sites, while possessing non-linear effects and interactions.

The risk models for the artificial sites possessed a underlying trend equal to half that of a good logistic model for LUNGSQ, and one of three more complex effects: FREQ, a frequent non-linear (threshold) effect (BWK > 1) affecting 4,334 of the 9,562 subjects; RARE, a rare threshold effect (BWK > 10), affecting 1,550 subjects; and INTER, an interaction (BYR · GYR) affecting 482 subjects. For three of the artificial sites the complex effect was weak (LO), and for the other three it was strong (HI). For each subject and each artificial site, a random choice as to whether that subject was a positive case for that site was made, based on probability given by the model for the artificial site. Models were fitted to these sites in the same way as to other sites and only subjects without cancer at a smoking related site were used as controls.

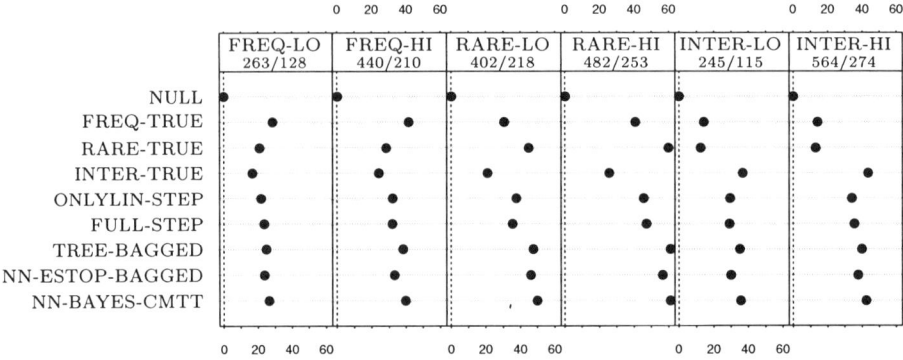

Figure 2: Percent improvement in deviance on test data for the artificial sites.

For comparison purposes, logistic models containing the true set of variables, including non-linearities and interactions, were fitted to the artificial data. For example, the model RARE-TRUE contained the continuous variables AGE, AGESQ, CDAY, CYR, and CYQUIT, and the binary variables SMOKE and BWK> 10.

Figure 2 shows performance on the artificial data. The neural networks and bagged trees were very effective at detecting non-linearities and interactions. Their performance was at the same level as the appropriate true models, while the performance of simple models lacking the ability to fit the complexities (e.g., FULL-STEP) was considerably worse.

6 Conclusions

For predicting the risk of cancer in our data, neural networks with Bayesian estimation of regularization parameters to control overfitting performed consistently but only slightly better than logistic regression models. This appeared to be due to the lack of complex relationships in the data: on artificial data with complex relationships they performed markedly better than logistic models. Good control of overfitting is essential for this task, as shown by the poor performance of neural networks with the number of hidden units chosen by cross-validation.

Given their ability to not overfit while still identifying complex relationships we expect that neural networks could prove useful in epidemiological data-analysis by providing a method for checking that a simple statistical model is not missing important complex relationships.

Acknowledgments

This research was funded by grants from the Workers Compensation Board of British Columbia, NSERC, and IRIS, and conducted at the BC Cancer Agency.

References

Baxt, W. G. 1995. Application of artificial neural networks to clinical medicine. *The Lancet*, 346:1135–1138.

Breiman, L. 1996. Bagging predictors. *Machine Learning*, 26(2):123–140.

Breiman, L., Friedman, J., Olshen, R., and Stone, C. 1984. *Classification and Regression Trees*. Wadsworth, Belmont, CA.

Burke, H., Rosen, D., and Goodman, P. 1995. Comparing the prediction accuracy of artificial neural networks and other statistical methods for breast cancer survival. In Tesauro, G., Touretzky, D. S., and Leen, T. K., editors, *Advances in Neural Information Processing Systems 7*, pages 1063–1067, Cambridge, MA. MIT Press.

Hastie, T. J. and Tibshirani, R. J. 1990. *Generalized additive models*. Chapman and Hall, London.

Jefferson, M. F., Pendleton, N., Lucas, S., and Horan, M. A. 1995. Neural networks (letter). *The Lancet*, 346:1712.

Lippmann, R., Lee, Y., and Shahian, D. 1995. Predicting the risk of complications in coronary artery bypass operations using neural networks. In Tesauro, G., Touretzky, D. S., and Leen, T. K., editors, *Advances in Neural Information Processing Systems 7*, pages 1055–1062, Cambridge, MA. MIT Press.

MacKay, D. J. C. 1995. Probable networks and plausible predictions - a review of practical Bayesian methods for supervised neural networks. *Network: Computation in Neural Systems*, 6:469–505.

Michie, D., Spiegelhalter, D., and Taylor, C. 1994. *Machine Learning, Neural and Statistical Classification*. Ellis Horwood, Hertfordshire, UK.

StatSci 1995. *S-Plus Guide to Statistical and Mathematical Analyses, Version 3.3*. StatSci, a division of MathSoft, Inc, Seattle.

Wyatt, J. 1995. Nervous about artificial neural networks? (commentary). *The Lancet*, 346:1175–1177.

Reinforcement Learning for Dynamic Channel Allocation in Cellular Telephone Systems

Satinder Singh
Department of Computer Science
University of Colorado
Boulder, CO 80309-0430
baveja@cs.colorado.edu

Dimitri Bertsekas
Lab. for Info. and Decision Sciences
MIT
Cambridge, MA 02139
bertsekas@lids.mit.edu

Abstract

In cellular telephone systems, an important problem is to dynamically allocate the communication resource (channels) so as to maximize service in a stochastic caller environment. This problem is naturally formulated as a dynamic programming problem and we use a reinforcement learning (RL) method to find dynamic channel allocation policies that are better than previous heuristic solutions. The policies obtained perform well for a broad variety of call traffic patterns. We present results on a large cellular system with approximately 49^{49} states.

In cellular communication systems, an important problem is to allocate the communication resource (bandwidth) so as to maximize the service provided to a set of mobile callers whose demand for service changes stochastically. A given geographical area is divided into mutually disjoint cells, and each cell serves the calls that are within its boundaries (see Figure 1a). The total system bandwidth is divided into channels, with each channel centered around a frequency. Each channel can be used simultaneously at different cells, provided these cells are sufficiently separated spatially, so that there is no interference between them. The minimum separation distance between simultaneous reuse of the same channel is called the *channel reuse constraint*.

When a call requests service in a given cell either a free channel (one that does not violate the channel reuse constraint) may be assigned to the call, or else the call is blocked from the system; this will happen if no free channel can be found. Also, when a mobile caller crosses from one cell to another, the call is "handed off" to the cell of entry; that is, a new free channel is provided to the call at the new cell. If no such channel is available, the call must be dropped/disconnected from the system.

One objective of a channel allocation policy is to allocate the available channels to calls so that the number of blocked calls is minimized. An additional objective is to minimize the number of calls that are dropped when they are handed off to a busy cell. These two objectives must be weighted appropriately to reflect their relative importance, since dropping existing calls is generally more undesirable than blocking new calls.

To illustrate the qualitative nature of the channel assignment decisions, suppose that there are only two channels and three cells arranged in a line. Assume a channel reuse constraint of 2, i.e., a channel may be used simultaneously in cells 1 and 3, but may not be used in channel 2 if it is already used in cell 1 or in cell 3. Suppose that the system is serving one call in cell 1 and another call in cell 3. Then serving both calls on the same channel results in a better channel usage pattern than serving them on different channels, since in the former case the other channel is free to be used in cell 2. The purpose of the channel assignment and channel rearrangement strategy is, roughly speaking, to create such favorable usage patterns that minimize the likelihood of calls being blocked.

We formulate the channel assignment problem as a dynamic programming problem, which, however, is too complex to be solved exactly. We introduce approximations based on the methodology of reinforcement learning (RL) (e.g., Barto, Bradtke and Singh, 1995, or the recent textbook by Bertsekas and Tsitsiklis, 1996). Our method learns channel allocation policies that outperform not only the most commonly used policy in cellular systems, but also the best heuristic policy we could find in the literature.

1 CHANNEL ASSIGNMENT POLICIES

Many cellular systems are based on a *fixed assignment* (FA) channel allocation; that is, the set of channels is partitioned, and the partitions are permanently assigned to cells so that all cells can use all the channels assigned to them simultaneously without interference (see Figure 1a). When a call arrives in a cell, if any pre-assigned channel is unused; it is assigned, else the call is blocked. No rearrangement is done when a call terminates. Such a policy is static and cannot take advantage of temporary stochastic variations in demand for service. More efficient are *dynamic channel allocation* policies, which assign channels to different cells, so that every channel is available to every cell on a need basis, unless the channel is used in a nearby cell and the reuse constraint is violated.

The best existing dynamic channel allocation policy we found in the literature is Borrowing with Directional Channel Locking (BDCL) of Zhang & Yum (1989). It numbers the channels from 1 to N, partitions and assigns them to cells as in FA. The channels assigned to a cell are its nominal channels. If a nominal channel is available when a call arrives in a cell, the smallest numbered such channel is assigned to the call. If no nominal channel is available, then the largest numbered free channel is borrowed from the neighbour with the most free channels. When a channel is borrowed, careful accounting of the directional effect of which cells can no longer use that channel because of interference is done. The call is blocked if there are no free channels at all. When a call terminates in a cell and the channel so freed is a nominal channel, say numbered i, of that cell, then if there is a call in that cell on a borrowed channel, the call on the smallest numbered borrowed channel is reassigned to i and the borrowed channel is returned to the appropriate cell. If there is no call on a borrowed channel, then if there is a call on a nominal channel numbered larger than i, the call on the highest numbered nominal channel is reassigned to i. If the call just terminated was itself on a borrowed channel, the call on the smallest numbered borrowed channel is reassigned to it and that channel is returned to the cell from which it was borrowed. Notice that when a borrowed channel is returned to its original cell, a nominal channel becomes free in that cell and triggers a reassignment. Thus, in the worst case a call termination in one cell can sequentially cause reassignments in arbitrarily far away cells — making BDCL somewhat impractical.

BDCL is quite sophisticated and combines the notions of channel-ordering, nominal channels, and channel borrowing. Zhang and Yum (1989) show that BDCL is superior to its competitors, including FA. Generally, BDCL has continued to be highly regarded in the literature as a powerful heuristic (Enrico et.al., 1996). In this paper, we compare the performance of dynamic channel allocation policies learned by RL with both FA and BDCL.

1.1 DYNAMIC PROGRAMMING FORMULATION

We can formulate the dynamic channel allocation problem using dynamic programming (e.g., Bertsekas, 1995). State transitions occur when channels become free due to call departures, or when a call arrives at a given cell and wishes to be assigned a channel, or when there is a handoff, which can be viewed as a simultaneous call departure from one cell and a call arrival at another cell. The state at each time consists of two components:

(1) The list of occupied and unoccupied channels at each cell. We call this the configuration of the cellular system. It is *exponential* in the number of cells.

(2) The event that causes the state transition (arrival, departure, or handoff). This component of the state is uncontrollable.

The decision/control applied at the time of a call departure is the rearrangement of the channels in use with the aim of creating a more favorable channel packing pattern among the cells (one that will leave more channels free for future assignments). Unlike BDCL, our RL solution will restrict this rearrangement to the cell with the current call departure. The control exercised at the time of a call arrival is the assignment of a free channel, or the blocking of the call if no free channel is currently available. In general, it may also be useful to do *admission control*, i.e., to allow the possibility of not accepting a new call even when there exists a free channel to minimize the dropping of ongoing calls during handoff in the future. We address admission control in a separate paper and here restrict ourselves to always accepting a call if a free channel is available. The objective is to learn a policy that assigns decisions (assignment or rearrangement depending on event) to each state so as to *maximize*

$$J = E\left\{\int_0^\infty e^{-\beta t} c(t) dt\right\},$$

where $E\{\cdot\}$ is the expectation operator, $c(t)$ is the number of ongoing calls at time t, and β is a discount factor that makes immediate profit more valuable than future profit. Maximizing J is equivalent to minimizing the expected (discounted) number of blocked calls over an infinite horizon.

2 REINFORCEMENT LEARNING SOLUTION

RL methods solve optimal control (or dynamic programming) problems by learning good approximations to the optimal value function, J^*, given by the solution to the Bellman optimality equation which takes the following form for the dynamic channel allocation problem:

$$J(x) = E_e \left\{ \max_{a \in A(x,e)} [E_{\Delta t}\{c(x, a, \Delta t) + \gamma(\Delta t)J(y)\}] \right\}, \tag{1}$$

where x is a configuration, e is the random event (a call arrival or departure), $A(x, e)$ is the set of actions available in the current state (x, e), Δt is the random time until the next event, $c(x, a, \Delta t)$ is the effective immediate payoff with the discounting, and $\gamma(\Delta t)$ is the effective discount for the next configuration y.

RL learns approximations to J^* using Sutton's (1988) temporal difference (TD(0)) algorithm. A fixed feature extractor is used to form an approximate compact representation of the exponential configuration of the cellular array. This approximate representation forms the input to a function approximator (see Figure 1) that learns/stores estimates of J^*. No partitioning of channels is done; all channels are available in each cell. On each event, the estimates of J^* are used both to make decisions and to update the estimates themselves as follows:

Call Arrival: When a call arrives, evaluate the next configuration for each free channel and assign the channel that leads to the configuration with the largest estimated value. If there is no free channel at all, no decision has to be made.

Call Termination: When a call terminates, one by one each ongoing call in that cell is considered for reassignment to the just freed channel; the resulting configurations are evaluated and compared to the value of not doing any reassignment at all. The action that leads to the highest value configuration is then executed.

On call arrival, as long as there is a free channel, the number of ongoing calls and the time to next event do not depend on the free channel assigned. Similarly, the number of ongoing calls and the time to next event do not depend on the rearrangement done on call departure. Therefore, both the sample immediate payoff which depends on the number of ongoing calls and the time to next event, and the effective discount factor which depends only on the time to next event are independent of the choice of action. Thus one can choose the current best action by simply considering the estimated values of the next configurations. The next configuration for each action is deterministic and trivial to compute.

When the next random event occurs, the sample payoff and the discount factor become available and are used to update the value function as follows: on a transition from configuration x to y on action a in time Δt,

$$J_{new}(\tilde{x}) = (1 - \alpha)J_{old}(\tilde{x}) + \alpha \left(c(x, a, \Delta t) + \gamma(\Delta t)J_{old}(\tilde{y}) \right) \tag{2}$$

where $\tilde{x}$ is used to indicate the approximate feature-based representation of x. The parameters of the function approximator are then updated to best represent $J_{new}(\tilde{x})$ using gradient descent in mean-squared error $(J_{new}(\tilde{x}) - J_{old}(\tilde{x}))^2$.

3 SIMULATION RESULTS

Call arrivals are modeled as Poisson processes with a separate mean for each cell, and call durations are modeled with an exponential distribution. The first set of results are on the 7 by 7 cellular array of Figure ??a with 70 channels (roughly 70^{49} configurations) and a channel reuse constraint of 3 (this problem is borrowed from Zhang and Yum's (1989) paper on an empirical comparison of BDCL and its competitors). Figures 2a, b & c are for uniform call arrival rates of 150, 200, and 350 calls/hr respectively in each cell. The mean call duration for all the experiments reported here is 3 minutes. Figure 2d is for non-uniform call arrival rates. Each curve plots the cumulative empirical blocking probability as a function of simulated time. Each data point is therefore the percentage of system-wide calls that were blocked up until that point in time. All simulations start with no ongoing calls.

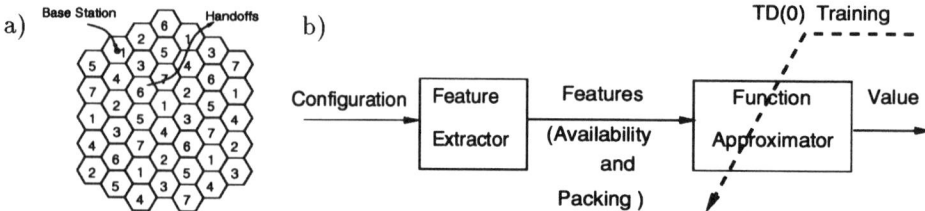

Figure 1: a) Cellular Array. The market area is divided up into cells, shown here as hexagons. The available bandwidth is divided into channels. Each cell has a base station responsible for calls within its area. Calls arrive randomly, have random durations and callers may move around in the market area creating handoffs. The channel reuse constraint requires that there be a minimum distance between simultaneous reuse of the same channel. In a fixed assignment channel allocation policy (assuming a channel reuse constraint of 3), the channels are partitioned into 7 lots labeled 1 to 7 and assigned to the cells in the compact pattern shown here. Note that the minimum distance between cells with the same number is at least three. b) A block diagram of the RL system. The exponential configuration is mapped into a feature-based approximate representation which forms the input to a function approximation system that learns values for configurations. The parameters of the function approximator are trained using gradient descent on the squared TD(0) error in value function estimates (c.f. Equation 2).

The RL system uses a linear neural network and two sets of features as input: one availability feature for each cell and one packing feature for each cell-channel pair. The availability feature for a cell is the number of free channels in that cell, while the packing feature for a cell-channel pair is the number of times that channel is used in a 4 cell radius. Other packing features were tried but are not reported because they were insignificant. The RL curves in Figure 2 show the empirical blocking probability whilst learning. Note that learning is quite rapid. As the mean call arrival rate is increased the relative difference between the 3 algorithms decreases. In fact, FA can be shown to be optimal in the limit of infinite call arrival rates (see McEliece and Sivarajan, 1994). With so many customers in every cell there are no short-term fluctuations to exploit. However, as demonstrated in Figure 2, for practical traffic rates RL consistently gives a big win over FA and a smaller win over BDCL.

One difference between RL and BDCL is that while the BDCL policy is independent of call traffic, RL adapts its policy to the particulars of the call traffic it is trained on and should therefore be less sensitive to different patterns of non-uniformity of call traffic across cells. Figure 3b presents multiple sets of bar-graphs of asymptotic blocking probabilities for the three algorithms on a 20 by 1 cellular array with 24 channels and a channel reuse constraint of 3. For each set, the average per-cell call arrival rate is the same (120 calls/hr; mean duration of 3 minutes), but the pattern of call arrival rates across the 20 cells is varied. The patterns are shown on the left of the bar-graphs and are explained in the caption of Figure 3b. From Figure 3b it is apparent that RL is much less sensitive to varied patterns of non-uniformity than both BDCL and FA.

We have showed that RL with a linear function approximator is able to find better dynamic channel allocation policies than the BDCL and FA policies. Using nonlinear neural networks as function approximators for RL did in some cases improve

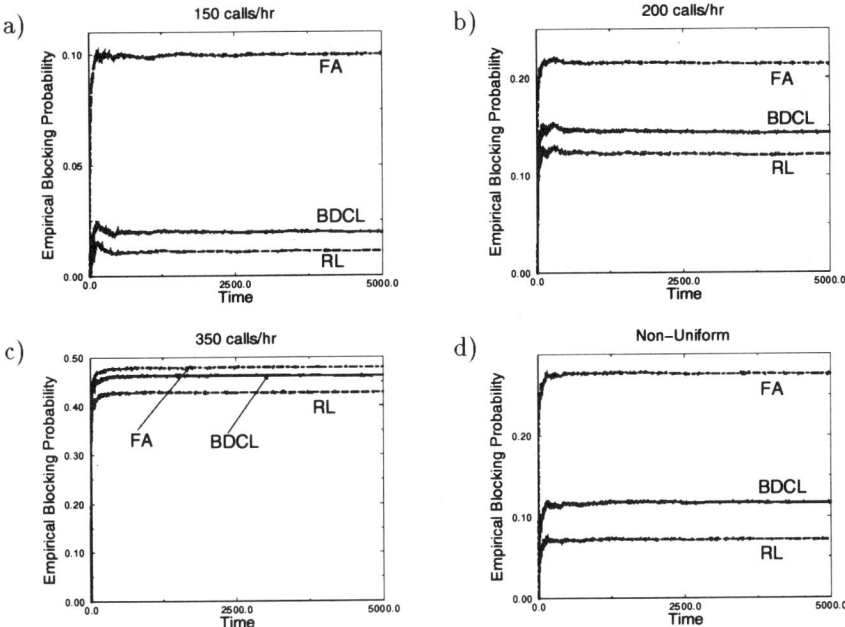

Figure 2: a), b), c) & d) These figures compare performance of RL, FA, and BDCL on the 7 by 7 cellular array of Figure 1a. The means of the call arrival (Poisson) processes are shown in the graph titles. Each curve presents the cumulative empirical blocking probability as a function of time elapsed in minutes. All simulations start with no ongoing calls and therefore the blocking probabilities are low in the early minutes of the performance curves. The RL curves presented here are for a linear function approximator and show performance while learning. Note that learning is quite rapid.

performance over linear networks by a small amount but at the cost of a big increase in training time. We chose to present results for linear networks because they have the advantage that even though training is centralized, the policy so learned is decentralized because the features are local and therefore just the weights from the local features in the trained linear network can be used to choose actions in each cell. For large cellular arrays, training itself could be decentralized because the choice of action in a particular cell has a minor effect on far away cells. We will explore the effect of decentralized training in future work.

4 CONCLUSION

The dynamic channel allocation problem is naturally formulated as an optimal control or dynamic programming problem, albeit one with very large state spaces. Traditional dynamic programming techniques are computationally infeasible for such large-scale problems. Therefore, knowledge-intensive heuristic solutions that ignore the optimal control framework have been developed. Recent approximations to dynamic programming introduced in the reinforcement learning (RL) community make it possible to go back to the channel assignment problem and solve it as an optimal control problem, in the process finding better solutions than previously available. We presented such a solution using Sutton's (1988) TD(0) with a feature-based linear network and demonstrated its superiority on a problem with approximately 70^{49} states. Other recent examples of similar successes are the game

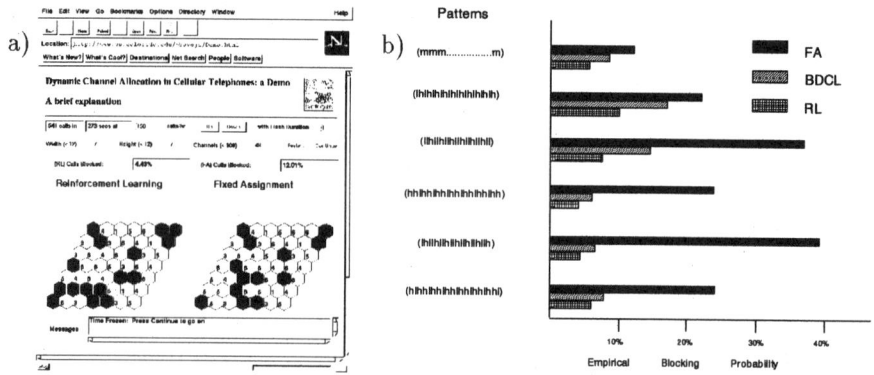

Figure 3: a) Screen dump of a Java Demonstration available publicly at http://www.cs.colorado.edu/~baveja/Demo.html b) Sensitivity of channel assignment methods to non-uniform traffic patterns. This figure plots asymptotic empirical blocking probability for RL, BDCL, and FA for a linear array of cells with different patterns (shown at left) of mean call arrival rates — chosen so that the average per cell call arrival rate is the same across patterns. The symbol l is for low, m for medium, and h for high. The numeric values of l, h, and m are chosen separately for each pattern to ensure that the average per cell rate of arrival is 120 calls/hr. The results show that RL is able to adapt its allocation strategy and thereby is better able to exploit the non-uniform call arrival rates.

of backgammon (Tesauro, 1992), elevator-scheduling (Crites & Barto, 1995), and job-shop scheduling (Zhang & Dietterich, 1995). The neuro-dynamic programming textbook (Bertsekas and Tsitsiklis, 1996) presents a variety of related case studies.

References

Barto, A.G., Bradtke, S.J. & Singh, S. (1995) Learning to act using real-time dynamic programming. *Artificial Intelligence*, 72:81–138.

Bertsekas, D.P. (1995) *Dynamic Programming and Optimal Control: Vols 1 and 2.* Athena-Scientific, Belmont, MA.

Bertsekas, D.P. & Tsitsiklis, J. (1996) *Neuro-Dynamic Programming* Athena-Scientific, Belmont, MA.

Crites, R.H. & Barto, A.G. (1996) Improving elevator performance using reinforcement learning. In *Advances is Neural Information Processing Systems 8*.

Del Re, W., Fantacci, R. & Ronga, L. (1996) A dynamic channel allocation technique based on Hopfield Neural Networks. *IEEE Transactions on Vehicular Technology*, 45:1.

McEliece, R.J. & Sivarajan, K.N. (1994), Performance limits for channelized cellular telephone systems. *IEEE Trans. Inform. Theory*, pp. 21–34, Jan.

Sutton, R.S. (1988) Learning to predict by the methods of temporal differences. *Machine Learning*, 3:9–44.

Tesauro, G.J. (1992) Practical issues in temporal difference learning. *Machine Learning*, 8(3/4):257–277.

Zhang, M. & Yum, T.P. (1989) Comparisons of Channel-Assignment Strategies in Cellular Mobile Telephone Systems. *IEEE Transactions on Vehicular Technology* Vol. 38, No. 4.

Zhang, W. & Dietterich, T.G. (1996) High-performance job-shop scheduling with a time-delay TD(lambda) network. In *Advances is Neural Information Processing Systems 8*.

Spectroscopic Detection of Cervical Pre-Cancer through Radial Basis Function Networks

Kagan Tumer
kagan@pine.ece.utexas.edu
Dept. of Electrical and Computer Engr.
The University of Texas at Austin

Nirmala Ramanujam
nimmi@ccwf.cc.utexas.edu
Biomedical Engineering Program
The University of Texas at Austin

Rebecca Richards-Kortum
kortum@mail.utexas.edu
Biomedical Engineering Program
The University of Texas at Austin

Joydeep Ghosh
ghosh@ece.utexas.edu
Dept. of Electrical and Computer Engr.
The University of Texas at Austin

Abstract

The mortality related to cervical cancer can be substantially reduced through early detection and treatment. However, current detection techniques, such as Pap smear and colposcopy, fail to achieve a concurrently high sensitivity and specificity. *In vivo* fluorescence spectroscopy is a technique which quickly, non-invasively and quantitatively probes the biochemical and morphological changes that occur in pre-cancerous tissue. RBF ensemble algorithms based on such spectra provide automated, and near real-time implementation of pre-cancer detection in the hands of non-experts. The results are more reliable, direct and accurate than those achieved by either human experts or multivariate statistical algorithms.

1 Introduction

Cervical carcinoma is the second most common cancer in women worldwide, exceeded only by breast cancer (Ramanujam et al., 1996). The mortality related to cervical cancer can be reduced if this disease is detected at the pre-cancerous state, known as squamous intraepithelial lesion (SIL). Currently, a Pap smear is used to screen for cervical cancer (Kurman et al., 1994). In a Pap test, a large number of cells obtained by scraping the cervical epithelium are smeared onto a slide which is then fixed and stained for cytologic examination. The Pap smear is unable to achieve a concurrently high sensitivity[1] and high specificity[2] due to both sampling and reading errors (Fahey et al., 1995). Furthermore, reading Pap smears is extremely labor intensive and requires highly trained professionals. A patient with a Pap smear interpreted as indicating the presence of SIL is followed up by a diagnostic procedure called colposcopy. Since this procedure involves biopsy, which requires histologic evaluation, diagnosis is not immediate.

In vivo fluorescence spectroscopy is a technique which has the capability to quickly, non-invasively and quantitatively probe the biochemical and morphological changes that occur as tissue becomes neoplastic. The measured spectral information can be correlated to tissue histo-pathology, the current "gold standard" to develop clinically effective screening and diagnostic algorithms. These mathematical algorithms can be implemented in software thereby, enabling automated, fast, non-invasive and accurate pre-cancer screening and diagnosis in hands of non-experts.

A screening and diagnostic technique for human cervical pre-cancer based on laser induced fluorescence spectroscopy has been developed recently (Ramanujam et al., 1996). Screening and diagnosis was achieved using a multivariate statistical algorithm (MSA) based on principal component analysis and logistic discrimination of tissue spectra acquired *in vivo*. Furthermore, we designed Radial Basis Function (RBF) network ensembles to improve the accuracy of the multivariate statistical algorithm, and to simplify the decision making process. Section 2 presents the data collection/processing techniques. In Section 3, we discuss the MSA, and describe the neural network based methods. Section 4 contains the experimental results and compares the neural network results to both the results of the MSA and to current clinical detection methods. A discussion of the results is given in Section 5.

2 Data Collection and Processing

A portable fluorimeter consisting of two nitrogen pumped-dye lasers, a fiber-optic probe and a polychromator coupled to an intensified diode array controlled by an optical multi-channel analyzer was utilized to measure fluorescence spectra from the cervix *in vivo* at three excitation wavelengths: 337, 380 and 460 nm (Ramanujam et al., 1996). Tissue biopsies were obtained only from abnormal sites identified by colposcopy and subsequently analyzed by the probe to comply with routine patient care procedure. Hemotoxylin and eosin stained sections of each biopsy specimen were evaluated by a panel of four board certified pathologists and a consensus diagnosis was established using the Bethesda classification system. Samples were classified as normal squamous (NS), normal columnar (NC), low grade (LG) SIL and high grade (HG) SIL. Table 1 provides the number of samples in the training (calibration) and test sets. Based on this data set, a clinically useful algorithm needs to discriminate SILs from the normal tissue types.

Figure 1 illustrates average fluorescence spectra per site acquired from cervical sites at 337 nm excitation from a typical patient. Evaluation of the spectra at 337 nm ex-

---

[1]Sensitivity is the correct classification percentage on the pre-cancerous tissue samples.
[2]Specificity is the correct classification percentage on normal tissue samples.

Table 1: Histo-pathologic classification of samples.

Histo-pathology	Training Set	Test Set
Normal	107 (SN: 94; SC: 13)	108 (SN: 94; SC: 14)
SIL	58 (LG: 23; HG: 35)	59 (LG: 24; HG: 35)

citation highlights one of the classification difficulties, namely that the fluorescence intensity of SILs (LG and HG) is less than that of the corresponding normal squamous tissue and greater than that of the corresponding normal columnar tissue over the entire emission spectrum[3]. Fluorescence spectra at all three excitation wavelengths comprise of a total of 161 excitation-emission wavelengths pairs. However, there is a significant cost penalty for using all 161 values. To alleviate this concern, a more cost-effective fluorescence imaging system was developed, using component loadings calculated from principal component analysis. Thus, the number of required fluorescence excitation-emission wavelength pairs were reduced from 161 to 13 with a minimal drop in classification accuracy (Ramanujam et al., 1996).

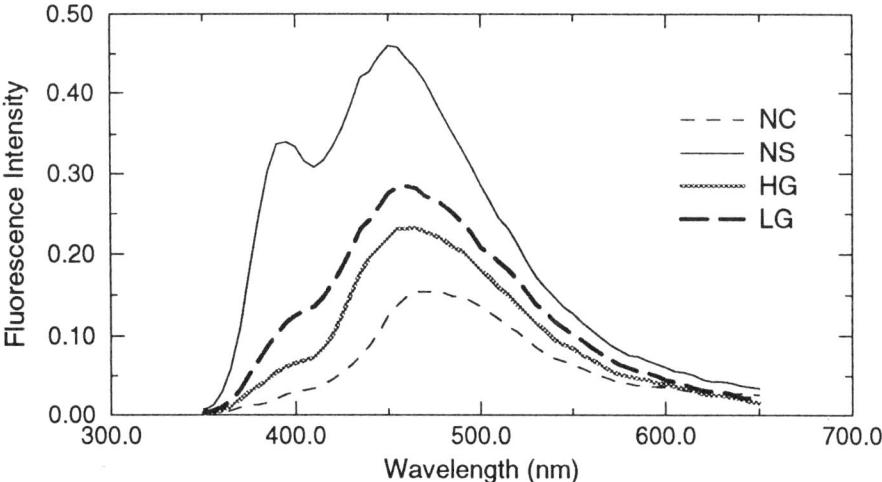

Figure 1: Fluorecsence spectra from a typical patient at 337 nm excitation.

3 Algorithm Development

3.1 Multivariate Statistical Algorithms

The multivariate statistical algorithm development described in (Ramanujam et al., 1996) consists of the following five steps: (1) pre-processing to reduce inter-patient and intra-patient variation of spectra from a tissue type, (2) dimension reduction of the pre-processed tissue spectra using Principal Component Analysis (PCA), (3) selection of diagnostically relevant principal components, (4) development of a classification algorithm based on logistic discrimination, and finally (5) retrospective and prospective evaluation of the algorithm's accuracy on a training (calibration) and test (prediction) set, respectively. Discrimination between SILs and the two normal tissue types could not be achieved effectively using MSA. Therefore two

---

[3]Spectral features observed in Figure 1 are representative of those measured at 380 nm and 460 nm excitation (not shown here).

constituent algorithms were developed: algorithm (1), to discriminate between SILs and normal squamous tissues, and algorithm (2), to discriminate between SILs and normal columnar tissues (Ramanujam et al., 1996).

3.2 Algorithms based on Neural Networks

The second stage of algorithm development consists of evaluating the applicability of neural networks to this problem. Initially, both Multi-Layered Perceptrons (MLPs) and Radial Basis function (RBF) networks were considered. However, MLPs failed to improve upon the MSA results for both algorithms (1) and (2), and frequently converged to spurious solutions. Therefore, our study focuses on RBF networks and RBF network ensembles.

Radial Basis Function Networks: The first step in applying RBF networks to this problem consisted of retracing the two-step process outlined for the multivariate statistical algorithm. For *constituent* algorithm (1) the kernels were initialized using a k-means clustering algorithm on the training set containing NS tissue samples and SILs. The RBF networks had 10 kernels, whose locations and spreads were adjusted during training. For *constituent* algorithm (2), we selected 10 kernels, half of which were fixed to patterns from the columnar normal class, while the other half were initialized using a k-means algorithm. Neither the kernel locations nor their spreads were adjusted during training. This process was adopted to rectify the large discrepancy between the samples from each category (13 for columnar normal vs. 58 for SILs). For each algorithm, the training time was estimated by maximizing the performance on one validation set. Once the stopping time was established, 20 cases were run for each algorithm[4].

Linear and Order statistics Combiners: There were significant variations among different runs of the RBF networks for all three algorithms. Therefore, selecting the "best" classifier was not the ideal choice. First, the definition of "best" depends on the selection of the validation set, making it difficult to ascertain whether one network will outperform all others given a different test set, as the validation sets are small. Second, selecting only one classifier discards a large amount of potentially relevant information. In order to use all the available data, and to increase both the performance and the reliability of the methods, the outputs of RBF networks were pooled before a classification decision was made.

The concept of combining classifier outputs[5] has been explored in a multitude of articles (Hansen and Salamon, 1990; Wolpert, 1992). In this article we use the median combiner, which belongs to the class order statistics combiners introduced in (Tumer and Ghosh, 1995), and the averaging combiner, which performs an arithmetic average of the corresponding outputs.

4 Results

Two-step algorithm: The ensemble results reported are based on pooling 20 different runs of RBF networks, initialized and trained as described in the previous section. This procedure was repeated 10 times to ascertain the reliability of the

---

[4] Each run has a different initialization set of kernels/spreads/weights.
[5] An extensive bibliography is available in (Tumer and Ghosh, 1996).

result and to obtain the standard deviations. For an application such as pre-cancer detection, the cost of a misclassification varies greatly from one class to another. Erroneously labeling a healthy tissue as pre-cancerous can be corrected when further tests are performed. Labeling a pre-cancerous tissue as healthy however, can lead to disastrous consequences. Therefore, for algorithm (1), we have increased the cost of a misclassified SIL until the sensitivity[6] reached a satisfactory level. The sensitivity and specificity values for *constituent* algorithm (1) based on both MSA and RBF ensembles are provided in Table 2. Table 3 presents sensitivity and specificity values for *constituent* algorithm (2) obtained from MSA and RBF ensembles[7]. For both algorithms (1) and (2), the RBF based combiners provide higher specificity than the MSA. The median combiner provides results similar to those of the average combiner, except for algorithm (2) where it provides better specificity. In order to obtain the final discrimination between normal tissue and SILs, *constituent* algorithms (1) and (2) are used sequentially, and the results are reported in Table 4.

Table 2: Accuracy of *constituent* algorithm (1) for differentiating SILs and normal squamous tissues, using MSA and RBF ensembles.

Algorithm	Specificity	Sensitivity
MSA	63%	90%
RBF-ave	66% ±1%	90% ±0%
RBF-med	66% ±1%	90% ±1%

Table 3: Accuracy of *constituent* algorithm (2) for differentiating SILs and normal columnar tissues, using MSA and RBF ensembles.

Algorithm	Specificity	Sensitivity
MSA	36%	97%
RBF-ave	37% ±5%	97% ±0%
RBF-med	44% ±7%	97% ±0%

One-step algorithm: The results presented above are based on the multi-step algorithm specifically developed for the MSA, which could not consolidate algorithms (1) and (2) into one step. Since the ultimate goal of these two algorithms is to separate SILs from normal tissue samples, a given pattern has to be processed through both algorithms. In order to simplify this decision process, we designed a one step RBF network to perform this separation. Because the pre-processing for algorithms (1) and (2) is different[8], the input space is now 26-dimensional. We initialized 10 kernels using a k-means algorithm on a trimmed[9] version of the training set. The kernel locations and spreads were not adjusted during training. The cost of a misclassified SIL was set at 2.5 times the cost of a misclassified normal tissue

---

[6]In this case, the cost of misclassifying a SIL was three times the cost of misclassifying a normal tissue sample.

[7]In this case, there was no need to increase the cost of a misclassified SIL, because of the high prominence of SILs in the training set.

[8]Normalization vs. normalization followed by mean scaling.

[9]The trimmed set has the same number of patterns from each class. Thus, it forces each class to have a similar number of kernels. This set is used *only* for initializing the kernels.

sample, in order to provide the best sensitivity/specificity pair. The average and median combiner results are obtained by pooling 20 RBF networks[10].

Table 4: One step RBF algorithm compared to multi-step MSA and clinical methods for differentiating SILs and normal tissue samples.

Algorithm	Specificity	Sensitivity
2-step MSA	63%	83%
2-step RBF-ave	65% ±2%	87% ±1%
2-step RBF-med	67% ±2%	87% ±1%
RBF-ave	67% ±.75%	91% ±1.5%
RBF-med	65.5% ±.5%	91% ±1%
Pap smear (human expert)	68% ±21%	62% ±23%
Colposcopy (human expert)	48%±23 %	94% ±6%

The results of both the two-step and one-step RBF algorithms and the results of the two-step MSA are compared to the accuracy of Pap smear screening and colposcopy in expert hands in Table 4. A comparison of one-step RBF algorithms to the two-step RBF algorithms indicates that the one-step algorithms have similar specificities, but a moderate improvement in sensitivity relative to the two-step algorithms. Compared to the MSA, the one-step RBF algorithms have a slightly decreased specificity, but a substantially improved sensitivity. In addition to the improved sensitivity, the one step RBF algorithms simplify the decision making process. A comparison between the one step RBF algorithms and Pap smear screening indicates that the RBF algorithms have a nearly 30% improvement in sensitivity with no compromise in specificity; when compared to colposcopy in expert hands, the RBF ensemble algorithms maintain the sensitivity of expert colposcopists, while improving the specificity by almost 20%. Figure 2 shows the trade-off between specificity and sensitivity for clinical methods, MSA and RBF ensembles, obtained by changing the misclassification cost. The RBF ensembles provide better sensitivity and higher reliability than any other method for a given specificity value.

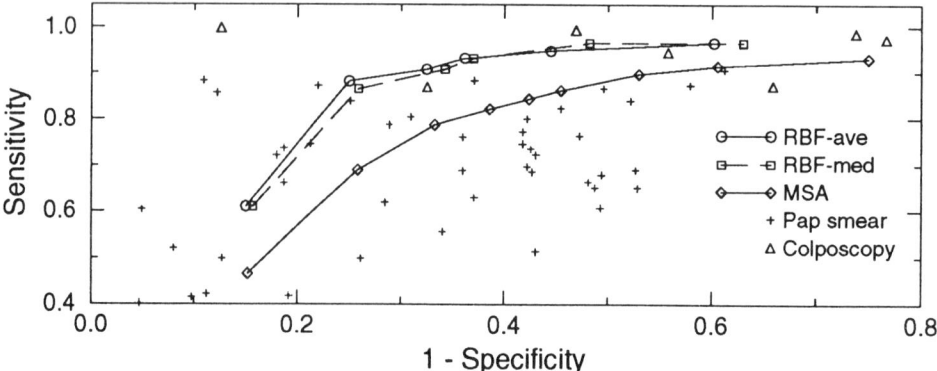

Figure 2: Trade-off between sensitivity and specifity for MSA and RBF ensembles. For reference, Pap smear and colposcopy results from the literature are included (Fahey et al., 1995).

---

[10]This procedure is repeated 10 times, in order to determine the standard deviation.

5 Discussion

The classification results of both the multivariate statistical algorithms and the radial basis function network ensembles demonstrate that significant improvement in classification accuracy can be achieved over current clinical detection modalities using cervical tissue spectral data obtained from *in vivo* fluorescence spectroscopy. The one-step RBF algorithm has the potential to significantly reduce the number of pre-cancerous cases missed by Pap smear screening and the number of normal tissues misdiagnosed by expert colposcopists.

The qualitative nature of current clinical detection modalities leads to a significant variability in classification accuracy. For example, estimates of the sensitivity and specificity of Pap smear screening have been shown to range from 11-99% and 14-97%, respectively (Fahey et al., 1995). This limitation can be addressed by the RBF network ensembles which demonstrate a significantly smaller variability in classification accuracy therefore enabling more reliable classification. In addition to demonstrating a superior sensitivity, the RBF ensembles simplify the decision making process of the two-step algorithms based on MSA into a single step that discriminates between SILs and normal tissues. We note that for the given data set, both MSA and MLP were unable to provide satisfactory solutions in one step.

The one-step algorithm development process can be readily implemented in software, enabling automated detection of cervical pre-cancer. It provides near real time implementation of pre-cancer detection in the hands of non-experts, and can lead to wide-scale implementation of screening and diagnosis and more effective patient management in the prevention of cervical cancer. The success of this application will represent an important step forward in both medical laser spectroscopy and gynecologic oncology.

Acknowledgements: This research was supported in part by NSF grant ECS 9307632, AFOSR contract F49620-93-1-0307, and Lifespex, Inc.

References

Fahey, M. T., Irwig, L., and Macaskill, P. (1995). Meta-analysis of pap test accuracy. *American Journal of Epidemiology*, 141(7):680–689.

Hansen, L. K. and Salamon, P. (1990). Neural network ensembles. *IEEE Transactions on Pattern Analysis and Machine Intelligence*, 12(10):993–1000.

Kurman, R. J., Henson, D. E., Herbst, A. L., Noller, K. L., and Schiffman, M. H. (1994). Interim guidelines of management of abnormal cervical cytology. *Journal of American Medical Association*, 271:1866–1869.

Ramanujam, N., Mitchell, M. F., Mahadevan, A., Thomsen, S., Malpica, A., Wright, T., Atkinson, N., and Richards-Kortum, R. R. (1996). Cervical pre-cancer detecion using a multivariate statistical algorithm based on fluorescence spectra at multiple excitation wavelengths. *Photochemistry and Photobiology*, 64(4):720–735.

Tumer, K. and Ghosh, J. (1995). Order statistcs combiners for neural classifiers. In *Proceedings of the World Congress on Neural Networks*, pages I:31–34, Washington D.C. INNS Press.

Tumer, K. and Ghosh, J. (1996). Error correlation and error reduction in ensemble classifiers. *Connection Science*. (to appear).

Wolpert, D. H. (1992). Stacked generalization. *Neural Networks*, 5:241–259.

Interpolating Earth-science Data using RBF Networks and Mixtures of Experts

E. Wan   D. Bone
Division of Information Technology
Canberra Laboratory, CSIRO
GPO Box 664, Canberra, ACT, 2601, Australia
{ernest, don}@cbr.dit.csiro.au

Abstract

We present a mixture of experts (ME) approach to interpolate sparse, spatially correlated earth-science data. Kriging is an interpolation method which uses a global covariation model estimated from the data to take account of the spatial dependence in the data. Based on the close relationship between kriging and the radial basis function (RBF) network (Wan & Bone, 1996), we use a mixture of generalized RBF networks to partition the input space into statistically correlated regions and learn the local covariation model of the data in each region. Applying the ME approach to simulated and real-world data, we show that it is able to achieve good partitioning of the input space, learn the local covariation models and improve generalization.

1. INTRODUCTION

Kriging is an interpolation method widely used in the earth sciences, which models the surface to be interpolated as a stationary random field (RF) and employs a linear model. The value at an unsampled location is evaluated as a weighted sum of the sparse, spatially correlated data points. The weights take account of the spatial correlation between the available data points and between the unknown points and the available data points. The spatial dependence is specified in the form of a global covariation model. Assuming global stationarity, the kriging predictor is the best unbiased linear predictor of the unsampled value when the true covariation model is used, in the sense that it minimizes the squared error variance under the unbiasedness constraint. However, in practice, the covariation of the data is unknown and has to be estimated from the data by an initial spatial data analysis. The analysis fits a covariation model to a covariation measure of the data such as the sample variogram or the sample covariogram, either graphically or by means of various least squares (LS) and maximum likelihood (ML) approaches. Valid covariation models are all radial basis functions.

Optimal prediction is achieved when the true covariation model of the data is used. In general, prediction (or generalization) improves as the covariation model used more closely matches the true covariation of the data. Nevertheless, estimating the covariation model from earth-science data has proved to be difficult in practice due to the sparseness of data samples. Furthermore for many data sets the global stationarity assumption is not valid. To address this, data sets are commonly manually partitioned into smaller regions within which the stationarity assumption is valid or approximately so.

In a previous paper, we showed that there is a close, formal relationship between kriging and RBF networks (Wan & Bone, 1996). In the equivalent RBF network formulation of kriging, the input vector is a coordinate and the output is a scalar physical quantity of interest. We pointed out that, under the stationarity assumption, the radial basis function used in an RBF network can be viewed as a covariation model of the data. We showed that an RBF network whose RBF units share an adaptive norm weighting matrix, can be used to estimate the parameters of the postulated covariation model, outperforming more conventional methods. In the rest of this paper we will refer to such a generalization of the RBF network as a generalized RBF (GRBF) network.

In this paper, we discuss how a mixture of GRBF networks can be used to partition the input space into statistically correlated regions and learn the local covariation model of each region. We demonstrate the effectiveness of the ME approach with a simulated data set and an aero-magnetic data set. Comparisons are also made of prediction accuracy of a single GRBF network and other more traditional RBF networks.

2 MIXTURE OF GRBF EXPERTS

Mixture of experts (Jacobs et al , 1991) is a modular neural network architecture in which a number of expert networks augmented by a gating network compete to learn the data. The gating network learns to assign probability to the experts according to their performance over various parts of the input space, and combines the outputs of the experts accordingly. During training, each expert is made to focus on modelling the local mapping it performs best, improving its performance further. Competition among the experts achieves a soft partitioning of the input space into regions with each expert network learning a separate local mapping. An hierarchical generalization of ME, the hierarchical mixture of experts (HME), in which each expert is allowed to expand into a gating network and a set of sub-experts, has also been proposed (Jordan & Jacobs, 1994).

Under the global stationarity assumption, training a GRBF network by minimizing the mean squared prediction error involves adjusting its norm weighting matrix. This can be interpreted as an attempt to match the RBF to the covariation of the data. It then seems natural to use a mixture of GRBF networks when only local stationarity can be assumed. After training, the gating network soft partitions the input space into statistically correlated regions and each GRBF network provides a model of the covariation of the data for a local region. Instead of an ME architecture, an HME architecture can be used. However, to simplify the discussion we restrict ourselves to the ME architecture.

Each expert in the mixture is a GRBF network. The output of expert i is given by:

$$\hat{y}_i(\mathbf{x}; \boldsymbol{\theta}_i) = \sum_{j=1}^{n_i} w_{ij} \phi(\mathbf{x}; \mathbf{c}_{ij}, \mathbf{M}_i) + w_{i0} \qquad (2.1)$$

where n_i is the number of RBF units, $\boldsymbol{\theta}_i = \{\{w_{ij}\}_{j=0}^{n_i}, \{\mathbf{c}_{ij}\}_{j=1}^{n_i}, \mathbf{M}_i\}$ are the parameters of the expert and $\phi(\mathbf{x};\mathbf{c},\mathbf{M}) = \phi(\|\mathbf{x}-\mathbf{c}\|_\mathbf{M})$. Assuming zero-mean Gaussian error and common variance σ_i^2, the conditional probability of y given $\mathbf{x}$ and $\boldsymbol{\theta}_i$ is given by:

$$P(y|\mathbf{x},\boldsymbol{\theta}_i) = \frac{1}{\sqrt{2\pi}\sigma_i} \exp\left(-\frac{1}{2\sigma_i^2}(y - \hat{y}_i(\mathbf{x};\boldsymbol{\theta}_i))^2\right). \qquad (2.3)$$

Since the radial basis functions we used have compact support and each expert only learns a local covariation model, small GRBF networks spanning overlapping regions can be used to reduce computation at the expense of some resolution in locating the boundaries of the regions. Also, only the subset of data within and around the region spanned by a GRBF network is needed to train it, further reducing computational effort.

With m experts, the ith output of the gating network gives the probability of selecting the expert i and is given by the normalized function:

$$g_i(\mathbf{x};\upsilon) = P(i|\mathbf{x},\upsilon) = \alpha_i \exp(q(\mathbf{x};\upsilon_i)) \Big/ \sum_{j=1}^{m} \alpha_j \exp(q(\mathbf{x};\upsilon_j)) \qquad (2.4)$$

where $\upsilon = \{\{\alpha_i\}_{i=1}^m, \{\upsilon_i\}_{i=1}^m\}$. Using $q(\mathbf{x};\upsilon_i) = \upsilon_i^T [\mathbf{x}^T \ 1]^T$ and setting all α_i's to 1, the gating network implements the softmax function and partitions the input space into a smoothed planar tessellation. Alternatively, with $q(\mathbf{x};\upsilon_i) = -\|\mathbf{T}_i(\mathbf{x}-\mathbf{u}_i)\|^2$ (where $\upsilon_i = \{\mathbf{u}_i, \mathbf{T}_i\}$ consists of a location vector and an affine transformation matrix) and restricting the α_i's to be non-negative, the gating network divides the input space into packed anisotropic ellipsoids. These two partitionings are quite convenient and adequate for most earth-science applications where $\mathbf{x}$ is a 2D or 3D coordinate.

The output of the experts are combined to give the overall output of the mixture:

$$\hat{y}(\mathbf{x};\boldsymbol{\theta}) = \sum_{i=1}^{m} P(i|\mathbf{x},\upsilon)\hat{y}_i(\mathbf{x};\boldsymbol{\theta}_i) = \sum_{i=1}^{m} g_i(\mathbf{x};\upsilon)\hat{y}_i(\mathbf{x};\boldsymbol{\theta}_i) \qquad (2.5)$$

where $\boldsymbol{\theta} = \{\upsilon, \{\boldsymbol{\theta}_i\}_{i=1}^m\}$ and the conditional probability of observing y given $\mathbf{x}$ and $\boldsymbol{\theta}$ is:

$$P(y|\mathbf{x},\boldsymbol{\theta}) = \sum_{i=1}^{m} P(i|\mathbf{x},\upsilon) P(y|\mathbf{x},\boldsymbol{\theta}_i). \qquad (2.6)$$

3 THE TRAINING ALGORITHM

The Expectation-Maximization (EM) algorithm of Jordan and Jacobs is used to train the mixture of GRBF networks. Instead of computing the ML estimates, we extend the algorithm by including priors on the parameters of the experts and compute the maximum a posteriori (MAP) estimates. Since an expert may be focusing on a small subset of the data, the priors help to prevent over-fitting and improve generalization.

Jordan & Jacobs introduced a set of indicator random variables $Z = \{z^{(t)}\}_{t=1}^N$ as missing data to label the experts that generate the observable data $D = \{(\mathbf{x}^{(t)}, y^{(t)})\}_{t=1}^N$. The log joint probability of the complete data $D_c = \{D, Z\}$ and parameters $\boldsymbol{\theta}$ can be written as:

$$\ln P(D_c, \boldsymbol{\theta}|\lambda) = \ln\left\{ P(\boldsymbol{\theta}|\lambda) \prod_{t=1}^{N} \prod_{i=1}^{m} \left\{ P(i|\mathbf{x}^{(t)},\upsilon) P(y^{(t)}|\mathbf{x}^{(t)},\boldsymbol{\theta}_i) \right\}^{z_i^{(t)}} \right\} \qquad (3.1)$$

where λ is a set of hyperparameters. Assuming separable priors on the parameters of the model i.e. $P(\boldsymbol{\theta}|\lambda) = P(\upsilon|\lambda_0) \prod_{i=1}^{m} P(\boldsymbol{\theta}_i|\lambda_i)$ with $\lambda = \{\lambda_i\}_{i=0}^m$, (3.1) can be rewritten as:

$$\begin{aligned}\ln P(D_c, \boldsymbol{\theta}|\lambda) = &\sum_{t=1}^{N}\sum_{i=1}^{m} z_i^{(t)} \ln P(i|\mathbf{x}^{(t)},\upsilon) + \ln P(\upsilon|\lambda_0) \\ &+ \sum_{i=1}^{m}\left\{\sum_{t=1}^{N} z_i^{(t)} \ln P(y^{(t)}|\mathbf{x}^{(t)},\boldsymbol{\theta}_i) + \ln P(\boldsymbol{\theta}_i|\lambda_i)\right\}\end{aligned} \qquad (3.2)$$

Since the posterior probability of the model parameters is proportional to the joint probability, maximizing (3.2) is equivalent to maximizing the log posterior. In the E-step, the observed data and the current network parameters are used to compute the expected value of the complete-data log joint probability:

$$Q(\theta|\theta^{(k)}) = \sum_{t=1}^{N}\sum_{i=1}^{m} h_i^{(k)}(t) \ln P(i|\mathbf{x}^{(t)}, \upsilon) + \ln P(\upsilon|\lambda_0)$$
$$+ \sum_{i=1}^{m}\left\{\sum_{t=1}^{N} h_i^{(k)}(t) \ln P(y^{(t)}|\mathbf{x}^{(t)}, \theta_i) + \ln P(\theta_i|\lambda_i)\right\} \quad (3.3)$$

where $\quad h_i^{(k)}(t) = E\left[z_i^{(t)}|D, \theta^{(k)}\right] = P(i|\mathbf{x}^{(t)}, y^{(t)}) = \dfrac{P(i|\mathbf{x}^{(t)}, \upsilon^{(k)}) P(y^{(t)}|\mathbf{x}^{(t)}, \theta_i^{(k)})}{\sum_{j=1}^{m} P(j|\mathbf{x}^{(t)}, \upsilon^{(k)}) P(y^{(t)}|\mathbf{x}^{(t)}, \theta_j^{(k)})}$ (3.4)

In the M-step, $Q(\theta|\theta^{(k)})$ is maximized with respect to θ to obtain $\theta^{(k+1)}$. As a result of the use of the indicator variables, the problem is decoupled into a separate set of interim MAP estimations:

$$\upsilon^{(k+1)} = \arg\max_{\upsilon} \sum_{t=1}^{N}\sum_{i=1}^{m} h_i^{(k)}(t) \ln P(i|\mathbf{x}^{(t)}, \upsilon) + \ln P(\upsilon|\lambda_0) \quad (3.5)$$

$$\theta_i^{(k+1)} = \arg\max_{\theta_i} \sum_{t=1}^{N} h_i^{(k)}(t) \ln P(y^{(t)}|\mathbf{x}^{(t)}, \theta_i) + \ln P(\theta_i|\lambda_i) \quad (3.6)$$

We assume a flat prior for the gating network parameters and the prior $P(\theta_i|\lambda_i) = \exp(-\tfrac{1}{2}\lambda_i \sum_{r=1}^{n_i}\sum_{s=1}^{n_i} w_{ir} w_{is} \phi(\mathbf{c}_{ir} - \mathbf{c}_{is})) / Z_R(\lambda_i)$ where $Z_R(\lambda_i)$ is a normalization constant, for the experts. This smoothness prior is used on the GRBF networks because it can be derived from regularization theory (Girosi & Poggio, 1990) and at the same time is consistent with the interpretation of the radial basis function as a covariation model. Hence, maximizing θ_i with (3.6) is equivalent to minimizing the cost function:

$$E_i = \sum_{t=1}^{N} h_i^{(k)}(t) \left(y(\mathbf{x}_j) - \hat{y}_i(\mathbf{x}_j)\right)^2 + \lambda_i^* \sum_{r=1}^{n_i}\sum_{s=1}^{n_i} w_{ir} w_{is} \phi(\mathbf{c}_{ir} - \mathbf{c}_{is}) \quad (3.7)$$

where $\lambda_i^* = \lambda_i \sigma_i^2$. The value of the effective regularization parameter, λ_i^*, can be set by generalized cross validation (GCV) (Orr, 1995) or by the 'evidence' method of (Mackay, 1991) using re-estimation formulas. However, in the simulations, for simplicity, we preset the value of the regularization parameter to a fixed value.

4 SIMULATION RESULTS

Using the Cholesky decomposition method (Cressie, 1993), we generate four 2D data sets using the four different covariation models shown in Figure 1. The four data set are then joined together to form a single 64x64 data set. Figure 3a shows the original data set and the hard boundaries of the 4 statistically distinct regions. We randomly sample the data to obtain a 400 sample training set and use the rest of the data for validation.

Two GRBF networks, with 64 and 144 adaptive anistropic spherical[1] units respectively, are used to learn the postulated global covariation model and the mapping. A 2-level

---

[1] The spherical model is widely used in geostatistics and when used as a covariance function is defined as $\varphi(\mathbf{h};a) = 1 - \{\tfrac{3}{2}(\tfrac{|\mathbf{h}|}{a}) - \tfrac{1}{2}(\tfrac{|\mathbf{h}|}{a})^3\}$ for $0 \leq \|\mathbf{h}\| \leq a$ and $\varphi(\mathbf{h};a) = 0$ for $\|\mathbf{h}\| > a$. Spherical does NOT mean isotropic.

HME with 4 GRBF network experts each with 36 spherical units are used to learn the local covariation models and the mapping. Softmax gating networks are used and each expert is somewhat 'localized' in each quadrant of the input space. The units of the experts are located at the same locations as the units of the 64-unit GRBF network with 24 overlapping units between any two of the experts. The design ensures that the HME does not have an advantage over the 64-unit GRBF network if the data is indeed globally stationary. Figure 2 shows the local covariation models learned by the HME with the smoothness priors and Figure 3b shows the interpolant generated and the partitioning.

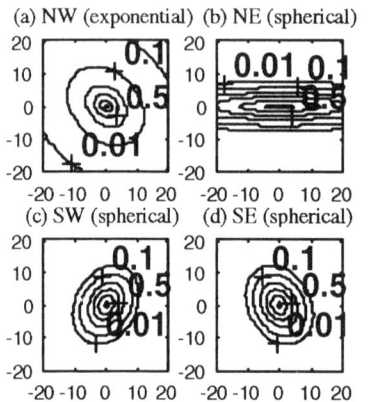

Figure 1: The profile of the true local covariation models of the simulated data set. Exponential and spherical models are used.

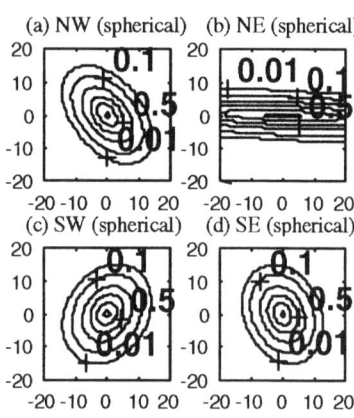

Figure 2: The profile of the local covariation models learned by the HME.

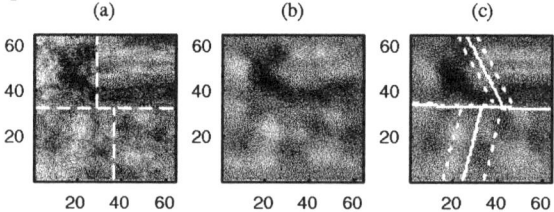

Figure 3: (a) Simulated data set and true partitions. (b) Interpolant generated by the 144 spherical unit GRBFN. (c) The HME interpolant and the soft partitioning learned (0.5, 0.9 probability contours of the 4 experts shown in solid and dotted lines respectively)

Table 1: Normalized mean squared prediction error for the simulated data set.

Network	RBF unit	NMSE
RBFN *(isotropic RBF units with width set to the distance to the nearest neighbor)*	64, Gaussian	0.761
	144, Gaussian	0.616
	400, Gaussian	0.543
RBFN *(identical isotropic RBF units with adaptive width)*	64, Gaussian	0.477
	144, Gaussian	0.475
GRBFN *(identical RBF units with adaptive norm weighting matrix)*	64, spherical	0.506
	144, spherical	0.431
HME *(2 levels, 4 GRBFN experts) without priors*	4x36, spherical	0.938
HME *(2 levels, 4 GRBFN experts) with priors*	4x36, spherical	0.433
kriging predictor *(using true local models)*		0.372

For comparison, a number of ordinary RBF networks are also used to learn the mapping. In all cases, the RBF units of networks of the same size share the same locations which are preset by a Kohonen map. Table 1 summarizes the normalized mean squared prediction error (NMSE)- the squared prediction error divided by the variance of the validation set - for each network. With the exception of HME, all results listed are obtained with a smoothness prior and a regularization parameter of 0.1. Ordinary weight decay is used for RBF networks with units of varying widths and the smoothness prior discussed in section 3 are used for the remaining networks. The NMSE of the kriging predictor that uses the true local models is also listed as a reference.

Similar experiments are also conducted on a real aero-magnetic data set. The flight paths along which the data is collected are divided into a 740 data points training set and a 1690 points validation set. The NMSE for each network is summarized in Table 2, the local covariation models learned by the HME is shown in Figure 4, and the interpolant generated by the HME and the partitioning is shown in Figure 5b.

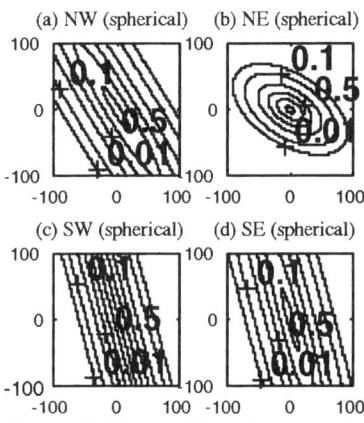

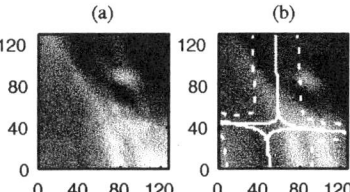

Figure 5: (a) Thin-plate interpolant of the entire aero-magnetic data set. (b) The HME interpolant and the soft partitioning (0.5, 0.9 probability contours of the 4 experts shown in solid and dotted lines respectively).

Figure 4: The profile of the local covariation models of the aero-magnetic data set learned by the HME.

Table 2: Normalized mean squared prediction error for the aero-magnetic data set.

Network	RBF units	NMSE
RBFN *(isotropic RBF units with width set to the distance to the nearest neighbor)*	49, Gaussian	1.158
	100, Gaussian	1.256
RBFN *(isotropic RBF units with width set to the mean distance to the 8 nearest neighbors)*	49, Gaussian	0.723
	100, Gaussian	0.699
RBFN *(identical isotropic RBF units with adaptive width)*	49, Gaussian	0.692
	100, Gaussian	0.614
GRBFN *(identical RBF units with adaptive norm weighting matrix)*	49, spherical	0.684
	100, spherical	0.612
HME *(2 levels, 4 GRBFN experts) without priors*	4x25, spherical	0.389
HME *(2 levels, 4 GRBFN experts) with priors*	4x25, spherical	0.315

5 DISCUSSION

The ordinary RBF networks perform worst with both the simulated data and the aero-magnetic data. As neither data set is globally stationary, the GRBF networks do not improve prediction accuracy over the corresponding RBF networks that use isotropic Gaussian units. In both cases, the hierarchical mixture of GRBF networks improves the prediction accuracy when the smoothness priors are used. Without the priors, the ML estimates of the HME parameters lead to improbably high and low predictions.

The improvement in prediction accuracy is more significant for the aero-magnetic data set than for the simulated data set due to some apparent global covariation of the simulated data which only becomes evident when the directional variograms of the data are plotted. However, despite the similar NMSE, Figure 3 shows that the interpolant generated by the 144-unit GRBF network does not contain the structural information that is captured by the HME interpolant and is most evident in the north-east region.

In the case of the simulated data set, the HME learns the local covariation models accurately despite the fact that the bottom level gating networks fail to partition the input space precisely along the north-south direction. The availability of more data and the straight east-west discontinuity allows the upper gating network to partition the input space precisely along the east-west direction. In the north-west region, although the class of function the expert used is different from that of the true model, the model learned still resembles the true model especially in the inner region where it matters most.

In the case of the aero-magnetic data set, the RBF and GRBF networks perform poorly due to the considerable extrapolation that is required in the prediction and the absence of global stationarity. However, the HME whose units capture the local covariation of the data interpolates and extrapolates significantly better. The partitioning as well as the local covariation model learned by the HME seems to be reasonably accurate and leads to the construction of prominent ridge-like structures in the north-west and south-east which are only apparent in the thin-plate interpolant of the entire data set of Figure 5a.

6 CONCLUSIONS

We show that a mixture of GRBF networks can be used to learn the local covariation of spatial data and improve prediction (or generalization) when the data is approximately locally stationary - a viable assumption in many earth-science applications. We believe that the improvement will be even more significant for data sets with larger spatial extent especially if the local regions are more statistically distinct. The estimation of the local covariation models of the data and the use of these models in producing the interpolant helps to capture the structural information in the data which, apart from accuracy of the prediction, is of critical importance to many earth-science applications.

The ME approach allows the objective and automatic partitioning of the input space into statistically correlated regions. It also allows the use of a number of small local GRBF networks each trained on a subset of the data making it scaleable to large data sets.

The mixture of GRBF networks approach is motivated by the statistical interpolation method of kriging. The approach therefore has a very sound physical interpretation and all the parameters of the network have clear statistical and/or physical meanings.

References

Cressie, N. A. (1993). *Statistics for Spatial Data*. Wiley, New York.

Jacobs, R. A., Jordan, M. I., Nowlan, S. J. & Hinton, G. E. (1991). Adaptive Mixtures of Local Experts. *Neural Computation* 3, pp. 79-87.

Jordan, M. I. & Jacobs, R. A. (1994). Hierarchical Mixtures of Experts and the EM Algorithm. *Neural Computation* 6, pp. 181-214.

MacKay, D. J. (1992). Bayesian Interpolation. *Neural Computation* 4, pp. 415-447.

Orr, M. J. (1995). Regularization in the Selection of Radial Basis Function Centers. *Neural Computation* 7, pp. 606-623.

Poggio, T. & Girosi, F. (1990). Networks for Approximation and Learning. In *Proceedings of the IEEE* 78, pp. 1481-1497.

Wan, E. & Bone, D. (1996). A Neural Network Approach to Covariation Model Fitting and the Interpolation of Sparse Earth-science Data. In *Proceedings of the Seventh Australian Conference on Neural Networks*, pp. 121-126.

Multi-effect Decompositions for Financial Data Modeling

Lizhong Wu & John Moody
Oregon Graduate Institute, Computer Science Dept.,
PO Box 91000, Portland, OR 97291
also at:
Nonlinear Prediction Systems,
PO Box 681, University Station, Portland, OR 97207

Abstract

High frequency foreign exchange data can be decomposed into three components: the inventory effect component, the surprise information (news) component and the regular information component. The presence of the inventory effect and news can make analysis of trends due to the diffusion of information (regular information component) difficult.

We propose a neural-net-based, independent component analysis to separate high frequency foreign exchange data into these three components. Our empirical results show that our proposed multi-effect decomposition can reveal the intrinsic price behavior.

1 Introduction

Tick-by-tick, high frequency foreign exchange rates are extremely noisy and volatile, but they are not simply pure random walks (Moody & Wu 1996). The price movements are characterized by a number of "stylized facts" [1], including the following two properties: (1) short term, weak oscillations on a time scale of several ticks and (2) erratic occurrence of turbulence lasting from minutes to tens of minutes. Property (1) is most likely caused by the market makers' inventory effect (O'Hara 1995), and property (2) is due to surprise information, such as news, rumors, or major economic announcements. The price changes due to property (1) are referred to as the inventory effect component, and the changes due to property (2) are referred to as the surprise information component. The price changes due to other information is referred to as the regular information component.

---

[1] This terminology is borrowed from the financial economics literature. For additional properties of high frequency foreign exchange price series, see (Guilaumet, Dacorogna, Dave, Muller, Olsen & Pictet 1994).

Due to the inventory effect, price changes show strong negative correlations on short time scales (Moody & Wu 1995). Because of the surprise information effect, distributions of price changes are non-normal (Mandelbrot 1963). Since both the inventory effect and the surprise information effect are short term and temporary, their corresponding price components are independent of the fundamental price changes. However, their existence will seriously affect data analysis and modeling (Moody & Wu 1995). Furthermore, the most reliable component of price changes, for forecasting purposes, is the long term trend. The presence of high frequency oscillations and short periods of turbulence make it difficult to identify and predict the changes in such trends, if they occur.

In this paper, we propose a novel approach with the following price model:

$$q(t) = c_1 p_1(t) + c_2 p_2(t) + c_3 p_3(t) + \varepsilon(t) . \tag{1}$$

In this model, $q(t)$ is the observed price series and $p_1(t)$, $p_2(t)$ and $p_3(t)$ correspond respectively to the regular information component, the surprise information component and the inventory effect component. $p_1(t)$, $p_2(t)$ and $p_3(t)$ are mutually independent and may individually be either iid or correlated. $\varepsilon(t)$ is process noise, and c_1, c_2 and c_3 are scale constants. Our goal is to find $p_1(t)$, $p_2(t)$ and $p_3(t)$ given $q(t)$.

The outline of the paper is as follows. We describe our approach for multi-effect decomposition in Section 2. In Section 3, we analyze the decomposed price components obtained for the high frequency foreign exchange rates and characterize their stochastic properties. We conclude and discuss the potential applications of our multi-effect decomposition in Section 4.

2 Multi-effect Decomposition

2.1 Independent Source Separation

The task of decomposing the observed price quotes into a regular information component, a surprise information component and an inventory effect component can be exactly fitted into the framework of independent source separation. Independent source separation can be described as follows:

> Assume that $X = \{x_i, i = 1, 2, \ldots, n\}$ are the sensor outputs which are some superposition of unknown independent sources $S = \{s_i, i = 1, 2, \ldots, m\}$. The task of independent source separation is to find a mapping $Y = f(X)$, so that $Y \approx AS$, where A is an $m \times m$ matrix in which each row and column contains only one non-zero element.

Approaches to separate statistically-independent components in the inputs include

- Blind source separation (Jutten & Herault 1991),
- Information maximization (Linsker 1989), (Bell & Sejnowski 1995),
- Independent component analysis, (Comon 1994), (Amari, Cichocki & Yang 1996),
- Factorial coding (Barlow 1961).

All of these approaches can be implemented by artificial neural networks. The network architectures can be linear or nonlinear, multi-layer perceptrons, recurrent networks or other context sensitive networks (Pearlmutter & Parra 1997). We can choose a training criterion to minimize the energy in the output units, to maximize the information transferred in the network, to reduce the redundancies between the outputs, or to use the Edgeworth expansion or Gram-Charlier expansion of a probability distribution, which leads to an analytic expression of the entropy in terms of measurable higher order cumulants.

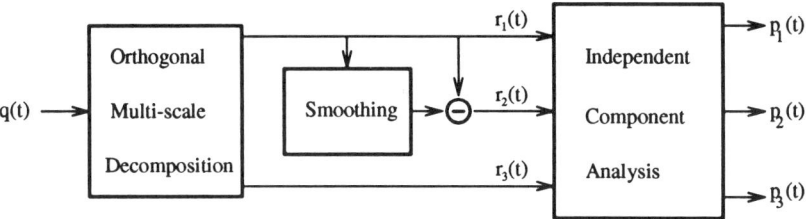

Figure 1: System diagram of multi-effect decomposition for high frequency foreign exchange rates. $q(t)$ are original price quotes, $r_i(t)$ are the reference inputs, and $p_i(t)$ are the decomposed components.

For our price decomposition problem, the non-Gaussian nature of price series requires that the transfer function of the decomposition system be nonlinear. In general, the nonlinearities in the transfer function are able to pick up higher order moments of the input distributions and perform higher order statistical redundancy reduction between outputs.

2.2 Reference input selection

In traditional approaches to blind source separation, nothing is assumed to be known about the inputs, and the systems adapt on-line and without a supervisor. This works only if the number of sensors is not less than the number of independent sources. If the number of sensors is less than that of sources, the sources can, in theory, be separated into disjoint groups (Cao & Liu 1996). However, the problem is ill-conditioned for most of the above practical approaches which only consider the case where the number of sensors is equal to the number of sources.

In our task to decompose the multiple components of price quotes, the problem can be divided into two cases. If the prices are sampled at regular intervals, we can use price quotes observed in different markets, and have the number of sensors be equal to the number of price components. However, in the high frequency markets, the price quotes are not regularly spaced in time. Price quotes from different markets will not appear at the same time, so we cannot apply the price quotes from different markets to the system. In this case, other reference inputs are needed.

Motivated by the use of reference inputs for noise canceling (Widrow, Glover, McCool, Kaunitz, Williams, Hearn, Zeidler, Dong & Goodlin 1975), we generate three reference inputs from original price quotes. They are the estimates of the three desired components. In the following, we briefly describe our procedure for generating the reference inputs.

By modeling the price quotes using a *"True Price"* state space model (Moody & Wu 1996)

$$q(t) = r_1(t) + r_3(t), \qquad (2)$$

where $r_1(t)$ is an estimate of the information component (*True Price*) and $r_3(t)$ is an estimate of the inventory effect component (additive noise), and by assuming that the *True Price* $r_1(t)$ is a fractional Brownian motion (Mandelbrot & Van Ness 1968), we can estimate $r_1(t)$ and $r_3(t)$ with given $q(t)$, (Moody & Wu 1996), as

$$r_1(t) = \sum_{m,n} S(m,\theta) Q_n^m \psi_n^m(t) \qquad (3)$$

$$r_3(t) = q(t) - r_1(t) \qquad (4)$$

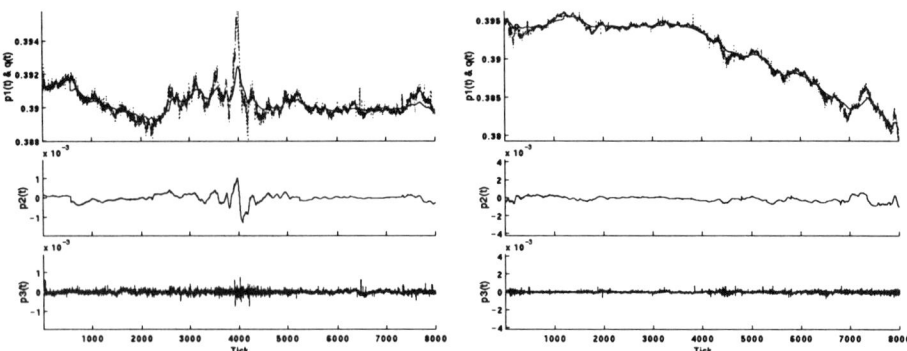

Figure 2: Multi-effect decompositions for two segments of the DEM/USD (log prices) extracted from September 1995. The three panels in each segment display the observed prices (the dotted curve in upper panel), the regular information component (solid curve in upper panel), the surprise information component (mid panel) and the inventory effect component (lower panel).

where $\psi_n^m(t)$ is an orthogonal wavelet function, Q_n^m is the coefficient of the wavelet transform of $q(t)$, m is the index of the scales and n is the time index of the components in the wavelet transfer, $S(m, \theta)$ is a smoothing function, and its parameters can be estimated using the EM algorithm (Wornell & Oppenheim 1992).

We then estimate the surprise information component as the residual between the information component and its moving average:

$$r_2(t) = r_1(t) - s(t) . \qquad (5)$$

$s(t)$ is an exponential moving average of $r_1(t)$ and

$$s(t) = (1 + \alpha)r_1(t) - \alpha s(t - 1) \qquad (6)$$

where α is a factor. Although it can be optimized based on the training data, we set $\alpha = -0.9$ in our current work.

Our system diagram for multi-effect decomposition is shown in Figure 1. Using multi-scale decomposition Eqn(3) and smoothing techniques Eqn(6), we obtain three reference inputs. We can then separate the reference inputs into three independent components via independent component analysis using an artificial neural network. Figure 2 presents multi-effect decompositions for two segments of the DEM/USD rates. The first segment contains some impulses, and the corresponding surprise information component is able to catch such volatile movements. The second segment is basically down trending, so its surprise information component is comparatively flat.

3 Empirical Analysis

3.1 Mutually Independent Analysis

Mutual independence of the variables is satisfied if the joint probability density function equals the product of the marginal densities, or equivalently, the characteristic function splits into the sum of marginal characteristic functions: $g(X) = \sum_{i=1}^{n} g_i(x_i)$. Taking the Taylor expansion of both sides of the above equation, products between different variables x_i in the left-hand side must be zero since there are no such terms in the right-hand side.

Table 1: Comparisons between the correlation coefficients ρ (normalized) and the cross-cumulants Γ (unnormalized) of order 4 before and after independent component analysis (ICA). The DEM/USD quotes for September 1995 is divided into 147 sub-sets of 1024 ticks. The results presented here are the median values. The last column is the absolute ratio of before ICA and after ICA. We note that all ratios are greater than 1, indicating that after ICA, the components become more independent.

Components pairs	Cross-Cumulants	Before ICA	After ICA	Absolute ratio
$p_1(t) \sim p_2(t)$	ρ_{12}	0.56	0.14	4.1
	Γ_{13}	2.7e-14	7.8e-17	342.2
	Γ_{22}	-5.6e-15	9.2e-16	6.0
	Γ_{31}	2.0e-11	1.3e-13	148.5
$p_1(t) \sim p_3(t)$	ρ_{13}	0.15	0.03	4.7
	Γ_{13}	2.1e-15	1.6e-17	128.9
	Γ_{22}	-2.0e-15	-4.5e-16	4.5
	Γ_{31}	5.9e-12	6.9e-14	84.5
$p_2(t) \sim p_3(t)$	ρ_{23}	0.17	0.04	4.3
	Γ_{13}	9.1e-16	-5.0e-19	1806.0
	Γ_{22}	1.2e-15	4.9e-17	24.3
	Γ_{31}	3.6e-15	3.0e-17	119.6

We observe the cross-cumulants of order 4:

$$\Gamma_{13} = M_{13} - 3M_{20}M_{11} \tag{7}$$
$$\Gamma_{22} = M_{22} - M_{20}M_{02} - 2M_{11}^2 \tag{8}$$
$$\Gamma_{31} = M_{31} - 3M_{02}M_{11} \tag{9}$$

where $M_{kl} = E\{x_i^k x_j^l\}$ denote the moments of order $k+l$. If x_i and x_j are independent, then their cross-cumulants must be zero (Comon 1994). Table 1 compares the cross-cumulants before and after independent component analysis (ICA) for the DEM/USD in September 1995. For reference, the correlation coefficients before and after ICA are also listed in the table. We see that after ICA, the components have become less correlated and thus more independent.

3.2 Autocorrelation Analysis

Figure 3 depicts the autocorrelation functions of the changes in individual components and compares them to the original returns. We compute the short-run autocorrelations for the lags up to 50. Figure 3 gives the means and standard deviations for September 1995. From the figure, we can see that both the inventory effect component and the original returns show very similar autocorrelation functions, which are dominated by the significant negative, first-order autocorrelations. The mean values for the other orders are basically equal to zero. The autocorrelations of the regular information component and the surprise information component show positive correlations except at first order. These non-zero autocorrelations are hidden by noise in the original series. The autocorrelation function of the surprise information component decays faster than that of the regular information component. On average, it is below the 95% confidence band for lags larger than 20 ticks.

The above autocorrelation analysis suggests the following. (1) Price changes due to the information effects are slightly trending on tick-by-tick time scales. The trend in the surprise information component is shorter term than that in the regular information component.

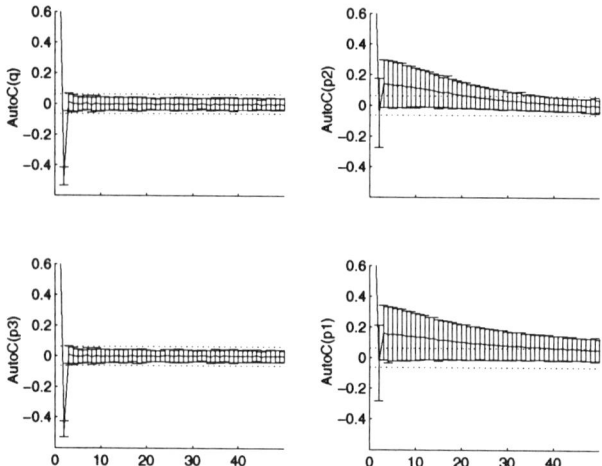

Figure 3: Comparison of autocorrelation functions of the changes in the original observed prices (the upper-left panel), the inventory effect component (the lower-left panel), the regular information component (the upper-right panel) and the surprise information component (the lower-right panel). The results presented are means and standard deviations, and the horizontal dotted lines represent the 95% confidence band. The DEM/USD in September 1995 is divided into 293 sub-sets of 1024 ticks with overlapping of 512 ticks.

(2) The autocorrelation function of original returns reflects only the price changes due to the inventory effect. This further confirms that the existence of short term memory can mislead the analysis of dependence on longer time scales. Subsequently, we can see the usefulness of the multi-effect decomposition. Our empirical results should be viewed as preliminary, since they may depend upon the choice of *True Price* model. Additional studies are ongoing.

4 Conclusion and Discussion

We have developed a neural-net-based independent component analysis (ICA) for the multi-effect decomposition of high frequency financial data. Empirical results with foreign exchange rates have demonstrated that the decomposed components are mutually independent. The obtained regular information component has recovered the trending behavior of the intrinsic price movements.

Potential applications for multi-effect decompositions include:
(1) outlier detection and filtering: Filtering techniques for removing various noisy effects and identifying long term trends have been widely studied (see for example Assimakopoulos (1995)). Multi-effect decompositions provide us with an alternative approach. As demonstrated in Section 3, the regular information component can, in most cases, catch relatively stable and longer term trends originally embedded in the price quotes.
(2) devolatilization: Price series are heteroscedastic (Bollerslev, Chou & Kroner 1992). Devolatilization has been widely studied (see, for example, Zhou (1995)). The regular information component obtained from our multi-effect decomposition appears less volatile, and furthermore, its volatility changes more smoothly compared to the original prices.
(3) mixture of local experts modeling: In most cases, one might be interested in only stable, long term trends of price movements. However, the surprise information and inventory effect components are not totally useless. By decomposing the price series into three mutually

independent components, the prices can be modeled by a mixture of local experts (Jacobs, Jordan & Barto 1990), and better modeling performances can be expected.

References

Amari, S., Cichocki, A. & Yang, H. (1996), A new learning algorithm for blind signal separation, in D. Touretzky, M. Mozer & M. Hasselmo, eds, 'Advances in Neural Information Processing Systems 8', MIT Press: Cambridge, MA.

Assimakopoulos, V. (1995), 'A successive filtering technique for identifying long-term trends', *Journal of Forecasting* **14**, 35–43.

Barlow, H. (1961), Possible principles underlying the transformation of sensory messages, in W. Rosenblith, ed., 'Sensory Communication', MIT Press: Cambridge, MA, pp. 217–234.

Bell, A. & Sejnowski, T. (1995), 'An information-maximization approach to blind separation and blind deconvolution', *Neural Computation* **7**(6), 1129–1159.

Bollerslev, T., Chou, R. & Kroner, K. (1992), 'ARCH modelling in finance: A review of the theory and empirical evidence', *Journal of Econometrics* **8**, 5–59.

Cao, X. & Liu, R. (1996), 'General approach to blind source separation', *IEEE Transactions on Signal Processing* **44**(3), 562–569.

Comon, P. (1994), 'Independent component analysis, a new concept?', *Signal Process* **36**, 287–314.

Guilaumet, D., Dacorogna, M., Dave, R., Muller, U., Olsen, R. & Pictet, O. (1994), From the bird's eye to the microscope, a survey of new stylized facts of the intra-daily foreign exchange markets, Technical Report DMG.1994-04-06, Olsen & Associates, Zurich, Switzerland.

Jacobs, R., Jordan, M. & Barto, A. (1990), Task decomposition through competition in a modular connectionist architecture: The what and where vision tasks, Technical Report COINS 90-27, Department of Brain & Cognitive Sciences, Massachusetts Institute of Technology, Cambridge, MA.

Jutten, C. & Herault, J. (1991), 'Blind separation of sources, part I: An adaptive algorithm based on neuromimetic architecture', *Signal Process* **24**(1), 1–10.

Linsker, R. (1989), An application of the principle of maximum information preservation to linear systems, in D. Touretzky, ed., 'Advances in Neural Information Processing Systems 1', Morgan Kaufmann Publishers, San Francisco, CA.

Mandelbrot, B. (1963), 'The variation of certain speculative prices', *Journal of Business* **36**, 394–419.

Mandelbrot, B. & Van Ness, J. (1968), 'Fractional Brownian motion, fractional noise, and applications', *SIAM Review* **10**.

Moody, J. & Wu, L. (1995), Statistical analysis and forecasting of high frequency foreign exchange rates, in 'The First International Conference on High Frequency Data in Finance', Zurich, Switzerland.

Moody, J. & Wu, L. (1996), What is the 'True Price'? – state space models for high frequency financial data, in S. Amari, L. Xu, L. Chan, I. King & K. Leung, eds, 'Progress in Neural Information Processing (Proceedings of ICONIPS*96, Hong Kong)', Springer-Verlag, Singapore, pp. 697–704, Vol.2.

O'Hara, M. (1995), *Market Microstructure Theory*, Blackwell Business.

Pearlmutter, B. A. & Parra, L. (1997), Maximum likelihood blind source separation: a context-sensitive generalization of ICA, in M. Mozer, M. Jordan & T. Petsche, eds, 'Advances in Neural Information Processing Systems 9', MIT Press: Cambridge, MA.

Widrow, B., Glover, J., McCool, J., Kaunitz, J., Williams, C., Hearn, R., Zeidler, J., Dong, E. & Goodlin, R. (1975), 'Adaptive noise cancelling: principles and applications', *Proceedings of IEEE* **63**(12), 1692–1716.

Wornell, G. & Oppenheim, A. (1992), 'Estimation of fractal signals from noisy measurements using wavelets', *IEEE Transactions on Signal Processing* **40**(3), 611–623.

Zhou, B. (1995), Forecasting foreign exchange rates series subject to de-volatilization, in 'The First International Conference on High Frequency Data in Finance', Zurich, Switzerland.

PART IX
CONTROL, NAVIGATION AND PLANNING

Multidimensional Triangulation and Interpolation for Reinforcement Learning

Scott Davies
scottd@cs.cmu.edu
Department of Computer Science, Carnegie Mellon University
5000 Forbes Ave, Pittsburgh, PA 15213

Abstract

Dynamic Programming, Q-learning and other discrete Markov Decision Process solvers can be applied to continuous d-dimensional state-spaces by quantizing the state space into an array of boxes. This is often problematic above two dimensions: a coarse quantization can lead to poor policies, and fine quantization is too expensive. Possible solutions are variable-resolution discretization, or function approximation by neural nets. A third option, which has been little studied in the reinforcement learning literature, is interpolation on a coarse grid. In this paper we study interpolation techniques that can result in vast improvements in the online behavior of the resulting control systems: multilinear interpolation, and an interpolation algorithm based on an interesting regular triangulation of d-dimensional space. We adapt these interpolators under three reinforcement learning paradigms: (i) offline value iteration with a known model, (ii) Q-learning, and (iii) online value iteration with a previously unknown model learned from data. We describe empirical results, and the resulting implications for practical learning of continuous non-linear dynamic control.

1 GRID-BASED INTERPOLATION TECHNIQUES

Reinforcement learning algorithms generate functions that map states to "cost-to-go" values. When dealing with continuous state spaces these functions must be approximated. The following approximators are frequently used:

- **Fine grids** may be used in one or two dimensions. Above two dimensions, fine grids are too expensive. Value functions can be discontinuous, which (as we will see) can lead to suboptimalities even with very fine discretization in two dimensions.

- **Neural nets** have been used in conjunction with TD [Sutton, 1988] and Q-learning [Watkins, 1989] in very high dimensional spaces [Tesauro, 1991, Crites and Barto, 1996]. While promising, it is not always clear that they produce the accurate value functions that might be needed for fine near-optimal control of dynamic systems, and the most commonly used methods of applying value iteration or policy iteration with a neural-net value function are often unstable. [Boyan and Moore, 1995].

Interpolation over points on a coarse grid is another potentially useful approximator for value functions that has been little studied for reinforcement learning. This paper attempts to rectify this omission. Interpolation schemes may be particularly attractive because they are local *averagers*, and convergence has been proven in such cases for offline value iteration [Gordon, 1995].

All of the interpolation methods discussed here split the state space into a regular grid of d-dimensional boxes; data points are associated with the centers or the corners of the resulting boxes. The value at a given point in the continuous state space is computed as a weighted average of neighboring data points.

1.1 MULTILINEAR INTERPOLATION

When using multilinear interpolation, data points are situated at the corners of the grid's boxes. The interpolated value within a box is an appropriately weighted average of the 2^d datapoints on that box's corners. The weighting scheme assures global continuity of the interpolated surface, and also guarantees that the interpolated value at any grid corner matches the given value of that corner.

In one-dimensional space, multilinear interpolation simply involves piecewise linear interpolations between the data points. In a higher-dimensional space, a recursive (though not terribly efficient) implementation can be described as follows:

- Pick an arbitrary axis. Project the query point along this axis to each of the two opposite faces of the box containing the query point.

- Use two $(d-1)$-dimensional multilinear interpolations over the 2^{d-1} datapoints on each of these two faces to calculate the values at both of these projected points.

- Linearly interpolate between the two values generated in the previous step.

Multilinear interpolation processes 2^d data points for every query, which becomes prohibitively expensive as d increases.

1.2 SIMPLEX-BASED INTERPOLATION

It is possible to interpolate over $d+1$ of the data points for any given query in only $O(d \log d)$ time and still achieve a continuous surface that fits the datapoints exactly. Each box is broken into $d!$ hyperdimensional triangles, or *simplexes*, according to the *Coxeter-Freudenthal-Kuhn* triangulation [Moore, 1992].

Assume that the box is the unit hypercube, with one corner at $(x_1, x_2, \ldots, x_d) = (0, 0, \ldots, 0)$, and the diagonally opposite corner at $(1, 1, \ldots, 1)$. Then, each simplex in the Kuhn triangulation corresponds to one possible permutation p of $(1, 2, \ldots, d)$, and occupies the set of points satisfying the equation

$$0 \leq x_{p(1)} \leq x_{p(2)} \leq \ldots \leq x_{p(d)} \leq 1.$$

Triangulating each box into $d!$ simplexes in this manner generates a *conformal mesh*: any two elements with a $(d-1)$-dimensional surface in common have entire faces in common, which ensures continuity across element boundaries when interpolating.

We use the Kuhn triangulation for interpolation as follows:

- Translate and scale to a coordinate system in which the box containing the query point is the unit hypercube. Let the new coordinate of the query point be $(x'_1, \ldots, x'_d)$.

- Use a sorting algorithm to rank x'_1 through x'_d. This tells us the simplex of the Kuhn triangulation in which the query point lies.

- Express $(x'_1, \ldots, x'_d)$ as a convex combination of the coordinates of the relevant simplex's $(d+1)$ corners.
- Use the coefficients determined in the previous step as the weights for a weighted sum of the data values stored at the corresponding corners.

At no point do we explicitly represent the $d!$ different simplexes. All of the above steps can be performed in $O(d)$ time except the second, which can be done in $O(d \log d)$ time using conventional sorting routines.

2 PROBLEM DOMAINS

CAR ON HILL: In the Hillcar domain, the goal is to park a car near the top of a one-dimensional hill. The hill is steep enough that the driver needs to back up in order to gather enough speed to get to the goal. The state space is two-dimensional (position,velocity). See [Moore and Atkeson, 1995] for further details, but note that our formulation is harder than the usual formulation in that the goal region is restricted to a narrow range of velocities around 0, and trials start at random states. The task is specified by a reward of -1 for any action taken outside the goal region, and 0 inside the goal. No discounting is used, and two actions are available: maximum thrust backwards, and maximum thrust forwards.

ACROBOT: The Acrobot is a two-link planar robot acting in the vertical plane under gravity with a weak actuator at its elbow joint joint. The shoulder is unactuated. The goal is to raise the hand to at least one link's height above the unactuated pivot [Sutton, 1996]. The state space is four-dimensional: two angular positions and two angular velocities. Trials always start from a stationary position hanging straight down. This task is formulated in the same way as the car-on-the-hill. The only actions allowed are the two extreme elbow torques.

3 APPLYING INTERPOLATION: THREE CASES

3.1 CASE I: OFFLINE VALUE ITERATION WITH A KNOWN MODEL

First, we precalculate the effect of taking each possible action from each state corresponding to a datapoint in the grid. Then, as suggested in [Gordon, 1995], we use these calculations to derive a *completely discrete* MDP. Taking any action from any state in this MDP results in c possible successor states, where c is the number of datapoints used per interpolation. Without interpolation, c is 1; with multilinear interpolation, 2^d; with simplex-based interpolation, $d+1$.

We calculate the optimal policy for this derived MDP offline using *value iteration* [Ross, 1983]; because the value iteration can be performed on a completely discrete MDP, the calculations are much less computationally expensive than they would have been with many other kinds of function approximators. The value iteration gives us values for the datapoints of our grid, which we may then use to interpolate the values at other states during online control.

3.1.1 Hillcar Results: value iteration with known model

We tested the two interpolation methods on a variety of quantization levels by first performing value iteration offline, and then starting the car from 1000 random states and averaging the number of steps taken to the goal from those states. We also recorded the number of backups required before convergence, as well as the execution time required for the entire value iteration on a 85 MHz Sparc 5. See Figure 1 for the results. All steps-to-goal values are means with an expected error of 2 steps.

Interpolation Method	Grid size			
	11^2	21^2	51^2	301^2
None				
Steps to Goal:	237	131	133	120
Backups:	2.42K	15.4K	156K	14.3M
Time (sec):	0.4	1.0	4.1	192
MultiLin				
Steps to Goal:	134	116	108	107
Backups:	4.84K	18.1K	205K	17.8M
Time (sec):	0.6	1.3	7.1	405
Simplex				
Steps to Goal:	134	118	109	107
Backups:	6.17K	18.1K	195K	17.9M
Time (sec):	0.5	1.2	5.7	328

Figure 1: Hillcar: value iteration with known model

Interpolation Method	Grid size							
	8^4	9^4	10^4	11^4	12^4	13^4	14^4	15^4
None								
Steps to Goal:	-	-	44089	-	26952	-	> 100000	-
Backups:	-	-	280K	-	622K	-	1.42M	-
Time (sec):	-	-	15	-	30	-	53	-
MultiLin								
Steps to Goal:	3340	2006	1136	3209	1300	1820	1518	1802
Backups:	233K	1.01M	730K	2.01M	2.03M	3.74M	4.45M	6.78M
Time (sec):	17	43	42	83	99	164	197	284
Simplex								
Steps to Goal:	4700	8007	2953	3209	4663	2733	1742	9613
Backups:	196K	1.16M	590K	2.28M	1.62M	4.03M	3.65M	6.73M
Time (sec):	9	24	22	47	47	86	93	142

Figure 2: Acrobot: value iteration with known model

The interpolated functions require more backups for convergence, but this is amply compensated by dramatic improvement in the policy. Surprisingly, both interpolation methods provide improvements even at extremely high grid resolutions – the noninterpolated grid with 301 datapoints along each axis fared no better than the interpolated grids with only 21 datapoints along each axis(!).

3.1.2 Acrobot Results: value iteration with known model

We used the same value iteration algorithm in the acrobot domain. In this case our test trials always began from the same start state, but we ran tests for a larger set of grid sizes (Figure 2).

Grids with different resolutions place grid cell boundaries at different locations, and these boundary locations appear to be important in this problem — the performance varies unpredictably as the grid resolution changes. However, in all cases, interpolation was necessary to arrive at a satisfactory solution; without interpolation, the value iteration often failed to converge at all. With relatively coarse grids it may be that any trajectory to the goal passes through some grid box more than once, which would immediately spell disaster for any algorithm associating a constant value over that entire grid box.

Controllers using multilinear interpolation consistently fared better than those employing the simplex-based interpolation; the smoother value function provided by multilinear interpolation seems to help. However, value iteration with the simplex-based interpolation was about twice as fast as that with multilinear interpolation. In higher dimensions this speed ratio will increase.

3.2 CASE II: Q-LEARNING

Under a second reinforcement learning paradigm, we do not use any model. Rather, we learn a *Q-function* that directly maps state-action pairs to long-term rewards [Watkins, 1989]. Does interpolation help here too?

In this implementation we encourage exploration by optimistically initializing the Q-function to zero everywhere. After travelling a sufficient distance from our last decision point, we perform a single backup by changing the grid point values according to a perceptron-like update rule, and then we greedily select the action for which the interpolated Q-function is highest at the current state.

3.2.1 Hillcar Results: Q-Learning

We used Q-Learning with a grid size of 11^2. Figure 3 shows learning curves for three learners using the three different interpolation techniques.

Both interpolation methods provided a significant improvement in both initial and final online performance. The learner without interpolation achieved a final average performance of about 175 steps to the goal; with multilinear interpolation, 119; with simplex-based interpolation, 122. Note that these are all significant improvements over the corresponding results for offline value iteration with a known model. Inaccuracies in the interpolated functions often cause controllers to enter cycles; because the Q-learning backups are being performed online, however, the Q-learning controller can escape from these control cycles by depressing the Q-values in the vicinities of such cycles.

3.2.2 Acrobot Results: Q-Learning

We used the same algorithms on the acrobot domain with a grid size of 15^4; results are shown in Figure 3.

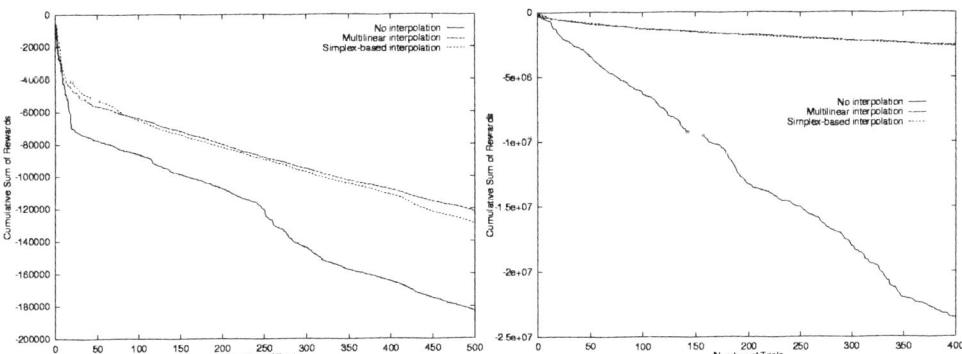

Figure 3: Left: Cumulative performance of Q-learning hillcar on an 11^2 grid. (Multilinear interpolation comes out on top; no interpolation on the bottom.) Right: Q-learning acrobot on a 15^4 grid. (The two interpolations come out on top with nearly identical performance.) For each learner, the y-axis shows the sum of rewards for all trials to date. The better the average performance, the shallower the gradient. Gradients are always negative because each state transition before reaching the goal results in a reward of -1.

Both Q-learners using interpolation improved rapidly, and eventually reached the goal in a relatively small number of steps per trial. The learner using multilinear interpolation eventually achieved an average of 1,529 steps to the goal per trial; the learner using simplex-based interpolation achieved 1,727 steps per trial. On the other hand, the learner not using any interpolation fared much worse, taking an average of more than 27,000 steps per trial. (A controller that chooses actions randomly typically takes about the same number of steps to reach the goal.)

Simplex-based interpolation provided on-line performance very close to that provided by multilinear interpolation, but at roughly half the computational cost.

3.3 CASE III: VALUE ITERATION WITH MODEL LEARNING

Here, we use a model of the system, but we do not assume that we have one to start with. Instead, we learn a model of the system as we interact with it; we assume this model is adequate and calculate a value function via the same algorithms we would use if we knew the true model. This approach may be particularly beneficial for tasks in which data is expensive and computation is cheap. Here, models are learned using very simple grid-based function approximators without interpolation for both the reward and transition functions of the model. The same grid resolution is used for the value function grid and the model approximator. We strongly encourage exploration by initializing the model so that every state is initially assumed to be an absorbing state with zero reward.

While making transitions through the state space, we update the model and use prioritized sweeping [Moore and Atkeson, 1993] to concentrate backups on relevant parts of the state space. We also occasionally stop to recalculate the effects of all actions under the updated model and then run value iteration to convergence. As this is fairly time-consuming, it is done rather rarely; we rely on the updates performed by prioritized sweeping to guide the system in the meantime.

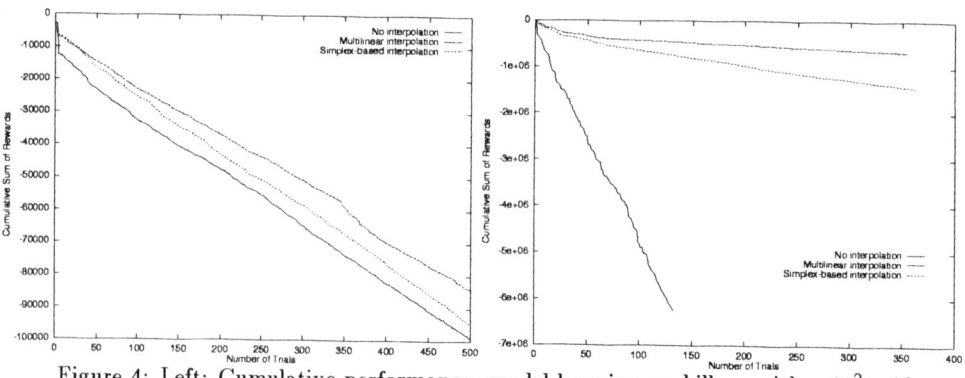

Figure 4: Left: Cumulative performance, model-learning on hillcar with a 11^2 grid. Right: Acrobot with a 15^4 grid. In both cases, multilinear interpolation comes out on top, while no interpolation winds up on the bottom.

3.3.1 Hillcar Results: value iteration with learned model

We used the algorithm described above with an 11-by-11 grid. An average of about two prioritized sweeping backups were performed per transition; the complete recalculations were performed every 1000 steps throughout the first two trials and every 5000 steps thereafter. Figure 4 shows the results for the first 500 trials.

Over the first 500 trials, the learner using simplex-based interpolation didn't fare much better than the learner using no interpolation. However, its performance on trials 1500-2500 (not shown) was close to that of the learner using multilinear interpolation, taking an average of 151 steps to the goal per trial while the learner using multilinear interpolation took 147. The learner using no interpolation did significantly worse than the others in these later trials, taking 175 steps per trial.

The model-learners' performance improved more quickly than the Q-learners' over the first few trials; on the other hand, their final performance was significantly worse that the Q-learners'.

3.3.2 Acrobot Results: value iteration with learned model

We used the same algorithm with a 15^4 grid on the acrobot domain, this time performing the complete recalculations every 10000 steps through the first two trials and every 50000 thereafter. Figure 4 shows the results. In this case, the learner using no interpolation took so much time per trial that the experiment was aborted early; after 100 trials, it was still taking an average of more than 45,000 steps to reach the goal. The learners using interpolation, however, fared much better. The learner using multilinear interpolation converged to a solution taking 938 steps per trial; the learner using simplex-based interpolation averaged about 2450 steps. Again, as the graphs show, these three learners initially improve significantly faster than did the Q-Learners using similar grid sizes.

4 CONCLUSIONS

We have shown how two interpolation schemes—one based on a weighted average of the 2^d points in a square cell, the other on a d-dimensional triangulation—may be used in three reinforcement learning paradigms: Optimal policy computation with a known model, Q-learning, and online value iteration while learning a model. In each case our empirical studies demonstrate interpolation resoundingly decreasing the quantization level necessary for a satisfactory solution. Future extensions of this research will explore the use of variable resolution grids and triangulations, multiple low-dimensional interpolations in place of one high-dimension interpolation in a manner reminiscent of CMAC [Albus, 1981], memory-based approximators, and more intelligent exploration.

This research was funded in part by a National Science Foundation Graduate Fellowship to Scott Davies, and a Research Initiation Award to Andrew Moore.

References

[Albus, 1981] J. S. Albus. *Brains, Behaviour and Robotics*. BYTE Books, McGraw-Hill, 1981.

[Boyan and Moore, 1995] J. A. Boyan and A. W. Moore. Generalization in Reinforcement Learning: Safely Approximating the Value Function. In *Neural Information Processing Systems 7*, 1995.

[Crites and Barto, 1996] R. H. Crites and A. G. Barto. Improving Elevator Performance using Reinforcement Learning. In D. Touretzky, M. Mozer, and M. Hasselmo, editors, *Neural Information Processing Systems 8*, 1996.

[Gordon, 1995] G. Gordon. Stable Function Approximation in Dynamic Programming. In *Proceedings of the 12th International Conference on Machine Learning*. Morgan Kaufmann, June 1995.

[Moore and Atkeson, 1993] A. W. Moore and C. G. Atkeson. Prioritized Sweeping: Reinforcement Learning with Less Data and Less Real Time. *Machine Learning*, 13, 1993.

[Moore and Atkeson, 1995] A. W. Moore and C. G. Atkeson. The Parti-game Algorithm for Variable Resolution Reinforcement Learning in Multidimensional State-spaces. *Machine Learning*, 21, 1995.

[Moore, 1992] D. W. Moore. Simplical Mesh Generation with Applications. PhD. Thesis. Report no. 92-1322, Cornell University, 1992.

[Ross, 1983] S. Ross. *Introduction to Stochastic Dynamic Programming*. Academic Press, New York, 1983.

[Sutton, 1988] R. S. Sutton. Learning to Predict by the Methods of Temporal Differences. *Machine Learning*, 3:9–44, 1988.

[Sutton, 1996] R. S. Sutton. Generalization in Reinforcement Learning: Successful Examples Using Sparse Coarse Coding. In D. Touretzky, M. Mozer, and M. Hasselmo, editors, *Neural Information Processing Systems 8*, 1996.

[Tesauro, 1991] G. J. Tesauro. Practical Issues in Temporal Difference Learning. RC 17223 (76307), IBM T. J. Watson Research Center, NY, 1991.

[Watkins, 1989] C. J. C. H. Watkins. Learning from Delayed Rewards. PhD. Thesis, King's College, University of Cambridge, May 1989.

Efficient Nonlinear Control with Actor-Tutor Architecture

Kenji Doya*
ATR Human Information Processing Research Laboratories
2-2 Hikaridai, Seika-cho, Soraku-gun, Kyoto 619-02, Japan.

Abstract

A new reinforcement learning architecture for nonlinear control is proposed. A direct feedback controller, or the actor, is trained by a value-gradient based controller, or the tutor. This architecture enables both efficient use of the value function and simple computation for real-time implementation. Good performance was verified in multi-dimensional nonlinear control tasks using Gaussian softmax networks.

1 INTRODUCTION

In the study of temporal difference (TD) learning in continuous time and space (Doya, 1996b), an optimal nonlinear feedback control law was derived using the gradient of the value function and the local linear model of the system dynamics. It was demonstrated in the simulation of a pendulum swing-up task that the value-gradient based control scheme requires much less learning trials than the conventional "actor-critic" control scheme (Barto et al., 1983).

In the actor-critic scheme, the actor, a direct feedback controller, improves its control policy stochastically using the TD error as the effective reinforcement (Figure 1a). Despite its relatively slow learning, the actor-critic architecture has the virtue of simple computation in generating control command. In order to train a direct controller while making efficient use of the value function, we propose a new reinforcement learning scheme which we call the "actor-tutor" architecture (Figure 1b).

---

*Current address: Kawato Dynamic Brain Project, JSTC. 2-2 Hikaridai, Seika-cho, Soraku-gun, Kyoto 619-02, Japan. E-mail: doya@erato.atr.co.jp

In the actor-tutor scheme, the optimal control command based on the current estimate of the value function is used as the target output of the actor. With the use of supervised learning algorithms (e.g., LMSE), learning of the actor is expected to be faster than in the actor-critic scheme, which uses stochastic search algorithms (e.g., A_{RP}). The simulation result below confirms this prediction. This hybrid control architecture provides a model of functional integration of motor-related brain areas, especially the basal ganglia and the cerebellum (Doya, 1996a).

2 CONTINUOUS TD LEARNING

First, we summarize the theory of TD learning in continuous time and space (Doya, 1996b), which is basic to the derivation of the proposed control scheme.

2.1 CONTINUOUS TD ERROR

Let us consider a continuous-time, continuous-state dynamical system

$$\frac{d\mathbf{x}(t)}{dt} = f(\mathbf{x}(t), \mathbf{u}(t)) \tag{1}$$

where $\mathbf{x} \in X \subset \mathbf{R}^n$ is the state and $\mathbf{u} \in U \subset \mathbf{R}^m$ is the control input (or the action). The reinforcement is given as the function of the state and the control

$$r(t) = r(\mathbf{x}(t), \mathbf{u}(t)). \tag{2}$$

For a given control law (or a policy)

$$\mathbf{u}(t) = \mu(\mathbf{x}(t)), \tag{3}$$

we define the "value function" of the state $\mathbf{x}(t)$ as

$$V^\mu(\mathbf{x}(t)) = \int_t^\infty \frac{1}{\tau} e^{-\frac{s-t}{\tau}} r(\mathbf{x}(s), \mathbf{u}(s)) ds, \tag{4}$$

where $\mathbf{x}(s)$ and $\mathbf{u}(s)$ ($t \le s < \infty$) follow the system dynamics (1) and the control law (3). Our goal is to find an optimal control law μ^* that maximizes $V^\mu(\mathbf{x})$ for any state $\mathbf{x} \in X$. Note that τ is the time constant of imminence-weighting, which is related to the discount factor γ of the discrete-time TD as $\gamma = 1 - \frac{\Delta t}{\tau}$.

By differentiating (4) by t, we have a local consistency condition for the value function

$$\tau \frac{d}{dt} V^\mu(\mathbf{x}(t)) = V^\mu(\mathbf{x}(t)) - r(t). \tag{5}$$

Let $P(\mathbf{x}(t))$ be the prediction of the value function $V^\mu(\mathbf{x}(t))$ from $\mathbf{x}(t)$ by a neural network, or some function approximator that has enough capability of generalization. The prediction should be adjusted to minimize the inconsistency

$$\hat{r}(t) = r(t) - P(\mathbf{x}(t)) + \tau \frac{dP(\mathbf{x}(t))}{dt}, \tag{6}$$

which is a continuous version of the TD error. Because the boundary condition for the value function is given on the attractor set of the state space, correction of $P(\mathbf{x}(t))$ should be made backward into time. The correspondence between continuous-time TD algorithms and discrete-time TD(λ) algorithms (Sutton, 1988) is shown in (Doya, 1996b).

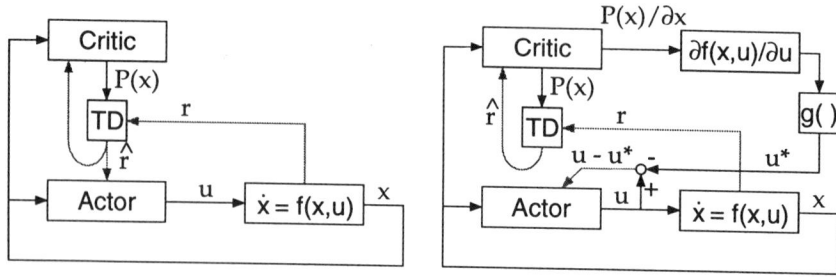

Figure 1: (a) Actor-critic (b) Actor-tutor

2.2 OPTIMAL CONTROL BY VALUE GRADIENT

According to the principle of dynamic programming (Bryson and Ho, 1975), the local constraint for the value function V^* for the optimal control law μ^* is given by the Hamilton-Jacobi-Bellman equation

$$V^*(t) = \max_{\mathbf{u}(t) \in U} \left[r(\mathbf{x}(t), \mathbf{u}(t)) + \tau \frac{\partial V^*(\mathbf{x}(t))}{\partial \mathbf{x}} f(\mathbf{x}(t), \mathbf{u}(t)) \right]. \tag{7}$$

The optimal control μ^* is given by solving the maximization problem in the HJB equation, i.e.,

$$\frac{\partial r(\mathbf{x}, \mathbf{u})}{\partial \mathbf{u}} + \tau \frac{\partial V^*(\mathbf{x})}{\partial \mathbf{x}} \frac{\partial f(\mathbf{x}, \mathbf{u})}{\partial \mathbf{u}} = 0. \tag{8}$$

When the cost for each control variable is given by a convex potential function $G_j()$

$$r(\mathbf{x}, \mathbf{u}) = R(\mathbf{x}) - \sum_j G_j(u_j), \tag{9}$$

equation (8) can be solved using a monotonic function $g_j(x) = (G'_j)^{-1}(x)$ as

$$u_j = g_j \left(\tau \frac{\partial V^*(\mathbf{x})}{\partial \mathbf{x}} \frac{\partial f(\mathbf{x}, \mathbf{u})}{\partial u_j} \right). \tag{10}$$

If the system is linear with respect to the input, which is the case with many mechanical systems, $\partial f(\mathbf{x}, \mathbf{u})/\partial u_j$ is independent of $\mathbf{u}$ and the above equation gives a closed-form optimal feedback control law $\mathbf{u} = \mu^*(\mathbf{x})$.

In practice, the optimal value function is unknown and we replace $V^*(\mathbf{x})$ with the current estimate of the value function $P(\mathbf{x})$

$$\mathbf{u} = g \left(\tau \frac{\partial P(\mathbf{x})}{\partial \mathbf{x}} \frac{\partial f(\mathbf{x}, \mathbf{u})}{\partial \mathbf{u}} \right). \tag{11}$$

While the system evolves with the above control law, the value function $P(\mathbf{x})$ is updated to minimize the TD error (6). In (11), the vector $\partial P(\mathbf{x})/\partial \mathbf{x}$ represents the desired motion direction in the state space and the matrix $\partial f(\mathbf{x}, \mathbf{u})/\partial \mathbf{u}$ transforms it into the action space. The function g, which is specified by the control cost, determines the amplitude of control output. For example, if the control cost G is quadratic, then (11) reduces to a linear feedback control. A practically important case is when g is a sigmoid, because this gives a feedback control law for a system with limited control amplitude, as in the examples below.

3 ACTOR-TUTOR ARCHITECTURE

It was shown in a task of a pendulum swing-up with limited torque (Doya, 1996b) that the above value-gradient based control scheme (11 can learn the task in much less trials than the actor-critic scheme. However, computation of the feedback command by (11) requires an on-line calculation of the gradient of the value function $\partial P(\mathbf{x})/\partial \mathbf{x}$ and its multiplication with the local linear model of the system dynamics $\partial f(\mathbf{x}, \mathbf{u})/\partial \mathbf{u}$, which can be too demanding for real-time implementation.

One solution to this problem is to use a simple direct controller network, as in the case of the actor-critic architecture. The training of the direct controller, or the actor, can be performed by supervised learning instead of trial-and-error learning because the target output of the controller is explicitly given by (11). Although computation of the target output may involve a processing time that is not acceptable for immediate feedback control, it is still possible to use its output for training the direct controller provided that there is some mechanism of short-term memory (e.g., eligibility trace in the connection weights).

Figure 1(b) is a schematic diagram of this "actor-tutor" architecture. The critic monitors the performance of the actor and estimates the value function. The "tutor" is a cascade of the critic, its gradient estimator, the local linear model of the system, and the differential model of control cost. The actor is trained to minimize the difference between its output and the tutor's output.

4 SIMULATION

We tested the performance of the actor-tutor architecture in two nonlinear control tasks; a pendulum swing-up task (Doya, 1996b) and the global version of a cart-pole balancing task (Barto et al., 1983).

The network architecture we used for both the actor and the critic was a Gaussian soft-max network. The output of the network is given by

$$y = \sum_{k=1}^{K} w_k b_k(\mathbf{x}),$$

$$b_k(\mathbf{x}) = \frac{\exp[-\sum_{i=1}^{n}(\frac{x_i - c_{ki}}{s_{ki}})^2]}{\sum_{l=1}^{K} \exp[-\sum_{i=1}^{n}(\frac{x_i - c_{li}}{s_{li}})^2]},$$

where $(c_{k1}, ..., c_{kn})$ and $(s_{k1}, ..., s_{kn})$ are the center and the size of the k-th basis function. It is in general possible to adjust the centers and sizes of the basis function, but in order to assure predictable transient behaviors, we fixed them in a grid. In this case, computation can be drastically reduced by factorizing the activation of basis functions in each input dimension.

4.1 PENDULUM SWING-UP TASK

The first task was to swing up a pendulum with a limited torque $|T| \leq T^{\max}$, which was about one fifth of the torque that was required to statically bring the pendulum up (Figure 2 (a)). This is a nonlinear control task in which the controller has to swing the pendulum several times at the bottom to build up enough momentum.

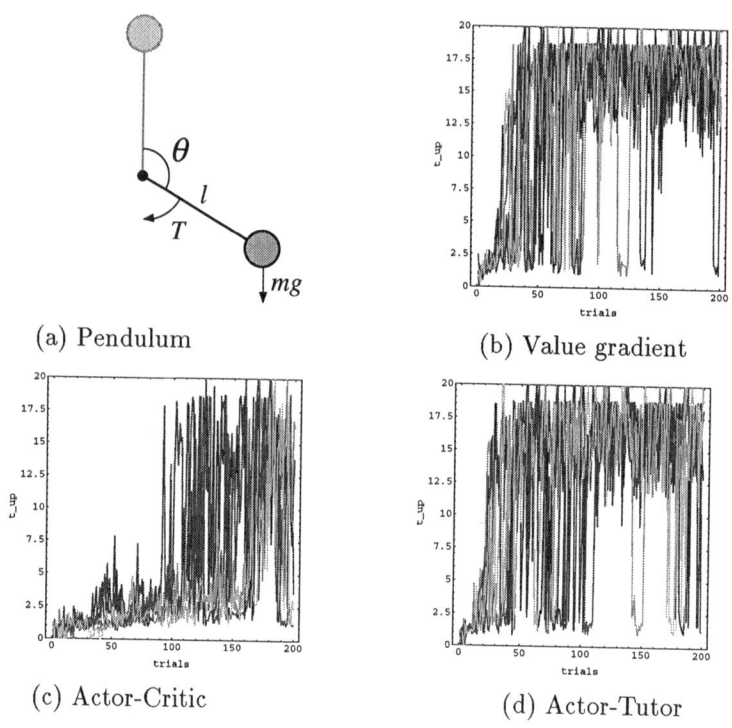

Figure 2: Pendulum swing-up task. The dynamics of the pendulum (a) is given by $ml\ddot{\theta} = -\mu\dot{\theta} + mgl\sin\theta + T$. The parameters were $m = l = 1$, $g = 9.8$, $\mu = 0.01$, and $T^{\max} = 2.0$. The learning curves for value-gradient based optimal control (b), actor-critic (c), and actor-tutor (d); t_up is time during which $|\theta| < 45°$.

The state space for the pendulum $\mathbf{x} = (\theta, \omega)$ was 2D and we used 12×12 basis functions to cover the range $|\theta| \leq 180°$ and $|\omega| \leq 180°/s$. The reinforcement for the state was given by the height of the tip of the pendulum, i.e., $R(\mathbf{x}) = \cos\theta$ and the cost for control G and the corresponding output sigmoid function g were selected to match the maximal output torque $T^{\max}$.

Figures 2 (b), (c), and (d) show the learning curves for the value-gradient based control (11), actor critic, and actor-tutor control schemes, respectively. As we expected, the learning of the actor-tutor was much faster than that of the actor-critic and was comparable to the value-gradient based optimal control schemes.

4.2 CART-POLE SWING-UP TASK

Next we tested the learning scheme in a higher-dimensional nonlinear control task, namely, a cart-pole swing-up task (Figure 3). In the pioneering work of , the actor-critic system successfully learned the task of balancing the pole within $\pm 12°$ of the upright position while avoiding collision with the end of the cart track. The task we chose was to swing up the pole from an arbitrary angle and to balance it upright. The physical parameters of the cart-pole were the same as in (Barto et al., 1983) except that the length of the track was doubled to provide enough room for swinging.

Efficient Nonlinear Control with Actor-Tutor Architecture

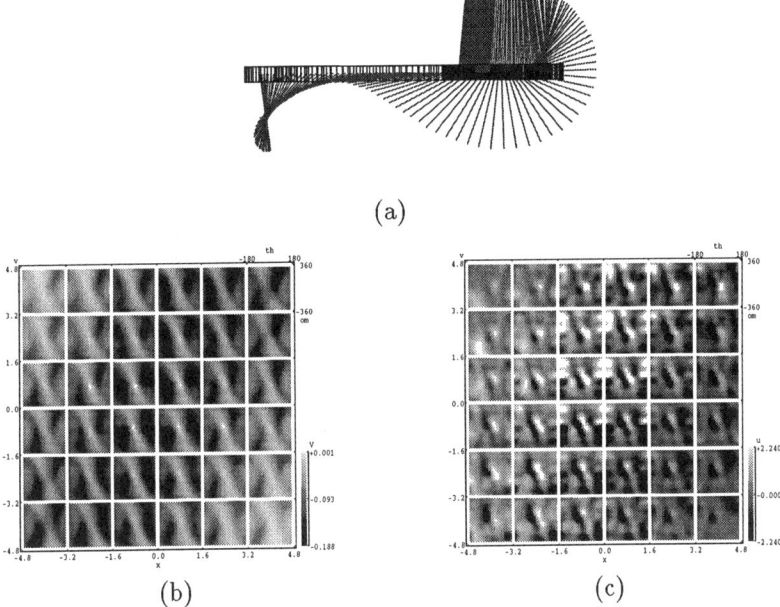

Figure 3: Cart-pole swing-up task. (a) An example of a swing-up trajectory. (b) Value function learned by the critic. (c) Feedback force learned by the actor. Each square in the plot shows a slice of the 4D state space parallel to the (θ, ω) plane.

Figure 3 (a) shows an example of a successful swing up after 1500 learning trials with the actor-tutor architecture. We could not achieve a comparable performance with the actor-critic scheme within 3000 learning trials. Figures 3 (b) and (c) show the value function and the feedback force field, respectively, in the 4D state space $\mathbf{x} = (x, v, \theta, \omega)$, which were implemented in $6 \times 6 \times 12 \times 12$ Gaussian soft-max networks. We imposed symmetric constraints on both actor and critic networks to facilitate generalization. It can be seen that the paths to the upright position in the center of the track are represented as ridges in the value function.

5 DISCUSSION

The biggest problem in applying TD or DP to real-world control tasks is the curse of dimensionality, which makes both the computation for each data point and the numbers of data points necessary for training very high. The actor-tutor architecture provides a partial solution to the former problem in real-time implementation. The grid-based Gaussian soft-max basis function network was successfully used in a 4D state space. However, a more flexible algorithm that allocates basis functions only in the relevant parts of the state space may be necessary for dealing with higher-dimension systems (Schaal and Atkeson, 1996).

In the above simulations, we assumed that the local linear model of the system dynamics $\partial f(\mathbf{x}, \mathbf{u})/\partial \mathbf{u}$ was available. In preliminary experiments, it was verified that the critic, the system model, and the actor can be trained simultaneously.

The actor-tutor architecture resembles "feedback error learning" (Kawato et al., 1987) in the sense that a nonlinear controller is trained by the output of anther controller. However, the actor-tutor scheme can be applied to a highly nonlinear control task to which it is difficult to prepare a simple linear feedback controller.

Motivated by the performance of the actor-tutor architecture and the recent physiological and fMRI experiments on the brain activity during the course of motor learning (Hikosaka et al., 1996; Imamizu et al., 1996), we proposed a framework of functional integration of the basal ganglia, the cerebellum, and cerebral motor areas (Doya, 1996a). In this framework, the basal ganglia learns the value function $P(\mathbf{x})$ (Houk et al., 1994) and generates the desired motion direction based on its gradient $\partial P(\mathbf{x})/\partial \mathbf{x}$. This is transformed into a motor command by the "transpose model" of the motor system $(\partial f(\mathbf{x}, \mathbf{u})/\partial \mathbf{u})^T$ in the lateral cerebellum (cerebrocerebellum). In early stages of learning, this output is used for control, albeit its feedback latency is long. As the subject repeats the same task, a direct controller is constructed in the medial and intermediate cerebellum (spinocerebellum) with the above motor command as the teacher. The direct controller enables quick, near-automatic performance with less cognitive load in other parts of the brain.

References

Barto, A. G., Sutton, R. S., and Anderson, C. W. (1983). Neuronlike adaptive elements that can solve difficult learning control problems. *IEEE Transactions on Systems, Man, and Cybernetics*, 13:834–846.

Bryson, Jr., A. E. . and Ho, Y.-C. (1975). *Applied Optimal Control*. Hemisphere Publishing, New York, 2nd edition.

Doya, K. (1996a). An integrated model of basal ganglia and cerebellum in sequential control tasks. *Society for Neuroscience Abstracts*, 22:2029.

Doya, K. (1996b). Temporal difference learning in continuous time and space. In Touretzky, D. S., Mozer, M. C., and Hasselmo, M. E., editors, *Advances in Neural Information Processing Systems 8*, pages 1073–1079. MIT Press, Cambridge, MA.

Hikosaka, O., Miyachi, S., Miyashita, K., and Rand, M. K. (1996). Procedural learning in monkeys — Possible roles of the basal ganglia. In Ono, T., McNaughton, B. L., Molotchnikoff, S., Rolls, E. T., and Nishijo, H., editors, *Perception, Memory and Emotion: Frontiers in Neuroscience*, pages 403–420. Pergamon, Oxford.

Houk, J. C., Adams, J. L., and Barto, A. G. (1994). A model of how the basal ganglia generate and use neural signals that predict reinforcement. In Houk, J. C., Davis, J. L., and Beiser, D. G., editors, *Models of Information Processing in the Basal Ganglia*, pages 249–270. MIT Press, Cambrigde, MA.

Imamizu, H., Miyauchi, S., Sasaki, Y., Takino, R., Putz, B., and Kawato, M. (1996). A functional MRI study on internal models of dynamic transformations during learning a visuomotor task. *Society for Neuroscience Abstracts*, 22:898.

Kawato, M., Furukawa, K., and Suzuki, R. (1987). A hierarchical neural network model for control and learning of voluntary movement. *Biological Cybernetics*, 57:169–185.

Schaal, S. and Atkeson, C. C. (1996). From isolation to cooperation: An alternative view of a system of experts. In Touretzky, D. S., Mozer, M. C., and Hasselmo, M. E., editors, *Advances in Neural Information Processing Systems 8*, pages 605–611. MIT Press, Cambridge, MA, USA.

Sutton, R. S. (1988). Learning to predict by the methods of temporal difference. *Machine Learning*, 3:9–44.

Local Bandit Approximation for Optimal Learning Problems

Michael O. Duff Andrew G. Barto
Department of Computer Science
University of Massachusetts
Amherst, MA 01003
{duff,barto}@cs.umass.edu

Abstract

In general, procedures for determining Bayes-optimal adaptive controls for Markov decision processes (MDP's) require a prohibitive amount of computation—the optimal learning problem is intractable. This paper proposes an approximate approach in which bandit processes are used to model, in a certain "local" sense, a given MDP. Bandit processes constitute an important subclass of MDP's, and have optimal learning strategies (defined in terms of Gittins indices) that can be computed relatively efficiently. Thus, one scheme for achieving approximately-optimal learning for general MDP's proceeds by taking actions suggested by strategies that are optimal with respect to local bandit models.

1 INTRODUCTION

Watkins [1989] has defined *optimal learning* as: "... the process of collecting and using information during learning in an optimal manner, so that the learner makes the best possible decisions at all stages of learning: learning itself is regarded as a multistage decision process, and learning is optimal if the learner adopts a strategy that will yield the highest possible return from actions over the whole course of learning."

For example, suppose a decision-maker is presented with two biased coins (the decision-maker does not know precisely how the coins are biased) and asked to allocate twenty flips between them so as to maximize the number of observed heads. Although the decision-maker is certainly interested in determining which coin has a higher probability of heads, his principle concern is with optimizing performance *en route* to this determination. An optimal learning strategy typically intersperses "exploitation" steps, in which the coin currently thought to have the highest proba-

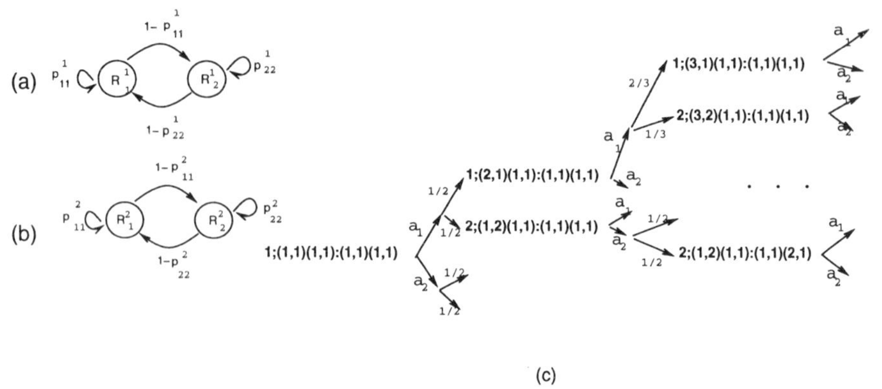

Figure 1: A simple example: dynamics/rewards under (a) action 1 and (b) action 2. (c) The decision problem in hyperstate space.

bility of heads is flipped, with "exploration" steps in which, on the basis of observed flips, a coin that would be deemed inferior is flipped anyway to further resolve its true potential for turning up heads. The coin-flip problem is a simple example of a (two-armed) *bandit problem*. A key feature of these problems, and of adaptive control processes in general, is the so-called "exploration-versus-exploitation trade-off" (or problem of "dual control" [Fel'dbaum, 1965]).

As an another example, consider the MDP depicted in Figures 1(a) and (b). This is a 2-state/2-action process; transition probabilities label arcs, and quantities within circles denote expected rewards for taking particular actions in particular states. The goal is to assign actions to states so as to maximize, say, the expected infinite horizon discounted sum of rewards (the value function) over all states. For the case considered in this paper, the transition probabilites are not known. Given that the process is in some state, one action may be optimal with respect to currently-perceived point-estimates of unknown parameters, while another action may result in greater information gain. Optimal learning is concerned with striking a balance between these two criteria.

While reinforcement learning approaches *have* recognized the dual-effects of control, at least in the sense that one must occasionally deviate from a greedy policy to ensure a search of sufficient breadth, many exploration procedures appear not to be motivated by real notions of optimal learning; rather, they aspire to be practical schemes for avoiding unrealistic levels of sampling and search that would be required if one were to strictly adhere to the theoretical sufficient conditions for convergence—that all state-action pairs must be considered infinitely many times.

If one is willing to adopt a Bayesian perspective, then the exploration-versus-exploitation issue has already been resolved, in principle. A solution was recognized by Bellman and Kalaba nearly fo rty years ago [Bellman & Kalaba, 1959]; their dynamic programming algorithm for computing Bayes-optimal policies begins by regarding "state" as an ordered pair, or "hyperstate," $(x, \mathcal{I})$, where x is a point in phase-space (Markov-chain state) and $\mathcal{I}$ is the "information pattern," which summarizes past history as it relates to modeling the transitional dynamics of x. Computation grows increasingly burdensome with problem size, however, so one is compelled to seek approximate solutions, some of which ignore the effects of information gain entirely. In contrast, the approach suggested in this paper explicitly acknowledges that there is an information-gain component to the optimal learning problem; if certain salient aspects of the value of information can be captured, even approximately, then one may be led to a reasonable method for approximating optimal learning policies.

Here is the basic idea behind the approach suggested in this paper: First note that there exists a special class of problems, namely multi-armed bandit problems, in which the information pattern is the sole component of the hyperstate. These special problems have the important feature that their optimal policies can be defined concisely in terms of "Gittins indices," and these indices can be computed in a relatively efficient way. This paper is an attempt to make use of the fact that this special subclass of MDP's has tractably-computable optimal learning strategies. Actions for general MDP's are derived by, first, attaching to a given general MDP in a given state a "local" n-armed bandit process that captures some aspect of the value of information gain as well as explicit reward. Indices for the local bandit model can be computed relatively efficiently; the largest index suggests the best action in an optimal-learning sense. The resulting algorithm has a receding-horizon flavor in that a new local-bandit process is constructed after each transition; it makes use of a mean-process model as in some previously-suggested approximation schemes, but here the value of information gain is explicitly taken into account, in part, through index calculations.

2 THE BAYES-BELLMAN APPROACH FOR ADAPTIVE MDP'S

Consider the two-state, two-action process shown in Figure 1, and suppose that one is uncertain about the transition probabilities. If the process is in a given state and an action is taken, then the result is that the process either stays in the state it is in or jumps to the other state—one observes a Bernoulli process with unknown parameter—just as in the coin-flip example. But in this case one observes *four* Bernoulli processes: the result of taking action 1 in state 1, action 1 in state 2, action 2 in state 1, action 2 in state 2. So if the prior probability for staying in the current state, for each of these state-action pairs, is represented by a beta distribution (the appropriate conjugate family of distributions with regard to Bernoulli sampling; i.e., a Bayesian update of a beta prior remains beta), then one may perform dynamic programming in a space of "hyperstates," in which the components are four pairs of parameters specifying the beta distributions describing the uncertainty in the transition probabilities, along with the Markov chain state: $\langle x, (\alpha_1^1, \beta_1^1), (\alpha_2^1, \beta_2^1)(\alpha_1^2, \beta_1^2), (\alpha_2^2, \beta_2^2)\rangle$, where for example (α_1^1, β_1^1) denotes the parmeters specifying the beta distribution that represents uncertainty in the transition probability p_{11}^1. Figure 1(c) shows part of the associated decision tree; an optimality equation may be written in terms of the hyperstates. MDP's with more than two states pose no special problem (there exists an appropriate generalization of the beta distribution). What *is* a problem is what Bellman calls the "problem of the expanding grid:" the number of hyperstates that must be examined grows exponentially with the horizon.

How does one proceed if one is constrained to practical amounts of computation and is willing to settle for an approximate solution? One could truncate the decision tree at some shorter and more manageable horizon, compute approximate terminal values by replacing the distributions with their means, and proceed with a receding-horizon approach: Starting from the approximate terminal values at the horizon, perform a backward sweep of dynamic programming, computing an optimal policy. Take the initial action of the policy, then shift the entire computational window forward one level and repeat. One can imagine a sort of limiting, degenerate version of this receding horizon approach in which the horizon is zero; that is, use the means of the current distributions to calculate an optimal policy, take an "optimal" action, observe a transition, perform a Bayesian modification of the prior, and repeat. This (certainty-equivalence) heuristic was suggested by [Cozzolino et al., 1965], and has recently reappeared in [Dayan & Sejnowski, 1996]. However, as was noted in [Cozzolino et al., 1965] "...the trade-off between immmediate gain and information does not exist in this heuristic. There is no mechanism which explicitly forces unexplored policies to be observed in early stages. Therefore, if it should happen that there is some very good policy which *a priori* seemed quite bad, it is entirely possible that this heuristic will never provide the information needed to recognize the policy as being better than originally thought..." This comment and others seem to refer to what is now regarded as a problem of "identifiability" associated with certainty-equivalence controllers in which a closed-loop system evolves identically for both true and false values of the unknown parameters; that is, certainty-equivalence control may make some of the unknown parameters invisible to the identification process and lead one to repeatedly choose the wrong action (see [Borkar & Varaiya, 1979], and also Watkins' discussion of "metastable policies" in [Watkins, 1989]).

3 BANDIT PROBLEMS AND INDEX COMPUTATION

One basic version of the bandit problem may be described as follows: There are some number of statistically independent reward processes—Markov chains with an imposed reward structure associated with the chain's arcs. At each discrete time-step, a decision-maker selects one of these processes to activate. The activated process yields an immediate reward and then changes state. The other processes remain frozen and yield no reward. The goal is to splice together the individual reward streams into one sequence having maximal expected discounted value.

The special Cartesian structure of the bandit problem turns out to imply that there are functions that map process-states to scalars (or "indices"), such that optimal policies consist simply of activating the task with the largest index. Consider one of the reward processes, let S be its state space, and let $\mathcal{B}$ be the set of all subsets of S. Suppose that $x(k)$ is the state of the process at time k and, for $B \in \mathcal{B}$, let $\tau(B)$ be the number of transitions until the process first enters the set B. Let $\nu(i; B)$ be the expected discounted reward per unit of discounted time starting from state i until the stopping time $\tau(B)$:

$$\nu(i; B) = \frac{E\left\{\sum_{k=0}^{\tau(B)-1} \gamma^k R(x(k))|x(0)=i\right\}}{E\left\{\sum_{k=0}^{\tau(B)-1} \gamma^k |x(0)=i\right\}}.$$

Then the Gittins index of state i for the process under consideration is

$$\nu(i) = \max_{B \in \mathcal{B}} \nu(i; B). \tag{1}$$

[Gittins & Jones, 1979] shows that the indices may be obtained by solving a set of functional equations. Other algorithms that have been suggested include those by Beale (see the discussion section following [Gittins & Jones, 1979]), [Robinsion, 1981], [Varaiya et al., 1985], and [Katehakis & Veinott, 1987]. [Duff, 1995] provides a reinforcement learning approach that gradually learns indices through online/model-free interaction with bandit processes. The details of these algorithms would require more space than is available here. The algorithm proposed in the next section makes use of the approach of [Varaiya et al., 1985].

4 LOCAL BANDIT APPROXIMATION AND AN APPROXIMATELY-OPTIMAL LEARNING ALGORITHM

The most obvious difference between the optimal learning problem for an MDP and the multi-armed bandit problem is that the MDP has a phase-space component (Markov chain state) to its hyperstate. A first step in bandit-based approximation, then, proceeds by "removing" this phase-space component. This can be achieved by viewing the process on a time-scale defined by the recurrence time of a given state. That is, suppose the process is in some state, x. In response to some given action, two things can happen: (1) The process can transition, in one time-step, into x again with some immediate reward, or (2) The process can transition into some state that is not x and experience some "sojourn" path of states and rewards before returning to x. On a time-scale defined by sojourn-time, one can view the process in a sort of "state-x-centric" way (if state x never recurs, then the sojourn-time is "infinite" and there is no value-of-information component of the local bandit model to acknowledge). From this perspective, the process appears to have only one state, and is *semi*-Markov; that is, the time between transitions is a random variable. Some other action taken in state x would give rise to a different sojourn reward process. For both processes (sojourn-processes initiated by different actions applied to state x), the sojourn path/reward will depend upon the policy for states encountered along sojourn paths, but suppose that this policy is fixed for the moment. By viewing the original process on a time-scale of sojourn-time, one has effectively collapsed the phase-space component of the hyperstate. The new process has one state, x, and the problem of choosing an action, given that one is uncertain about the transition probabilities, presents itself as a semi-Markov bandit problem.

The preceding discussion suggests an algorithm for approximately-optimal learning:

(0) Given that the uncertainty in transition probabilities is expressed in terms of sufficient statistics $<\vec{\alpha},\vec{\beta}>$, and the process is currently in state x_t.

(1) Compute the optimal policy for the mean process, $\pi^*[\bar{P}(\vec{\alpha},\vec{\beta})]$; that is, compute the policy that is optimal for the MDP whose transition probabilities are taken to be the mean values associated with $<\vec{\alpha},\vec{\beta}>$—this defines a nominal (certainty-equivalent) policy for sojourn states.

(2) Construct a local bandit model at state x_t; that is, the decision-maker must choose between some number (the number of admissible actions) of sojourn reward processes—this is a semi-Markov multi-armed bandit problem.

(3) Compute the Gittins indices for the local bandit model.

(4) Take the action with the largest index.

(5) Observe a transition to x_{t+1} in the underlying MDP.

(6) Update $<\vec{\alpha},\vec{\beta}>$ accordingly (Bayes update).

(7) Go to step (1)

The local semi-Markov bandit process associated with **state 1 / action 1** for the 2-state example MDP of Figure 1 is shown in Figure 2. The sufficient statistics for p_{11}^1 are denoted by (α,β), and $\frac{\alpha}{\alpha+\beta}$ and $\frac{\beta}{\alpha+\beta}$ are the expected probabilities for transition into **state 1** and **state 2**, respectively. Γ and R_{121} are random variables signifying sojourn time and reward.

The goal is to compute the index for the root information-state labeled $<\alpha,\beta>$ and to compare it with that computed for a similar diagram associated with the bandit

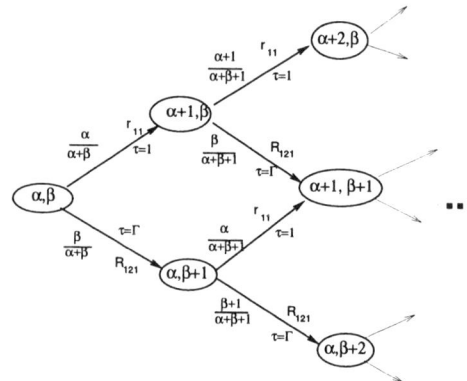

Figure 2: A local semi-Markov bandit process associated with state 1 / action 1 for the 2-state example MDP of Figure 1.

process for taking action 2. The approximately-optimal action is suggested by the process having the largest root-node index. Indices for semi-Markov bandits can be obtained by considering the bandits as Markov, but performing the optimization in Equation 1 over a restricted set of stopping times. The algorithm suggested in [Tsitsiklis, 1993], which in turn makes use of methods described in [Varaiya et al., 1985], proceeds by "reducing" the graph through a sequence of node-excisions and modifications of rewards and transition probabilities; [Duff, 1997] details how these steps may be realized for the special semi-Markov processes associated with problems of optimal learning.

5 Discussion

In summary, this paper has presented the problem of optimal learning, in which a decision-maker is obliged to enjoy or endure the consequences of its actions in quest of the asymptotically-learned optimal policy. A Bayesian formulation of the problem leads to a clear concept of a solution whose computation, however, appears to entail an examination of an intractably-large number of hyperstates. This paper has suggested extending the Gittins index approach (which applies with great power and elegance to the special class of multi-armed bandit processes) to general adaptive MDP's. The hope has been that if certain salient features of the value of information could be captured, even approximately, then one could be led to a reasonable method for avoiding certain defects of certainty-equivalence approaches (problems with identifiability, "metastability"). Obviously, positive evidence, in the form of empirical results from simulation experiments, would lend support to these ideas— work along these lines is underway.

Local bandit approximation is but one approximate computational approach for problems of optimal learning and dual control. Most prominent in the literature of control theory is the "wide-sense" approach of [Bar-Shalom & Tse, 1976], which utilizes local quadratic approximations about nominal state/control trajectories. For certain problems, this method has demonstrated superior performance compared to a certainty-equivalence approach, but it is computationally very intensive and unwieldy, particularly for problems with controller dimension greater than one.

One could revert to the view of the bandit problem, or general adaptive MDP, as simply a very large MDP defined over hyperstates, and then consider a somewhat direct approach in which one performs approximate dynamic programming with function approximation over this domain—details of function-approximation, feature-selection, and "training" all become important design issues. [Duff, 1997] provides further discussion of these topics, as well as a consideration of action-elimination procedures [MacQueen, 1966] that could result in substantial pruning of the hyperstate decision tree.

Acknowledgements

This research was supported, in part, by the National Science Foundation under grant ECS-9214866 to Andrew G. Barto.

References

Bar-Shalom, Y. & Tse, E. (1976) Caution, probing and the value of information in the control of uncertain systems, *Ann. Econ. Soc. Meas.* 5:323-337.

R. Bellman & R. Kalaba, (1959) On adaptive control processes. *IRE Trans.*, 4:1-9.

Bokar, V. & Varaiya, P.P. (1979) Adaptive control of Markov chains I: finite parameter set. *IEEE Trans. Auto. Control* 24:953-958.

Cozzolino, J.M., Gonzalez-Zubieta, R., & Miller, R.L. (1965) Markov decision processes with uncertain transition probabilities. *Tech. Rpt. 11, Operations Research Center, MIT.*

Dayan, P. & Sejnowski, T. (1996) Exploration Bonuses and Dual Control. *Machine Learning* (in press).

Duff, M.O. (1995) Q-learning for bandit problems. in *Machine Learning: Proceedings of the Twelfth International Conference on Machine Learning*: pp. 209-217.

Duff, M.O. (1997) Approximate computational methods for optimal learning and dual control. *Technical Report*, Deptartment of Computer Science, Univ. of Massachusetts, Amherst.

Fel'dbaum, A. (1965) *Optimal Control Systems*, Academic Press.

Gittins, J.C. & Jones, D. (1979) Bandit processes and dynamic allocation indices (with discussion). *J. R. Statist. Soc. B* **41**:148-177.

Katehakis, M.H. & Veinott, A.F. (1987) The multi-armed bandit problem: decomposition and computation *Math. OR* **12**: 262-268.

MacQueen, J. (1966). A modified dynamic programming method for Markov decision problems, *J. Math. Anal. Appl.*, 14:38-43.

Robinsion, D.R. (1981) Algorithms for evaluating the dynamic allocation index. *Research Report No. 80/DRR/4, Manchester-Sheffield School of Probability and Statistics.*

Tsitsiklis, J. (1993) A short proof of the Gittins index theorem. *Proc. 32nd Conf. Dec. and Control*: 389-390.

Varaiya, P.P., Walrand, J.C., & Buyukkoc, C. (1985) Extensions of the multiarmed bandit problem: the discounted case. *IEEE Trans. Auto. Control* **30**(5):426-439.

Watkins, C. (1989) *Learning from Delayed Rewards* Ph.D. Thesis, Cambidge University.

Reinforcement Learning for Mixed Open-loop and Closed-loop Control

Eric A. Hansen, Andrew G. Barto, and Shlomo Zilberstein
Department of Computer Science
University of Massachusetts
Amherst, MA 01003
{hansen,barto,shlomo}@cs.umass.edu

Abstract

Closed-loop control relies on sensory feedback that is usually assumed to be free. But if sensing incurs a cost, it may be cost-effective to take sequences of actions in open-loop mode. We describe a reinforcement learning algorithm that learns to combine open-loop and closed-loop control when sensing incurs a cost. Although we assume reliable sensors, use of open-loop control means that actions must sometimes be taken when the current state of the controlled system is uncertain. This is a special case of the hidden-state problem in reinforcement learning, and to cope, our algorithm relies on short-term memory. The main result of the paper is a rule that significantly limits exploration of possible memory states by pruning memory states for which the estimated value of information is greater than its cost. We prove that this rule allows convergence to an optimal policy.

1 Introduction

Reinforcement learning (RL) is widely-used for learning closed-loop control policies. Closed-loop control works well if the sensory feedback on which it relies is accurate, fast, and inexpensive. But this is not always the case. In this paper, we address problems in which sensing incurs a cost, either a direct cost for obtaining and processing sensory data or an indirect opportunity cost for dedicating limited sensors to one control task rather than another. If the cost for sensing is significant, exclusive reliance on closed-loop control may make it impossible to optimize a performance measure such as cumulative discounted reward. For such problems, we describe an RL algorithm that learns to combine open-loop and closed-loop control. By learning to take open-loop sequences of actions between sensing, it can optimize a tradeoff between the cost and value of sensing.

The problem we address is a special case of the problem of hidden state or partial observability in RL (e.g., Whitehead & Lin, 1995; McCallum, 1995). Although we assume sensing provides perfect information (a significant limiting assumption), use of open-loop control means that actions must sometimes be taken when the current state of the controlled system is uncertain. Previous work on RL for partially observable environments has focused on coping with sensors that provide imperfect or incomplete information, in contrast to deciding whether or when to sense. Tan (1991) addressed the problem of sensing costs by showing how to use RL to learn a cost-effective sensing procedure for state identification, but his work addressed the question of which sensors to use, not when to sense, and so still assumed closed-loop control.

In this paper, we formalize the problem of mixed open-loop and closed-loop control as a Markov decision process and use RL in the form of Q-learning to learn an optimal, state-dependent sensing interval. Because there is a combinatorial explosion of open-loop action sequences, we introduce a simple rule for pruning this large search space. Our most significant result is a proof that Q-learning converges to an optimal policy even when a fraction of the space of possible open-loop action sequences is explored.

2 Q-learning with sensing costs

Q-learning (Watkins, 1989) is a well-studied RL algorithm for learning to control a discrete-time, finite state and action Markov decision process (MDP). At each time step, a controller observes the current state x, takes an action a, and receives an immediate reward r with expected value $r(x, a)$. With probability $p(x, a, y)$ the process makes a transition to state y, which becomes the current state on the next time step. A controller using Q-learning learns a state-action value function, $\hat{Q}(x, a)$, that estimates the expected total discounted reward for taking action a in state x and performing optimally thereafter. Each time step, $\hat{Q}$ is updated for state-action pair (x, a) after receiving reward r and observing resulting state y, as follows:

$$\hat{Q}(x, a) \leftarrow \hat{Q}(x, a) + \alpha \left[r + \gamma \hat{V}(y) - \hat{Q}(x, a) \right],$$

where $\alpha \in (0, 1]$ is a learning rate parameter, $\gamma \in [0, 1)$ is a discount factor, and $\hat{V}(y) = \max_b \hat{Q}(y, b)$. Watkins and Dayan (1992) prove that $\hat{Q}$ converges to an optimal state-action value function Q (and $\hat{V}$ converges to an optimal state value function V) with probability one if all actions continue to be tried from all states, the state-action value function is represented by a lookup-table, and the learning rate is decreased in an appropriate manner.

If there is a cost for sensing, acting optimally may require a mixed strategy of open-loop and closed-loop control that allows a controller to take open-loop sequences of actions between sensing. This possibility can be modeled by an MDP with two kinds of actions: *control actions* that have an effect on the current state but do not provide information, and a *sensing action* that reveals the current state but has no other effect. We let o (for observation) denote the sensing action and assume it provides perfect information about the underlying state. Separating control actions and the sensing action gives an agent control over when to receive sensory feedback, and hence, control over sensing costs.

When one control action follows another without an intervening sensing action, the second control action is taken without knowing the underlying state. We model this by including "memory states" in the state set of the MDP. Each memory state represents memory of the last observed state and the open-loop sequence of control actions taken since; because we assume sensing provides perfect information,

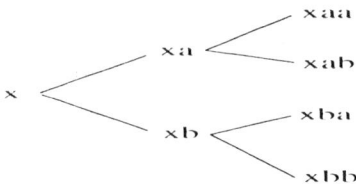

Figure 1: A tree of memory states rooted at observed state x. The set of control actions is {a,b} and the length bound is 2.

remembering this much history provides a *sufficient statistic* for action selection (Monahan, 1982). Possible memory states can be represented using a tree like the one shown in Figure 1, where the root represents the last observed state and the other nodes represent memory states, one for each possible open-loop action sequence. For example, let xa denote the memory state that results from taking control action a in state x. Similarly, let xab denote the memory state that results from taking control action b in memory state xa. Note that a control action causes a deterministic transition to a subsequent memory state, while a sensing action causes a stochastic transition to an observed state – the root of some tree. There is a tree like the one in figure 1 for each observable state.

This problem is a special case of a partially observable MDP and can be formalized in an analogous way (Monahan, 1982). Given a state-transition and reward model for a core MDP with a state set that consists only of the underlying states of a system (which for this problem we also call observable states), we can define a state-transition and reward model for an MDP that includes memory states in its state set. As a convenient notation, let $p(x, a_1..a_k, y)$ denote the probability that taking an open-loop action sequence $a_1..a_k$ from state x results in state y, where both x and y are states of the underlying system. These probabilities can be computed recursively from the single-step state-transition probabilities of the core MDP as follows:

$$p(x, a_1..a_k, y) = \sum_z p(x, a_1..a_{k-1}, z) p(z, a_k, y).$$

State-transition probabilities for the sensing action can then be defined as

$$p(xa_1..a_k, o, y) = p(x, a_1..a_k, y),$$

and a reward function for the generalized MDP can be similarly defined as

$$r(xa_1..a_{k-1}, a_k) = \sum_y p(x, a_1..a_{k-1}, y) r(y, a_k),$$

where the cost of sensing in state x of the core MDP is $r(x, o)$.

If we assume a bound on the number of control actions that can be taken between sensing actions (i.e., a bound on the depth of each tree) and also assume a finite number of underlying states, the number of possible memory states is finite. It follows that the MDP we have constructed is a well-defined finite state and action MDP, and all of the theory developed for Q-learning continues to apply, including its convergence proof. (This is not true of partially observable MDPs in general.) Therefore, Q-learning can in principle find an optimal policy for interleaving control actions and sensing, assuming sensing provides perfect information.

3 Limiting Exploration

A problem with including memory states in the state set of an MDP is that it increases the size of the state set exponentially. The combinatorial explosion of state-action values to be learned raises doubt about the computational feasibility of this generalization of RL. We present a solution in the form of a rule for pruning each tree of memory states, thereby limiting the number of memory states that must be explored. We prove that even if some memory states are never explored, Q-learning converges to an optimal state-action value function. Because the state-action value function is left undefined for unexplored memory states, we must carefully define what we mean by an optimal state-action value function.

Definition: *A state-action value function is optimal if it is sufficient for generating optimal behavior and the values of the state-action pairs visited when behaving optimally are optimal.*

A state-action value function that is undefined for some states is optimal, by this definition, if a controller that follows it behaves identically to a controller with a complete, optimal state-action value function. This is possible if the states for which the state-action value function is undefined are not encountered when an agent acts optimally. Barto, Bradtke, and Singh (1995) invoke a similar idea for a different class of problems.

Let $g(xa_1..a_k)$ denote the expected reward for taking actions $a_1..a_k$ in open-loop mode after observing state x:

$$g(xa_1..a_k) = r(x, a_1) + \sum_{i=1}^{k-1} \gamma^i r(xa_1..a_i, a_{i+1}).$$

Let $h(xa_1..a_k)$ denote the discounted expected value of perfect information after reaching memory state $xa_1..a_k$, which is equal to the discounted Q-value for sensing in memory state $xa_1..a_k$ minus the cost for sensing in this state:

$$h(xa_1..a_k) = \gamma^k \sum_y p(xa_1..a_k, o, y) V(y) = \gamma^k (Q(xa_1..a_k, o) - r(xa_1..a_k, o)).$$

Both g and h are easily learned during Q-learning, and we refer to the learned estimates as $\hat{g}$ and $\hat{h}$. These are used in the pruning rule, as follows:

Pruning rule: *If $\hat{g}(xa_1..a_k) + \hat{h}(xa_1..a_k) \leq \hat{V}(x)$, then memory states that descend from $xa_1..a_k$ do not need to be explored. A controller should immediately execute a sensing action when it reaches one of these memory states.*

The intuition behind the pruning rule is that a branch of a tree of memory states can be pruned after reaching a memory state for which the value of information is greater than or equal to its cost. Because pruning is based on estimated values, memory states that are pruned at one point during learning may later be explored as learned estimates change. The net effect of pruning, however, is to focus exploration on a subset of memory states, and as Q-learning converges, the subset of unpruned memory states becomes stable. The following theorem is proved in an appendix.

Theorem: *Q-learning converges to an optimal state-action value function with probability one if, in addition to the conditions for convergence given by Watkins and Dayan (1992), exploration is limited by the pruning rule.*

This result is closely related to a similar result for solving this class of problems using dynamic programming (Hansen, 1997), where it is shown that pruning can assure convergence to an optimal policy even if no bound is placed on the length of open-loop action sequences – under the assumption that it is optimal to sense at finite intervals. This additional result can be extended to Q-learning as well, although we do not present the extension in this paper. An artificial length bound can be set as low or high as desired to ensure a finite set of memory states.

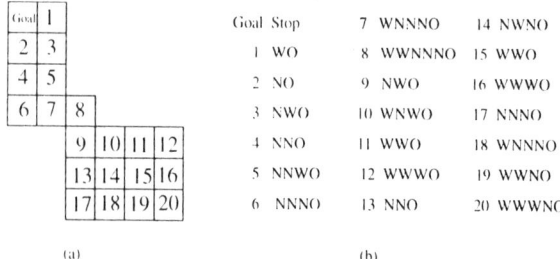

Figure 2: (a) Grid world with numbered states (b) Optimal policy

We use the notation g and h in our statement of the pruning rule to emphasize its relationship to pruning in heuristic search. If we regard the root of a tree of memory states as the start state and the memory state that corresponds to the best open-loop action sequence as the goal state, then g can be regarded as the cost-to-arrive function and the value of perfect information h can be regarded as an upper bound on the cost-to-go function.

4 Example

We describe a simple example to illustrate the extent of pruning possible using this rule. Imagine that a "robot" must find its way to a goal location in the upper left-hand corner of the grid shown in Figure 2a. Each cell of the grid corresponds to a state, with the states numbered for convenient reference. The robot has five control actions; it can move north, east, south, or west, one cell at a time, or it can stop. The problem ends when the robot stops. If it stops in the goal state it receives a reward of 100, otherwise it receives no reward. The robot must execute a sequence of actions to reach the goal state, but its move actions are stochastic. If the robot attempts to move in a particular direction, it succeeds with probability 0.8. With probability 0.05 it moves in a direction 90 degrees off to one side of its intended direction, with probability 0.05 it moves in a direction 90 degrees off to the other side, and with probability 0.1 it does not move at all. If the robot's movement would take it outside the grid, it remains in the same cell. Because its progress is uncertain, the robot must interleave sensing and control actions to keep track of its location. The reward for sensing is -1 (i.e., a cost of 1) and for each move action it is -4. To optimize expected total reward, the robot must find its way to the goal while minimizing the combined cost of moving and sensing.

Figure 2b shows the optimal open-loop sequence of actions for each observable state. If the bound on the length of an open-loop sequence of control actions is five, the number of possible memory states for this problem is over 64,000, a number that grows explosively as the length bound is increased (to over 16 million when the bound is nine). Using the pruning rule, Q-learning must explore just less than 1000 memory states (and no deeper than nine levels in any tree) to converge to an optimal policy, even when there is no bound on the interval between sensing actions.

5 Conclusion

We have described an extension of Q-learning for MDPs with sensing costs and a rule for limiting exploration that makes it possible for Q-learning to converge to an optimal policy despite exploring a fraction of possible memory states. As already pointed out, the problem we have formalized is a partially observable MDP, although one that is restricted by the assumption that sensing provides perfect information. An interesting direction in which to pursue this work would be to explore its relationship to work on RL for partially observable MDPs, which has so far focused on the problem of sensor uncertainty and hidden state. Because some of this work also makes use of tree representations of the state space and of learned state-action values (e.g., McCallum, 1995), it may be that a similar pruning rule can constrain exploration for such problems.

Acknowledgements

Support for this work was provided in part by the National Science Foundation under grants ECS-9214866 and IRI-9409827 and in part by Rome Laboratory, USAF, under grant F30602-95-1-0012.

References

Barto, A.G.; Bradtke, S.J.; & Singh, S.P. (1995) Learning to act using real-time dynamic programming. *Artificial Intelligence* 72(1/2):81-138.

Hansen, E.A. (1997) Markov decision processes with observation costs. University of Massachusetts at Amherst, Computer Science Technical Report 97-01.

McCallum, R.A. (1995) Instance-based utile distinctions for reinforcement learning with hidden state. In Proc. 12th Int. Machine Learning Conf. Morgan Kaufmann.

Monahan, G.E. (1982) A survey of partially observable Markov decision processes: Theory, models, and algorithms. *Management Science* 28:1-16.

Tan, M. (1991) Cost-sensitive reinforcement learning for adaptive classification and control. In Proc. 9th Nat. Conf. on Artificial Intelligence. AAAI Press/MIT Press.

Watkins, C.J.C.H. (1989) Learning from delayed rewards. Ph.D. Thesis, University of Cambridge, England.

Watkins, C.J.C.H. & Dayan, P. (1992) Technical note: Q-learning. *Machine Learning* 8(3/4):279-292.

Whitehad, S.D. & Lin, L.-J.(1995) Reinforcement learning of non-Markov decision processes. *Artificial Intelligence* 73:271-306.

Appendix

Proof of theorem: Consider an MDP with a state set that consists only of the memory states that are not pruned. We call it a "pruned MDP" to distinguish it from the original MDP for which the state set consists of all possible memory states. Because the pruned MDP is a finite state and action MDP, Q-learning with pruning converges with probability one. What we must show is that the state-action values to which it converges include every state-action pair visited by an optimal controller for the original MDP, and that for each of these state-action pairs the learned state-action value is equal to the optimal state-action value for the original MDP.

Let $\hat{Q}$ and $\hat{V}$ denote the values that are learned by Q-learning when its exploration is limited by the pruning rule, and let Q and V denote value functions that are optimal when the state set of the MDP includes all possible memory states. Because an MDP has an optimal stationary policy and each control action causes a deterministic transition to a subsequent memory state, there is an optimal path through each tree of memory states. The learned value of the root state of each tree is optimal if and only if the learned value of each memory state along this path is also optimal.

Therefore to show that Q-learning with pruning converges to an optimal state-action value function, it is sufficient to show that $\hat{V} = V$ for every observable state x. Our proof is by induction on the number of control actions that can be taken between one sensing action and the next. We use the fact that if Q-learning has converged, then $\hat{g}(xa_1..a_i) = g(xa_1..a_i)$ and $\hat{h}(xa_1..a_i) = \sum_y p(x, a_1..a_i, y)\hat{V}(y)$ for every memory state $xa_1..a_i$.

First note that if $\hat{g}(xa_1) + \gamma r(xa_1, o) + \hat{h}(xa_1) > \hat{V}(x)$, that is, if $\hat{V}$ for some observable state x can be improved by exploring a path of a single control action followed by sensing, then it is contradictory to suppose Q-learning with pruning has converged because single-depth memory states in a tree are never pruned. Now, make the inductive hypothesis that Q-learning with pruning has not converged if $\hat{V}$ can be improved for some observable state by exploring a path of less than k control actions before sensing. We show that it has not converged if $\hat{V}$ can be improved for some observable state by exploring a path of k control actions before sensing.

Suppose $\hat{V}$ for some observable state x can be improved by exploring a path that consists of taking the sequence of control actions $a_1..a_k$ before sensing, that is,

$$\hat{g}(xa_1..a_k) + \gamma^k r(xa_1..a_k, o) + \hat{h}(xa_1..a_k) > \hat{V}(x),$$

Since only pruning can prevent improvement in this case, let $xa_1..a_i$ be the memory state at which application of the pruning rule prevents $xa_1..a_k$ from being explored. Because the tree has been pruned at this node, $\hat{V}(x) \geq \hat{g}(xa_1..a_i) + \hat{h}(xa_1..a_i)$, and so

$$\hat{g}(xa_1..a_k) + \gamma^k r(xa_1..a_k, o) + \hat{h}(xa_1..a_k) > \hat{g}(xa_i..a_i) + \hat{h}(xa_1..a_i).$$

We can expand this inequality as follows:

$$\hat{g}(xa_1..a_i) + \gamma^i \sum_y p(x, a_1..a_i, y) \left[\hat{g}(ya_{i+1}..a_k) + \gamma^{k-i} r(ya_{i+1}..a_k, o) + \hat{h}(ya_{i+1}..a_k) \right]$$

$$> \hat{g}(xa_1..a_i) + \hat{h}(xa_1..a_i).$$

Simplification and expansion of $\hat{h}$ yields

$$\sum_{y \in S} p(x, a_1..a_i, y) \left[\hat{g}(ya_{i+1}..a_k) + \gamma^{k-i} r(ya_{i+1}..a_k, o) + \gamma^{k-i} \sum_z p(y, a_{i+1}..a_k, z)\hat{V}(z) \right]$$

$$> \sum_y p(x, a_1..a_i, y)\hat{V}(y).$$

Therefore, there is some observable state, y, such that

$$\hat{g}(ya_{i+1}..a_k) + \gamma^{k-i} r(ya_{i+1}..a_k, o) + \gamma^{k-i} \sum_z p(y, a_{i+1}..a_k, z)\hat{V}(z) > \hat{V}(y).$$

Because the value of observable state y can be improved by taking less than k control actions before sensing, by the inductive hypothesis Q-learning has not yet converged. □

The proof provides insight into how pruning works. If a state-action pair along some optimal path is temporarily pruned, it must be possible to improve the value of some observable state by exploring a shorter path of memory states that has not been pruned. The resulting improvement of the value function changes the threshold for pruning and the state-action pair that was formerly pruned may no longer be so, making further improvement of the learned value function possible.

Multi-Grid Methods for Reinforcement Learning in Controlled Diffusion Processes

Stephan Pareigis
stp@numerik.uni-kiel.de
Lehrstuhl Praktische Mathematik
Christian-Albrechts-Universität Kiel
Kiel, Germany

Abstract

Reinforcement learning methods for discrete and semi-Markov decision problems such as Real-Time Dynamic Programming can be generalized for Controlled Diffusion Processes. The optimal control problem reduces to a boundary value problem for a fully nonlinear second-order elliptic differential equation of Hamilton-Jacobi-Bellman (HJB-) type. Numerical analysis provides multi-grid methods for this kind of equation. In the case of Learning Control, however, the systems of equations on the various grid-levels are obtained using observed information (transitions and local cost). To ensure consistency, special attention needs to be directed toward the type of time and space discretization during the observation. An algorithm for multi-grid observation is proposed. The multi-grid algorithm is demonstrated on a simple queuing problem.

1 Introduction

Controlled Diffusion Processes (CDP) are the analogy to Markov Decision Problems in continuous state space and continuous time. A CDP can always be discretized in state space and time and thus reduced to a Markov Decision Problem. Algorithms like Q-learning and RTDP as described in [1] can then be applied to produce controls or optimal value functions for a fixed discretization.

Problems arise when the discretization needs to be refined, or when multi-grid information needs to be extracted to accelerate the algorithm. The relation of time to state space discretization parameters is crucial in both cases. Therefore a mathematical model of the discretized process is introduced, which reflects the properties of the converged empirical process. In this model, transition probabilities of the discrete process can be expressed in terms of the transition probabilities of the continuous process. Recent results in numerical methods for stochastic control problems in continuous time can be applied to give assumptions that guarantee a local consistency condition which is needed for convergence. The same assumptions allow application of multi-grid methods.

In section 2 Controlled Diffusion Processes are introduced. A model for the discretized process is suggested in section 3 and the main theorem is stated. Section 4 presents an algorithm for multi-grid observation according to the results in the preceding section. Section 5 shows an application of multi-grid techniques for observed processes.

2 Controlled Diffusion Processes

Consider a Controlled Diffusion Process (CDP) $\xi(t)$ in some bounded domain $\Omega \subset \mathbb{R}^n$ fulfilling the diffusion equation

$$d\xi(t) = b(\xi(t), u(t))dt + \sigma(\xi(t))dw. \tag{1}$$

The control $u(t)$ takes values in some finite set U. The immediate reinforcement (cost) for state $\xi(t)$ and control $u(t)$ is

$$r(t) = r(\xi(t), u(t)). \tag{2}$$

The control objective is to find a feedback control law

$$u(t) = \mathbf{u}(\xi(t)), \tag{3}$$

that minimizes the total discounted cost

$$J(x, u) = \mathbb{E}_x^u \int_0^\infty e^{-\beta t} r(\xi(t), u(t))dt, \tag{4}$$

where $\mathbb{E}_x^u$ is the expectation starting in $x \in \Omega$ and applying the control law $u(.)$. $\beta > 0$ is the discount.

The transition probabilities of the CDP are given for any initial state $x \in \Omega$ and subset $A \subset \Omega$ by the stochastic kernels

$$P_t^u(x, A) := \text{prob}\{\xi(t) \in A \,|\, \xi(0) = x, u\}. \tag{5}$$

It is known that the kernels have the properties

$$\int_\Omega (y - x) P_t^u(x, dy) = t \cdot b(x, u) + o(t) \tag{6}$$

$$\int_\Omega (y - x)(y - x)^T P_t^u(x, dy) = t \cdot \sigma(x)\sigma(x)^T + o(t). \tag{7}$$

For the optimal control it is sufficient to calculate the optimal value function $V : \Omega \to \mathbb{R}$

$$V(x) := \inf_{u(.)} J(x, u). \tag{8}$$

Under appropriate smoothness assumptions V is a solution of the Hamilton-Jacobi-Bellman (HJB-) equation

$$\min_{\alpha \in U} \{\mathcal{L}^\alpha V(x) - \beta V(x) + r(x,\alpha)\} = 0, \quad x \in \Omega. \tag{9}$$

Let $a(x) = \sigma(x)\sigma(x)^T$ be the diffusion matrix, then $\mathcal{L}^\alpha$, $\alpha \in U$ is defined as the elliptic differential operator

$$\mathcal{L}^\alpha := \sum_{i,j=1}^n a_{ij}(x)\partial_{x_i}\partial_{x_j} + \sum_{i=1}^n b_i(x,\alpha)\partial_{x_i}. \tag{10}$$

3 A Model for Observed CDP's

Let Ω_{h_i} be the centers of cells of a cell-centered grid on Ω with cell sizes h_0, $h_1 = h_0/2$, $h_2 = h_1/2$, ... For any $x \in \Omega_{h_i}$ we shall denote by $A(x)$ the cell of x. Let $\Delta t > 0$ be a parameter for the time discretization.

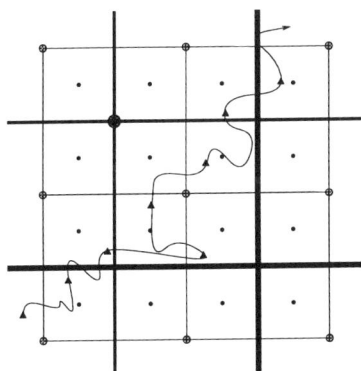

Figure 1: The picture depicts three cell-centered grid levels and the trajectory of a diffusion process. The approximating value function is represented locally constant on each cell. The triangles on the path denote the position of the diffusion at sample times $0, \Delta t, 2\Delta t, 3\Delta t, \ldots$. Transitions between respective cells are then counted in matrices Q_i^a, for each control a and grid i.

By counting the transitions between cells and calculating the empirical probabilities as defined in (20) we obtain empirical processes on every grid. By the law of great numbers the empirical processes will converge towards observed CDPs as subsequently defined.

Definition 1 *An observed process $\xi_{h_i,\Delta t_i}(t)$ is a Controlled Markov Chain (i.e. discrete state-space and discrete time) on Ω_{h_i} and interpolation time Δt_i with the transition probabilities*

$$\begin{aligned} p_{h_i,\Delta t_i}^u(x,y) &:= \mathrm{prob}\{\xi(\Delta t_i) \in A(y) | \xi(0) \in A(x), u\} \\ &= \frac{1}{h_i^n} \int_{A(x)} P_{\Delta t_i}^u(z, A(y))dz, \end{aligned} \tag{11}$$

where $x, y \in \Omega_{h_i}$ and $\xi(t)$ is a solution of (1). Also define the observed reinforcement ρ as

$$\rho_{h_i,\Delta t_i}(x,u) := \frac{1}{h_i^n} \int_{A(x)} \mathbb{E}_z^u \int_0^{\Delta t_i} r(\xi(\tau), u(\tau))d\tau dz. \tag{12}$$

On every grid Ω_{h_i} the respective process $\xi_{h_i,\Delta t_i}$ has its own value function $V_{h_i,\Delta t_i}$. By theorem 10.4.1. in Kushner, Dupuis ([5], 1992) it holds, that

$$V_{h_i,\Delta t_i}(x) \to V(x) \text{ for all } x \in \Omega, \tag{13}$$

if the following local consistency conditions hold.

Definition 2 *Let* $\Delta \xi_{h,\Delta t} = \xi_{h,\Delta t}(\Delta t) - \xi_{h,\Delta t}(0)$. $\xi_{h,\Delta t}$ *is called locally consistent to a solution* $\xi(.)$ *of (1), iff*

$$\mathbb{E}_x^u \Delta \xi_{h,\Delta t} = b(x,a)\Delta t + o(\Delta t) \tag{14}$$
$$\mathbb{E}_x^u [\Delta \xi_{h,\Delta t} - \mathbb{E}_x^u \Delta \xi_{h,\Delta t}][\Delta \xi_{h,\Delta t} - \mathbb{E}_x^u \Delta \xi_{h,\Delta t}]^T = a(x)\Delta t + o(\Delta t) \tag{15}$$
$$\sup_n |\Delta \xi_{h,\Delta t}(n\Delta t)| \to 0 \text{ as } h \to 0. \tag{16}$$

To verify these conditions for the observed CDP, the expectation and variance can be calculated. For the expectation we get

$$\mathbb{E}_x^u \Delta \xi_{h_i,\Delta t_i} = \sum_{y \in \Omega_{h_i}} p_{h_i,\Delta t_i}^u(x,y)(y-x)$$
$$= \frac{1}{h_i^n} \sum_{y \in \Omega_{h_i}} \int_{A(x)} (y-x) P_{\Delta t_i}^u(z, A(y)) dz. \tag{17}$$

Recalling properties (6) and (7) and doing a similar calculation for the variance we obtain the following theorem.

Theorem 3 *For observed CDPs* $\xi_{h_i,\Delta t_i}$ *let* h_i *and* Δt_i *be such that*

$$h_i/\Delta t_i \to 0 \text{ as } \Delta t_i \to 0. \tag{18}$$

Furthermore, $\xi_{h_i,\Delta t_i}$ *shall be truncated at some radius* R, *such that* $R \to 0$ *for* $h_i \to 0$ *and expectation and variance of the truncated process differ only in the order* $o(\Delta t)$ *from expectation and variance of* $\xi_{h_i,\Delta t_i}$. *Then the observed processes* $\xi_{h_i,\Delta t_i}$ *truncated at* R *are locally consistent to the diffusion process* $\xi(.)$ *and therefore the value functions* $V_{h_i,\Delta t_i}$ *converge to the value function* V.

4 Identification by Multi-Grid Observation

The condition in Theorem 3 provides information as how to choose parameters in the algorithm with empirical data. Choose discretization values h_0, Δt_0 for the coarsest grid Ω_0. Δt_0 should typically be of order $\|b\|_{sup}/h_0$. Then choose for the finer grids

grid	0	1	2	3	4	5	...
space	h_0	$\frac{h_0}{2}$	$\frac{h_0}{4}$	$\frac{h_0}{8}$	$\frac{h_0}{16}$	$\frac{h_0}{32}$	...
time	Δt_0	$\frac{\Delta t_0}{2}$	$\frac{\Delta t_0}{2}$	$\frac{\Delta t_0}{4}$	$\frac{\Delta t_0}{4}$	$\frac{\Delta t_0}{8}$	...

$$\tag{19}$$

The sequences verify the assumption (18). We may now formulate the algorithm for Multi-Grid Observation of the CDP $\xi(.)$. Note that only observation is being carried out. The actual calculation of the value function may be done separately as described in the next section. The choice of the control is assumed to be done by a separate controller. Let Ω_k be the finest grid, i.e. Δt_k and h_k the finest discretizations. Let $U_l = U^{\Delta t_l / \Delta t_k} = U \times \ldots \times U$, $\Delta t_l / \Delta t_k$ times. $Q_l^{a_l}$ is a $|\Omega_l| \times |\Omega_l|$-matrix ($a_l \in U_l$), containing the number of transitions between cells in Ω_l. $R_l^{a_l}$ is a $|\Omega_l|$-vector containing the empirical cost for every cell in Ω_l. The immediate cost is given by the system as $r_l = \int_0^{\Delta t_l} e^{-\beta t} r(\xi(t), a_l) dt$. T denotes current time.

---

0. **Initialize** Ω_l, $Q_l^{a_l}$, $R_l^{a_l}$ for all $a_l \in U_l$, $l = 0, \ldots, k$
1. **repeat** {
2.   **choose** $a = a(T) \in U$ and apply a constantly on $[T; T + \Delta t_k]$
3. $T := T + \Delta t_k$
4.   **for** $l = 0$ **to** k **do** {
5.   **determine cell** $x_l \in \Omega_l$ with $\xi(T - \Delta t_l) \in A(x_l)$
6.   **determine cell** $y_l \in \Omega_l$ with $\xi(T) \in A(y_l)$
7.   **if** $\|x_k - y_k\| \geq R$ (truncation radius) **then goto** 2. **else**
8. $a_l := (a(T - \Delta t_l), a(T + \Delta t_k - \Delta t_l), \ldots, a(T - \Delta t_k))$
9.   **receive immediate cost** r_l
10. $Q_l^{a_l}(x_l, y_l) := Q_l^{a_l}(x_l, y_l) + 1$
11. $R_l^{a_l}(x_l) := \left(r_l + R_l^{a_l}(x_l) \cdot \sum_{z \in \Omega_l} Q_l^{a_l}(x_l, z)\right) / \left(1 + \sum_{z \in \Omega_l} Q_l^{a_l}(x_l, z)\right)$
    } (for-do)
  } (repeat)

Before applying a multi-grid algorithm for the calculation of the value function on the basis of the observations, one should make sure that every box has at least some data for every control. Especially in the early stages of learning only the two coarsest grids Ω_0, Ω_1 could be used for computation of the optimal value function and finer grids may be added (possibly locally) as learning evolves.

5 Application of Multi-Grid Techniques

The identification algorithm produces matrices $Q_l^{a_l}$ containing the number of transitions between boxes in Ω_l. We will calculate from the matrices Q the transition matrices P by the formula

$$P_l^{a_l}(x, y) = Q_l^{a_l}(x, y) / \left(\sum_{z \in \Omega_l} Q_l^{a_l}(x, z)\right), \quad x, y \in \Omega_l, \ a_l \in U_l, \ l = 0, \ldots, k. \quad (20)$$

Now we define matrices A and right hand sides f as

$$A_l^{a_l} := (\beta_l P_l^{a_l} - I)/\Delta t_l \quad f_l^{a_l} := R_l^{a_l}/\Delta t_l, \quad (21)$$

where $\beta_l = e^{-\beta \Delta t_l}$. The discrete Bellman equation takes the following form

$$\min_{a_l \in U_l} \{A_l^{a_l} V_l(x) - f_l^{a_l}(x)\} = 0. \quad (22)$$

The problem is now in a form to which the multi-grid method due to Hoppe, Bloß ([2], 1989) can be applied. For prolongation and restriction we choose bilinear interpolation and full weighted restriction for cell-centered grids. We point out, that for any cell $x \in \Omega_l$ only those neighboring cells shall be used for prolongation and restriction for which the minimum in (22) is attained for the same control as the minimizing control in x (see [2], 1989 and [3], 1996 for details). On every grid

Ω_l the defect in equation (22) is calculated and used for a correction on grid Ω_{l-1}. As a smoother nonlinear Gauss-Seidel iteration applied to (22) is used.

Our approach differs from the algorithm in Hoppe, Bloß ([2], 1989) in the special form of the matrices $A_l^{a_i}$ in equation (22). The stars are generally larger than nine-point, in fact the stars grow with decreasing h although the matrices remain sparse. Also, when working with empirical information the relationship between the matrices $A_l^{a_i}$ on the various grids is based on observation of a process, which implies that coarse grid corrections do not always correct the equation of the finest grid (especially in the early stages of learning). However, using the observed transition matrices $A_l^{a_i}$ on the coarse grids saves the computing time which would otherwise be needed to calculate these matrices by the Galerkin product (see Hackbusch [4], 1985).

6 Simulation with precomputed transitions

Consider a homogeneous server problem with two servers holding data $(x_1, x_2) \in [0,1] \times [0,1]$. Two independent data streams arrive, one at each server. A controller has to decide to which server to route. The modeling equation for the stream shall be

$$dx = b(x, u)dt + \sigma(x)dw, \quad u \in \{1, 2\} \quad (23)$$

with

$$b(x,1) = \begin{pmatrix} 1 \\ -1 \end{pmatrix} \quad b(x,2) = \begin{pmatrix} -1 \\ 1 \end{pmatrix} \quad \sigma = \begin{pmatrix} 1 & 0 \\ 0 & 1 \end{pmatrix} \quad (24)$$

The boundaries at $x_1 = 0$ and $x_2 = 0$ are reflecting. The exceeding data on either server $x_1, x_2 > 1$ is rejected from the system and penalized with $g(x_1, 1) = g(1, x_2) = 10$, $g = 0$ otherwise. The objective of the control policy shall be to minimize

$$\mathbb{E} \int_0^\infty e^{-\beta t}(x_1(t) + x_2(t) + g(x_1, x_2))dt. \quad (25)$$

The plots of the value function show, that in case of high load (i.e. x_1, x_2 close to 1) a maximum of cost is assumed. Therefore it is cheaper to overload a server and pay penalty than to stay close to the diagonal as is optimal in the low load case.

For simulation we used precomputed (i.e. converged heuristic) transition probabilities to test the multi-grid performance. The discount β was set to .7. The multi-grid algorithm reduces the error in each iteration by a factor 0.21, using 5 grid levels and a V-cycle and two smoothing iterations on the coarsest grid. For comparison, the iteration on the finest grid converges with a reduction factor 0.63.

7 Discussion

We have given a condition for sampling controlled diffusion processes such that the value functions will converge while the discretization tends to zero. Rigorous numerical methods can now be applied to reinforcement learning algorithms in continuous-time, continuous-state as is demonstrated with a multi-grid algorithm for the HJB-equation. Ongoing work is directed towards adaptive grid refinement algorithms and application to systems that include hysteresis.

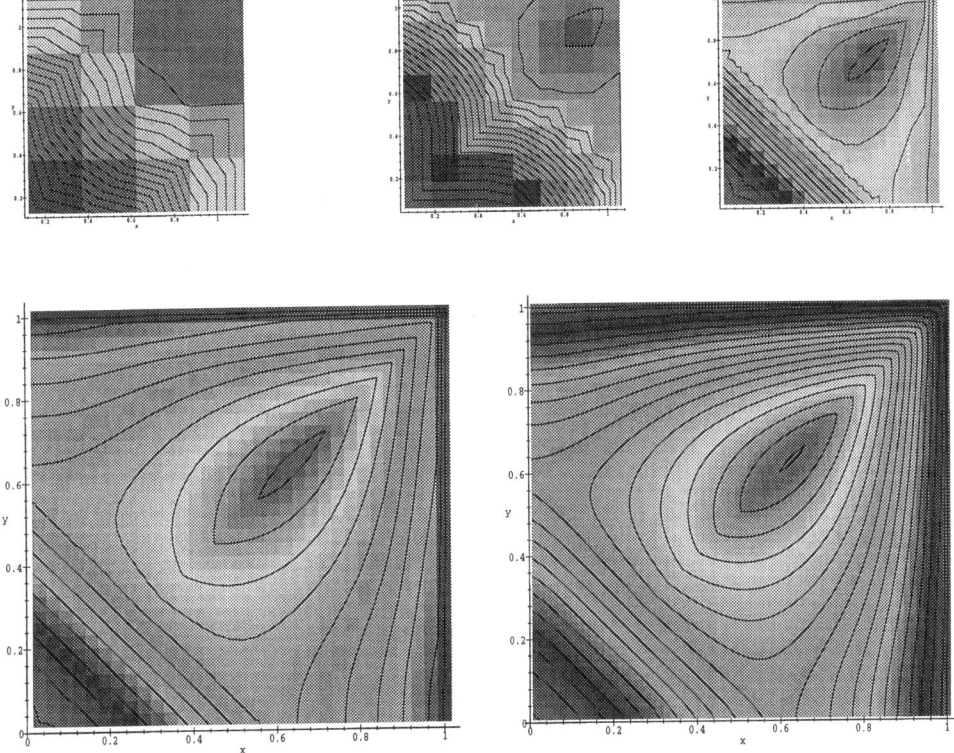

Figure 2: Contour plots of the predicted reward in a homogeneous server problem with nonlinear costs are shown on different grid levels. On the coarsest 4×4 grid a sampling rate of one second is used with 9-point-star transition matrices. At the finest grid (64×64) a sampling rate of $\frac{1}{4}$ second is used with observation on 81-point-stars. Inside the egg-shaped area the value function assumes its maximum.

References

[1] A. Barto, S. Bradtke, S. Singh. *Learning to Act using Real-Time Dynamic Programming*, AI Journal on Computational Theories of Interaction and Agency, 1993.

[2] M. Bloß and R. Hoppe. *Numerical Computation of the Value Function of Optimally Controlled Stochastic Switching Processes by Multi-Grid Techniques*, Numer Funct Anal And Optim 10(3+4), 275-304, 1989.

[3] S. Pareigis. *Lernen der Lösung der Bellman-Gleichung durch Beobachtung von kontinuierlichen Prozessen*, PhD Thesis, 1996.

[4] W. Hackbusch. *Multi-Grid Methods and Applications*, Springer-Verlag, 1985.

[5] H. Kushner and P. Dupuis. *Numerical Methods for Stochastic Control Problems in Continuous Time*, Springer-Verlag, 1992.

Learning From Demonstration

Stefan Schaal
sschaal@cc.gatech.edu; http://www.cc.gatech.edu/fac/Stefan.Schaal

College of Computing, Georgia Tech, 801 Atlantic Drive, Atlanta, GA 30332-0280
ATR Human Information Processing, 2-2 Hikaridai, Seiko-cho, Soraku-gun, 619-02 Kyoto

Abstract

By now it is widely accepted that learning a task from scratch, i.e., without any prior knowledge, is a daunting undertaking. Humans, however, rarely attempt to learn from scratch. They extract initial biases as well as strategies how to approach a learning problem from instructions and/or demonstrations of other humans. For learning control, this paper investigates how learning from demonstration can be applied in the context of reinforcement learning. We consider priming the Q-function, the value function, the policy, and the model of the task dynamics as possible areas where demonstrations can speed up learning. In general nonlinear learning problems, only model-based reinforcement learning shows significant speed-up after a demonstration, while in the special case of linear quadratic regulator (LQR) problems, all methods profit from the demonstration. In an implementation of pole balancing on a complex anthropomorphic robot arm, we demonstrate that, when facing the complexities of real signal processing, model-based reinforcement learning offers the most robustness for LQR problems. Using the suggested methods, the robot learns pole balancing in just a *single* trial after a 30 second long demonstration of the human instructor.

1. INTRODUCTION

Inductive supervised learning methods have reached a high level of sophistication. Given a data set and some prior information about its nature, a host of algorithms exist that can extract structure from this data by minimizing an error criterion. In learning control, however, the learning task is often less well defined. Here, the goal is to learn a policy, i.e., the appropriate actions in response to a perceived state, in order to steer a dynamical system to accomplish a task. As the task is usually described in terms of optimizing an arbitrary performance index, no direct training data exist which could be used to learn a controller in a supervised way. Even worse, the performance index may be defined over the long term behavior of the task, and a problem of temporal credit assignment arises in how to credit or blame actions in the past for the current performance. In such a setting, typical for reinforcement learning, learning a task from scratch can require a prohibitively time-consuming amount of exploration of the state-action space in order to find a good policy.

On the other hand, learning without prior knowledge seems to be an approach that is rarely taken in human and animal learning. Knowledge how to approach a new task can be transferred from previously learned tasks, and/or it can be extracted from the performance of a teacher. This opens the questions of how learning control can profit from these kinds of information in order to accomplish a new task more quickly. In this paper we will focus on learning from demonstration.

Learning from demonstration, also known as "programming by demonstration", "imitation learning", and "teaching by showing" received significant attention in automatic robot assembly over the last 20 years. The goal was to replace the time-consuming manual pro-

Learning from Demonstration

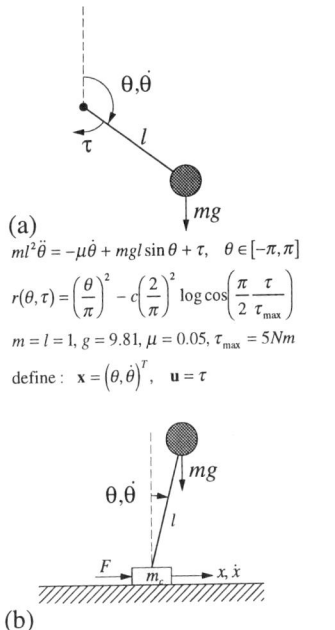

(a)
$ml^2\ddot{\theta} = -\mu\dot{\theta} + mgl\sin\theta + \tau, \quad \theta \in [-\pi, \pi]$

$r(\theta,\tau) = \left(\dfrac{\theta}{\pi}\right)^2 - c\left(\dfrac{2}{\pi}\right)^2 \log\cos\left(\dfrac{\pi}{2}\dfrac{\tau}{\tau_{max}}\right)$

$m = l = 1, g = 9.81, \mu = 0.05, \tau_{max} = 5Nm$

define: $\mathbf{x} = (\theta, \dot{\theta})^T, \quad \mathbf{u} = \tau$

(b)
$ml\ddot{x}\cos\theta + ml^2\ddot{\theta} - mgl\sin\theta = 0$

$(m + m_c)\ddot{x} + ml\ddot{\theta}\cos\theta - ml\dot{\theta}^2\sin\theta = F$

define: $\mathbf{x} = (x, \dot{x}, \theta, \dot{\theta})^T, \quad \mathbf{u} = F$

$r(\mathbf{x}, \mathbf{u}) = \mathbf{x}^T\mathbf{Q}\mathbf{x} + \mathbf{u}^T\mathbf{R}\mathbf{u}$

$l = 0.75m, m = 0.15kg, m_c = 1.0kg$

$\mathbf{Q} = diag(1.25, 1, 12, 0.25), \mathbf{R} = 0.01$

Figure 1: a) pendulum swing up, b) cart pole balancing

gramming of a robot by an automatic programming process, solely driven by showing the robot the assembly task by an expert. In concert with the main stream of Artificial Intelligence at the time, research was driven by symbolic approaches: the expert's demonstration was segmented into primitive assembly actions and spatial relationships between manipulator and environment, and subsequently submitted to symbolic reasoning processes (e.g., Lozano-Perez, 1982; Dufay & Latombe, 1983; Segre & DeJong, 1985). More recent approaches to programming by demonstration started to include more inductive learning components (e.g., Ikeuchi, 1993; Dillmann, Kaiser, & Ude, 1995). In the context of human skill learning, teaching by showing was investigated by Kawato, Gandolfo, Gomi, & Wada (1994) and Miyamoto et al. (1996) for a complex manipulation task to be learned by an anthropomorphic robot arm. An overview of several other projects can be found in Bakker & Kuniyoshi (1996).

In this paper, the focus lies on reinforcement learning and how learning from demonstration can be beneficial in this context. We divide reinforcement learning into two categories: reinforcement learning for nonlinear tasks (Section 2) and for (approximately) linear tasks (Section 3), and investigate how methods like Q-learning, value-function learning, and model-based reinforcement learning can profit from data from a demonstration. In Section 2.3, one example task, pole balancing, is placed in the context of using an actual, anthropomorphic robot to learn it, and we reconsider the applicability of learning from demonstration in this more complex situation.

2. REINFORCEMENT LEARNING FROM DEMONSTRATION

Two example tasks will be the basis of our investigation of learning from demonstration. The nonlinear task is the "pendulum swing-up with limited torque" (Atkeson, 1994; Doya, 1996), as shown in Figure 1a. The goal is to balance the pendulum in an upright position starting from hanging downward. As the maximal torque available is restricted such that the pendulum cannot be supported against gravity in all states, a "pumping" trajectory is necessary, similar as in the mountain car example of Moore (1991), but more delicately in its timing since building up too much momentum during pumping will overshoot the upright position. The (approximately) linear example, Figure 1b, is the well-known cart-pole balancing problem (Widrow & Smith, 1964; Barto, Sutton, & Anderson, 1983). For both tasks, the learner is given information about the one-step reward r (Figure 1), and both tasks are formulated as continuous state and continuous action problems. The goal of each task is to find a policy which minimizes the infinite horizon discounted reward:

$$V(\mathbf{x}(t)) = \int_t^\infty e^{-\frac{(s-t)}{\tau}} r(\mathbf{x}(s), \mathbf{u}(s)) ds \quad \text{or} \quad V(\mathbf{x}(t)) = \sum_{i=t}^\infty \gamma^{i-t} r(\mathbf{x}(i), \mathbf{u}(i)) \quad (1)$$

where the left hand equation is the continuous time formulation, while the right hand equation is the corresponding discrete time version, and where $\mathbf{x}$ and $\mathbf{u}$ denote a n-dimensional state vector and a m-dimensional command vector, respectively. For the Swing-Up, we assume that a teacher provided us with 5 successful trials starting from different initial conditions. Each trial consists of a time series of data vectors $(\theta, \dot{\theta}, \tau)$ sampled at 60Hz. For the Cart-Pole, we have a 30 second demonstration of successful balancing, represented as a 60Hz time series of data vectors $(x, \dot{x}, \theta, \dot{\theta}, F)$. How can these demonstrations be used to speed up reinforcement learning?

2.1 THE NONLINEAR TASK: SWING-UP

We applied reinforcement learning based on learning a value function (V-function) (Dyer & McReynolds, 1970) for the Swing-Up task, as the alternative method, Q-learning (Watkins, 1989), has yet received very limited research for continuous state-action spaces. The V–function assigns a scalar reward value $V(\mathbf{x}(t))$ to each state $\mathbf{x}$ such that the entire V–function fulfills the consistency equation:

$$V(\mathbf{x}(t)) = \arg\min_{\mathbf{u}(t)} \left(r(\mathbf{x}(t), \mathbf{u}(t)) + \gamma V(\mathbf{x}(t+1)) \right) \quad (2)$$

For clarity, this equation is given for a discrete state-action system; the continuous formulation can be found, e.g., in Doya (1996). The optimal policy, $\mathbf{u} = \pi(\mathbf{x})$, chooses the action $\mathbf{u}$ in state $\mathbf{x}$ such that (2) is fulfilled. Note that this computation involves an optimization step that includes knowledge of the subsequent state $\mathbf{x}(t+1)$. Hence, it requires a model of the dynamics of the controlled system, $\mathbf{x}(t+1) = f(\mathbf{x}(t), \mathbf{u}(t))$. From the viewpoint of learning from demonstration, V-function learning offers three candidates which can be primed from a demonstration: the value function $V(\mathbf{x})$, the policy $\pi(\mathbf{x})$, and the model $f(\mathbf{x}, \mathbf{u})$.

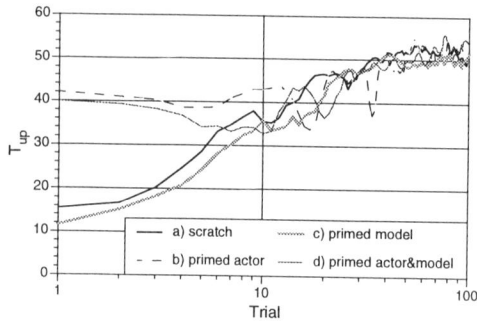

Figure 2: Smoothed learning curves of the average of 10 learning trials for the learning conditions a) to d) (see text). Good performance is characterized by $T_{up} > 45s$; below this value the system is usually able to swing up properly but it does not know how to stop in the upright position.

2.1.1 V-Learning

In order to assess the benefits of a demonstration for the Swing-Up, we implemented V–learning as suggested in Doya's (1996) continuous TD (CTD) learning algorithm. The V–function and the dynamics model were incrementally learned by a nonlinear function approximator, Receptive Field Weighted Regression (RFWR) (Schaal & Atkeson (1996)). Differing from Doya's (1996) implementation, we used the optimal action suggested by CTD to learn a model of the policy π (an "actor" as in Barto et al. (1983)), again represented by RFWR. The following learning conditions were tested empirically:

a) *Scratch*: Trial by trial learning of value function V, model f, and actor π from scratch.
b) *Primed Actor*: Initial training of π from the demonstration, then trial by trial learning.
c) *Primed Model*: Initial training of f from the demonstration, then trial by trial learning.
d) *Primed Actor&Model*: Priming of π and f as in b) and c), then trial by trial learning.

Figure 2 shows the results of learning the Swing-Up. Each trial lasted 60 seconds. The time T_{up} the pole spent in the interval $\theta \in [-\pi/2, \pi/2]$ during each trial was taken as the performance measure (Doya, 1996). Comparing conditions a) and c), the results demonstrate that learning the pole model from the demonstration did not speed up learning. This is not surprising since learning the V–function is significantly more complicated than learning the model, such that the learning process is dominated by V–function learning. Interestingly, priming the actor from the demonstration had a significant effect on the initial performance (condition a) vs. b)). The system knew right away how to pump up the pendulum, but, in order to learn how to balance the pendulum in the upright position, it finally took the same amount of time as learning from scratch. This behavior is due to the fact that, theoretically, the *V*–function can only be approximated correctly if the entire state-action space is explored densely. Only if the demonstration covered a large fraction of the entire state space one would expect that *V*–learning can profit from it. We also investigated using the demonstration to prime the *V*–function by itself or in combination with the other functions. The results were qualitatively the same as is shown in Figure 2: if the policy was included in the priming, the learning traces were like b) and d), otherwise like a) and c). Again, this is not totally surprising. Approximating a *V*-function is not just supervised learning as for π and f, it requires an iterative procedure to ensure the validity of (2) and amounts to a complicated nonstationary function approximation process. Given the limited amount of data from the demonstration, it is generally very unlikely to approximate a good value function.

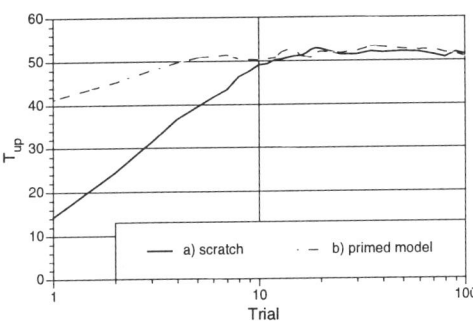

Figure 3: Smoothed learning curves of the average of 10 learning trials for the learning conditions a) and b) (see text) of the Swing-Up problem using "mental simulations". See Figure 2 for explanations how to interpret the graph.

2.1.2 Model-Based *V*-Learning

If learning a model f is required, one can make more powerful use of it. According to the certainty equivalence principle, f can substitute the real world, and planning can be run in "mental simulations" instead of interaction with the real world. In reinforcement learning, this idea was originally pursued by Sutton's (1990) DYNA algorithms for discrete state-action spaces. Here we will explore in how far a continuous version of DYNA, DYNA-CTD, can help in learning from demonstration. The only difference compared to CTD in Section 2.1.1 is that after every real trial, DYNA-CTD performs five "mental trials" in which the model of the dynamics acquired so far replaces the actual pole dynamics. Two learning conditions we be explored:

a) *Scratch*: Trial by trial learning of *V*, model f, and policy π from scratch.
b) *Primed Model*: Initial training of f from the demonstration, then trial by trial learning.

Figure 3 demonstrates that in contrast to *V*–learning in the previous section, learning from demonstration can make a significant difference now: after the demonstration, it only takes about 2-3 trials to accomplish a good swing-up with stable balancing, indicated by T_{up} >45s. Note that also learning from scratch is significantly faster than in Figure 2.

2.2 THE LINEAR TASK: CART-POLE BALANCING

One might argue that applying reinforcement learning from demonstration to the Swing-Up task is premature, since reinforcement learning with nonlinear function approximators has yet to obtain appropriate scientific understanding. Thus, in this section we turn to an easier task: the cart-pole balancer. The task is approximately linear if the pole is started in a close to upright position, and the problem has been well studied in the dynamic programming literature in the context of linear quadratic regulation (LQR) (Dyer & McReynolds, 1970).

2.2.1 Q–Learning

In contrast to *V*-learning, *Q*–learning (Watkins, 1989; Singh & Sutton, 1996) learns a more complicated value function, $Q(\mathbf{x}, \mathbf{u})$, which depends both on the state and the command. The analogue of the consistency equation (2) for *Q*–learning is:

$$Q(\mathbf{x}(t), \mathbf{u}(t)) = r(\mathbf{x}(t), \mathbf{u}(t)) + \gamma \arg\min_{\mathbf{u}(t+1)} \left(Q(\mathbf{x}(t+1), \mathbf{u}(t+1)) \right) \quad (3)$$

At every state **x**, picking the action **u** which minimizes Q is the optimal action under the reward function (1). As an advantage, evaluating the Q–function to find the optimal policy *does not* require a model the dynamical system f that is to be controlled; only the value of the one-step reward r is needed. For learning from demonstration, priming the Q–function and/or the policy are the two candidates to speed up learning.

For LQR problems, Bradtke (1993) suggested a Q–learning method that is ideally suited for learning from demonstration, based on extracting a policy. He observed that for LQR the Q–function is quadratic in the states and commands:

$$Q(\mathbf{x},\mathbf{u}) = \left[\mathbf{x}^T, \mathbf{u}^T\right] \begin{bmatrix} \mathbf{H}_{11} & \mathbf{H}_{12} \\ \mathbf{H}_{21} & \mathbf{H}_{22} \end{bmatrix} \left[\mathbf{x}^T, \mathbf{u}^T\right]^T, \; \mathbf{H}_{11} = n \times n, \; \mathbf{H}_{22} = m \times m, \; \mathbf{H}_{12} = \mathbf{H}_{21}^T = n \times m \quad (4)$$

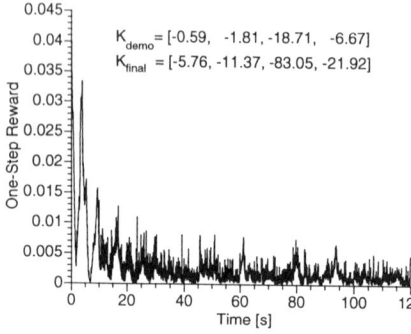

Figure 4: Typical learning curve of a noisy simulation of the cart-pole balancer using Q-learning. The graph shows the value of the one-step reward over time for the first learning trial. The pole is never dropped.

and that the (linear) policy, represented as a gain matrix **K**, can be extracted from (4) as:

$$u_{opt} = -\mathbf{K}\mathbf{x} = -\mathbf{H}_{22}^{-1}\mathbf{H}_{21}\mathbf{x} \quad (5)$$

Conversely, given a stabilizing initial policy $\mathbf{K}_{demo}$, the current Q–function can be approximated by a recursive least squares procedure, and it can be optimized by a policy iteration process with guaranteed convergence (Bradkte, 1993). As a demonstration allows one to extract an initial policy $\mathbf{K}_{demo}$ by linearly regressing the observed command **u** against the corresponding observed states **x**, one-shot learning of pole balancing is achievable. As shown in Figure 4, after about 120 seconds (12 policy iteration steps), the policy is basically indistinguishable from the optimal policy. A caveat of this Q–learning, however, is that it cannot not learn *without* a *stabilizing* initial policy.

2.2.2 Model-based V–Learning

Learning an LQR task by learning the V-function is one of the classic forms of dynamic programming (Dyer & McReynolds, 1970). Using a stabilizing initial policy $\mathbf{K}_{demo}$, the current V–function can be approximated by recursive least squares in analogy with Bradtke (1993). Similarly as for $\mathbf{K}_{demo}$, a (linear) model f_{demo} of the cart-pole dynamics can be extracted from a demonstration by linear regression of the cart-pole state **x**(t) vs. the previous state and command vector (**x**(t-1), **u**(t-1)), and the model can be refined with every new data point experienced during learning. The policy update becomes:

$$\mathbf{K} = \gamma\left(R + \gamma \mathbf{B}^T \mathbf{H} \mathbf{B}\right)^{-1} \mathbf{B}^T \mathbf{H} \mathbf{A}, \text{ where } V(\mathbf{x}) = \mathbf{x}^T \mathbf{H} \mathbf{x}, \; f_{demo} = [\mathbf{A} \, \mathbf{B}], \; \mathbf{A} = n \times n, \mathbf{B} = n \times m \quad (6)$$

Thus, a similar process as in Bradtke (1993) can be used to find the optimal policy **K**, and the system accomplishes one shot learning, qualitatively indistinguishable from Figure 4.

Again, as pointed out in Section 2.1.2, one can make more efficient use of the learned model by performing mental simulations. Given the model f_{demo}, the policy **K** can be calculated by off-line policy iteration from an initial estimate of **H**, e.g., taken to be the identity matrix (Dyer & McReynolds, 1970). Thus, no initial (stabilizing) policy is required, but rather an estimate of the task dynamics. Also this method achieves one shot learning.

2.3 POLE BALANCING WITH AN ACTUAL ROBOT

As a result of the previous section, it seems that there are no real performance differences between V-learning, Q-learning, and model-based V-learning for LQR problems. To explore the usefulness of these methods in a more realistic framework, we implemented learning from demonstration of pole balancing on an anthropomorphic robot arm. The robot is equipped with a 60 Hz video-based stereo vision. The pole is marked by two color blobs which can be tracked in real-time. A 30 second long demonstration of pole balancing was is provided by a human standing in front of the two robot cameras.

There are a few crucial differences in comparison with the simulations. First, as the demonstration is vision-based, only kinematic variables can be extracted from the demonstration. Second, visual signal processing has about 120ms time delay. Third, a command given to the robot is not executed with very high accuracy due to unknown nonlinearities of the robot. And lastly, humans use internal state for pole balancing, i.e., their policy is partially based on non-observable variables. These issues have the following impact:

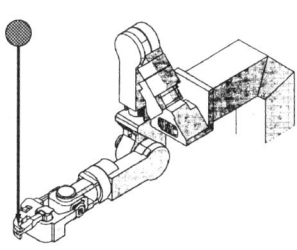

Kinematic Variables: In this implementation, the robot arm replaces the cart of the Cart-Pole problem. Since we have an estimate of the inverse dynamics and inverse kinematics of the arm, we can use the acceleration of the finger in Cartesian space as command input to the task. The arm is also much heavier than the pole which allows us to neglect the interaction forces the pole exerts on the arm. Thus, the pole balancing dynamics of Figure 1b can be reformulated as:

$$uml\cos\theta + \ddot{\theta}ml^2 - mgl\sin\theta = 0, \quad \ddot{x} = u \qquad (7)$$

Figure 5: Sketch of SARCOS anthropomorphic robot arm

All variables in this equation can be extracted from a demonstration. We omit the 3D extension of these equations.

Delayed Visual Information: There are two possibilities of dealing with delayed variables. Either the state of the system is augmented by delayed commands corresponding to $7*1/60s \approx 120s$ delay time, $\mathbf{x}^T = (x, \dot{x}, \theta, \dot{\theta}, u_{t-1}, u_{t-2}, \ldots, u_{t-7})$, or a state predictive controller is employed. The former method increases the complexity of a policy significantly, while the latter method requires a model f.

Inaccuracies of Command Execution: Given an acceleration command u, the robot will execute something close to u, but not u exactly. Thus, learning a function which includes u, e.g., the dynamics model (7), can be dangerous since the mapping $(x, \dot{x}, \theta, \dot{\theta}, u) \rightarrow (\ddot{x}, \ddot{\theta})$ is contaminated by the nonlinear dynamics of the robot arm. Indeed, it turned out that we could not learn such a model reliably. This could be remedied by "observing" the command u, i.e., by extracting $u = \ddot{x}$ from visual feedback.

Internal State in Demonstrated Policy: Investigations with human subjects have shown that humans use internal state in pole balancing. Thus, a policy cannot be observed that easily anymore as claimed in Section 2.2: a regression analysis for extracting the policy of a teacher must find the appropriate time-alignment of observed current state and command(s) in the past. This can become a numerically involved process as regressing a policy based on delayed commands is endangered by singular regression matrices. Consequently, it easily happens that one extracts a *nonstabilizing* policy from the demonstration, which prevents the application of Q-learning and V-learning as described in Section 2.2.

As a result of these considerations, the most trustworthy item to extract from a demonstration is the model of the pole dynamics. In our implementation it was used in two ways, for calculating the policy as in (6), and in state-predictive control with a Kalman filter to overcome the delays in visual information processing. The model was learned incrementally in real-time by an implementation of RFWR (Schaal & Atkeson 1996). Figure 6 shows the results of learning from scratch and learning from demonstration of the actual robot. Without a demonstration, it took about 10-20 trials before learning succeeded in reliable performance longer than one minute. With a 30 second long demonstration, learning was reliably accomplished in one *single* trial, using a large variety of physically different poles and using demonstrations from arbitrary people in the laboratory.

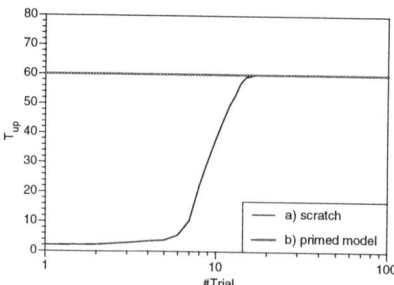

Figure 6: Smoothed average of 10 learning curves of the robot for pole balancing. The trials were aborted after successful balancing of 60 seconds. We also tested long term performance of the learning system by running pole balancing for over an hour—the pole was never dropped.

3. CONCLUSION

We discussed learning from demonstration in the context of reinforcement learning, focusing on Q–learning, value function learning, and model based reinforcement learning. Q–learning and value function learning can theoretically profit from a demonstration by extracting a policy, by using the demonstration data to prime the Q/value function, or, in the case of value function learning, by extracting a predictive model of the world. Only in the special case of LQR problems, however, could we find a significant benefit of priming the learner from the demonstration. In contrast, model-based reinforcement learning was able to greatly profit from the demonstration by using the predictive model of the world for "mental simulations". In an implementation with an anthropomorphic robot arm, we illustrated that even in LQR problems, model-based reinforcement learning offers larger robustness towards the complexity in real learning systems than Q–learning and value function learning. Using a model-based strategy, our robot learned pole-balancing from a demonstration in a *single* trial with great reliability. The important message of this work is that not every learning approach is equally suited to allow knowledge transfer and/or the incorporation of biases. This issue may serve as a critical additional constraint to evaluate artificial and biological models of learning.

Acknowledgments

Support was provided by the ATR Human Information Processing Labs, the German Research Association, the Alexander v. Humboldt Foundation, and the German Scholarship Foundation.

References

Atkeson, C. G. (1994). "Using local trajectory optimizers to speed up global optimization in dynamic programming." In: Moody, Hanson, & Lippmann (Ed.), *Adv. in Neural Inf. Proc. Sys. 6*. Morgan Kaufmann.

Bakker, P., & Kuniyoshi, Y. (1996). "Robot see, robot do: An overview of robot imitation.", Autonomous Systems Section, Electrotechnical Laboratory, Tsukuba Science City, Japan.

Barto, A. G., Sutton, R. S., & Anderson, C. W. (1983). "Neuronlike adaptive elements that can solve difficult learning control problems." *IEEE Transactions on Systems, Man, and Cybernetics*, **SMC-13**, 5.

Bradtke, S. J. (1993). "Reinforcement learning applied to linear quadratic regulation." In: Hanson, J. S., Cowan, J. D., & Giles, C. L. (Eds.), *Advances in Neural Inf. Processing Systems 5*, pp.295-302. Morgan Kaufmann.

Dillmann, R., Kaiser, M., & Ude, A. (1995). "Acquisition of elementary robot skills from human demonstration." In: *International Symposium on Intelligent Robotic Systems (SIRS'95)*, Pisa, Italy.

Doya, K. (1996). "Temporal difference learning in continuous time and space." In: Touretzky, D. S., Mozer, M. C., & Hasselmo, M. E. (Eds.), *Advances in Neural Information Processing Systems 8*. MIT Press.

Dufay, B., & Latombe, J.-C. (1984). "An approach to automatic robot programming based on inductive learning." In: Brady, M., & Paul, R. (Eds.), *Robotics Research*, pp.97-115. Cambridge, MA: MIT Press.

Dyer, P., & McReynolds, S. R. (1970). *The computation and theory of opitmal control*. NY: Academic Press.

Ikeuchi, K. (1993b). "Assembly plan from observation.", School of Computer Science, Carnegie Mellon University, Pittsburgh, PA.

Kawato, M., Gandolfo, F., Gomi, H., & Wada, Y. (1994b). "Teaching by showing in kendama based on optimization principle." In: *Proceedings of the International Conference on Artificial Neural Networks (ICANN'94)*, **1**, pp.601-606.

Lozano-Perez, T. (1982). "Task-Planning." In: Brady, M., Hollerbach, J. M., Johnson, T. L., Lozano-P_rez, T., & Mason, M. T. (Eds.), , pp.473-498. MIT Press.

Miyamoto, H., Schaal, S., Gandolfo, F., Koike, Y., Osu, R., Nakano, E., Wada, Y., & Kawato, M. (in press). "A Kendama learning robot based on bi-directional theory." *Neural Networks*.

Moore, A. (1991a). "Fast, robust adaptive control by learning only forward models." In: Moody, J. E., Hanson, S. J., & and Lippmann, R. P. (Eds.), *Advances in Neural Inf. Proc. Systems 4*. Morgan Kaufmann.

Schaal, S., & Atkeson, C. G. (1996). "From isolation to cooperation: An alternative of a system of experts." In: Touretzky, D. S., Mozer, M. C., & Hasselmo, M. E. (Eds.), *Advances in Neural Information Processing Systems 8*. Cambridge, MA: MIT Press.

Segre, A. B., & DeJong, G. (1985). "Explanation-based manipulator learning: Acquisition of planning ability through observation." In: *Conference on Robotics and Automation*, pp.555-560.

Singh, S. P., & Sutton, R. S. (1996). "Reinforcement learning with eligibility traces." *Machine Learning*.

Sutton, R. S. (1990). "Integrated architectures for learning, planning, and reacting based on approximating dynamic programming." In: *Proceedings of the International Machine Learning Conference*.

Watkins, C. J. C. H. (1989). "Learning with delayed rewards." Ph.D. thesis, Cambridge University (UK), .

Widrow, B., & Smith, F. W. (1964). "Pattern recognizing control systems." In: *1963 Comp. and Inf. Sciences (COINS) Symp. Proc.*, 288-317, Washington: Spartan.

Exploiting Model Uncertainty Estimates for Safe Dynamic Control Learning

Jeff G. Schneider
The Robotics Institute
Carnegie Mellon University
Pittsburgh, PA 15213
schneide@cs.cmu.edu

Abstract

Model learning combined with dynamic programming has been shown to be effective for learning control of continuous state dynamic systems. The simplest method assumes the learned model is correct and applies dynamic programming to it, but many approximators provide uncertainty estimates on the fit. How can they be exploited? This paper addresses the case where the system must be prevented from having catastrophic failures during learning. We propose a new algorithm adapted from the dual control literature and use Bayesian locally weighted regression models with dynamic programming. A common reinforcement learning assumption is that aggressive exploration should be encouraged. This paper addresses the converse case in which the system has to reign in exploration. The algorithm is illustrated on a 4 dimensional simulated control problem.

1 Introduction

Reinforcement learning and related grid-based dynamic programming techniques are increasingly being applied to dynamic systems with continuous valued state spaces. Recent results on the convergence of dynamic programming methods when using various interpolation methods to represent the value (or cost-to-go) function have given a sound theoretical basis for applying reinforcement learning to continuous valued state spaces [Gordon, 1995]. These are important steps toward the eventual application of these methods to industrial learning and control problems.

It has also been reported recently that there are significant benefits in data and computational efficiency when data from running a system is used to build a model, rather than using it once for single value function updates (as Q-learning would do) and discarding it [Sutton, 1990, Moore and Atkeson, 1993, Schaal and Atkeson, 1993, Davies, 1996]. Dynamic programming sweeps can then be done on the learned model either off-line or on-line. In its vanilla form, this method assumes the model is correct and does deterministic dynamic programming using the model. This assumption is often not correct, especially in the early stages of learning. When learning simulated or software systems, there may be no harm in the fact that this assumption does not hold. However, in real, physical systems there are often states that really are catastrophic and must be avoided even during learning. Worse yet, learning may have to occur during normal operation of the system in which case its performance during learning must not be significantly degraded.

The literature on adaptive and optimal linear control theory has explored this problem considerably under the names stochastic control and dual control. Overviews can be found in [Kendrick, 1981, Bar-Shalom and Tse, 1976]. The control decision is based on three components call the *deterministic, cautionary,* and *probing* terms. The deterministic term assumes the model is perfect and attempts to control for the best performance. Clearly, this may lead to disaster if the model is inaccurate. Adding a cautionary term yields a controller that considers the uncertainty in the model and chooses a control for the best expected performance. Finally, if the system learns while it is operating, there may be some benefit to choosing controls that are suboptimal and/or risky in order to obtain better data for the model and ultimately achieve better long-term performance. The addition of the probing term does this and gives a controller that yields the best long-term performance.

The advantage of dual control is that its strong mathematical foundation can provide the optimal learning controller under some assumptions about the system, the model, noise, and the performance criterion. Dynamic programming methods such as reinforcement learning have the advantage that they do not make strong assumptions about the system, or the form of the performance measure. It has been suggested [Atkeson, 1995, Atkeson, 1993] that techniques used in global linear control, including caution and probing, may also be applicable in the local case. In this paper we propose an algorithm that combines grid based dynamic programming with the *cautionary* concept from dual control via the use of a Bayesian locally weighted regression model.

Our algorithm is designed with industrial control applications in mind. A typical scenario is that a production line is being operated conservatively. There is data available from its operation, but it only covers a small region of the state space and thus can not be used to produce an accurate model over the whole potential range of operation. Management is interested in improving the line's response to changes in setpoints or disturbances, but can not risk much loss of production during the learning process. The goal of our algorithm is to collect new data and optimize the process while explicitly minimizing the risk.

2 The Algorithm

Consider a system whose dynamics are given by $x^{k+1} = f(x^k, u^k)$. The state, x, and control, u, are real valued vectors and k represents discrete time increments. A model of f is denoted as $\hat{f}$. The task is to minimize a cost functional of the form $J = \sum_{k=0}^{N} L(x^k, u^k, k)$ subject to the system dynamics. N may or may not be fixed depending on the problem. L is given, but f must be learned. The goal is to acquire data to learn f in order to minimize J without incurring huge penalties in J during learning. There is an implicit assumption that the cost function defines catastrophic states. If it were known that there were no disasters to avoid, then simpler, more aggressive algorithms would likely outperform the one presented here. The top level algorithm is as follows:

1. Acquire some data while operating the system from an existing controller.
2. Construct a model from the data using Bayesian locally weighted regression.
3. Perform DP with the model to compute a value function and a policy.
4. Operate the system using the new policy and record additional data.

5. Repeat to step 2 while there is still some improvement in performance.

In the rest of this section we describe steps 2 and 3.

2.1 Bayesian locally weighted regression

We use a form of locally weighted regression [Cleveland and Delvin, 1988, Atkeson, 1989, Moore, 1992] called Bayesian locally weighted regression [Moore and Schneider, 1995] to build a model from data. When a query, x_q, is made, each of the stored data points receives a weight $w_i = \exp(-\|x_i - x_q\|^2/K)$. K is the *kernel width* which controls the amount of localness in the regression. For Bayesian LWR we assume a wide, weak normal-gamma prior on the coefficients of the regression model and the inverse of the noise covariance. The result of a prediction is a t distribution on the output that remains well defined even in the absence of data (see [Moore and Schneider, 1995] and [DeGroot, 1970] for details).

The distribution of the prediction in regions where there is little data is crucial to the performance of the DP algorithm. As is often the case with learning through search and experimentation, it is at least as important that a function approximator predicts its own ignorance in regions of no data as it is how well it interpolates in data rich regions.

2.2 Grid based dynamic programming

In dynamic programming, the optimal value function, V, represents the cost-to-go from each state to the end of the task assuming that the optimal policy is followed from that point on. The value function can be computed iteratively by identifying the best action from each state and updating it according to the expected results of the action as given by a model of the system. The update equation is:

$$V^{k+1}(x) = \min_{u \in U} L(x,u) + V^k(\hat{f}(x,u)) \qquad (1)$$

In our algorithm, updates to the value function are computed while considering the probability distribution on the results of each action. If we assume that the output of the real system at each time step is an independent random variable whose probability density function is given by the uncertainty from the model, the update equation is as follows:

$$V^{k+1}(x) = \min_{u \in U} L(x,u) + E[V^k(f(x,u))|\hat{f}] \qquad (2)$$

Note that the independence assumption does not hold when reasonably smooth system dynamics are modeled by a smooth function approximator. The model error at one time step along a trajectory is highly correlated with the model error at the following step assuming a small distance traveled during the time step.

Our algorithm for DP with model uncertainty on a grid is as follows:

1. Discretize the state space, X, and the control space, U.

2. For each state and each control cache the cost of taking this action from this state. Also compute the probability density function on the next state from the model and cache the information. There are two cases which are shown graphically in fig. 1:
   - If the distribution is much narrower than the grid spacing, then the model is confident and a deterministic update will be done according to eq. 1. Multilinear interpolation is used to compute the value function at the mean of the predicted next state [Davies, 1996].
   - Otherwise, a stochastic update will be done according to eq. 2. The pdf of each of the state variables is stored, discretized at the same intervals as the grid representing the value function. Output independence is

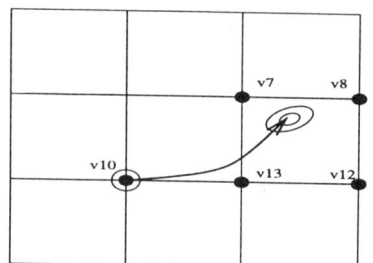 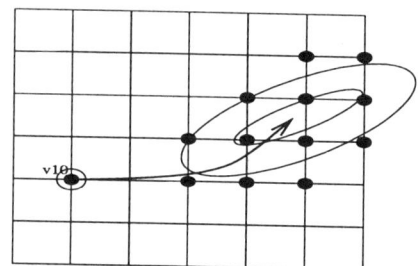

High Confidence Next State   **Low Confidence Next State**

Figure 1: Illustration of the two kinds of cached updates. In the high confidence scenario the transition is treated as deterministic and the value function is computed with multilinear interpolation: $V_{10}^{k+1} = L(x, u) + 0.4V_7^k + 0.3V_8^k + 0.2V_{11}^k + 0.1V_{12}^k$. In the low confidence scenario the transition is treated stochastically and the update takes a weighted sum over all the vertices of significant weight as well as the probability mass outside the grid: $V_{10}^{k+1} = L(x, u) + \frac{\sum_{\{x'|p(x')>\epsilon\}} p(x'|\hat{f}, x, u) V^k(x')}{\sum_{\{x'|p(x')>\epsilon\}} p(x'|\hat{f}, x, u)}$.

> assumed and later the pdf of each grid point will be computed as the product of the pdfs for each dimension and a weighted sum of all the grid points with significant weight will be computed. Also the total probability mass outside the bounds of the grid is computed and stored.

3. For each state, use the cached information to estimate the cost of choosing each action from that state. Update the value function at that state according to the cost of the best action found.

4. Repeat 3 until the value function converges, or the desired number of steps has been reached in finite step problems.

5. Record the best action (policy) for each grid point.

3 Experiments: Minimal Time Cart-Pole Maneuvers

The inverted pendulum is a well studied problem. It is easy to learn to stabilize it in a small number of trials, but not easy to learn quick maneuvers. We demonstrate our algorithm on the harder problem of moving the cart-pole stably from one position to another as quickly as possible. We assume we have a controller that can balance the pole and would like to learn to move the cart quickly to new positions, but never drop the pole during the learning process. The simulation equations and parameters are from [Barto et al., 1983] and the task is illustrated at the top of fig. 2. The state vector is $x = $ [pole angle (θ), pole angular velocity ($\dot{\theta}$), cart position (ρ), cart velocity ($\dot{\rho}$)]. The control vector, u, is the one dimensional force applied to the cart. x_0 is [0 0 17 0] and the cost function is $J = \sum_{i=0}^{N} x^T x + 0.01 u^T u$. N is not fixed. It is determined by the amount of time it takes for the system to reach a goal region about the target state, [0 0 0 0]. If the pole is dropped, the trial ends and an additional penalty of 10^6 is incurred.

This problem has properties similar to familiar process control problems such as cooking, mixing, or cooling, because it is trivial to stabilize the system and it can be moved slowly to a new desired position while maintaining the stability by slowly changing positional setpoints. In each case, the goal is to learn how to respond faster without causing any disasters during, or after, the learning process.

3.1 Learning an LQR controller

We first learn a linear quadratic regulator that balances the pole. This can be done with minimal data. The system is operated from the state, [0 0 0 0] for 10 steps of length 0.1 seconds with a controller that chooses u randomly from a zero mean gaussian with standard deviation 0.5. This is repeated to obtain a total of 20 data points. That data is used to fit a global linear model mapping x onto x'. An LQR controller is constructed from the model and the given cost function following the derivation in [Dyer and McReynolds, 1970].

The resulting linear controller easily stabilizes the pole and can even bring the system stably (although very inefficiently as it passes through the goal several times before coming to rest there) to the origin when started as far out as $x = [0\ 0\ 10\ 0]$. If the cart is started further from the origin, the controller crashes the system.

3.2 Building the initial Bayesian LWR model

We use the LQR controller to generate data for an initial model. The system is started at $x = [0\ 0\ 1\ 0]$ and controlled by the LQR controller with gaussian noise added as before. The resulting 50 data points are stored for an LWR model that maps $[\theta, \dot{\theta}, u] \to [\ddot{\theta}, \ddot{p}]$. The data in each dimension of the state and control space is scaled to [0 1]. In this scaled space, the LWR kernel width is set to 1.0.

Next, we consider the deterministic DP method on this model. The grid covers the ranges: [±1.0 ±4.0 ±21.0 ±20.0] and is discretized to [11 9 11 9] levels. The control is ±30.0 discretized to 15 levels. Any state outside the grid bounds is considered failure and incurs the 10^6 penalty. If we assume the model is correct, we can use deterministic DP on the grid to generate a policy. The computation is done with fixed size steps in time of 0.25 seconds. We observe that this policy is able to move the system safely from an initial state of [0 0 12 0], but crashes if it is started further out. Failure occurs because the best path generated using the model strays far from the region of the data (in variables θ and $\dot{\theta}$) used to construct the model.

It is disappointing that the use of LWR for nonlinear modeling didn't improve much over a globally linear model and an LQR controller. We believe this is a common situation. It is difficult to build better controllers from naive use of nonlinear modeling techniques because the available data models only a narrow region of operation and safely acquiring a wider range of data is difficult.

3.3 Cautionary dynamic programming

At this point we are ready to test our algorithm. Step 3 is executed using the LWR model from the data generated by the LQR controller as before. A trace of the system's operation when started at a distance of 17 from the goal is shown at the top of fig. 2. The controller is extremely conservative with respect to the angle of the pole. The pole is never allowed to go outside ±0.13 radians. Even as the cart approaches the goal at a moderate velocity the controller chooses to overshoot the goal considerably rather than making an abrupt action to brake the system.

The data from this run is added to the model and the steps are repeated. Traces of the runs from three iterations of the algorithm are shown in fig. 2. At each trial, the controller becomes more aggressive and completes the task with less cost. After the third iteration, no significant improvement is observed. The costs are summarized and compared with the LQR and deterministic DP controllers in table 1.

Fig. 3 is another illustration of how the policy becomes increasingly aggressive. It plots the pole angle vs. the pole angular velocity for the original LQR data and the executions at each of the following three trials. In summary, our algorithm is able

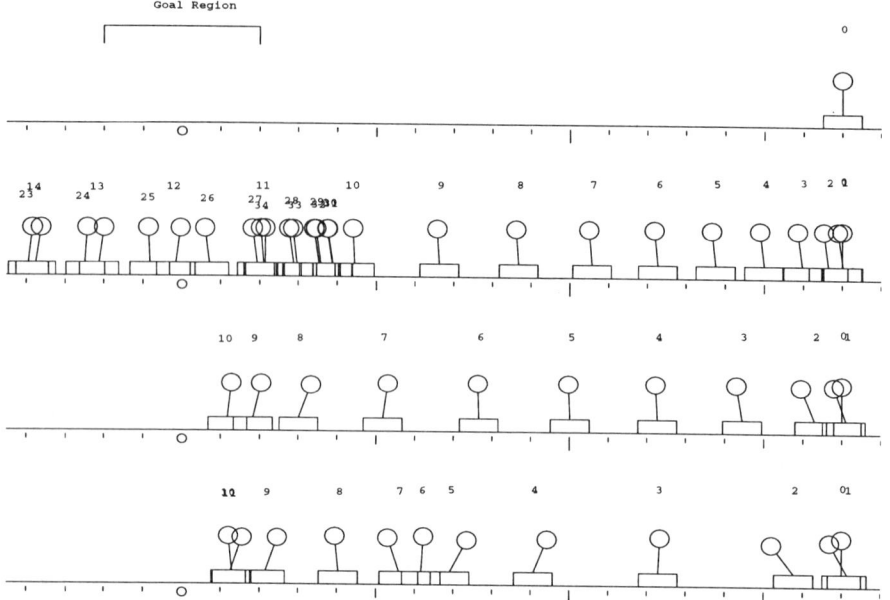

Figure 2: The task is to move the cart to the origin as quickly as possible without dropping the pole. The bottom three pictures show a trace of the policy execution obtained after one, two, and three trials (shown in increments of 0.5 seconds)

Controller	Number of data points used to build the controller	Cost from initial state 17
LQR	20	failure
Deterministic DP	50	failure
Stochastic DP trial 1	50	12393
Stochastic DP trial 2	221	7114
Stochastic DP trial 3	272	6270

Table 1: Summary of experimental results

to start from a simple controller that can stabilize the pole and learn to move it aggressively over a long distance without ever dropping the pole during learning.

4 Discussion

We have presented an algorithm that uses Bayesian locally weighted regression models with dynamic programming on a grid. The result is a cautionary adaptive control algorithm with the flexibility of a non-parametric nonlinear model instead of the more restrictive parametric models usually considered in the dual control literature. We note that this algorithm presents a viewpoint on the exploration vs exploitation issue that is different from many reinforcement learning algorithms, which are devised to encourage exploration (as in the *probing* concept in dual control). However, we argue that modeling the data first with a continuous function approximator and then doing DP on the model often leads to a situation where exploration must be *inhibited* to prevent disasters. This is particularly true in the case of real, physical systems.

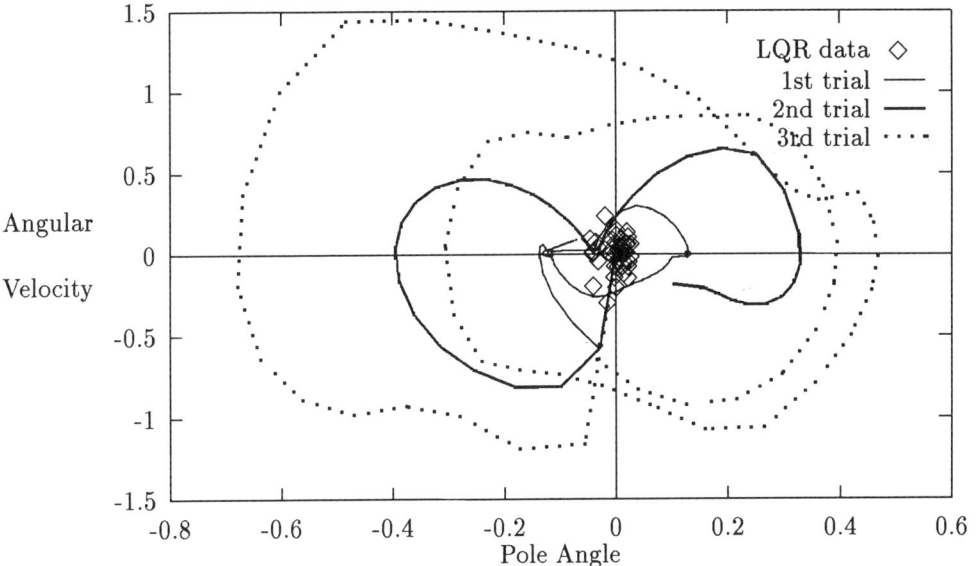

Figure 3: Execution trace. At each iteration, the controller is more aggressive.

References

[Atkeson, 1989] C. Atkeson. Using local models to control movement. In *Advances in Neural Information Processing Systems*, 1989.

[Atkeson, 1993] C. Atkeson. Using local trajectory optimizers to speed up global optimization in dynamic programming. In *Advances in Neural Information Processing Systems (NIPS-6)*, 1993.

[Atkeson, 1995] C. Atkeson. Local methods for active learning. Invited talk at AAAI Fall Symposium on Active Learning, 1995.

[Bar-Shalom and Tse, 1976] Y. Bar-Shalom and E. Tse. *Concepts and Methods in Stochastic Control*. Academic Press, 1976.

[Barto et al., 1983] A. Barto, R. Sutton, and C. Anderson. Neuronlike adaptive elements that can solve difficult learning control problems. *IEEE Transactions on Systems, Man, and Cybernetics*, 1983.

[Cleveland and Delvin, 1988] W. Cleveland and S. Delvin. Locally weighted regression: An approach to regression analysis by local fitting. *Journal of the American Statistical Association*, pages 596–610, September 1988.

[Davies, 1996] S. Davies. Applying grid-based interpolation to reinforcement learning. In *Neural Information Processing Systems 9*, 1996.

[DeGroot, 1970] M. DeGroot. *Optimal Statistical Decisions*. McGraw-Hill, 1970.

[Dyer and McReynolds, 1970] P. Dyer and S. McReynolds. *The Computation and Theory of Optimal Control*. Academic Press, 1970.

[Gordon, 1995] G. Gordon. Stable function approximation in dynamic programming. In *The 12th International Conference on Machine Learning*, 1995.

[Kendrick, 1981] D. Kendrick. *Stochastic Control for Economic Models*. McGraw-Hill, 1981.

[Moore and Atkeson, 1993] A. Moore and C. Atkeson. Prioritized sweeping: Reinforcement learning with less data and less real time. *Machine Learning*, 13(1):103–130, 1993.

[Moore and Schneider, 1995] A. Moore and J. Schneider. Memory based stochastic optimization. In *Advances in Neural Information Processing Systems (NIPS-8)*, 1995.

[Moore, 1992] A. Moore. Fast, robust adaptive control by learning only forward models. In *Advances in Neural Information Processing Systems 4*, 1992.

[Schaal and Atkeson, 1993] S. Schaal and C. Atkeson. Assessing the quality of learned local models. In *Advances in Neural Information Processing Systems (NIPS-6)*, 1993.

[Sutton, 1990] R. Sutton. First results with dyna, an intergrated architecture for learning, planning, and reacting. In *AAAI Spring Symposium on Planning in Uncertain, Unpredictable, or Changing Environments*, 1990.

Analytical Mean Squared Error Curves in Temporal Difference Learning

Satinder Singh
Department of Computer Science
University of Colorado
Boulder, CO 80309-0430
baveja@cs.colorado.edu

Peter Dayan
Brain and Cognitive Sciences
E25-210, MIT
Cambridge, MA 02139
bertsekas@lids.mit.edu

Abstract

We have calculated analytical expressions for how the bias and variance of the estimators provided by various temporal difference value estimation algorithms change with offline updates over trials in absorbing Markov chains using lookup table representations. We illustrate classes of learning curve behavior in various chains, and show the manner in which TD is sensitive to the choice of its step-size and eligibility trace parameters.

1 INTRODUCTION

A reassuring theory of asymptotic convergence is available for many reinforcement learning (RL) algorithms. What is not available, however, is a theory that explains the finite-term learning curve behavior of RL algorithms, e.g., what are the different kinds of learning curves, what are their key determinants, and how do different problem parameters effect rate of convergence. Answering these questions is crucial not only for making useful comparisons between algorithms, but also for developing hybrid and new RL methods. In this paper we provide preliminary answers to some of the above questions for the case of absorbing Markov chains, where mean square error between the estimated and true predictions is used as the quantity of interest in learning curves.

Our main contribution is in deriving the analytical update equations for the two components of MSE, bias and variance, for popular Monte Carlo (MC) and TD(λ) (Sutton, 1988) algorithms. These derivations are presented in a larger paper. Here we apply our theoretical results to produce analytical learning curves for TD on two specific Markov chains chosen to highlight the effect of various problem and algorithm parameters, in particular the definite trade-offs between step-size, α, and eligibility-trace parameter, λ. Although these results are for specific problems, we

2 ANALYTICAL RESULTS

A random walk, or trial, in an absorbing Markov chain with only terminal payoffs produces a sequence of states terminated by a payoff. The prediction task is to determine the expected payoff as a function of the start state i, called the optimal value function, and denoted $\mathbf{v}^*$. Accordingly, $v_i^* = E\{r|s_1 = i\}$, where s_t is the state at step t, and r is the random terminal payoff. The algorithms analysed are iterative and produce a sequence of estimates of $\mathbf{v}^*$ by repeatedly combining the result from a new trial with the old estimate to produce a new estimate. They have the form: $v_i(t) = v_i(t-1) + \alpha(t)\delta_i(t)$ where $\mathbf{v}(t) = \{v_i(t)\}$ is the estimate of the optimal value function after t trials, $\delta_i(t)$ is the result for state i based on random trial t, and the step-size $\alpha(t)$ determines how the old estimate and the new result are combined. The algorithms differ in the δs produced from a trial.

Monte Carlo algorithms use the final payoff that results from a trial to define the $\delta_i(t)$ (e.g., Barto & Duff, 1994). Therefore in MC algorithms the estimated value of a state is unaffected by the estimated value of any other state. The main contribution of TD algorithms (Sutton, 1988) over MC algorithms is that they update the value of a state based not only on the terminal payoff but also on the the estimated values of the intervening states. When a state is first visited, it initiates a short-term memory process, an eligibility trace, which then decays exponentially over time with parameter λ. The amount by which the value of an intervening state combines with the old estimate is determined in part by the magnitude of the eligibility trace at that point.

In general, the initial estimate $\mathbf{v}(0)$ could be a random vector drawn from some distribution, but often $\mathbf{v}(0)$ is fixed to some initial value such as zero. In either case, subsequent estimates, $\mathbf{v}(t); t > 0$, will be random vectors because of the random δs. The random vector $\mathbf{v}(t)$ has a bias vector $\mathbf{b}(t) \stackrel{def}{=} E\{\mathbf{v}(t) - \mathbf{v}^*\}$ and a covariance matrix $C(t) \stackrel{def}{=} E\{(\mathbf{v}(t) - E\{\mathbf{v}(t)\})(\mathbf{v}(t) - E\{\mathbf{v}(t)\})^T\}$. The scalar quantity of interest for learning curves is the weighted MSE as a function of trial number t, and is defined as follows:

$$\text{MSE}(t) = \sum_i p_i(E\{(v_i(t) - v_i^*)^2\}) = \sum_i p_i(b_i^2(t) + C_{ii}(t)),$$

where $p_i = (\mu^T[I - Q]^{-1})_i / \sum_j (\mu^T[I - Q]^{-1})_j$ is the weight for state i, which is the expected number of visits to i in a trial divided by the expected length of a trial[1] (μ_i is the probability of starting in state i; Q is the transition matrix of the chain).

In this paper we present results just for the standard TD(λ) algorithm (Sutton, 1988), but we have analysed (Singh & Dayan, 1996) various other TD-like algorithms (e.g., Singh & Sutton, 1996) and comment on their behavior in the conclusions. Our analytical results are based on two non-trivial assumptions: first that lookup tables are used, and second that the algorithm parameters α and λ are functions of the trial number alone rather than also depending on the state. We also make two assumptions that we believe would not change the general nature of the results obtained here: that the estimated values are updated offline (after the end of each trial), and that the only non-zero payoffs are on the transitions to the terminal states. With the above caveats, our analytical results allow rapid computation of *exact* mean square error (MSE) learning curves as a function of trial number.

---

[1] Other reasonable choices for the weights, p_i, would not change the nature of the results presented here.

2.1 BIAS, VARIANCE, And MSE UPDATE EQUATIONS

The analytical update equations for the bias, variance and MSE are complex and their details are in Singh & Dayan (1996) — they take the following form in outline:

$$\mathbf{b}(t) = \mathbf{a}^m + B^m \mathbf{b}(t-1) \tag{1}$$

$$C(t) = A^S + B^S C(t-1) + f^S(\mathbf{b}(t-1)) \tag{2}$$

where matrix B^m depends linearly on $\alpha(t)$ and B^S and f^S depend at most quadratically on $\alpha(t)$. We coded this detail in the C programming language to develop a software tool[2] whose rapid computation of exact MSE error curves allowed us to experiment with many different algorithm and problem parameters on many Markov chains. Of course, one could have averaged together many empirical MSE curves obtained via simulation of these Markov chains to get approximations to the analytical MSE error curves, but in many cases MSE curves that take minutes to compute analytically take days to derive empirically on the same computer for five significant digit accuracy. Empirical simulation is particularly slow in cases where the variance converges to non-zero values (because of constant step-sizes) with long tails in the asymptotic distribution of estimated values (we present an example in Figure 1c). Our analytical method, on the other hand, computes exact MSE curves for L trials in $O(|state\ space|^3 L)$ steps regardless of the behavior of the variance and bias curves.

2.2 ANALYTICAL METHODS

Two consequences of having the analytical forms of the equations for the update of the mean and variance are that it is possible to optimize schedules for setting α and λ and, for fixed λ and α, work out terminal rates of convergence for $\mathbf{b}$ and C.

Computing one-step optimal α's: Given a particular λ, the effect on the MSE of a single step for any of the algorithms is quadratic in α. It is therefore straightforward to calculate the value of α that minimises $\text{MSE}(t)$ at the next time step. This is called the *greedy* value of α. It is not clear that if one were interested in minimising $\text{MSE}(t+t')$, one would choose successive $\alpha(u)$ that greedily minimise $\text{MSE}(t); \text{MSE}(t+1); \ldots$. In general, one could use our formulæ and dynamic programming to optimise a whole schedule for $\alpha(u)$, but this is computationally challenging.

Note that this technique for setting greedy α assumes complete knowledge about the Markov chain and the initial bias and covariance of $\mathbf{v}(0)$, and is therefore not directly applicable to realistic applications of reinforcement learning. Nevertheless, it is a good analysis tool to approximate omniscient optimal step-size schedules, eliminating the effect of the choice of α when studying the effect of the λ.

Computing one-step optimal λ's: Calculating analytically the λ that would minimize $\text{MSE}(t)$ given the bias and variance at trial $t-1$ is substantially harder because terms such as $[I - \lambda(t)Q]^{-1}$ appear in the expressions. However, since it is possible to compute $\text{MSE}(t)$ for any choice of λ, it is straightforward to find to any desired accuracy the $\lambda_g(t)$ that gives the lowest resulting $\text{MSE}(t)$. This is possible only because $\text{MSE}(t)$ can be computed very cheaply using our analytical equations.

The caveats about greediness in choosing $\alpha_g(t)$ also apply to $\lambda_g(t)$. For one of the Markov chains, we used a stochastic gradient ascent method to optimise $\lambda(u)$ and

---

[2] The analytical MSE error curve software is available via anonymous ftp from the following address: ftp.cs.colorado.edu /users/baveja/AMse.tar.Z

Analytical MSE Curves for TD Learning

$\alpha(u)$ to minimise $\text{MSE}(t+t')$ and found that it was not optimal to choose $\lambda_g(t)$ and $\alpha_g(t)$ at the first step.

Computing terminal rates of convergence: In the update equations 1 and 2, $\mathbf{b}(t)$ depends linearly on $\mathbf{b}(t-1)$ through a matrix B^m; and $C(t)$ depends linearly on $C(t-1)$ through a matrix B^S. For the case of fixed α and λ, the maximal and minimal eigenvalues of B^m and B^S determine the fact and speed of convergence of the algorithms to finite endpoints. If the modulus of the real part of any of the eigenvalues is greater than 1, then the algorithms will not converge in general. We observed that the mean update is more stable than the mean square update, i.e., appropriate eigenvalues are obtained for larger values of α (we call the largest feasible α the largest learning rate for which TD will converge). Further, we know that the mean converges to $\mathbf{v}^*$ if α is sufficiently small that it converges at all, and so we can determine the terminal covariance. Just like the delta rule, these algorithms converge at best to an ϵ-ball for a constant finite step-size. This amounts to the MSE converging to a fixed value, which our equations also predict. Further, by calculating the eigenvalues of B^m, we can calculate an estimate of the rate of decrease of the bias.

3 LEARNING CURVES ON SPECIFIC MARKOV CHAINS

We applied our software to two problems: a symmetric random walk (SRW), and a Markov chain for which we can control the frequency of returns to each state in a single run (we call this the *cyclicity* of the chain).

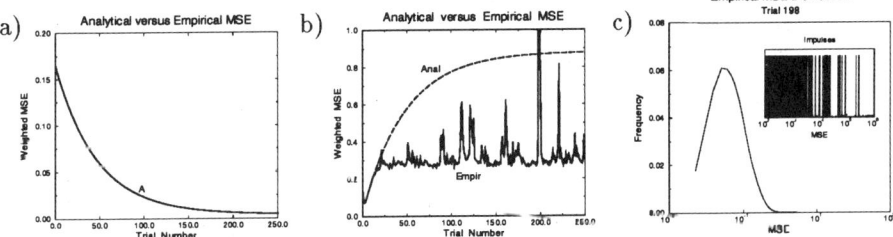

Figure 1: Comparing Analytical and Empirical MSE curves. a) analytical and empirical learning curves obtained on the 19 state SRW problem with parameters $\alpha = 0.01$, $\lambda = 0.9$. The empirical curve was obtained by averaging together more than three million simulation runs, and the analytical and empirical MSE curves agree up to the fourth decimal place; b) a case where the empirical method fails to match the analytical learning curve after more than 15 million runs on a 5 state SRW problem. The empirical learning curve is very spiky. c) Empirical distribution plot over 15.5 million runs for the MSE at trial 198. The inset shows impulses at actual sample values greater than 100. The largest value is greater than 200000.

Agreement: First, we present empirical confirmation of our analytical equations on the 19 state SRW problem. We ran TD(λ) for specific choices of α and λ for more than three million simulation runs and averaged the resulting empirical weighted MSE error curves. Figure 1a shows the analytical and empirical learning curves, which agree to within four decimal places.

Long-Tails of Empirical MSE distribution: There are cases in which the agreement is apparently much worse (see Figure 1b). This is because of the surprisingly *long tails* for the empirical MSE distribution – Figure 1c shows an example for a 5 state SRW. This points to interesting structure that our analysis is unable to reveal.

Effect of α and λ: Extensive studies on the 19 state SRW that we do not have space to describe fully show that: H1) for each algorithm, increasing α while holding λ fixed increases the asymptotic value of MSE, and similarly for increasing λ whilst holding α constant; H2) larger values of α or λ (except λ very close to 1) lead to faster convergence to the asymptotic value of MSE if there exists one; H3) in general, for each algorithm as one decreases λ the reasonable range of α shrinks, i.e., larger α can be used with larger λ without causing excessive MSE. The effect in H3 is counter-intuitive because larger λ tends to amplify the effective step-size and so one would expect the opposite effect. Indeed, this increase in the range of feasible α is not strictly true, especially very near $\lambda = 1$, but it does seem to hold for a large range of λ.

MC versus TD(λ): Sutton (1988) and others have investigated the effect of λ on the empirical MSE at small trial numbers and consistently shown that TD is better for some $\lambda < 1$ than MC ($\lambda = 1$). Figure 2a shows substantial changes as a function of trial number in the value of λ that leads to the lowest MSE. This effect is consistent with hypotheses $H1$-$H3$. Figure 2b confirms that this remains true even if greedy choices of α tailored for each value of λ are used. Curves for different values of λ yield minimum MSE over different trial number segments. We observed these effects on several Markov chains.

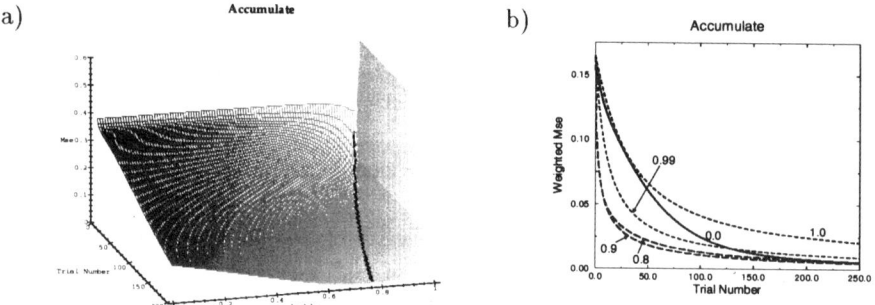

Figure 2: U-shaped Curves. a) Weighted MSE as a function of λ and trial number for fixed $\alpha = 0.05$ (minimum in λ shown as a black line). This is a 3-d version of the U-shaped curves in Sutton (1988), with trial number being the extra axis. b) Weighted MSE as a function of trial number for various λ using greedy α. Curves for different values of λ yield minimum MSE over different trial number segments.

Initial bias: Watkins (1989) suggested that λ trades off bias for variance, since $\lambda \sim 1$ has low bias, but potentially high variance, and conversely for $\lambda \sim 0$. Figure 3a confirms this in a problem which is a little like a random walk, except that it is highly cyclic so that it returns to each state many times in a single trial. If the initial bias is high (low), then the initial greedy value of λ is high (low). We had expected the asymptotic greedy value of λ to be 0, since once $\mathbf{b}(t) \sim 0$, then $\lambda = 0$ leads to lower variance updates. However, Figure 3a shows a non-zero asymptote – presumably because larger learning rates can be used for $\lambda > 0$, because of covariance. Figure 3b shows, however, that there is little advantage in choosing λ cleverly except in the first few trials, at least if good values of α are available.

Eigenvalue stability analysis: We analysed the eigenvalues of the covariance update matrix B^S (c.f. Equation 2) to determine maximal fixed α as a function of λ. Note that larger α tends to lead to faster learning, provided that the values converge. Figure 4a shows the largest eigenvalue of B^S as a function of λ for various

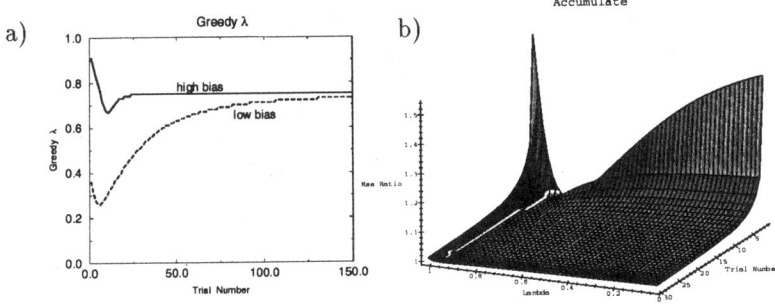

Figure 3: Greedy λ for a highly cyclic problem. a) Greedy λ for high and low initial bias (using greedy α). b) Ratio of MSE for given value of λ to that for greedy λ at each trial. The greedy λ is used for every step.

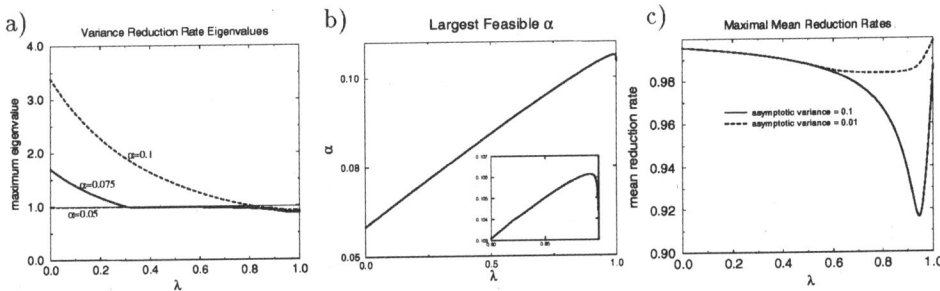

Figure 4: Eigenvalue analysis of covariance reduction. a) Maximal modulus of the eigenvalues of B^S. These determine the rate of convergence of the variance. Values greater than 1 lead to instability. b) Largest α such that the covariance is bounded. The inset shows a blowup for $0.9 \leq \lambda \leq 1$. Note that $\lambda = 1$ is not optimal. c) Maximal bias reduction rates as a function of λ, after controlling for asymptotic variance (to 0.1 and 0.01) by choosing appropriate α's. Again, $\lambda < 1$ is optimal.

α. If this eigenvalue is larger than 1, then the algorithm will diverge – a behavior that we observed in our simulations. The effect of hypothesis H3 above is evident – for larger λ, only smaller α can be used. Figure 4b shows this in more graphic form, indicating the largest α that leads to stable eigenvalues for B^S. Note the reversal very close to $\lambda = 1$, which provides more evidence against the pure MC algorithm. The choice of α and λ control both rate of convergence and the asymptotic MSE. In Figure 4c we control for the asymptotic variance by choosing appropriate αs as a function of λ and plot maximal eigenvalues of B^m (c.f. Equation 1; it controls the terminal rate of convergence of the bias to zero) as a function of λ. Again, we see evidence for TD over MC.

4 CONCLUSIONS

We have provided analytical expressions for calculating how the bias and variance of various TD and Monte Carlo algorithms change over iterations. The expressions themselves seem not to be very revealing, but we have provided many illustrations of their behavior in some example Markov chains. We have also used the analysis to calculate one-step optimal values of the step-size α and eligibility trace λ parameters. Further, we have calculated terminal mean square errors and maximal bias reduction rates. Since all these results depend on the precise Markov chains chosen, it is hard to make generalisations.

We have posited four general conjectures: H1) for constant λ, the larger α, the larger the terminal MSE; H2) the larger α or λ (except for λ very close to 1), the faster the convergence to the asymptotic MSE, provided that this is finite; H3) the smaller λ, the *smaller* the range of α for which the terminal MSE is not excessive; H4) higher values of λ are good for cases with high initial biases. The third of these is somewhat surprising, because the effective value of the step-size is really $\alpha/(1-\lambda)$. However, the lower λ, the more the value of a state is based on the value estimates for nearby states. We conjecture that with small λ, large α can quickly lead to high correlation in the value estimates of nearby states and result in runaway variance updates.

Two main lines of evidence suggest that using values of λ other than 1 (i.e., using a temporal difference rather than a Monte-Carlo algorithm) can be beneficial. First, the *greedy* value of λ chosen to minimise the MSE at the end of the step (whilst using the associated greedy α) remains away from 1 (see Figure 3). Second, the eigenvalue analysis of B^S showed that the largest value of α that can be used is higher for $\lambda < 1$ (also the asymptotic speed with which the bias can be guaranteed to decrease fastest is higher for $\lambda < 1$).

Although in this paper we have only discussed results for the standard TD(λ) algorithm (called Accumulate), we have also analysed Replace TD(λ) of Singh & Sutton (1996) and various others. This analysis clearly provides only an early step to understanding the course of learning for TD algorithms, and has focused exclusively on prediction rather than control. The analytical expressions for MSE might lend themselves to general conclusions over whole classes of Markov chains, and our graphs also point to interesting unexplained phenomena, such as the apparent long tails in Figure 1c and the convergence of greedy values of λ in Figure 3. Stronger analyses such as those providing large deviation rates would be desirable.

References

Barto, A.G. & Duff, M. (1994). Monte Carlo matrix inversion and reinforcement learning. NIPS 6, pp 687-694.

Singh, S.P. & Dayan, P. (1996). Analytical mean squared error curves in temporal difference learning. *Machine Learning*, submitted.

Singh, S.P. & Sutton, R.S. (1996). Reinforcement learning with replacing eligibility traces. *Machine Learning*, to appear.

Sutton, R.S. (1988). Learning to predict by the methods of temporal difference. *Machine Learning*, **3**, pp 9-44.

Watkins, C.J.C.H. (1989). *Learning from Delayed Rewards*. PhD Thesis. University of Cambridge, England.

Learning Decision Theoretic Utilities Through Reinforcement Learning

Magnus Stensmo
Computer Science Division
University of California
Berkeley, CA 94720, U.S.A.
magnus@cs.berkeley.edu

Terrence J. Sejnowski
Howard Hughes Medical Institute
The Salk Institute
10010 North Torrey Pines Road
La Jolla, CA 92037, U.S.A.
terry@salk.edu

Abstract

Probability models can be used to predict outcomes and compensate for missing data, but even a perfect model cannot be used to make decisions unless the utility of the outcomes, or preferences between them, are also provided. This arises in many real-world problems, such as medical diagnosis, where the cost of the test as well as the expected improvement in the outcome must be considered. Relatively little work has been done on learning the utilities of outcomes for optimal decision making. In this paper, we show how temporal-difference reinforcement learning (TD(λ)) can be used to determine decision theoretic utilities within the context of a mixture model and apply this new approach to a problem in medical diagnosis. TD(λ) learning of utilities reduces the number of tests that have to be done to achieve the same level of performance compared with the probability model alone, which results in significant cost savings and increased efficiency.

1 INTRODUCTION

Decision theory is normative or prescriptive and can tell us how to be rational and behave optimally in a situation [French, 1988]. Optimal here means to maximize the value of the expected future outcome. This has been formalized as the *maximum expected utility principle* by [von Neumann and Morgenstern, 1947]. Decision theory can be used to make optimal choices based on probabilities and utilities. Probability theory tells us how probable different future states are, and how to reason with and represent uncertainty information.

Utility theory provides values for these states so that they can be compared with each other. A simple form of a utility function is a *loss function*. Decision theory is a combination of probability and utility theory through expectation.

There has previously been a lot of work on learning probability models (neural networks, mixture models, probabilistic networks, *etc.*) but relatively little on representing and reasoning about preference and learning utility models. This paper demonstrates how both linear utility functions (*i.e.*, loss functions) and non-linear ones can be learned as an alternative to specifying them manually.

Automated fault or medical diagnosis is an interesting and important application for decision theory. It is a sequential decision problem that includes complex decisions (What is the most optimal test to do in a situation? When is it no longer effective to do more tests?), and other important problems such as missing data (both during diagnosis, *i.e.*, tests not yet done, and in the database which learning is done from). We demonstrate the power of the new approach by applying it to a real-world problem by learning a utility function to improve automated diagnosis of heart disease.

2 PROBABILITY, UTILITY AND DECISION THEORY MODELS

The system has separate probability and decision theory models. The probability model is used to predict the probabilities for the different outcomes that can occur. By modeling the joint probabilities these predictions are available no matter how many or few of the input variables are available at any instant. Diagnosis is a missing data problem because of the question-and-answer cycle that results from the sequential decision making process.

Our decision theoretic automated diagnosis system is based on hypotheses and deductions according to the following steps:

1. Any number of observations are made. This means that the values of one or several observation variables of the probability model are determined.

2. The system finds probabilities for the different possible outcomes using the joint probability model to calculate the conditional probability for each of the possible outcomes given the current observations.

3. Search for the next observation that is expected to be most useful for improving the diagnosis according to the Maximum Expected Utility principle.

    Each possible next variable is considered. The expected value of the system prediction with this variable observed minus the current maximum value before making the additional observation and the cost of the observation is computed and defined as the net *value of information* for this variable [Howard, 1966]. The variable with the maximum of all of these is then the best next observation to make.

4. The steps 1–3 above are repeated until further improvements are not possible. This happens when none of the net value of information values in step 3 is positive. They can be negative since a positive cost has been subtracted.

Note that we only look ahead one step (called a *myopic* approximation [Gorry and Barnett, 1967]). This is in principle suboptimal, however, the reinforcement learning procedure described below can compensate for this. The optimal solution is to consider all possible sequences, but the search tree grows exponentially in the number of unobserved variables.

Joint probabilities are modeled using *mixture models* [McLachlan and Basford, 1988]. Such models can be efficiently trained using the *Expectation-Maximization* (EM) *algorithm* [Dempster et al., 1977], which has the additional benefit that missing variable values in the training data also can be handled correctly. This is important since most real-world data sets are incomplete. More detail on the probability model can be found in [Stensmo and Sejnowski, 1995; Stensmo, 1995]. This paper is concerned with the utility function part of the decision theoretic model.

The utilities are values assigned to different states so that their usefulness can be compared and actions are chosen to maximize the expected future utility. Utilities are represented as preferences when a certain disease has been classified but the patient in reality has another one [Howard, 1980; Heckerman et al., 1992]. For each pair of diseases there is a utility value between 0 and 1, where a 0 means maximally bad and a 1 means maximally good. This is a $d \times d$ matrix for d diseases, and the matrix can be interpreted as a kind of a loss function. The notation is natural and helps for acquiring the values, which is a non-trivial problem. Preferences are subjective contrary to probabilities which are objective (for the purposes of this paper). For example, a doctor, a patient and the insurance company may have different preferences, but the probabilities for the outcomes are the same.

Methods have been devised to convert perceived risk to monetary values [Howard, 1980]. Subjects were asked to answer questions such as: "How much would you have to be paid to accept a one in a millionth chance of instant painless death?" The answers are recorded for various low levels of risk. It has been empirically found that people are relatively consistent and that perceived risk is linear for low levels of probability. Howard defined the unit *micromort* (mmt) to mean *one in 1 millionth chance of instant painless death* and [Heckerman et al., 1992] found that one subject valued 1 micromort to $20 (in 1988 US dollars) linearly to within a factor of two. We use this to convert utilities in [0,1] units to dollar values and vice versa.

Previous systems asked experts to supply the utility values, which can be very complicated, or used some simple approximation. [Heckerman et al., 1992] used a utility value of 1 for misclassification penalty when both diseases are malign or both are benign, and 0 otherwise (see Figure 4, left). They claim that it worked in their system but this approximation should reduce accuracy. We show how to adapt and learn utilities to find better ones.

3 REINFORCEMENT LEARNING OF UTILITIES

Utilities are adapted using a type of *reinforcement learning*, specifically the method of *temporal differences* [Sutton, 1988]. This method is capable of adjusting the utility values correctly even though a reinforcement signal is only received after each full sequence of questions leading to a diagnosis.

The temporal difference algorithm (TD(λ)) learns how to predict future values from past experience. A sequence of observations is used, in our case they are the results of the medical tests that have been done. We used TD(λ) to learn how to predict the expected utility of the final diagnosis.

Using the notation of Sutton, the function P_t predicts the expected utility at time t. P_t is a vector of expected utilities, one for each outcome. In the linear form described above, $P_t = P(x_t, w_t) = w_t x_t$, where w_t is a matrix of utility values and x_t is the vector of probabilities of the outcomes, our state description. The objective is to learn the utility matrix w_t.

We use an intra-sequence version of the TD(λ) algorithm so that learning can occur during normal operation of the system [Sutton, 1988]. The update equation is

$$w_{t+1} = w_t + \alpha[P(x_{t+1}, w_t) - P(x_t, w_t)] \sum_{k=1}^{t} \lambda^{t-k} \nabla_w P(x_k, w_t), \tag{1}$$

where α is the learning rate and λ is a discount factor. With $P_k = P(x_k, w_t) = x_k w_t$ and $e_t = \sum_{k=1}^{t} \lambda^{t-k} \nabla_w P(x_k, w_t) = \sum_{k=1}^{t} \lambda^{t-k} x_k$, (1) becomes the two equations

$$w_{t+1} = w_t + \alpha w_t [x_{t+1} - x_t] e_t$$
$$e_{t+1} = x_{t+1} + \lambda e_t,$$

starting with $e_1 = x_1$. These update equations were used after each question was answered. When the diagnosis was done, the reinforcement signal z (considered to be observation P_{t+1}) was obtained and the weights were updated: $w_{t+1} = w_t + \alpha w_t [z - x_t] e_t$. A final update of e_t was not necessary. Note that this method allows for the use of any differentiable utility function, specifically a neural network, in the place of $P(x_k, w_t)$.

Preference is subjective. In this paper we investigated two examples of reinforcement. One was to simply give the highest reinforcement ($z = 1$) on correct diagnosis and the lowest ($z = 0$) for errors. This yielded a linear utility function or loss function that was the unity matrix which confirmed that the method works. When applied to a non-linear utility function the result is non-trivial.

In the second example the reinforcement signal was modified by a penalty for the use of a high number questions by multiplying each z above with $(\max_q - q)/(\max_q - \min_q)$, where q is the number of questions used for the diagnostic sequence, and the minimum and maximum number of questions are $\min_q$ and $\max_q$, respectively. The results presented in the next section used this reinforcement signal.

4 RESULTS

The publicly available Cleveland heart-disease database was used to test the method. It consists of 303 cases where the disorder is one of four types of heart-disease or its absence. There are fourteen variables as shown in Figure 1. Continuous variables were converted into a *1-of-N* binary code based on their distributions among the cases in the database. Nominal and categorical variables were coded with one unit per value. In total 96 binary variables coded the 14 original variables.

To find the parameter values for the mixture model that was used for probability estimation, the EM algorithm was run until convergence [Stensmo and Sejnowski, 1995; Stensmo, 1995]. The classification error was 16.2%. To get this result all of the observation variables were set to their correct values for each case. Note that all this information might not be available in a real situation, and that the decision theory model was not needed in this case.

To evaluate how well the complete sequential decision process system does, we went through each case in the database and answered the questions that came up according to the correct values for the case. When the system completed the diagnosis sequence, the result was compared to the actual disease that was recorded in the database. The number of questions that were answered for each case was also recorded (q above). After all of the cases had been processed in this way, the average number of questions needed, its standard

	Observ.	Description	Values	Cost (mmt)	Cost ($)
1	age	Age in years	continuous	0	0
2	sex	Sex of subject	male/female	0	0
3	cp	Chest pain	four types	20	400
4	trestbps	Resting blood pressure	continuous	40	800
5	chol	Serum cholesterol	continuous	100	2000
6	fbs	Fasting blood sugar	<, or > 120 mg/dl	100	2000
7	restecg	Resting electrocardiographic result	five values	100	2000
8	thalach	Maximum heart rate achieved	continuous	100	2000
9	exang	Exercise induced angina	yes/no	100	2000
10	oldpeak	ST depression induced by exercise relative to rest	continuous	100	2000
11	slope	Slope of peak exercise ST segment	up/flat/down	100	2000
12	ca	Number major vessels colored by flouroscopy	0-3	100	2000
13	thal	Defect type	normal/fixed/reversible	100	2000

	Disorder	Description	Values
14	num	Heart disease	No disease/ four types

Figure 1: The Cleveland Heart Disease database. The database consists of 303 cases described by 14 variables. Observation costs are somewhat arbitrarily assigned and are given in both dollars and converted to micromorts (mmt) in [0,1] units based on $20 per micromort (one in 1 millionth chance of instant painless death).

deviation, and the number of errors were calculated. If the system had several best answers, one was selected randomly.

Observation costs were assigned to the different variables according to Figure 1. Using the full utility/decision model and the 0/1-approximation for the utility function (left part of Figure 4), there were 29.4% errors. The results are summarized in Figure 2. Over the whole data set an average of 4.42 questions were used with a standard deviation of 2.02. Asking about 4–5 questions instead of 13 is much quicker but unfortunately less accurate. This was before the utilities were adapted.

With TD(λ) learning (Figure 3), the number of errors decreased to 16.2% after 85 repeated presentations of all of the cases in random order. We varied λ from 0 to 1 in increments of 0.1, and α over several orders of magnitude to find the reported results. The resulting average number of questions were 6.05 with a standard deviation of 2.08. The utility matrix after 85 iterations is shown in Figure 4 with $\alpha=0.0005$ and $\lambda=0.1$.

The price paid for increased robustness was an increase in the average number of questions from 4.42 to 6.05, but the same accuracy was achieved using only less than half of them on average. Many people intuitively think that half of the questions should be enough. There is, however, no reason for this; furthermore there is no procedure to stop asking questions if observations are chosen randomly.

In this paper a simple state description has been used, namely the predicted probabilities of the outcomes. We have also tried other representations by including the test results in the state description. On this data set similar results were obtained.

Model	Errors	# Questions	St. Dev.
Probability model only	16.2%	13	—
0/1 approximation	29.4%	4.42	2.02
After 85 iterations of TD(λ) learning	16.2%	6.05	2.08

Figure 2: Results on the Cleveland Heart Disease Database. The three methods are described in the text. The first method does not use a utility model. The 0/1 approximation use the matrix in Figure 4, left. The utility matrix that was learned by TD(λ) is shown in Figure 4, right.

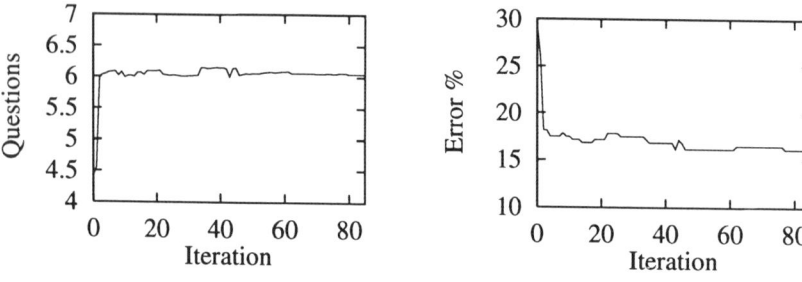

Figure 3: Learning graphs with discount-rate parameter $\lambda=0.1$, and learning rate $\alpha=0.0005$ for the TD(λ) algorithm. One iteration is a presentation of all of the cases in random order.

5 SUMMARY AND DISCUSSION

We have shown how utilities or preferences can be learned for different expected outcomes in a complex system for sequential decision making based on decision theory. Temporal-differences reinforcement learning was efficient and effective.

This method can be extended in several directions. Utilities are usually modeled linearly in decision theory (as with the misclassification utility matrix), since manual specification and interpretation of the utility values then is quite straight-forward. There are advantages with non-linear utility functions and, as indicated above, our method can be used for any utility function that is differentiable.

	Initial					After 85 iterations			
1	0	0	0	0	0.8179	0.0698	0.0610	0.0435	0.0505
0	1	1	1	1	0.0579	0.6397	0.2954	0.3331	0.6308
0	1	1	1	1	0.0215	0.1799	0.6305	0.3269	0.6353
0	1	1	1	1	0.0164	0.1430	0.2789	0.7210	0.6090
0	1	1	1	1	0.0058	0.1352	0.2183	0.2742	0.8105

Figure 4: Misclassification utility matrices. The disorder *no disease* is listed in the first row and column, followed by the four types of heart disease. **Left:** Initial utility matrix. **Right:** After TD learning with discount-rate parameter $\lambda=0.1$ and learning rate $\alpha=0.0005$. Element U_{ij} (row i, column j) is the utility when outcome i has been chosen but when it actually is j. Maximally good has value 1, and maximally bad has value 0.

An alternative to learning the utility or value function is to directly learn the optimal actions to take in each state, as in Q-learning [Watkins and Dayan, 1992]. This would require one to learn which question to ask in each situation instead of the utility values but would not be directly analyzable in terms of maximum expected utility.

Acknowledgements

Financial support for M.S. was provided by the Wenner-Gren Foundations and the Foundation Blanceflor Boncompagni-Ludovisi, née Bildt. The heart-disease database is from the University of California, Irvine Repository of Machine Learning Databases and originates from R. Detrano, Cleveland Clinic Foundation. Stuart Russell is thanked for discussions.

References

Dempster, A. P., Laird, N. M. and Rubin, D. B. (1977). Maximum likelihood from incomplete data via the EM algorithm. *Journal of the Royal Statistical Society, Series, B.*, **39**, 1–38.

French, S. (1988). *Decision Theory: An Introduction to the Mathematics of Rationality*. Ellis Horwood, Chichester, UK.

Gorry, G. A. and Barnett, G. O. (1967). Experience with a model of sequential diagnosis. *Computers and Biomedical Research*, **1**, 490–507.

Heckerman, D. E., Horvitz, E. J. and Nathwani, B. N. (1992). Toward normative expert systems: Part I. The Pathfinder project. *Methods of Information in Medicine*, **31**, 90–105.

Howard, R. A. (1966). Information value theory. *IEEE Transactions on Systems Science and Cybernetics*, **SSC-2**, 22–26.

Howard, R. A. (1980). On making life and death decisions. In Schwing, R. C. and Albers, Jr., W. A., editors, *Societal risk assessment: How safe is safe enough?* Plenum Press, New York, NY.

McLachlan, G. J. and Basford, K. E. (1988). *Mixture Models: Inference and Applications to Clustering*. Marcel Dekker, Inc., New York, NY.

Stensmo, M. (1995). *Adaptive Automated Diagnosis*. PhD thesis, Royal Institute of Technology (Kungliga Tekniska Högskolan), Stockholm, Sweden.

Stensmo, M. and Sejnowski, T. J. (1995). A mixture model system for medical and machine diagnosis. In Tesauro, G., Touretzky, D. S. and Leen, T. K., editors, *Advances in Neural Information Processing Systems*, vol. 7, pp 1077–1084. MIT Press, Cambridge, MA.

Sutton, R. S. (1988). Learning to predict by the method of temporal differences. *Machine Learning*, **3**, 9–44.

von Neumann, J. and Morgenstern, O. (1947). *Theory of Games and Economic Behavior*. Princeton University Press, Princeton, NJ.

Watkins, C. J. and Dayan, P. (1992). Q-learning. *Machine Learning*, **8**, 279–292.

On-line Policy Improvement using Monte-Carlo Search

Gerald Tesauro
IBM T. J. Watson Research Center
P. O. Box 704
Yorktown Heights, NY 10598

Gregory R. Galperin
MIT AI Lab
545 Technology Square
Cambridge, MA 02139

Abstract

We present a Monte-Carlo simulation algorithm for real-time policy improvement of an adaptive controller. In the Monte-Carlo simulation, the long-term expected reward of each possible action is statistically measured, using the initial policy to make decisions in each step of the simulation. The action maximizing the measured expected reward is then taken, resulting in an improved policy. Our algorithm is easily parallelizable and has been implemented on the IBM SP1 and SP2 parallel-RISC supercomputers.

We have obtained promising initial results in applying this algorithm to the domain of backgammon. Results are reported for a wide variety of initial policies, ranging from a random policy to TD-Gammon, an extremely strong multi-layer neural network. In each case, the Monte-Carlo algorithm gives a substantial reduction, by as much as a factor of 5 or more, in the error rate of the base players. The algorithm is also potentially useful in many other adaptive control applications in which it is possible to simulate the environment.

1 INTRODUCTION

Policy iteration, a widely used algorithm for solving problems in adaptive control, consists of repeatedly iterating the following policy improvement computation (Bertsekas, 1995): (1) First, a value function is computed that represents the long-term expected reward that would be obtained by following an initial policy. (This may be done in several ways, such as with the standard dynamic programming algorithm.) (2) An improved policy is then defined which is greedy with respect to that value function. Policy iteration is known to have rapid and robust convergence properties, and for Markov tasks with lookup-table state-space representations, it is guaranteed to convergence to the optimal policy.

In typical uses of policy iteration, the policy improvement step is an extensive off-line procedure. For example, in dynamic programming, one performs a sweep through all states in the state space. Reinforcement learning provides another approach to policy improvement; recently, several authors have investigated using RL in conjunction with nonlinear function approximators to represent the value functions and/or policies (Tesauro, 1992; Crites and Barto, 1996; Zhang and Dietterich, 1996). These studies are based on following actual state-space trajectories rather than sweeps through the full state space, but are still too slow to compute improved policies in real time. Such function approximators typically need extensive off-line training on many trajectories before they achieve acceptable performance levels.

In contrast, we propose an on-line algorithm for computing an improved policy in real time. We use Monte-Carlo search to estimate $V_P(x, a)$, the expected value of performing action a in state x and subsequently executing policy P in all successor states. Here, P is some given arbitrary policy, as defined by a "base controller" (we do not care how P is defined or was derived; we only need access to its policy decisions). In the Monte-Carlo search, many simulated trajectories starting from (x, a) are generated following P, and the expected long-term reward is estimated by averaging the results from each of the trajectories. (Note that Monte-Carlo sampling is needed only for non-deterministic tasks, because in a deterministic task, only one trajectory starting from (x, a) would need to be examined.) Having estimated $V_P(x, a)$, the improved policy P' at state x is defined to be the action which produced the best estimated value in the Monte-Carlo simulation, i.e., $P'(x) = \arg\max_a V_P(x, a)$.

1.1 EFFICIENT IMPLEMENTATION

The proposed Monte-Carlo algorithm could be very CPU-intensive, depending on the number of initial actions that need to be simulated, the number of time steps per trial needed to obtain a meaningful long-term reward, the amount of CPU per time step needed to make a decision with the base controller, and the total number of trials needed to make a Monte-Carlo decision. The last factor depends on both the variance in expected reward per trial, and on how close the values of competing candidate actions are.

We propose two methods to address the potentially large CPU requirements of this approach. First, the power of parallelism can be exploited very effectively. The algorithm is easily parallelized with high efficiency: the individual Monte-Carlo trials can be performed independently, and the combining of results from different trials is a simple averaging operation. Hence there is relatively little communication between processors required in a parallel implementation.

The second technique is to continually monitor the accumulated Monte-Carlo statistics during the simulation, and to prune away both candidate actions that are sufficiently unlikely (outside some user-specified confidence bound) to be selected as the best action, as well as candidates whose values are sufficiently close to the value of the current best estimate that they are considered equivalent (i.e., choosing either would not make a significant difference). This technique requires more communication in a parallel implementation, but offers potentially large savings in the number of trials needed to make a decision.

2 APPLICATION TO BACKGAMMON

We have initially applied the Monte-Carlo algorithm to making move decisions in the game of backgammon. This is an absorbing Markov process with perfect state-space information, and one has a perfect model of the nondeterminism in the system, as well as the mapping from actions to resulting states.

In backgammon parlance, the expected value of a position is known as the "equity" of the position, and estimating the equity by Monte-Carlo sampling is known as performing a "rollout." This involves playing the position out to completion many times with different random dice sequences, using a fixed policy P to make move decisions for both sides. The sequences are terminated at the end of the game (when one side has borne off all 15 checkers), and at that time a signed outcome value (called "points") is recorded. The outcome value is positive if one side wins and negative if the other side wins, and the magnitude of the value can be either 1, 2, or 3, depending on whether the win was normal, a gammon, or a backgammon. With normal human play, games typically last on the order of 50-60 time steps. Hence if one is using the Monte-Carlo player to play out actual games, the Monte-Carlo trials will on average start out somewhere in the middle of a game, and take about 25-30 time steps to reach completion.

In backgammon there are on average about 20 legal moves to consider in a typical decision. The candidate plays frequently differ in expected value by on the order of .01. Thus in order to resolve the best play by Monte-Carlo sampling, one would need on the order of 10K or more trials per candidate, or a total of hundreds of thousands of Monte-Carlo trials to make one move decision. With extensive statistical pruning as discussed previously, this can be reduced to several tens of thousands of trials. Multiplying this by 25-30 decisions per trial with the base player, we find that about a million base-player decisions have to be made in order to make one Monte-Carlo decision. With typical human tournament players taking about 10 seconds per move, we need to parallelize to the point that we can achieve at least 100K base-player decisions per second.

Our Monte-Carlo simulations were performed on the IBM SP1 and SP2 parallel-RISC supercomputers at IBM Watson and at Argonne National Laboratories. Each SP node is equivalent to a fast RS/6000, with floating-point capability on the order of 100 Mflops. Typical runs were on configurations of 16-32 SP nodes, with parallel speedup efficiencies on the order of 90%.

We have used a variety of base players in our Monte-Carlo simulations, with widely varying playing abilities and CPU requirements. The weakest (and fastest) of these is a purely random player. We have also used a few single-layer networks (i.e., no hidden units) with simple encodings of the board state, that were trained by back-propagation on an expert data set (Tesauro, 1989). These simple networks also make fast move decisions, and are much stronger than a random player, but in human terms are only at a beginner-to-intermediate level. Finally, we used some multi-layer nets with a rich input representation, encoding both the raw board state and many hand-crafted features, trained on self-play using the TD(λ) algorithm (Sutton, 1988; Tesauro, 1992). Such networks play at an advanced level, but are too slow to make Monte-Carlo decisions in real time based on full rollouts to completion. Results for all these players are presented in the following two sections.

2.1 RESULTS FOR SINGLE-LAYER NETWORKS

We measured the game-playing strength of three single-layer base players, and of the corresponding Monte-Carlo players, by playing several thousand games against a common benchmark opponent. The benchmark opponent was TD-Gammon 2.1 (Tesauro, 1995), playing on its most basic playing level (1-ply search, i.e., no lookahead). Table 1 shows the results. Lin-1 is a single-layer neural net with only the raw board description (number of White and Black checkers at each location) as

Network	Base player	Monte-Carlo player	Monte-Carlo CPU
Lin-1	-0.52 ppg	-0.01 ppg	5 sec/move
Lin-2	-0.65 ppg	-0.02 ppg	5 sec/move
Lin-3	-0.32 ppg	+0.04 ppg	10 sec/move

Table 1: Performance of three simple linear evaluators, for both initial base players and corresponding Monte-Carlo players. Performance is measured in terms of expected points per game (ppg) vs. TD-Gammon 2.1 1-ply. Positive numbers indicate that the player here is better than TD-Gammon. Base player stats are the results of 30K trials (std. dev. about .005), and Monte-Carlo stats are the results of 5K trials (std. dev. about .02). CPU times are for the Monte-Carlo player running on 32 SP1 nodes.

input. Lin-2 uses the same network structure and weights as Lin-1, plus a significant amount of random noise was added to the evaluation function, in order to deliberately weaken its playing ability. These networks were highly optimized for speed, and are capable of making a move decision in about 0.2 msec on a single SP1 node. Lin-3 uses the same raw board input as the other two players, plus it has a few additional hand-crafted features related to the probability of a checker being hit; there is no noise added. This network is a significantly stronger player, but is about twice as slow in making move decisions.

We can see in Table 1 that the Monte-Carlo technique produces dramatic improvement in playing ability for these weak initial players. As base players, Lin-1 should be regarded as a bad intermediate player, while Lin-2 is substantially worse and is probably about equal to a human beginner. Both of these networks get trounced by TD-Gammon, which on its 1-ply level plays at strong advanced level. Yet the resulting Monte-Carlo players from these networks appear to play about equal to TD-Gammon 1-ply. Lin-3 is a significantly stronger player, and the resulting Monte-Carlo player appears to be clearly better than TD-Gammon 1-ply. It is estimated to be about equivalent to TD-Gammon on its 2-ply level, which plays at a strong expert level.

The Monte-Carlo benchmarks reported in Table 1 involved substantial amounts of CPU time. At 10 seconds per move decision, and 25 move decisions per game, playing 5000 games against TD-Gammon required about 350 hours of 32-node SP machine time. We have also developed an alternative testing procedure, which is much less expensive in CPU time, but still seems to give a reasonably accurate measure of performance strength. We measure the average equity loss of the Monte-Carlo player on a suite of test positions. We have a collection of about 800 test positions, in which every legal play has been extensively rolled out by TD-Gammon 2.1 1-ply. We then use the TD-Gammon rollout data to grade the quality of a given player's move decisions.

Test set results for the three linear evaluators, and for a random evaluator, are displayed in Table 2. It is interesting to note for comparison that the TD-Gammon 1-ply base player scores 0.0120 on this test set measure, comparable to the Lin-1 Monte-Carlo player, while TD-Gammon 2-ply base player scores 0.00843, comparable to the Lin-3 Monte-Carlo player. These results are exactly in line with what we measured in Table 1 using full-game benchmarking, and thus indicate that the test-set methodology is in fact reasonably accurate. We also note that in each case, there is a huge error reduction of potentially a factor of 4 or more in using the Monte-Carlo technique. In fact, the rollouts summarized in Table 2 were done using fairly aggressive statistical pruning; we expect that rolling out decisions more

Evaluator	Base loss	Monte-Carlo loss	Ratio
Random	0.330	0.131	2.5
Lin-1	0.040	0.0124	3.2
Lin-2	0.0665	0.0175	3.8
Lin-3	0.0291	0.00749	3.9

Table 2: Average equity loss per move decision on an 800-position test set, for both initial base players and corresponding Monte-Carlo players. Units are ppg; smaller loss values are better. Also computed is ratio of base player loss to Monte-Carlo loss.

extensively would give error reduction ratios closer to factor of 5, albeit at a cost of increased CPU time.

2.2 RESULTS FOR MULTI-LAYER NETWORKS

Using large multi-layer networks to do full rollouts is not feasible for real-time move decisions, since the large networks are at least a factor of 100 slower than the linear evaluators described previously. We have therefore investigated an alternative Monte-Carlo algorithm, using so-called "truncated rollouts." In this technique trials are not played out to completion, but instead only a few steps in the simulation are taken, and the neural net's equity estimate of the final position reached is used instead of the actual outcome. The truncated rollout algorithm requires much less CPU time, due to two factors: First, there are potentially many fewer steps per trial. Second, there is much less variance per trial, since only a few random steps are taken and a real-valued estimate is recorded, rather than many random steps and an integer final outcome. These two factors combine to give at least an order of magnitude speed-up compared to full rollouts, while still giving a large error reduction relative to the base player.

Table 3 shows truncated rollout results for two multi-layer networks: TD-Gammon 2.1 1-ply, which has 80 hidden units, and a substantially smaller network with the same input features but only 10 hidden units. The first line of data for each network reflects very extensive rollouts and shows quite large error reduction ratios, although the CPU times are somewhat slower than acceptable for real-time play. (Also we should be somewhat suspicious of the 80 hidden unit result, since this was the same network that generated the data being used to grade the Monte-Carlo players.) The second line of data shows what happens when the rollout trials are cut off more aggressively. This yields significantly faster run-times, at the price of only slightly worse move decisions.

The quality of play of the truncated rollout players shown in Table 3 is substantially better than TD-Gammon 1-ply or 2-ply, and it is also substantially better than the full-rollout Monte-Carlo players described in the previous section. In fact, we estimate that the world's best human players would score in the range of 0.005 to 0.006 on this test set, so the truncated rollout players may actually be exhibiting superhuman playing ability, in reasonable amounts of SP machine time.

3 DISCUSSION

On-line search may provide a useful methodology for overcoming some of the limitations of training nonlinear function approximators on difficult control tasks. The idea of using search to improve in real time the performance of a heuristic controller

Hidden Units	Base loss	Truncated Monte-Carlo loss	Ratio	M-C CPU
10	0.0152	0.00318 (11-step, thorough)	4.8	25 sec/move
		0.00433 (11-step, optimistic)	3.5	9 sec/move
80	0.0120	0.00181 (7-step, thorough)	6.6	65 sec/move
		0.00269 (7-step, optimistic)	4.5	18 sec/move

Table 3: Truncated rollout results for two multi-layer networks, with number of hidden units and rollout steps as indicated. Average equity loss per move decision on an 800-position test set, for both initial base players and corresponding Monte-Carlo players. Again, units are ppg, and smaller loss values are better. Also computed is ratio of base player loss to Monte-Carlo loss. CPU times are for the Monte-Carlo player running on 32 SP1 nodes.

is an old one, going back at least to (Shannon, 1950). Full-width search algorithms have been extensively studied since the time of Shannon, and have produced tremendous success in computer games such as chess, checkers and Othello. Their main drawback is that the required CPU time increases exponentially with the depth of the search, i.e., $T \sim B^D$, where B is the effective branching factor and D is the search depth. In contrast, Monte-Carlo search provides a tractable alternative for doing very deep searches, since the CPU time for a full Monte-Carlo decision only scales as $T \sim N \cdot B \cdot D$, where N is the number of trials in the simulation.

In the backgammon application, for a wide range of initial policies, our on-line Monte-Carlo algorithm, which basically implements a single step of policy iteration, was found to give very substantial error reductions. Potentially 80% or more of the base player's equity loss can be eliminated, depending on how extensive the Monte-Carlo trials are. The magnitude of the observed improvement is surprising to us: while it is known theoretically that each step of policy iteration produces a strict improvement, there are no guarantees on how much improvement one can expect. We have also noted a rough trend in the data: as one increases the strength of the base player, the ratio of error reduction due to the Monte-Carlo technique appears to increase. This could reflect superlinear convergence properties of policy iteration.

In cases where the base player employs an evaluator that is able to estimate expected outcome, the truncated rollout algorithm appears to offer favorable tradeoffs relative to doing full rollouts to completion. While the quality of Monte-Carlo decisions is not as good using truncated rollouts (presumably because the neural net's estimates are biased), the degradation in quality is fairly small in at least some cases, and is compensated by a great reduction in CPU time. This allows more sophisticated (and thus slower) base players to be used, resulting in decisions which appear to be both better and faster.

The Monte-Carlo backgammon program as implemented on the SP offers the potential to achieve real-time move decision performance that exceeds human capabilities. In future work, we plan to augment the program with a similar Monte-Carlo algorithm for making doubling decisions. It is quite possible that such a program would be by far the world's best backgammon player.

Beyond the backgammon application, we conjecture that on-line Monte-Carlo search may prove to be useful in many other applications of reinforcement learning and adaptive control. The main requirement is that it should be possible to simulate the environment in which the controller operates. Since basically all of the recent successful applications of reinforcement learning have been based on training in simulators, this doesn't seem to be an undue burden. Thus, for example, Monte-

Carlo search may well improve decision-making in the domains of elevator dispatch (Crites and Barto, 1996) and job-shop scheduling (Zhang and Dietterich, 1996).

We are additionally investigating two techniques for training a controller based on the Monte-Carlo estimates. First, one could train each candidate position on its computed rollout equity, yielding a procedure similar in spirit to TD(1). We expect this to converge to the same policy as other TD(λ) approaches, perhaps more efficiently due to the decreased variance in the target values as well as the easily parallelizable nature of the algorithm. Alternately, the base position – the initial position from which the candidate moves are being made – could be trained with the best equity value from among all the candidates (corresponding to the move chosen by the rollout player). In contrast, TD(λ) effectively trains the base position with the equity of the move chosen by the base controller. Because the improved choice of move achieved by the rollout player yields an expectation closer to the true (optimal) value, we expect the learned policy to differ from, and possibly be closer to optimal than, the original policy.

Acknowledgments

We thank Argonne National Laboratories for providing SP1 machine time used to perform some of the experiments reported here. Gregory Galperin acknowledges support under Navy-ONR grant N00014-96-1-0311.

References

D. P. Bertsekas, Dynamic Programming and Optimal Control. Athena Scientific, Belmont, MA (1995).

R. H. Crites and A. G. Barto, "Improving elevator performance using reinforcement learning." In: D. Touretzky et al., eds., Advances in Neural Information Processing Systems 8, 1017-1023, MIT Press (1996).

C. E. Shannon, "Programming a computer for playing chess." *Philosophical Magazine* **41**, 265-275 (1950).

R. S. Sutton, "Learning to predict by the methods of temporal differences." *Machine Learning* **3**, 9-44 (1988).

G. Tesauro, "Connectionist learning of expert preferences by comparison training." In: D. Touretzky, ed., Advances in Neural Information Processing Systems 1, 99-106, Morgan Kaufmann (1989).

G. Tesauro, "Practical issues in temporal difference learning." *Machine Learning* **8**, 257-277 (1992).

G. Tesauro, "Temporal difference learning and TD-Gammon." *Comm. of the ACM*, **38:3**, 58-67 (1995).

W. Zhang and T. G. Dietterich, "High-performance job-shop scheduling with a time-delay TD(λ) network." In: D. Touretzky et al., eds., Advances in Neural Information Processing Systems 8, 1024-1030, MIT Press (1996).

Analysis of Temporal-Difference Learning with Function Approximation

John N. Tsitsiklis and Benjamin Van Roy
Laboratory for Information and Decision Systems
Massachusetts Institute of Technology
Cambridge, MA 02139
e-mail: jnt@mit.edu, bvr@mit.edu

Abstract

We present new results about the temporal-difference learning algorithm, as applied to approximating the cost-to-go function of a Markov chain using linear function approximators. The algorithm we analyze performs on-line updating of a parameter vector during a single endless trajectory of an aperiodic irreducible finite state Markov chain. Results include convergence (with probability 1), a characterization of the limit of convergence, and a bound on the resulting approximation error. In addition to establishing new and stronger results than those previously available, our analysis is based on a new line of reasoning that provides new intuition about the dynamics of temporal-difference learning. Furthermore, we discuss the implications of two counter-examples with regards to the significance of on-line updating and linearly parameterized function approximators.

1 INTRODUCTION

The problem of predicting the expected long-term future cost (or reward) of a stochastic dynamic system manifests itself in both time-series prediction and control. An example in time-series prediction is that of estimating the net present value of a corporation, as a discounted sum of its future cash flows, based on the current state of its operations. In control, the ability to predict long-term future cost as a function of state enables the ranking of alternative states in order to guide decision-making. Indeed, such predictions constitute the *cost-to-go function* that is central to dynamic programming and optimal control (Bertsekas, 1995).

Temporal-difference learning, originally proposed by Sutton (1988), is a method for approximating long-term future cost as a function of current state. The algorithm is recursive, efficient, and simple to implement. Linear combinations of fixed basis functions are used to approximate the mapping from state to future cost. The weights of the linear combination are updated upon each observation of a state transition and the associated cost. The objective is to improve approximations of long-term future cost as more and more state transitions are observed. The trajectory of states and costs can be generated either by a physical system or a simulated model. In either case, we view the system as a Markov chain. Adopting terminology from dynamic programming, we will refer to the function mapping states of the Markov chain to expected long-term cost as the cost-to-go function.

In this paper, we introduce a new line of analysis for temporal-difference learning. In addition to providing new intuition about the dynamics of the algorithm, this approach leads to a stronger convergence result than previously available, as well as an interpretation of the limit of convergence and bounds on the resulting approximation error, neither of which have been available in the past. Aside from the statement of results, we maintain the discussion at an informal level, and make no attempt to present a complete or rigorous proof. The formal and more general analysis based on our line of reasoning can found in (Tsitsiklis and Van Roy, 1996), which also discusses the relationship between our results and other work involving temporal-difference learning.

The convergence results assume the use of both on-line updating and linearly parameterized function approximators. To clarify the relevance of these requirements, we discuss the implications of two counter-examples that are presented in (Tsitsiklis and Van Roy, 1996). These counter-examples demonstrate that temporal-difference learning can diverge in the presence of either nonlinearly parameterized function approximators or arbitrary (instead of on-line) sampling distributions.

2 DEFINITION OF TD(λ)

In this section, we define precisely the nature of temporal-difference learning, as applied to approximation of the cost-to-go function for an infinite-horizon discounted Markov chain. While the method as well as our subsequent results are applicable to Markov chains with fairly general state spaces, including continuous and unbounded spaces, we restrict our attention in this paper to the case where the state space is finite. Discounted Markov chains with more general state spaces are addressed in (Tsitsiklis and Van Roy, 1996). Application of this line of analysis to the context of undiscounted absorbing Markov chains can be found in (Bertsekas and Tsitsiklis, 1996) and has also been carried out by Gurvits (personal communication).

We consider an aperiodic irreducible Markov chain with a state space $S = \{1, \ldots, n\}$, a transition probability matrix P whose (i,j)th entry is denoted by p_{ij}, transition costs $g(i,j)$ associated with each transition from a state i to a state j, and a discount factor $\alpha \in (0,1)$. The sequence of states visited by the Markov chain is denoted by $\{i_t \mid t = 0, 1, \ldots\}$. The cost-to-go function $J^* : S \mapsto \Re$ associated with this Markov chain is defined by

$$J^*(i) \triangleq E\left[\sum_{t=0}^{\infty} \alpha^t g(i_t, i_{t+1}) \mid i_0 = i\right].$$

Since the number of dimensions is finite, it is convenient to view J^* as a vector instead of a function.

We consider approximations of J^* using a function of the form

$$\tilde{J}(i, r) = (\Phi r)(i).$$

Here, $r = (r(1), \ldots, r(K))$ is a parameter vector and Φ is a $n \times K$. We denote the ith row of Φ as a (column) vector $\phi(i)$.

Suppose that we observe a sequence of states i_t generated according to the transition probability matrix P and that at time t the parameter vector r has been set to some value r_t. We define the temporal difference d_t corresponding to the transition from i_t to i_{t+1} by

$$d_t = g(i_t, i_{t+1}) + \alpha \tilde{J}(i_{t+1}, r_t) - \tilde{J}(i_t, r_t).$$

We define a sequence of *eligibility vectors* z_t (of dimension K) by

$$z_t = \sum_{k=0}^{t} (\alpha \lambda)^{t-k} \phi(i_k).$$

The TD(λ) updates are then given by

$$r_{t+1} = r_t + \gamma_t d_t z_t,$$

where r_0 is initialized to some arbitrary vector, γ_t is a sequence of scalar step sizes, and λ is a parameter in $[0, 1]$. Since temporal-difference learning is actually a continuum of algorithms, parameterized by λ, it is often referred to as TD(λ). Note that the eligibility vectors can be updated recursively according to $z_{t+1} = \alpha \lambda z_t + \phi(i_{t+1})$, initialized with $z_{-1} = 0$.

3   ANALYSIS OF TD(λ)

Temporal-difference learning originated in the field of reinforcement learning. A view commonly adopted in the original setting is that the algorithm involves "looking back in time and correcting previous predictions." In this context, the eligibility vector keeps track of how the parameter vector should be adjusted in order to appropriately modify prior predictions when a temporal-difference is observed. Here, we take a different view which involves examining the "steady-state" behavior of the algorithm and arguing that this characterizes the long-term evolution of the parameter vector. In the remainder of this section, we introduce this view of TD(λ) and provide an overview of the analysis that it leads to. Our goal in this section is to convey some intuition about how the algorithm works, and in this spirit, we maintain the discussion at an informal level, omitting technical assumptions and other details required to formally prove the statements we make. These technicalities are addressed in (Tsitsiklis and Van Roy, 1996), where formal proofs are presented.

We begin by introducing some notation that will make our discussion here more concise. Let $\pi(1), \ldots, \pi(n)$ denote the steady-state probabilities for the process i_t. We assume that $\pi(i) > 0$ for all $i \in S$. We define an $n \times n$ diagonal matrix D with diagonal entries $\pi(1), \ldots, \pi(n)$. We define a weighted norm $\|\cdot\|_D$ by

$$\|J\|_D = \sqrt{\sum_{i \in S} \pi(i) J^2(i)}.$$

We define a "projection matrix" Π by

$$\Pi J = \arg \min_{\bar{J} = \Phi r} \|J - \bar{J}\|_D.$$

It is easy to show that $\Pi = \Phi (\Phi' D \Phi)^{-1} \Phi' D$.

We define an operator $T^{(\lambda)} : \Re^n \mapsto \Re^n$, indexed by a parameter $\lambda \in [0, 1)$ by

$$(T^{(\lambda)} J)(i) = (1 - \lambda) \sum_{m=0}^{\infty} \lambda^m E \left[\sum_{t=0}^{m} \alpha^t g(i_t, i_{t+1}) + \alpha^{m+1} J(i_{m+1}) \mid i_0 = i \right].$$

For $\lambda = 1$ we define $(T^{(1)}J)(i) = J^*(i)$, so that $\lim_{\lambda\uparrow 1}(T^{(\lambda)}J)(i) = (T^{(1)}J)(i)$. To interpret this operator in a meaningful manner, note that, for each m, the term

$$E\left[\sum_{t=0}^{m} \alpha^t g(i_t, i_{t+1}) + \alpha^{m+1} J(i_{m+1}) \mid i_0 = i\right]$$

is the expected cost to be incurred over m transitions plus an approximation to the remaining cost to be incurred, based on J. This sum is sometimes called the "m-stage truncated cost-to-go." Intuitively, if J is an approximation to the cost-to-go function, the m-stage truncated cost-to-go can be viewed as an improved approximation. Since $T^{(\lambda)}J$ is a weighted average over the m-stage truncated cost-to-go values, $T^{(\lambda)}J$ can also be viewed as an improved approximation to J^*. A property of $T^{(\lambda)}$ that is instrumental in our proof of convergence is that $T^{(\lambda)}$ is a contraction of the norm $\|\cdot\|_D$. It follows from this fact that the composition $\Pi T^{(\lambda)}$ is also a contraction with respect to the same norm, and has a fixed point of the form Φr^* for some parameter vector r^*.

To clarify the fundamental structure of TD(λ), we construct a process $X_t = (i_t, i_{t+1}, z_t)$. It is easy to see that X_t is a Markov process. In particular, z_{t+1} and i_{t+1} are deterministic functions of X_t and the distribution of i_{t+2} only depends on i_{t+1}. Note that at each time t, the random vector X_t, together with the current parameter vector r_t, provides all necessary information for computing r_{t+1}. By defining a function s with $s(r, X) = (g(i,j) + \alpha \tilde{J}(j,r) - \tilde{J}(i,r))z$, where $X = (i, j, z)$, we can rewrite the TD(λ) algorithm as

$$r_{t+1} = r_t + \gamma_t s(r_t, X_t).$$

For any r, $s(r, X_t)$ has a "steady-state" expectation, which we denote by $E_0[s(r, X_t)]$. Intuitively, once X_t reaches steady-state, the TD(λ) algorithm, in an "average" sense, behaves like the following deterministic algorithm:

$$\bar{r}_{\tau+1} = \bar{r}_\tau + \gamma_\tau E_0[s(\bar{r}_\tau, X_t)].$$

Under some technical assumptions, a theorem from (Benveniste, et al., 1990) can be used to deduce convergence TD(λ) from that of the deterministic counterpart. Our study centers on an analysis of this deterministic algorithm. A theorem from (Benveniste, et al, 1990) is used to formally deduce convergence of the stochastic algorithm.

It turns out that

$$E_0[s(r, X_t)] = \Phi' D\Big(T^{(\lambda)}(\Phi r) - \Phi r\Big).$$

Using the contraction property of $T^{(\lambda)}$,

$$\begin{aligned}(r - r^*)' E_0[s(r, X_t)] &= (\Phi r - \Phi r^*)' D\Big(\Pi T^{(\lambda)}(\Phi r) - \Phi r^* + (\Phi r^* - \Phi r)\Big) \\ &\leq \|\Phi r - \Phi r^*\|_D \cdot \|\Pi T^{(\lambda)}(\Phi r) - \Phi r^*\|_D - \|\Phi r^* - \Phi r\|_D^2 \\ &\leq (\alpha - 1)\|\Phi r - \Phi r^*\|_D^2.\end{aligned}$$

Since $\alpha < 1$, this inequality shows that the steady state expectation $E_0[s(r, X_t)]$ generally moves the parameter vector towards r^*, the fixed point of $\Pi T^{(\lambda)}$, where "closeness" is measured in terms of the norm $\|\cdot\|_D$. This provides the main line of reasoning behind the proof of convergence provided in (Tsitsiklis and Van Roy, 1996). Some illuminating interpretations of this deterministic algorithm, which are useful in developing an intuitive understanding of temporal difference learning, are also discussed in (Tsitsiklis and Van Roy, 1996).

4 CONVERGENCE RESULT

We now present our main result concerning temporal-difference learning. A formal proof is provided in (Tsitsiklis and Van Roy, 1996).

Theorem 1 *Let the following conditions hold:*
(a) The Markov chain i_t has a unique invariant distribution π that satisfies $\pi' P = \pi'$, with $\pi(i) > 0$ for all i.
(b) The matrix Φ has full column rank; that is, the "basis functions" $\{\phi_k \mid k = 1, \ldots, K\}$ are linearly independent.
(c) The step sizes γ_t are positive, nonincreasing, and predetermined. Furthermore, they satisfy $\sum_{t=0}^{\infty} \gamma_t = \infty$, and $\sum_{t=0}^{\infty} \gamma_t^2 < \infty$.
We then have:
(a) For any $\lambda \in [0,1]$, the TD(λ) algorithm, as defined in Section 2, converges with probability 1.
(b) The limit of convergence r^* is the unique solution of the equation

$$\Pi T^{(\lambda)}(\Phi r^*) = \Phi r^*.$$

(c) Furthermore, r^* satisfies

$$\|\Phi r^* - J^*\|_D \leq \frac{1 - \lambda\alpha}{1 - \alpha} \|\Pi J^* - J^*\|_D.$$

Part (b) of the theorem leads to an interesting interpretation of the limit of convergence. In particular, if we apply the TD(λ) operator to the final approximation Φr^*, and then project the resulting function back into the span of the basis functions, we get the same function Φr^*. Furthermore, since the composition $\Pi T^{(\lambda)}$ is a contraction, repeated application of this composition to any function would generate a sequence of functions converging to Φr^*.

Part (c) of the theorem establishes that a certain desirable property is satisfied by the limit of convergence. In particular, if there exists a vector r such that $\Phi r = J^*$, then this vector will be the limit of convergence of TD(λ), for any $\lambda \in [0, 1]$. On the other hand, if no such parameter vector exists, the distance between the limit of convergence Φr^* and J^* is bounded by a multiple of the distance between the projection ΠJ^* and J^*. This latter distance is amplified by a factor of $(1 - \lambda\alpha)/(1 - \alpha)$, which becomes larger as λ becomes smaller.

5 COUNTER-EXAMPLES

Sutton (1995) has suggested that on-line updating and the use of linear function approximators are both important factors that make temporal-difference learning converge properly. These requirements also appear as assumptions in the convergence result of the previous section. To formalize the fact that these assumptions are relevant, two counter-examples were presented in (Tsitsiklis and Van Roy, 1996).

The first counter-example involves the use of a variant of TD(0) that does not sample states based on trajectories. Instead, the states i_t are sampled independently from a distribution $q(\cdot)$ over S, and successor states j_t are generated by sampling according to $\Pr[j_t = j|i_t] = p_{i_t,j}$. Each iteration of the algorithm takes on the form

$$r_{t+1} = r_t + \gamma_t \phi(i_t)\big(g(i_t, j_t) + \alpha\phi'(j_t)r_t - \phi'(i_t)r_t\big).$$

We refer to this algorithm as q–sampled TD(0). Note that this algorithm is closely related to the original TD(λ) algorithm as defined in Section 2. In particular, if i_t is generated by the Markov chain and $j_t = i_{t+1}$, we are back to the original algorithm. It is easy to show, using a subset of the arguments required to prove Theorem 1, that this algorithm converges when $q(i) = \pi(i)$ for all i, and the Assumptions of Theorem 1 are satisfied. However, results can be very different when $q(\cdot)$ is arbitrary. In particular, the counter-example presented in (Tsitsiklis an Van Roy, 1996) shows that for any sampling distribution $q(\cdot)$ that is different from $\pi(\cdot)$ there exists a Markov chain with steady-state probabilities $\pi(\cdot)$ and a linearly parameterized function approximator for which q-sampled TD(0) diverges. A counter-example with similar implications has also been presented by Baird (1995).

A generalization of temporal difference learning is commonly used in conjunction with nonlinear function approximators. This generalization involves replacing each vector $\phi(i_t)$ that is used to construct the eligibility vector with the vector of derivatives of $\tilde{J}(i_t, \cdot)$, evaluated at the current parameter vector r_t. A second counter-example in (Tsitsiklis and Van Roy, 1996), shows that there exists a Markov chain and a nonlinearly parameterized function approximator such that both the parameter vector and the approximated cost-to-go function diverge when such a variant of TD(0) is applied. This nonlinear function approximator is "regular" in the sense that it is infinitely differentiable with respect to the parameter vector. However, it is still somewhat contrived, and the question of whether such a counter-example exists in the context of more standard function approximators such as neural networks remains open.

6 CONCLUSION

Theorem 1 establishes convergence with probability 1, characterizes the limit of convergence, and provides error bounds, for temporal-difference learning. It is interesting to note that the margins allowed by the error bounds are inversely proportional to λ. Although this is only a bound, it strongly suggests that higher values of λ are likely to produce more accurate approximations. This is consistent with the examples that have been constructed by Bertsekas (1994).

The sensitivity of the error bound to λ raises the question of whether or not it ever makes sense to set λ to values less than 1. Many reports of experimental results, dating back to Sutton (1988), suggest that setting λ to values less than one can often lead to significant gains in the rate of convergence. A full understanding of how λ influences the rate of convergence is yet to be found, though some insight in the case of look-up table representations is provided by Dayan and Singh (1996). This is an interesting direction for future research.

Acknowledgments

We thank Rich Sutton for originally making us aware of the relevance of on-line state sampling, and also for pointing out a simplification in the expression for the error bound of Theorem 1. This research was supported by the NSF under grant DMI-9625489 and the ARO under grant DAAL-03-92-G-0115.

References

Baird, L. C. (1995). "Residual Algorithms: Reinforcement Learning with Function Approximation," in Prieditis & Russell, eds. Machine Learning: Proceedings of the Twelfth International Conference, 9-12 July, Morgan Kaufman Publishers, San Francisco, CA.

Bertsekas, D. P. (1994) "A Counter-Example to Temporal-Difference Learning,"

Neural Computation, vol. 7, pp. 270-279.

Bertsekas, D. P. (1995) *Dynamic Programming and Optimal Control*, Athena Scientific, Belmont, MA.

Bertsekas, D. P. & Tsitsiklis, J. N. (1996) *Neuro-Dynamic Programming*, Athena Scientific, Belmont, MA.

Benveniste, A., Metivier, M., & Priouret, P., (1990) *Adaptive Algorithms and Stochastic Approximations*, Springer-Verlag, Berlin.

Dayan, P. D. & Singh, S. P (1996) "Mean Squared Error Curves in Temporal Difference Learning," preprint.

Gurvits, L. (1996) personal communication.

Sutton, R. S., (1988) "Learning to Predict by the Method of Temporal Differences," Machine Learning, vol. 3, pp. 9-44.

Sutton, R.S. (1995) "On the Virtues of Linear Learning and Trajectory Distributions," Proceedings of the Workshop on Value Function Approximation, Machine Learning Conference 1995, Boyan, Moore, and Sutton, Eds., p. 85. Technical Report CMU-CS-95-206, Carnegie Mellon University, Pittsburgh, PA 15213.

Tsitsiklis, J. N. & Van Roy, B. (1996) "An Analysis of Temporal-Difference Learning with Function Approximation," to appear in the *IEEE Transactions on Automatic Control*.

Approximate Solutions to Optimal Stopping Problems

John N. Tsitsiklis and Benjamin Van Roy
Laboratory for Information and Decision Systems
Massachusetts Institute of Technology
Cambridge, MA 02139
e-mail: jnt@mit.edu, bvr@mit.edu

Abstract

We propose and analyze an algorithm that approximates solutions to the problem of optimal stopping in a discounted irreducible aperiodic Markov chain. The scheme involves the use of linear combinations of fixed basis functions to approximate a Q–function. The weights of the linear combination are incrementally updated through an iterative process similar to Q–learning, involving simulation of the underlying Markov chain. Due to space limitations, we only provide an overview of a proof of convergence (with probability 1) and bounds on the approximation error. This is the first theoretical result that establishes the soundness of a Q–learning–like algorithm when combined with arbitrary linear function approximators to solve a sequential decision problem. Though this paper focuses on the case of finite state spaces, the results extend naturally to continuous and unbounded state spaces, which are addressed in a forthcoming full-length paper.

1 INTRODUCTION

Problems of sequential decision–making under uncertainty have been studied extensively using the methodology of dynamic programming [Bertsekas, 1995]. The hallmark of dynamic programming is the use of a *value function*, which evaluates expected future reward, as a function of the current state. Serving as a tool for predicting long-term consequences of available options, the value function can be used to generate optimal decisions.

A number of algorithms for computing value functions can be found in the dynamic programming literature. These methods compute and store one value per state in a state space. Due to the curse of dimensionality, however, states spaces are typically intractable, and the practical applications of dynamic programming are severely limited.

The use of function approximators to "fit" value functions has been a central theme in the field of reinforcement learning. The idea here is to choose a function approximator that has a tractable number of parameters, and to tune the parameters to approximate the value function. The resulting function can then be used to approximate optimal decisions.

There are two preconditions to the development an effective approximation. First, we need to choose a function approximator that provides a "good fit" to the value function for some setting of parameter values. In this respect, the choice requires practical experience or theoretical analysis that provides some rough information on the shape of the function to be approximated. Second, we need effective algorithms for tuning the parameters of the function approximator.

Watkins (1989) has proposed the Q–learning algorithm as a possibility. The original analyses of Watkins (1989) and Watkins and Dayan (1992), the formal analysis of Tsitsiklis (1994), and the related work of Jaakkola, Jordan, and Singh (1994), establish that the algorithm is sound when used in conjunction with exhaustive look-up table representations (i.e., without function approximation). Jaakkola, Singh, and Jordan (1995), Tsitsiklis and Van Roy (1996a), and Gordon (1995), provide a foundation for the use of a rather restrictive class of function approximators with variants of Q–learning. Unfortunately, there is no prior theoretical support for the use of Q–learning–like algorithms when broader classes of function approximators are employed.

In this paper, we propose a variant of Q–learning for approximating solutions to optimal stopping problems, and we provide a convergence result that established its soundness. The algorithm approximates a Q–function using a linear combination of arbitrary fixed basis functions. The weights of these basis functions are iteratively updated during the simulation of a Markov chain. Our result serves as a starting point for the analysis of Q–learning–like methods when used in conjunction with classes of function approximators that are more general than piecewise constant. In addition, the algorithm we propose is significant in its own right. Optimal stopping problems appear in practical contexts such as financial decision making and sequential analysis in statistics. Like other problems of sequential decision making, optimal stopping problems suffer from the curse of dimensionality, and classical dynamic programming methods are of limited use. The method we propose presents a sound approach to addressing such problems.

2 OPTIMAL STOPPING PROBLEMS

We consider a discrete-time, infinite-horizon, Markov chain with a finite state space $S = \{1, \ldots, n\}$ and a transition probability matrix P. The Markov chain follows a trajectory $x_0, x_1, x_2, \ldots$ where the probability that the next state is y given that the current state is x is given by the (x, y)th element of P, and is denoted by p_{xy}. At each time $t \in \{0, 1, 2, \ldots\}$ the trajectory can be stopped with a terminal reward of $G(x_t)$. If the trajectory is not stopped, a reward of $g(x_t)$ is obtained. The objective is to maximize the expected infinite-horizon discounted reward, given by

$$E\left[\sum_{t=0}^{\tau-1} \alpha^t g(x_t) + \alpha^\tau G(x_\tau)\right],$$

where $\alpha \in (0, 1)$ is a discount factor and τ is the time at which the process is stopped. The variable τ is defined by a stopping policy, which is given by a sequence of mappings $\mu_t : S^{t+1} \mapsto \{\text{stop}, \text{continue}\}$. Each μ_t determines whether or not to terminate, based on $x_0, \ldots, x_t$. If the decision is to terminate, then $\tau = t$.

We define the value function to be a mapping from states to the expected discounted future reward, given that an optimal policy is followed starting at a given state. In particular, the value function $J^* : S \mapsto \Re$ is given by

$$J^*(x) = \inf_{\{\mu_1, \mu_2, \ldots\}} E\left[\sum_{t=0}^{\tau-1} \alpha^t g(x_t) + \alpha^\tau G(x_\tau) | x_0 = x\right],$$

where τ is the stopping time given by the policy $\{\mu_t\}$. It is well known that the value function is the unique solution to Bellman's equation:

$$J^*(x) = \max\left[G(x), g(x) + \alpha \sum_{y \in S} p_{xy} J^*(y)\right].$$

Furthermore, there is always an optimal policy that is stationary (i.e., of the form $\{\mu_t = \mu^*, \forall t\}$) and defined by

$$\mu^*(x) = \begin{cases} \text{stop}, & \text{if } G(x) \geq V^*(x), \\ \text{continue}, & \text{otherwise}. \end{cases}$$

Following Watkins (1989), we define the Q-function as the function $Q^* : S \mapsto \Re$ given by

$$Q^*(x) = g(x) + \alpha \sum_{y \in S} p_{xy} V^*(y).$$

It is easy to show that the Q-function uniquely satisfies

$$Q^*(x) = g(x) + \alpha \sum_{y \in S} p_{xy} \max[G(y), Q^*(y)], \quad \forall x \in S. \tag{1}$$

Furthermore, an optimal policy can be defined by

$$\mu^*(x) = \begin{cases} \text{stop}, & \text{if } G(x) \geq Q^*(x), \\ \text{continue}, & \text{otherwise}. \end{cases}$$

3 APPROXIMATING THE Q-FUNCTION

Classical computational approaches to solving optimal stopping problems involve computing and storing a value function in a tabular form. The most common way for doing this is through use of an iterative algorithm of the form

$$J_{k+1}(x) = \max\left[G(x), g(x) + \alpha \sum_{y \in S} p_{xy} J_k(y)\right].$$

When the state space is extremely large, as is the typical case, two difficulties arise. The first is that computing and storing one value per state becomes intractable, and the second is that computing the summation on the right hand side becomes intractable. We will present an algorithm, motivated by Watkins' Q-learning, that addresses both these issues, allowing for approximate solution to optimal stopping problems with large state spaces.

3.1 LINEAR FUNCTION APPROXIMATORS

We consider approximations of Q^* using a function of the form

$$\tilde{Q}(x,r) = \sum_{k=1}^{K} r(k)\phi_k(x).$$

Here, $r = \big(r(1),\ldots,r(K)\big)$ is a parameter vector and each ϕ_k is a fixed scalar function defined on the state space S. The functions ϕ_k can be viewed as basis functions (or as vectors of dimension n), while each $r(k)$ can be viewed as the associated weight. To approximate the Q-function, one usually tries to choose the parameter vector r so as to minimize some error metric between the functions $\tilde{Q}(\cdot,r)$ and $Q^*(\cdot)$.

It is convenient to define a vector-valued function $\phi : S \mapsto \Re^K$, by letting $\phi(x) = (\phi_1(x),\ldots,\phi_K(x))$. With this notation, the approximation can also be written in the form $\tilde{Q}(x,r) = (\Phi r)(x)$, where Φ is viewed as a $|S| \times K$ matrix whose ith row is equal to $\phi(x)$.

3.2 THE APPROXIMATION ALGORITHM

In the approximation scheme we propose, the Markov chain underlying the stopping problem is simulated to produce a single endless trajectory $\{x_t | t = 0, 1, 2, \ldots\}$. The algorithm is initialized with a parameter vector r_0, and after each time step, the parameter vector is updated according to

$$r_{t+1} = r_t + \gamma_t \phi(x_t) \Big(g(x_t) + \alpha \max\Big[\phi'(x_{t+1})r_t, G(x_{t+1})\Big] - \phi'(x_t)r_t\Big),$$

where γ_t is a scalar stepsize.

3.3 CONVERGENCE THEOREM

Before stating the convergence theorem, we introduce some notation that will make the exposition more concise. Let $\pi(1),\ldots,\pi(n)$ denote the steady-state probabilities for the Markov chain. We assume that $\pi(x) > 0$ for all $x \in S$. Let D be an $n \times n$ diagonal matrix with diagonal entries $\pi(1),\ldots,\pi(n)$. We define a weighted norm $\|\cdot\|_D$ by

$$\|J\|_D = \sqrt{\sum_{x \in S} \pi(x) J^2(x)}.$$

We define a "projection matrix" Π that induces a weighted projection onto the subspace $\mathcal{X} = \{\Phi r \mid r \in \Re^K\}$ with projection weights equal to the steady-state probabllilities. In particular,

$$\Pi J = \arg\min_{\bar{J} \in \mathcal{X}} \|J - \bar{J}\|_D.$$

It is easy to show that Π is given by $\Pi = \Phi(\Phi'D\Phi)^{-1}\Phi'D$.

We define an operator $F : \Re^n \mapsto \Re^n$ by

$$FJ = g + \alpha P \max\Big[\Phi r_t, G\Big],$$

where the max denotes a componentwise maximization.

We have the following theorem that ensures soundness of the algorithm:

Theorem 1 Let the following conditions hold:
(a) The Markov chain has a unique invariant distribution π that satisfies $\pi' P = \pi'$, with $\pi(x) > 0$ for all $x \in S$.
(b) The matrix Φ has full column rank; that is, the "basis functions" $\{\phi_k \mid k = 1, \ldots, K\}$ are linearly independent.
(c) The step sizes γ_t are nonnegative, nonincreasing, and predetermined. Furthermore, they satisfy $\sum_{t=0}^{\infty} \gamma_t = \infty$, and $\sum_{t=0}^{\infty} \gamma_t^2 < \infty$.
We then have:
(a) The algorithm converges with probability 1.
(b) The limit of convergence r^* is the unique solution of the equation

$$\Pi F(\Phi r^*) = \Phi r^*.$$

(c) Furthermore, r^* satisfies

$$\|\Phi r^* - Q^*\|_D \leq \frac{\|\Pi Q^* - Q^*\|_D}{1 - \alpha}.$$

3.4 OVERVIEW OF PROOF

The proof of Theorem 1 involves an analysis in a Euclidean space where the operator F and projection Π serve as tools for interpreting the algorithm's dynamics. The ideas for this type of analysis can be traced back to Van Roy and Tsitsiklis (1996) and have since been used to analyze Sutton's temporal-difference learning algorithm (Tsitsiklis and Van Roy, 1996b). Due to space limitations, we only provide an overview of the proof.

We begin by establishing that, with respect to the norm $\|\cdot\|_D$, P is a nonexpansion and F is a contraction. In the first case, we apply Jensen's inequality to obtain

$$\begin{aligned}
\|PJ\|_D^2 &= \sum_{x \in S} \pi(x) \left(\sum_{y \in S} p_{xy} J(y) \right)^2 \\
&\leq \sum_{x \in S} \pi(x) \sum_{y \in S} p_{xy} J^2(y) \\
&= \sum_{y \in S} \sum_{x \in S} \pi(x) p_{xy} J^2(y) \\
&= \sum_{y \in S}^{n} \pi(y) J^2(y) \\
&= \|J\|_D^2.
\end{aligned}$$

The fact that F is a contraction now follows from the fact that

$$|(FJ)(x) - (F\bar{J})(x)| \leq \alpha |(PJ)(x) - (P\bar{J})(x)|,$$

for any $J, \bar{J} \in \Re^n$ and any state $x \in S$.

Let $s : \Re^m \mapsto \Re^m$ denote the "steady-state" expectation of the steps taken by the algorithm:

$$s(r) = E_0 \Big[\phi(x_t) \left(g(x_t) + \alpha \max \left[\phi'(x_{t+1}) r, G(x_{t+1}) \right] - \phi'(x_t) r \right) \Big],$$

where $E_0[\cdot]$ denotes the expectation with respect to steady-state probabilities. Some simple algebra gives

$$s(r) = \Phi' D \Big(F(\Phi r) - \Phi r \Big).$$

We focus on analyzing a deterministic algorithm of the form

$$\bar{r}_{t+1} = \bar{r}_t + \gamma_t s(\bar{r}_t).$$

The convergence of the stochastic algorithm we have proposed can be deduced from that of this deterministic algorithm through use of a theorem on stochastic approximation, contained in (Benveniste, et al., 1990).

Note that the composition $\Pi F(\cdot)$ is a contraction with respect to $\|\cdot\|_D$ with contraction coefficient α since projection is nonexpansive and F is a contraction. It follows that $\Pi F(\cdot)$ has a fixed point of the form Φr^* for some $r^* \in \Re^m$ that uniquely satisfies

$$\Phi r^* = \Pi F(\Phi r^*).$$

To establish convergence, we consider the potential function $U(r) = \frac{1}{2}\|r - r^*\|_D^2$. We have

$$\begin{aligned}(\nabla U(r))'s(r) &= \left(r - r^*\right)' \Phi' D \left(F(\Phi r) - \Phi r \right) \\ &= \left(r - r^*\right)' \Phi' D \left(\Pi F(\Phi r) - (I - \Pi)F(\Phi r) - \Phi r \right) \\ &= \left(\Phi r - \Phi r^*\right)' D \left(\Pi F(\Phi r) - \Phi r \right),\end{aligned}$$

where the last equality follows because $\Phi' D \Pi = \Phi' D$. Using the contraction property of F and the nonexpansion property of projection, we have

$$\begin{aligned}\|\Pi F(\Phi r) - \Phi r^*\|_D &= \|\Pi F(\Phi r) - \Pi F(\Phi r^*)\|_D \\ &\leq \alpha \|\Phi r - \Phi r^*\|_D,\end{aligned}$$

and it follows from the Cauchy-Schwartz inequality that

$$\begin{aligned}(\nabla U(r))'s(r) &= \left(\Phi r - \Phi r^*\right)' D \left(\Pi F(\Phi r) - \Phi r^* + \Phi r^* - \Phi r \right) \\ &\leq \|\Phi r - \Phi r^*\|_D \|\Pi F(\Phi r) - \Phi r^*\|_D - \|\Phi r - \Phi r^*\|_D^2 \\ &\leq (\alpha - 1)\|\Phi r - \Phi r^*\|_D^2.\end{aligned}$$

Since Φ has full column rank, it follows that $(\nabla U(r))'s(r) \leq -\epsilon U(r)$, for some fixed $\epsilon > 0$, and $\bar{r}_t$ converges to r^*.

We can further establish the desired error bound:

$$\begin{aligned}\|\Phi r^* - Q^*\|_D &\leq \|\Phi r^* - \Pi Q^*\|_D + \|\Pi Q^* - Q^*\|_D \\ &= \|\Pi F(\Phi r^*) - \Pi Q^*\|_D + \|\Pi Q^* - Q^*\|_D \\ &\leq \alpha \|\Phi r^* - Q^*\|_D + \|\Pi Q^* - Q^*\|_D,\end{aligned}$$

and it follows that

$$\|\Phi r^* - Q^*\|_D \leq \frac{\|\Pi Q^* - Q^*\|_D}{1 - \alpha}.$$

4 CONCLUSION

We have proposed an algorithm for approximating Q-functions of optimal stopping problems using linear combinations of fixed basis functions. We have also presented a convergence theorem and overviewed the associated analysis. This paper has served a dual purpose of establishing a new methodology for solving difficult optimal stopping problems and providing a starting point for analyses of Q-learning-like algorithms when used in conjunction with function approximators.

The line of analysis presented in this paper easily generalizes in several directions. First, it extends to unbounded continuous state spaces. Second, it can be used to analyze certain variants of Q-learning that can be used for optimal stopping problems where the underlying Markov processes are not irreducible and/or aperiodic. Rigorous analyses of some extensions, as well as the case that was discussed in this paper, are presented in a forthcoming full-length paper.

Acknowledgments

This research was supported by the NSF under grant DMI-9625489 and the ARO under grant DAAL-03-92-G-0115.

References

Benveniste, A., Metivier, M., & Priouret, P. (1990) *Adaptive Algorithms and Stochastic Approximations*, Springer-Verlag, Berlin.

Bertsekas, D. P. (1995) *Dynamic Programming and Optimal Control.* Athena Scientific, Belmont, MA.

Gordon, G. J. (1995) Stable Function Approximation in Dynamic Programming. Technical Report: CMU-CS-95-103, Carnegie Mellon University.

Jaakkola, T., Jordan M. I., & Singh, S. P. (1994) "On the Convergence of Stochastic Iterative Dynamic Programming Algorithms," Neural Computation, Vol. 6, No. 6.

Jaakkola T., Singh, S. P., & Jordan, M. I. (1995) "Reinforcement Learning Algorithms for Partially Observable Markovian Decision Processes," in *Advances in Neural Information Processing Systems 7*, J. D. Cowan, G. Tesauro, and D. Touretzky, editors, Morgan Kaufmann.

Sutton, R. S. (1988) Learning to Predict by the Method of Temporal Differences. *Machine Learning*, 3:9-44.

Tsitsiklis, J. N. (1994) "Asynchronous Stochastic Approximation and Q-Learning," Machine Learning, vol. 16, pp. 185-202.

Tsitsiklis, J. N. & Van Roy, B. (1996a) "Feature-Based Methods for Large Scale Dynamic Programming," Machine Learning, Vol. 22, pp. 59-94.

Tsitsiklis, J. N. & Van Roy, B. (1996b) An Analysis of Temporal-Difference Learning with Function Approximation. Technical Report: LIDS-P-2322, Laboratory for Information and Decision Systems, Massachusetts Institute of Technology.

Van Roy, B. & Tsitsiklis, J. N. (1996) "Stable Linear Approximations to Dynamic Programming for Stochastic Control Problems with Local Transitions," in *Advances in Neural Information Processing Systems 8*, D. S. Touretzky, M. C. Mozer, and M. E. Hasselmo, editors, MIT Press.

Watkins, C. J. C. H. (1989) Learning from Delayed Rewards. Doctoral dissertation, University of Cambridge, Cambridge, United Kingdom.

Watkins, C. J. C. H. & Dayan, P. (1992) "Q-learning," Machine Learning, vol. 8, pp. 279-292.

Index of Authors

Abramowicz, Halina, 925
Abu-Mostafa, Yaser S., 634
Adler, Robert J., 309
Amari, Shun-ichi, 127, 599
Apsel, Alyssa, 685
Archie, Kevin A., 83
Attias, H., 27

Bös, Siegfried, 141
Bair, Wyeth, 34
Baluja, Shumeet, 319
Band, Pierre, 967
Baram, Yoram, 326
Barber, David, 274, 333, 340
Bartels, Andreas M., 111
Bartlett, Marian Stewart, 817
Bartlett, Peter L., 134
Barto, Andrew G., 3, 1019, 1026
Becker, Suzanna, 824
Bell, Anthony J., 758, 831
Bengio, Yoshua, 946
Bert, Joel, 967
Bertsekas, Dimitri, 974
Bienenstock, Elie, 838
Bishop, Christopher M., 333, 347, 354
Bisio, Giacomo M., 104
Blair, Alan D., 10
Blake, A., 361
Bone, Don, 988
Bradley, P. S., 368
Bregler, Christoph, 845
Bricolo, Emanuela, 41
Brightwell, G., 148
Brown, Timothy X., 932
Burges, Chris J.C., 155, 375
Burgess, A. Neil, 382

Callan, James P., 3
Caruana, Rich, 389
Cauwenberghs, Gert, 734
Cavanaugh, James R., 34
Chatterjee, Chanchal, 396
Chiang, Yu-Ming, 699
Clouse, Daniel S., 403
Coetzee, Frans M., 410
Cohn, David A., 417, 939
Cook, Gary, 800
Cooper, Gregory F., 578
Cottrell, Garrison W., 403, 894
Cowan, Jack D., 536, 852, 887

Davies, Scott, 1005

Dayan, Peter, 17, 48, 676, 1054
Deco, Gustavo, 76
DeWeerth, Stephen P., 706
de Bonet, Jeremy S., 424
de Sa, Virginia R., 389
Dimitrov, Alexander, 852, 887
Dodier, Robert H., 953
Dong, Dawei W., 859
Doya, Kenji, 1012
Drucker, Harris, 155
Duff, Michael O., 1019
Dunmur, A. P., 431

Edwards, R. Timothy, 734
Elisseeff, André, 162
Ernst, Udo, 90
Etienne-Cummings, Ralph, 685

Ferrá, H., 190
Ferrée, Thomas C., 55
Finch, Andrew M., 438
Finke, Michael, 459
Finkel, Leif H., 915
Flexer, Arthur, 445
Fragnière, Eric, 741
Freeman, William T., 662
Frey, Brendan J., 452
Fritsch, Juergen, 459

Gabbiani, Fabrizio, 62
Galperin, Gregory R., 1068
Gautrais, Jacques, 901
Geisel, Theo, 90
Geman, Stuart, 838
Ghahramani, Zoubin, 501
Ghosh, Joydeep, 981
Ghosn, Joumana, 946
Giles, C. Lee, 403
Gold, Steven, 620
Golowich, Steven E., 281
Grace, John, 967
Gray, Michael S., 751, 866
Grier, David G., 536
Grossberg, Stephen, 873

Häfliger, Philipp, 692
Halkjær, Søren, 169
Hancock, Edwin R., 438, 880
Hansen, Eric A., 1026
Harris, John G., 699
Hasler, Paul, 720
Heskes, Tom, 176, 466

Hochreiter, Sepp, 473
Horiuchi, Timothy, 706
Horn, David, 925
Horne, Bill G., 403
Hornik, Kurt, 522
Hyvärinen, Aapo, 480

Iizuka, Kunihiko, 713
Isard, M., 361
Isbell, Jr., Charles L., 424

Jaakkola, Tommi S., 487
Ji, Chuanyi, 494
Jordan, Michael I., 267, 487, 501, 557

Kamimura, Ryotaro, 508
Kang, Kukjin, 183
Kaufman, Linda, 155
Kenyon, C., 148
Koch, Christof, 62, 706, 720
Kowalczyk, A., 190
Kruger, W. Fritz, 720
Krzyżak, Adam, 197

Lambert, Russell H., 758
Laskey, Kathryn, 76
Lazzaro, John, 727
Lee, D. D., 515
Lee, Te-Won, 758
Leen, Todd K., 606
Leisch, Friedrich, 522
Leite, J. A. F., 880
Lewicki, Michael S., 529
Li, Zhaoping, 69
Lin, Juan K., 536
Linder, Tamás, 197
Lippmann, Richard, 727
Littlestone, Nick, 204
Lockery, Shawn R., 55
Logothetis, Nikos, 41
Lowe, David, 543
Lyon, Richard, 807

Müller, Klaus-Robert, 599
Ma, Sheng, 494
Maass, Wolfgang, 211, 218
Mahowald, Misha, 692
Malik, Jitendra, 845
Mangasarian, O. L., 368
Marcotte, Ben A., 55
Martignon, Laura, 76
Mathieson, Mark, 550
Matić, Nada P., 765
Matsui, Hirofumi, 713
Meilă, Marina, 557
Meir, Ron, 309
Mel, Bartlett W., 83

Merz, Christopher J., 564
Mesterharm, Chris, 204
Metzner, Walter, 62
Miller, David J., 571
Minch, Bradley A., 720
Miyamoto, Masayuki, 713
Mjolsness, Eric, 620
Monti, Stefano, 578
Moody, John E., 585, 995
Morciniec, Michal, 253
Morris, Tonia G., 706
Movellan, Javier R., 751
Movshon, J. Anthony, 34
Mozer, Michael C., 953
Mueller, Paul, 685
Mundel, Trevor, 887
Munro, Paul W., 592
Murata, Noboru, 599

Nabney, Ian T., 288
Naftaly, Ury, 925
Nakano, Ryohei, 627
Nelson, Alex T., 793
Neukirchen, C., 772
Neuneier, Ralph, 669
Niranjan, Mahesan, 960
Noda, Hideki, 246
Nowlan, Steven J., 866

Oh, Jong-Hoon, 183
Oja, Erkki, 480
Opper, Manfred, 141, 225
Orponen, Pekka, 218
Orr, Genevieve B., 232, 606

Padgett, Curtis, 894
Papka, Ron, 3
Parberry, Ian, 239
Pareigis, Stephan, 1033
Parmanto, Bambang, 592
Parra, Lucas C., 613
Paugam-Moisy, Hélène, 148, 162
Pawelzik, Klaus R., 90
Pazzani, Michael J., 564
Pearlmutter, Barak A., 613
Peper, Ferdinand, 246
Pineda, Fernando J., 734
Plate, Tony, 967
Platt, John C., 765
Poggio, Tomaso, 41
Pollack, Jordan B., 10
Potter, Daniel, 838
Pouget, Alexandre, 97, 676, 866

Qazaz, Cazhaow S., 347

Röbel, Alex, 779

Index of Authors

Rögnvaldsson, Thorsteinn S., 585
Ramanujam, Nirmala, 981
Rangarajan, Anand, 620
Richards-Kortum, Rebecca, 981
Riedmiller, Martin, 655
Riesenhuber, Maximilian, 17
Rigoll, G., 772
Rohwer, Richard, 253
Roychowdhury, Vwani P., 396
Ruderman, Daniel L., 83

Saad, David, 260, 288
Sabatini, Silvio P., 104
Sahar-Pikielny, Carmit, 925
Saito, Kazumi, 627
Saul, Lawrence K., 267, 501
Schölkopf, B., 375
Schaal, Stefan, 1040
Schmidhuber, Jürgen, 473
Schneider, Jeff G., 1047
Schreiner, C. E., 27
Sejnowski, Terrence J., 111, 529, 751, 817, 831, 866, 1061
Seung, H. S., 515
Siapas, Athanassios, 118
Sill, Joseph, 634
Singer, Yoram, 641
Singh, Satinder, 939, 974, 1054
Smola, Alex, 155, 281
Smyth, Padhraic, 648
Solari, Fabio, 104
Solla, Sara A., 260
Sollich, Peter, 274
Somers, David, 118
Sona, Diego, 786
Sperduti, Alessandro, 786
Stahlberger, Achim, 655
Starita, Antonina, 786
Stensmo, Magnus, 1061
Stonick, Virginia L., 410
Street, W. N., 368
Svensén, Markus, 354

Takahashi, Naomi, 685
Tang, Akaysha C., 111
Tenenbaum, Joshua B., 662
Tesauro, Gerald, 1068
Thorpe, Simon J., 901
Tipping, Michael E., 543
Titterington, D. M., 431
Todorov, Emanuel, 118
Tresp, Volker, 669
Tseng, Hung-Li, 239
Tsitsiklis, John N., 1075, 1082
Turner, Kagan, 981

Uyar, Hasan S., 571

Vaadia, Eilon, 76
van der Spiegel, Jan, 685
Van Roy, Benjamin, 1075, 1082
van Schaik, André, 741
Vapnik, Vladimir, 155, 281
Vidmar, Lucky, 953
Viola, Paul, 424
Vittoz, Eric, 741

Waibel, Alex, 459
Wan, Eric A., 793
Wan, Ernest, 988
Warmuth, Manfred K., 641
Waterhouse, Steve, 800
Watts, Lloyd, 692
Wawrzynek, John, 727
Webb, Brandyn, 807
Weiss, Yair, 908
Wessel, Ralf, 62
West, Ansgar H. L., 288
Williams, Christopher K. I., 295, 340, 354
Williamson, James R., 873
Wilson, Richard C., 438
Winther, Ole, 169, 225
Wolf, Fred, 90
Wong, K. Y. Michael, 302
Wu, Lizhong, 995

Yaeger, Larry, 807
Yen, Shih-Cheng, 915
Yuille, Alan, 620

Zeevi, Assaf J., 309
Zemel, Richard S., 676, 866
Zhang, Kechen, 97
Ziehe, Andreas, 599
Zilberstein, Shlomo, 1026
Zimmermann, Hans Georg, 669

Keyword Index

access control, 932
acetylcholine, 111
acoustic processing, 734
acoustic signals, 599
action potentials, 692
active learning, 417
actor-tutor, 1012
adaptation, 111, 720, 765
adaptive batch, 232
adaptive control, 713
adaptive filters, 599, 758, 831
adaptive learning constant, 127
adaptive momentum, 606
air temperature regulation, 953
analog computation, 218
analog neural networks, 685
analog VLSI, 685, 692, 706, 713, 727, 734, 741
analogy, 662
analytical MSE curves, 1054
anisotropic diffusion, 873
annealing, 232
annealing schedules, 606
appearance models, 845
approximation, 309
architecture, 148, 162
arcing, 522
area MT, 34
area V1, 34
asynchronous transfer mode (ATM), 932
asynchrony, 901
attention, 17
attractor networks, 817
attractors, 90
auditory modeling, 741
auditory scene analysis, 27
auditory system, 27
auto-zeroing, 720
autoassociator, 676

backgammon, 10, 1068
backpropagation, 389
bagging, 522, 967
batch learning, 232
Baum-Welch, 641
Bayes statistics, 225, 438
Bayesian belief networks, 578, 908
Bayesian decision theory, 838
Bayesian inference, 253, 295, 340, 347, 361, 529
Bayesian learning, 204
Bayesian model averaging, 76
Bayesian model-selection, 333
Bayesian regression, 1047
Bayesian regularization, 967
belief networks, 48, 452, 529, 557

bias, 932, 1054
bias initialization, 288
bias minimization, 417
biased estimators, 347
bilinear programming, 368
binding problem, 838
binocular rivalry, 48
binocular vision, 866
biomechanics, 55
biomedical applications, 967
blind signal processing, 536
blind signal separation, 127, 599, 758
Boltzmann machines, 487
boosting, 800
bootstrapping, 176, 466

cancer, 967
cavity field, 431
cavity method, 302
cellular telephones, 974
central pattern generator, 55
cervical cancer, 981
chaining, 333
character recognition, 807
chemotaxis, 55
choppers, 741
classification, 326, 340, 550, 662
classifiers, 522
clustering, 368, 824
CMOS VLSI, 713
co-evolution, 10
coarse code, 97
cochlear nucleus, 741
coding, 901
collective information, 508
combinations of classifiers, 494
combinatorial optimization, 319
combining, 981
combining estimators, 676
combining generalizers, 564
committee tree, 302
committees, 592
comparison, 967
competing experts, 824
competitive committee, 592
competitive learning, 592, 824
competitive network, 713
complex cells, 83
complexity regularization, 197, 669
componential model, 529
compositional probability distribution, 838
compositionality, 838
computational complexity, 211, 239
computational power, 218

computer vision, 361
concave, 368
confidence intervals, 932
constant error flow, 473
constructive learning algorithm, 459, 765, 786, 873
context, 90, 824
continuous TD, 1012
contour enhancement, 69, 880
contour integration, 69
contour suppression and segmentation, 69
contours, 915
control, 953, 1026
controlled diffusion process, 1033
convergence performance, 627
convergence properties, 169, 197, 606
correlated features, 169, 389
correlation, 692, 734
cortex dynamics, 90
cortical circuitry, 824
cortical dynamics, 69
cost estimation, 253
covariance function, 295, 340
covariation model, 988
credit applications, 634
cross-correlation, 866
cross-validation, 648
crossover, 319

data perturbation, 382
data transformations, 169
decision rule complexity, 375
decision theory, 1061
decision trees, 501, 939
decomposition, 396
degrees of freedom, 382
dendrites, 83
density estimation, 529, 536, 613
density model, 354
deterministic annealing, 620
diagnosis, 368, 1061
diffusion processes, 1033
direction selectivity, 104
discrete relaxation, 438
discriminant functions, 786
disparity energy, 866
doubly stochastic matrix, 557, 620
dual control, 1019
dynamic channel allocation, 974
dynamic features, 751
dynamic programming, 1005, 1047
    real time, 1033
dynamic resource allocation, 974
dynamical systems, 218, 779

early stopping, 141, 669
edge detectors, 852
efficiency of learning, 127
eigen-decomposition, 396

eigenvalue spectrum, 169
electroreceptors, 62
electrosensory system, 62
EM algorithm, 354, 431, 452, 571, 620, 641, 648, 845, 880
ensemble methods, 176, 466, 592, 800
entropy, 758, 831
equivalent kernels, 382
error bars, 176
error emphasis, 807
error rates, 190
error surface, 410
estimations, 97
Ethernet, 932
Euler-Lagrange equations, 267
evidence approximation, 333
evolutionary computation, 10
exact learning, 148, 162
expectation-maximization, see EM algorithm
experiment design, 417
exploration, 417
exploration vs. exploitation, 1019
exponentiated gradient descent, 3
extra outputs, 389

face emotion, 894
faces, 817
facilitation, 915
factorial codes, 613
factorial learning, 431, 662
fast pruning, 655
feature extraction, 246, 480, 543, 655
feature relevance, 389
feedback, 529, 713
feedforward networks, 134, 141, 176, 466
feedforward processing, 901
filter banks, 845
financial criterion, 946
financial modeling, 960, 995
finite dataset, 274
finite-state machine, 403
first-order algorithm, 627
Fisher linear discriminant, 62
fixed architecture, 925
floating gate, 720
free energy, 333
frequency balancing, 807
function approximation, 281
function estimation, 197, 281, 309

gain fields, 17
game-playing, 10
Gaussian classifier, 571
Gaussian processes, 253, 295, 340
generalization, 134, 183, 375, 389, 543
generalization properties, 627
generalized additive models, 967
generative model, 48, 354

Keyword Index

genetic algorithms, 319, 424
Gibbs sampling, 529
Gittins indices, 1019
global optimization, 410
graded-potential neurons, 55
gradient autocorrelator, 852
gradient descent, 260
graph embedding, 239
graph matching, 438
graphical models, 487, 501

Hamming distance, 438
handwriting recognition, 765, 786, 807
head injury, 550
Hebbian learning, 246, 480, 692
Helmholtz machine, 48
HEP detectors, 925
hidden Markov models, 459, 501, 641, 648, 727, 751, 772
hidden state, 1026
hierarchical classifiers, 459
hierarchical mixtures of experts, 459
hierarchical modeling, 838
hierarchical network, 529
hierarchical structures, 17
higher-order statistics, 480, 831
higher-order units, 83
hill-climbing, 319
hints, 634
homotopy, 410
Hopfield network, 239
horizontal connections, 90
Hough transform, 925
hybrid architectures, 953
hybrid HMM/ANN systems, 772
Hybrid Monte Carlo, 340
hybrid speech recognition, 459
hyperparameters, 295, 340

image classification, 873
image interpretation, 908
image processing, 901
image representation, 894
imitation learning, 1040
incomplete examples, 550
incremental learning, 319
independent component analysis, 480, 536, 613, 817, 995
individual information, 508
inferotemporal cortex, 41
infomax, 831
information content, 246
information controller, 508
information geometry, 127
information retrieval, 3
information theory, 758, 772, 831
information value, 1019
infra-red imagery, 880

input-dependent noise, 347
inputs vs. outputs, 389
integrate-and-fire neurons, 901
intelligent sensing, 1026
interpolation, 267, 988, 1005
intra-cortical neural interactions, 69
inventory effects, 995
IT, 17

Kalman filter, 793, 960
Kohonen networks, 445
kriging, 988
Kullback-Leibler divergence, 620

language induction, 403
Laplace approximation, 340
Laplace's sixth principle, 838
latent structure, 431
latent variable, 354, 452
lateral connectivity, 97, 852
lateral inhibition, 104
learning, 10, 281, 424, 786
learning algorithm, 3, 578
learning bias, 403
learning curves, 141, 183, 190
learning dynamics, 274, 288, 1047
learning from demonstration, 1040
learning of learning, 599
learning rate, 141, 274
learning rate schedules, 606
learning theory, 134
lifetime prediction, 939
line identification, 925
linear discriminant analysis, 396
linear model, 104, 274
linear perceptron, 169
linear-threshold algorithms, 204
lipreading, 751
LMS, 232
local minima, 410
local optimization, 239
local splines, 880
locally weighted learning, 1040
locally weighted regression, 417, 1047
loglinear models, 76
long short term memory, 473
long-range connections, 915
long-term dependencies, 473
look up table, 953
lower bounds, 211
Lyapunov function, 97

machine learning, 634
Markov chain, 76, 309
Markov decision process, 1026
maximum expected utility, 1061
maximum likelihood, 97, 347, 613, 824
MC3, 76

MCMC, 340
mean field, 225, 431, 452, 501
mean field theory, 302
mean-field annealing, 438
mean-field methods, 48
medical application, 169
medical diagnosis, 634
memory management, 939
memory-based learning, 1047
metastable states, 302
micropower circuits, 727
microscopic equations, 302
minimization, 368
minimum description length, 838
missing data, 550, 571
misspecification, 309
mistake bounds, 204
mistake-driven algorithms, 204
mixture models, 267, 309, 648, 662, 873
mixture of experts, 183, 309, 571, 800, 845, 866, 988
model comparison, 333
model composition, 76
model noise, 260
model selection, 648
model uncertainty, 1047
momentum, 606
monotonicity, 634
Monte Carlo, 333, 452
Monte Carlo model, 76
Monte Carlo search, 1068
motion, 34
motion detection, 706
multi-armed bandit, 1019
multi-effect decompositions, 995
multi-grid method, 1033
multi-phase pipeline, 354
multi-task learning, 389, 592, 946
multi-unit recordings, 76
multidimensional scaling, 445
multilayer networks, 148, 162, 225
multiplicative updates, 204
multiscale representation, 880
music, 779
mutual information, 508, 772

natural gradient, 127
natural images, 859
natural language queries, 3
natural scenes, 831
natural sounds, 27
negative training, 807
nematode, 55
network ensembles, 981
neural coding, 97, 676
neural fields, 104
neural networks, 564, 578, 599, 634, 772, 894, 960
neural synchrony, 69
neuro-dynamic programming, 1075, 1082

neuromodulation, 111
neuromorphic, 706
news effects, 995
Newton, 807
NMDA channels, 83
noise, 97, 218
noise cancellation, 995
noise reduction, 793
noisy examples, 260
non-negative least squares, 515
non-stationary signals, 599
nonlinear control, 1012
nonlinear dynamics, 246
nonlinear phenomena, 118
nonparametric statistics, 382
nonstationary systems, 779
nonuniformity correction, 699
normalized error, 807

object recognition, 17, 41, 824, 838, 845
OBS, 655
Occam's razor, 669
offset correction, 699
on-line learning, 127, 204, 232, 260, 274, 288, 599, 606, 873
optical flow, 751
optimal brain damage, 669
optimal control, 953
optimal junction tree, 557
optimal learning, 1019
optimal parameters, 274
optimal stopping, 1082
optimization, 319, 424, 908
options pricing, 960
order statistics, 981
order-parameter function, 274
ordered classes, 550
ordinal regression, 550
orientation, 55
orientation preference, 90
orientation selectivity, 925
orientation tuning, 83, 887
output adaptation, 765
overfitting, 141, 669, 967

parameter estimation, 641
parameter sharing, 946
partially observable, 1026
path functional, 267
pattern importance, 522
pattern recognition, 326, 515, 634, 662
PCA, 751
penalty term, 627
perceptron, 141, 204
permutation matrix, 557
personal digital assistant, 807
phase transition, 183
phoneme classification, 800

Keyword Index

pitch detection, 741
PLS-completeness, 239
pole balancing, 1040
policy improvement, 1068, 1075
pop-out, 887
population codes, 676
portfolio management, 946
power law, 27
power spectrum, 27
pre-attentive search, 915
prediction, 309, 793, 1075
primary visual cortex, 887
principal components, 246, 564, 817
probabilistic inference, 487, 676
probabilistic reasoning, 1061
probability bounds, 487
probability estimators, 578
process fluctuation, 713
processes, 908
prognosis, 368
pruning, 669
psychophysics, 859
pyramidal cells, 62

Q-learning, 1005, 1082
quadratic assignment, 620
quadratic programming, 515

radial basis functions, *see* RBF networks
RAMnets, 253
random dot stereograms, 866
random guessing, 473
random sampling, 361
random search, 424
RBF networks, 41, 197, 543, 765, 779, 981, 988
receptive fields, 90, 104
recognition, 817, 894
reconstruction, 779
recurrent interactions, 118
recurrent networks, 104, 218, 473, 515
redundant features, 389
regression, 155, 176, 347, 382, 466, 564
regularization, 260, 382, 669
regularization term, 627
reinforcement learning, 10, 974, 1005, 1012, 1026,
    1033, 1040, 1054, 1061, 1075, 1082
relative entropy, 641
relaxation, 880, 908
replica method, 302
resampling, 522
Resource Allocating Network, 765
response function, 169
Riccati equation, 692
ridge regression, 967
Riemannian space, 127
risk minimization, 197
robot learning, 1040
rollout, 1068

saccades, 706
saliency, 720, 915
Sammon mapping, 445, 543
sample aggregation, 932
scene adaptation, 699
scene interpretation, 838
scene labeling, 838
search engines, 3
second moments, 845
second-order algorithm, 627
selection mechanism, 866
selective attention, 706
self similarity, 27
self-amplification, 620
self-organization, 758, 831, 873
self-organizing maps, 354, 445, 536
semi-Markov bandit process, 1019
sensor calibration, 699
sensory coding, 831
separation of sources, 480
separation results, 211
sequence clustering, 648
sequential estimation, 960
sequential experiment design, 417
shot-noise processes, 295
sigmoid belief networks, 487
sigmoid nonlinearity, 246
sigmoidal neurons, 211
signal estimation, 793
signal processing, 734
silicon cochlea, 727
silicon model, 741
simulated annealing, 55, 424
simulation, 550
slice sampling, 452
smooth pursuit, 706
softassign, 620
softmax, 340
source separation, 995
    acoustic, 613
    blind, 613
space-complexity, 494
spatial decorrelation, 852
spatiotemporal feature extraction, 685
spatiotemporal statistics, 859
spectroscopy, 981
speech, 734, 779
speech processing, 793
speech recognition, 772, 800
speechreading, 751
spike timing, 111
spiking neurons, 211, 218, 741, 901
stability parameter, 302
stable state, 239
stacking, 765
state decoding, 727
state-space, 793
statistical intervals, 176
statistical mechanics, 183, 225, 260, 274, 288

statistical methods, 772
statistical physics, 438
stereopsis, 866
stimulus reconstruction, 34
stochastic learning, 232, 606
stock selection, 946
stroke warping, 807
structural representation, 17
style, 662
suboptimal phase, 288
subsampling, 932
supervised learning, 225, 389, 501, 571, 655
support vector machine, 281, 375
support vectors, 155
surrogates, 76
survival curves, 368
symmetric phase, 288
symmetry breaking, 183
synchronization, 76, 915
system model, 779

tangent distance, 786
TDNN, 403
temperature regulation, 953
template matching, 734
temporal coding, 62, 211
temporal correlation, 27, 692
temporal differences, 974, 1054
temporal patterns, 76
temporal-difference learning, 1061, 1075
texture, 845
texture segmentation, 873
thermodynamic limit, 190
threshold units, 148
tilt illusion, 887
time series, 309, 501, 648, 779, 793
time-complexity, 494
time-frequency representations, 734
time-series prediction, 953
top-down feedback, 69
topographic, 354
topographic mapping, 543
tracking, 706
trading module, 946
training, 807
training process, 141
transfer, 662
translation invariance, 83, 824
trees, 967
triangular binding, 838
triangulation, 557, 1005
2D cortical motion detection, 685

uniform convergence, 134
universal approximator, 211, 288
unlabeled features, 571
unsupervised learning, 368, 452, 515, 529, 571,
    613, 676, 817, 824

user adaptation, 765
utility theory, 1061

V4, 17
value function approximation, 1082
value iteration, 1005
value of information, 1061
vanishing gradient, 473
variance, 1054
variance minimization, 417
variational methods, 501
variational principle, 267
VC dimension, 190, 218
vector quantization, 445
vertex elimination, 557
vision, 361, 751, 824, 901, 908
visual coding, 859
visual cortex, 34, 83, 90, 104, 118, 852, 915
visual motion, 685
visual system, 41
VLSI motion detection, 685
voting classifier, 522

wake-sleep, 17
weak classifiers, 494
weight decay, 134, 543
weight initialization, 288
weight magnitudes, 134
weight normalization, 692
weight pruning, 669
weight vector length, 246
white noise, 34, 62
Wiener-Kolmogorov filtering, 62
winner-take-all, 713, 720
Winnow, 204
wordspotting, 727

XOR, 410